MW00836973

Wasserman & Whipp's

Principles of Exercise Testing and Interpretation

SIXTH EDITION

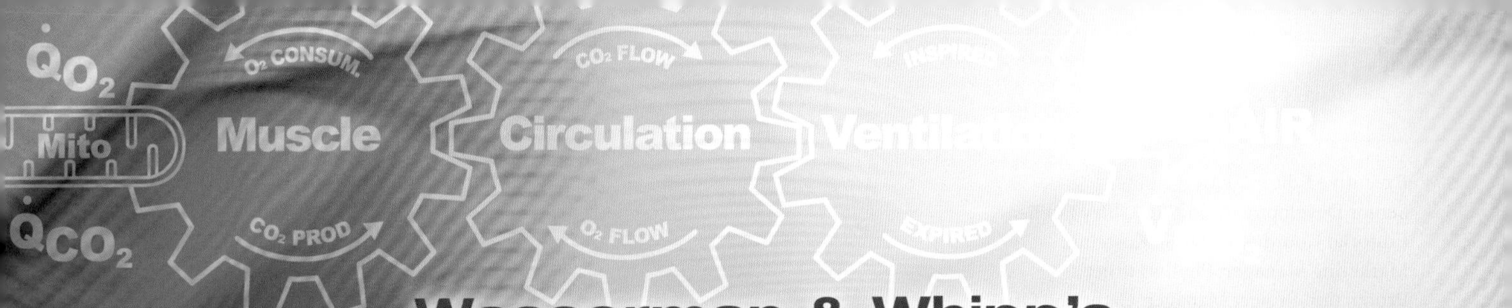

Wasserman & Whipp's Principles of Exercise Testing AND Interpretation

SIXTH EDITION

Kathy E. Sietsema, MD
Emeritus Professor of Medicine
David Geffen School of Medicine, UCLA
Division of Respiratory and
Critical Care Physiology and Medicine
The Lundquist Institute for Biomedical Innovation
Harbor-UCLA Medical Center
Torrance, California

Darryl Y. Sue, MD
Emeritus Professor of Medicine
David Geffen School of Medicine, UCLA
Division of Respiratory and
Critical Care Physiology and Medicine
The Lundquist Institute for Biomedical Innovation
Harbor-UCLA Medical Center
Torrance, California

William W. Stringer, MD, FACP, FCCP
Professor of Medicine
David Geffen School of Medicine, UCLA
Division Chief
Division of Respiratory and
Critical Care Physiology and Medicine
The Lundquist Institute for Biomedical Innovation
Harbor-UCLA Medical Center
Torrance, California

Susan A. Ward, DPhil
Emeritus Professor
University of Leeds
Leeds, United Kingdom
Human Bio-Energetics Research Centre
Crickhowell, United Kingdom

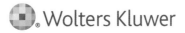

Wolters Kluwer

Philadelphia • Baltimore • New York • London
Buenos Aires • Hong Kong • Sydney • Tokyo

Executive Editor: Sharon Zinner
Senior Development Editor: Ashley Fischer
Editorial Coordinator: Julie Kostelnik
Marketing Manager: Phyllis Hitner
Production Project Manager: Catherine Ott
Design Coordinator: Stephen Druding
Manufacturing Coordinator: Kathy Brown
Prepress Vendor: Absolute Service, Inc.

Sixth edition

9 8 7 6 5 4 3 2 1

Printed in China

Library of Congress Cataloging-in-Publication Data
ISBN: 978-1-975136-43-7
Library of Congress Control Number: 2020905821

shop.lww.com

CCS0720

Preface

This sixth edition of *Principles of Exercise Testing and Interpretation* has been retitled by the current editors to acknowledge its unique legacy evolved from the long-standing collaboration between Karlman Wasserman and Brian J. Whipp. Beginning in the 1950s, Karl Wasserman embarked on a career of research in the physiology of breathing, cardiovascular function, and exercise, seeking to apply principles established from studies of normal exercise responses to understand and quantify alterations in function resulting from chronic disease. Over more than six decades, he shared his unabashed enthusiasm for this subject with scores of research collaborators across a range of disciplines and inspired colleagues, trainees, and mentees around the globe. Among these, his association with Brian J. Whipp, starting in the early 1960s at Stanford University, was foundational to the conception and development of novel rapid-response sensors and algorithms which opened the way to real-time, breath-by-breath analysis of pulmonary gas exchange during exercise. These technical advances were paralleled by the development of clinically relevant protocols for performing exercise tests and establishment of systematic approaches to characterizing, modeling, and interpreting the resulting physiological data. This work has had a major role in shaping the way cardiopulmonary exercise testing is now performed in clinical practice.

In response to requests from clinicians seeking practical education in this area, Drs. Wasserman and Whipp, along with Dr. James Hansen and other colleagues in the Respiratory Division at Harbor-UCLA Medical Center, established a live-learning course on exercise testing in 1985, and the first edition of this book followed soon thereafter. Exercise science and the practice of clinical exercise testing have expanded substantially over subsequent years, and a thorough representation of these topics would extend far beyond the scope of this text. *Wasserman and Whipp's Principles of Exercise Testing and Interpretation*, sixth edition, is intended to provide the reader with a rigorous approach to conducting cardiopulmonary exercise testing and a solid physiological rationale for understanding and interpreting the results. It is written from the perspective of authors who are each pleased to identify as (in the words of the late BJW) "'et al' . . . as in *Wasserman et al*," and the book adopts that body of work as its framework. With the scope of the content so defined, the sixth edition has been updated to reflect relevant advances in exercise physiology and clinical applications of exercise testing, and the compendium of clinical case examples has been supplemented with contemporary cases from our practices.

The premise of the book continues to be that the most important requirement for exercise performance is transport of oxygen to support the bioenergetic processes in the involved muscle cells (including, of course, the heart) and elimination of the carbon dioxide and protons formed as metabolic byproducts. Thus, appropriate cardiovascular and ventilatory responses are required to match those of muscle respiration in meeting the energy demands of exercise. This is depicted by the iconic "gears" logo which has graced the book cover of each edition of *Principles of Exercise Testing and Interpretation*, illustrating that normal exercise performance entails an efficient coupling of external to internal (cellular) respiration. Any defect in the systems between the muscle cell and the environment—whether in the lungs, heart, peripheral, or pulmonary circulations, the muscles themselves, or some combination of these—can result in a reduction in the capacity of the system as a whole or in the efficiency of its component parts, that is, exercise intolerance. Thus, we can quantify exercise capacity or, conversely, exercise impairment, in terms of the capacity for gas transport and exchange. Furthermore, we can describe pathophysiology in terms of how it affects the responses of individual components of the systems coupling internal to external gas exchange. The symptoms of exercise intolerance, most commonly dyspnea and/or fatigue at inappropriately low levels of exercise, can often be traced to the effects of disease on the response patterns of these component systems. And this, fortunately, can often be identified from noninvasive measures. As Karl has so often avowed, it is likely that no test in medicine is as informative and cost-effective as cardiopulmonary exercise testing for distinguishing among the broad spectrum of disorders causing symptoms of exercise intolerance. Without it, the evaluation of patients with exercise intolerance may be too narrowly focused by the physician working within the diagnostic spectrum of his or her particular subspecialty.

Increasingly, cardiopulmonary exercise testing is used for quantifying impairment and/or risk in patients with known diagnoses. In these contexts, the multiplicity of variables resulting from a cardiopulmonary exercise test could seem excessive or unnecessarily complicated. However, it is precisely the breadth of information provided by such testing that allows the examiner to confirm whether the patient's limitation is in fact attributable to the clinical condition of interest rather than to a different or coexisting disorder.

This, of course, can have profound impact on diagnostic classification and treatment decisions.

The focus of this book is on characterizing exercise function in terms of standardized measurements and expressions of the gas exchange and related variables which are most central to cardiopulmonary exercise testing. There are additional measurements that are uniquely valuable in specific clinical contexts, such as hemodynamics, cardiac imaging, or visualizing the upper airway, but thorough discussions of these are outside the scope of this book. There are also populations for which exercise testing is of demonstrated value, including children and athletes, which are not fully represented herein, as work with these populations extends beyond the expertise of the authors. Finally, there are measures that are integral to exercise testing, notably interpretation of the exercise electrocardiogram (ECG), that are also not detailed. This should not be taken to mean that we do not view the ECG as an essential component of exercise testing, only that ECG interpretation has been thoroughly described elsewhere. We therefore include the interpretation of the ECG in the case discussions in Chapter 10 but not images of the tracings or the approach to their interpretation.

The book is organized to progress from essential background information to practical applications. Chapters 1 through 9 discuss normal human exercise physiology, the effects of pathophysiology on exercise responses, pragmatic issues related to conducting tests and reporting data, and uses of testing in clinical practice. The bulk of the text comprises Chapter 10, which is a compendium of clinical cases drawn from the authors' experiences. These sample a wide range of normal and abnormal physiology and illustrate a variety of applications of exercise testing as well as approaches to interpreting and utilizing the results.

We hope that the content of this book will be useful as a guide for those who wish to conduct cardiopulmonary exercise testing and also to inform those who simply wish to effectively use test results in decision making for their patients or clients. In either case, an understanding of the physiological rationale for the measurements and how they are made is essential. Our goal, therefore, was to write a comprehensive yet practical book that would serve multiple purposes and be of use to a range of exercise scientists, clinicians, and technical staff interested in understanding and quantifying functional capacity.

Acknowledgments

We are grateful to the innumerable individuals who have contributed indirectly to this project, including colleagues, our former fellows and students, and the many physicians and scientists who have participated in our postgraduate course (practicum) in exercise testing and interpretation over the last four decades. This sixth edition, like its predecessors, benefits from many thoughtful discussions with course participants who generously shared their insights and expertise with us.

We are indebted also to the many technical staff who have worked in our laboratories over the years, caring for the safety and comfort of our patients, and keeping us honest.

Finally, we of course acknowledge Karl Wasserman and Brian Whipp for their unstinting intellectual leadership, guidance and collegiality. We equally treasure the wisdom, humor, and gentle but firm candor of James E. Hansen who we were fortunate to know as a mentor, colleague and friend. The purpose, format, and core content of this book originated from their individual and collective visions.

Contributors

Harry B. Rossiter, PhD
Professor of Medicine
David Geffen School of Medicine, UCLA
Division of Respiratory and
Critical Care Physiology and Medicine
The Lundquist Institute for Biomedical Innovation
Harbor-UCLA Medical Center
Torrance, California

Janos Porszasz, MD, PhD
Professor of Medicine
David Geffen School of Medicine, UCLA
Division of Respiratory and
Critical Care Physiology and Medicine
The Lundquist Institute for Biomedical Innovation
Harbor-UCLA Medical Center
Torrance, California

Contents

To view this case please access the eBook bundled with this text. Instructions are located on the inside front cover.

CHAPTER 1

Exercise Testing and Interpretation

WHAT IS CARDIOPULMONARY EXERCISE TESTING?

Cardiopulmonary exercise testing (CPET) is an examination that allows the investigator to simultaneously study the responses of the cardiovascular and ventilatory systems to a defined progressive (or incremental) exercise stress performed to the limit of tolerance. This is possible because gas exchange measured at the airway is a consequence both of the metabolic work of the exercising muscle and of the multiple integrated systems that link those metabolic processes to external gas exchange (**Fig. 1.1**). Thus, the adequacy and efficiency of the heart, lungs, circulating blood, pulmonary blood flow, and peripheral oxygen (O_2) extraction are reflected in the pattern of O_2 uptake ($\dot{V}O_2$), carbon dioxide (CO_2) output ($\dot{V}CO_2$), and minute ventilation ($\dot{V}E$) at the lungs, and in their relationships to other vital signs.

During CPET, serial (typically breath-by-breath) measurements of gas exchange are accompanied by measurements of electrocardiogram (ECG), heart rate, and blood pressure. Importantly, gas exchange variables add meaning to the ECG and blood pressure responses by relating them to the actual rather than estimated energy expended during the task being performed. They also provide a basis for inferring important information about unmeasured aspects of the exercise response, such as the cardiac stroke volume and arterial-venous oxygen content difference, reflected in the O_2 extracted from each heartbeat (oxygen pulse), and ventilation to perfusion ($\dot{V}/\dot{Q}$) matching in the lung reflected in the level of $\dot{V}E$ relative to $\dot{V}O_2$ and $\dot{V}CO_2$.

CELL RESPIRATION AND BIOENERGETICS

The energy to support life across a wide range of levels of physical activity is obtained predominantly from the oxidation of metabolic substrate. O_2 is the key that unlocks the energy from substrate by serving as the ultimate proton acceptor for oxidative processes that yield high-energy compounds. The energy is located in the chemical bonds of phosphate anions (~P) of the high-energy compounds adenosine triphosphate (ATP) and phosphocreatine (PCr). The ATP is the immediate source of energy used in muscular work, required as the source of energy powering the interaction between actin and myosin filaments that cause muscle to contract. The splitting of high-energy phosphate bonds of ATP at the myofibril thus transduces chemical energy into mechanical energy of muscular work.

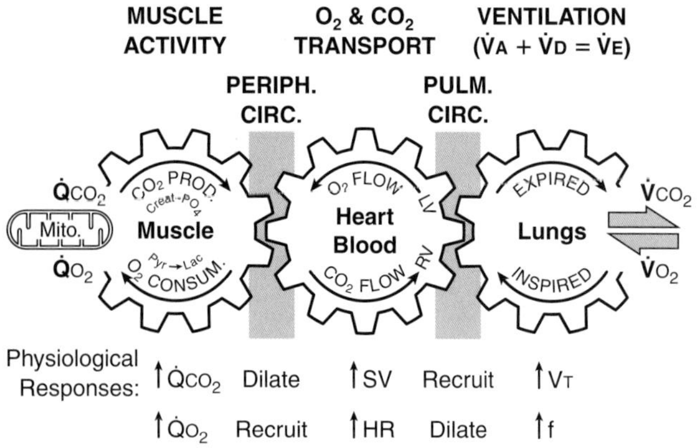

FIGURE 1.1. Gas transport mechanisms for coupling cellular (internal) to pulmonary (external) respiration. The gears represent the functional interdependence of the physiologic components of the system. The large increase in oxygen (O_2) use by the muscles ($\dot{Q}O_2$) is achieved by increased extraction of O_2 from the blood perfusing the muscles, the dilatation of selected peripheral vascular beds, an increase in cardiac output (stroke volume and heart rate), an increase in pulmonary blood flow by recruitment and vasodilatation of pulmonary blood vessels, and, finally, an increase in ventilation. Oxygen is taken up ($\dot{V}O_2$) from the alveoli in proportion to the pulmonary blood flow and degree of O_2 desaturation of hemoglobin in the pulmonary capillary blood. In the steady state, $\dot{V}O_2 = \dot{Q}O_2$. Minute ventilation ($\dot{V}E$) [tidal volume [V_T] × breathing frequency [f]] increases in relation to the newly produced CO_2 ($\dot{Q}CO_2$) arriving at the lungs and the drive to achieve arterial CO_2 and hydrogen ion homeostasis. These variables are related in the following way: $\dot{V}CO_2 = \dot{V}A \times PaCO_2/PB$, where $\dot{V}CO_2$ is minute CO_2 output, $\dot{V}A$ is minute alveolar ventilation, $PaCO_2$ is arterial or ideal alveolar CO_2 partial pressure, and PB is barometric pressure. The $\dot{V}O_2$, $\dot{V}CO_2$, $\dot{Q}O_2$, and $\dot{Q}CO_2$ are expressed as standard temperature and pressure dry. $\dot{V}E$, $\dot{V}A$, and dead space ventilation ($\dot{V}D$) are expressed as body temperature and pressure saturated. The representation of uniformly sized gears is not intended to imply equal changes in each of the components of the coupling. For instance, the increase in cardiac output is relatively small for the increase in metabolic rate. This implies an increased extraction of O_2 from and CO_2 loading into the blood by the muscles. In contrast, at moderate work intensities, $\dot{V}E$ increases in approximate proportion to the new CO_2 brought to the lungs by the venous return. The development of metabolic acidosis at heavy and very heavy work intensities accelerates the increase in ventilation to provide respiratory compensation for the metabolic acidosis.

The reserve of ATP in the muscle cell is small relative to potential needs and must be regenerated from other chemical sources as it is used. As detailed in Chapter 2, there are three bioenergetic processes responsible for the generation of ATP in the muscle (**Fig. 1.2**). These are aerobic (O_2-requiring) oxidation of substrates (primarily glycogen and fatty acids), anaerobic hydrolysis of PCr, and anaerobic (non-O_2-requiring) catabolism of glycogen or glucose to yield lactic acid or, more precisely, the lactate ion and its associated proton (H^+). Each of these processes is critically important for the normal exercise response, and each plays a different role in the overall bioenergetic response.

PCr represents an immediate source of ~P to regenerate ATP and prevent its rapid depletion, but PCr stores in muscle are also limited, so ATP production from energy stored in fat and carbohydrate substrate must increase rapidly if exercise is to be sustained. Because most ATP production for sustained exercise comes from aerobic processes and there is a relatively precise quantitative relationship between the O_2 consumption and ~P production, the rate of muscle O_2 consumption ($\dot{Q}O_2$) can be used as a measure of the rate of ATP expended for physical work.

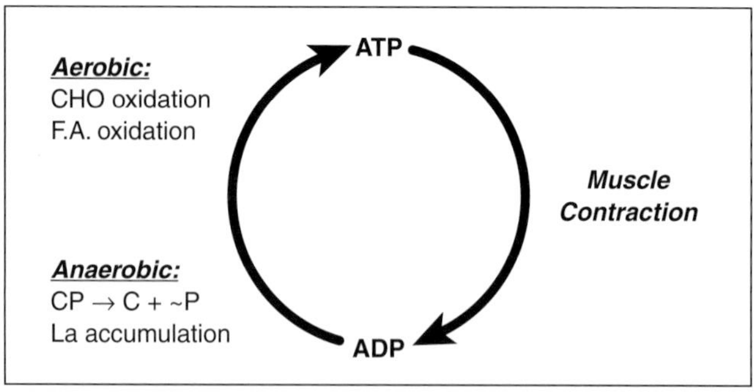

FIGURE 1.2. Sources of energy for adenosine triphosphate (ATP) regeneration from adenosine diphosphate (ADP). Abbreviations: CHO, carbohydrate; CP, creatine phosphate; FA, fatty acid.

The aerobic oxidation of carbohydrates and fatty acids provides the major source of ATP regeneration for sustained exercise, becoming the unique source in the steady state of moderate-intensity (ie, aerobic) exercise. In a normally nourished individual, about 80% of the energy comes from aerobic oxidation of carbohydrate and about 20% comes from fatty acid oxidation. To comfortably sustain a given level of exercise, the cardiorespiratory responses must be adequate to deliver enough O_2 to regenerate all the ATP from adenosine diphosphate needed for the physical task through these aerobic pathways. Intramuscular stores of PCr support ATP regeneration early in exercise before aerobic mechanisms have been fully recruited; that is, PCr is rapidly hydrolyzed by creatine kinase to creatine (Cr) and inorganic phosphate (Pi), with release of a ~P moiety (**Fig. 1.3**).

Whereas aerobic oxidation of carbohydrate and fatty acids is the source of ATP regeneration during moderate-intensity exercise, and 85% to 90% of high-energy phosphate

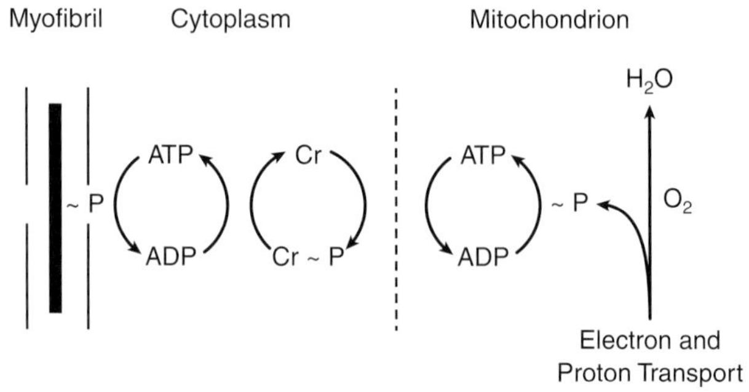

FIGURE 1.3. Scheme by which phosphocreatine (creatine phosphate, PCr or Cr ~ P) supplies high-energy phosphate (~P) to adenosine diphosphate (ADP) at the myofibril. Because of its quantity in resting muscle, PCr serves as a reservoir of readily available ~P as well as a shuttle mechanism to translocate ~P from mitochondria to the myofibril contractile sites. Abbreviations: ATP, adenosine; triphosphate; H_2O, water; O^2, oxygen.

is still produced aerobically, even at peak exercise, aerobic ATP production may be insufficient to fully account for all of the needs of more intense exercise. During high-intensity exercise, therefore, anaerobic catabolism of glucose and glycogen (glycolysis) also plays a role, but with a number of consequences. First, the amount of ATP produced by anaerobic glycolysis is relatively small per unit of glycogen and glucose consumed, so substrate may be depleted. Second, two lactate anions are produced with the anaerobic consumption of each six-carbon moiety of glycogen or glucose molecule. Because an H^+ ion is produced with each lactate ion, anaerobic glycolysis has important implications with respect to acid-base balance, gas exchange, ventilation, dyspnea, and fatigue during exercise.

The relationship between the responses of $\dot{V}O_2$ and $\dot{V}CO_2$ varies with each of the three sources of ATP generation. For instance, when the generation of ATP is entirely aerobic, the proportion of $\dot{Q}O_2$ and CO_2 production ($\dot{Q}CO_2$) depends on the ratio of carbohydrate to fatty acid in the substrate being oxidized in the muscle cells. On the other hand, when PCr is split, it is converted to Cr and Pi. Because PCr reacts like a relatively strong acid, whereas Cr is neutral in water, the splitting of PCr decreases cell acidity.[1,2] This reaction, therefore, consumes some CO_2 produced from cellular metabolism by its conversion to bicarbonate (HCO_3^-) in the tissues, reducing $\dot{V}CO_2$ relative to $\dot{V}O_2$. This contributes to a dissociation of the $\dot{V}CO_2$ kinetics relative to those of $\dot{V}O_2$ early in exercise (to be discussed more thoroughly in Chapter 2).[3,4] Finally, when ~P is generated from anaerobic glycolysis, the H^+ produced with lactate is buffered predominantly by HCO_3^-, thereby "consuming" HCO_3^- and adding CO_2 to that produced by aerobic metabolism. Not only does this cause a metabolic acidosis to develop, but elimination of this additional CO_2 results in a disproportionately higher $\dot{V}CO_2$ than $\dot{V}O_2$, and a greater increase in $\dot{V}E$.

Because these different mechanisms of ATP regeneration have different effects on gas exchange, study of the gas exchange responses to exercise can reveal information regarding the relative contributions of aerobic respiration, PCr hydrolysis, and anaerobic glycolysis to the total bioenergetic response.

NORMAL COUPLING OF EXTERNAL TO CELLULAR RESPIRATION

Figure 1.1 schematizes the coupling of pulmonary ($\dot{V}O_2$ and $\dot{V}CO_2$) to cellular ($\dot{Q}O_2$ and $\dot{Q}CO_2$) respiration by the circulation.[5] Clearly, the circulation must increase at a rate that is adequate to meet the O_2 requirement ($\dot{Q}O_2$) of the cells, and cardiac output increases in proportion to the $\dot{Q}O_2$ and $\dot{V}O_2$ (a 5-6 to 1 ratio). If $\dot{V}O_2$ fails to increase at a rate appropriate for $\dot{Q}O_2$, such as seen in diseases of the cardiovascular system,[6,7] lactic acidosis may occur at an abnormally low work rate.

To regulate arterial pH and PCO_2 at physiologic levels during exercise, the ventilatory control mechanism(s) must increase $\dot{V}E$ at a rate closely linked to the requirements to clear CO_2 at the lungs and compensate for the degree of lactic acidosis. $\dot{V}E$ must therefore increase at a greater rate, relative to work rate, when lactic acidosis is superimposed on the aerobic respiratory acid (CO_2) load. Further, to constrain the fall in pH resulting from the metabolic acidosis, $\dot{V}E$ must increase at an even greater rate than $\dot{V}CO_2$ in order to reduce arterial PCO_2.[8] This hyperventilation response typically results in only partial respiratory compensation for the metabolic acidemia of high-intensity exercise.

WHY MEASURE GAS EXCHANGE TO EVALUATE CARDIORESPIRATORY FUNCTION AND CELLULAR RESPIRATION?

Physical exercise requires the interaction of physiological control mechanisms to facilitate coupling of the cardiovascular and ventilatory systems to support their common function—that of meeting the increased metabolic demands ($\dot{Q}O_2$ and $\dot{Q}CO_2$) of the contracting muscles (see **Fig. 1.1**). Thus, both systems are stressed during exercise by the requirement to meet the increased need for delivery of O_2 to the contracting muscles and for removal of metabolic CO_2. Therefore, by studying *external* respiration in response to exercise, it is possible to address the functional competence or "health" of the several organ systems coupling *cellular* to external respiration.

Cardiopulmonary exercise testing offers the investigator the unique opportunity to study the cellular, cardiovascular, and ventilatory system responses simultaneously under precisely controlled conditions of metabolic stress. Exercise tests in which gas exchange is not determined cannot completely evaluate the ability of these systems to subserve their common major function, which is support of cellular respiration. A CPET allows the investigator to distinguish between a normal and an abnormal response characteristic of disease(s), grade the adequacy of the coupling mechanisms, and assess the effect of therapy on a diseased organ system(s). This is in contrast to more narrowly targeted exercise tests performed specifically to identify exercise-induced myocardial ischemia.

CARDIAC STRESS TESTS AND PULMONARY STRESS TESTS

It is, of course, impossible to stress only the heart or lungs during exercise. Both the heart and lungs are needed to support the respiration/metabolism of all living cells of the body and to maintain their energy requirements. The function of the heart, the lungs, and the peripheral and pulmonary circulations needs to be coordinated in order to meet the increased cellular respiratory demands of exercise. Cardiac abnormalities can result in abnormalities in lung gas exchange during exercise.[9-12] Similarly, pulmonary disorders can alter the cardiovascular responses to exercise by limiting cardiac filling, either because of increased pulmonary vascular resistance or extreme changes in intrathoracic pressure during breathing.[13,14] The term *cardiopulmonary exercise test* reflects recognition that exercise stimulates multiple integrated systems supporting gas exchange and that the measurements derived from the test similarly reflect the integrated function of those multiple systems.

PATTERNS OF CHANGE IN EXTERNAL RESPIRATION ($\dot{V}O_2$ AND $\dot{V}CO_2$) AS RELATED TO FUNCTION, FITNESS, AND DISEASE

This book is devoted largely to describing patterns of gas exchange that relate to organ system function, fitness, and features found in disease. As described earlier, increases in external respiration ($\dot{V}O_2$ and $\dot{V}CO_2$) need to be intimately coupled to the increases in cellular respiration ($\dot{Q}O_2$ and $\dot{Q}CO_2$). The proportional contributions of aerobic and anaerobic regeneration of ATP during exercise can often be inferred from measurements of external respiration. For example, $\dot{V}O_2$ and $\dot{V}CO_2$ kinetics in response to exercise differ depending on whether work is performed above or below the anaerobic threshold (*AT*), ie, with or without lactate accumulation (**Fig. 1.4**). For work performed below the *AT* (without a lactic acidosis), oxidative metabolism is sufficient for regeneration of all the required ATP in the steady state, and the patterns of $\dot{V}O_2$ and $\dot{V}CO_2$ increase as shown in the right side of the *Without Lactic Acidosis* panel of **Figure 1.4**. In contrast, if the O_2 supply or use is inadequate to meet the total ATP production need, lactic acidosis develops and the patterns of increase in $\dot{V}O_2$ and $\dot{V}CO_2$ change as shown in the right side of the *With Lactic Acidosis* panel of **Figure 1.4**. In the former condition, work can be performed in a true steady state in which $\dot{V}O_2$ is equal to $\dot{Q}O_2$ and $\dot{V}CO_2$ is equal to $\dot{Q}CO_2$. In the latter state, the oxygen delivery and use systems fail to meet the metabolic energy requirements, $\dot{V}O_2$ does not reach a steady state, and work is performed with development of lactic acidosis. Consequently, $\dot{V}CO_2$ increases in excess of $\dot{V}O_2$ due to the CO_2 released from HCO_3^- as it buffers lactic acid.

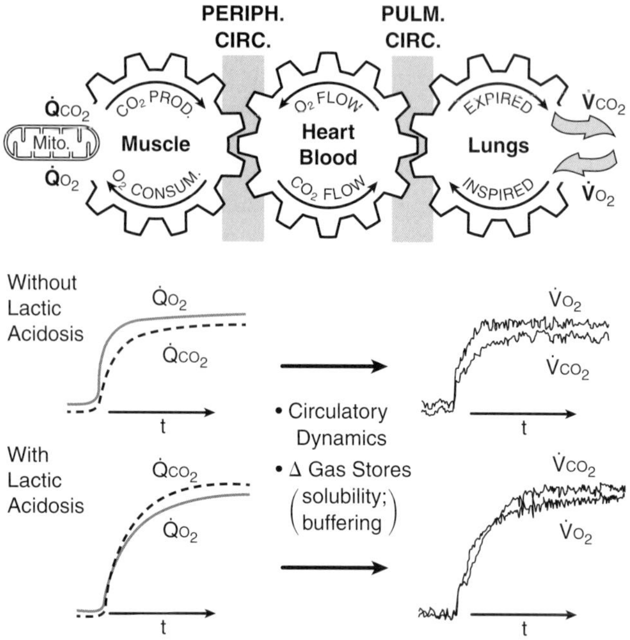

FIGURE 1.4. Scheme of coupling of external to cellular respiration for constant work rate exercise. The right side of the figure shows breath-by-breath data for 6 minutes of constant work rate exercise for work rates with and without lactic acidosis. Each study is an overlay of four repetitions to reduce random noise in the data and enhance the physiological features. Measurements of external respiration (right) can be used as a basis for reconstructing the changes in muscle cellular respiration. The left side of the figure shows, schematically, the changes in muscle cellular respiration that would account for the observed changes in external respiration. The factors that modulate the relationship between cellular respiration and external respiration are shown in the center. At the start of exercise, there is normally a brief step-like increase in both oxygen uptake ($\dot{V}O_2$) and carbon dioxide output ($\dot{V}CO_2$) consequent to the abrupt increase in pulmonary blood flow due to an immediate increase in heart rate and stroke volume. After an approximate 15-second delay, $\dot{V}O_2$ and $\dot{V}CO_2$ increase further when venous blood formed after exercise started, arrives at the lungs. At this early time, $\dot{V}CO_2$ increases more slowly than $\dot{V}O_2$. The slower rise in $\dot{V}CO_2$ than $\dot{V}O_2$ is accounted for by use of carbon dioxide (CO_2) in the production of bicarbonate (HCO_3^-) associated with release of potassium (K^+) by the muscle cell associated with the splitting of phosphocreatine and perhaps other chemical reactions in the tissues that store some of the metabolic CO_2. For work rates without a lactic acidosis, $\dot{V}O_2$ normally reaches a steady state by approximately 3 minutes and $\dot{V}CO_2$ by 4 minutes. For work rates with a lactic acidosis, $\dot{V}O_2$ does not reach a steady state by 3 minutes and may not reach a steady state before the subject fatigues. In contrast, $\dot{V}CO_2$ kinetics remain relatively unchanged, although with the level of $\dot{V}CO_2$ exceeding $\dot{V}O_2$ after the first several minutes of heavy-intensity exercise (see Chapter 2 for discussion of mechanisms). Abbreviations: $\dot{Q}CO_2$, produced CO_2; $\dot{Q}O_2$, muscle O_2 consumption.

FACTORS LIMITING EXERCISE

Common symptoms that stop individuals from performing exercise include fatigue, dyspnea, and/or pain (eg, angina or claudication). Quantitative exercise testing in which large muscle groups are stressed (walking, running, or cycling) can identify if exercise tolerance is reduced compared to normal individuals and, if so, whether abnormal cardiovascular, ventilatory, or metabolic responses to exercise account for that reduction and reproduce the patient's symptoms.

Fatigue

A muscle is considered to fatigue when its force output decreases for a given stimulus. However, the exact mechanisms of muscle fatigue remain a topic of debate, with candidate mediators including decreased cellular pH, increased Pi, increased levels of free radicals and their related redox-active derivatives, and decreased ATP. However, regardless of the precise mechanisms, the consistent physiological signal for impending fatigue during exercise is the failure of $\dot{V}O_2$ to reach a steady state and therefore to match the cellular O_2 requirement. A number of investigators have measured $\dot{V}O_2$ during incremental exercise in both patients with heart failure and normal individuals and observed that $\dot{V}O_2$ increases more slowly, relative to the increase in work rate, before the onset of fatigue.[6,7,15] This places further demands on anaerobic mechanisms of ATP regeneration. Although this phenomenon can be seen as work rate is increased toward maximal $\dot{V}O_2$ in normal individuals, it is particularly notable in heart failure patients as they approach their symptom-limited maximum.

Dyspnea

Dyspnea is a common exercise-induced symptom of multiple disease states. It occurs in patients with pathophysiology that results in inefficient gas exchange due to $\dot{V}/\dot{Q}$ mismatching (high physiological dead space), lactic acidosis occurring at low work rates (eg, low cardiac output response to exercise), exercise-induced arterial hypoxemia, and disorders associated with impaired lung mechanics. These pathophysiological changes can occur singly, but more commonly they occur in combinations. For example, patients with chronic obstructive pulmonary disease (COPD) have a combination of impaired ventilatory mechanics that limit their maximal ability to ventilate their lungs, along with $\dot{V}/\dot{Q}$ mismatching that causes $\dot{V}E$ to be inefficient in eliminating CO_2. In addition, they may have exercise-induced arterial hypoxemia that further stimulates ventilatory drive.

Dyspnea also occurs in patients with left ventricular failure. These patients have lactic acidosis occurring at a low work rate as well as inefficient lung gas exchange due to $\dot{V}/\dot{Q}$ mismatching (high physiologic dead space). Both of these mechanisms stimulate $\dot{V}E$ consequent to the inefficient elimination of CO_2. Any pathophysiology that increases ventilatory drive can cause or exacerbate dyspnea.

Arterial hypoxemia is a common disorder in lung and pulmonary vascular diseases. If arterial PO_2 decreases sufficiently during exercise, it stimulates the carotid body chemoreceptors to increase $\dot{V}E$, which, in turn, can contribute to dyspnea. This is exacerbated above the *AT*, as the carotid chemoreceptors are also stimulated by arterial acidemia during exercise.[16] Mechanisms of dyspnea in health and disease are discussed further in later chapters.

Pain

Pain in the chest, arm, or neck is a common symptom of myocardial ischemia (angina pectoris) brought on by exercise in patients with coronary artery disease. This is a reflection of an inadequate myocardial O_2 supply relative to demand. Reducing the O_2 demand by decreasing myocardial work or increasing myocardial O_2 supply can delay or eliminate anginal pain. Successful treatment of myocardial ischemia by medications or revascularization can be documented with CPET.

Claudication results from an O_2 supply–demand imbalance in the muscles of the exercising extremities. Walking at a normal pace requires an increase in $\dot{Q}O_2$ of the muscles of locomotion of approximately 20-fold compared to rest. Therefore, the ability of muscle blood flow to increase appropriately is critically important to enable walking without ischemic pain. Stenosis in the conducting vessels to the lower extremity due to atherosclerosis may limit the increase in leg blood flow in response to exercise, and result in regional O_2 supply–demand imbalance. Critically low levels of O_2 in the affected muscles[17] cause local K^+, lactate, and H^+ accumulation secondary to the ischemia, which are likely mediators of the exercise-induced leg pain. The impaired blood supply will be reflected in slowed $\dot{V}O_2$ kinetics.[18]

EVIDENCE OF SYSTEMIC DYSFUNCTION UNIQUELY REVEALED BY INTEGRATIVE CARDIOPULMONARY EXERCISE TESTING

Recent reviews and guidelines have emphasized the unique indications for CPET in certain patient populations.[19,20] These include evaluation of aerobic fitness in normal individuals, evaluation of unexplained exertional dyspnea, assessment of severity of COPD and interstitial lung diseases, assessment of perioperative risk, interrogation of valvular heart disease and dysfunction, prognostication of patients with chronic heart failure or pulmonary hypertension, and assessment and prescription for cardiopulmonary rehabilitation. In addition, there are compelling data for using CPET in the assessment of congenital heart diseases, cystic fibrosis, idiopathic pulmonary fibrosis, and for monitoring of therapy in heart failure. The following are some examples of how CPET has been used for diagnosis, staging, and prognosis in a number of medical conditions.

Diagnosis of Exercise Intolerance, Especially Exertional Dyspnea and Myocardial Ischemia

Obligatory changes in the normal exercise gas exchange responses occur when diseases of the cardiovascular or ventilatory systems, or both, impair their functioning. Thus, the gas exchange responses to exercise could indicate which systems are functioning poorly and which are functioning well. CPET can help not only to distinguish between lung and cardiovascular disease but also often to distinguish one cardiovascular disease from another as the cause of exercise limitation. For instance, coronary artery disease, chronic heart failure, and peripheral vascular disease have abnormal patterns of exercise gas exchange somewhat distinct from each other.[21] Gas exchange measurements can confirm ischemia-induced left ventricular dysfunction during exercise and identify the metabolic rate at which the ischemia and dysfunction take place, improving sensitivity and specificity for myocardial ischemia over that seen when only the ECG is used.[22] A CPET may also identify findings characteristic of pulmonary vasculopathy leading to pulmonary hypertension early in the course of disease, and identify the presence of an exercise-induced right-to-left shunt.[23]

A test in which exercise gas exchange is measured with the 12-lead ECG should be among the most sensitive tests to evaluate causes of exercise intolerance because exercise amplifies the abnormal manifestations of the organs that couple external to cellular respiration. Also, no test is likely to be capable of objectively quantifying improvement or worsening of these functions with greater sensitivity than a CPET. Thus, CPET—with gas exchange, ECG, blood pressure, and spirometry—early in the evaluation of the patient with exercise limitation could reduce use of less sensitive diagnostic tests.

To facilitate recognition of the patterns of disease that are useful in diagnostic assessments, we believe that the data collected during a CPET should be displayed graphically. Over time from our practice experience, we developed a nine-panel graphical display that allows ready identification of response patterns characteristic of common medical conditions. This approach is discussed in Chapters 6 and 9 and illustrated in Chapter 10 in the presentation of CPET data from patients with a large variety of diseases.

Cardiopulmonary Exercise Testing and Prognosis in Patients With Known Disorders

Many of the clinical applications of CPET in patient populations are related to the prognostic significance of exercise capacity. This is exemplified in the experience of patients with chronic heart failure, for which CPET has essentially revolutionized assessment. Beginning in the late 1980s, the connection between peak $\dot{V}O_2$ during exercise and patient survival was firmly established, with additional prognostic value of $\dot{V}O_2$ at the *AT*. Subsequently, multiple studies validated the additional and independent value of "excess ventilation" during CPET as a marker of prognosis. The latter, expressed often as the slope of the $\dot{V}E$-$\dot{V}CO_2$ relationship or as the nadir (minimum) value of the ventilatory equivalent for CO_2 ($\dot{V}E/\dot{V}CO_2$) response at or near the *AT*, has provided both prognostic information and additional insights into the pathophysiology of exercise intolerance in this disorder. Other useful gas exchange measurements during exercise include the end-tidal PCO_2 and the oxygen uptake efficiency slope, a measurement relating $\dot{V}E$ to $\dot{V}O_2$ that may be useful during submaximal exercise. Much of the early data in this latter area came from studies of patients with reduced ejection fraction heart failure, but the observations have extended to include those with preserved ejection fraction. Evidence that CPET can yield reliable information on prognosis in clinical populations has been demonstrated in its effective use in decision making regarding advanced therapies such as transplantation.[24] Of note, as medical management of heart failure has greatly improved prognosis over the last several decades, gas exchange indices appear to reflect this change. For example, one analysis suggests that the peak $\dot{V}O_2$ that corresponded to a given prognosis 20 years ago is now considerably lower for the same clinical outcome.[25]

Cardiopulmonary Exercise Testing and Preoperative Assessment

The metabolic demand associated with the perioperative period demonstrates similarities to the "stress" of exercise, and CPET can be helpful in determining the overall capacity of the heart, lungs, and systemic and pulmonary circulations to adapt to these challenges. However, contrasting the capacity of the patient with demands in the operative and postoperative period has rarely been evaluated. Instead, measurements of exercise capacity have been correlated with risks of perioperative complications, such as the ability to be liberated from mechanical ventilation, postoperative infections, wound dehiscence, long-term impairment, and mortality. Studies have been performed prior to abdominal and thoracic surgery as well as for multiple types of other surgeries.[26-28] Of note is the special case of lung resection, in which postoperative lung capacity is expected to be incrementally reduced, often on a baseline of existing chronic lung disease (eg, COPD). In this situation, CPET has proven useful for helping determine if a given patient has adequate pulmonary reserve to undergo the contemplated resection.[29]

SUMMARY

Organ dysfunction that limits exercise can usually be detected by evidence of an abnormality in the coupling of external (pulmonary) respiration to cellular respiration. The CPET provides new insights into disease manifestation, degree of functional impairment, and prognosis of patients with known conditions, particularly in those patients with cardiovascular diseases. Exercise "amplifies" the functional manifestation of a basic disease process, which may be subtle or difficult to identify from resting measures. Further, integrative CPET, in which gas exchange is measured dynamically at the airway over the range of achievable work, rather than as a single steady-state measurement, can usually identify the pathophysiology of reduced exercise tolerance when its underlying cause is unknown. Discerning the pathophysiology of the intolerance, in turn, is often sufficient to make an anatomical diagnosis. If not, it can narrow the diagnostic choices among diverse processes causing similar symptoms and suggest the most appropriate line of additional testing. When the cause of the patient's exercise intolerance is not clinically obvious, therefore, we believe that it may be cost-effective to perform a CPET before proceeding with more invasive and expensive testing. Because so many organ systems are involved in meeting and coordinating the normal responses to exercise, CPET is relevant to the assessment of a wide range of clinical conditions and likely covers a broader range of potential diagnoses than any other test in medicine. As stated by the European Society of Cardiology, "The full potentials of CPET in the clinical and research setting still remain largely underused."[30]

REFERENCES

1. Piiper J. Production of lactic acid in heavy exercise and acid-base balance. In: Moret PR, Weber J, Haissly J, et al, eds. *Lactate: Physiologic, Methodologic and Pathologic Approach*. New York, NY: Springer; 1980:35-45.
2. Wasserman K, Stringer W, Casaburi R, Zhang YY. Mechanism of the exercise hyperkalemia: an alternate hypothesis. *J Appl Physiol*. 1997; 83:631-643.

3. Chuang ML, Ting H, Otsuka T, et al. Aerobically generated CO(2) stored during early exercise. *J Appl Physiol (1985)*. 1999;87(3):1048-1058.
4. Wasserman K, Stringer W, Sun X-G, et al. Circulatory coupling of external to muscle respiration during exercise. In: Wasserman K, ed. *Cardiopulmonary Exercise Testing and Cardiovascular Health*. Armonk, NY: Futura Publishing; 2002:3-26.
5. Wasserman K. Coupling of external to cellular respiration during exercise: the wisdom of the body revisited. *Am J Physiol*. 1994;266:E519-E539.
6. Kitzman DW, Higginbotham MB, Cobb FR, Sheikh KH, Sullivan MJ. Exercise intolerance in patients with heart failure and preserved left ventricular systolic function: failure of the Frank-Starling mechanism. *J Am Coll Cardiol*. 1994;17:1065-1072.
7. Wilson JR, Ferraro N, Weber KT. Respiratory gas analysis during exercise as a noninvasive measure of lactate concentration in chronic congestive heart failure. *Am J Cardiol*. 1983;51:1639-1643.
8. Wasserman K, Van Kessel A, Burton GG. Interaction of physiological mechanisms during exercise. *J Appl Physiol*. 1967;22:71-85.
9. Kleber F, Reindl I, Wernecke K, et al. Dyspnea in heart failure. In: Wasserman K, ed. *Exercise Gas Exchange in Heart Disease*. Armonk, NY: Futura Publishing; 1996:95-107.
10. Metra M, Raccagni D, Carini G, et al. Ventilatory and arterial blood gas changes during exercise in heart failure. In: Wasserman K, ed. *Exercise Gas Exchange in Heart Disease*. Armonk, NY: Futura Publishing; 1996:125-143.
11. Sullivan MJ, Higginbotham MB, Cobb FR. Increased exercise ventilation in patients with chronic heart failure: intact ventilatory control despite hemodynamic and pulmonary abnormalities. *Circulation*. 1988; 77:552-559.
12. Wasserman K, Zhang YY, Gitt A, et al. Lung function and exercise gas exchange in chronic heart failure. *Circulation*. 1997;96:2221-2227.
13. Butler J, Schrijen F, Henriquez A, Polu JM, Albert RK. Cause of the raised wedge pressure on exercise in chronic obstructive pulmonary disease. *Am Rev Respir Dis*. 1988;138:350-354.
14. Hansen JE, Wasserman K. Pathophysiology of activity limitation in patients with interstitial lung disease. *Chest*. 1996;109:1566-1576.
15. Sullivan MJ, Knight JD, Higginbotham MB, Cobb FR. Relation between central and peripheral hemodynamics during exercise in patients with chronic heart failure. Muscle blood flow is reduced with maintenance of arterial perfusion pressure. *Circulation*. 1989;80:769-781.
16. Wasserman K, Whipp BJ, Koyal SN, Cleary M. Effect of carotid body resection on ventilatory and acid-base control during exercise. *J Appl Physiol*. 1975;39:354-358.
17. Bylund-Fellenius AC, Walker PM, Elander A, Holms S, Holm J, Scherstén T. Energy metabolism in relation to oxygen partial pressure in human skeletal muscle during exercise. *Biochem J*. 1981;200:247-255.
18. Auchincloss JH, Ashutosh K, Rana S, et al. Effect of cardiac, pulmonary, and vascular disease on one-minute oxygen uptake. *Chest*. 1976; 70:486-493.
19. Guazzi M, Arena R, Halle M, Piepoli MF, Myers J, Lavie CJ. 2016 Focused update: clinical recommendations for cardiopulmonary exercise testing data assessment in specific patient populations. *Circulation*. 2016;133:e694-e711.
20. Palange P, Laveneziana P, Neder JA, Ward SA. Introduction: CPET in clinical practice. Recent advances, current challenges and future directions. In: Palange P, Laveneziana P, Neder JA, et al, eds. *Clinical Exercise Testing (ERS Monograph)*. Sheffield, United Kingdom: European Respiratory Society; 2018:x-xxv.
21. Wasserman K. Diagnosing cardiovascular and lung pathophysiology from exercise gas exchange. *Chest*. 1997;112:1091-1101.
22. Belardinelli R, Lacalaprice F, Tiano L, Muçai A, Perna GP. Cardiopulmonary exercise testing is more accurate than ECG-stress testing in diagnosing myocardial ischemia in subjects with chest pain. *Int J Cardiol*. 2014;174:337-342.
23. Sun XG, Hansen JE, Oudiz R, Wasserman K. Gas exchange detection of exercise-induced right-to-left shunt in patients with primary pulmonary hypertension. *Circulation*. 2002;105(1):54-60.
24. Mancini DM, Eisen H, Kussmaul W, Mull R, Edmunds LH Jr, Wilson JR. Value of peak exercise oxygen consumption for optimal timing of cardiac transplantation in ambulatory patients with heart failure. *Circulation*. 1991;83(3):778-786.
25. Paolillo S, Veglia F, Salvioni E, et al; for MECKI Score Research Group. Heart failure prognosis over time: how the prognostic role of oxygen consumption and ventilatory efficiency during exercise has changed in the last 20 years. *Eur J Heart Fail*. 2019;21:208-217.
26. Older PO, Levett DZH. Cardiopulmonary exercise testing and surgery. *Ann Am Thorac Soc*. 2017;14(suppl 1):S74-S83.
27. Levett DZH, Jack S, Swart M, et al; for Perioperative Exercise Testing and Training Society (POETTS). Perioperative cardiopulmonary exercise testing (CPET): consensus clinical guidelines on indications, organization, conduct, and physiological interpretation. *Br J Anaesth*. 2018;120:484-500.
28. Harvie D, Levett DZH. Exercise testing for pre-operative evaluation. In: Palange P, Laveneziana P, Neder JA, et al, eds. *Clinical Exercise Testing (ERS Monograph)*. Sheffield, United Kingdom: European Respiratory Society; 2018:251-227.
29. Brunelli A, Kim AW, Berger KI, Addrizzo-Harris DJ. Physiologic evaluation of the patient with lung cancer being considered for resectional surgery: diagnosis and management of lung cancer, 3rd ed: American College of Chest Physicians evidence-based clinical practice guidelines. *Chest*. 2013;143(suppl 5):e166S-e190S.
30. Mezzani A, Agostoni P, Cohen-Solal A, et al. Standards for the use of cardiopulmonary exercise testing for the functional evaluation of cardiac patients: a report from the exercise physiology section of the European Association for Cardiovascular Prevention and Rehabilitation. *Eur J Cardiovasc Prev Rehabil*. 2009;16:249-267.

CHAPTER 2

Physiology of Exercise

The performance of muscular work necessitates the physiological responses of the cardiovascular and ventilatory systems to be coupled with the increase in metabolic rate; efficient coupling minimizing the stress to the component mechanisms supporting the energy transformations. In other words, cellular respiratory (internal respiration) requirements can only be met by the interaction of physiological mechanisms that link gas exchange between the cells and the atmosphere (external respiration) (see **Fig. 1.1**). Inefficient coupling increases the stress to these systems and, when sufficiently severe, can result in symptoms that impair or limit work performance. Efficient gas exchange between the cells and the environment requires the following:

- Appropriate intracellular structure, energy substrate, and enzyme concentrations
- An effective system of blood vessels that can selectively distribute blood flow to match local tissue gas exchange requirements for O_2 delivery and removal of CO_2 and, at higher work rates, lactate
- A heart capable of pumping the quantity of oxygenated blood needed to sustain the energy transformations
- Blood with normal hemoglobin of adequate concentration
- An effective pulmonary circulation through which the regional blood flow is matched to its ventilation
- Normal lung and chest wall mechanics
- Ventilatory control mechanisms capable of regulating arterial blood CO_2 and O_2 partial pressures and hydrogen ion or proton (H^+) concentration

The response of each of the coupling links in the gas exchange process is usually quite predictable and can be used as a frame of reference for considerations of

The authors wish to acknowledge the seminal contributions of Drs. Brian J. Whipp and Karlman Wasserman in their original authorship of this chapter.

impaired function. This chapter reviews the essentials of skeletal muscle physiology, including the relationship between structure and function, cellular respiration, substrate metabolism, and the effect of an inadequate O_2 supply. After considering internal (cellular) respiration, it examines the circulatory and ventilatory links between internal and external respiration, including the factors that determine the magnitude and time course of the cardiovascular, pulmonary gas exchange and ventilatory responses, and how they are coupled to the metabolic stress of exercise and determine exercise tolerance. Thus, this chapter is comprehensive and serves as the underpinning of the interpretation of the clinical problems to follow in subsequent chapters. Related historical perspectives can be found in the recent publications edited by Tipton.[1,2]

SKELETAL MUSCLE: MECHANICAL PROPERTIES AND FIBER TYPES

Human skeletal muscles consist of two basic fiber types: types I and II (**Table 2.1**). These fiber types are classified on the basis of both their contractile and biochemical properties.[3-5] Type I (slow-twitch) fibers take a longer time to develop peak tension (approximately 80 ms) and longer time to half relaxation following their activation than type II (fast-twitch) fibers (approximately 30 ms). The slow contractile properties of type I fibers appear to result largely from the relatively low activity of the myosin ATPase at the myofibril that catalyzes the splitting of the terminal high-energy phosphate of adenosine triphosphate (ATP), the lower calcium (Ca^{++}) activity of the regulatory protein troponin, and the slower rate of Ca^{++} uptake by sarcoplasmic reticulum. These same properties appear to confer a relatively high resistance to fatigue on the type I fibers.

Biochemical differences between the two basic fiber types focus chiefly on their capacity for oxidative and glycolytic activities. Type I slow-twitch fibers, being especially rich in myoglobin, are classified as red fibers, whereas type II fast-twitch fibers, which contain considerably less myoglobin, are classified as white fibers. The type I fibers tend to have significantly greater activities of oxidative enzymes than the type II fibers, which typically have a more glycolytic activity and enzyme profile. The type II fibers are further classified into type IIa and type IIx (formerly classified as type IIb).[5] Type IIa fibers have greater oxidative and lesser glycolytic potential compared with the type IIx fibers (see **Table 2.1**). With respect to substrate stores, muscle glycogen concentration is similar in type I and type II fibers, but the triglyceride content is two to three times greater in type I fibers. Also, the phosphocreatine (PCr) concentration is approximately 20% lower in type I fibers than type II.[6] Rodent studies suggest that type I fibers may be more efficient than the type II fibers, using less substrate energy to fuel muscle contractions, especially at lower force generation or slower shortening velocity.[7,8] Considerable potential for change by specific training exists in the enzyme concentrations of a particular fiber. For example, a type IIa fiber in an endurance-trained athlete could have higher concentrations of oxidative enzymes than type I fiber of a chronically sedentary individual.[9] These structural and functional differences between fiber types depend to a large extent on their neural innervation. A single motor neuron supplies numerous individual muscle fibers; this functional assembly being termed a motor unit. These fibers are distributed throughout the muscle rather than being spatially contiguous. Fibers comprising a motor unit are characteristically of the same fiber type, and substrate depletion occurs rather uniformly within each fiber of the contracting unit.

Fiber type distribution within human skeletal muscle varies from muscle to muscle. For example, the soleus muscle typically has a much higher density of type I fibers (>80%) than the gastrocnemius muscle (approximately 50%) or the triceps brachii (approximately 20% to 50%). The vastus lateralis muscle (approximately 50% type I fibers) has been used widely for analysis of fiber type characteristics in humans. Its basic fiber type pattern varies within the muscle and among individuals. Thus, type I fibers are preferentially expressed in deeper muscle regions compared to near the surface, and deeper muscle regions have greater capillary density. Elite endurance athletes typically have a high percentage of type I fibers in this muscle (>70% is not uncommon) compared with untrained control individuals (approximately 50%) or elite sprinters (20%-30%).

Whereas basic fiber type pattern is genetically determined, it is greatly influenced by the neural characteristics of the efferent motor neuron. When the motor nerves innervating a predominantly slow-twitch muscle are cut and cross-spliced to a predominantly fast-twitch muscle, the contractile and biochemical characteristics of the muscle begin to resemble the features of the muscle originally

TABLE 2.1 Characteristics of Muscle Fiber Types

	Slow oxidative (type I)	Fast oxidative (type IIa)	Fast glycolytic (type IIx)
Contraction	Slow twitch	Fast twitch	Fast twitch
Fiber size	Small	Intermediate	Large
Color	Red	Red	White
Myoglobin concentration	High	High	Low
Mitochondrial content	High	High	Low

innervated by the nerve.[10] Thus, an important trophic influence on muscle function is conferred by its nerve supply. Although phenotypic changes within a muscle fiber are influenced by training status, a typical program of exercise training does not result in dramatic interchanges between fractional expression of type I and type II myosin heavy chains, contrasting with the large adaptations observed in oxidative or glycolytic enzyme activities. Aging results in increased type I fiber expression, via selective loss of innervation of type II fibers. This process may contribute to age-associated muscle atrophy. Evidence is also accumulating that long-term muscle inactivity (eg, muscle denervation, complete bed rest, spaceflight, or chronic disease) results in a shift toward a greater percentage of type II fibers and loss of muscle oxidative capacity.

The pattern of activation of fiber types depends on the form of exercise. For low-intensity exercise, the type I fibers tend to be predominantly recruited, whereas the type II fibers (which produce greater force) are recruited at higher work rates, especially above 60% to 80% of the maximal aerobic power.[4,11,12] It should be noted that although endurance training increases the oxidative capacity of activated muscle fibers and detraining reduces it, it is difficult to discern a specific pathophysiology in the overall response to detraining, other than an increase in anaerobic metabolism at a lower work rate.

BIOENERGETICS

Skeletal muscle may be considered to be a machine that is fueled by the chemical energy of substrates derived from ingested food and stored predominantly as carbohydrates and lipids throughout the body, as well as PCr and ATP stored in the muscle. Although protein is a perfectly viable energy source, it is not used to fuel the energy needs of the body to any appreciable extent, except under conditions of starvation. Lactate is a carbohydrate moiety that is preferentially used as a fuel in place other carbohydrates or fats under conditions when blood lactate concentration exceeds cellular concentration. The interested reader is referred to the references for additional details on this section.[13-19]

The free energy of the substrate (ie, that fraction of the total chemical energy that is capable of doing work) is not used directly for muscle contraction. It must first be converted into and stored as the terminal phosphate bond of ATP. This terminal phosphate bond therefore has a high free energy of hydrolysis (ΔG) and is designated as a high-energy phosphate ($\sim P$) bond. Estimates of ΔG per $\sim P$ bond for physiological conditions such as those occurring in contracting muscle are approximately −65 to −70 kJ/mol. The activation energy of myosin ATPase is approximately 40 kJ/mol,[20] meaning that the free energy from $\sim P$ bond cleavage to activate the myosin head after unbinding with actin is likely well in excess of that needed across the wide variety of conditions in which muscle fatigue occurs.[21]

Therefore, muscle is ultimately a digital device operating in discrete multiple units of $\sim P$ bond energy, with one $\sim P$ bond thought to be cleaved per myosin cross-bridge linkage to, and subsequent release from, actin.[22,23] The muscle uses this energy for the conformational changes, manifested externally by shortening and/or increasing tension. Thus, muscular exercise depends on the structural characteristics of muscle and on the body's physiological support systems, which operate to maintain a physicochemical milieu for adequate ATP regeneration. Although whole-body metabolic rate increases by approximately 15 to 20 times the resting value (in an active healthy individual), the exercising muscle increases ATP use by approximately 100 times between rest (approximately 1 mM/kg/min) and maximal exercise (approximately 100 mM/kg/min). However, because the resting intramuscular [ATP] is low (i.e., approximately 8 mM/kg), a continual and proportional resynthesis of ATP from adenosine diphosphate (ADP) during exercise is required if rapid ATP depletion is to be avoided. Indeed, [ATP] typically remains unchanged during exercise, although decreases have been reported under extreme conditions of ischemia, hypoxia, and very severe intensity muscle contractions.

Sources of High-Energy Phosphate and Cellular Respiration

Energy for muscular contraction is obtained predominantly through the oxidation in the mitochondria of three-carbon (pyruvate) and two-carbon (acetyl-CoA) metabolic intermediaries from carbohydrate and fatty acid catabolitsm (**Fig. 2.1**) and, in nutritionally deficient states, certain amino acids. A small additional amount of energy comes from the Embden-Meyerhof pathway (glycolysis) in the cell cytoplasm that catabolizes glucose and glycosyl units (from glycogen) to pyruvate (see **Fig. 2.1**). Both the mitochondrial and cytosolic sources of energy are transformed into high-energy phosphate compounds, predominantly PCr and ATP. During the splitting of $\sim P$ from these compounds, energy is released for cellular reactions such as biosynthesis, active transport, and muscle contraction. Exercise entails an acceleration of these energy-yielding reactions in the muscles to regenerate $\sim P$ at the increased rates needed for the energy expenditure of physical work. Thus, the cellular consumption of O_2 is increased, which must be matched by an increased delivery of O_2 from the atmosphere to the mitochondria. Simultaneously, CO_2, a major catabolic end product of exercise, is removed from the cell by muscle blood flow and eliminated from the body by ventilating the pulmonary blood flow.

In the mitochondrial tricarboxylic acid (TCA) cycle, acetyl-CoA reacts with oxaloacetate to form citrate (see **Fig. 2.1**). A series of catabolic reactions in the TCA cycle results in CO_2 formation and the transfer of protons (H^+) and their associated electrons to the mitochondrial electron transport system. Electrons flow down the energy gradient of the electron transport system to the terminal electron acceptor: O_2. This process pumps H^+ ions out of the mitochondrial matrix, producing an electrochemical gradient across the inner mitochondrial membrane. The resulting potential energy is harnessed via ATP synthase

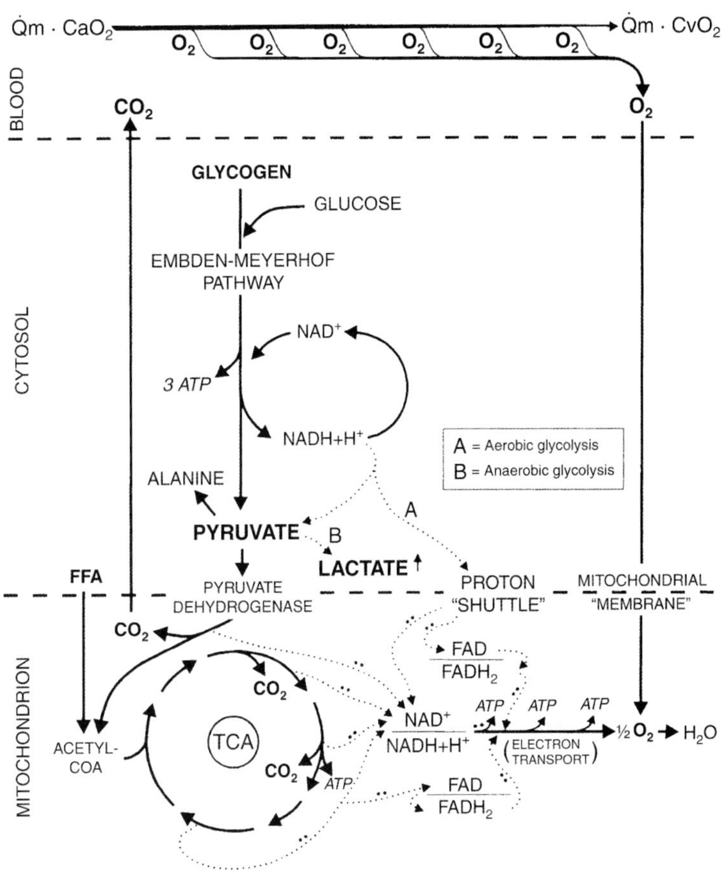

FIGURE 2.1. Scheme of the major biochemical pathways for production of adenosine triphosphate (ATP). Pathway A, theoretical maximum high ATP yield from carbohydrate catabolism by aerobic glycolysis and free fatty acid (FFA) oxidation, via the "shuttle" of H^+ ions from the cytosol to the mitochondrion and the transfer of H^+ and electrons to O_2 by the mitochondrial electron transport system, which is supported by O_2 flow from the blood to the mitochondrion. Pathway B, low ATP yield from carbohydrate catabolism by anaerobic glycolysis, when O_2 flow to mitochondria becomes inadequate, with cytosolic NADH + H^+ being reoxidized to NAD^+ via the conversion of pyruvate to lactate.

(complex V) for the resynthesis of ATP from ADP and inorganic phosphate (Pi). In this way, ATP resynthesis is coupled to the consumption of O_2 (ie, oxidative phosphorylation). At the end of the electron transport system, cytochrome oxidase catalyzes the reaction of a pair of H^+ ions and electrons with an atom of O_2 (½O_2) to form a molecule of water. For each transfer of a pair of H^+ ions and electrons down the electron transport system, the maximum ATP yield is three molecules if the electron transport process begins at nicotinamide adenine dinucleotide (NAD^+) (complex I), but only two if it begins at flavin adenine dinucleotide (FAD) (complex III) (see **Fig. 2.1**). However, the actual ATP yields are likely lower (ie, approximately 2.5 and 1.5 ATP molecules,[24] respectively), reflecting factors such as H^+ losses due to leaky inner mitochondrial membranes and active transport of ADP and Pi from the cytoplasm into the mitochondrial matrix.[25,26] The precise stoichiometry is therefore difficult to establish.

There is a net gain of 7 ATP molecules during the cytosolic catabolism of glycogen to pyruvate via glycolysis, if the reduced nicotinamide adenine dinucleotide (NADH + H^+) in the cytosol is reoxidized in the mitochondria (see **Fig. 2.1**, pathway A).[24] The number of ATP molecules produced in this way falls to 5 if $FADH_2$ is used (see **Fig. 2.1**, pathway A).[24] Of the ATP molecules regenerated by this mechanism, three are formed in the cytosol by glycolysis, and the remainder in the electron transport system during the coupled reoxidation of cytosolic NADH + H^+. Mitochondrial shuttles accept H^+ ions from the cytosolic NADH + H^+ and transfer them to NAD^+ or FAD in the mitochondrion (see **Fig. 2.1**). This method of regenerating oxidized NAD^+ in the cytosol maintains the cytosolic redox state and enables glycolysis to continue. Because O_2 is the ultimate recipient of the H^+ ions that are generated by glycolysis and transported into the mitochondria, this glycolysis is aerobic (see **Fig. 2.1**, pathway A).

The formation of acetyl-CoA from pyruvate and its subsequent entry into the TCA cycle yields a total of four reduced mitochondrial NADH + H^+ and one $FADH_2$. Because the reoxidation of each NADH + H^+ by the electron transport chain yields 2.5 ATP molecules and $FADH_2$ yields 1.5, there is a net gain of 11.5 ATP molecules. However, two molecules of acetyl-CoA are formed from each glycogen molecule, so the total net gain is 23 ATP molecules from these reactions. When added to the net gain of up to 7 from aerobic glycogenolysis (see **Fig. 2.1**), the complete oxidation of glycogen yields 30 ATP molecules. Because 6 molecules of O_2 are used for glucose oxidation and 30 high-energy phosphate bonds are formed, the ratio of ~P to O_2 (~P:O_2) is 5 for glycogen (**Table 2.2**). Six molecules of CO_2 and H_2O are catabolic end products of these reactions (Equation 3).

Under conditions in which the mitochondrial proton shuttles fail to reoxidize the NADH + H^+ generated by glycolysis at a rate sufficient to keep cytosolic [NADH + H^+]/[NAD^+] normal (see **Fig. 2.1**), the redox state of the cytosol

TABLE 2.2 Theoretical Maximal and Actual Estimates of High-Energy Phosphate Yield From Carbohydrate and Free Fatty Acid Oxidation for a Standardized Exercise Bout Requiring an O_2 Uptake of 1 L/min

	RQ	$\dot{V}O_2$ (L/min)	$\dot{V}CO_2$ (L/min)	~P:O_2 (max)	~P:CO_2 (max)	~P:O_2 (actual)	~P:CO_2 (actual)
Carbohydrate (glucose)	1.0	1.0	1.0	6.00	6.00	4.80	4.80
Free fatty acid (palmitate)	0.7	1.0	0.7	5.65	8.13	4.35	6.25

Abbreviation: CO_2, carbon dioxide; O_2, oxygen; ~P, high-energy phosphate; RQ, respiratory quotient; $\dot{V}CO_2$, CO_2 output; $\dot{V}O_2$, O_2 uptake.

is lowered. Because NADH + H^+ accumulates in the cytosol at the expense of NAD^+, glycolysis would slow if it were not for an alternate pathway capable of reoxidizing cytosolic NADH + H^+. When NADH + H^+ accumulates, pyruvate can reoxidize the NADH + H^+ back to NAD^+. However, by its acceptance of the two H^+ ions, pyruvate is reduced to lactate (see **Fig. 2.1**, pathway B). Thus, pyruvate oxidation of NADH + H^+ results in lactate accumulation. Because the breakdown of glycogen to lactate occurs without use of O_2, it is termed anaerobic glycolysis. The substrate price for the production of energy from this reaction is expensive compared with the complete oxidation of glycogen to CO_2 and H_2O. The net gain in ATP is only 3 from each glycosyl unit instead of 30. For the same work rate, therefore, this pathway causes glycogen to be used at a considerably faster rate than when the production of ~P is wholly aerobic.

Moreover, the two lactate anions, along with their associated protons, that accumulate when each glycosyl unit undergoes anaerobic metabolism disturb acid-base balance in the cell and blood (**Fig. 2.2**). That the "turn-on" of anaerobic ATP production does not signal the "turn-off" of aerobic ATP production deserves emphasis. Both aerobic and anaerobic mechanisms share a common pathway (glycosyl breakdown to pyruvate) and therefore share in energy generation at high work rates, with the anaerobic mechanism providing an increasing proportion of energy as the work rate is increased.

Phosphocreatine Breakdown

Muscular O_2 consumption during exercise is inextricably linked to increased rates of ~P utilization. Oxidative phosphorylation is the major source of resynthesis of ATP, which is used to fuel muscular contraction and active transport during exercise. However, PCr, with an intracellular concentration some 3 to 4 times greater than that of ATP, can also serve as a mediator of ATP resynthesis through the creatine kinase reaction; that is,

$$PCr + ADP + \beta H^+ \leftrightarrow Cr + ATP \quad (1)$$

Note that the breakdown of PCr produces an alkalinizing reaction, the degree of which depends on a variable stoichiometry as indicated by the β in Equation 1 (see "Buffering the Exercise-Induced Lactic Acidosis" and "Carbon Dioxide Output Kinetics" below).

Kushmerick and Conley[27] called PCr a "chemical capacitor" for ATP. That is, it acts as a spatial and temporal energy buffer within the muscle cell to prevent a fall of [ATP] during times of increased energy demand.[28] For example, a decrease in [PCr] contributes to energy provision during the initial stages of constant work rate exercise when $\dot{V}O_2$ has not yet attained steady state levels, thus creating an "O_2 deficit"; that is, a reduction in bodily stores of energy equivalents that is replenished through oxidative processes only once recovery from exercise is complete. The PCr contribution to the O_2 deficit is proportionally greater than the slower the time course of the $\dot{V}O_2$ increase (see "Oxygen Deficit" below). For moderate-intensity (ie, aerobic) exercise (see "Arterial Lactate Increase as a Function of Time" below), the sum of the utilization of PCr and O_2 stores is sufficient to account for the entire O_2 deficit.

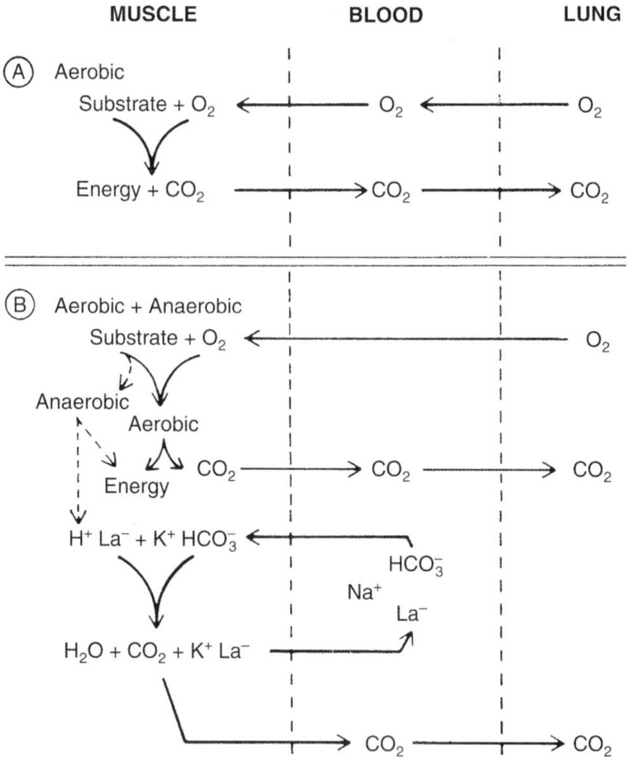

FIGURE 2.2. Gas exchange during aerobic (A) and aerobic plus anaerobic (B) exercise. The acid-base consequence of the latter is a net increase in cell hydrogen (H^+) and lactate (La^-) production. The buffering of the accumulating H^+ takes place in the cell at the site of formation by bicarbonate (HCO_3^-). This mechanism will increase the carbon dioxide (CO_2) production of the cell by approximately 22 mL/mEq for each millimole of H^+ buffered by HCO_3^-. The increase in cell [lactate] and decrease in cell [HCO_3^-] will result in chemical concentration gradients, causing lactate to be transported out of and HCO_3^- to be transported into the cell. Abbreviations: H_2O, water; K, potassium; Na, sodium; O_2, oxygen.

At higher work rates, however, anaerobic energy transfer from glycogenolysis to form lactate supplements these stored resources.

In addition to serving as an "energy buffer," PCr is also thought to play an important role in the control of oxidative phosphorylation, likely through its relationship to local ADP:

$$[ADP] = ([ATP][Cr])/([PCr][H^+]\,Keq) \quad (2)$$

where Keq is the equilibrium constant of the creatine kinase reaction. Thus, [ADP] increases as [PCr] and $[H^+]$ decrease. The ADP accumulation is damped by PCr breakdown but provides an important signal for triggering the increase in mitochondrial O_2 consumption to supply ATP to the cytosol at a higher rate.[28-31] In fact, the time course of the change in [PCr] during constant work rate exercise (measured by phosphorus-31 nuclear magnetic resonance spectroscopy) is essentially indistinguishable from that of $\dot{V}O_2$ (and, by extension, cellular O_2 consumption) in exercising humans.[31] These reactions are reversed in early recovery and constitute part of the repayment of the O_2 debt.

Substrate Utilization

At this point, several terms need to be clarified for precision and to avoid possible confusion (see **Fig. 1.1**). The symbol $\dot{V}O_2$ indicates O_2 uptake by the lungs per minute. It is distinguished from O_2 consumption by the cells, which is symbolized by $\dot{Q}O_2$. The symbol $\dot{V}CO_2$ indicates CO_2 output by the lungs per minute, distinguished from CO_2 production by the cells, which is symbolized by $\dot{Q}CO_2$. Thus, the substrate mixture undergoing oxidation is characterized by the net rates of O_2 consumption ($\dot{Q}O_2$) and CO_2 yield or production ($\dot{Q}CO_2$). The ratio $\dot{V}CO_2/\dot{V}O_2$ as measured at the mouth (ie, the respiratory exchange ratio, R) reflects $\dot{Q}CO_2/\dot{Q}O_2$, the metabolic respiratory quotient (RQ), *only* when there is a steady state in $\dot{V}CO_2$ and $\dot{V}O_2$; that is, when there is no further removal of CO_2 from and no further addition of O_2 to the body, the CO_2 stores and O_2 stores are constant. Thus, in the new exercise steady state, $\dot{V}CO_2$ and $\dot{V}O_2$ are equal to $\dot{Q}CO_2$ and $\dot{Q}O_2$, respectively.

During acute hyperventilation (eg, resulting from acute hypoxia, pain, anxiety, or volitional influences), considerably more CO_2 is unloaded from the body CO_2 stores than O_2 is loaded into the O_2 stores. This is because hemoglobin (Hb), at sea level, is almost completely saturated with O_2 at the end of the pulmonary capillaries and the physical solubility of O_2 in blood is low, meaning that increases in alveolar O_2 partial pressure (PO_2) will have minimal effects on increasing O_2 stores. On the other hand, appreciable amounts of CO_2 can be unloaded from blood and tissue stores as alveolar ventilation ($\dot{V}A$) is increased and arterial PCO_2 ($PaCO_2$) is reduced. Thus, with acute hyperventilation, R will exceed the metabolic RQ until the CO_2 stores have stabilized at the new lower level (ie, with $\dot{V}CO_2$ equaling $\dot{Q}CO_2$). Similarly, during the acute metabolic (largely lactic) acidosis of exercise, "extra" CO_2 is evolved when bicarbonate (HCO_3^-) buffers the acidosis (see **Fig. 2.2**). This will also result in R exceeding RQ until a new lower steady state in CO_2 stores is attained, when $\dot{V}CO_2$ again equals $\dot{Q}CO_2$ and R again equals RQ. Differences between R and RQ will also occur during acute hypoventilation and recovery from the metabolic acidosis but in the opposite direction.

As seen in the following equations, carbohydrate (eg, glycogen or glucose) is oxidized with RQ equal to 1.0 (ie, six CO_2 molecules produced and six O_2 molecules consumed) and has an actual $\sim P{:}O_2$ in the range of 4.83 to 5.00, depending on whether glucose or glycogen is the substrate (see **Table 2.2**):

$$C_6H_{12}O_6 + 6\,O_2 \rightarrow 6\,CO_2 + 6\,H_2O + 29 \text{ or } 30\,ATP \quad (3)$$

Lipid (eg, palmitate) is oxidized with RQ equal to 0.71 (ie, 16 CO_2 molecules produced to 23 O_2 consumed) and has a $\sim P{:}O_2$ of 4.35 (ie, 100 ATP/23 O_2):

$$C_{16}H_{32}O_2 + 23\,O_2 \rightarrow 16\,CO_2 + 16\,H_2O + 100\,ATP \quad (4)$$

Slightly more ATP is generated per molecule of O_2 used (ie, $\sim P{:}O_2$ is greater) when carbohydrate is the substrate compared with a fatty acid such as palmitic acid (ie, about 6%-10% more, depending on the involved fatty acids). Consequently, steady-state $\dot{V}O_2$ is slightly increased (and steady-state $\dot{V}CO_2$ is slightly reduced) for a given work rate when fatty acids are the predominant substrate (**Fig. 2.3**, left panel).[32,33] Intermediate steady-state RQ values reflect different proportions of carbohydrate and fat being used (**Fig. 2.4**). With respect to storage economy, however, fat is the more efficient energy source.

When a steady state of gas exchange exists, R provides an accurate reflection of whole-body RQ. During exercise, the muscle RQ can be estimated from the steady-state increase in $\dot{V}CO_2$ relative to the increase in $\dot{V}O_2$ over the range of moderate-intensity work rates. It should be noted that muscle RQ makes a progressively greater contribution to R with increasing work rate, in proportion to the increase in the active muscle mass. Because muscle RQ is high relative to that of most other organs (with the exception of the nervous system), the total body RQ increases from a resting value of approximately 0.8 (on an average Western diet) toward approximately 0.95 with increasing work rate over the moderate-intensity range (**Fig. 2.5**). An RQ of 0.95 indicates that about 84% of the substrate during exercise is derived from carbohydrate (see **Fig. 2.4**). Although the fuel mixture for the total body derives proportionally more from carbohydrate than from lipid stores as work rate increases (see **Fig. 2.5**), R decreases slowly over time during prolonged constant work rate exercise (particularly at higher work rates) (**Fig. 2.6**), reflecting a decrease in the proportional utilization of carbohydrate as muscle glycogen stores decline.

When muscle glycogen stores become depleted, as occurs in prolonged exercise at higher work rates associated with a metabolic acidosis, fatigue ensues, although prior

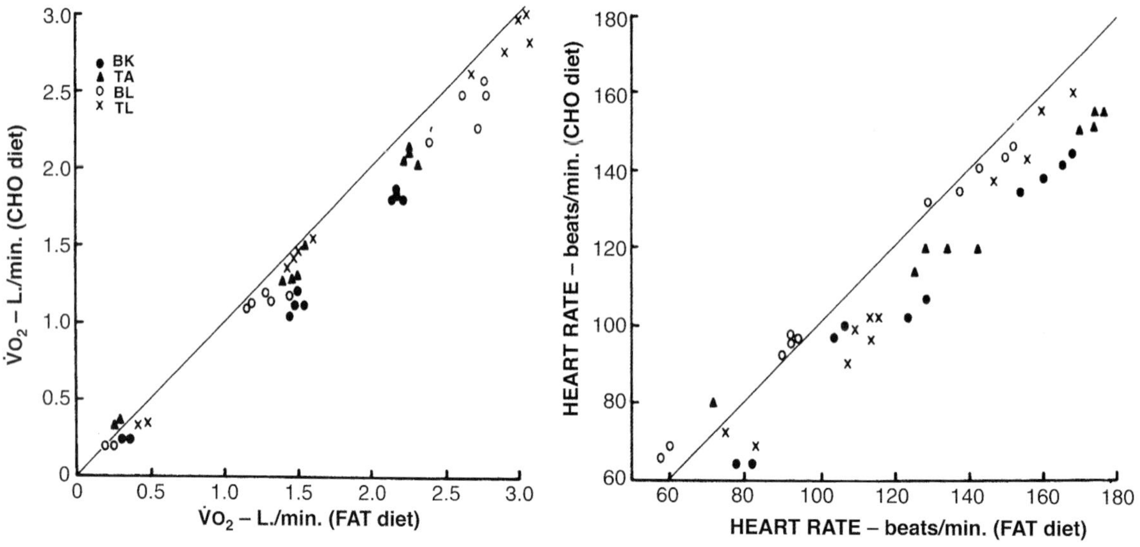

FIGURE 2.3. Effect of dietary substrate on group-mean (n = 4) O_2 uptake ($\dot{V}O_2$) (left panel) and heart rate (right panel) at rest and during two different moderate constant cycle ergometer work rates after 3 days on a high-carbohydrate diet (resting respiratory quotient [RQ] = 0.97) and after 3 days on a high-fat diet (resting RQ = 0.75). $\dot{V}O_2$ is higher on the high-fat diet than on the high-carbohydrate diet for both work rates. This is consistent with the biochemical evidence that the high-energy phosphate yield from fat is less than that from carbohydrate for a given O_2 cost. Heart rate during exercise is higher on the high-fat diet than on the high-carbohydrate diet, reflecting the link between cardiac output and O_2 consumption.

muscle glycogen supplementation strategies and acute ingestion of glucose can prolong exercise time.[34,35] The rate of decrease in muscle glycogen during prolonged exercise can be slowed by raising blood glucose levels with a continued infusion of glucose.[36] The importance of muscle glycogen in exercise tolerance was well described in the early experiments of Bergström et al,[37] who demonstrated a strong positive correlation between the tolerable duration of high-intensity exercise and the preexercise muscle glycogen content.

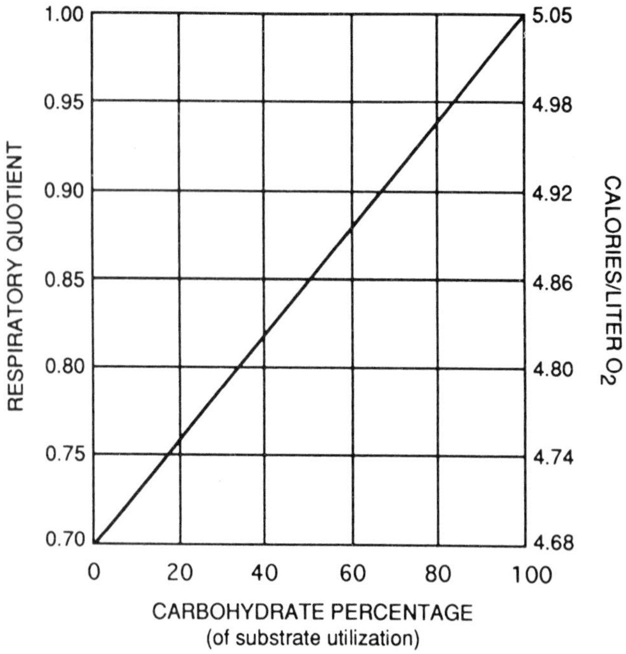

FIGURE 2.4. The percentage of carbohydrate substrate in the diet estimated from the respiratory quotient measurement. The calories of energy obtained per liter of O_2 consumed for each combination is given on the right ordinate. *(Reprinted from Lusk G.* The Elements of the Science of Nutrition. *New York, NY: Johnson Reprint Corp; 1976. Copyright © 1976 Elsevier. With permission.)*

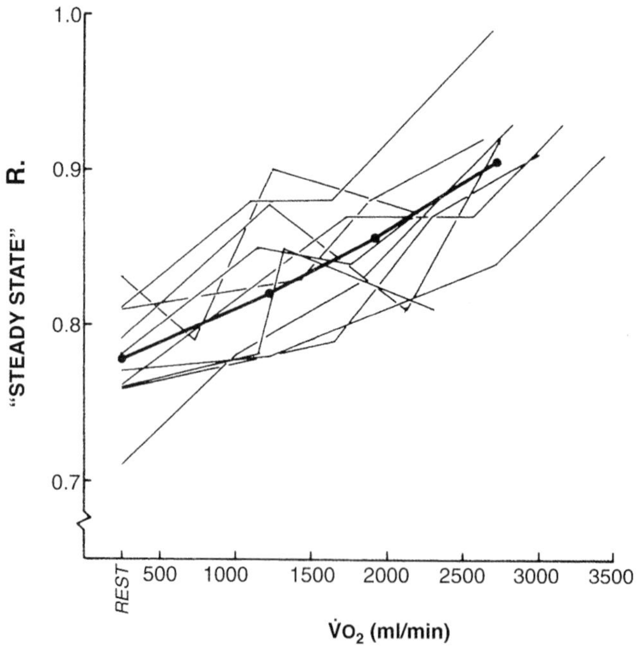

FIGURE 2.5. Group-mean (n = 10) steady-state gas exchange ratio (R, equal to the respiratory quotient) for prolonged constant work rate cycle ergometer exercise (target duration = 50 min) of moderate, heavy, and very heavy intensities, determined as the ratio of steady-state carbon dioxide output to O_2 uptake ($\dot{V}O_2$).

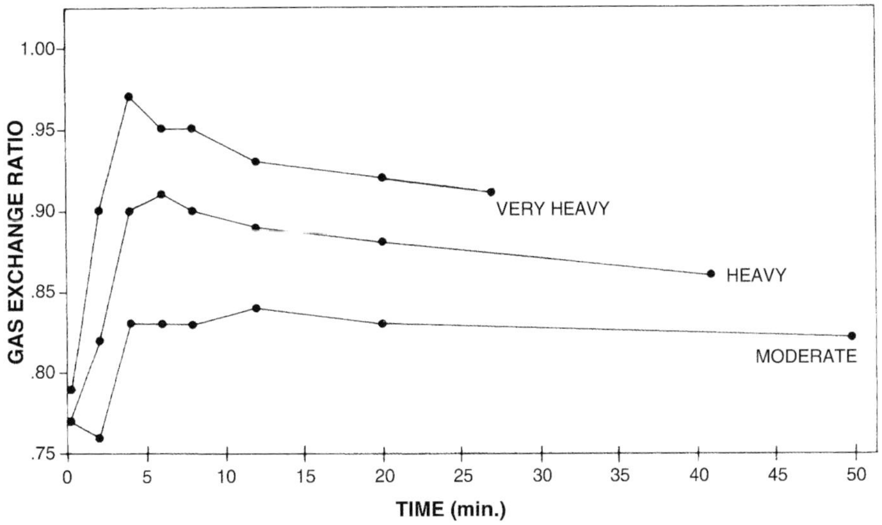

FIGURE 2.6. Gas exchange ratio (R) as a function of time for constant work rate cycle ergometer exercise of moderate, heavy, and very heavy intensities in a normal individual. Note that R is (1) higher as exercise intensity increases, largely reflective of a higher carbohydrate to fat ratio, and (2) slowly declines with time after the initial increase, likely resulting from a slow depletion of muscle carbohydrate stores.

Physical fitness, in the sense of the capacity for sustained activity, affects the substrate utilization pattern. An individual with greater cardiorespiratory fitness uses a greater proportion of fatty acids for energy than an unfit individual, both at rest and during submaximal exercise.[14,16,19,38,39] This mechanism conserves glycogen, allowing more work to be performed before glycogen depletion ensues, with consequent intolerance. The specific contribution of different substrates during exercise is considered in the following sections.

Carbohydrates

Skeletal muscle in humans contains, on average, 80 to 100 mmol (15-18 g) glucose per kilogram of wet weight stored as glycogen. For a 70-kg man, this amounts to approximately 400 g of muscle glycogen.[37] However, a contracting muscle can draw only on its own glycogen reserves and not on the pools in noncontracting muscles.

Normally, approximately 4 to 5 g of glucose are available in the blood (approximately 100 mg/100 mL). Although muscle uptake of blood glucose increases considerably during exercise, the blood concentration does not fall because of an increased rate of glucose release from the liver. The liver represents a highly labile glycogen reserve, in the range of 50 to 90 g. This glycogen is broken down into glucose by glycogenolysis and released into the blood. Glucose can also be produced in the liver (gluconeogenesis) from lactate, pyruvate, glycerol, and alanine precursors. The rate of glucose release from the liver into the circulation depends on both the blood glucose concentration and a complex interaction of hormones such as insulin, glucagon, and the catecholamines epinephrine and norepinephrine.[19] As exercise intensity and duration increase, the circulating levels of catecholamines and glucagon increase,[19,40,41] contributing to blood glucose homeostasis despite its increased utilization by the exercising muscles. These regulatory processes maintain physiologically adequate concentrations of glucose, except when muscle and liver glycogen stores become greatly depleted.

Lipids

Skeletal muscles have access to their own intramuscular store of lipids, averaging 20 g of triglycerides per kilogram of wet weight. This source accounts for a considerable proportion of the total energy required by the muscles, depending on the cardiorespiratory fitness of the individual, the duration and intensity of exercise, and the rate of muscle glycogen depletion.[16,18,38,39]

Extramuscular lipid sources are also used during exercise. These stores are large—in a 70-kg male, approximately 15 kg of triglycerides, which is equivalent to about 135 000 kcal of energy. Triglyceride hydrolysis in adipose tissue yields glycerol and free fatty acids (mainly palmitic, stearic, oleic, and linoleic acids). The free fatty acids are transported in the blood, bound predominantly to albumin, although accounting for only a small proportion (usually less than 5%) of the total plasma fatty acid pool; triglycerides accounting for the remainder.

Resting plasma free fatty acid concentrations are approximately 0.5 mmol/L, increasing during exercise to approximately 2 mmol/L. The turnover rate of the plasma free fatty acid pool is high, with a half-time of 2 to 3 minutes at rest and less during exercise. As a consequence, the flux of free fatty acids to the exercising muscle (ie, plasma flow × plasma free fatty acid concentration) is an important determinant of skeletal muscle uptake.

The sympathetic nervous system, along with catecholamines from the adrenal medulla, controls adipose tissue lipolysis during exercise.[16,18,19,38] Epinephrine and norepinephrine increase the local concentration of cyclic 3′,5′-AMP through activation of adenyl cyclase. This leads to increased rates of hydrolysis of the stored adipose tissue triglycerides. Other factors reduce the rate of adipose tissue lipolysis during exercise, including increased blood [lactate] and exogenous glucose loads.

Interestingly, the plasma concentration of free fatty acids does not increase with physical training and may even decrease slightly. Therefore, the increased proportional contribution of free fatty acid oxidation to exercise energetics, when measured at a specific work rate after training, may reflect increased utilization from intramuscular sources.

Amino Acids

Amino acid oxidation is not normally a significant contributor to intramuscular ATP production during exercise (contributing less than 10% at most), although it may become more important when glycogen depletion occurs.[16,38] Only a small number of amino acids are capable of undergoing oxidation, of which the branched-chain amino acids leucine and isoleucine are the most significant as they can be converted to acetyl-CoA (see "Sources of High-Energy Phosphate and Cellular Respiration" above).

OXYGEN COST OF WORK

The O_2 cost of performing work depends on the work rate. **Figure 2.7** shows the time course of $\dot{V}O_2$ from unloaded cycling for various levels of constant work rate cycle ergometer exercise in a normal individual.[42] Note that, in this individual, a steady state is reached within 3 minutes up to a work rate of 150 W. At higher work rates, $\dot{V}O_2$ continued to increase above the 3-minute value; and, above 250 W, the individual was unable to complete the 10-minute task duration. The end-exercise $\dot{V}O_2$ for each work rate above 250 W was the same, thereby identifying the individual's maximum $\dot{V}O_2$ ($\dot{V}O_2max$); that is, defined as no further increase in $\dot{V}O_2$ despite further increases in work rate.[43,44] Note that the higher the work rate, the earlier $\dot{V}O_2max$ is reached, thus signifying that the level of intolerance was reached earlier (exercise not being sustainable at $\dot{V}O_2max$). The relationship between work rate and the tolerable duration (in this case, determined by the time at which $\dot{V}O_2max$ was reached for the three work rates above 250 W) characterizes the individual's power-duration relationship (see "Power-Duration Curve and Critical Power" below). The $\dot{V}O_2$ kinetic profiles shown in **Figure 2.7** are generally typical of all individuals, but the work rate at which the nonsteady-state pattern of $\dot{V}O_2$ emerges differs depending on the individual's cardiorespiratory fitness (see "Oxygen Uptake Kinetics" below).

$\dot{V}O_2$ Steady State and Work Efficiency

When plotting the steady-state $\dot{V}O_2$ values for those cycle ergometer work rates in which a steady state is achieved (ie, in the moderate-intensity domain), such as shown for 50 W, 100 W, and 150 W in **Figure 2.7**, a linear relationship between $\dot{V}O_2$ and work rate is obtained (**Fig. 2.8**). The slope of this relationship ($\Delta\dot{V}O_2/\Delta WR$ or the $\dot{V}O_2$ response "gain") is relatively invariant in normal individuals (approximately 9-11 mL/min/W for cycle ergometry), regardless of age, sex, or training status. Because substrate utilization is relatively invariant during short duration exercise, the energy equivalent of the increase in $\dot{V}O_2$ required to perform a particular work rate increment (ie, the work efficiency) also does not vary widely among individuals.[38,45,46]

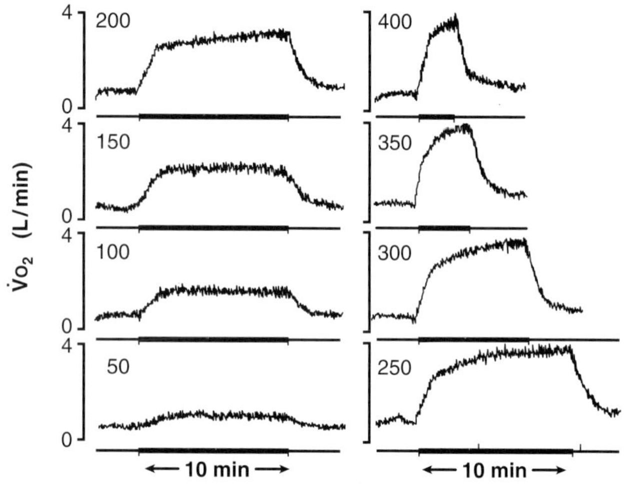

FIGURE 2.7. O_2 uptake ($\dot{V}O_2$) as a function of time for eight different constant work rate cycle ergometer tests, each starting from unloaded cycling, for a normal individual. The work rate (watts) for each test is shown in the respective panel. The bar on the x-axis indicates the period of the imposed work rate. The $\dot{V}O_2$ asymptote (steady state) is significantly delayed for exercise above the anaerobic threshold. *(Reprinted from Whipp BJ, Mahler M. Dynamics of pulmonary gas exchange during exercise. In: West JB, ed.* Pulmonary Gas Exchange. *New York, NY: Academic Press; 1980:33-96. Copyright © 1980 Elsevier. With permission.)*

This is a manifestation of the work efficiency: the constancy of the energy transfer processes within the active musculature reflecting the basic biochemical energy-yielding reactions needed for muscle contraction. However, there are also reports of work efficiency being higher (ie, lower $\Delta\dot{V}O_2/\Delta WR$) in individuals having a high proportion of type I fibers in their locomotor muscles.[45,47]

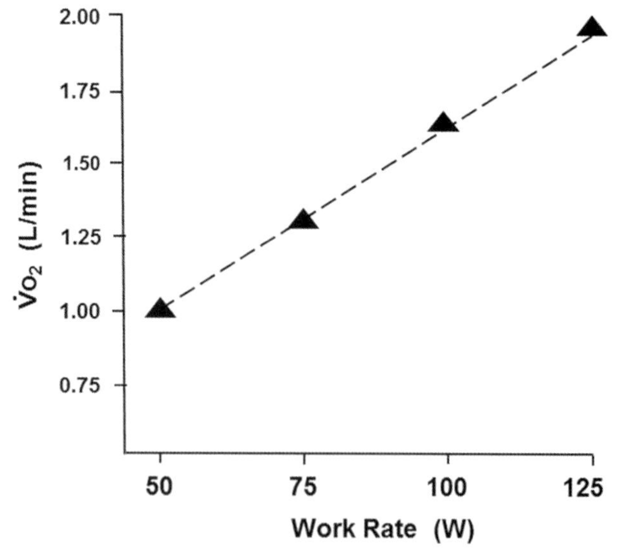

FIGURE 2.8. The steady-state relationship between O_2 uptake ($\dot{V}O_2$) and work rate for moderate cycle ergometer exercise, for a normal individual. This relationship is quite predictable for cycle ergometer exercise regardless of age, gender, or training. *(Data from Whipp BJ, Wasserman K. Oxygen uptake kinetics for various intensities of constant load work.* J Appl Physiol. *1972;33:351-356.)*

It is important to recognize that the $\dot{V}O_2$ of the "unloaded" cycle ergometer can vary considerably from one individual to another because of differences in the actual energy transfer of the "unloaded" cycling that depends on the characteristics of the ergometer, pedal frequency, and body weight because of the additional work rate generated as a result of moving the lower extremities[48] and pedaling cadence.[49] For obese individuals, the additional $\dot{V}O_2$ cost corresponds to an upward displacement of the $\dot{V}O_2$-work rate relationship of approximately 5.8 mL/min per kilogram of body weight, as long as pedaling frequency is constrained to be relatively constant; with the predicted $\dot{V}O_2$ (mL/min) for a given work rate being given by 5.8 × body wt (kg) + 151 + 10.1 × WR (watts).[48] This effect is more pronounced on the treadmill because movement of the entire body necessitates a greater additional energy cost. However, the work efficiency and $\Delta\dot{V}O_2/\Delta WR$ are essentially unchanged in obesity, again reflecting the constancy of the intramuscular energy transfer processes.

$\Delta\dot{V}O_2/\Delta WR$ is consequently much more uniform among individuals than $\dot{V}O_2/WR$. This accounts for gross and net efficiencies increasing with work rate as these are calculated, respectively, using the total $\dot{V}O_2$ associated with a particular work rate (ie, including resting and unloaded components) and the $\dot{V}O_2$ from a resting baseline (ie, including the unloaded component).[38,48-50] These fixed $\dot{V}O_2$ baseline corrections impose a progressively smaller influence on the total $\dot{V}O_2$ as work rate increases such that, unlike work efficiency, gross and net efficiency increase. Care must be taken not to confuse changes in skill or motor efficiency due to practice with changes in work efficiency. To measure work efficiency, relatively simple tasks should be employed that do not depend on technique and for which the work output can be measured (eg, cycling). To calculate work efficiency, the caloric equivalent of the steady-state $\dot{V}O_2$ (4.98 Cal/L $\dot{V}O_2$ at RQ = 0.95) (see **Fig. 2.4**) and the external power (0.014 Cal/min/W) for at least two measured work rates must be known. For cycle ergometry, normal individuals have a work efficiency of approximately 28%.[38,48-50]

$\dot{V}O_2$ Nonsteady State

For moderate constant work rate exercise, $\dot{V}O_2$ typically rises exponentially to attain a new steady state within about 2 to 3 minutes in healthy young individuals (see **Fig. 2.7**). For work rates that are accompanied by a metabolic acidosis, the continued slow increase in $\dot{V}O_2$ reflects an additional "slow component" that is superimposed on the primary exponential response (see **Fig. 2.7**). For such work rates, the magnitude of increase in $\dot{V}O_2$ between 3 and 6 minutes (a useful practical index for quantifying the magnitude of the $\dot{V}O_2$ slow component) correlates with the increase in arterial [lactate] over the same time interval in healthy individuals[51,52] and patients with heart disease (**Fig. 2.9**).[53] The characteristics of the $\dot{V}O_2$ slow component and its control mechanisms are considered in greater detail below (see "Oxygen Uptake Kinetics" below).

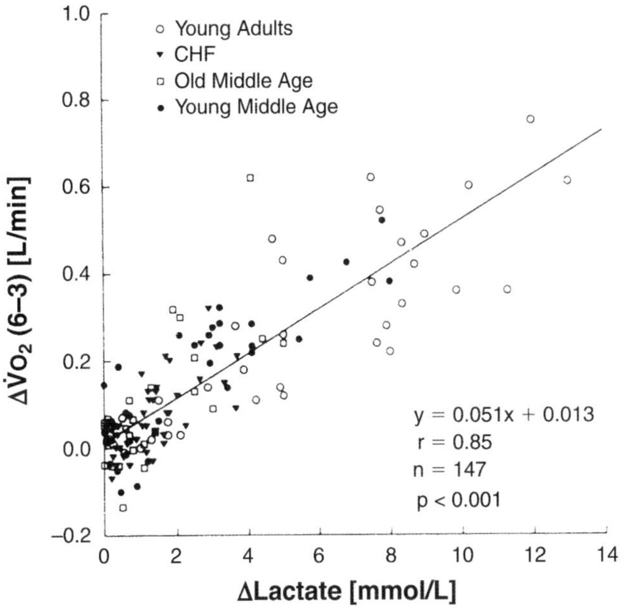

FIGURE 2.9. Arterial blood [lactate] above resting value (ΔLactate) as a function of the difference in O_2 uptake ($\dot{V}O_2$) between 3 and 6 minutes of moderate and suprathreshold constant work rate cycle ergometer exercise ($\Delta\dot{V}O_2$ [6 − 3]) in normal young (○), middle-aged (●), and late middle-aged (□) individuals and in patients with heart failure (▼). Normally, $\dot{V}O_2$ does not increase beyond 3 minutes when the exercise is performed at or below the anaerobic threshold (ie, $\Delta\dot{V}O_2$ [6 − 3] = 0). CHF, cardiac heart failure. *(Data from Roston WL, Whipp BJ, Davis JA, Cunningham DA, Effros RM, Wasserman K. Oxygen uptake kinetics and lactate concentration during exercise in humans.* Am Rev Respir Dis. *1987;135:1080-1084; Zhang YY, Wasserman K, Sietsema KE, et al.* O_2 *uptake kinetics in response to exercise. A measure of tissue anaerobiosis in heart failure.* Chest. *1993;103:735-741; and unpublished data on late middle-aged adults.)*

ARTERIAL LACTATE INCREASE

Arterial Lactate Increase as a Function of Work Rate

Figure 2.10 shows arterial [lactate] as related to $\dot{V}O_2$ in three groups of individuals performing incremental cycle ergometer exercise (ie, a stepped work rate increase or a continuous ramp exercise where the work rate is changed as a linear function of time): normal individuals who are relatively active, sedentary normal individuals, and patients with heart disease.[54] All show similar resting and low-level exercise arterial [lactate]. The pattern of [lactate] increase is qualitatively similar for each group, but the $\dot{V}O_2$ (and hence work rate) at which the [lactate] starts to increase differs. Arterial [lactate] does not start to increase in the young, active individuals until $\dot{V}O_2$ is increased to as much as 10 times resting. In contrast, the $\dot{V}O_2$ at which [lactate] starts to increase in the sedentary individuals is about 4 times the resting level (equivalent to the $\dot{V}O_2$ required for adults to walk at a normal pace). In the cardiac patients with a low, symptom-limited peak $\dot{V}O_2$, arterial [lactate] increases at exceedingly low work rates, perhaps less than twice resting metabolic rate, or can even be raised at rest.

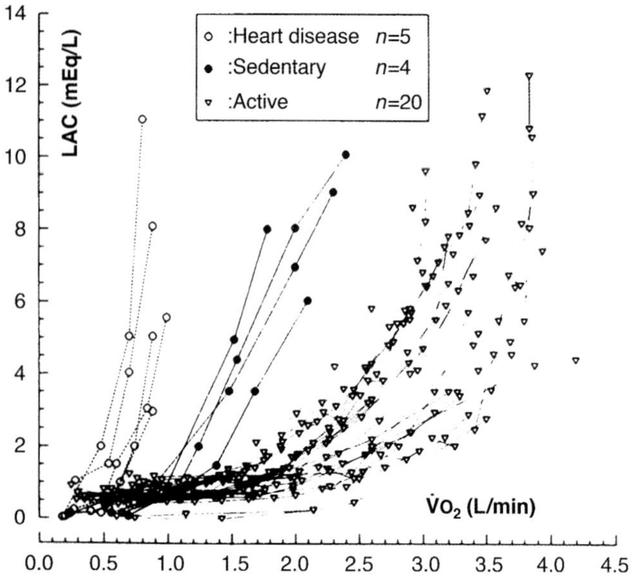

FIGURE 2.10. Arterial [lactate] as a function of O_2 uptake ($\dot{V}O_2$) for incremental cycle ergometer exercise in active (∇) and sedentary (●) healthy individuals and in patients with heart disease (○). Lactate concentration rises from approximately the same resting value to approximately similar levels at maximal exercise in each of the three groups. The fitter the individual for aerobic exercise, the higher the $\dot{V}O_2$ before [lactate] starts to increase significantly above resting levels. *(Modified from Wasserman K. Coupling of external to cellular respiration during exercise: the wisdom of the body revisited.* Am J Physiol. *1994;266[4 pt 1]:E519-E539.)*

The $\dot{V}O_2$ at which arterial [lactate] starts to increase is termed the *lactate threshold* (*LT*) and is generally synonymous with what has been termed the *lactic acidosis threshold* (*LAT*), the *anaerobic threshold* (*AT*), and the *gas exchange threshold* (*GET*). The *AT*, *LT*, *LAT*, and *GET* describe events deriving from the onset of a metabolic acidosis in exercising muscle. The distinction in terminology reflects the method of measurement.[55-57] Although these terms are often used interchangeably, we regard the technically correct definitions to be as follows (see also Chapter 3, "Anaerobic (Lactate, Lactic Acidosis) Threshold"):

- **Anaerobic threshold:** the exercise $\dot{V}O_2$ above which anaerobically produced ~P supplements the aerobically produced ~P, with consequent lowering of the cytosolic redox state, increasing the [lactate]/[pyruvate] (L/P) ratio, and lactate production at the site of cellular anaerobiosis
- **Lactate threshold:** the exercise $\dot{V}O_2$ above which a sustained increase in arterial [lactate] is observed, accompanied by an increase in arterial L/P ratio
- **Lactic acidosis threshold:** the exercise $\dot{V}O_2$ above which arterial standard (Std) HCO_3^- (the principal buffer of the metabolically produced H^+) is observed to decrease because of a net increase in H^+ accumulation
- **Gas exchange threshold:** the exercise $\dot{V}O_2$ above which a systematic increase in $\dot{V}CO_2$ is observed, assumed to reflect the onset of HCO_3^- buffering of the metabolic acidosis

Thus, the *LAT* contrasts with the *LT* in methodology only. The latter is determined from actual measurements of arterial [lactate] increase, whereas the former is determined by the decrease in arterial [HCO_3^-] due to its buffering of the newly accumulating metabolic proton load. The *LT* and *LAT* are systematically related and conceptually interchangeable, but there is a small quantitative (and functionally insignificant) difference between them.

In normal individuals, the *AT* is, on average, about 50% to 60% of their $\dot{V}O_2$max, but with a range extending from 40% to more than 80% (see Chapter 7). As an individual ages, the *AT* becomes a higher fraction of $\dot{V}O_2$max because $\dot{V}O_2$max decreases at a proportionately faster rate than the *AT*.[58] The *AT* (and $\dot{V}O_2$max) is increased in individuals with high cardiorespiratory fitness and with endurance training, and appears to be a good discriminator of the highest work rate that can be endured for a prolonged period of exercise (eg, the marathon).[59,60]

There is still considerable debate about the best-fit mathematical model to describe the arterial [lactate] response as a function of increasing work rate.[61] It should be noted that the considerable complexity in the multiple kinetic processes involved with lactate production and clearance means that the profile of this response is different if measured during independent constant work rate tests compared with incremental work rate tests. The former typically results in "threshold-like" behavior, whereas in the latter, both continuous-exponential and threshold models have been tested.[55,57,62-64] To obtain a better understanding of the pattern of change in arterial [lactate] during incremental exercise, a group-mean plot of arterial [lactate] against the simultaneously measured $\dot{V}O_2$ was obtained by overlaying the individual plots of 17 physically active, healthy young males.[55,57] These [lactate]-$\dot{V}O_2$ plots were normalized along the $\dot{V}O_2$ axis by (1) anchoring each plot to the $\dot{V}O_2$ corresponding to the individual *LT* and then (2) scaling the $\dot{V}O_2$ axis so that each plot had the same span below and above the *LT* (**Fig. 2.11**). Because [lactate] increases steeply with little further increase in $\dot{V}O_2$ as $\dot{V}O_2$max is approached, the analysis was restricted to the region of interest (ie, from resting [lactate] to an exercise [lactate] of 4.5 mmol/L).

As illustrated in **Figure 2.11** (upper panel), a monoexponential (ie, "continuous") model of [lactate] increase from rest as a function of $\dot{V}O_2$ does not describe the data well. In contrast, the points distribute evenly around the two components of the threshold model (see **Fig. 2.11**, lower panel). This threshold denotes the *LT*. Although neither the threshold nor the monoexponential model provides a perfect fit to the [lactate]-$\dot{V}O_2$ relationship at all work rates, the data in the region of interest (ie, below 4.5 mmol/L) clearly fit the threshold model better than the exponential model. Supporting the threshold model are numerous muscle biopsy studies demonstrating that muscle [lactate] does not increase at work rates within the moderate-intensity domain,[65-68] coinciding with the $\dot{V}O_2$ at which arterial [lactate] begins to increase.[68]

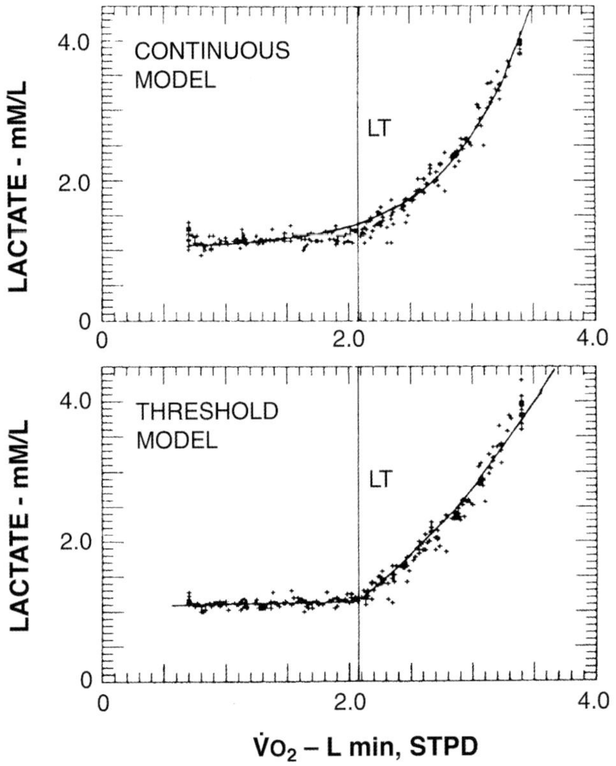

FIGURE 2.11. Evaluating threshold behavior of group-mean (n = 17) arterial [lactate] as a function of O_2 uptake ($\dot{V}O_2$) for incremental cycle ergometer exercise (active healthy individuals from Fig. 2.10), using a continuous exponential model (upper panel) and a threshold model (lower panel). Data are plotted only over the region of interest for model evaluation (ie, up to a [lactate] of 4.5 mmol/L). For averaging, individual responses were normalized along the $\dot{V}O_2$ axis by anchoring each plot to the $\dot{V}O_2$ at the lactate threshold (*LT*) and then scaling the $\dot{V}O_2$ axis so that each plot had the same span below and above the *LT*. Upper panel, The solid curve is the best-fit continuous exponential to the averaged data. The [lactate] values lie above the exponential model curve at the lowest $\dot{V}O_2$ but are below the model curve in the region of the *LT*. Lower panel, the solid lines are the best-fit threshold model to the same data, which provides a better fit to the data. The vertical solid line shows the group-mean *LT*. Abbreviation: STP, standard temperature pressure dry. *(Data from a smaller number of individuals are presented in Wasserman K, Beaver WL, Whipp BJ. Gas exchange theory and the lactic acidosis (anaerobic) threshold.* Circulation. *1990;81[suppl 1]:II14-II30.)*

Arterial Lactate Increase as a Function of Time

Although a given work rate may be stressful for one individual and thus cause early intolerance, it may not be a significant physical stress for an individual with greater cardiorespiratory fitness. Therefore, adjectives such as *moderate, heavy,* and *very heavy* are used to describe the degree of metabolic strain during exercise and are based on the temporal response profile of arterial [lactate] and $\dot{V}O_2$[69,70] during constant work rate exercise (see "Oxygen Uptake Kinetics" below). Because *AT* and $\dot{V}O_2$max are highly variable among individuals, the [lactate] and $\dot{V}O_2$ profiles provide a more reliable index of relative intensity than, for example, a given percentage of heart rate or $\dot{V}O_2$max.[70]

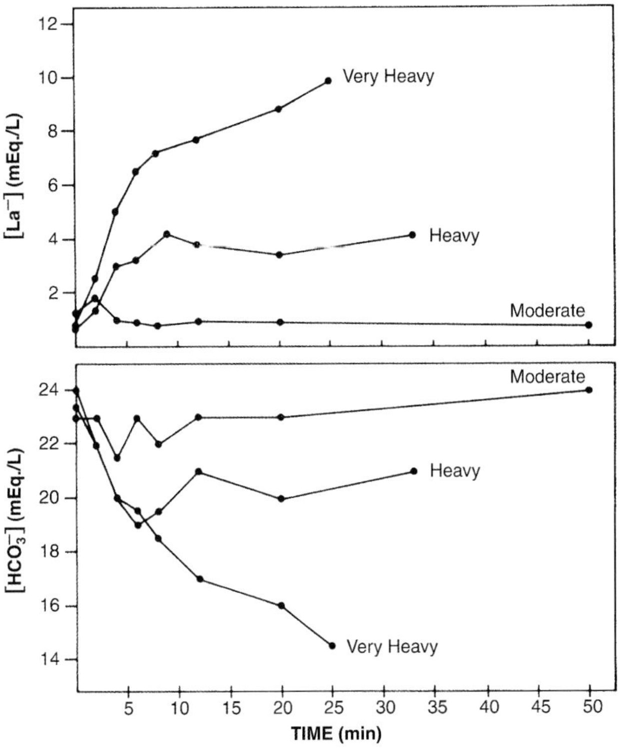

FIGURE 2.12. Arterial [lactate] and [bicarbonate] as a function of time for prolonged constant work rate cycle ergometer exercise (target duration = 50 min) of moderate, heavy, and very heavy intensities in a normal individual. The increase in [lactate] and decrease in [bicarbonate] were quantitatively similar. Note that the tolerance time was reduced for the heavy and very heavy work rates.

Thus, for constant work rate cycle ergometer exercise, three patterns of arterial [lactate] increase are typically observed (**Fig. 2.12**).[69] The first pattern is one in which either no increase in [lactate] is observed or [lactate] rises transiently and then returns to its resting value (or lower) as $\dot{V}O_2$ reaches a steady state. This is defined as *moderate-intensity* exercise, which extends up to the *AT*, for which the exercise is relatively comfortable and can be sustained for many hours in a steady state.

Heavy-intensity exercise is defined as a sustained increase in arterial [lactate], reflecting the presence of a metabolic acidosis, that can be stabilized with time. This results from the rate of lactate utilization by the liver and other actively metabolizing organs, such as the heart, rising more slowly than the rate of lactate production by the exercising muscle, although a balance is eventually reached at a new, raised level of arterial [lactate].[71,72] Exercise in this domain cannot be sustained for prolonged periods (see **Fig. 2.12**) for reasons that include accelerated muscle glycogen depletion when a metabolic rate is sustained that demands a high rate of anaerobic glycolysis. This intensity domain extends from the *AT* to critical power (CP) (see "Power-Duration Curve and Critical Power" below).

At higher work rates, arterial [lactate] cannot stabilize, continuing to increase with time to the point of intolerance (see **Fig. 2.12**); this is termed *very heavy exercise* (see "Power-Duration Curve and Critical Power" below). At these work rates, arterial [lactate] in normal individuals can achieve levels as great as 10 mmol/L or more at end exercise. Exercise in this domain is characterized by a continuous non-steady state, and as such, is typically limited by the attainment of $\dot{V}O_2$max (in healthy individuals) and/or by limiting symptoms (in paticnts).

Mechanisms of Arterial Lactate Increase

The mechanistic basis of the arterial [lactate] increase during exercise, and therefore the *AT*, remain contentious.[13,71,73-75] Several mechanisms have the potential to yield increases in muscular lactate production as $\dot{V}O_2$ increases during exercise, as well as mechanisms that contribute to the rate of lactate clearance from the blood. Ultimately, arterial [lactate] increase depends on the balance among production, transport, and clearance. Lactate is a preferential substrate, meaning it will be taken up from the blood and favored for oxidation in place of carbohydrates or fatty acids, even during exercise. This can occur as long as the extracellular [lactate] is greater than the concentration within the cell. Therefore, understanding the behavior of arterial [lactate] requires consideration of both production (and appearance in the blood) and utilization (and clearance from the blood). These are described in the following sections.

Increasing Glycolytic Flux and Exercise Intensity

Glycolysis and glycogenolysis are activated extremely rapidly at the onset of muscular contractions, following increases in intramuscular [Ca^{++}] and [ADP] among other factors. Lactate is considered by some as the terminal product of glycolysis[76] because lactate dehydrogenase (LDH), the enzyme that catalyses the reaction of pyruvate and NADH + H^+ to lactate and NAD^+, is near equilibrium with an equilibrium constant that strongly favors lactate and has a high activity relative to other glycolytic enzymes.[77] Resting muscle L/P ratio is approximately 10:1 to 20:1, meaning that an increase in glycolytic flux will lead to an increase in lactate formation, regardless of local PO_2.[76] Increasing exercise intensity strengthens the activation of glycolytic enzymes, the rate of glycolysis and glycogenolysis, and the formation of cytosolic NADH + H^+. Lactate formation is greater at higher exercise intensities, but whether or not the lactate formed actually accumulates is dependent on variables such as muscle fiber type, pyruvate dehydrogenase (PDH) activity, the size of the available mitochondrial pool, and the mitochondrial PO_2.

Sequential Recruitment of Type II Muscle Fibers

Another mechanism proposed for the increase in [lactate] during exercise is the increased recruitment of type II muscle fibers above the *AT*.[78] These fibers contain high levels of glycogen and PCr, but also glycolytic enzyme activity is greater and oxidative enzyme activity is lower (especially in type IIx fibers). This may lead to a mismatch between lactate formation and pyruvate and NADH + H^+ oxidation, resulting in elevated [lactate] and net lactate efflux, such as in "Warburg" cancer cells or in patients with chronic muscular deconditioning. In young heathy individuals, 20 minutes of constant work rate cycling below *AT* did not deplete glycogen or PCr in type II fibers (only in type I fibers), whereas glycogen and PCr depletion was evident in type II muscle fibers when working above the *AT*.[11] This observation supports the concept that a greater reliance on muscle activity in less oxidative, type II fibers during exercise above *AT* contributes to increasing arterial [lactate].

Pyruvate Dehydrogenase Activity

Lactate can accumulate in the muscle during exercise if glycolysis proceeds at a rate faster than pyruvate can be used by the mitochondrial TCA cycle (see **Fig. 2.1**). PDH plays a major role in the transport of pyruvate across the mitochondrial inner membrane with subsequent conversion to acetyl-CoA followed by entry into the TCA cycle and oxidation. The relative activities of PDH and LDH therefore have an important role in determining the rate of lactate formation. PDH is activated slowly at exercise onset, and the speed of this activation may decline with age.[79,80] Increasing PDH activity by pharmacological intervention with dichloroacetate infusion reduces muscle acidification and arterial lactate accumulation during high-intensity exercise.[81] There are other potential fates of pyruvate that may influence the rate of lactate formation, such as efflux from the cell, conversion to alanine, or even gluconeogenesis requiring "reversal of glycolysis." However, these pathways play a small to no role during exercise.

Change in Cytosolic Redox State Limiting Mitochondrial Proton Shuttles

As discussed above (see "Sources of High-Energy Phosphate and Cellular Respiration" in the previous section), in the process of glycolysis (see **Fig. 2.1**), the oxidized form of cytosolic NAD^+ is converted into the reduced form NADH + H^+. It is subsequently reoxidized back to NAD^+ (or FAD) by mitochondrial membrane proton shuttles (see **Fig. 2.1**, pathway A). Conditions of low mitochondrial density, low expression of the proton shuttle, low activity of the electron transport system, or inadequate O_2 availability in the mitochondria will cause the cytosolic [NADH + H^+]/[NAD^+] ratio to increase. With this change in redox state, reoxidation of cytosolic NADH + H^+ can take place by pathway B of Figure 2.1 (pyruvate + NADH + H^+ → lactate + NAD^+). Thus, in poorly oxidative muscles or when O_2 cannot be supplied at a sufficiently rapid rate to regenerate cytosolic NAD^+ by pathway A, pathway B will be favored. The cell redox state is therefore lowered (increased [NADH + H^+]/[NAD^+]), forcing an increase in the L/P ratio (**Fig. 2.13**).

Figure 2.13 shows arterial [lactate], [pyruvate], and L/P ratio as functions of $\dot{V}O_2$, expressed logarithmically, for incremental exercise in a single individual who was representative of the average response of a group of 10 healthy individuals.[82] Below the *AT*, [lactate] increased very slightly as did [pyruvate], such that the L/P ratio did not increase until the *AT* was reached. Pyruvate concentration also

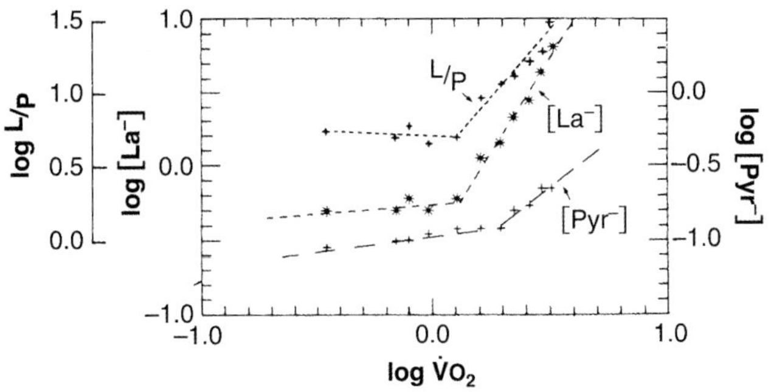

FIGURE 2.13. Log arterial [lactate] (La^-), log arterial [pyruvate] (Pyr^-), and log [lactate]-to-[pyruvate] ratio (L/P) as a function of log O_2 uptake ($\dot{V}O_2$) for incremental cycle ergometer exercise in a normal individual. The log-log transform of the [lactate]-$\dot{V}O_2$ and [pyruvate]-$\dot{V}O_2$ relationships allows easy detection of the [lactate] and [pyruvate] inflection points. The [pyruvate] inflection point is at a higher $\dot{V}O_2$ than the [lactate] inflection point. Because the pre-threshold [pyruvate] slope is the same as the [lactate] slope, the L/P ratio does not increase until the [lactate] inflection point (ie, the lactate threshold). *(Reproduced with permission from Wasserman K, Beaver WL, Davis JA, Pu JZ, Heber D, Whipp BJ. Lactate, pyruvate, and lactate-to-pyruvate ratio during exercise and recovery.* J Appl Physiol. *1985;59[3]:935-940. Copyright © 1985 American Physiological Society. All rights reserved.)*

increased steeply but not until a $\dot{V}O_2$ that was well above the *AT*. Also, as [pyruvate] increased at a slower rate than [lactate] above the *AT*, the L/P ratio continued to increase until $\dot{V}O_2$peak. A similar phenomenon has been observed in the muscle cells of humans.[83,84]

Although the rate of lactate formation with increasing work rate is a necessity of mass action resulting from increased glycolysis, the accumulation of intramuscular and arterial lactate is not. The increase in arterial [lactate] with an increase in L/P ratio indicates that the increase in [lactate] results from a shift in equilibrium between lactate and pyruvate as a result of change in the [NADH + H^+]/[NAD^+] ratio (see **Fig. 2.1**). The conversion of pyruvate to lactate results in the reoxidation of cytosolic NADH + H^+, providing NAD^+ for continued glycolysis even under anaerobic conditions. Because no O_2 is used in the reoxidation of pathway B (see **Fig. 2.1**), this glycolysis is anaerobic. Simultaneously, reoxidation of cytosolic NADH + H^+ can take place aerobically, in mitochondrial-rich or better-oxygenated contracting muscle cells, by pathway A; this is aerobic glycolysis (see **Fig. 2.1**).

The exercise-induced rise in arterial [lactate] may continue into the recovery phase at a slowed rate for several minutes before it starts to decrease (**Fig. 2.14**).[82] Pyruvate

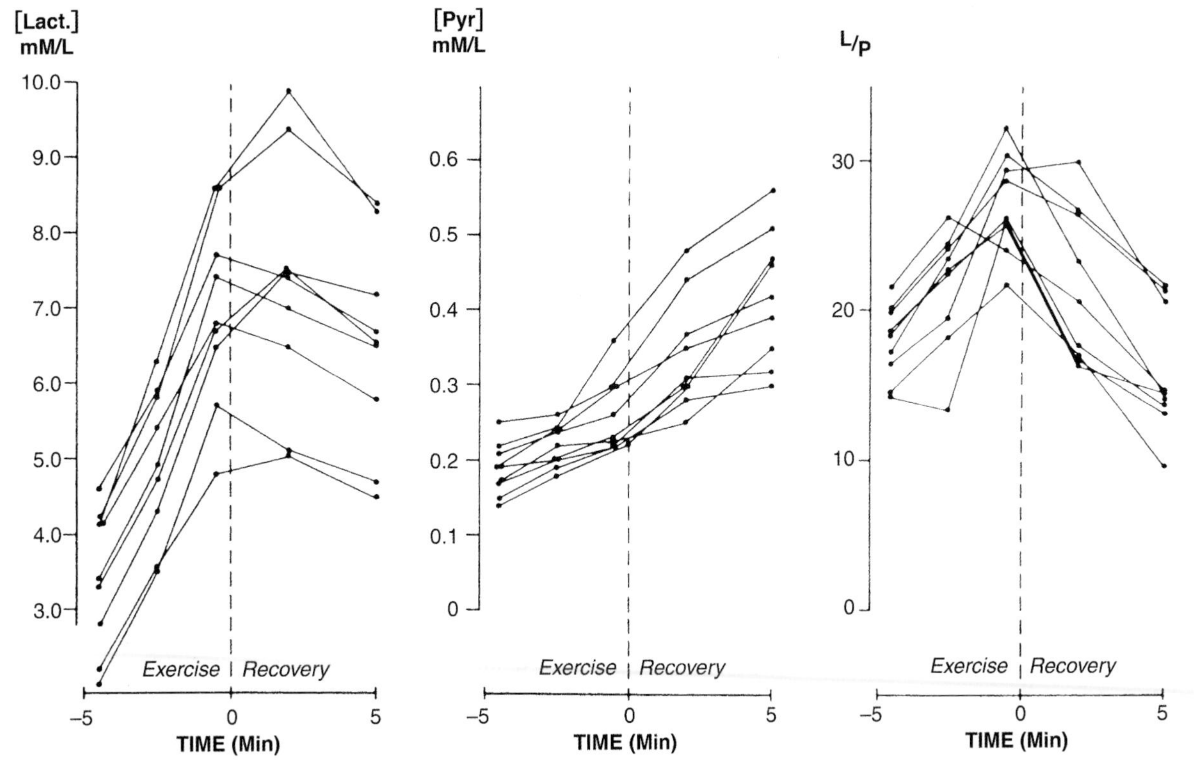

FIGURE 2.14. As for the study depicted in Fig. 2.13, arterial [lactate] (Lact.), [pyruvate] (Pyr), and [lactate]-to-[pyruvate] ratio (L/P) as a function of time during the last 5 minutes of incremental cycle ergometer exercise and first 5 minutes of recovery, for 10 individuals. [lactate] either increases or decreases slightly by 2 minutes of recovery, with all individuals showing a decrease by 5 minutes of recovery. In contrast, [pyruvate] continues to rise through the first 5 minutes of recovery. As a consequence, L/P ratio decreases by 2 minutes of recovery and continues to decrease toward control value by 5 minutes of recovery. *(Reproduced with permission from Wasserman K, Beaver WL, Davis JA, Pu JZ, Heber D, Whipp BJ. Lactate, pyruvate, and lactate-to-pyruvate ratio during exercise and recovery.* J Appl Physiol. *1985;59[3]:935-940. Copyright © 1985 American Physiological Society. All rights reserved.)*

concentration, on the other hand, actually increases more rapidly at the start of recovery. Thus, as soon as exercise stops (and the O_2 requirement decreases), the L/P ratio reverses, which supports the exercise-induced [lactate] increase at the *AT* not simply being a mass action effect consequent to [pyruvate] increase.

Lactate Production and Clearance

As the product of glycolysis and the preferred substrate for mitochondrial oxidation, lactate has been regarded as the link between glycolytic and aerobic metabolism.[73,85] As previously described, below the *AT* lactate is formed during increasing glycolytic flux. Lactate may be exchanged among cells for delivery of oxidative and gluconeogenic substrates as well as for cell-to-cell signaling. Examples of the cell-cell lactate shuttles include lactate exchanges between type II and type I fibers within a working muscle and between working skeletal muscle and heart, brain, liver, kidneys, astrocytes, and neurons.[71,73]

The primary mechanism for lactate and H^+ movement out of the muscle cell is via 1:1 monocarboxylate (MCT)-mediated sarcolemmal co-transport, with contributions also from Na^+/H^+ and Na^+/HCO_3^- co-transport.[86-88] The MCTs are bidirectional, allowing both lactate release and uptake, depending on the relative concentration and pH differences across the membrane in question.[89] Lactate transport appears to be accelerated by the H^+ gradient across the sarcolemmal membrane, based on studies with cardiac sarcolemmal vesicles.[90] At the cellular level, this will be established primarily by the $[HCO_3^-]$ gradient. Lactate efflux from muscle was found to be highly influenced by the $[HCO_3^-]$ of the muscle perfusate.[91,92] The reciprocal changes of [lactate] and $[HCO_3^-]$ in the extracellular fluid during heavy exercise suggest that permeation of lactate across the sarcolemmal membrane is a coupled HCO_3^--lactate antiport carrier mechanism. This is supported by the study of Korotzer et al,[93] which showed that intravenous injection of the carbonic anhydrase inhibitor acetazolamide prior to performing heavy exercise significantly attenuates the increase in arterial [lactate] and decrease in $[HCO_3^-]$. Replacing the intracellular HCO_3^-, which is consumed when it buffers newly produced H^+, with HCO_3^- from the bloodstream minimizes the decrease in intracellular pH.

Lactate release from muscle occurs when contractions start. This is followed by lactate uptake as muscle $\dot{V}O_2$ reaches a new steady state. At low work rates in healthy individuals, when blood flow is raised above baseline, the rate of lactate uptake by muscle can actually exceeds its production, and arterial [lactate] may fall below resting levels.[69,94] During incremental exercise, however, studies using radiolabeled carbon tracers show that the rate of lactate clearance falls behind lactate appearance in the arterial blood as work rate increases, meaning that arterial lactate begins to accumulate.[95] Variables that affect both appearance and disappearance of lactate from the arterial blood, such as muscle fiber type, LDH and PDH activity, intramuscular PO_2 and perfusion of working and nonworking tissues during exercise will therefore influence the occurrence of the *AT*.

In summary, it is difficult to attribute the increase in arterial [lactate] for heavy exercise, with an increase in L/P ratio, solely to any one mechanism. Experimental studies support the concept that the major mechanism accounting for the increase in lactate production at the *AT* is the lowering of cytosolic redox state induced by a net increase in anaerobic glycolysis. If this is not matched by a net uptake of lactate from the arterial blood, then arterial [lactate] increases.

Oxygen Supply and Critical Capillary PO_2

In well-oxygenated muscle, O_2 is consumed by active muscle cells for the aerobic regeneration of ATP (see **Fig. 2.1**). Wittenberg and Wittenberg[96] demonstrated that isolated mitochondria can respire and rephosphorylate ADP to ATP at a PO_2 of 2 mm Hg or less. However, the capillary PO_2 must be appreciably greater than 2 mm Hg to provide a PO_2 diffusion gradient sufficient to sustain mitochondrial respiration during exercise. The critical level of capillary PO_2 (ie, the lowest capillary PO_2 that allows the muscle mitochondria to sustain exercise aerobically) has been estimated to be approximately 15 to 20 mm Hg.[96-99] To maintain a muscle end-capillary PO_2 of 15 mm Hg requires a muscle blood flow ($\dot{Q}m$) of at least 6 L/min for a muscle $\dot{Q}O_2$ of 1 L/min, assuming [Hb] = 15 g/dL, and an SaO_2 of at least 95%. This predicts that approximately 17% (ie, $\dot{Q}m/\dot{Q}O_2$) of the O_2 inflow into the muscle capillary bed would remain at the venous end of the bed (or a muscle O_2 "extraction" of 83%).

Figure 2.15 schematizes the effects of nonuniformity of muscle blood flow relative to muscle O_2 consumption ($\dot{Q}m/\dot{Q}O_2$) on the PO_2 profile along a muscle capillary for physiological rates of O_2 delivery and utilization. This model allows for the Bohr effect resulting from aerobic metabolism (ie, a decreasing pH in the capillary, resulting from increasing aerobic CO_2 production, that facilitates O_2 unloading from Hb) but not for anaerobic glycolysis. It illustrates that at a $\dot{Q}m/\dot{Q}O_2$ ratio of 5, muscle capillary PO_2 would fall below the critical level before the blood reached the venous end of the capillary bed, thus limiting O_2 diffusion and oxidative phosphorylation. A $\dot{Q}m/\dot{Q}O_2$ ratio of 6, on the other hand, is sufficient to maintain PO_2 above approximately 15 mm Hg at the end of the capillary. Therefore, a $\dot{Q}m/\dot{Q}O_2$ ratio <6 is expected to promote lactate formation to maintain cytosolic redox state in the face of high glycolytic flux, and thus [lactate] would increase in the muscle.

The capillary PO_2 cannot decrease below the critical capillary PO_2 because the mitochondrial PO_2 would be too low for O_2 consumption. That the critical capillary PO_2 was reached would be evidenced by the failure of end-capillary or femoral venous PO_2 to decrease further despite increasing work rate (see **Fig. 2.15**). This model also illustrates that the capillary PO_2 is heterogeneous—both longitudinally along the capillary and across capillaries in regions with differing $\dot{Q}m/\dot{Q}O_2$ ratios. Rather than considering a single mean

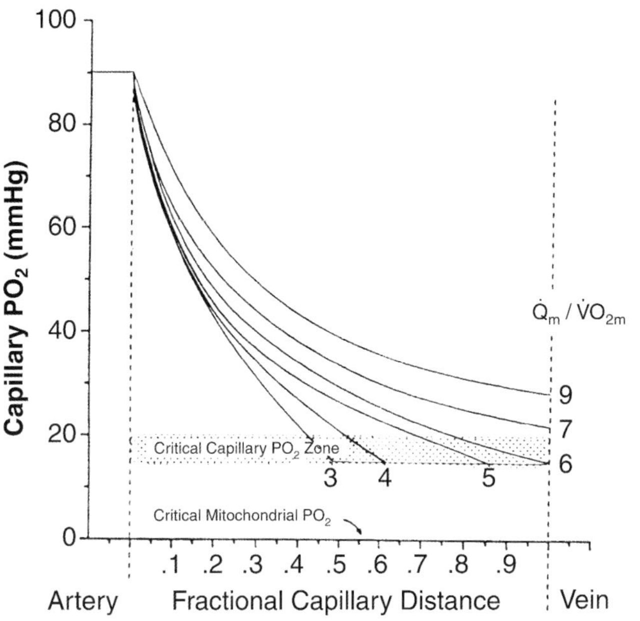

FIGURE 2.15. Model of the effects of nonuniformity in the ratio of muscle blood flow to muscle O_2 consumption ($\dot{Q}m/\dot{V}O_{2m}$) on the profile of muscle capillary O_2 partial pressure (PO_2) as blood travels from artery to vein. The model assumes: [hemoglobin] = 15 g/dL, arterial PO_2 = 90 mm Hg, a linear O_2 consumption along the capillary, and a Bohr effect resulting from aerobic carbon dioxide production decreasing capillary pH. The capillary PO_2 declines along the capillary bed even with a homogenous $\dot{Q}m/\dot{V}O_{2m}$ value (ie, 6). The rate of decline of capillary PO_2 is more rapid with lower values $\dot{Q}m/\dot{V}O_{2m}$. The end-capillary PO_2 cannot decrease below the critical capillary PO_2. Any muscle unit with a $\dot{Q}m/\dot{V}O_{2m}$ value less than 6 will have increased anaerobic metabolism and lactate production. See text for application of model. *(Reproduced with permission from Wasserman K. Coupling of external to cellular respiration during exercise: the wisdom of the body revisited.* Am J Physiol. *1994;266[4 pt 1]:E519-E539. Copyright © 1994 American Physiological Society. All rights reserved.)*

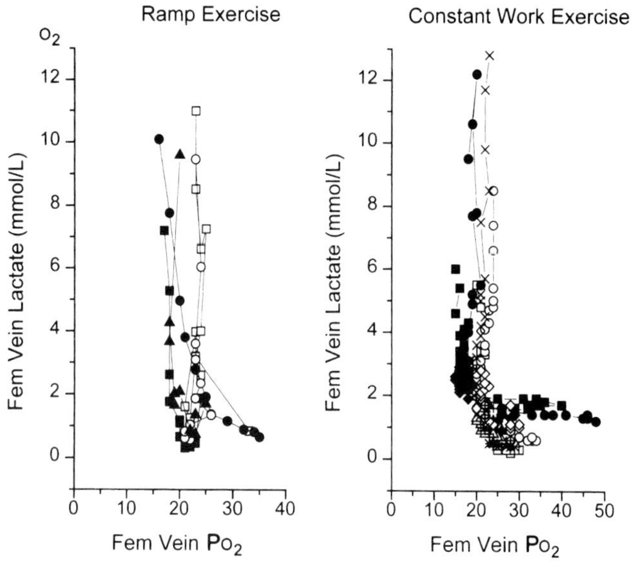

FIGURE 2.16. Group-mean (n = 5, each represented by different symbols) femoral venous [lactate] as function of femoral venous PO_2 for ramp incremental cycle ergometer exercise (left panel) and 10 constant work rate exercise tests (5 below and 5 above the anaerobic threshold) (right panel). The highest PO_2 values occur at exercise onset. *(Modified from Stringer WW, Wasserman K, Casaburi R, Pórszász J, Maehara K, French W. Lactic acidosis as a facilitator of oxyhemoglobin dissociation during exercise.* J Appl Physiol. *1994;76:1462-1467.)*

capillary PO_2 value for the muscle circulation as a whole, the question could better be asked whether regional $\dot{Q}m$ and therefore, capillary PO_2 are sufficiently high at a given $\dot{Q}O_2$ to prevent an acceleration of lactate formation.[100]

Major factors determining the PO_2 gradient between the capillary and the muscle mitochondrion are the resistances to O_2 diffusion by the red cell membrane, plasma, capillary endothelium, interstitial space, and sarcolemma.[101] By measuring oxymyoglobin saturation in human muscle using magnetic resonance spectroscopy, Molé et al[102] and Richardson et al[103] independently estimated the intramuscular PO_2 to be about 5 mm Hg for all metabolic rates above 50% $\dot{V}O_2$max (ie, PO_2 is above the critical mitochondrial value of approximately 2 mm Hg to maintain oxidative phosphorylation).[13] The implication is that diffusional conductance, and not intracellular PO_2, is the limiting factor in vivo for the maximal rate of intramuscular oxidation during exercise.[99] However, with a widely heterogeneous muscle structure, and mean mitochondrial PO_2 values from myoglobin spectroscopy deriving from a large volume of muscle, we cannot yet rule out that oxidative phosphorylation in some regions of active muscle may become O_2 limited when mean PO_2 reaches its lowest values around the *AT*.[13]

Experimental support for the critical capillary PO_2 concept was provided by the studies of Stringer et al[98] and Koike et al[104] in which femoral venous PO_2 and [lactate] were measured during cycle ergometry in normal individuals and patients with chronic heart failure, respectively. During incremental exercise, femoral venous PO_2 reached its lowest value of 15 to 20 mm Hg at approximately 50% of the individuals' work capacity and remained relatively constant thereafter. As would be predicted from the critical capillary PO_2 concept, femoral venous [lactate] then started to increase (**Fig. 2.16**). This was the case whether incremental or heavy constant work rate exercise was performed. The net increase in lactate efflux from the muscle is demonstrated by the greater [lactate] in femoral venous than arterial blood (**Fig. 2.17**). This is in agreement with prior studies on lactate balance across the exercising extremity.[104-107]

Additional observations support a role for O_2 delivery in lactate accumulation during exercise. For example, arterial [lactate] can be reduced or increased as a result of increases or decreases, respectively, in arterial oxygenation.[108-111] Koike et al[112,113] also demonstrated that the *AT* is sensitive to O_2 delivery, using controlled carbon monoxide inhalation to impair O_2 binding by Hb and thus decrease arterial O_2 content (by approximately 10% and 20% prior to incremental exercise) (**Fig. 2.18**). The *AT* and peak $\dot{V}O_2$ were reduced by percentages consistent with the percentage reductions in arterial O_2 content. Although elevated

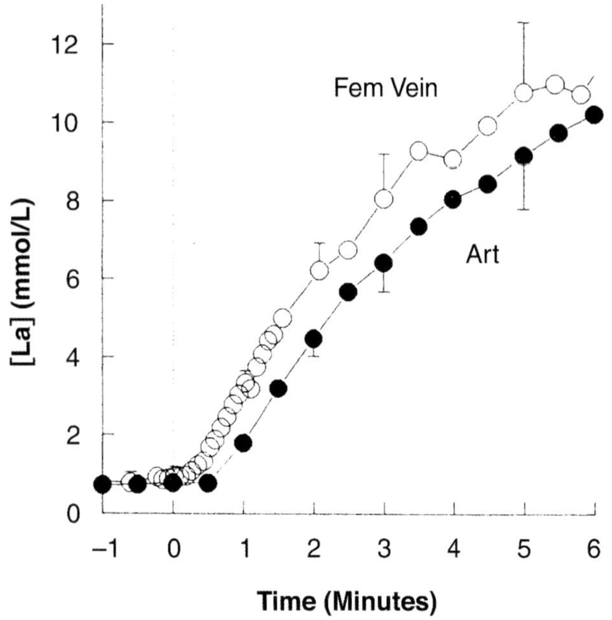

FIGURE 2.17. Group-mean (n = 5) femoral venous [lactate] (o) and arterial [lactate] (●) as a function of time for heavy constant work rate cycle ergometer exercise. Note that the increase in femoral venous [lactate] precedes the increase in arterial [lactate]. Vertical bars on points are standard errors of the mean.

carboxyhemoglobin had no effect on the $\dot{V}O_2$ response below the *AT*, $\dot{V}O_2$ was reduced above the *AT* (see **Fig. 2.18**).

pH Change and Oxyhemoglobin Dissociation Above the Anaerobic Threshold

To further investigate the mechanisms of O_2 transport and utilization above and below *AT*, femoral venous blood sampling was conducted during moderate and heavy constant work rate exercise in healthy individuals.[98] Femoral venous PO_2 decreased to its lowest value (15-20 mm Hg) by 60 seconds after exercise onset for both the moderate and heavy exercise intensities and remained unchanged thereafter as the exercise continued; that is, femoral venous PO_2 was not different above or below *AT*, despite the large difference in work rate and $\dot{V}O_2$ (**Fig. 2.19**, left panel). The greater $\dot{V}O_2$ during heavy exercise above *AT* was facilitated, at least in part, by increased O_2 extraction. This was evidenced by the continued fall in femoral venous oxyhemoglobin saturation past the time when the end-capillary PO_2 became constant, for the entire 6 minutes of exercise (see **Fig. 2.19**, middle panel). This continued O_2 extraction during supra-*AT* exercise followed the decrease in femoral venous pH (see **Fig. 2.19**, right panel).

The femoral venous oxyhemoglobin desaturation which was not accounted for by the PO_2 decrease could be completely accounted for by the pH decrease via the Bohr effect (see "Oxygen Supply and Critical Capillary PO_2" above). To illustrate this, the data shown in **Figure 2.19** were replotted, with femoral venous oxyhemoglobin saturation values plotted against the independently measured femoral venous PO_2 values (**Fig. 2.20**); pH isopleths are overlaid on these data. It is apparent from this plot that the decrease in femoral venous oxyhemoglobin saturation below 25% could be accounted for by the decrease in arterial pH and not a decrease in PO_2.

This mechanism maintains the capillary PO_2 while facilitating progressive O_2 dissociation from Hb to maintain oxidative metabolism for ATP regeneration.[54] Thus, in McArdle syndrome or other disorders of glycolysis in which [lactate] cannot increase, it is not possible to extract O_2 to the extent seen in normal individuals during maximal exercise. This has been experimentally demonstrated by the reduced arterial-mixed venous O_2 difference for the work rate at which the patient with muscle phosphofructokinase deficiency is forced to stop exercise due to muscle pain or fatigue.[114] Although femoral venous PO_2 remains constant above the *AT* in healthy individuals, femoral venous oxyhemoglobin saturation continues to decrease in accordance with the pH decrease. Thus, for normal O_2 extraction

FIGURE 2.18. O_2 uptake ($\dot{V}O_2$) responses to three ramp incremental cycle ergometer tests from unloaded cycling in a normal individual: one air breathing test (control, ●) and two tests of air plus carbon monoxide breathing that resulted in carboxyhemoglobin (COHb) levels of 10.1% (∇) and 17.6% (o), respectively, and conducted in randomized sequence. Ramp phase starts at 0. There was no effect of increased [COHb] on $\dot{V}O_2$ until the anaerobic threshold (*AT*, arrow) of the respective test was surpassed; then the increase in $\dot{V}O_2$ was slower the higher the [COHb]. The *AT* and peak $\dot{V}O_2$ were systematically decreased as [COHb] was increased. The difference between the $\dot{V}O_2$ of the control and COHb tests represents the reduction in $\dot{V}O_2$ caused by the reduced blood O_2 content. *(Reproduced with permission from Koike A, Weiler-Ravell D, McKenzie DK, Zanconato S, Wasserman K. Evidence that the metabolic acidosis threshold is the anaerobic threshold.* J Appl Physiol. *1990;68[6]:2521-2526. Copyright © 1990 American Physiological Society. All rights reserved.)*

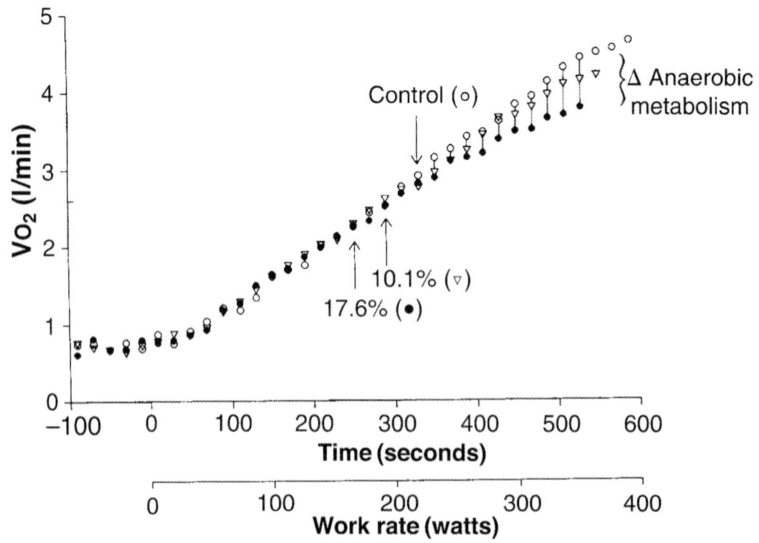

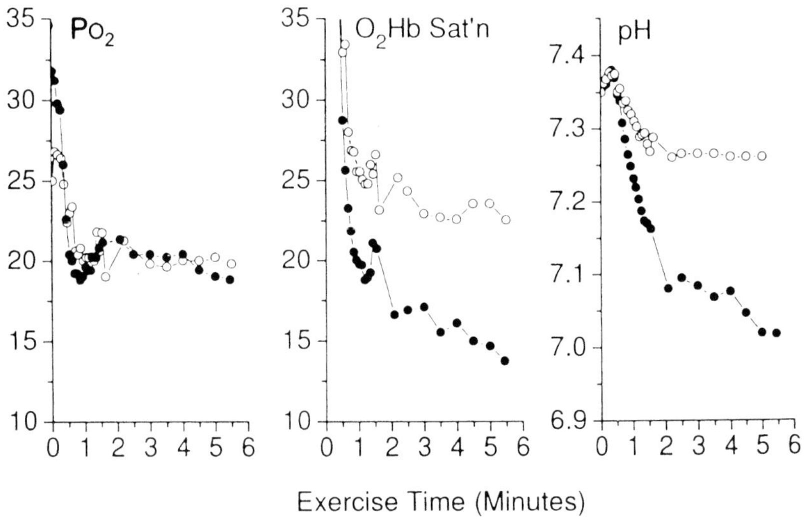

FIGURE 2.19. Group-mean (n = 5) femoral venous Po_2 (left panel), oxyhemoglobin saturation (O_2Hb Sat'n) (center panel), and pH (right panel) as a function of time for two constant work rate cycle ergometer tests: one below (o) and one above (●) the anaerobic threshold (*AT*). The below- and above-*AT* work rates averaged 113 and 265 W, respectively. Note that O_2Hb saturation is lower during the higher intensity exercise despite identical Po_2 values, which reflects the Bohr effect resulting from the decreasing pH. *(Modified from Stringer WW, Wasserman K, Casaburi R, Pórszász J, Maehara K, French W. Lactic acidosis as a facilitator of oxyhemoglobin dissociation during exercise.* J Appl Physiol. *1994;76:1462-1467.)*

by the exercising muscles, two factors—decreasing capillary Po_2 and increasing capillary $[H^+]$—demand consideration. The former plays a more important role in oxyhemoglobin dissociation below the *AT*, whereas the latter has a major role above it (see **Fig. 2.20**).

The biochemical interactions between capillary blood and muscle cell for optimizing the O_2 supply to mitochondria during heavy exercise are summarized in **Figure 2.21**. As the blood transits the muscle capillary bed from arteriole to venule, capillary Po_2 decreases leading to oxyhemoglobin dissociation and O_2 diffusion into the muscle cell. When capillary Po_2 reaches its critical value toward the end of the capillary, O_2 transfer is compromised, leading to anaerobic metabolism with lactate formation. The lactate anion is transported out of the muscle cell with a proton, leading to a decrease in capillary pH. Thus, although intracellular buffering of the acidosis by HCO_3^- minimizes the change in cell pH, it acidifies blood more quickly than if a non-HCO_3^- buffer neutralized the cellular acidosis. The HCO_3^- is drawn into the acidifying muscle cell, and the evolved CO_2 readily diffuses out into the blood, which further facilitates oxyhemoglobin dissociation via the Haldane effect. That is, the dissociation of O_2 from Hb as blood traverses the exercising muscle capillary bed simultaneously facilitates the binding of molecular CO_2 (as carbamino CO_2, Equation 13 below)

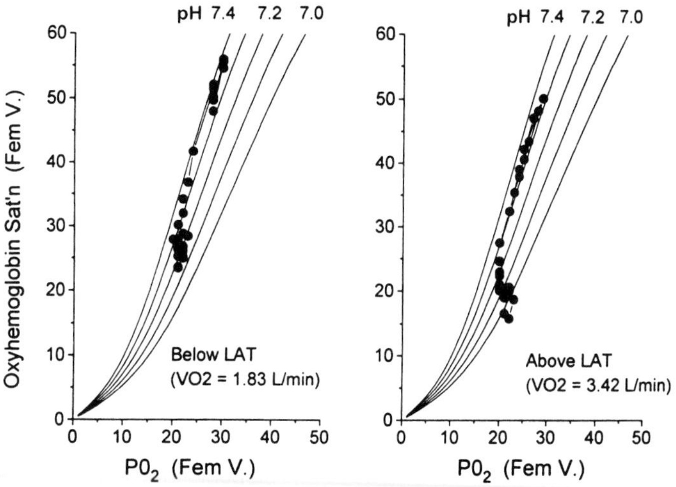

FIGURE 2.20. As for the study depicted in Figure 2.19, group-mean (n = 5) femoral venous oxyhemoglobin saturation (see Fig. 2.19, center panel) as a function of femoral venous Po_2 (see Fig. 2.19, left panel) for two constant work rate cycle ergometer tests: one below (o) and one above (●) the anaerobic or lactic acidosis threshold (*LAT*) (left and right panels, respectively). Superimposed are venous pH isopleths for oxyhemoglobin dissociation ranging from 7.0 to 7.4, calculated from equations reported by Severinghaus (Severinghaus JW. Simple accurate equations for human blood O_2 dissociation computations. *J Appl Physiol.* 1979;46:599-602.). The highest femoral venous oxyhemoglobin saturation values occurred at exercise onset, with progressive decreases as exercise continued but falling along pH isopleths in agreement with measured pH (see Fig. 2.19, right panel). Thus, the entire decrease in O_2Hb saturation that took place after Po_2 reached its lowest value could be accounted for by the Bohr effect. *(Reproduced with permission from Stringer WW, Wasserman K, Casaburi R, Pórszász J, Maehara K, French W. Lactic acidosis as a facilitator of oxyhemoglobin dissociation during exercise.* J Appl Physiol. *1994;76[4]:1462-1467. Copyright © 1994 American Physiological Society. All rights reserved.)*

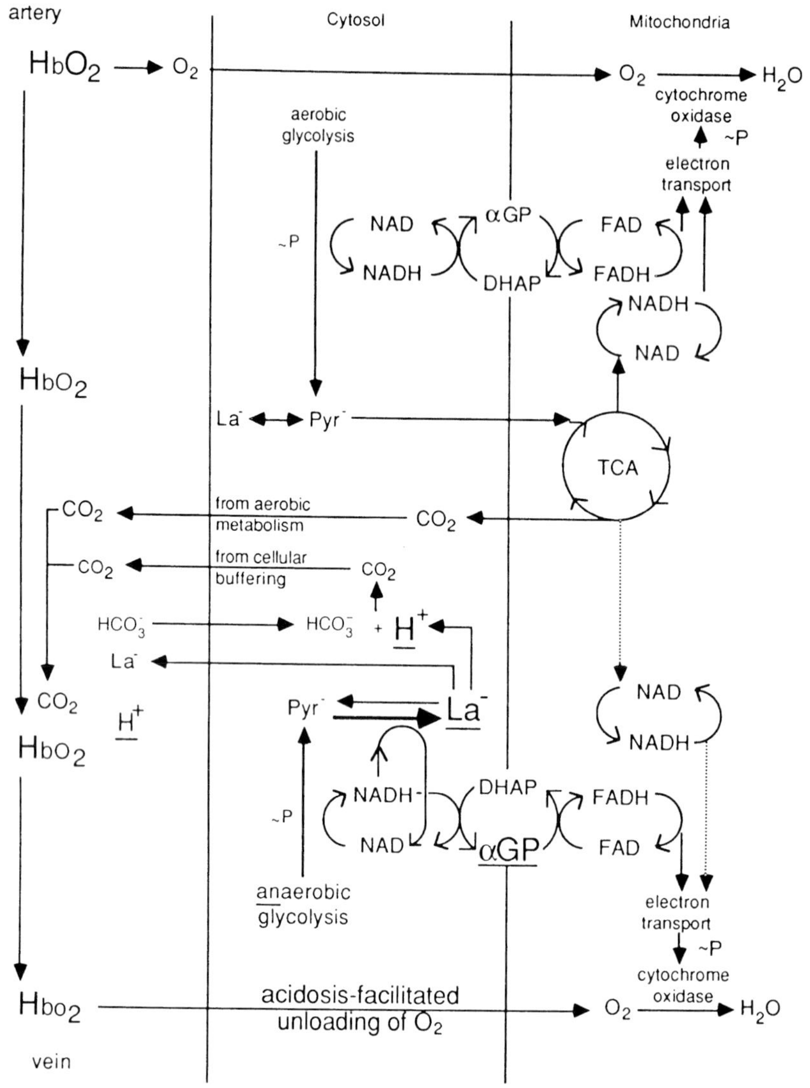

FIGURE 2.21. Scheme of changing muscle capillary oxyhemoglobin (HbO_2) saturation during blood transit from artery to vein during heavy intensity exercise. At the arterial end of the capillary, HbO_2 dissociates primarily due to decrease in P_{O_2}. Glycolysis proceeds aerobically, without an increase in [lactate] (La^-), because mitochondrial membrane redox shuttles (eg, the glycerol-3-phosphate shuttle that converts dihydroxyacetone phosphate [DHAP] to glycerol 3-phosphate [αGP]) dictate cytosolic redox state NADH + H^+/NAD^+ (NADH/NAD). The primary substrate for the tricarboxylic acid (TCA) cycle is pyruvate (Pyr). As pyruvate is metabolized in the mitochondria, protons and electrons flow through the electron transport system to O_2, generating high-energy phosphate (~P) with water (H_2O) and carbon dioxide (CO_2) as by-products. As blood reaches the venous end of the capillary, where P_{O_2} may become critically low at higher work rates, mitochondrial membrane redox shuttles fails to reoxidize NADH to NAD^+ at an adequate rate. Thus, the NADH + H^+/NAD^+ ratio increases. Accordingly, pyruvate is converted to La^-, and DHAP is converted to αGP in proportion to the change in cell redox state. The effect is an increase in cell [La^-] with a stoichiometric increase in [H^+]. The latter is immediately buffered by HCO_3^- in the cell. Decreasing cellular [HCO_3^-] and increasing cellular [La^-] results in intracellular-extracellular La^- and HCO_3^- exchange (see Fig. 2.2). Simultaneously, CO_2 formed during intracellular buffering leaves the cell. The sum of aerobically and anaerobically produced CO_2 (from aerobic glycolysis and buffering of the metabolic acidosis, respectively), along with decreasing blood [HCO_3^-] (see Fig. 2.2), further acidifies the capillary blood toward the venous end of the capillary, enhancing dissociation of HbO_2 (Bohr effect). This acidosis-facilitated dissociation of HbO_2 allows aerobic metabolism to proceed at a rate proportional to the rate of acidification of blood, without a further reduction in capillary P_{O_2}. *(Modified from Wasserman K. Coupling of external to cellular respiration during exercise: the wisdom of the body revisited.* Am J Physiol. *1994;266[4 pt 1]:E519-E539.)*

and H^+ ions produced by carbonic acid (H_2CO_3) dissociation (Equation 11 below) and, above the *AT*, by anaerobic glycolysis. The metabolic acidosis–facilitated oxyhemoglobin dissociation ensures a greater O_2 extraction from capillary blood, thereby supporting a higher maximal $\dot{V}O_2$ than would otherwise be possible.

BUFFERING THE EXERCISE-INDUCED LACTIC ACIDOSIS

Lactic acid, produced fleetingly from lactate ions and their associated protons, is the predominant fixed acid produced during exercise. It has a dissociation constant (pK) of approximately 3.9 and is therefore essentially totally dissociated at the pH of the muscle cell (approximately 7.0 at rest). The major intramuscular buffer of this proton load is HCO_3^-, which is a volatile buffer. This process yields H_2CO_3 and therefore CO_2 (see Equation 11 and "Arterial and Venous P_{CO_2} and Carbon Dioxide Content" below), the latter being readily removed from the intracellular environment; that is, thereby removing H^+ and constraining the fall of pH.

Because the net increase in intracellular $[H^+]$ during exercise is buffered by intracellular HCO_3^-, additional CO_2 is produced in the muscle over that expected from aerobic metabolism as H_2CO_3 dissociates. This results in an increase in end-capillary P_{CO_2} without a further fall in P_{O_2} (**Fig. 2.22**, lower curve). Simultaneously, the decrease in intracellular $[HCO_3^-]$ results in a decrease in extracellular $[HCO_3^-]$ and therefore in femoral venous $[HCO_3^-]$ (see **Fig. 2.22**, upper curve). Both the decrease in femoral venous $[HCO_3^-]$ and the simultaneous increase in P_{CO_2} reflect acidification of the capillary blood of the muscle cells producing lactate and H^+.[107,115]

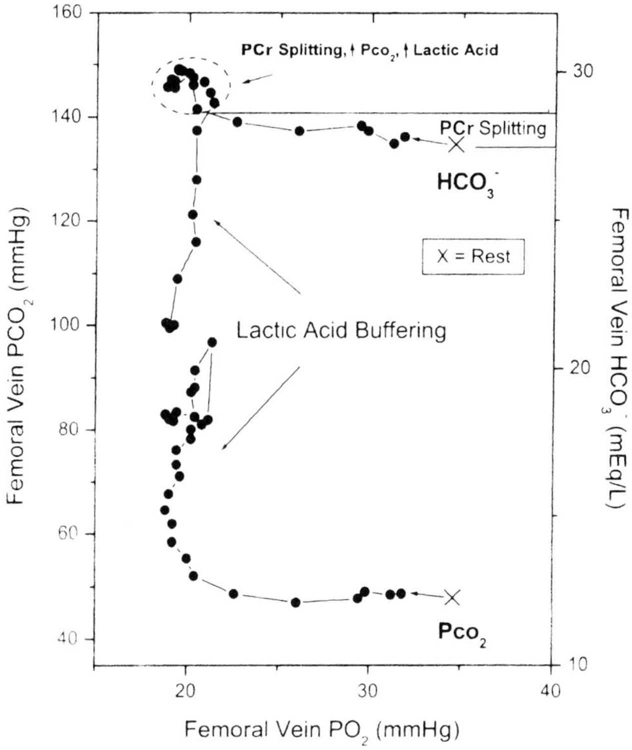

FIGURE 2.22. Group-mean (n = 5) femoral venous P_{CO_2} (lower panel) and [bicarbonate] (HCO_3^-) (upper panel) as a function of femoral venous P_{O_2} for heavy constant work rate cycle ergometer exercise (see Fig. 2.19), with blood sampled at 5-second intervals. The direction of change during the exercise is leftward from the rest (X). The increase in femoral venous $[HCO_3^-]$ during the first 30 seconds of exercise occurs without an increase in femoral venous P_{CO_2}; that is, a true metabolic alkalosis, likely resulting from the splitting of phosphocreatine (PCr) (see text). The onset of the lactic acidosis starts after the minimal (critical) capillary P_{O_2} is reached (about 18 mm Hg), after which femoral venous $[HCO_3^-]$ decreases and femoral venous P_{CO_2} increases due to the HCO_3^- buffering of H^+ in the exercising muscle, without a further fall in femoral venous P_{O_2}. *(Reproduced with permission from Stringer W, Wasserman K, Casaburi R, Pórszász J, Maehara K, French W. Lactic acidosis as a facilitator of oxyhemoglobin dissociation during exercise.* J Appl Physiol. *1994;76[4]:1462-1467. Copyright © 1994 American Physiological Society. All rights reserved)*

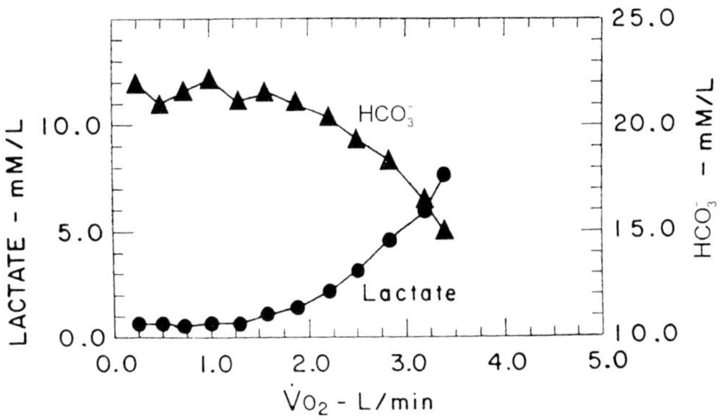

FIGURE 2.23. Arterial [lactate] and standard $[HCO_3^-]$ as a function of O_2 uptake ($\dot{V}O_2$) for incremental cycle ergometer exercise in a normal individual. *(Modified from Wasserman K, Beaver WL, Davis JA, Pu JZ, Heber D, Whipp BJ. Lactate, pyruvate, and lactate-to-pyruvate ratio during exercise and recovery.* J Appl Physiol. *1985;59:935-940.)*

Nonaerobic CO_2 production by the muscle cell increases at a rate commensurate with the rate of HCO_3^- buffering of metabolically produced protons. Approximately 22.3 mL CO_2 will be produced over that generated from aerobic metabolism for each mmol of H^+ buffered by HCO_3^- (see **Fig. 2.2**). The resulting increase in arterial [lactate] and decrease in arterial $[HCO_3^-]$ are matched almost millimoles per liter for millimoles per liter, once [lactate] has increased by about 0.5 to 1.0 mmol/L (**Figs. 2.23, 2.24** and **2.25**).[57,69,107,115-118]

To better appreciate the dynamics of lactate and HCO_3^- movement between muscle cells and perfusing blood, arterial [lactate] and Std $[HCO_3^-]$ were measured every 7.5 seconds during the first 3 minutes and then every 30 seconds during the remaining 3 minutes of a 6-minute constant work rate exercise at three different intensities: moderate, heavy, and very heavy (see **Fig. 2.25**).[107] For the latter two exercise intensities, [lactate] started to increase at about 40 seconds after exercise onset and Std $[HCO_3^-]$ started to decrease at about 50 seconds. Thereafter, [lactate] and Std $[HCO_3^-]$ changed reciprocally.

The initial H^+ buffering following exercise onset is accomplished primarily via the concomitant breakdown of PCr (Equation 1) which causes muscle cell pH to become alkaline (**Fig. 2.26**) (see "Phosphocreatine Breakdown" above).[119-123] This alkalinizing effect occurs during the first minute or so of exercise, when PCr hydrolysis is rapid, until it is more than offset by the acidifying effects of increased aerobic CO_2 production and, above the *AT*, lactic acidosis. Furthermore, because PCr is a highly dissociated acid at muscle cell pH while creatine is neutral, the intracellular concentration of nondiffusible anions decreases when PCr breaks down. Thus, a state of intracellular cation (largely potassium ions, K^+) excess and H^+ depletion is created. It has been proposed that K^+ therefore transfers out of the

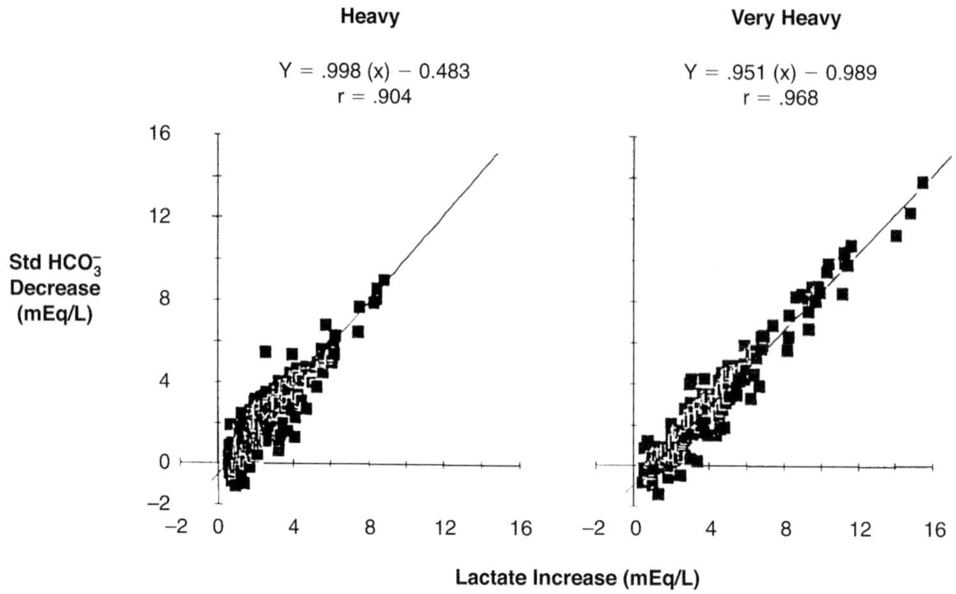

FIGURE 2.24. Arterial standard (Std) [bicarbonate] [HCO$_3^-$] decrease as a function of arterial [lactate] increase from resting values for the heavy (left panel) and very heavy (right panel) exercise intensities shown in Figure 2.25. The fall in Std [HCO$_3^-$] is delayed until after [lactate] has started to increase, after which the changes are approximately equal and opposite: heavy (n = 181): slope = 0.998 (confidence interval [CI], 0.92 to 1.06), intercept = −0.48 (CI, −0.71 to −0.26); very heavy (n = 141): slope = 0.951 (CI, 0.92 to 0.98), intercept = −0.99 (CI, −1.12 to −0.78). *(Reproduced with permission from Stringer W, Casaburi R, Wasserman K. Acid-base regulation during exercise and recovery in humans.* J Appl Physiol. *1992;72[3]:954-961. Copyright © 1992 American Physiological Society. All rights reserved.)*

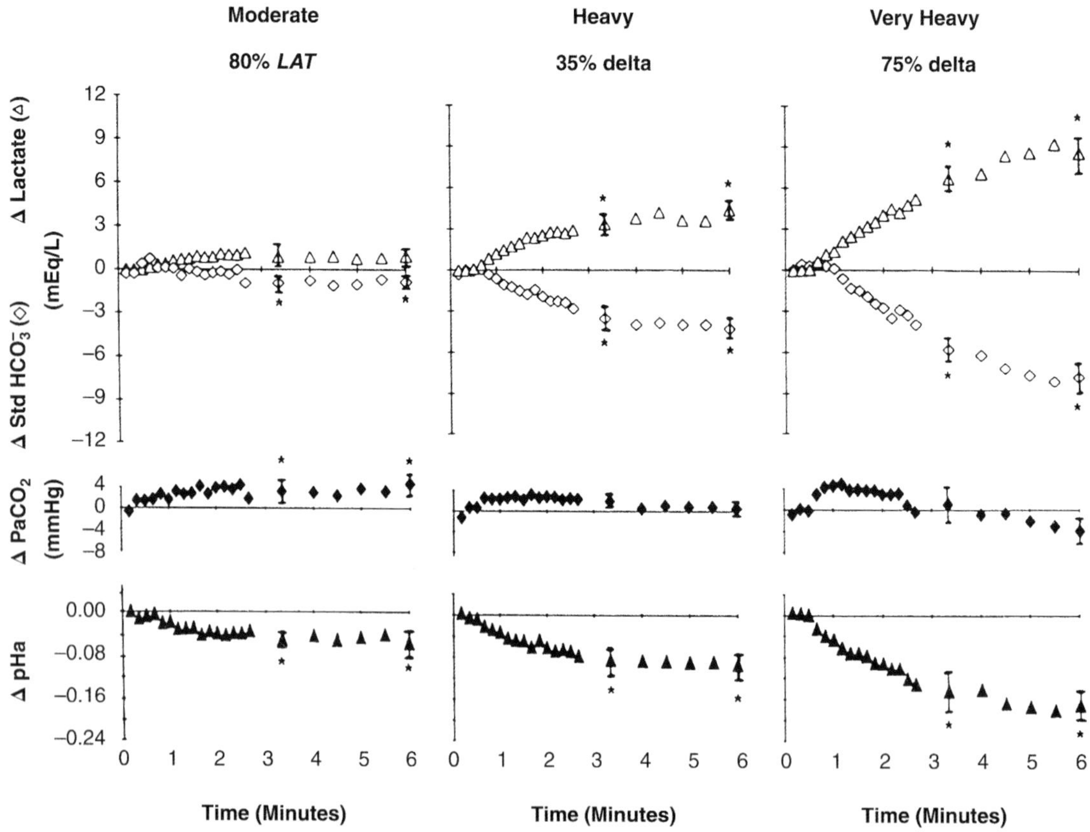

FIGURE 2.25. Group-mean (n = 8) arterial [lactate], standard [bicarbonate] (Std [HCO$_3^-$]), P_{CO_2}, and pH as change from resting for moderate (left panel), heavy (center panel), and very heavy (right panel) constant work rate cycle ergometer exercise. Resting values for arterial pH, P_{CO_2}, standard [HCO$_3^-$], [lactate], and hemoglobin are 7.40 ± 0.03 (standard deviation), 39.8 ± 3.1 mm Hg, 24.5 ± 1.3 mEq/L, 0.89 ± 0.47 mEq/L, and 14.2 g/dL, respectively. Significant differences from baseline (zero time) are shown at 3 and 6 minutes (*$P < .05$ from rest). *(Reproduced with permission from Stringer W, Casaburi R, Wasserman K. Acid-base regulation during exercise and recovery in humans.* J App Physiol. *1992;72[3]:954-961. Copyright © 1992 American Physiological Society. All rights reserved.)*

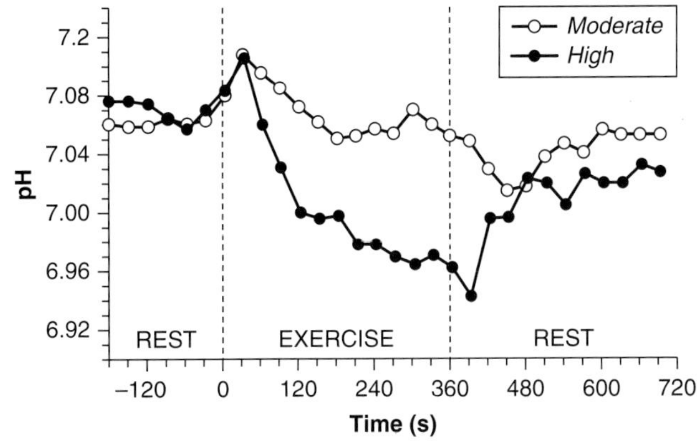

FIGURE 2.26. Quadriceps muscle pH as a function of time for prone moderate- (o) and high-intensity (●) constant work rate knee-extension exercise in a normal individual, measured by phosphorus-31 nuclear magnetic resonance spectroscopy. *(From Rossiter HB, Ward SA, Kowalchuk JM, Howe FA, Griffiths JR, Whipp BJ. Dynamic asymmetry of phosphocreatine concentration and O_2 uptake between the on- and off-transients of moderate- and high-intensity exercise in humans.* J Physiol. *2002;541[pt 3]:991-1002. Copyright © 2002 The Physiological Society. Reprinted by permission of John Wiley & Sons, Inc.)*

muscle cell into interstitial fluid and blood (**Fig. 2.27**)[124]; ionic balance within the muscle cell being maintained by uptake of cations (i.e., H^+) and anion formation (ie, HCO_3^-) from H_2CO_3 dissociation. The net effect of this latter reaction is the fixation of metabolic CO_2 as HCO_3^- within the muscle cell early in exercise (see "Carbon Dioxide Output Kinetics" below). The increase in [HCO_3^-] balancing [K^+] efflux from the muscle cell is reflected in the exercising muscle venous effluent, with femoral venous pH, [HCO_3^-], and [K^+] increasing concurrently.[124] The new HCO_3^- produced by the events associated with PCr splitting account for the failure of arterial [HCO_3^-] to decrease until [lactate] has increased by approximately 0.5 to 1.0 mmol/L (see **Figs. 2.24** and **2.25**). As this early exercise-induced metabolic alkalosis initially masks the metabolic acidosis related to the increase in [lactate], the *LT* slightly precedes the *LAT* and the decrease in arterial Std [HCO_3^-].[107,115]

CARDIOVASCULAR RESPONSES TO EXERCISE

Cardiac output, together with the arterial-mixed venous O_2 content difference ($C(a - \bar{v})O_2$), quantifies the $\dot{V}O_2$ response during exercise:

$$\dot{V}O_2 = \text{cardiac output} \times C(a - \bar{v})O_2 \quad (5)$$

Cardiac output increases at the start of exercise in the upright position through increases in stroke volume and heart rate. Heart rate increases initially as vagal tone decreases with a subsequent increase in sympathetic stimulation. Stroke volume increases as a result of increased venous return resulting from the rhythmic compression of veins by contracting muscles (muscle pump), decreased intrathoracic pressure accompanying increased depth of breathing, and increased cardiac inotropy. As work rate is

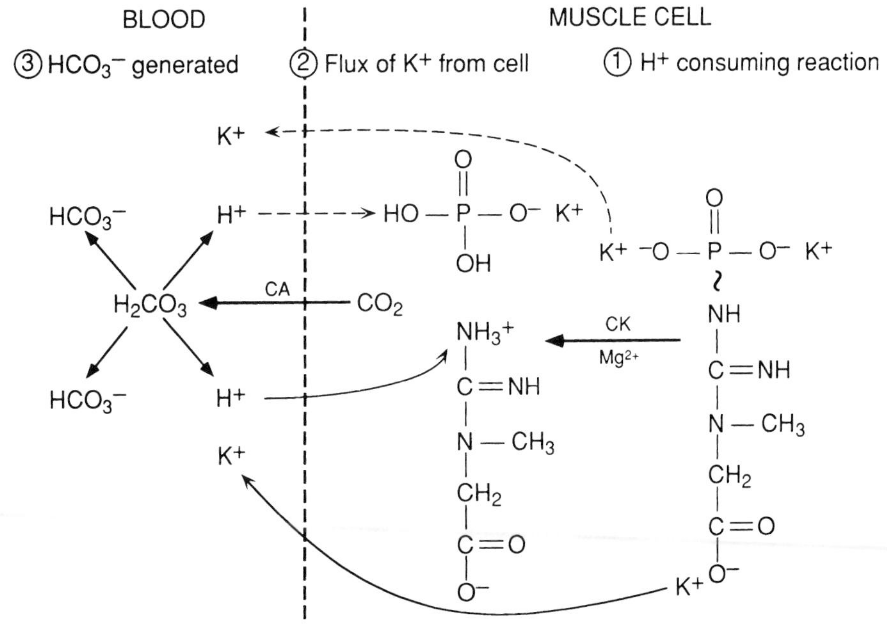

FIGURE 2.27. Hypothesis describing the mechanism for early changes in femoral venous pH, [bicarbonate] [HCO_3^-], and [potassium] [K^+] in response to exercise. Step 1 shows that when phosphocreatine (PCr) is hydrolyzed into creatine and inorganic phosphate (Pi), hydrogen ions (H^+) are consumed, resulting in a reduction of negative charges in the cell and an alkalinizing reaction. Step 2 illustrates that the excess in intracellular cation and shortage of H^+ causes K^+ to leave the cell and H^+ to enter the cell. Step 3 shows that the resulting efflux of K^+ from the cell is balanced by newly formed HCO_3^- in the interstitial fluid and therefore the effluent blood of the muscle. Thus, metabolic carbon dioxide, when hydrated, becomes H_2CO_3, which dissociates into H^+ (which is taken up by the alkaline muscle cell) and HCO_3^- anion (which serves to balance the positive charge of K^+). *(Reproduced with permission from Wasserman K, Stringer W, Casaburi R, Zhang YY. Mechanism of the exercise hyperkalemia: an alternate hypothesis.* J Appl Physiol. *1997;83[2]:631-643. Copyright © 1997 American Physiological Society. All rights reserved.)*

increased, further increases in cardiac output are achieved predominantly by increasing heart rate, with stroke volume remaining relatively constant (although see "Cardiac Output" below).

The pulmonary vascular bed dilates at the start of exercise in concert with the increase in right ventricular output and pulmonary artery pressure. This dilatation results in the perfusion of previously unperfused and underperfused lung units in the normal pulmonary vascular bed, accounting for the fact that there is only a small increase in pulmonary artery pressure in the normal lung as pulmonary blood flow increases. A low pulmonary vascular resistance is essential for the normal exercise response of the left ventricle. Without it, the weakly muscled right ventricle could not readily pump the venous blood through the pulmonary circulation to the left side of the heart at a rate fast enough to achieve the increase in cardiac output needed to support cellular respiration.

Because the proportional increases in cardiac output and muscle blood flow are less than that of $\dot{V}O_2$, the extraction of O_2 from (and addition of CO_2 to) the muscle capillary blood must increase. The falling capillary PO_2 and the Bohr effect allow extraction of 75% to 85% of the O_2 going through the capillary bed of maximally working muscle (see "Oxygen Supply and Critical Capillary PO_2" above).

The O_2 supply to the muscle cells during exercise is dependent on several factors: cardiac output and its peripheral distribution, arterial O_2 content, arterial PO_2 (PaO_2), the characteristics of oxyhemoglobin dissociation, and [Hb]. As previously stated, the transport of O_2 from blood to mitochondria is dependent on maintaining an adequate diffusion gradient for O_2 as the blood travels through the contracting muscle capillary bed. The PO_2 gradient between blood and cell is high at the arterial end of the capillary but decreases as the blood approaches the venous end of the capillary, depending on the ratio of muscle blood flow to metabolic rate ($\dot{Q}m/\dot{Q}O_2$) (see **Fig. 2.15**). The critical capillary PO_2 normally limiting diffusion during exercise appears to be about 15-20 mm Hg.[96-99]

Cardiac Output

The cardiac output obviously must play a key role in the O_2 supply to the cells. Normal peak values of cardiac output are typically in the range of 25 to 30 L/min but lower in less fit and elderly individuals and appreciably higher in highly fit young endurance athletes (>40 L/min); these differences are reflective of activity-related adaptations in stroke volume. Over the tolerable work rate range, cardiac output is generally agreed to increase reasonably linearly with $\dot{V}O_2$, having a slope for cycle ergometry of approximately 5 to 6 (when cardiac output and $\dot{V}O_2$ are reported in the same units) and an intercept on the cardiac output axis of approximately 5 L/min.[125-129]

Despite extensive research, there is no general agreement on exactly how the central circulatory responses to exercise are initiated and sustained during exercise, although there are likely to be broad similarities with those involved in ventilatory control. In particular, neural feedforward drives from (1) "central command," whereby descending locomotor influences from higher regions of the central nervous system elicit parallel activation of ponto-medullary circulatory- (and respiratory-) integrating regions, and (2) reflex stimulation of group III and IV mechanoreceptor and chemoreceptor afferents in the exercising muscles appear of major importance (see "Ventilatory Control" below).[126,130-134] In turn, these mechanisms adjust autonomic inotropic and chronotropic drives to the heart and vasoconstrictor drives to resistance vessels, eliciting increases in cardiac output and arterial blood pressure (the latter under the modulating influence of the arterial baroreflex) and thence increases muscle blood flow and perfusion pressure.

As schematized in **Figure 2.28**, the form of response, for which the relationship between two primary variables (eg, *y*, *x*) is linear and does not project through the origin (0,0), yields a derived response (y/x) at any particular x-value that is equal to the slope of the dashed line projecting from that point back to the origin (see **Fig. 2.28**, left panels). Not only does the derived response y/x increase as x increases but it does so in a hyperbolic fashion, declining when the y-axis intercept is positive and increasing when the y-axis intercept is negative (see **Fig. 2.28**, right panels). In the limit (ie, at very high values of x), the slope value of the primary linear relationship will equal to the asymptotic value of the derived hyperbolic relationship.

Therefore, when $\dot{V}O_2$ is plotted as a function of cardiac output (primary variables), at any particular work rate the slope of the line joining the $\dot{V}O_2$, cardiac output locus to the origin (ie, the ratio of $\dot{V}O_2$ to cardiac output [see **Fig. 2.28**, panel c, left: dashed line]) equals $C(a - \bar{v})O_2$ (derived variable) at that work rate (Equation 5). And because of the negative intercept on the $\dot{V}O_2$ axis, $C(a - \bar{v})O_2$ will increase hyperbolically as work rate and $\dot{V}O_2$ increase (see **Fig. 2.28**, panel c, right). The maximum (or asymptotic) $C(a - \bar{v})O_2$ value achieved (S_c) will, in the limit, equal the slope of the primary $\dot{V}O_2$-cardiac output relationship.

As arterial O_2 content normally does not decrease significantly with increasing work rate (although this may not be the case for highly fit endurance athletes[135-137]), this implies that $C(a - \bar{v})O_2$ increases as the mirror image of mixed venous O_2 content; that is, normally from approximately 5 mL/100 mL at rest to approximately 15 to 18 mL/100 mL at peak exercise (**Fig. 2.29E**).[125-128,138] As peak work rates are approached, arterial O_2 content can demonstrate a slight increase as a result of hemoconcentration (see "Hemoglobin" below), while blood acidification contributes to the decrease in femoral venous and mixed venous O_2 contents (Bohr effect) (see **Figs. 2.20** and **2.30B**) (see "pH Change and Oxyhemoglobin Dissociation Above the Anaerobic Threshold" above).[98,107]

It should be noted, however, that instances of a more curvilinear cardiac output profile as peak work rates are

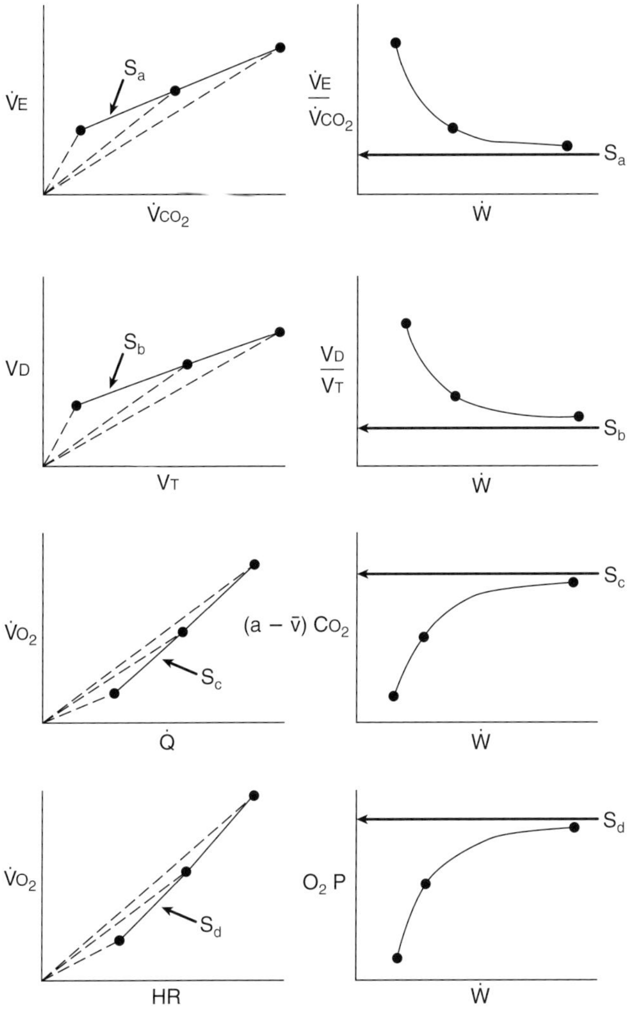

FIGURE 2.28. Schematized key physiological relationships in response to increasing work rate ($\dot{W}$). Left panels, For a primary relationship between two variables *x* and *y* that is linear with an intercept on the y-axis (positive or negative), the derived response at any particular work rate is equal to the ratio of the corresponding responses of the primary variables *x*/*y* (ie, the slope of the dashed lines that project back to the origin). Right panels, Such derived responses will demonstrate a hyperbolic profile, decreasing when the y-axis intercept is positive and increasing when the y-axis intercept is negative. The asymptotic values of these hyperbolic relationships (S_A, S_B, S_C, and S_D) are equal the slope values of the corresponding primary linear relationships. Ventilation ($\dot{V}E$), CO_2 output ($\dot{V}CO_2$), ventilatory equivalent for CO_2 ($\dot{V}E/\dot{V}CO_2$), physiological dead space (V_D), tidal volume (V_T), physiological dead space fraction of the breath (V_D/V_T), O_2 uptake ($\dot{V}O_2$), cardiac output ($\dot{Q}_T$), arterial-mixed venous O_2 content difference ([a − v̄]O_2), heart rate (HR), O_2 pulse (O_2-P). *(Reprinted from Whipp BJ. The bioenergetic and gas exchange basis of exercise testing.* Clin Chest Med. *1994;15[2]:173-192. Figure 4. Copyright © 1994 Elsevier. With permission.)*

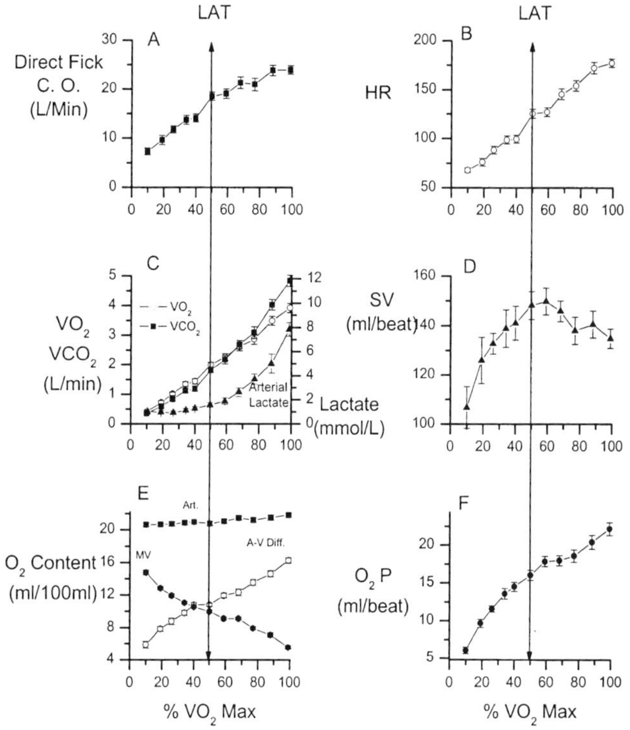

FIGURE 2.29. Group-mean (n = 5, 10 tests, mean ± standard error) cardiac output (CO, L/min) (A); heart rate (HR, beats/min) (B); O_2 uptake ($\dot{V}O_2$, L/min), carbon dioxide output ($\dot{V}CO_2$, L/min), and arterial [lactate] (mmol/L) (C); stroke volume (mL/beat) (D); arterial (Art., mL/100 mL) and mixed venous (MV, mL/100 mL) O_2 contents and arterial-mixed venous O_2 content difference (A-V Diff., mL/100 mL) (E); and O_2 pulse (O_2P, mL O_2/beat) (F), as a function of percentage maximal O_2 uptake (%$\dot{V}O_2$max) for ramp incremental cycle ergometer exercise. Vertical arrows at 50% $\dot{V}O_2$max mark the mean lactic acidosis threshold (*LAT*). *(Reproduced with permission from Stringer W, Hansen J, Wasserman K. Cardiac output estimated noninvasively from oxygen uptake during exercise.* J Appl Physiol. *1997;82[3]:908-912. Copyright © 1997 American Physiological Society. All rights reserved.)*

approached have been reported for nonsteady state (ie, incremental) exercise (see **Fig. 2.29A**).[138,139] As a result, C(a − v̄)O_2 may exhibit a more linear profile of response (see **Fig. 2.29E**).[138] Based on this behavior, a noninvasive method for estimating the cardiac output and stroke volume (with knowledge of heart rate) during exercise is presented in Chapter 3, although it should be emphasized that the assumption of an approximately linear C(a − v̄)O_2 response profile (see **Fig. 2.29E**)[138] may be protocol and subject dependent (as discussed above).

In the upright posture, stroke volume normally increases abruptly at exercise onset from resting values of approximately 60 to 70 mL (although these are higher for exercise performed in the supine posture because blood does not pool in the dependent lower limbs) to attain values in the region of approximately 90 to 120 mL at peak exercise and appreciably higher in endurance-trained individuals.[125-129,132] However, stroke volume has also been reported to continue to increase (see **Fig. 2.29D**) or even to start to decrease as peak work rates are approached, possibly reflective of factors such as exercise protocol, fitness, posture, and blood volume.[127,138-142]

Regardless, increasing heart rate is the predominant support for the further cardiac output increases at higher work rates, typically increasing relatively linearly with $\dot{V}O_2$ (see **Fig. 2.29B**; see the case studies of normal individuals in Chapter 10) to attain peak values of ≥200 beats/min in healthy young individuals.[125-129,132] Although peak heart rate is independent of fitness, it is age-dependent, declining by

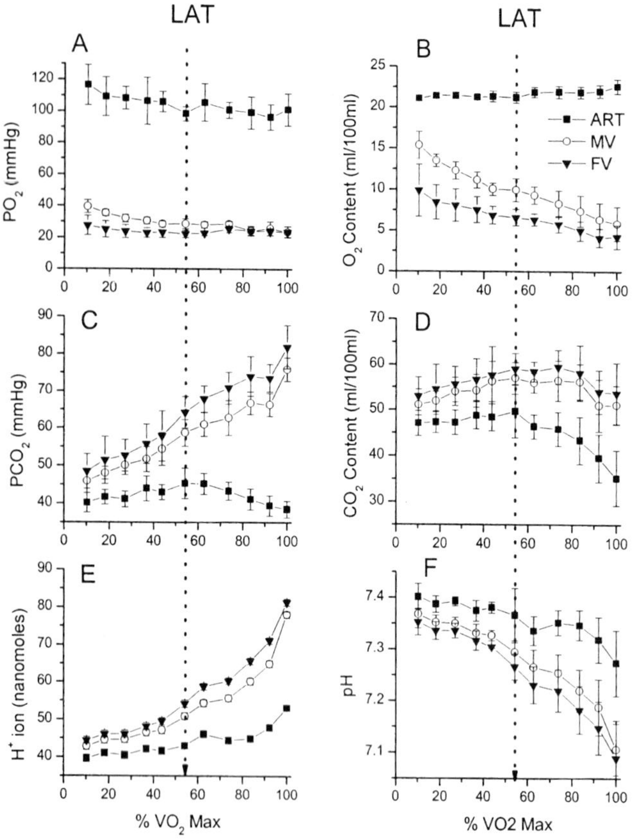

FIGURE 2.30. As for the study depicted in Figure 2.29, group-mean (n = 5, mean ± standard deviation) P_{O_2} (A), O_2 content (B), P_{CO_2} (C), carbon dioxide (CO_2) content (D), hydrogen (H^+) concentration (E), and pH (F) in arterial (■, ART), mixed venous (○, MV), and femoral vein (▼, FV) blood as a function of percentage maximal O_2 uptake (%$\dot{V}O_2$max) during ramp incremental cycle ergometer exercise. Lactic acidosis threshold (*LAT*) (average = 54% of $\dot{V}O_{2max}$) is shown by the vertical dashed line. *(Reproduced with permission from Stringer W, Hansen J, Wasserman K. Cardiac output estimated noninvasively from oxygen uptake during exercise.* J Appl Physiol. *1997;82[3]:908-912. Copyright © 1997 American Physiological Society. All rights reserved.)*

approximately 10 beats/min per decade. Normally, peak heart rate is close to the predicted maximum heart rate, which is typically estimated as (220 − age in years; having a standard deviation of the order of ≥10 beats/min). Thus, the heart rate reserve, which is the difference between the predicted maximum and actual peak heart rates, will be essentially zero, although premature cessation of the exercise test because of poor effort or exacerbated symptoms will be reflected in a positive heart rate reserve.

The rate-pressure product, the product of heart rate and systolic blood pressure, increases during exercise, becoming steeper above the *AT*.[143] This may reflect increasing catecholamine levels and could be a mechanism for enhancing O_2 delivery to exercising muscle when there is an imbalance between O_2 demand and O_2 supply.

Because heart rate increases linearly with $\dot{V}O_2$, the higher $\dot{V}O_2$ required for a given work rate when fatty acids are the predominant substrate (see "Substrate Utilization" above) should predictably demand a greater heart rate and cardiac output, compared with carbohydrate (see **Fig.2.3**, right panel).

Oxygen Pulse

The ratio of $\dot{V}O_2$ to heart rate (HR) provides a useful index, the O_2 pulse, which represents the volume of O_2 extracted from each heartbeat.[144] Its determinants are evident from a rearrangement of the Fick principle:

$$\dot{V}O_2/HR = SV \cdot C(a - \bar{v})O_2 \quad (6)$$

where SV is stroke volume. As the heart rate-$\dot{V}O_2$ relationship is linear with a positive intercept on the heart rate axis (see **Fig. 2.28**, panel d, left), the normal O_2 pulse profile is predictably hyperbolic (see **Figs. 2.28**, panel d, right and **2.29F**). The higher stroke volume in endurance-trained individuals results in the O_2 pulse at a given $\dot{V}O_2$ being increased. However, interpreting an O_2 pulse profile during exercise solely in terms of stroke volume can be potentially misleading, unless $C(a - \bar{v})O_2$ can reasonably be assumed not to be changing.[144] This may apply in phase I of constant work rate exercise (see "Oxygen Uptake Kinetics" and "Carbon Dioxide Output Kinetics" below), the initial period following exercise onset when the composition of blood entering the pulmonary circulation has yet to be influenced by the increased metabolic rate in muscles, and therefore, for which, $C(a - \bar{v})O_2$ is still at resting values. As a result, the initial increase in stroke volume will be reflected in a corresponding increase in the O_2 pulse. However, once $C(a - \bar{v})O_2$ starts to increase, this will contribute to the O_2 pulse response. Unambiguous interpretation of an O_2 pulse profile in terms of its determinants, stroke volume and $C(a - \bar{v})O_2$, therefore requires actual measurement of one or other of these.

Distribution of Peripheral Blood Flow

During exercise, the fraction of the cardiac output diverted to the skeletal muscles increases progressively with work rate (from approximately 15%-20% at rest to approximately 85%-90% at peak exercise), while the fraction perfusing organs such as the kidney, liver, and gastrointestinal tract decreases.[128,129,145-147] The increase in blood flow through the working muscles ($\dot{Q}$m), and a small fraction through the skin to eliminate some of the heat generated during exercise, accounts for almost all of the increase in cardiac output that takes place during exercise. As a result, $\dot{Q}$m increases essentially linearly over the tolerable work rate range, from approximately 1.5 to 2 L/min at rest to approximately 20 L/min at peak exercise in normal individuals and as high as 35 to 40 L/min in elite endurance athletes.

The mechanisms controlling muscle blood flow during exercise are multifactorial.[132,145-149] At the onset of exercise, muscle blood flow initially benefits from recruitment of the muscle pump. Thus, not only is venous return increased, but the associated reduction in venous pressure may increase flow through upstream arterial (ie, resistance) vessels as a result of a widened arteriovenous pressure gradient. Also, rhythmic compression of arterioles and consequent decreasing of transmural pressure could lead to myogenic vasodilatation of resistance vessels. In addition, there may be rapid-onset local vasodilation, mediated by autonomic vasodilator nerve activation, acetylcholine spill-over from motor nerves, and/or local humoral mediation (eg, involving nitric oxide and vascular smooth muscle K^+ channels).

Subsequently, however, increases in skeletal muscle vascular conductance develop that are the result of the global increase in reflex sympathetic vasoconstrictor drive (particularly to gastrointestinal and renal beds) being overridden by locally mediated arteriolar vasodilatation mediated by factors such as PO_2, PCO_2, H^+, ATP, adenosine, Pi, K^+, osmolarity, endothelial release of nitric oxide and prostaglandins, reactive O_2 species, flow-related vessel wall shear stress, and ATP release from red cells.[145-147,150-152] This functional sympatholysis thus favors distribution of the increased cardiac output to the regions of the exercising muscles in which metabolism is most disturbed (ie, matching local blood flow to local metabolic demands, $\dot{Q}m/\dot{Q}O_2$). At higher work rates, however, further increases in muscle blood flow are influenced to a progressively greater extent by the increasing arterial blood pressure. In addition, a potential conflict can arise at near maximal work rates if these are associated with excessively high ventilatory requirements (eg, in elite endurance athletes and patients with lung or heart disease), as the metabolic requirements of the respiratory muscles may result in their perfusion demands being sufficiently high so as to compromise those of the exercising limb muscles. Thus, a proportion of the blood flow that would normally reach the exercising limbs is reflexly diverted to the respiratory muscles (termed respiratory muscle steal).[153-155]

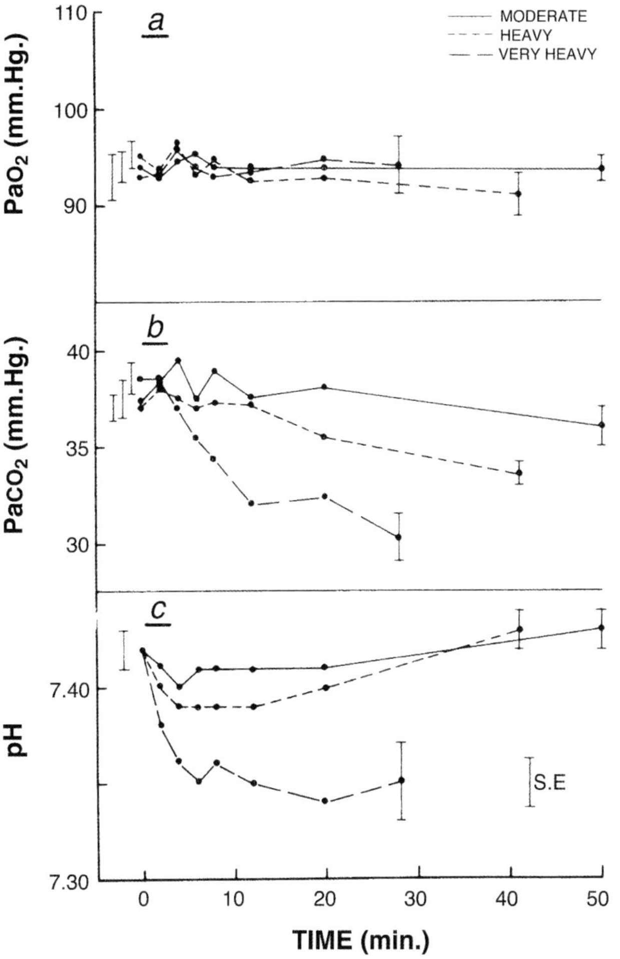

FIGURE 2.31. Group-mean (n = 10) arterial PO_2 (PaO_2), arterial PCO_2 ($PaCO_2$), and pH for prolonged constant work rate cycle ergometer exercise (target duration = 50 min) of moderate, heavy, and very heavy intensities. *(Reproduced with permission from Wasserman K, VanKessel AL, Burton GG. Interaction of physiological mechanisms during exercise.* J Appl Physiol. *1967;22[1]:71-85. Copyright © 1967 American Physiological Society. All rights reserved.)*

Arterial PO_2

In the normal individual at sea level, PaO_2 is a function of mean alveolar PO_2 (PAO_2). For an idealized lung (all lung units having the same alveolar ventilation-perfusion ratio [$\dot{V}A/\dot{Q}$] and no diffusion impairment) where R is assumed to be 0.8 and $PACO_2$ to be equal to 40 mm Hg, PAO_2 would equal approximately 100 mm Hg. However, reductions in PaO_2 relative to the ideal PAO_2 are due to one or more of the following mechanisms: a right-to-left shunt, O_2 diffusion disequilibrium at the alveolar-capillary interface, or $\dot{V}A/\dot{Q}$ maldistribution. Normal young adults have a PaO_2 of about 90 mm Hg (**Fig. 2.31**) with an alveolar-arterial PO_2 difference [$P(A - a)O_2$] of approximately 10 mm Hg during moderate exercise at sea level.[69,137,156,157] This difference between PAO_2 and PaO_2 can be attributed to a small right-to-left shunt (possibly the thebesian blood vessels in the heart and the bronchial circulation) and the lack of total regional uniformity of $\dot{V}A/\dot{Q}$. In highly fit individuals, the development of diffusion impairments and $\dot{V}A/\dot{Q}$ mismatching have also been described at very high work rates with $P(A - a)O_2$ exceeding 30 mm Hg.[135-137]

Oxyhemoglobin Dissociation

The O_2 content of blood as a function of PO_2—the oxyhemoglobin dissociation curve—has a sigmoid relationship (**Fig. 2.32**), with a plateau value for arterial blood of approximately 20 mL/100 mL in normal adults (assuming [Hb] = 15 g/dL). The P_{50}, or the PO_2 at which Hb is 50% saturated with O_2, is approximately 28 mm Hg at pH of 7.40, PCO_2 of 40, and temperature of 37°C. The remarkable characteristic of blood is the increase in O_2 content, above that physically dissolved (only 0.3 mL per 100 mL at a PO_2 of 100 mm Hg), which is related to the strong O_2-binding properties of the Hb molecule.

Altered Hb affinity for O_2, either congenitally or acquired, may impair muscle O_2 supply.[158,159] This might be due to either the effect on the arterial O_2 content or on oxyhemoglobin P_{50}. For example, genetic defects causing a shift in the oxyhemoglobin dissociation curve to the left (low P_{50}) can impair O_2 extraction by the exercising muscle, leading to the minimal capillary PO_2 needed for diffusion being attained earlier with consequent impairment of O_2 diffusion (see "Oxygen Supply and Critical Capillary PO_2" above). This has the potential to reduce $\dot{V}O_2$ and might also induce polycythemia in compensation. In contrast, hemoglobinopathies that shift the oxyhemoglobin dissociation curve to the right (high P_{50}) allow O_2 to

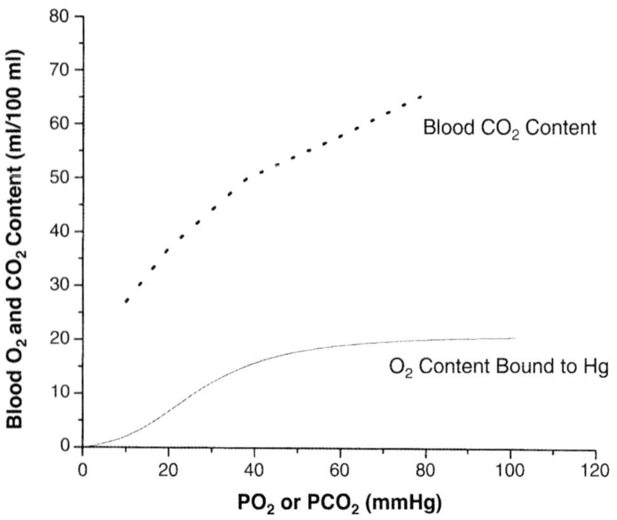

FIGURE 2.32. Blood carbon dioxide (CO_2) (dashed line) and O_2 (solid line) dissociation curves; that is, content as a function of partial pressure (pH = 7.4, temperature = 37°C, P_{50} = 28 mm Hg, [hemoglobin] = 15 g/100 mL). The arterial O_2 content is primarily related to O_2 bound to hemoglobin, as the dissolved O_2 content is small (0.3 mL/100 mL at a Po_2 of 100 mm Hg). In the physiological range, the CO_2 dissociation curve is steep, relative to the O_2 dissociation curve. *(CO_2 content data are from Christiansen J, Douglas CG, Haldane JS. The dissociation of CO_2 by human blood.* J Appl Physiol. *1913;47:ii.)*

unload from Hb more readily and are generally associated with anemia.

Shifts in P_{50} are common even in normal individuals. For example, a rightward shift of the oxyhemoglobin dissociation curve (increased P_{50}) resulting from acidosis (Bohr effect), increased temperature, or high levels of 2,3-diphosphoglycerate favors diffusion of O_2 from the capillaries into the mitochondria. This contrasts with the leftward shift (decreased P_{50}) resulting from alkalosis, carbon monoxide toxicity, or low 2,3-diphosphoglycerate concentrations, where the Po_2 diffusion gradient is reduced. Therefore, O_2 affinity for Hb increases as blood transits the pulmonary capillary bed, and $[H^+]$ and Pco_2 decrease. In contrast, O_2 affinity for Hb decreases in the peripheral capillary blood as muscle $[H^+]$ and Pco_2 increase consequent to the increased metabolic rate. Hence, the characteristics of the oxyhemoglobin dissociation curve are not static but are subject to constant change depending on the local environmental and metabolic factors throughout the round trip from central to peripheral circulations. During exercise, factors such as these assist normal O_2 loading in the pulmonary circulation and unloading in the exercising muscles (see "pH Change and Oxyhemoglobin Dissociation Above the Anaerobic Threshold" above).

Hemoglobin Concentration

Hemoconcentration during exercise has been widely demonstrated and reflects a shift of plasma into extracellular fluid compartments and thence into exercising muscle cells, consequent to increases in both intracapillary hydrostatic pressure and intramuscular osmolality (**Figs. 2.33** and **2.34**).[160-164] It is more marked above the *AT* because of the intracellular increase in osmotically active species such as lactate, which is reflected in more marked increases in the plasma concentrations of cations and anions (see **Figs. 2.33** and **2.34**).[161,164] Also, increases in red cell concentration increase the arterial O_2 content, providing more O_2 delivery unit cardiac output (see **Fig. 2.34**). Localized hemoconcentration within the exercising muscle capillaries provides further benefit. Thus, when blood flow is increased (as with increasing work rate), the distance between adjacent red blood cells decreases, thereby increasing the capillary

FIGURE 2.33. Group-mean (n = 10) arterial plasma concentrations of sodium (Na^+), potassium (K^+), calcium (Ca^{++}), and total measured cations (left panel), and chloride (Cl^-), bicarbonate (HCO_3^-), lactate (La^-), and total measured anions (right panel) for incremental cycle ergometer exercise. The vertical bars on points are the standard errors of means. The vertical line is the average lactate threshold (*LT*).

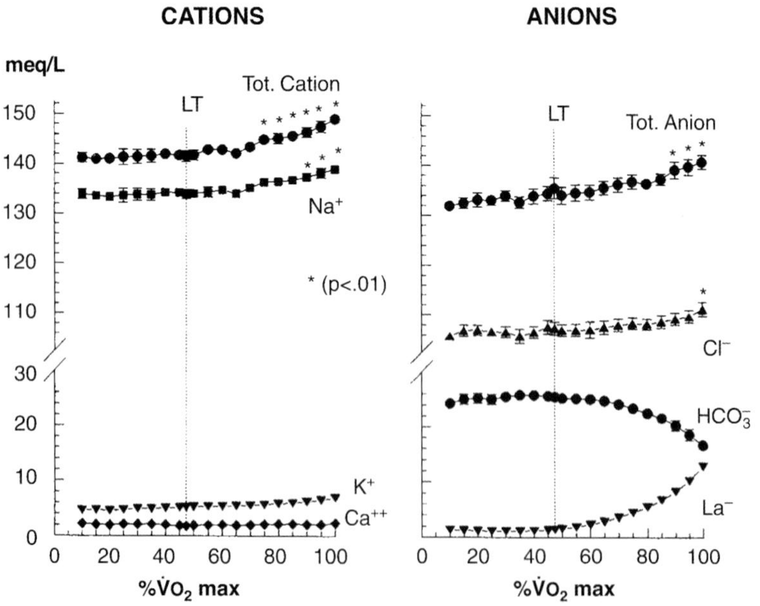

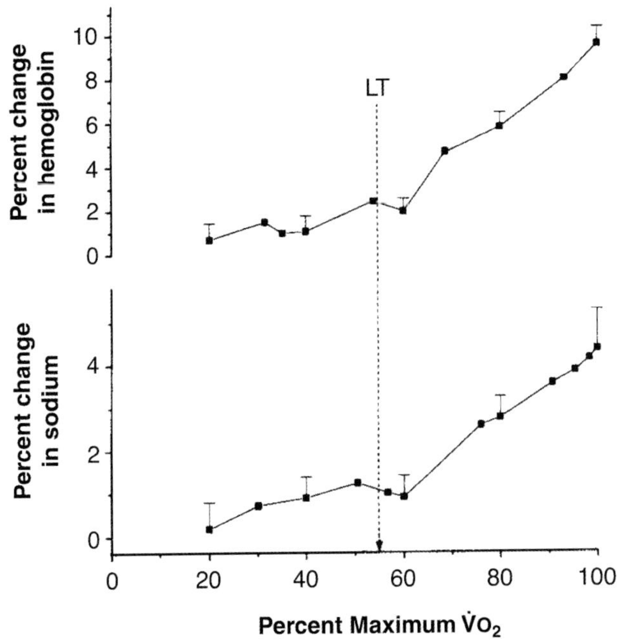

FIGURE 2.34. Group-mean (n = 10) changes in arterial [hemoglobin] and plasma [sodium] during incremental cycle ergometer exercise. The vertical bars on points are the standard errors of means. The vertical line is the average lactate threshold (*LT*), with a standard deviation of ±4.8%.

hematocrit and promoting diffusional transfer of O_2 from the capillary to the muscle mitochondrion.[165] These effects could benefit the individual during exercise in which the O_2 supply limits exercise performance.

Arterial Oxygen Content

The arterial O_2 content (CaO_2) depends on PaO_2, the [Hb] that is free to take up O_2, and the total volume of arterial blood. The CaO_2 can be calculated from [Hb], SaO_2, and PaO_2, as shown in the following equation[166]:

$$CaO_2\ (mL\ O_2/100\ mL) = [Hb]\ (g/dL) \times SaO_2 \times 1.34\ mL\ O_2/g\ Hb + (0.003 \times PaO_2)\ (7)$$

Anemia, resulting in a decreased CaO_2, can thus compromise the supply of O_2 to the exercising muscles. The Hb that is inactive (as in methemoglobin) or has carbon monoxide on the O_2-binding sites (as in cigarette smokers) will also result in a reduced CaO_2. Each of these conditions will result in a more rapid decrease in muscle capillary PO_2 than normal, such that the minimal capillary PO_2 needed for diffusion will be reached at a lower metabolic rate than if all of the Hb were available for O_2 transport (see **Figs. 2.15** and **2.21**). In the presence of anemia or increased concentration of inactive Hb, the blood flow–metabolic rate ratio of the muscle ($\dot{Q}m/\dot{Q}O_2$) must increase to support a given level of cellular respiration.

GAS EXCHANGE KINETICS

As discussed in Chapter 1, the typical response profiles of $\dot{V}O_2$ and $\dot{V}CO_2$ for moderate constant work rate exercise (ie, exercise that does not engender a metabolic acidosis) and heavy-intensity constant work rate exercise (ie, exercise that results in a sustained metabolic acidosis) are qualitatively different (see **Fig. 1.4**).[31,165,167,168]

This makes it possible to discern if a particular work rate is above or below the *AT* simply from gas exchange measurements. Thus, in the absence of metabolic acidosis, $\dot{V}O_2$ in healthy individuals reaches a steady state by 3 minutes, whereas $\dot{V}CO_2$ increases more slowly because of CO_2 storage, reaching a steady state in about 4 to 5 minutes (see **Fig. 2.35A**). The steady-state $\dot{V}CO_2$ is slightly lower than $\dot{V}O_2$, as the whole-body RQ and therefore R are less than 1.0. In contrast, for constant work rate exercise above the *AT*, the overall $\dot{V}O_2$ kinetics are slow compared with exercise performed below the *AT* (see **Fig. 2.35B**), and a steady state in $\dot{V}O_2$ is often not reached before intolerance is reached. Also, $\dot{V}CO_2$ rises more rapidly and to higher levels than $\dot{V}O_2$ (see **Figs. 2.35B,C** and **2.36**), reflecting the excess CO_2 generated when HCO_3^- buffers the lactic acidosis (see **Fig. 2.2**) and also by CO_2 unloading from body stores due to the compensatory hyperventilation for the metabolic acidosis that decreases $PaCO_2$ (see "Ventilatory Responses to Exercise" below). As a result, exercise above *AT* is associated with a rapid increase in R above 1.0; that is, within about a minute after exercise onset.

Gas exchange kinetics are typically discerned using a constant work rate exercise test (ie, having an abrupt step-increase in work rate). Dynamic discrimination of responses is typically optimized by employing multiple repetitions of a test in a given individual. An averaged response profile can then be obtained by interpolating individual breath-by-breath data sets (eg, each second) and then time aligning the several interpolated data sets to time zero (ie, exercise onset) and time averaging them (e.g. each second) to reduce random breath-to-breath fluctuations or "noise."[169,170]

The $\dot{V}O_2$ and $\dot{V}CO_2$ responses following the onset of constant work rate exercise from rest can be characterized by three time-related phases (**Fig. 2.37**).[167,170,171]

Phase I is the period following the onset of constant work rate exercise before the products of exercise metabolism to reach the lungs from the exercising muscles and is normally about 15 to 20 seconds in duration.[170,172-174] During this period, therefore, the mixed venous blood entering the pulmonary capillary bed has not yet changed its composition from that at rest. However, because of the abrupt increase in cardiac output and pulmonary blood flow that occurs at exercise onset (see "Cardiac Output" above), $\dot{V}O_2$ and $\dot{V}CO_2$ both increase abruptly[173-176]; that is,

$$\dot{V}O_2 = \dot{Q}p \cdot (CaO_2 - C\bar{v}O_2)\ (8)$$

$$\dot{V}CO_2 = \dot{Q}p \cdot (C\bar{v}CO_2 - CaCO_2)\ (9)$$

where $\dot{Q}p$ is pulmonary blood flow (normally equal to cardiac output). During phase I, as $C\bar{v}O_2$ and $C\bar{v}CO_2$ have yet to change, the gas exchange response increments ($\Delta\dot{V}O_2$, $\Delta\dot{V}CO_2$) will be directly proportional to the phase I

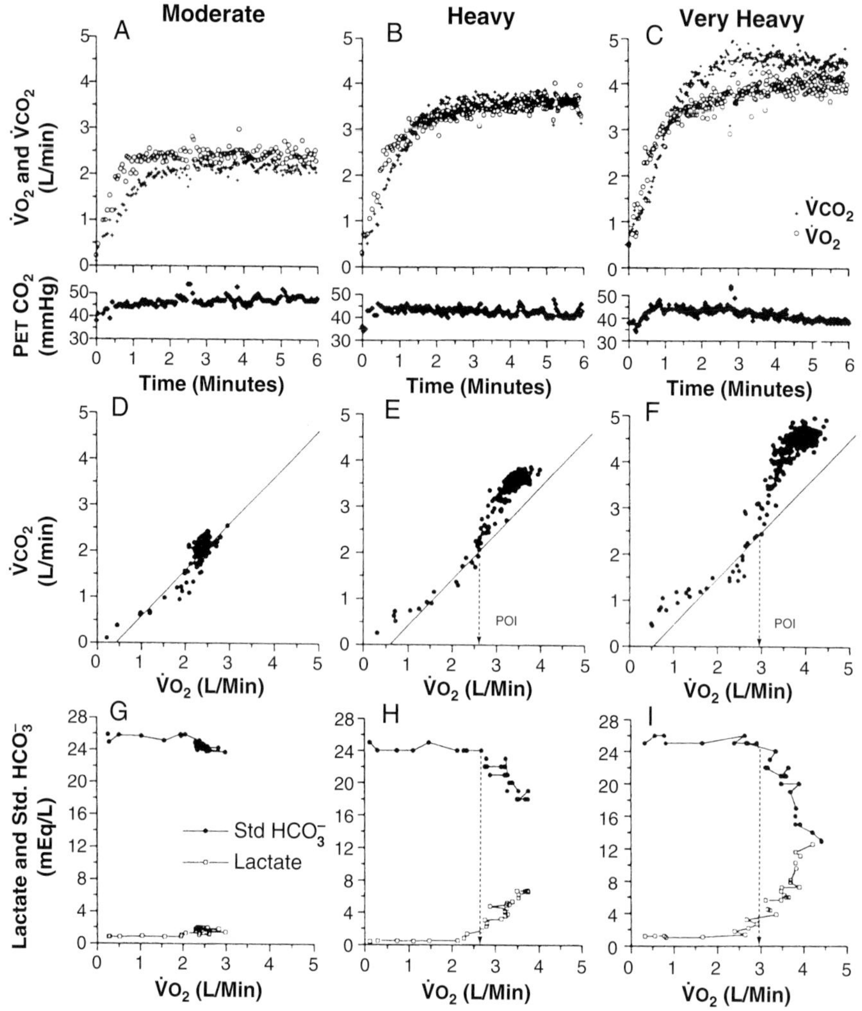

FIGURE 2.35. Group-mean (n = 8) O_2 uptake ($\dot{V}O_2$), carbon dioxide output ($\dot{V}CO_2$), and end-tidal P_{CO_2} (P_{ETCO_2}) as a function of time (A-C), and $\dot{V}CO_2$, arterial [lactate], and standard [bicarbonate] (Std HCO_3^-) as a function of $\dot{V}O_2$ (D-I) for constant work rate cycle ergometer exercise of moderate, heavy, and very heavy intensities. Steepening of $\dot{V}CO_2$ relative to $\dot{V}O_2$ (arrow in E and F) occurs simultaneously with the increase in [lactate] and decrease in [HCO_3^-] (arrow in H and I) at point of inflection (POI), reflecting buffering of the lactic acidosis by HCO_3^-. *(Modified by permission from Springer: Stringer W, Wasserman K, Casaburi R. The $\dot{V}CO_2$/$\dot{V}O_2$ relationship during heavy, constant work rate exercise reflects the rate of lactate accumulation.* Eur J Appl Physiol. *1995;72:25-31. Copyright © 1995 Springer Nature.)*

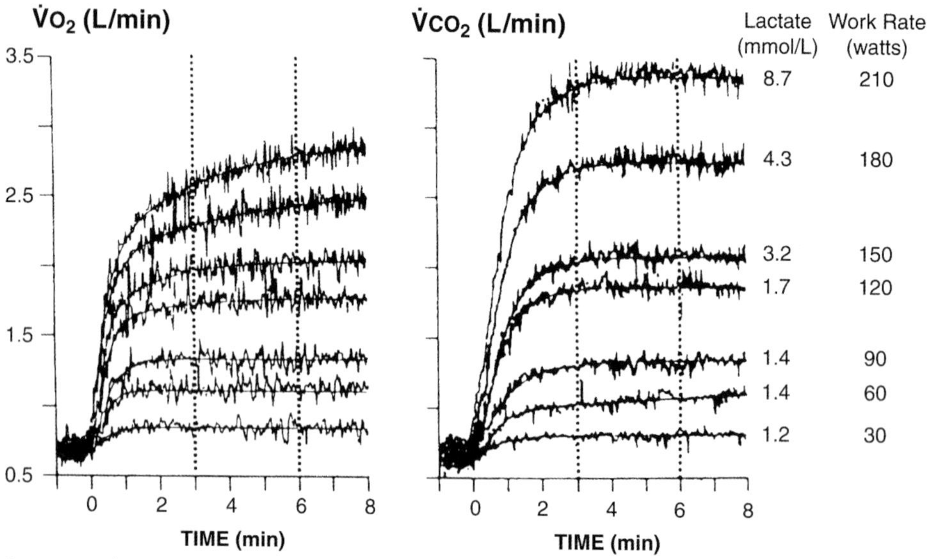

FIGURE 2.36. O_2 uptake ($\dot{V}O_2$) and carbon dioxide output ($\dot{V}CO_2$) as a function of time for constant work rate cycle ergometer exercise at seven different work rates for a normal individual. The three lowest work rates are below the individual's anaerobic threshold (*AT*), whereas the four highest work rates are above it. The $\dot{V}O_2$ continues to rise with time for the four work rates above the *AT*, the rate of rise being more marked the higher the work rate. In contrast, the $\dot{V}CO_2$ kinetics are relatively unchanged, reaching a constant level by 3 to 4 minutes in all seven tests. *(Modified from Casaburi R, Barstow TJ, Robinson T, Wasserman K. Influence of work rate on ventilatory and gas exchange kinetics.* J Appl Physiol. *1989;67:547-555.)*

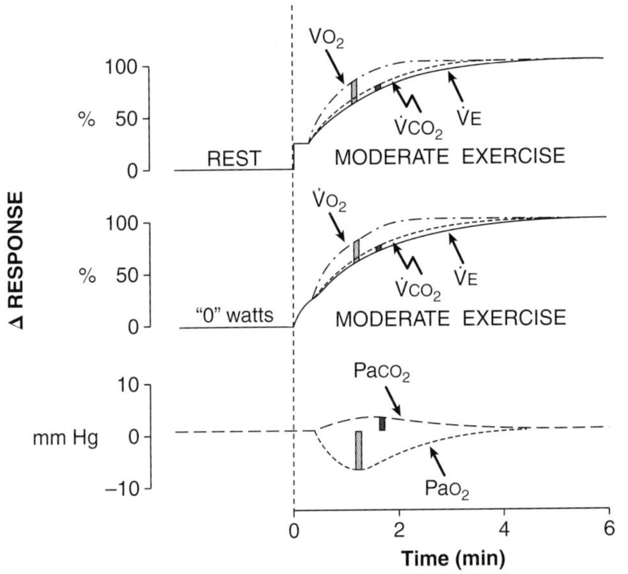

FIGURE 2.37. Schematic depiction of time course of O_2 uptake ($\dot{V}O_2$, — - —), carbon dioxide output ($\dot{V}CO_2$; ------), and ventilation ($\dot{V}E$; ——) in response to moderate constant work rate exercise from rest (upper panel) and unloaded cycling (middle panel), with corresponding profiles of arterial PCO_2 ($PaCO_2$; — — —) and PO_2 (PaO_2; — - - —) (lower panel). *(Reprinted with permission from Whipp BJ, Ward SA. Ventilatory control dynamics during muscular exercise in man.* Int J Sports Med. *1980;1[4]:146-159. Figure 2. Copyright © Georg Thieme Verlag KG.)*

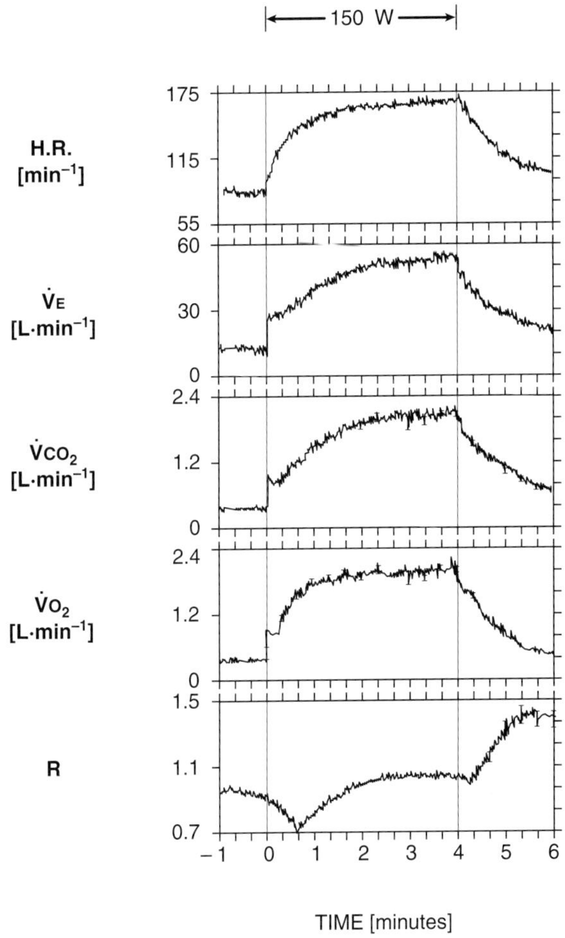

FIGURE 2.38. Averaged (six repetitions) heart rate (HR), ventilation ($\dot{V}E$), carbon dioxide output ($\dot{V}CO_2$), O_2 uptake ($\dot{V}O_2$), and the gas exchange ratio (R) for moderate constant work rate cycle ergometer exercise in a normal individual. The vertical bars are the standard errors of the mean. The abrupt increase in $\dot{V}E$, $\dot{V}CO_2$, and $\dot{V}O_2$ at exercise onset (zero time) is termed *phase I* and ascribed to the concomitant abrupt increase in pulmonary blood flow. The R is usually unchanged from rest for about the first 15 seconds of exercise. The start of phase II is signaled by a decrease in R and is the period of exponential-like increase in $\dot{V}O_2$, $\dot{V}CO_2$, and $\dot{V}E$ to their asymptotes (phase III). This is the period when increasing cellular respiration is reflected in lung gas exchange. The R decreases transiently during phase II because $\dot{V}O_2$ increases faster than $\dot{V}CO_2$ due to gas solubility differences in tissues and phosphocreatine splitting (see Fig. 2.27). It then increases to a value higher than rest because the respiratory quotient (RQ) of the exercising muscle substrate, being primarily glycogen, is higher than the average resting RQ.

increment in $\dot{Q}p$ ($\Delta\dot{Q}p$): that is, $\Delta\dot{V}O_2 \propto \Delta\dot{Q}p$ and $\Delta\dot{V}CO_2 \propto \Delta\dot{Q}p$, with R ($\dot{V}CO_2/\dot{V}O_2$) remaining at resting levels.[167,170,177] When the exercise is performed in the supine position or instituted from an active baseline (eg, unloaded pedaling) rather than rest, the phase I $\dot{V}O_2$ and $\dot{V}CO_2$ responses are smaller and more sluggish (see **Fig. 2.37**), reflecting the smaller $\dot{Q}p$ increase in the former for which baseline stroke volume is already increased above resting levels (see "Cardiac Output" above).

Phase II reflects the period of major increase in cellular respiration (mainly active locomotor muscle) that begins at the end of phase I and continues until a steady state is obtained and for which the changing mixed venous blood composition is expressed at the lungs. $\dot{V}O_2$ and $\dot{V}CO_2$ develop monoexponentially toward their new steady states, this being attained more rapidly for $\dot{V}O_2$ than for $\dot{V}CO_2$ (see **Figs. 2.37** and **2.38**). Phase III reflects the steady-state phase of gas exchange in which cardiac output and the mixed venous gas concentrations have stabilized at their new levels. For exercise below the *AT* (moderate intensity), the phase III or steady-state response results in a steady-state $\dot{V}O_2$ gain ($\Delta\dot{V}O_2/\Delta WR$) of approximately 10 mL/min/W (see "$\dot{V}O_2$ Steady State and Work Efficiency" above). For exercise above the *AT* (heavy or very heavy intensity), where a steady state is often not reached, the $\dot{V}O_2$ response gain can be as much as 14 mL/min/W.

Oxygen Uptake Kinetics

Moderate Exercise

The increase in $\dot{V}O_2$ during exercise reflects both cardiac output and $C(a - \bar{v})O_2$ responses. If, during phase I of moderate exercise, $\dot{V}O_2$ were to be double the resting value and $C(a - \bar{v})O_2$ did not increase, then cardiac output could be inferred to have increased 2-fold. For this reason, the phase I $\dot{V}O_2$ response has also been termed the cardiodynamic phase.[72] However, during upright exercise starting from seated rest, Casaburi et al[178] showed that about one-third of the phase I $\dot{V}O_2$ may be accounted for by an abrupt increase in $C(a - \bar{v})O_2$ at exercise onset. This is apparently due to blood stasis during rest in the upright resting posture; that is, if stasis is prevented with elastic wraps on the legs, this abrupt increase in $C(a - \bar{v})O_2$ is not evident.[179]

Changes in lung gas stores have relatively little effect on $\dot{V}O_2$ kinetics for two reasons: Alveolar O_2 (and CO_2) concentrations change very little, and, in normal individuals, any decrease in end-expiratory lung volume (EELV) is usually modest (i.e., typically less than 0.5 L) and occurs rather rapidly.[167-169,180] That is, because 0.5 L of alveolar gas contain about 75 mL of O_2, a change in EELV during phase I or II would have only a modest impact on gas exchange kinetics, even if it occurred rapidly.[168] However, breath-to-breath changes in EELV do contribute to breath-to-breath fluctuations observed in $\dot{V}O_2$ (and $\dot{V}CO_2$), making it more difficult to quantify accurately their kinetics (see above). Despite the relatively small changes in lung gas stores at exercise onset, an approach has been described to correct for both change in alveolar concentration and change in lung volume for study of $\dot{V}O_2$ and $\dot{V}CO_2$ kinetics.[181]

Studies of $\dot{V}O_2$ kinetics commonly focus on the predominant phase II component, which is why such studies are often conducted from an exercising baseline; that is, to reduce the influence of phase I. During phase II, $\dot{V}O_2$ is equal to the O_2 consumed by the cells plus the creditors of the O_2 debt. These include the decrease in O_2 content in venous blood, physically dissolved O_2, changes in [oxymyoglobin] in the contracting muscles, the decrease in muscle [PCr], anaerobic glycolysis that results in accumulation of lactate (even transiently), and any change in lung O_2 stores (see "Oxygen Deficit" below) (**Fig. 2.39**).

The resulting phase II $\dot{V}O_2$ response is well characterized by a single exponential function (**Fig. 2.40**), having a time constant (ie, the time to attain 63% of the final response) in healthy individuals of approximately 30 seconds.[167-170] A steady state in $\dot{V}O_2$ is achieved and can be sustained only when all of the cellular energy requirements are derived from reactions using O_2 transferred from the atmosphere. The time constant of the $\dot{V}O_2$ response can

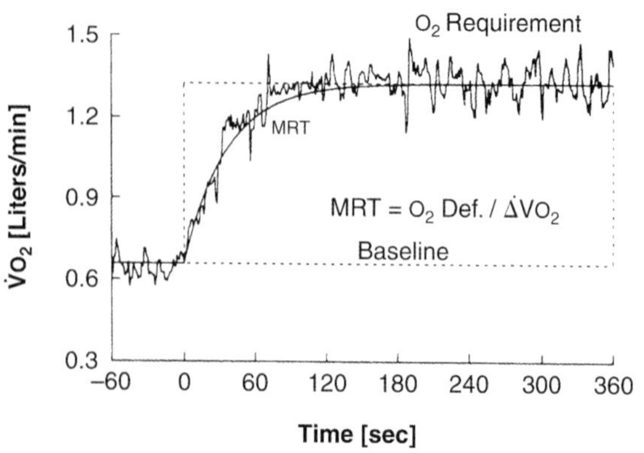

FIGURE 2.39. Illustration of method for calculating O_2 uptake ($\dot{V}O_2$) mean response time (MRT) for constant work rate cycle ergometer exercise. A single exponential best-fit curve is put through the data, and the time constant (63% of the asymptotic response) for the increase in $\dot{V}O_2$ above baseline is calculated. If there were no O_2 deficit, the $\dot{V}O_2$ would reach a steady state during the first breath, and the MRT would be 0. As shown in the equation, the O_2 deficit can be calculated from the MRT and the steady-state increase in $\dot{V}O_2$ above baseline.

be significantly increased (ie, kinetics slowed) in deconditioned individuals; the healthy elderly; and in chronic heart, lung, or renal disease.[31,165] The mechanisms leading to this slowed kinetic response may differ among these conditions, but they each result in a delayed attainment of steady state and therefore a greater O_2 deficit is accumulated for a given work rate. Slowed $\dot{V}O_2$ kinetics in aging or chronic disease place the engaged skeletal muscle in a lower energetic state for a given work rate because a large fraction of the O_2 deficit is composed of PCr breakdown. Endurance exercise training, to increase the oxidative capacity of skeletal muscle, reverses this effect, speeds $\dot{V}O_2$ kinetics, and reduces the O_2 deficit of the exercise.[31,165]

Normally, the phase II $\dot{V}O_2$ kinetics are largely determined by intramuscular processes, initiated at exercise onset with the splitting of high-energy phosphate bonds of preexisting ATP to support the immediate energy requirements of contracting muscle. The resulting ADP is immediately rephosphorylated to ATP through PCr breakdown.[29] [PCr] therefore rapidly decreases to a new level that is proportional to the work rate (see **Fig. 2.40**), returning to the preexercise resting level within the first few minutes of recovery.[182-185] The anaerobic mechanisms of ATP regeneration during moderate-intensity exercise—splitting of intramuscular PCr and, to a lesser extent, anaerobic glycolysis—operate only transiently until mitochondrial oxidative phosphorylation becomes fully recruited with a $\dot{V}O_2$ steady state being attained.[182,184] However, while PCr hydrolysis occurs immediately at exercise onset, the PCr stores are limited in quantity and are not replenished until the return to a resting state. The PCr is restored by aerobic (O_2-requiring) mechanisms in recovery and accounts for a major part of the O_2 debt (see "Oxygen Debt" below). Experimental evidence suggests that the increases in the intramuscular concentration of Pi and, in particular, of ADP stimulate oxidative phosphorylation, thereby replenishing ATP and maintaining muscle [ATP] at the resting level in all but the most extreme conditions.[30,186]

The phase II $\dot{V}O_2$ response strongly associates with the kinetics of muscle PCr breakdown (see **Fig. 2.40**).[31,182,184] This results in intramuscular accumulation of ADP and Pi, which are important signals for mitochondrial oxidative phosphorylation and therefore $\dot{Q}O_2$ and $\dot{V}O_2$ during exercise[28-31,186]; ATP is therefore replenished, keeping muscle [ATP] relatively constant. This $\dot{V}O_2$ response is appreciably speeded when PCr breakdown is inhibited by pharmacological blockade of creatine kinase, with ADP and Pi accumulating extremely rapidly.[187] Hence, mitochondrial oxidative capacity (the functional proxy of muscle mitochondrial content) is a key determinant of $\dot{V}O_2$ kinetics.[188] Thus, exercise that relies solely on type I fibers, with a greater mitochondrial content, results in faster $\dot{V}O_2$ kinetics than exercise that engages both type I and type II fibers. However, although delivery of the reducing equivalents $NADH + H^+$ and O_2 to the mitochondrial electron transport system each have the potential to limit the rate of

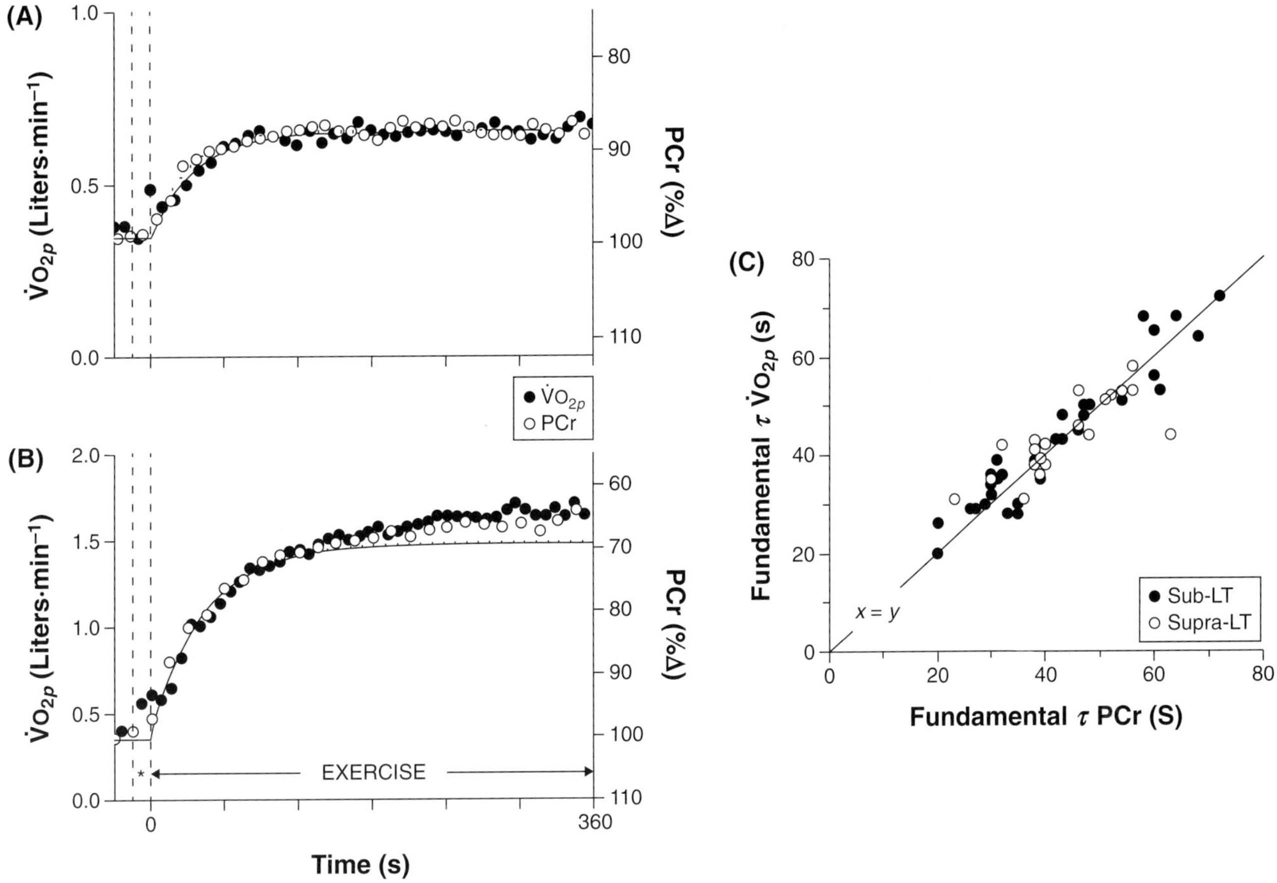

FIGURE 2.40. Simultaneously determined quadriceps muscle [phosphocreatine] (PCr, ○), measured by phosphorus-31 nuclear magnetic resonance spectroscopy, and O_2 uptake ($\dot{V}O_2p$, ●) as a function of time for prone moderate (A, upper left panel) and suprathreshold (B, lower left panel) constant work rate knee-extension exercise in a normal individual. The PCr scale is time aligned to account for the limb-to-lung transit delay (indicated by *) and inverted to illustrate the kinetic identity between the variables. Left dashed vertical line indicates exercise onset; right vertical line indicates the start of the phase II response. The phase II or (fundamental) $\dot{V}O_2p$ time constant (τ) as a function of the phase II τPCr for subthreshold (●) and suprathreshold (○) exercise for a group of normal individuals (C, right panel). The tightness of the scatter around the line of identity suggests that the phase II kinetics of $\dot{V}O_2p$ in health are closely related to intramuscular feedback processes within the phosphate system. *(From Rossiter HB. Exercise: kinetic considerations for gas exchange.* Compr Physiol. *2011;1(1):203-244. Figure 10. Copyright © 2011 American Physiological Society. Reprinted by permission of John Wiley & Sons, Inc.)*

increase in $\dot{V}O_2$ at exercise onset, their delivery normally appears to be in excess and not limiting to $\dot{V}O_2$ kinetics.[31,81,189,190] Nevertheless, these substrates *could* become limiting under certain conditions, for example, during aging where activation of PDH is slowed[79] or in heart failure where muscle capillary PO_2 falls rapidly at exercise onset.[191]

Supra-*AT* Exercise

During exercise above *AT*, $\dot{V}O_2$ kinetics become more complex (see **Figs. 2.7**, **2.36**, and **2.40**).[31,165,167-169] During heavy-intensity exercise (ie, somewhat above *AT*), $\dot{V}O_2$ can reach a steady state but does so with a very delayed time course. Thus, it may take up to 15 minutes for $\dot{V}O_2$ to stabilize, and with an increased steady-state amplitude (ie, with a gain of approximately 11-13 mL/min/W) (**Fig. 2.41**).[192,193] As described above (see "Arterial Lactate Increase as a Function of Time" above), exercise in this domain is characterized by a raised but stable arterial [lactate]. However, at higher work rates (in the very heavy intensity domain), steady states in $\dot{V}O_2$ and [lactate] are rarely attained, with the end-exercise $\dot{V}O_2$ gain reaching as high as 13 to 14 mL/min/W (see **Fig. 2.41**).[192,193]

The threshold that identifies whether a work rate can be sustained in a delayed steady state (heavy) or whether a steady state can never be reached (very heavy) is termed critical power (see "Power-Duration Curve and Critical Power" below).[193] The CP is a key functional threshold that has significant consequences for exercise tolerance.[194] In healthy individuals, exercise above CP causes $\dot{V}O_2$ to increase inexorably as long as the work rate is sustained. Under these conditions, $\dot{V}O_2$ will eventually reach $\dot{V}O_2$max, at which time the $\dot{V}O_2$ requirement continues to increase while $\dot{V}O_2$ itself is limited at the maximum: setting up the conditions for intolerance. However, even higher work rates for which the O_2 cost of exercise exceeds $\dot{V}O_2$max from the outset (severe exercise) are associated with a reduced

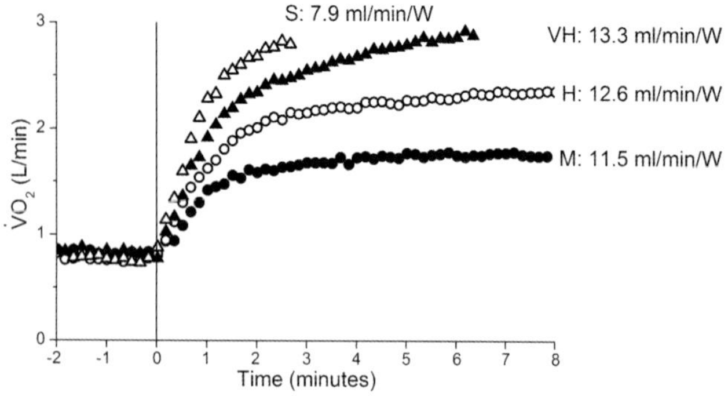

FIGURE 2.41. Averaged (three repetitions) O_2 uptake ($\dot{V}O_2$) as a function of time to severe (S, Δ), very heavy (VH, ▲), heavy (H, ○), and moderate (M, ●) constant work rate cycle ergometer exercise in a normal individual. The end-exercise $\dot{V}O_2$ gain (mL/min/W) values are displayed for each exercise intensity. Note that the gain is increased in heavy- and very heavy-intensity exercises due to the influence of the $\dot{V}O_2$ slow component. In severe intensity exercise, the gain is reduced because the subject reaches maximum $\dot{V}O_2$ prior to the $\dot{V}O_2$ response meeting its asymptotic gain. *(Modified from Özyener F, Rossiter HB, Ward SA, Whipp BJ. Influence of exercise intensity on the on- and off-transient kinetics of pulmonary oxygen uptake in humans.* J Physiol. *2001;533[pt 3]:891-902. Figure 1. Copyright © 2001 The Physiological Society. Reprinted by permission of John Wiley & Sons, Inc.)*

$\dot{V}O_2$ gain (see **Fig. 2.41**).[192] This is because $\dot{V}O_2$ is unable to project above the maximum value, and therefore can never reach its requirement. Such work rates are typically only sustainable for approximately 2-3 minutes.

The additional $\dot{V}O_2$ response that causes an increased, or "excess," O_2 cost of work has been termed the $\dot{V}O_2$ slow component because it is slow in its onset (it is only observed approximately 2-3 minutes after exercise onset) and develops slowly relative to phase II $\dot{V}O_2$ kinetics.[42,51,52] The rate of increase in $\dot{V}O_2$ during the slow component phase correlates with the magnitude of the corresponding arterial [lactate] increase (see **Fig. 2.9**).[51,52]

There is some debate regarding the mechanisms that contribute to the $\dot{V}O_2$ slow component.[31,165,168] It largely (ie, approximately 85%) reflects an increased O_2 cost of work in the active locomotor muscles,[195] with the remainder presumed to reflect increases in cardiac and ventilatory work, for example.[31,165,168] However, although the $\dot{V}O_2$ slow component is associated with lactate accumulation, lactate per se does not cause the slow component.[196] Rather, the most consistently supported candidate for the cause of the $\dot{V}O_2$ slow component is a reduced muscular efficiency consequent to the progressive recruitment of more low-efficiency fast-twitch muscle fibers as the exercise bout proceeds. Nevertheless, progressive type II fiber recruitment has been difficult to demonstrate, although studies of muscle imaging by magnetic resonance[197] and glycogen depletion in type II muscle fibers[11] support this proposal. Furthermore, muscle fatigue seems to be an obligatory requirement of the $\dot{V}O_2$ slow component, the magnitude of muscle fatigue correlating with the magnitude of the slow component.[198,199] Thus, the $\dot{V}O_2$ slow component likely reflects a progressive inefficiency of muscle contractions, resulting from muscle fatigue and additional muscle fiber recruitment to maintain the imposed work rate, causing an increase in ATP requirement but without the ability to meet the $\dot{V}O_2$ demands of the task in a steady state.

Particularly pertinent to cardiopulmonary exercise testing (CPET) is the consideration of how $\dot{V}O_2$ responds to the relatively rapid incremental work rate profile lasting 8 to 12 minutes (see Chapter 5, "Incremental Exercise Test to Symptom-Limited Maximum"). Thus, following a short delay-like phase, $\dot{V}O_2$ increases smoothly and linearly when work rate is increased relatively rapidly, in either a continuous ramp pattern or incrementally in equal steps of 1-minute duration (see Chapter 3, "Oxygen Uptake and Work Rate") (see **Figs. 2.52**, **3.2**, and **3.14**). The slope of the linear phase of the resulting relationship between $\dot{V}O_2$ and work rate ($\Delta\dot{V}O_2/\Delta WR$) is normally equal to about 10 mL/min/W (see **Fig. 3.2**) (see Chapter 7) and similar to the sub-*AT* steady-state $\dot{V}O_2$ gain (see "$\dot{V}O_2$ Steady State and Work Efficiency" above) (see **Fig. 2.41**). However, in the context of work efficiency computation, the numerical similarity of the steady state and ramp/incremental $\dot{V}O_2$ gains should be interpreted with caution. That is, calculation of the caloric equivalent of $\dot{V}O_2$ for a particular work rate requires both $\dot{V}O_2$ and $\dot{V}CO_2$ to have achieved steady states, which is not the case for ramp or incremental protocols (see "$\dot{V}O_2$ Steady State and Work Efficiency" above).

This lagged-linear behavior of $\dot{V}O_2$ with ramp or incremental exercise is predictable from the monoexponential kinetics of the predominant phase II $\dot{V}O_2$ response to moderate constant work rate exercise (see **Fig. 2.40**), such that $\dot{V}O_2$ lags the steady-state $\dot{V}O_2$ response by a constant interval (which is equal to the mean response time, MRT; see "Mean Response Time" below).[200] That the $\dot{V}O_2$ response retains its linear trajectory above the *AT* rather than becoming steeper is a reflection of the slow recruitment kinetics of the $\dot{V}O_2$ slow component (see above) (see **Figs. 2.7**, **2.36**, and **2.40**), relative to the imposed work rate incrementation rate. Thus, with very slow work rate incrementation rates, the $\dot{V}O_2$-WR relationship has been demonstrated to become steeper above the *AT*, as there is sufficient time for the $\dot{V}O_2$ slow component to develop.[42]

Mean Response Time

The MRT describes the time taken for a variable (eg, $\dot{V}O_2$) to reach 63% of its response amplitude. It provides an empirical expedient for quantifying the speed of the overall kinetics of the $\dot{V}O_2$ response while making no assumption about the character of the underlying phase I, phase II, or slow components.[169] The MRT therefore reflects an overall, "lumped" estimate of the speed of the $\dot{V}O_2$ kinetics, treated as if they were monoexponential from exercise onset (which, of course, is not the case). However, the value of the MRT is meaningful for calculation of the O_2 deficit (see "Oxygen Deficit" below).

The temporal response profiles of $\dot{V}O_2$, $\dot{V}CO_2$, and R for four different constant work rates are shown in **Figure 2.42**

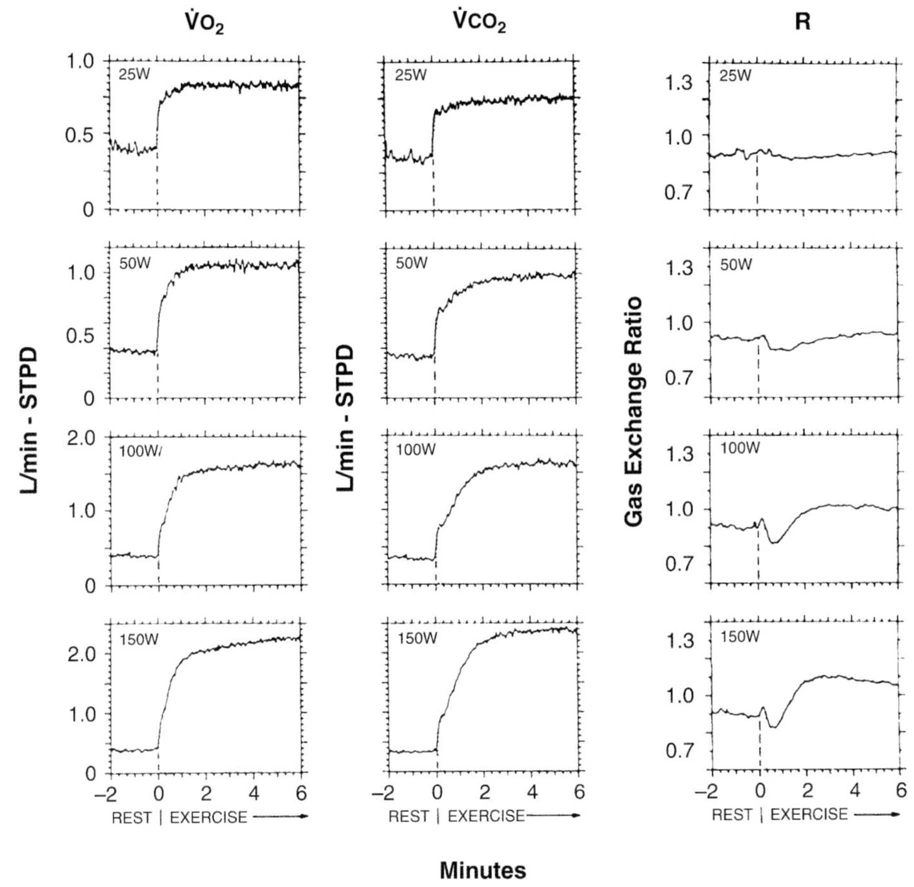

FIGURE 2.42. Averaged (four repetitions) O_2 uptake ($\dot{V}O_2$), carbon dioxide output ($\dot{V}CO_2$), and the gas exchange ratio (R) for constant work rate cycle ergometer exercise (6 min) at four different work rates, starting from rest, for a normal individual. The vertical dashed line indicates the time of start of exercise. Abbreviation: STPD, standard temperature pressure dry. *(Data taken from study reported in Sietsema K, Daly JA, Wasserman K. Early dynamics of O2 uptake and heart rate as affected by exercise work rate.* J Appl Physiol. *1989;67:2535-2541.)*

for a normal individual. He is below his *AT* at 50 W, with $\dot{V}O_2$ being in steady state by 3 minutes. However, he is clearly above his *AT* at 150 W; that is, $\dot{V}O_2$ continues to increase, and the $\dot{V}CO_2$ response increases beyond $\dot{V}O_2$. The fraction of the phase I contribution to the steady-state $\dot{V}O_2$ decreases at the higher work rates so that the phase II and slow component kinetics become more important in achieving the $\dot{V}O_2$ requirement. This influences the MRT and contributes to a slowing of the MRT as work rate increases.

The MRT is similar among individuals of differing fitness at very low work rates (eg, unloaded or zero watts cycling) because even unfit normal individuals can achieve a reasonably fully expressed phase I $\dot{V}O_2$ response during very light work. However, as work rate is increased, the discrimination in fitness becomes more obvious, those with the highest $\dot{V}O_2max$ typically having the lowest MRT for a given work rate.

Oxygen Deficit

The O_2 deficit is traditionally computed as the difference between the total volume of O_2 taken in during a constant work rate bout (equal to the integral under the $\dot{V}O_2$ response curve) and the total O_2 cost of the bout (equal to the product of the steady-state increment in $\dot{V}O_2$ [$\Delta\dot{V}O_2$] and the exercise duration) (see **Fig. 2.39**). A simplification in the O_2 deficit calculation that avoids the need to compute the integral under the $\dot{V}O_2$ response curve is given by[169]:

$$O_2 \text{ deficit} = \text{MRT} \cdot \Delta\dot{V}O_2 \ (10)$$

A justifiable estimate of the O_2 deficit can be obtained for sub-*AT* work rates, as a steady state is achieved.[52,168,169,201] This allows the steady-state O_2 cost of work to be clearly established, so that it can be extrapolated back to exercise onset and used as an estimate of the O_2 cost of exercise during phases I and II, where the O_2 cost is not directly known.[201] However, attempts to determine the actual O_2 cost of muscle contractions during the nonsteady state[202,203] suggest that this might be an over simplification and that early contractions may be more efficient than those occurring contractions that occur later in exercise. Nonetheless, this method provides a reasonable estimate of the O_2 deficit for sub-*AT* exercise. However, as described earlier ("Supra-*AT* Exercise" section), work efficiency above the *AT* decreases progressively as exercise is continued, reflecting the expression of the $\dot{V}O_2$ slow component. It is therefore not reasonable to assume a constant O_2 cost of exercise from the $\dot{V}O_2$ response asymptote (or any other single value measured during supra-*AT* the exercise). The assumptions underlying the calculation of the O_2 deficit become invalid above the *AT*.[168,169,204]

Oxygen Debt

The O_2 debt is observed during the recovery period and is the difference between the total volume of O_2 taken up that is in excess of the baseline $\dot{V}O_2$.[205] Once $\dot{V}O_2$ reaches a steady state during sub-*AT* constant work rate exercise, the O_2 debt no longer increases, regardless of the exercise duration.[206] In this instance, the O_2 debt will be repaid typically within approximately 5 minutes of recovery, and its size approximates that of the O_2 deficit.[201] For supra-*AT* exercise, however, the O_2 debt can be quite high (greater than the O_2 deficit) and may not be repaid for an hour or more. Its size is linked to the associated increase in blood [lactate].[207] As long as $\dot{V}O_2$ does not reach a steady state and [lactate] continues to rise during the exercise, the O_2 deficit and the O_2 debt will each continue to increase.

Carbon Dioxide Output Kinetics

Moderate Exercise

The $\dot{V}CO_2$ response features for moderate constant WR exercise are qualitatively similar to those of $\dot{V}O_2$. That is, in phase I, $\dot{V}CO_2$ increases immediately and abruptly and in proportion to the corresponding $\dot{V}O_2$ response (see **Figs. 2.37, 2.38**, and **2.42**), the consequence of the associated increase in pulmonary blood flow at exercise onset. In phase II, $\dot{V}CO_2$, having slower kinetics than $\dot{V}O_2$, is associated with a transient decline in R, which represents the uptake of a proportion of the metabolically produced CO_2 into body stores (see **Figs. 2.37, 2.38, 2.42**, and **2.43**); this is "repaid" at exercise cessation, when R exhibits a transient overshoot.[167,208-210] Consequently, R decreases during the first minute or so of moderate exercise (see **Figs. 2.38, 2.42**, and **2.43**).

As noted earlier (in the "Buffering the Exercise-Induced Lactic Acidosis" section), a major source of this transient CO_2 storage results from the intramuscular alkalosis associated with PCr breakdown early in the exercise (Equation 1) (see **Figs. 2.26** and **2.27**).[119-122,208] Thus, Chuang et al[208] concluded that the metabolic CO_2 retained as HCO_3^- in association with PCr hydrolysis contributes significantly (approximately 60%-70%) to the slower phase II $\dot{V}CO_2$ kinetics (see **Figs. 2.38, 2.42**, and **2.43**). Additional contributions accrue from increased CO_2 held in physical solution when muscle tissue P_{CO_2} increases, and an increasing CO_2 binding due to decreasing venous oxyhemoglobin saturation (see **Figs. 2.38, 2.42**, and **2.43**) (see "Arterial and Venous P_{CO_2} and Carbon Dioxide Content" above).[208,210] However, the increase in venous CO_2 content, other than that due to the Haldane effect (see "pH Change and Oxyhemoglobin Dissociation Above the Anaerobic Threshold" above), is not of major significance as it is closely offset by the concomitant unmeasured O_2 consumed from the venous blood O_2 stores.

Supra-*AT* Exercise

Above the *AT*, $\dot{V}CO_2$ response kinetics become more complex (see **Figs. 2.35** and **2.36**).[209-211] This reflects the summed contributions from several mechanisms, each having different temporal characteristics. For example, for constant work rate exercise, there is an underlying component related to aerobic metabolic CO_2 production, whose kinetics can be presumed to be reasonably similar to those for moderate constant work rate exercise, with the possibility of an additional slow component reflective of the $\dot{V}O_2$ slow component (**Fig. 2.44**, profile 1).[210] There is also the immediate demand placed on pulmonary CO_2 clearance by HCO_3^--mediated buffering of metabolically produced H^+, which is dictated by the *rate* (rather than the *amount*) at which muscle and blood $[HCO_3^-]$ decrease (see "Buffering the Exercise-Induced Lactic Acidosis" above) (see **Fig. 2.44**, profile 2). Subsequently, a component resulting from ventilatory compensation for the metabolic acidosis develops (see **Fig. 2.44**, profile 3), with $\dot{V}E$ increasing out of proportion to $\dot{V}CO_2$ such that Pa_{CO_2} falls to constrain the fall in arterial pH (see **Figs. 2.25** and **2.31**) (see "Ventilatory Responses

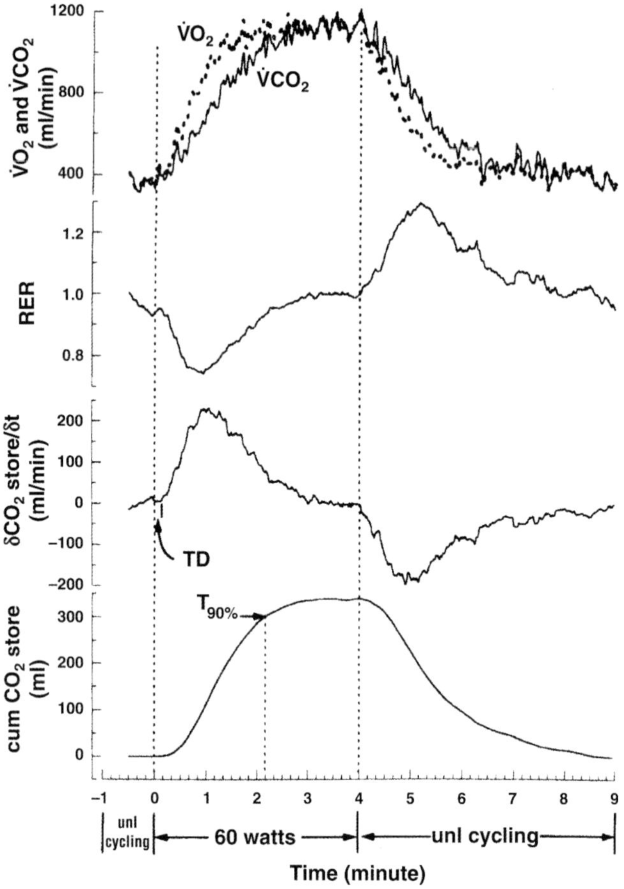

FIGURE 2.43. From above to below, O_2 uptake ($\dot{V}O_2$) and carbon dioxide output ($\dot{V}CO_2$), gas exchange ratio (RER), rate of change in CO_2 stores (δCO_2 store/δt), and the cumulative change in CO_2 stores (cum CO_2 store) in response to moderate constant work rate cycle ergometer exercise from unloaded cycling for a normal individual. Abbreviations: TD, time delay for increase in CO_2 stores to be reflected in pulmonary gas exchange; $T_{90\%}$, time for completion of 90% of CO_2 stores change. *(Reproduced with permission from Chuang ML, Ting H, Otsuka T, et al. Aerobically generated CO_2 stored during early exercise.* J Appl Physiol. *1999;87[3]:1048-1058. Copyright © 1999 American Physiological Society. All rights reserved.)*

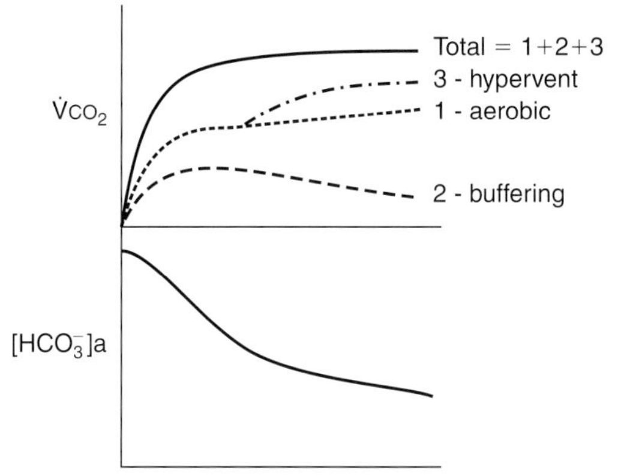

FIGURE 2.44. Schematic of the contributions to the carbon dioxide output ($\dot{V}CO_2$) response (above) and arterial [bicarbonate] (below) to suprathreshold constant work rate exercise. *(From Whipp BJ. Physiological mechanisms dissociating pulmonary CO_2 and O_2 exchange dynamics during exercise in humans. Exp Physiol. 2007;92[2]:347-355. Figure 3. Reprinted by permission of John Wiley & Sons, Inc.)*

to Exercise" below). The resulting $\dot{V}CO_2$ kinetics often have a monoexponential-like appearance, with $\dot{V}CO_2$ eventually appearing to stabilize (see **Fig. 2.36**).[209,210] This deceptively simple $\dot{V}CO_2$ response profile thus obscures a considerable degree of kinetic complexity.

Power-Duration Curve and Critical Power

The power-duration curve describes the time for which very heavy intensity, constant work rate exercise may be sustained to the limit of tolerance (t_{lim}). This relationship is demonstrably hyperbolic for work rates lasting between approximately 2 and 30 minutes, higher work rates being less sustainable than lower work rates (**Fig. 2.45**, upper panel).[193,212,213] It is characterized by two parameters: a power (ie, work rate) asymptote termed the critical power (CP) and a curvature constant of the hyperbola termed W′. The CP is a parameter related to aerobic function that represents the highest work rate for which $\dot{V}O_2$ can achieve a steady state.[193,214] Specifically, muscle [PCr], [Pi] and pH, $\dot{V}O_2$, and arterial [lactate] and [HCO_3^-] can each stabilize at work rates below but not above CP.[193,214] The W′ parameter is mathematically equivalent to a constant amount of work (ie, the product of the work rate and t_{lim}) that can be performed above CP.[193,213] Although W′ has been likened to an "anaerobic work capacity," this nomenclature is somewhat misleading as the parameter is a mathematical rather than a physiologic construct. When work rate (power) is plotted as a function of the reciprocal of time ($1/t_{lim}$), the relationship is highly linear (see **Fig. 2.45**, lower panel) with a slope equal to W′ and a power intercept equal to CP.[193]

Critical power is a highly significant threshold for endurance exercise performance, as it

1. Describes the limit between work rates that can be met in a $\dot{V}O_2$ steady state and those which cannot[193]
2. Partitions the supra-*AT* work rate range into its heavy and very heavy intensity domains[70]

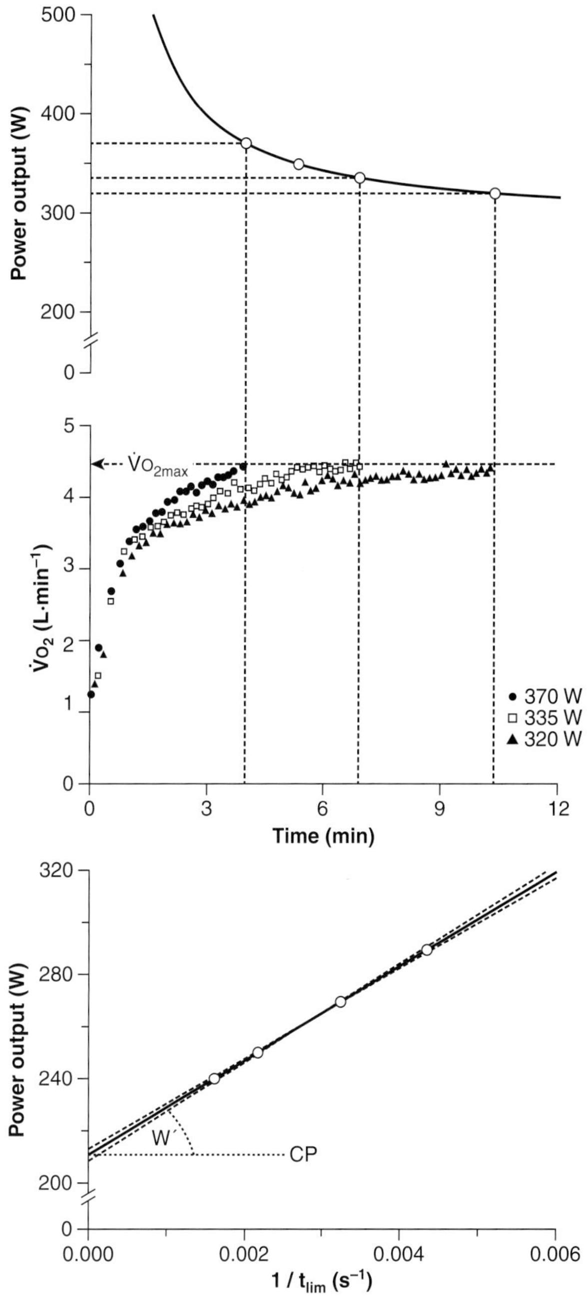

FIGURE 2.45. Upper panel, hyperbolic relationship between power output (or work rate) and time in a normal individual, established from four different high-intensity constant-power tests (o) each performed to the limit of tolerance (t_{lim}). Middle panel, the corresponding O_2 uptake ($\dot{V}O_2$) responses as a function of time illustrate that intolerance was achieved with $\dot{V}O_2$ at its maximum in each case (examples from only three tests are shown for clarity). Lower panel, extraction of critical power (CP) and W′ is facilitated by linear regression of power and $1/t_{lim}$ (solid line; with 95% confidence limits: dashed lines), for which CP is the y-axis intercept and W′ is the slope. *(Reproduced with permission from Murgatroyd SR, Ferguson C, Ward SA, Whipp BJ, Rossiter HB. Pulmonary O_2 uptake kinetics as a determinant of high-intensity exercise tolerance in humans.* J Appl Physiol. *2011;110[6]:1598-1606. Figure 1. Copyright © 2011 American Physiological Society. All rights reserved.)*

3. Is strongly associated with both *AT* and $\dot{V}O_2max$ but with an appreciable interindividual variability, between approximately 30% and 80% of the range between *AT* and $\dot{V}O_2max$ (equivalent to approximately 40%-90% $\dot{V}O_2max$)[194,215]
4. Is increased following endurance exercise training and reduced by hypoxia, chronic heart failure, or chronic obstructive pulmonary disease (COPD)[194,216]

When blood flow to working muscle is completely occluded by means of an inflatable cuff, CP falls to zero and the amount of work possible is wholly described by W′.[217] W′ is dramatically reduced (by up to 70%) in patients with chronic heart failure and COPD,[194] not because the capacity for anaerobic metabolism is more limited in these individuals but because their symptoms limit muscle recruitment and reduce overall activation of anaerobic energy pathways.[218,219]

In healthy individuals, the shape of the power-duration curve, and therefore t_{lim} at a given supra-CP work rate, is strongly dependent on $\dot{V}O_2$ kinetics, which determine how quickly $\dot{V}O_2max$ is reached after exercise onset (see **Fig. 2.45**, middle panel). Thus, individuals with fast phase II $\dot{V}O_2$ kinetics have a high CP; that is, they can perform high work rates in a steady state.[220] Also, those having a large $\dot{V}O_2$ slow component have a high W′.[220] Acute sojourn to high altitude reduces both CP and W′, the overall effect being a decreased tolerance to supra-CP exercise.[221] The reduction in CP at high altitude is not unexpected, as CP is strongly related to aerobic function. A reduction in W′, on the other hand, may reflect a hypoxic-induced shift toward ventilatory limitation rather than compromised anaerobic energy stores.[221] Therefore, although $\dot{V}O_2$ kinetics shape the power-duration curve in healthy individuals, the rate of attainment of other limiting variables may assume greater importance in patients with chronic disease.

The nonlinear, hyperbolic shape of the power-duration curve explains why a given increase in aerobic fitness leads to a much greater increase in exercise tolerance; that is, why the magnitude of improvement in t_{lim} following an intervention such as exercise training is appreciably greater than that of CP and $\dot{V}O_2peak$.[222,223] This is of significant impact for patients in response to therapy. For example, interventions designed to increase muscle oxidative function (and consequently increase CP), such as cardiac or pulmonary rehabilitation, may result in only approximately 5% to 10% in peak $\dot{V}O_2$ but increase tolerance for constant work rate exercise by 30% or more. This is because a small increase in CP results in a substantial increase in t_{lim}, owing to the curvature of the power-duration relationship.[222,223] Thus, a small increase in CP can convert a work rate that was previously intolerable into one that can be met into a steady state with considerably improved tolerance (ie, <CP). The approach of constant work rate testing above CP has therefore been extensively used to test the efficacy of therapeutics aimed at increasing exercise tolerance in patient groups because it is far more sensitive than incremental exercise at determining a meaningful improvement in physical function.[215,223,224]

VENTILATORY RESPONSES TO EXERCISE

The $\dot{V}E$ during exercise has the primary function of regulating arterial PCO_2 and pH for moderate-intensity exercise and mediating ventilatory compensation for the metabolic acidosis to constrain the fall of arterial pH at supra-*AT* work rates. That is, in order to remove the CO_2 produced during aerobic metabolism, the exercising muscles must be perfused by arterialized blood with a PCO_2 low enough to allow this CO_2 to diffuse into the muscle circulation at a sufficiently rapid rate (see **Fig. 1.1**). To rearterialize the blood, $\dot{V}E$ must increase appropriately to eliminate the exercise-related CO_2 load by preferentially responding to the demands for pulmonary CO_2 clearance (ie, $\dot{V}CO_2$). This, pari passu, ensures adequate replenishment of the O_2 consumed. Above the *AT*, however, $\dot{V}E$ increases out of proportion to $\dot{V}CO_2$ such that $PaCO_2$ falls to constrain the fall in arterial pH (see **Figs. 2.25** and **2.31**)

Arterial and Venous PCO_2 and Carbon Dioxide Content

The vast majority of CO_2 in arterial blood is carried as HCO_3^- (approximately 88%), with physically dissolved and carbamino CO_2 accounting for approximately 5% and approximately 7%, respectively.[225-227] CO_2 is more soluble than O_2 in blood when hydrated, forming H_2CO_3, which is a relatively strong acid (pK approximately 3.8). This hydration reaction is catalyzed in the red blood cells by the CA-I and CA-II isoforms of carbonic anhydrase (CA):

$$H_2O + CO_2 \overset{CA}{\leftrightarrow} H_2CO_3 \leftrightarrow HCO_3^- + H^+ \quad (11)$$

The logarithmic form of Equation 11 yields the more familiar Henderson-Hasselbalch equation:

$$pH = pK + \log\{[HCO_3^-]/(\alpha \cdot PCO_2)\} \quad (12)$$

where pK = 6.1 and α is the CO_2 solubility coefficient relating $PaCO_2$ to CO_2 content (0.0307 mM/mm Hg at 37°C in human plasma).

CO_2 also binds to Hb and other proteins to create reversible carbamino groups:

$$RNH_2 + CO_2 \leftrightarrow RNHCOOH \leftrightarrow RNHCOO^- + H^+ \quad (13)$$

In contrast to O_2 (see "Oxyhemoglobin Dissociation" above), the ability of venous blood to take up CO_2 is not limited over the physiological range. Thus, the CO_2 dissociation curve (the plot of CO_2 content against PCO_2) is relatively linear, only becoming somewhat less steep when PCO_2 rises to higher levels (see **Fig. 2.32**). As for O_2, the CO_2 dissociation curve can be influenced by factors whose influence changes with exercise, key being the Hb oxygenation status and blood pH.[225-227] As deoxygenated Hb is a better buffer than oxygenated Hb, the dissociation of O_2 from Hb as blood traverses the exercising-muscle capillary bed simultaneously facilitates CO_2 carriage through the Haldane effect, in an analogous fashion to the Bohr effect (see "pH Change and Oxyhemoglobin Dissociation Above the Anaerobic Threshold" above).

Below the *AT*, arterial P_{CO_2} and $[H^+]$ (and therefore CO_2 content) remain essentially constant in the steady state of constant work rate exercise,[69,134,171,228] although for rapid incremental (ie, nonsteady-state) exercise, they predictably trend toward a small but systematic increase (see **Fig. 2.30C,E**) (see "Ventilatory Control" below) reflecting the slightly slower kinetics of $\dot{V}_E$ relative to $\dot{V}_{CO_2}$.[209,229,230]

Above the *AT*, however, the beneficial result of the Haldane effect is more than offset by the influence of the falling blood pH that occurs (see **Fig. 2.30F**). That is, the progressively more marked metabolic acidosis that occurs with further increases in work rate requires a progressively greater degree of buffering by HCO_3^- to constrain the falling arterial pH (see **Fig. 2.30F**), such that mixed venous and femoral venous CO_2 contents level off and start to decline (see **Fig. 2.30D**) despite the trajectory of P_{CO_2} increase (see **Fig. 2.30C**). Therefore, the increase in the mixed venous-arterial CO_2 content difference ($C(\bar{v} - a)_{CO_2}$) during heavy exercise is primarily due to the decrease in arterial CO_2 content relative to the mixed venous CO_2 content, not due to an increase in mixed venous CO_2 content. This differs from the mechanism of increasing $C(a - \bar{v})_{O_2}$ (see "Cardiovascular Responses to Exercise" above), which is primarily due to the decrease in mixed venous O_2 content and only a small increase in arterial O_2 content.

It is instructive to view the influence of blood pH (as pH isopleths) on these arterial and mixed venous CO_2 content responses during incremental exercise, in the context of the CO_2 dissociation curve; that is, as a function of the corresponding blood P_{CO_2} (**Fig. 2.46**).[229] At rest, CO_2 content in the arterial and the mixed venous blood are approximately 21 mM and 23 mM, respectively. Both increase slightly during early exercise due to the associated increases in P_{CO_2} (see above). However, beyond the *AT*, as blood pH starts to fall progressively, arterial and mixed venous CO_2 content start to reverse. Although mixed venous CO_2 content returns very close to its resting value, the arterial CO_2 content attains values considerably below resting. Thus, the increase in $C(\bar{v} - a)_{CO_2}$ difference at work rates below the *AT* is primarily due to an increase in mixed venous CO_2 content, with little change in arterial values. In contrast, as exercise proceeds above the *AT*, the arterial CO_2 content is progressively driven downward, primarily accounting for the increase in $C(\bar{v} - a)_{CO_2}$ difference at maximal exercise. HCO_3^- is the dominant form in which CO_2 is transported and therefore accounts for the major increase in $C(\bar{v} - a)_{CO_2}$ at peak exercise, in contrast to carbamino, and dissolved CO_2 (**Fig 2.47**).[229] In summary, the changes in blood CO_2 content during incremental exercise are essentially fully explained by the changes related to blood pH, the influence of Hb oxygenation status (ie, the Haldane effect) being very small.

Ventilatory Determinants

Carbon Dioxide and H+ Elimination

At rest, the total H^+ in body water at rest is approximately 0.0034 mmol, comprising 0.0028 mmol intracellularly

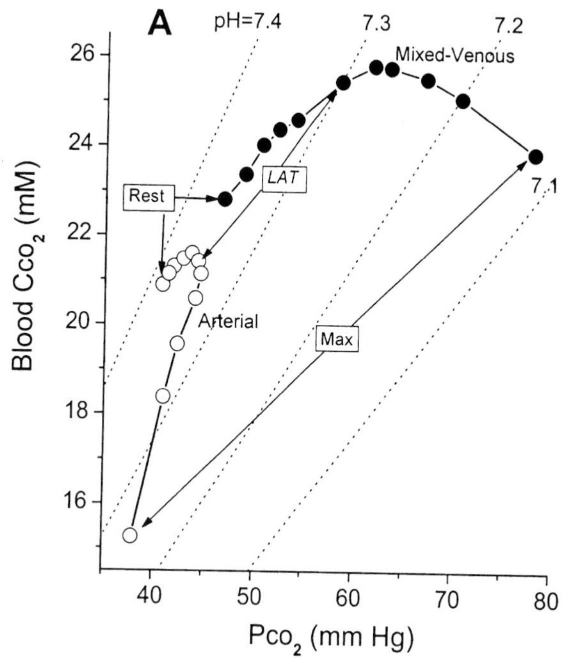

FIGURE 2.46. Arterial (○) and mixed venous (●) blood carbon dioxide (CO_2) contents as a function of P_{CO_2} (ie, CO_2 dissociation curve), for a range of pH isopleths (dashed lines), during ramp incremental cycle ergometer exercise. Above the lactic acidosis threshold (*LAT*), despite the continuing increase in mixed venous P_{CO_2}, the major mechanism accounting for increasing the mixed venous-arterial CO_2 content difference ($C(\bar{v} - a)_{CO_2}$) was the decrease in Pa_{CO_2} and Ca_{CO_2}. *(Reproduced with permission from Sun XG, Hansen JE, Stringer WW, Ting H, Wasserman K. Carbon dioxide pressure-concentration relationship in arterial and mixed venous blood during exercise.* J Appl Physiol. *2001;90[5]:1798-1810. Copyright © 2001 American Physiological Society. All rights reserved.)*

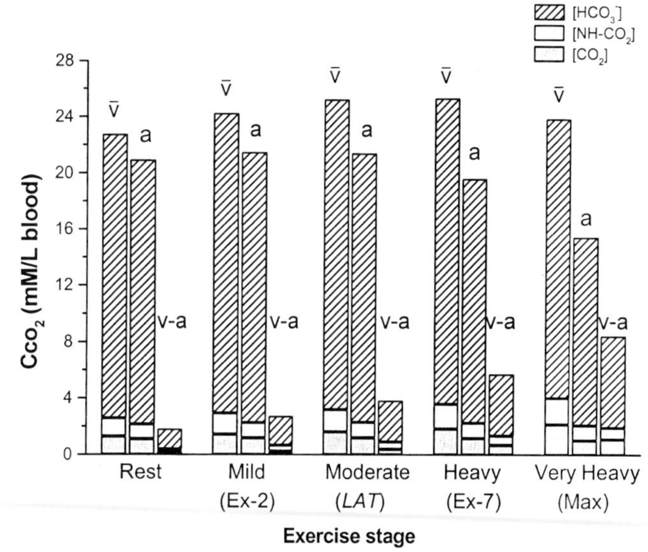

FIGURE 2.47. Blood carbon dioxide (CO_2) content components (bicarbonate, carbamino, and dissolved CO_2) in mixed venous CO_2 content ($\bar{v}$), arterial CO_2 content (a), and venous-arterial ($\bar{v}$ − a) CO_2 content difference at rest and for mild-, moderate-, heavy-, and very heavy-intensity constant work rate cycle ergometer exercise. *(Reproduced with permission from Sun XG, Hansen JE, Stringer WW, Ting H, Wasserman K. Carbon dioxide pressure-concentration relationship in arterial and mixed venous blood during exercise.* J Appl Physiol. *2001;90[5]:1798-1810. Copyright © 2001 American Physiological Society. All rights reserved.)*

(assuming, for a 70-kg individual, cell water = 28 L and $[H^+]$ = 0.0001 mmol/L at a pH of 7.0) and 0.00062 mmol extracellularly (assuming extracellular water = 14 L and $[H^+]$ = 0.000044 mmol/L at a pH of 7.36). For even the very mildest of aerobic exercise tasks (ie, without a metabolic acidosis) such as walking at 3.0 mph in a normal individual, the H^+ equivalents produced each minute from aerobic metabolism are extremely large compared to the H^+ content in the aqueous fluids of the body; that is, approximately 880 mL of CO_2/min or 40 mmol of respiratory H^+ per minute. Because the end products of the bioenergetic pathways for generating ~P are acidic (ie, volatile H_2CO_3 and nonvolatile lactic acid), $\dot{V}E$ during exercise must keep pace with the resulting CO_2-H^+ load if pH homeostasis of body fluids is to be preserved (see **Fig. 2.37**). This is accomplished through clearance of aerobically produced H^+ as CO_2 for sub-*AT* work rates and additional nonaerobic CO_2 from bicarbonate buffering of lactic acid for supra-*AT* work rates, and by mediating ventilatory compensation for the falling arterial pH.

As discussed earlier (see "Substrate Utilization"), CO_2 production for moderate exercise (ie, below *AT*) is related to exercising muscle $\dot{Q}O_2$ by the RQ of the metabolic substrate being catabolized (see **Table 2.2**). As discussed above (see "Substrate Utilization"), free fatty acids have a lower RQ than carbohydrate (see **Fig. 2.4**), and therefore $\dot{V}CO_2$ at a given work rate is higher when carbohydrate is the predominant substrate compared with fatty acids.[231,232] Thus, a low-carbohydrate diet reduced $\dot{V}CO_2$ and R at rest and during steady-state moderate exercise.[232] Interestingly, however, there was little effect on the rest-to-exercise increase in $\dot{V}CO_2$. This was suggested to reflect the exercising muscles using stored muscle glycogen as the major substrate during moderate exercise despite changes induced in substrate utilization by other tissues at rest.

Above the *AT*, for exercise at a work rate that causes arterial [lactate] to increase at a rate of 0.5 mmol/min, the associated increase in total body $[H^+]$ would be 15 mmol/min or 4400 times the content of H^+ in the aqueous fluids of the body (assuming a lactate volume of distribution of 30% of body weight [21 L]). Because the buffering of the lactic acidosis is mediated via HCO_3^-, this additional H^+ equivalent over that produced by aerobic metabolism can be eliminated from the body in the form of CO_2 (see **Figs. 2.35** and **2.36**); that is, 22.3 mL of CO_2 for each mmol of $[HCO_3^-]$ decrease. This CO_2 source is cleared at the lungs when the ventilatory control mechanism compensates for the metabolic acidosis by hyperventilation, although the compensatory hyperventilation in response to the increasing in arterial $[H^+]$ is relatively slow to develop (see "Ventilatory Control" below).

During recovery, these reactions reverse, with the speed of recovery being only a few minutes for exercise at or below the *AT*, as only the ventilatory excretion of the exercise-induced increase in CO_2 stores is required. Considerably longer is required for supra-*AT* exercise, depending on the rate of regeneration of HCO_3^-, which, in turn, is dependent on the rate of lactate metabolism.[72,107]

Patients with abnormal respiratory mechanics (eg, COPD or obesity) or impaired chemoreceptor function, or normal individuals breathing through high-resistive apparatus, can develop a significant respiratory acidosis due to CO_2 retention. However, respiratory alkalosis does not typically develop during exercise in normal individuals and is only rarely seen in pathophysiological states.

Alveolar Ventilation

The level of $\dot{V}A$ necessary to clear a given amount of CO_2 from the blood per unit time (ie, $\dot{V}CO_2$) depends on the fractional CO_2 concentration in the alveolar gas ($FACO_2$, = $PACO_2/PB$), where PB is the barometric pressure and $PACO_2$ is the "ideal" alveolar PCO_2 (which is equal to arterial PCO_2) (see "Arterial PO_2" above). Mass balance considerations dictate that, in an ideal lung, the $\dot{V}A/\dot{Q}$ ratios of all lung units are the same, thereby making the CO_2 concentration the same in all alveolar spaces. Thus,

$$\dot{V}CO_2 = \dot{V}A \times (PACO_2/PB) \quad (14)$$

and

$$\dot{V}A = \dot{V}CO_2/(PB/PACO_2) \quad (15)$$

Equation 15 derives the theoretical $\dot{V}A$ required for maximally efficient lungs to regulate $PACO_2$ at a given $\dot{V}CO_2$. This is usefully displayed through the $\dot{V}A$-$PACO_2$ relationship, upon which are superimposed isopleths of $\dot{V}CO_2$ (**Fig. 2.48**).

Dead Space Ventilation

However, not all respired air ventilates the lungs effectively. That is, some must ventilate the conducting airways, which are uninvolved in gas exchange (anatomical dead space), and some must ventilate nonperfused or underperfused alveoli (alveolar dead space); this combined dead space is termed the physiological dead space. The physiological

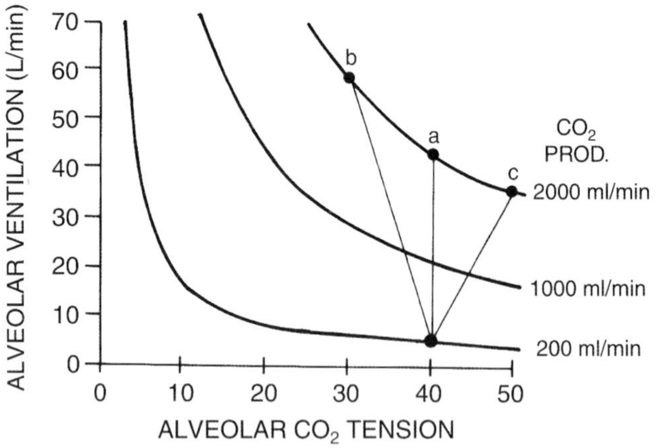

FIGURE 2.48. Effect of alveolar ventilation on ideal alveolar PCO_2 during exercise. The point on the carbon dioxide output (CO_2 PROD) isopleth of 200 mL/min represents the normal resting value. Points a, b, and c illustrate the alveolar ventilations required for isocapnia, hypocapnia (−10 mm Hg), and hypercapnia (+10 mm Hg) for an exercise CO_2 output of 2000 mL/min. *(From Wasserman K. Breathing during exercise.* N Engl J Med. *1978;298[14]:780-785. Copyright © 1978 Massachusetts Medical Society. Reprinted with permission from Massachusetts Medical Society.)*

dead space ventilation ($\dot{V}_D$) is equal to the difference between the total ventilation ($\dot{V}_E$) and the ideal $\dot{V}_A$. Uneven regional $\dot{V}_A$ relative to $\dot{Q}$ will result in an increase in the calculated physiological dead space to tidal volume ratio (V_D/V_T) for the lung as a whole and therefore an increase in the $\dot{V}_E$ required to clear a given level of $\dot{V}CO_2$. This is illustrated in **Figure 2.48**, where a $PaCO_2$ of 40 mm Hg has been established by admixture of equal blood flows from two differing but homogenous populations of acini yielding pulmonary venous PCO_2 values of 50 mm Hg (*c*) and 30 mm Hg (*b*). The corresponding average $\dot{V}_A$ from these two compartments will be greater than the $\dot{V}_A$ from a single homogeneous set of acini having a $PaCO_2$ of 40 mm Hg (*a*). Thus, when $\dot{V}_A$ and $\dot{Q}$ are regionally mismatched, the overall $\dot{V}_A$ will be dominated by the lung units with the low alveolar PCO_2 (ie, high $\dot{V}_A/\dot{Q}$ or overventilated lung units). This will be reflected in a relatively low mixed expired PCO_2 compared with that for an ideal lung in which $\dot{V}_A$ and $\dot{Q}$ are perfectly matched.

The physiological V_D can be calculated using Enghoff modification of the Bohr equation:

$$V_D = V_T\,(PaCO_2 - P\bar{E}CO_2)/PaCO_2 \quad (16)$$

where $P\bar{E}CO_2$ is the PCO_2 in the mixed expired gas and V_T is the tidal volume. Thus, the difference between the actual ventilation (ie, $\dot{V}_E$) and the theoretical $\dot{V}_A$ is dictated by V_D/V_T:

$$\dot{V}_A = \dot{V}_E\,(1 - V_D/V_T) \quad (17)$$

As the $\dot{V}_E$ response in the early stages of an incremental exercise test is normally accomplished largely through an increasing V_T (see "Breathing Pattern" below), the lung expansion will tend to also increase the anatomical V_D as the conducting airways are slightly compliant.[156,233,234]

In healthy individuals, V_D/V_T at rest is normally of the order of 0.3 and declines with increasing work rate.[69,156,157,233] This reflects the proportionally greater ventilation of the highly compliant alveoli relative to the poorly compliant conducting airways, coupled with an improved $\dot{V}_A/\dot{Q}$ distribution. Specifically, as the physiological V_D increases essentially linearly with V_T with a positive V_D-intercept (see **Fig. 2.28**, panel b, left),[234] the V_D/V_T decline will be hyperbolic (see **Fig. 2.28**, panel b, right).[235]

Total (or Expired) Ventilation

The actual ventilation ($\dot{V}_E$) is the sum of the $\dot{V}_A$ and the $\dot{V}_D$. To determine the $\dot{V}_E$ needed to eliminate a given quantity of CO_2, the term $\dot{V}_E\,(1 - V_D/V_T)$ can be substituted for $\dot{V}_A$ (Equation 17) in the $\dot{V}_A$ equation (Equation 15). This is displayed graphically in **Figure 2.49**. The resulting equation is

$$\dot{V}_E\,(BTPS) = 863\,\dot{V}CO_2\,(STPD)/PaCO_2\,(1 - V_D/V_T) \quad (18)$$

where 863 is a constant that accommodates the conversion of fractional concentration to partial pressure and the conventions of expressing $\dot{V}_E$ as body temperature pressure saturated (BTPS) and $\dot{V}CO_2$ as standard temperature pressure dry (STPD).

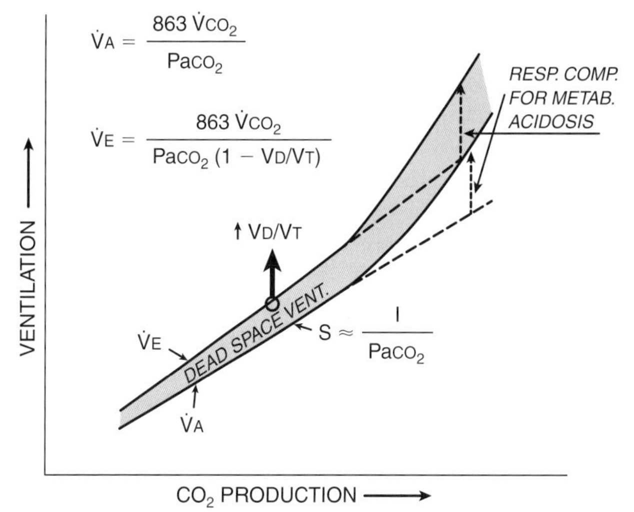

FIGURE 2.49. Determinants of the alveolar and total ventilation responses ($\dot{V}_A$ and $\dot{V}_E$, respectively) to increasing work rate, as functions of CO_2 output ($\dot{V}CO_2$); the corresponding equations are shown at the top of the figure. V_D/V_T is the physiological dead space to tidal volume ratio, and S is the slope of the $\dot{V}_A$-$\dot{V}CO_2$ relationship, which is the reciprocal of the arterial PCO_2 ($PaCO_2$). Respiratory compensation for the metabolic acidosis steepens the ventilatory response profiles, reducing $PaCO_2$. *(Modified from Wasserman K. Breathing during exercise.* N Engl J Med. *11978;298[14]:780-785. Copyright © 1978 Massachusetts Medical Society. Reprinted with permission from Massachusetts Medical Society.)*

Over a wide range of work rates up to the point at which ventilatory compensation for the metabolic acidosis develops, $\dot{V}_E$ normally increases linearly with $\dot{V}CO_2$ with a small positive $\dot{V}_E$ intercept (see **Fig. 2.28**, panel a, left), with allowance being made for breathing apparatus dead space (Appendix C)[236-238]:

$$\dot{V}_E = m \cdot \dot{V}CO_2 + c \quad (19)$$

where m is the $\dot{V}_E$-$\dot{V}CO_2$ slope (ie, $\Delta\dot{V}_E/\Delta\dot{V}CO_2$) and c is the $\dot{V}_E$-intercept.

Rearranging Equation 18 yields

$$\dot{V}_E/\dot{V}CO_2 = 863/[PaCO_2 \cdot (1 - V_D/V_T)] \quad (20)$$

Because of the $\dot{V}_E$-intercept on the $\dot{V}_E$-$\dot{V}CO_2$ relationship, the $\dot{V}_E/\dot{V}CO_2$ decline will be hyperbolic with an asymptotic (or nadir) value closely approximating the $\dot{V}_E$-$\dot{V}CO_2$ slope (see **Fig. 2.28**, panel a, right). Were the $\dot{V}_E$ intercept to be zero (ie, with the $\dot{V}_E$-$\dot{V}CO_2$ relationship passing through the origin), $\dot{V}_E/\dot{V}CO_2$ would remain unchanged at resting levels. The $\dot{V}_E/\dot{V}CO_2$ nadir typically occurs at or soon after the *AT* but prior to the onset of ventilatory compensation (ventilatory compensation point [VCP]).[235,237,238] Importantly, rearranging Equation 20 demonstrates that if the hyperbolic profiles of $\dot{V}_E/\dot{V}CO_2$ and V_D/V_T decline are matched, $PaCO_2$ regulation is ensured[235,237]:

$$PaCO_2 = 863/\{(\dot{V}_E/\dot{V}CO_2) \cdot (1 - V_D/V_T)\} \quad (21)$$

The $\dot{V}_E$-$\dot{V}CO_2$ slope and the $\dot{V}_E/\dot{V}CO_2$ nadir or $\dot{V}_E/\dot{V}CO_2$ at the *AT* have been termed indices of ventilatory efficiency and have considerable utility in CPET interpretation, not only diagnostically but also prognostically (see Chapter 8).[224,239,240]

These indices are increased in hyperventilatory conditions such as arterial hypoxemia and metabolic acidemia and also when V_D/V_T is high (eg, in lung disease and the elderly), reflecting the greater ventilatory requirement for Pa_{CO_2} regulation. In contrast, they are decreased in hypoventilatory conditions (eg, with diminished chemosensitivity). Interpretation of ventilatory efficiency therefore needs some caution, as an abnormally high ventilatory efficiency could reflect Pa_{CO_2} being low, V_D/V_T being high, or both. A further consideration relates to the $\dot{V}_E/\dot{V}_{CO_2}$ profile. That is, in poorly fit individuals for whom *AT* and VCP may occur on the still-declining $\dot{V}_E/\dot{V}_{CO_2}$ response, the minimum $\dot{V}_E/\dot{V}_{CO_2}$ attained would exceed its true nadir and therefore the $\dot{V}_E$-$\dot{V}_{CO_2}$ slope, with the latter therefore being the more valid index of ventilatory efficiency in such circumstances.[219] A corollary is that VCP identification may not require the demonstration of an actual increase in $\dot{V}_E/\dot{V}_{CO_2}$: ventilatory compensation could be achieved were $\dot{V}_E/\dot{V}_{CO_2}$ still to be declining but less markedly than Pa_{CO_2} regulation would require.[210]

Thus, as is evident from Equation 18 and **Figure 2.49**, the $\dot{V}_E$ required for a given work rate is defined by three factors: the $\dot{V}_{CO_2}$, the level or setpoint at which Pa_{CO_2} is regulated by the ventilatory control mechanisms, and the V_D/V_T. This is depicted quantitatively in **Figure 2.50**, for two individuals (*a* and *b*) exercising at a steady-state $\dot{V}_{O_2}$ of 2 L/min. Quadrant 2 of **Figure 2.50** ($\dot{V}_{CO_2}$ versus $\dot{V}_{O_2}$, with isopleths of the gas exchange ratio, R) shows that the $\dot{V}_{CO_2}$ for a given O_2 cost of exercise can be quite variable, depending on the gas exchange ratio (R) (ie, $\dot{V}_{CO_2} = R \times \dot{V}_{O_2}$). That is, the $\dot{V}_{CO_2}$ response will be greater when carbohydrate with an RQ and R of 1.0 is the substrate undergoing oxidation (*b*) than for fatty acid (eg, palmitate) oxidation (*a*) with RQ and R close to 0.7 (see **Table 2.2**). Thus, $\dot{V}_{CO_2}$ equals 2.0 L/min and 1.4 L/min, respectively. The R will also be increased, approaching or exceeding 1.0 (see "Buffering the Exercise-Induced Lactic Acidosis" above), for supra-*AT* work rates because of the supplemental $\dot{V}_{CO_2}$ deriving from HCO_3^- buffering of lactic acidosis. How the $\dot{V}_{CO_2}$ response influences $\dot{V}_A$ is dictated by the set-point for Pa_{CO_2} regulation (isopleths) (Equation 14) and is shown in quadrant 3 of **Figure 2.50**. In turn, quadrant 4 shows the translation of the $\dot{V}_A$ response into $\dot{V}_E$, dictated by V_D/V_T (isopleths). Assume individual *a* (*dotted trajectory*) has normal lung function and therefore a normal V_D/V_T of approximately 0.1 at this $\dot{V}_{O_2}$ but to be moderately hypoventilating with a Pa_{CO_2} of 50 mm Hg. This results in an exercise ventilation of 27 L/min. In contrast, assume that individual *b* (*dashed trajectory*) is a patient with severe COPD, having a Pa_{CO_2} of 30 mm Hg and an elevated V_D/V_T of 0.5. The high R, $\dot{V}_{CO_2}$, and V_D/V_T coupled with the low Pa_{CO_2} act collectively to increase the ventilatory requirement some 4-fold to 115 L/min; in a COPD patient, such a requirement is unlikely to be attainable because of respiratory-mechanical and respiratory-metabolic limits.[48,241,242]

Breathing Pattern

At low and moderate work rates, increases in $\dot{V}_E$ are primarily achieved by an increase in V_T and, to a lesser degree, respiratory frequency (f) until a critical lung volume (approximately 50%-60% of vital capacity) is reached (range 1) (**Fig. 2.51**), unless f entrains with locomotor cadence, which it frequently does).[216,242-244] The V_T response normally reflects an increasing end-inspiratory lung volume (EILV), resulting from inspiratory muscle stimulation, coupled with a decreasing EELV, consequent to expiratory muscle recruitment.[242,244-246] As lung expansion operates over the quasi-linear region of the lung compliance curve,

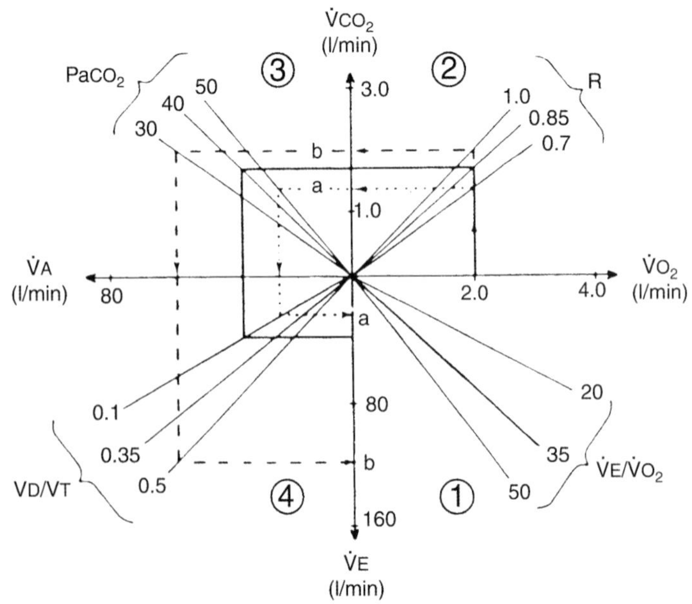

FIGURE 2.50. Graphic display of influence of the gas exchange ratio (R), arterial P_{CO_2} (Pa_{CO_2}), and physiological dead space fraction of the breath (V_D/V_T) on the ventilatory requirement ($\dot{V}_E$) for exercise requiring an O_2 uptake ($\dot{V}_{O_2}$) of 2 L/min. The ventilatory requirement can be significantly altered from normal response (solid line), with a particular combination of determining variables leading to a reduced (a, dotted trajectory) or markedly increased (b, dashed trajectory) $\dot{V}_E$. See text for details. Abbreviation: $\dot{V}_A$, alveolar ventilation. *(Modified from Whipp BJ, Pardy RL. Breathing during exercise. In:* Handbook of Physiology. *Vol. 3. Bethesda, MD: American Physiological Society; 1985:605.)*

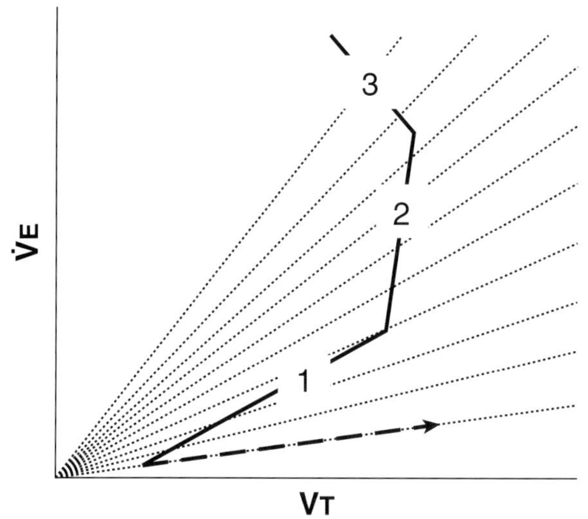

FIGURE 2.51. Ventilation (V̇E) as a function of tidal volume (V_T) during incremental exercise schematized for a typical individual (solid line) and an individual who entrains at a constant breathing frequency (dashed line). The fine dotted lines represent isofrequency isopleths. The numbers 1, 2, and 3 represent ranges 1, 2, and 3, respectively. *(Reprinted with permission from Ward SA. Regulation of breathing during exercise. In: Granger DN, Granger JP, eds.* Colloquium Series on Integrated Systems Physiology: The Respiratory System. *Princeton, NJ: Morgan & Claypool Life Sciences Publishers; 2014:1-91. Figure 9.)*

there is an optimal mechanical advantage for the inspiratory muscles and the elastic work of breathing.

The continuing stimulation of V̇E as work rate increases further (ie, into range 2) reflects f taking over from VT—both inspiratory duration (T_I) and expiratory duration (T_E) shortening. This results in a steepening of the V̇E-VT relationship (see **Fig. 2.51**). This constraint on further appreciable lung expansion beyond range 1 has been suggested to indicate a volume threshold for activation of tachypnea-effecting vagal pulmonary mechanoreceptors being surpassed.[243,246] As peak exercise is approached, the f response may become sufficiently striking that lung inflation becomes impaired and VT actually starts to fall, despite V̇E continuing to increase, causing the V̇E-VT relationship to develop a negative slope (range 3) (see **Fig. 2.51**). It is important to emphasize that the VT constraint at higher work rates is not a manifestation of the volume limitation seen in restrictive lung diseases, when EILV can encroach on inspiratory capacity (see Chapters 3 and 10). However, there can be parallels with obstructive lung diseases such as COPD. For example, in highly fit endurance athletes, despite normal respiratory mechanics at rest, expiratory flow limitation can develop near or at peak exercise consequent to the exceptionally high V̇E demands that compromise breathing reserve, as can "dynamic hyperinflation" consequent to extreme degrees of f increase and T_E shortening that cause the normal decline in EELV to be reversed.[242,244-248] This predisposes EILV to approach limiting levels, which would have the additional consequences of elevating the operational lung inflation range onto the flatter upper regions of the compliance curve and compromising inspiratory muscle function. Such effects are likely to be more prevalent in elderly physically active individuals because of age-related decreases in lung recoil.

Ventilatory Control

In humans, the primary operation for moderate-intensity exercise is regulation of arterial PCO_2 and pH through a matching of V̇E to V̇CO_2 (Equation 21), which shifts to arterial pH regulation for supra-*AT* work rates characterized by a metabolic acidosis. However, there is no general agreement on the mechanisms controlling ventilation during exercise, although some combination of feedback (eg, via central and peripheral chemoreception) and feedforward (eg, via central command and exercising-muscle mechanoreception and chemoreception) drives is generally invoked. The observation that $PaCO_2$, pH, and PO_2 are essentially unchanged during moderate-intensity exercise, despite considerable increases in CO_2 production and O_2 consumption, has been difficult to explain mechanistically within the framework of currently recognized stimuli and the manner by which they are thought to produce their effects on V̇E. Key considerations in this regard are the underlying ventilatory requirements of the task and the dynamic profiles of the V̇E responses achieved, in the context of the demands for CO_2 and H^+ clearance. The following is a brief review of these mechanisms; the interested reader is referred to the references for more detailed discussion.[72,134,171,209,228,230,244,249-251]

Moderate Exercise

For constant work rate exercise below *AT* initiated without prior warning to the subject, V̇E initially increases immediately and abruptly (phase I component), followed by a more dominant exponential phase II component that leads to the steady state normally within 5 to 6 minutes (phase III component) (see **Fig. 2.37**) (see "Gas Exchange Kinetics" above).

The phase I V̇E response develops in rather close proportion to the corresponding V̇O_2 and V̇CO_2 responses, such that R and arterial and end-tidal PO_2 and PCO_2 ($PETO_2$ and $PETCO_2$, respectively) remain relatively stable (see **Fig. 2.37**).[167,170,171,177]

Because of its immediacy, the primary candidate for mediating V̇E control in this phase is generally acknowledged to be neurogenic; that is, being initiated prior to the arrival of the products of exercise metabolism at known sites of chemoreception (the carotid and central chemoreceptors). This could be mediated through parallel activation of ponto-medullary respiratory-integrating regions (eg, ventrolateral medulla, nucleus tractus solitarius) by descending voluntary locomotor influences from higher regions of the central nervous system, in proportion to motor command required for the task (ie, central command).[134,228,244,250,252,253] Possible sites include the motor cortex, the paraventricular locomotor region or the fields of Forel in the hypothalamus, and the mesencephalic locomotor region and the periaqueductal grey in the midbrain.

Reflex stimulation originating within the exercising muscles and projecting centrally via the dorsal roots and dorsal horn of the spinal cord to supraspinal respiratory-integrating sites, and also broadly proportional to work rate (and therefore metabolic rate), has also been proposed.[134,244,250,252,254,255] Sources include (1) small-diameter myelinated group III afferents primarily by mechanical stimuli such as tendon stretch, light pressure, and distortion and (2) nonmyelinated group IV afferents primarily by exercise metabolites such as lactic acidosis, K^+, bradykinin, arachidonic acid and its cyclo-oxygenase metabolites, and ATP and also by local vascular distention.

However, a potential drawback of such mechanisms is that, unless the resulting hyperpnea is accompanied by a proportional increase in cardiac output, P_{ETCO_2} and Pa_{CO_2} will fall and P_{ETO_2} and Pa_{O_2} will rise,[177,235] which is not the case (see **Fig. 2.37**). Such proportional changes have been described,[256,257] with a role for cardiac afferents having been proposed.[72,177] However, this latter proposal is not supported by studies on heart-lung transplantation patients[258,259] or calves with implanted artificial hearts,[260] suggesting that the similarity of the phase I $\dot{V}_E$ and cardiac output responses may reflect parallel drives rather than cardiodynamic mediation.[230,235]

In phase II, the exponential increase in $\dot{V}_E$ lags slightly behind that of $\dot{V}_{CO_2}$ (and therefore appreciably more than $\dot{V}_{O_2}$), leading to a small transient overshoot of Pa_{CO_2} and a larger transient undershoot of Pa_{O_2} (see **Fig. 2.37**).[72,230] This kinetic disparity accounts for the small sustained increase in Pa_{CO_2} seen with incremental exercise (see **Fig. 2.30C**). This close dynamic coupling of $\dot{V}_E$ to $\dot{V}_{CO_2}$, retained for a range of work rate forcing functions (step, ramp, impulse, sinusoid) and when $\dot{V}_{CO_2}$ kinetics are deliberately manipulated by alterations of body CO_2 stores, has been suggested to reflect the operation of a mechanism linked to the demands for CO_2 clearance at the lung; that is, the kinetics of the associated $\dot{Q}_{O_2}$, $\dot{V}_{O_2}$, and $\dot{Q}_{CO_2}$ responses being appreciably faster.[72,171,230,251] These observations led to the proposal that $\dot{V}_E$ during both phase II and phase III is driven, largely if not entirely, by the "CO_2 flow to the lungs"; that is, the product of venous return (or cardiac output) and the mixed-venous CO_2 content ($C\bar{v}_{CO_2}$).[72] This was modified subsequently, with the recognition that a control mechanism proportional to the demands for pulmonary CO_2 clearance depends not on the CO_2 flow to the lungs but rather on the difference between the CO_2 flow *to* the lungs and the CO_2 flow *from* the lungs; that is, the product of cardiac output and ($C[\bar{v} - a]_{CO_2}$).[251] Although a receptor mechanism sensitive simply to mixed venous P_{CO_2}[261] is therefore not sufficiently robust,[72,230] the precise identity of such a CO_2-linked mechanism remains unclear, not the least because of the absence of a sustained Pa_{CO_2} error signal that could stimulate carotid and central chemoreceptors.[72,171,228,230,244,250,251] One potential stimulus that encodes elements of $\dot{V}_{CO_2}$ is the intrabreath oscillation of Pa_{CO_2},[72,171,228,230,243] the consequence of an intermittent ventilation of exchanging alveoli in the face of more nearly continuous pulmonary-capillary perfusion (see Chapter 3, "Arterial–End-Tidal P_{CO_2} Difference" and **Fig. 3.27**).[262]

The phase II $\dot{V}_E$ kinetics are modulated by carotid chemoreceptor activation status.[72,171,230,243,263,264] Considerable evidence in this regard (and also for other aspects of ventilatory control in exercise described below) has accrued from studies on asymptomatic asthmatic patients who had undergone bilateral surgical resection of their carotid bodies (BCBR) but with arterial baroreception preserved.[265] Thus, the phase II response was appreciably slower than normal following BCBR.[72,230,263,264] Also, acute hypoxia has been shown to speed the phase II kinetics in normal individuals, and hyperoxia to be associated with a slowing, consistent with observations in BCBR individuals that $\dot{V}_E$ did not increase in response to hypoxia nor did it decrease (even transiently) in response to acute hyperoxia.[72,230,264] The exact mechanisms remain to be elucidated, however, although several potential stimuli including increases in plasma $[K^+]$ and osmolarity have been proposed.[72,230,264,266]

What is evident is that the clear dissociation between work rate and $\dot{V}_E$ in phase II argues against an obligatory involvement of the central and peripheral neurogenic mechanisms described above. It also does not support an involvement of an additional source of central, nonsensory neural feedforward control, a "short-term modulation" (STM) mechanism with relatively slow exponential kinetics developing over several minutes, reflective of a respiratory neuronal after-discharge or memory.[134,228] However, although this is qualitatively reminiscent of the phase II hyperpnea, there are several differences. Thus, the phase II $\dot{V}_E$ kinetics are symmetrical for exercise onset and offset (ie, having similar time constants),[72,171,230] whereas those for STM are appreciably slower following stimulus removal than for stimulus application.[134,228] Also, STM kinetics are not influenced by carotid chemoreceptor activity and do not readily accommodate the demonstration that procedures designed to alter phase II $\dot{V}_{CO_2}$ kinetics lead to similar directional changes in the phase II $\dot{V}_E$ kinetics.[72,230,251]

It is generally assumed that the ventilatory control mechanisms recruited in phase I and phase II maintain their influence into the steady state (ie, phase III). For example, the carotid chemoreflex appears to contribute some 15% to 20% of the phase III response, as judged by the magnitude of the transient $\dot{V}_E$ decrease when the inspired gas is switched abruptly from air to 100% O_2 (Dejours O_2 test; see Chapter 3 "Carotid Body Contribution to Ventilation") (**Fig. 3.37**), this contribution being greater in patients who develop arterial hypoxemia during exercise.[263,264] Also, there is a broad evidence base that stimulation of putative mechanisms during phase III (eg, muscle reflexes, central command, carotid and central chemoreflexes, cardiac reflexes) can elicit an increased $\dot{V}_E$.[72,134,171,228,230,244,249,250,263,264]

In contrast is the lack of effect on the phase III $\dot{V}_E$ response when such putative influences are removed or are absent because of "accidents of nature"; for example, inactivation of carotid chemoreceptors by hyperoxia or

BCBR[72,171,230,251,263,264]; diminished or absent central chemosensitivity, as in congenital central hypoventilation syndrome, despite normal lung function[267]; disruption of muscle afferent traffic and descending central command projections following complete spinal cord transection[230,268-270]; and following heart-lung transplantation.[258,259] Such observations suggest that the ventilatory control system may possess a considerable degree of redundancy during exercise; that is, when one mechanism is inactivated, others can presumably take over.[72,228,249,255,271] There is a contrary observation in this regard, however, that supports a contribution from muscle reflex drive to the phase III $\dot{V}_E$: intrathecal lumbar administration of fentanyl to effect partial blockade of lower limb muscle afferents causing a reduction of $\dot{V}_E$.[244,250]

That the group of mechanisms which apparently are obligatory for mediating the dynamic and steady-state $\dot{V}_E$ responses to moderate exercise appears to be small, and that there is an absence of classical humoral steady-state error signals, has led to the formulation of less conventional control schemes.[72,171,272-274] For example, brainstem respiratory-integrating sites would establish the $\dot{V}_E$ response necessary to regulate Pa_{CO_2} during exercise by "optimizing" the "cost" of Pa_{CO_2} regulation with that of mechanically generating the $\dot{V}_E$ response,[275,276] or linking the $\dot{V}_E$ response to resting ventilatory drive via a serotonergic STM mechanism (see above) to ensure isocapnia in the face of influences that might alter the resting Pa_{CO_2} setpoint.[272] Furthermore, longer term modulation or plasticity has the potential to alter $\dot{V}_E$ during exercise, elicited by the memory of a concomitantly imposed additional ventilatory stimulus (eg, repetitive hypoxic or external dead space exposures) whose effect is maintained for a prolonged period following removal of the stimulus.[249,272,277-279] This could have potential significance when ventilatory control is perturbed, as in pulmonary disease. Whether such schemes are key elements of the normal ventilatory control process during exercise in humans is presently unclear, however.

Supra-*AT* Exercise

Additional ventilatory drives related to the metabolic acidemia, and also possibly exercise-induced arterial hypoxemia and augmented central command and muscle reflex drives, are recruited above the *AT*, with $\dot{V}_E$ steady states typically not being attained. Thus, $\dot{V}_E$ is caused to increase at a greater rate relative to $\dot{V}_{CO_2}$ than for sub-*AT* work rates (**Fig. 2.52**), with the consequent hypocapnia serving to constrain the falling pHa (ie, ventilatory compensation) (see **Fig. 2.30C**).[72,209,228,280] Substituting for Pa_{CO_2} from Equation 18 into the Henderson-Hasselbalch equation (Equation 12) usefully yields

$$pHa = pK + \log\{\underbrace{([HCO_3^-]a/25.9)}\cdot\underbrace{(\dot{V}_E/\dot{V}_{CO_2})}\cdot\underbrace{(1 - V_D/V_T)}\} \quad (22)$$

where the bracketed terms (from left to right) represent metabolic acid-base "setpoint," "ventilatory control" operator, and gas-exchange "efficiency" elements, respectively.

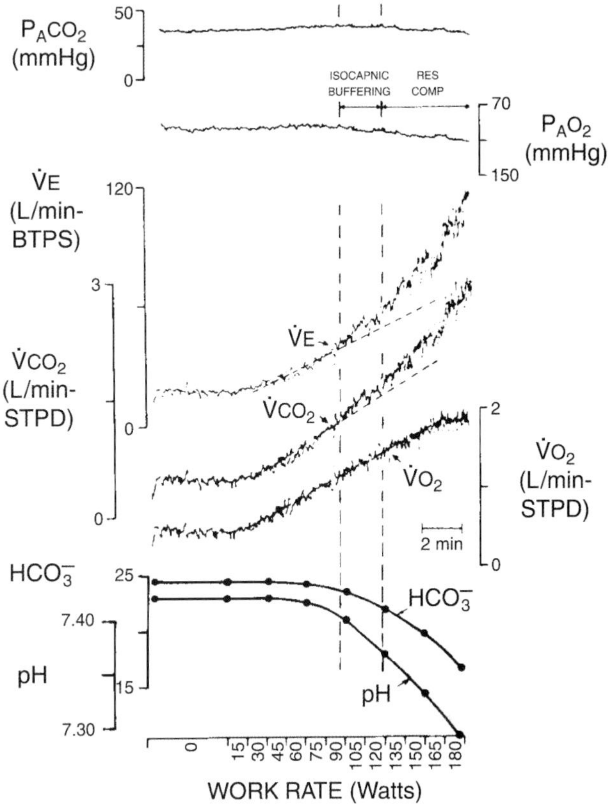

FIGURE 2.52. Alveolar end-tidal P_{CO_2} and P_{O_2} (P_{ACO_2}, P_{AO_2}), ventilation ($\dot{V}_E$), CO_2 output ($\dot{V}_{CO_2}$), O_2 uptake ($\dot{V}_{O_2}$), arterial bicarbonate concentration ($[HCO_3^-]$) and arterial pH as a function of work rate for an incremental cycle-ergometer exercise test. The anaerobic threshold (*AT*) occurs when arterial $[HCO_3^-]$ starts to fall, reflecting buffering of the metabolic acidosis; $\dot{V}_{CO_2}$ therefore begins to accelerate (*left vertical dashed line*). $\dot{V}_E$ continues to respond in proportion to $\dot{V}_{CO_2}$ beyond the *AT*, ensuring stability of P_{ACO_2} until the onset of respiratory compensation for the metabolic acidosis (*right vertical dashed line*). However, as $\dot{V}_E$ increases at a greater rate than $\dot{V}_{O_2}$ above the *AT*, P_{AO_2} rises. *Isocapnic buffering* refers to the period between *AT* and the onset of respiratory compensation. Beyond the respiratory compensation point, $\dot{V}_E$ increases at a greater rate than $\dot{V}_{CO_2}$, causing P_{ACO_2} therefore to decrease (i.e. respiratory compensation).

The effectiveness of ventilatory compensation thus depends not simply on $\dot{V}_E/\dot{V}_{CO_2}$ increasing but also on $\dot{V}_E/\dot{V}_{CO_2}$ increasing relative to V_D/V_T.

Based largely on studies on BCBR patients and O_2 breathing in normal individuals, the carotid chemoreceptors are thought to mediate much, if not all, of the supra-*AT* ventilatory compensation in humans (although alternative views have been expressed),[228,281] responding to blood-borne stimuli such as $[H^+]$, $[K^+]$, catecholamines, osmolarity, and, possibly, angiotensin II.[72,171,209,228,230,263,264,266] However, the kinetics of the ventilatory compensation are relatively slow.[72,171,209,230,263,282]

Thus, despite the developing metabolic acidosis, $\dot{V}_E$ initially continues to increase with its sub-*AT* proportion to $\dot{V}_{CO_2}$ during incremental exercise of the kind used in CPET. This gives rise to a phase of "isocapnic buffering" between the *AT* and VCP, within which P_{ETCO_2} and Pa_{CO_2} do not evidence any systematic decline (see **Fig. 2.52**).[72] This contrasts with slow incremental exercise, for which the *AT* and VCP are coincident (ie, there has been sufficient time for the compensation to be evident at the *AT*). These slow kinetics may reflect the existence of an amplitude- or time-related threshold for H^+ detection at the carotid chemoreceptor, perhaps involving slow intracellular expression of the metabolic acidemia and/or slow H^+ signal transduction.[230,249]

It is generally assumed that the central chemoreceptors, although sensitive to local increases in $[H^+]$, do not contribute to the supra-*AT* ventilatory compensation because the impermeability of the blood-brain barrier prevents migration of metabolically produced H^+ ions from arterial blood into the cerebrospinal fluid.[228] Interestingly, however, an even more slowly expressed compensatory $\dot{V}_E$ response has been demonstrated for prolonged supra-*AT* constant work rate exercise following suppression of carotid chemosensitivity by hyperoxic inhalations (ie, inspired $[O_2]$ approaching 100%), with arterial pH slowly, but systematically, being restored back toward normal despite the elevated arterial [lactate].[283] This $\dot{V}_E$ response was suggested to reflect central chemoreceptor stimulation consequent to a slowly developing "leak" of H^+ ions from arterial blood into the cerebrospinal fluid.[284]

With regard to ventilatory compensation, some have proposed that the VCP is a proxy for the CP (see "Power-Duration Curve and Critical Power" above). However, as discussed by Ward,[285] there is not a body of convincing evidence to support this contention; for example, unlike $\dot{V}O_2max$ or the *AT*, the VCP is influenced by factors such as the work rate incrementation rate, consistent with the relatively slow kinetics of the $\dot{V}_E$ response to the metabolic acidosis above *AT*.

On a practical note, the delayed ventilatory compensation for the metabolic acidosis of rapid ramp incremental exercise and the associated gas exchange responses are integral elements in the noninvasive estimation of the *AT*, as described in Chapter 3 ("Anaerobic (Lactate, Lactic Acidosis) Threshold") (see **Fig. 2.52**). Briefly, the point at which the accelerating $\dot{V}CO_2$ response, relative to $\dot{V}O_2$, is taken to reflect the additional CO_2 load generated by HCO_3^- buffering of the lactic acidosis (see "Buffering the Exercise-Induced Lactic Acidosis" above) and provides the V-slope index for estimating the *AT*.[56] This is supported by the demonstration of delayed ventilatory compensation, with the maintained proportion between $\dot{V}_E$ and $\dot{V}CO_2$ being reflected in $\dot{V}_E/\dot{V}CO_2$ not changing and P_{ETCO_2} therefore not falling. However, as $\dot{V}_E$ must therefore start to increase at a greater rate than $\dot{V}O_2$ beyond the *AT*, the ventilatory equivalent for O_2 ($\dot{V}_E/\dot{V}O_2$) starts to increase, as does P_{ETO_2}.

SUMMARY

The major physiological responses to exercise are summarized in **Figure 1.1**. Approximately 25% to 30% of the calories generated during work are transformed into useful external work, while the remainder is lost primarily as heat. The oxidative energy obtained from O_2 creditors (Hb, myoglobin, PCr, and pyruvate conversion to lactate) during the O_2 deficit period, which must be repaid during the recovery period of exercise as the O_2 debt, varies with the work rate. If an individual is very fit for a particular work rate, the O_2 deficit and debt will be relatively small. That is, for moderate work rates, the pyruvate-to-lactate mechanism provides none or only a very small fraction of the creditors of the O_2 deficit. In contrast, for very heavy work rates, the pyruvate-to-lactate mechanism may account for upward of 80% of the total O_2 deficit.

Gas exchange during exercise should be considered from the standpoint of cellular respiration and how cardiovascular and ventilatory mechanisms are coupled to it. Not only does the magnitude of cellular respiration affect external respiration, but, importantly, the degree to which the work rate is above an individual's *AT* has a major influence on the cardiovascular and ventilatory responses to exercise. Thus, *AT* is reduced when the cardiovascular transport of O_2 is impaired. And, importantly, exercise above the *AT* increases CO_2 and H^+ production, with both being powerful ventilatory stimuli. The associated gas exchange kinetics are also altered, and exercise endurance is reduced.

The distribution of the cardiac output to exercising muscle depends on the work rate, through local humoral factors that optimize the O_2 (blood) flow–metabolic rate relationship. Presumably because of local control mechanisms, the $\dot{Q}O_2/\dot{Q}m$ ratio and thereby the end-capillary P_{O_2} in the exercising muscles are relatively uniform. The relative uniformity of the regional $\dot{Q}O_2$-$\dot{Q}m$ relationship enables the muscle end-capillary P_{O_2} to be sufficiently high in all muscle capillary beds to allow as much as 85%, on average, of the O_2 to be extracted from muscle blood flow during maximal exercise.

During exercise, $\dot{V}_E$ responds to the changing rate of CO_2 delivery to the lungs, including that generated by aerobic oxidation of energy substrate and that generated by the buffering of the lactic acidosis by HCO_3^-. In addition, the carotid bodies monitor arterial $[H^+]$, providing sufficient ventilatory drive to minimize the decrease in arterial pH that occurs above the *AT*. Exercise ventilation is also determined by the size of the physiological V_D and the level at which arterial P_{CO_2} is regulated. Pa_{O_2} normally remains relatively constant during exercise, despite increasing $\dot{V}O_2$.

Incremental exercise tests that measure $\dot{V}O_2$ and $\dot{V}CO_2$ breath by breath allow detection of the *AT* by gas exchange. Also, breath-by-breath measurements of $\dot{V}O_2$ and $\dot{V}CO_2$ during constant work rate exercise can be used to determine if the exercise is being performed with or without a metabolic acidosis and to estimate the magnitude of the arterial [lactate] increase at the work rate performed.

Breath-by-breath gas exchange measurements in response to appropriately chosen work rate protocols can therefore provide considerable insight into mechanisms of cardiovascular and ventilatory control and the state of cellular respiration.

REFERENCES

1. Tipton C, ed. *Exercise Physiology: People and Ideas*. Oxford, United Kingdom: Oxford University Press; 2003.
2. Tipton C, ed. *History of Exercise Physiology*. Champaign, IL: Human Kinetics; 2014.
3. Greising SM, Gransee HM, Mantilla CB, Sieck GC. Systems biology of skeletal muscle: fiber type as an organizing principle. *Wiley Interdiscip Rev Syst Biol Med*. 2012;4:457-473.
4. Saltin B, Gollnick PD. Skeletal muscle adaptability: significance for metabolism and performance. In: Peachey LD, Adrian RH, Greiger SR, eds. *Handbook of Physiology: Skeletal Muscle*. Bethesda, MD: American Physiology Society; 1983:555-631.
5. Schiaffino S, Reggiani C. Fiber types in mammalian skeletal muscles. *Physiol Rev*. 2011;91:1447-1531.
6. Tsintzas K, Williams C, Constantin-Teodosiu D, et al. Phosphocreatine degradation in type I and type II muscle fibres during submaximal exercise in man: effect of carbohydrate ingestion. *J Physiol*. 2001;537(pt 1):305-311.
7. Barclay CJ. Mechanical efficiency and fatigue of fast and slow muscles of the mouse. *J Physiol*. 1996;497(pt 3):781-794.
8. Gibbs CL, Gibson WR. Energy production of rat soleus muscle. *Am J Physiol*. 1972;223:864-871.
9. Henricksson J, Reitman IS. Quantitative measures of enzyme activities in type I and type II muscle fibres of man after training. *Acta Physiol Scand*. 1976;97:392-397.
10. Pette D. J.B. Wolffe memorial lecture. Activity-induced fast to slow transitions in mammalian muscle. *Med Sci Sports Exerc*. 1984;16:517-528.
11. Krustrup P, Söderlund K, Mohr M, Bangsbo J. The slow component of oxygen uptake during intense, sub-maximal exercise in man is associated with additional fibre recruitment. *Pflugers Arch*. 2004;447:855-866.
12. Petrofsky JS. Frequency and amplitude analysis of the EMG during exercise on the bicycle ergometer. *Eur J Appl Physiol Occup Physiol*. 1979;41:1-15.
13. Clanton TL, Hogan MC, Gladden LB. Regulation of cellular gas exchange, oxygen sensing, and metabolic control. *Compr Physiol*. 2013;3:1135-1190.
14. Gonzalez JT, Fuchs CJ, Betts JA, van Loon LJ. Liver glycogen metabolism during and after prolonged endurance-type exercise. *Am J Physiol Endocrinol Metab*. 2016;311:E543-E553.
15. Hargreaves MH, Snow R. Amino acids and endurance exercise. *Int J Sport Nutr Exerc Metab*. 2001;11:133-345.
16. Hargreaves M, Spriet LL. Exercise metabolism: fuels for the fire. *Cold Spring Harb Perspect Med*. 2018;8(8):a029744.
17. Jensen TE, Richter EA. Regulation of glucose and glycogen metabolism during and after exercise. *J Physiol*. 2012;590:1069-1076.
18. Jeukendrup AE, Saris WH, Wagenmakers AJ. Fat metabolism during exercise: a review. Part I: fatty acid mobilization and muscle metabolism. *Int J Sports Med*. 1998;19:231-244.
19. Trefts E, Williams AS, Wasserman DH. Exercise and the regulation of hepatic metabolism. *Prog Mol Biol Transl Sci*. 2015;135:203-225.
20. Sheetz MP, Chasan K, Spudich JA. ATP-dependent movement of myosin in vitro: characterization of a quantitative assay. *J Cell Biol*. 1984;99:1867-1871.
21. Grassi B, Rossiter HB, Zoladz JA. Skeletal muscle fatigue and decreased efficiency: two sides of the same coin? *Exerc Sport Sci Rev*. 2015;43:75-83.
22. Krebs HA, Kornberg HL. *Energy Transformations in Living Matter*. Berlin, Germany: Springer; 1957.
23. Wilkie DR, Woledge RC. The application of irreversible thermodynamics to muscular contraction. Comments on a recent theory by S. R. Caplan. *Proc R Soc Lond B Biol Sci*. 1967;169:17-29.
24. Stryer L. *Biochemistry*. 4th ed. New York, NY: W. H. Freeman & Company; 1995.
25. Jastroch M, Divakaruni AS, Mookerjee S, Treberg JR, Brand MD. Mitochondrial proton and electron leaks. *Essays Biochem*. 2010;47:53-67.
26. Taylor EB. Functional properties of the mitochondrial carrier system. *Trends Cell Biol*. 2017;27:633-644.
27. Kushmerick MJ, Conley KE. Energetics of muscle contraction: the whole is less than the sum of its parts. *Biochem Soc Trans*. 2002;30:227-231.
28. Meyer RA. A linear model of muscle respiration explains monoexponential phosphocreatine changes. *Am J Physiol*. 1988;254(4 pt 1):C548-C553.
29. Bessman SP, Geiger PJ. Transport of energy in muscle: the phosphorylcreatine shuttle. *Science*. 1981;211:448-452.
30. Chance B, Leigh J Jr, Clark B, et al. Control of oxidative metabolism and oxygen delivery in human skeletal muscle: a steady-state analysis of the work/energy cost transfer function. *Proc Natl Acad Sci U S A*. 1985;82:8384-8388.
31. Rossiter HB. Exercise: kinetic considerations for gas exchange. *Compr Physiol*. 2011;1:203-244.
32. Cathcart EP, Burnett WA. The influence of muscle work on metabolism in varying conditions of diet. *Proc Roy Soc (Biol)*. 1926;99:405-426.
33. Heigenhauser GJ, Sutton JR, Jones NL. Effect of glycogen depletion on the ventilatory response to exercise. *J Appl Physiol Respir Environ Exerc Physiol*. 1983;54:470-474.
34. Costill DL, Hargreaves M. Carbohydrate nutrition and fatigue. *Sports Med*. 1992;13:86-92.
35. Coyle EF. Carbohydrate supplementation during exercise. *J Nutr*. 1992;122(suppl 3):788-795.
36. Ahlborg B, Bergström J, Ekelund LG, Hultman E. Muscle glycogen and muscle electrolytes during prolonged physical exercise. *Acta Physiol Scand*. 1967;70:129-142.
37. Bergström J, Hermansen L, Hultman E, Saltin B. Diet, muscle glycogen and physical performance. *Acta Physiol Scand*. 1967;71:140-150.
38. Brooks GA. Bioenergetics of exercising humans. *Compr Physiol*. 2012;2:537-562.
39. Jeukendrup AE, Saris WH, Wagenmakers AJ. Fat metabolism during exercise: a review—part II: regulation of metabolism and the effects of training. *Int J Sports Med*. 1998;19:293-302.
40. Brenner I, Shek PN, Zamecnik J, Shephard RJ. Stress hormones and the immunological responses to heat and exercise. *Int J Sports Med*. 1998;19:130-143.
41. Weltman A, Wood CM, Womack CJ, et al. Catecholamine and blood lactate responses to incremental rowing and running exercise. *J Appl Physiol (1985)*. 1994;76:1144-1149.
42. Whipp BJ, Mahler M. Dynamics of pulmonary gas exchange during exercise. In: *Pulmonary Gas Exchange*. Vol 2. New York, NY: Academic Press; 1980:33-96.
43. Mitchell JH, Sproule BJ, Chapman CB. The physiological meaning of the maximal oxygen intake test. *J Clin Invest*. 1958;37:538-547.
44. Taylor HL, Buskirk E, Henschel A. Maximal oxygen intake as an objective measure of cardio-respiratory performance. *J Appl Physiol*. 1955;8:73-80.
45. Mogensen M, Bagger M, Pedersen PK, Fernström M, Sahlin K. Cycling efficiency in humans is related to low UCP3 content and to type I fibres but not to mitochondrial efficiency. *J. Physiol*. 2006;571(pt 3):669-681.
46. Ortega JD. Counterpoint: skeletal muscle mechanical efficiency does not increase with age. *J Appl Physiol (1985)*. 2013;114:1109-1111.
47. Coyle EF, Sidossis LS, Horowitz JF, Beltz JD. Cycling efficiency is related to the percentage of type I muscle fibers. *Med Sci Sports Exerc*. 1992;24:782-788.
48. Wasserman K, Whipp BJ. Exercise physiology in health and disease (state of the art). *Am Rev Respir Dis*. 1975;112:219-249.
49. Gaesser GA, Brooks GA. Muscular efficiency during steady-rate exercise: effects of speed and work rate. *J Appl Physiol*. 1975;38:1132-1139.
50. Whipp BJ, Wasserman K. Efficiency of muscular work. *J Appl Physiol*. 1969;26:644-648.
51. Roston WL, Whipp BJ, Davis JA, Cunningham DA, Effros RM, Wasserman K. Oxygen uptake kinetics and lactate concentration during exercise in humans. *Am Rev Respir Dis*. 1987;135:1080-1084.
52. Whipp BJ, Wasserman K. Oxygen uptake kinetics for various intensities of constant-load work. *J Appl Physiol*. 1972;33:351-356.

53. Zhang YY, Wasserman K, Sietsema KE, et al. O_2 uptake kinetics in response to exercise. A measure of tissue anaerobiosis in heart failure. *Chest*. 1993;103:735-741.
54. Wasserman K. Coupling of external to cellular respiration during exercise: the wisdom of the body revisited. *Am J Physiol*. 1994;266(4 pt 1):E519-E539.
55. Beaver WL, Wasserman K, Whipp BJ. Improved detection of lactate threshold during exercise using a log-log transformation. *J Appl Physiol (1985)*. 1985;59:1936-1940.
56. Beaver WL, Wasserman K, Whipp BJ. A new method for detecting anaerobic threshold by gas exchange. *J Appl Physiol (1985)*. 1986;60:2020-2027.
57. Wasserman K, Beaver WL, Whipp BJ. Gas exchange theory and the lactic acidosis (anaerobic) threshold. *Circulation*. 1990;81(suppl 1):II14-II30.
58. Paterson DH, Cunningham DA. The gas transporting systems: limits and modifications with age and training. *Can J Appl Physiol*. 1999;24:28-40.
59. Tanaka K, Matsuura Y, Matsuzaka A, et al. A longitudinal assessment of anaerobic threshold and distance-running performance. *Med Sci Sports Exerc*. 1984;16:278-282.
60. Zoladz JA, Sargeant AJ, Emmerich J, Stoklosa J, Zychowski A. Changes in acid-base status of marathon runners during incremental field test. Relationship to mean competitive marathon velocity. *Eur J Appl Physiol Occup Physiol*. 1993;67:71-76.
61. Jamnick NA, Botella J, Pyne DB, Bishop DJ. Manipulating graded exercise test variables affects the validity of the lactate threshold and $\dot{V}O_2$peak. *PLoS One*. 2018;13:e0199794.
62. Dennis SC, Noakes TD, Bosch AN. Ventilation and blood lactate increase exponentially during incremental exercise. *J Sports Sci* 1992; 10: 437-449.
63. Hughson RL, Weisiger KH, Swanson GD. Blood lactate concentration increases as a continuous function in progressive exercise. *J Appl Physiol (1985)*. 1987;62:1975-1981.
64. Yeh MP, Gardner RM, Adams TD, Yanowitz FG, Crapo RO. "Anaerobic threshold": problems of determination and validation. *J Appl Physiol Respir Environ Exerc Physiol*. 1983;55:1178-1186.
65. Chwalbinska-Moneta J, Robergs RA, Costillo DL, Fink WJ. Threshold for muscle lactate accumulation during progressive exercise. *J Appl Physiol*. 1989;66:2710-2716.
66. Jorfeldt L, Juhlin-Dannfelt A, Karlsson J. Lactate release in relation to tissue lactate in human skeletal muscle during exercise. *J Appl Physiol Respir Environ Exerc Physiol*. 1978;44:350-352.
67. Katz A, Sahlin K. Regulation of lactic acid production during exercise. *J Appl Physiol (1985)*. 1988;65:509-518.
68. Knuttgen HG, Saltin B. Muscle metabolites and oxygen uptake in short-term submaximal exercise in man. *J Appl Physiol*. 1972;32:690-694.
69. Wasserman K, Van Kessel A, Burton GG. Interaction of physiological mechanisms during exercise. *J Appl Physiol*. 1967;22:71-85.
70. Whipp B. Domains of aerobic function and their limiting parameters. In: Steinacker JM, Ward SA, eds. *The Physiology and Pathophysiology of Exercise Tolerance*. New York, NY: Plenum; 1996:83-89.
71. Brooks GA. Cell-cell and intracellular lactate shuttles. *J Physiol*. 2009;587(pt 23):5591-5600.
72. Wasserman K, Whipp BJ, Casaburi R. Respiratory control during exercise. In: Cherniack NS, Widdicombe G, eds. *Handbook of Physiology, Respiration (Control)*. Bethesda, MD: American Physiological Society; 1986:595-619.
73. Brooks GA. The science and translation of lactate shuttle theory. *Cell Metab*. 2018;27:757-785.
74. Ferguson BS, Rogatzki MJ, Goodwin ML, Kane DA, Rightmire Z, Gladden LB. Lactate metabolism: historical context, prior misinterpretations, and current understanding. *Eur J Appl Physiol*. 2018;118: 691-728.
75. Lindinger M, Whipp BJ. The anaerobic threshold: fact or misinterpretation. In: Taylor NAS, Groeller H, eds. *Physiological Bases of Human Performance During Work and Exercise*. Edinburgh, United Kingdom: Elsevier; 2008:191-199.
76. Rogatzki MJ, Ferguson BS, Goodwin ML, Gladden LB. Lactate is always the end product of glycolysis. *Front Neurosci*. 2015;9:22.
77. Lambeth MJ, Kushmerick MJ. A computational model for glycogenolysis in skeletal muscle. *Ann Biomed Eng*. 2002;30:808-827.
78. Ivy JL, Withers RT, Van Handel PJ, Elger DH, Costill DL. Muscle respiratory capacity and fiber type as determinants of the lactate threshold. *J Appl Physiol Respir Environ Exerc Physiol*. 1980;48:523 527.
79. Gurd BJ, Peters SJ, Heigenhauser GJ, et al. O_2 uptake kinetics, pyruvate dehydrogenase activity, and muscle deoxygenation in young and older adults during the transition to moderate-intensity exercise. *Am J Physiol Regul Integr Comp Physiol*. 2008;294:R577-R584.
80. Spriet LL, Heigenhauser GJ. Regulation of pyruvate dehydrogenase (PDH) activity in human skeletal muscle during exercise. *Exerc Sport Sci Rev*. 2002;30:91-95.
81. Rossiter HB, Ward SA, Howe FA, et al. Effects of dichloroacetate on $\dot{V}O_2$ and intramuscular ^{31}P metabolite kinetics during high-intensity exercise in humans. *J Appl Physiol (1985)*. 2003;95:1105-1115.
82. Wasserman K, Beaver WL, Davis JA, Pu JZ, Heber D, Whipp BJ. Lactate, pyruvate, and lactate-to-pyruvate ratio during exercise and recovery. *J Appl Physiol (1985)*. 1985;59:935-940.
83. Bylund-Fellenius AC, Walker PM, Elander A, Holm S, Holm J, Scherstén T. Energy metabolism in relation to oxygen partial pressure in human skeletal muscle during exercise. *Biochem J*. 1981;200:247-255.
84. Karlsson J. Pyruvate and lactate ratios in muscle tissue and blood during exercise in man. *Acta Physiol Scand*. 1971;81:455-458.
85. Gladden LB. Lactate metabolism: a new paradigm for the third millennium. *J Physiol*. 2004;558(pt 1):5-30.
86. Bonen A. The expression of lactate transporters (MCT_1 and MCT_4) in heart and muscle. *Eur J Appl Physiol*. 2001;86:6-11.
87. Juel C. Regulation of pH in human skeletal muscle: adaptations to physical activity. *Acta Physiol (Oxf)*. 2008;193:17-24.
88. Thomas C, Bishop DJ, Lambert K, Mercier J, Brooks GA. Effects of acute and chronic exercise on sarcolemmal MCT1 and MCT4 contents in human skeletal muscles: current status. *Am J Physiol Regul Integr Comp Physiol*. 2012;302:R1-R14.
89. Brown MA, Brooks GA. Trans-stimulation of lactate transport from rat sarcolemmal membrane vesicles. *Arch Biochem Biophys*. 1994;313:22-28.
90. Trosper TL, Philipson KD. Lactate transport by cardiac sarcolemmal vesicles. *Am J Physiol*. 1987;252(5 pt 1):C483-C489.
91. Hirsche H, Hombach V, Langhor VD, Wacker U, Busse J. Lactic acid permeation rate in working gastrocnemii of dogs during metabolic alkalosis and acidosis. *Pflugers Arch*. 1975;56:209-222.
92. Mainwood GW, Worsley-Brown P, Paterson RA. The metabolic changes in frog sartorius muscles during recovery from fatigue at different external bicarbonate concentrations. *Can J Physiol Pharmacol*. 1972;50:143-155.
93. Korotzer B, Jung T, Stringer W, et al. Effect of acetazolamide on lactate, lactate threshold and acid-base balance during exercise. *Am J Respir Crit Care Med*. 1997;155:A171.
94. Stanley WC, Gertz EW, Wisneski JA, Neese RA, Morris DL, Brooks GA. Lactate extraction during net lactate release in legs of humans during exercise. *J Appl Physiol (1985)*. 1986;60:1116-1120.
95. Stanley WC, Gertz EW, Wisneski JA, Morris DL, Neese RA, Brooks GA. Systemic lactate kinetics during graded exercise in man. *Am J Physiol*. 1985;249(6 pt 1):E595-E602.
96. Wittenberg BA, Wittenberg JB. Transport of oxygen in muscle. *Ann Rev Physiol*. 1989;51:857-878.
97. Grassi B, Poole DC, Richardson RS, Knight DR, Erickson BK, Wagner PD. Muscle O_2 uptake kinetics in humans: implications for metabolic control. *J Appl Physiol (1985)*. 1996;80:988-998.
98. Stringer W, Wasserman K, Casaburi R, Pórszász J, Maehara K, French W. Lactic acidosis as a facilitator of oxyhemoglobin dissociation during exercise. *J Appl Physiol (1985)*. 1994;76:1462-1467.
99. Wagner PD. Diffusive resistance to O_2 transport in muscle. *Acta Physiol Scand*. 2000;168:609-614.
100. Whipp BJ, Lamarra N, Ward SA. Obligatory anaerobiosis resulting from oxygen uptake-to-blood flow ratio dispersion in skeletal muscle: a model. *Eur J Appl Physiol Occup Physiol*. 1995;71: 147-152.

101. Gayeski TEJ, Honig CR. Intracellular PO_2 in long axis of individual fibers in working dog gracilis muscle. *Am J Physiol.* 1988;254(6 pt 2):H1179-H1186.
102. Molé PA, Chung Y, Tran TK, Sailasuta N, Hurd R, Jue T. Myoglobin desaturation with exercise intensity in human gastrocnemius muscle. *Am J Physiol.* 1999;277:R173-R180.
103. Richardson RS, Newcomer SC, Noyszewski EA. Skeletal muscle intracellular PO_2 assessed by myoglobin desaturation: Response to graded exercise. *J Appl Physiol (1985).* 2001;91:2679-2685.
104. Koike A, Wasserman K, Taniguichi K, Hiroe M, Marumo F. Critical capillary oxygen partial pressure and lactate threshold in patients with cardiovascular disease. *J Am Coll Cardiol.* 1994;23:1644-1650.
105. Andersen P, Saltin B. Maximal perfusion of skeletal muscle in man. *J Physiol.* 1985;366:233-249.
106. Donald KW, Gloster J, Harris AE, Reeves J, Harris P. The production of lactic acid during exercise in normal subjects and in patients with rheumatic heart disease. *Am Heart J.* 1961;62:494-510.
107. Stringer W, Casaburi R, Wasserman K. Acid-base regulation during exercise and recovery in humans. *J Appl Physiol (1985).* 1992;72:954-961.
108. Cooper DM, Wasserman DH, Vranic M, Wasserman K. Glucose turnover in response to exercise during high- and low-FIO_2 breathing in man. *Am J Physiol.* 1986;251(2 pt 1):E209-E214.
109. Lundin G, Strom G. The concentration of blood lactic acid in man during muscular work in relation to the partial pressure of oxygen of the inspired air. *Acta Physiol Scand.* 1947;13:253-266.
110. Vogel JA, Gleser MA. Effect of carbon monoxide on oxygen transport during exercise. *J Appl Physiol.* 1972;32:234-239.
111. Yoshida T, Udo M, Chida M, Ichioka M, Makiguchi K. Effect of hypoxia on arterial and venous blood levels of oxygen, carbon dioxide, hydrogen ions and lactate during incremental forearm exercise. *Eur J Appl Physiol Occup Physiol.* 1989;58:772-777.
112. Koike A, Weiler-Ravell D, McKenzie DK, Zanconato S, Wasserman K. Evidence that the metabolic acidosis threshold is the anaerobic threshold. *J Appl Physiol (1985).* 1990;68:2521-2526.
113. Koike A, Wasserman K, McKenzie DK, Zanconato S, Weiler-Ravell D. Evidence that diffusion limitation determines oxygen uptake kinetics during exercise in humans. *J Clin Invest.* 1990;86:1698-1706.
114. Lewis SF, Vora S, Haller RG. Abnormal oxidative metabolism and O_2 transport in muscle phosphofructokinase deficiency. *J Appl Physiol (1985).* 1991;70:391-398.
115. Beaver WL, Wasserman K, Whipp BJ. Bicarbonate buffering of lactic acid generated during exercise. *J Appl Physiol (1985).* 1986;60:472-478.
116. Bouhuys A, Pool J, Binkhorst RA, van Leeuwen P. Metabolic acidosis of exercise in healthy males. *J Appl Physiol.* 1966;21:1040-1046.
117. Owles WH. Alterations in the lactic acid content of the blood as a result of light exercise, and associated changes in the CO_2-combining power of the blood and in the alveolar CO_2 pressure. *J Physiol.* 1930;69:214-237.
118. Yoshida T, Udo M, Chida M, Makiguchi K, Ichioka M, Muraoka I. Arterial blood gases, acid-base balance, and lactate and gas exchange variables during hypoxic exercise. *Int J Sports Med.* 1989;10:279-285.
119. Kemp G. Lactate accumulation, proton buffering, and pH change in ischemically exercising muscle. *Am J Physiol Reg Integr Comp Physiol.* 2005;289:R895-R901.
120. Piiper J. Production of lactic acid in heavy exercise and acid-base balance. In: Moret PR, Weber J, Haissly J, Denolin H, eds. *Lactate: Physiologic, Methodologic and Pathologic Approach.* New York, NY: Springer; 1980.
121. Roussel M, Mattei JP, Le Fur Y, Ghattas B, Cozzone PJ, Bendahan D. Metabolic determinants of the onset of acidosis in exercising human muscle: a ^{31}P-MRS study. *J Appl Physiol (1985).* 2003;94:1145-1152.
122. Steinhagen C, Hirche HJ, Nestle HW, Bovenkamp U, Hosselmann I. The interstitial pH of the working gastrocnemius muscle of the dog. *Pflügers Archiv.* 1976;367:151-156.
123. Yoshida T, Watari H. Changes in intracellular pH during repeated exercise. *Eur J Appl Physiol Occup Physiol.* 1993;67:274-278.
124. Wasserman K, Stringer W, Casaburi R, Zhang YY. Mechanism of the exercise hyperkalemia: an alternate hypothesis. *J Appl Physiol (1985).* 1997;83:631-643.
125. Bevegård BS, Shepherd JT. Regulation of the circulation during exercise in man. *Physiol Rev* 1967;47:178-213.
126. Clausen JP. Effect of physical training on cardiovascular adjustments to exercise in man. *Physiol Rev.* 1977;57:779-815.
127. Janicki JS, Sheriff DD, Robotham JL, Wise RA. Cardiac output during exercise: contributions of the cardiac, circulatory and respiratory systems. In: Rowell LB, Shepherd JT, eds. *Handbook of Physiology, Section 12: Exercise: Regulation and Integration of Multiple Systems.* New York, NY: American Physiological Society; 1996:649-704.
128. Rowell LB. *Human Circulation Regulation during Physical Stress.* New York, NY: Oxford University Press; 1993.
129. Wade OL, Bishop JM. *Cardiac Output and Regional Blood Flow.* Oxford, United Kingdom: Blackwell; 1962.
130. Boushel R. Muscle metaboreflex control of the circulation during exercise. *Acta Physiol (Oxf).* 2010;199:367-383.
131. Murphy MN, Mizuno M, Mitchell JH, Smith SA. Cardiovascular regulation by skeletal muscle reflexes in health and disease. *Am J Physiol Heart Circ Physiol.* 2011;301:H1191-H1204.
132. Mueller PJ, Clifford PS, Crandall CG, Smith SA, Fadel PJ. Integration of central and peripheral regulation of the circulation during exercise: acute and chronic adaptations. *Compr Physiol.* 2017;8:103-151.
133. Rowell LB, O'Leary DS, Kellogg DL Jr. Integration of cardiovascular control systems in dynamic exercise. In: Rowell LB, Shepherd JT, eds. *Handbook of Physiology, Section 12: Exercise: Regulation and Integration of Multiple Systems.* New York, NY: American Physiological Society: 1996;770-838.
134. Waldrop TG, Eldridge FL, Iwamoto GA, Mitchell JH. Central neural control of respiration and circulation during exercise. In: Rowell LB, Shepherd JT, eds. *Handbook of Physiology, Section 12: Exercise: Regulation and Integration of Multiple Systems.* New York, NY: American Physiological Society; 1996:333-380.
135. Dempsey JA, Wagner PD. Exercise-induced arterial hypoxemia. *J Appl Physiol (1985).* 1999; 87:1997-2006.
136. Powers SK, Martin D, Dodd S. Exercise-induced hypoxaemia in elite endurance athletes. Incidence, causes and impact on $\dot{V}O_2$max. *Sports Med.* 1993;16:14-22.
137. Stickland MK, Lindinger MI, Olfert IM, Heigenhauser GJ, Hopkins SR. Pulmonary gas exchange and acid-base balance during exercise. *Compr Physiol.* 2013;3:693-739.
138. Stringer W, Whipp B, Wasserman K, Pórszász J, Christenson P, French WJ. Non-linear cardiac output dynamics during ramp-incremental cycle ergometry. *Eur J Appl Physiol.* 2005;93:634-639.
139. González-Alonso J. Point: stroke volume does/does not decline during exercise at maximal effort in healthy individuals. *J Appl Physiol (1985).* 2008;104:275-276.
140. Vella CA, Robergs RA. A review of the stroke volume response to upright exercise in healthy subjects. *Br J Sports Med.* 2005;39:190-195.
141. Vieira SS, Lemes B, de T C de Carvalho P, et al. Does stroke volume increase during an incremental exercise? A systematic review. *Open Cardiovasc Med J.* 2016;10:57-63.
142. Warburton DE, Gledhill N. Counterpoint: stroke volume does not decline during exercise at maximal effort in healthy individuals. *J Appl Physiol (1985).* 2008;104:276-278.
143. Riley M, Maehara K, Pórszász J, et al. Association between the anaerobic threshold and the break-point in the double product/work rate relationship. *Eur J Appl Physiol Occup Physiol.* 1997;75:14-21.
144. Henderson Y, Prince AL. The oxygen pulse and the systolic discharge. *Am J Physiol.* 1914;35:106-115.
145. Joyner MJ, Casey DP. Regulation of increased blood flow (hyperemia) to muscles during exercise: a hierarchy of competing physiological needs. *Physiol Rev.* 2015;95:549-601.
146. Laughlin MH, Davis MJ, Secher NH, et al. Peripheral circulation. *Compr Physiol.* 2012;2:321-447.
147. Laughlin MH, Korthuis RJ, Duncker DJ, Bache RJ. Control of blood flow to cardiac and skeletal muscle during exercise. In: Rowell LB, Shepherd JT, eds. *Handbook of Physiology, Section 12: Exercise: Regulation and Integration of Multiple Systems.* New York, NY: American Physiological Society; 1996:705-769.

148. Sheriff DD. Role of mechanical factors in governing muscle blood flow. *Acta Physiol.* 2010;199:385-391.
149. Tschakovsky ME, Sheriff DD. Immediate exercise hyperemia: contributions of the muscle pump vs. rapid vasodilation. *J Appl Physiol (1985).* 2004;97:739-747.
150. Davis MJ, Hill MA, Kuo L. Local regulation of microvascular perfusion. In: Tuma R, Duran W, Ley K, eds. *Handbook of Physiology: Microcirculation II, Regulation of Microvascular Blood Flow.* New York, NY: Elsevier; 2008:1-127.
151. Heinonen I, Koga S, Kalliokoski KK, Musch TI, Poole DC. Heterogeneity of muscle blood flow and metabolism: influence of exercise, aging, and disease states. *Exerc Sport Sci Rev.* 2015;43:117-124.
152. Mortensen SP, Saltin B. Regulation of the skeletal muscle blood flow in humans. *Exp Physiol.* 2014;99:1552-1558.
153. Borghi-Silva A, Oliveira CC, Carrascosa C, et al. Respiratory muscle unloading improves leg muscle oxygenation during exercise in patients with COPD. *Thorax* 2008;63:910-915.
154. Dempsey JA, Romer L, Rodman J, Miller J, Smith C. Consequences of exercise-induced respiratory muscle work. *Respir Physiol Neurobiol.* 2006;151:242-250.
155. Olson TP, Joyner MJ, Dietz NM, et al. Effects of respiratory muscle work on blood flow distribution during exercise in heart failure. *J Physiol.* 2010;588(pt 13):2487-2501.
156. Asmussen E. Muscular exercise. In: Fenn WO, Rahn H, eds. *Handbook of Physiology.* Vol 11. Washington, DC: American Physiological Society; 1965:939-978.
157. Whipp BJ, Wasserman K. Alveolar-arterial gas tension differences during graded exercise. *J Appl Physiol.* 1969;27:361-365.
158. Bunn HF, Forget BG. *Hemoglobin: Molecular, Genetic and Clinical Aspects.* Philadelphia, PA: W. B. Saunders; 1986.
159. Connes P, Machado R, Hue O, Reid H. Exercise limitation, exercise testing and exercise recommendations in sickle cell anemia. *Clin Hemorheol Microcirc.* 2011;49:151-163.
160. Van Beaumont W. Red cell volume with changes in plasma osmolarity during maximal exercise. *J Appl Physiol.* 1973;35:47-50.
161. Harrison MH. Effects on thermal stress and exercise on blood volume in humans. *Physiol Rev.* 1985;65:149-209.
162. Kaltreider N, Meneely G. The effect of exercise on the volume of the blood. *J Clin Invest.* 1940;19:627-634.
163. Senay LC Jr, Rogers G, Jooste P. Changes in blood plasma during progressive treadmill and cycle exercise. *J Appl Physiol.* 1980;49:59-65.
164. Sjøgaard G, Saltin B. Extra- and intracellular water spaces in muscles of man at rest and with dynamic exercise. *Am J Physiol.* 1982;243:R271-R280.
165. Poole DC, Jones AM. Oxygen uptake kinetics. *Compr Physiol.* 2012;2:933-996.
166. Finch C, Lenfant C. Oxygen transport in man. *N Engl J Med.* 1972;286:407-415.
167. Linnarsson D. Dynamics of pulmonary gas exchange and heart rate changes at start and end of exercise. *Acta Physiol Scand Suppl.* 1974;415:1-68.
168. Whipp BJ, Ward SA, Rossiter HB. Pulmonary O_2 uptake during exercise: conflating muscular and cardiovascular responses. *Med Sci Sports Exerc.* 2005;37:1574-1585.
169. Whipp BJ, Rossiter HB. The kinetics of oxygen uptake: physiological inferences from the parameters. In: Jones AM, Poole DC, eds. *Oxygen Uptake Kinetics in Health and Disease.* London, United Kingdom: Routledge; 2005:64-94.
170. Whipp BJ, Ward SA, Lamarra N, Davis JA, Wasserman K. Parameters of ventilatory and gas exchange dynamics during exercise. *J Appl Physiol Respir Environ Exerc Physiol.* 1982;52:1506-1513.
171. Whipp BJ. The control of exercise hyperpnea. In: Hornbein TF, ed. *Regulation of Breathing.* New York, NY: Marcel Dekker; 1981:1069-1139.
172. Barstow TJ, Lamarra N, Whipp BJ. Modulation of muscle and pulmonary O_2 uptakes by circulatory dynamics during exercise. *J Appl Physiol (1985).* 1990;68:979-989.
173. De Cort SC, Innes JA, Barstow TJ, Guz A. Cardiac output, oxygen consumption and arteriovenous oxygen difference following a sudden rise in exercise level in humans. *J Physiol.* 1991;441:501-512.
174. Krogh A, Lindhard J. The regulation of respiration and circulation during the initial stages of muscular work. *J Physiol.* 1913;47:112-136.
175. Jones PW, French W, Weissman ML, Wasserman K. Ventilatory responses to cardiac output changes in patients with pacemakers. *J Appl Physiol Respir Environ Exerc Physiol.* 1981;51:1103-1107.
176. Weissman ML, Jones PW, Oren A, Lamarra N, Whipp BJ, Wasserman K. Cardiac output increase and gas exchange at start of exercise. *J Appl Physiol Respir Environ Exerc Physiol.* 1982;52:236-244.
177. Wasserman K, Whipp BJ, Castagna J. Cardiodynamic hyperpnea: hyperpnea secondary to cardiac output increase. *J Appl Physiol.* 1974;36:457-464.
178. Casaburi R, Daly J, Hansen JE, Effros RM. Abrupt changes in mixed venous blood gas composition after the onset of exercise. *J Appl Physiol (1985).* 1989;67:1106-1112.
179. Casaburi R, Cooper CB, Effros RM, et al. Time course of mixed venous oxygen saturation following various modes of exercise transition. *FASEB J.* 1989;3:A849.
180. Wüst RC, Aliverti A, Capelli C, Kayser B. Breath-by-breath changes of lung oxygen stores at rest and during exercise in humans. *Respir Physiol Neurobiol.* 2008;164:291-299.
181. Beaver WL, Lamarra N, Wasserman K. Breath-by-breath measurement of true alveolar gas exchange. *J Appl Physiol Respir Environ Exerc Physiol.* 1981;51:1662-1675.
182. Barstow TJ, Buchthal S, Zanconato S, Cooper DM. Muscle energetics and pulmonary oxygen uptake kinetics during moderate exercise. *J Appl Physiol (1985).* 1994;74:1742-1749.
183. Mahler M. First-order kinetics of muscle oxygen consumption, and an equivalent proportionality between QO_2 and phosphorylcreatine level. Implications for the control of respiration. *J Gen Physiol.* 1985;86:135-165.
184. Rossiter HB, Ward SA, Doyle VL, Howe FA, Griffiths JR, Whipp BJ. Inferences from pulmonary O_2 uptake with respect to intramuscular [phosphocreatine] kinetics during moderate exercise in humans. *J Physiol.* 1999;518(pt 3):921-932.
185. Yoshida T, Watari H. ^{31}P-Nuclear magnetic resonance spectroscopy study of the time course of energy metabolism during exercise and recovery. *Eur J Appl Physiol Occup Physiol.* 1993;66:494-499.
186. Chance B, Mauriello G, Aubert XM. ADP arrival at muscle mitochondria following a twitch. In: Rodahl K, Horvath SM, eds. *Muscle as a Tissue.* New York, NY: McGraw-Hill; 1962.
187. Grassi B, Rossiter HB, Hogan MC, et al. Faster O_2 uptake kinetics in canine skeletal muscle in situ after acute creatine kinase inhibition. *J Physiol.* 2011;589 (pt 1):221-233.
188. Wüst RC, van der Laarse WJ, Rossiter HB. On–off asymmetries in oxygen consumption kinetics of single *Xenopus laevis* skeletal muscle fibres suggest higher-order control. *J Physiol.* 2013;591:731-744.
189. Hughson RL, Kowalchuk JM. Kinetics of oxygen uptake for submaximal exercise in hyperoxia, normoxia, and hypoxia. *Can J Appl Physiol.* 1995;20:198-210.
190. Koga S, Okushima D, Poole DC, Rossiter HB, Kondo N, Barstow TJ. Unaltered $\dot{V}O_2$ kinetics despite greater muscle oxygenation during heavy-intensity two-legged knee extension versus cycle exercise in humans. *Am J Physiol Regul Integr Comp Physiol.* 2019;317:R203-R213.
191. Sperandio PA, Oliveira MF, Rodrigues MK, et al. Sildenafil improves microvascular O_2 delivery-to-utilization matching and accelerates exercise O_2 uptake kinetics in chronic heart failure. *Am J Physiol Heart Circ Physiol.* 2012;303:H1474-H1480.
192. Özyener F, Rossiter HB, Ward SA, Whipp BJ. Influence of exercise intensity on the on- and off-transient kinetics of pulmonary oxygen uptake in humans. *J Physiol.* 2001;533(pt 3):891-902.
193. Poole DC, Ward SA, Gardner GW, Whipp BJ. Metabolic and respiratory profile of the upper limit for prolonged exercise in man. *Ergonomics.* 1988;31:1265-1279.
194. Poole DC, Burnley M, Vanhatalo A, Rossiter HB, Jones AM. Critical power: an important fatigue threshold in exercise physiology. *Med Sci Sports Exerc.* 2016;48:2320-2334.

195. Poole DC, Schaffartzik W, Knight DR, et al. Contribution of exercising legs to the slow component of oxygen uptake kinetics in humans. *J Appl Physiol (1985)*. 1991;71:1245-1260.
196. Poole DC, Gladden LB, Kurdak S, Hogan MC. L-(+)-lactate infusion into working dog gastrocnemius: no evidence lactate per se mediates $\dot{V}O_2$ slow component. *J Appl Physiol (1985)*. 1994;76:787-792.
197. Endo MY, Kobayakawa M, Kinugasa R, et al. Thigh muscle activation distribution and pulmonary VO_2 kinetics during moderate, heavy, and very heavy intensity cycling exercise in humans. *Am J Physiol Regul Integr Comp Physiol*. 2007;293:R812-R820.
198. Cannon DT, White AC, Andriano MF, Kolkhorst FW, Rossiter HB. Skeletal muscle fatigue precedes the slow component of oxygen uptake kinetics during exercise in humans. *J Physiol*. 2011;589(pt 3):727-739.
199. Keir DA, Copithorne DB, Hodgson MD, Pogliaghi S, Rice CL, Kowalchuk JM. The slow component of pulmonary O_2 uptake accompanies peripheral muscle fatigue during high-intensity exercise. *J Appl Physiol (1985)*. 2016;121:493-502.
200. Whipp BJ, Davis JA, Torres F, Wasserman K. A test to determine parameters of aerobic function during exercise. *J Appl Physiol Respir Environ Exerc Physiol*. 1981;50:217-221.
201. Whipp BJ, Seard C, Wasserman K. Oxygen deficit-oxygen debt relationships and efficiency of anaerobic work. *J Appl Physiol*. 1970;28:452-456.
202. Bangsbo J, Krustrup P, González-Alonso J, Saltin B. ATP production and efficiency of human skeletal muscle during intense exercise: effect of previous exercise. *Am J Physiol Endocrinol Metab*. 2001;280:E956-E964.
203. Wüst RC, Grassi B, Hogan MC, Howlett RA, Gladden LB, Rossiter HB. Kinetic control of oxygen consumption during contractions in self-perfused skeletal muscle. *J Physiol*. 2011;589:3995-4009.
204. Özyener F, Rossiter HB, Ward SA, Whipp BJ. Negative accumulated oxygen deficit during heavy and very heavy intensity cycle ergometry in humans. *Eur J Appl Physiol*. 2003;90:185-190.
205. Hill AV, Long CNH, Lupton H. Muscular exercise, lactic acid and the supply and utilisation of oxygen. Part VI. *Proc R Soc Lond*. 1924;97:127-137.
206. Schneider EG, Robinson S, Newton JL. Oxygen debt in aerobic work. *J Appl Physiol*. 1968;25:58-62.
207. Margaria R, Edwards HT, Dill DB. The possible mechanisms of contracting and paying the oxygen debt and the role of lactic acid in muscular contraction. *Am J Physiol*. 1933;106:689-715.
208. Chuang ML, Ting H, Otsuka T, et al. Aerobically generated CO_2 stored during early exercise. *J Appl Physiol (1985)*. 1999;87:1048-1058.
209. Wasserman K, Casaburi R. Acid-base regulation during exercise in humans. In: Whipp BJ, Wasserman K, eds. *Exercise: Pulmonary Physiology and Pathophysiology*. New York, NY: Decker; 1991:405-448.
210. Whipp BJ. Mechanisms dissociating pulmonary CO_2 and O_2 exchange dynamics during exercise. *Exp Physiol*. 2007;92:347-355.
211. Stringer WW, Wasserman K, Casaburi R. The Vco_2/Vo_2 relationship during heavy, constant work rate exercise reflects the rate of lactic acid accumulation. *Eur J Appl Physiol Occup Physiol*. 1995;72:25-31.
212. Monod H, Scherrer J. The work capacity of a synergic muscle group. *Ergonomics*. 1965;8:329-338.
213. Moritani T, Nagata A, deVries H, Muro M. Critical power as a measure of physical work capacity and anaerobic threshold. *Ergonomics*. 1981;24:339-350.
214. Jones AM, Wilkerson DP, DiMenna F, Fulford J, Poole DC. Muscle metabolic responses to exercise above and below the "critical power" assessed using ^{31}P-MRS. *Am J Physiol Regul Integr Comp Physiol*. 2008;294:R585-R593.
215. van der Vaart H, Murgatroyd SR, Rossiter HB, Chen C, Casaburi R, Porszasz J. Selecting constant work rates for endurance testing in COPD: the role of the power-duration relationship. *COPD*. 2014;11:267-276.
216. Ward SA. Discriminating features of responses in cardiopulmonary exercise testing. In: Ward SA, Palange P, eds. *Clinical Exercise Testing (ERS Monograph)*. Sheffield, United Kingdom: European Respiratory Society; 2007:36-68.
217. Broxterman RM, Craig JC, Smith JR, et al. Influence of blood flow occlusion on the development of peripheral and central fatigue during small muscle mass handgrip exercise. *J Physiol*. 2015;593:4043-4054.
218. Mezzani A, Corrà U, Giordano A, Colombo S, Psaroudaki M, Giannuzzi P. Upper intensity limit for prolonged aerobic exercise in chronic heart failure. *Med Sci Sports Exerc*. 2010;42:633-639.
219. Neder JA, Jones PW, Nery LE, Whipp BJ. Determinants of the exercise endurance capacity in patients with chronic obstructive pulmonary disease. The power-duration relationship. *Am J Respir Crit Care Med*. 2000;162(2 pt 1):497-504.
220. Murgatroyd SR, Ferguson C, Ward SA, Whipp BJ, Rossiter HB. Pulmonary O_2 uptake kinetics as a determinant of high-intensity exercise tolerance in humans. *J Appl Physiol (1985)*. 2011;110:1598-1606.
221. Valli G, Cogo A, Passino C, et al. Exercise intolerance at high altitude (5050 m): critical power and W′. *Respir Physiol Neurobiol*. 2011;177:333-341.
222. Poole DC, Ward SA, Whipp BJ. The effects of training on the metabolic and respiratory profile of high-intensity cycle ergometer exercise. *Eur J Appl Physiol Occup Physiol*. 1990;59:421-429.
223. Whipp BJ, Ward SA. Quantifying intervention-related improvements in exercise tolerance. *Eur Respir J*. 2009;33:1254-1260.
224. Puente-Maestu L, Palange P, Casaburi R, et al. Use of exercise testing in the evaluation of interventional efficacy: an official ERS statement. *Eur Respir J*. 2016;47:429-460.
225. Hsia CC. Respiratory function of hemoglobin. *N Engl J Med*. 1998;338:239-427.
226. Klocke RA. Carbon dioxide transport. In: Farhi LE, Tenney SM, eds. *Handbook of Physiology, Section 3: The Respiratory System, Vol IV: Gas Exchange*. Washington, DC: American Physiological Society; 1987:173-197.
227. Lindinger MI, Heigenhauser GJF. Effects of gas exchange on acid-base balance. *Compr Physiol*. 2012;2:2203-2254.
228. Forster HV, Haouzi P, Dempsey JA. Control of breathing during exercise. *Compr Physiol*. 2012;2:743-777.
229. Sun XG, Hansen JE, Stringer WW, Ting H, Wasserman K. Carbon dioxide pressure-concentration relationship in arterial and mixed venous blood during exercise. *J Appl Physiol (1985)*. 2001;90:1798-1810.
230. Whipp BJ, Ward SA. The coupling of ventilation to pulmonary gas exchange during exercise. In: Whipp BJ, Wasserman K, eds. *Exercise: Pulmonary Physiology and Pathophysiology*. New York, NY: Dekker; 1991:271-307.
231. Brown SE, Wiener S, Brown RA, Marcarelli PA, Light RW. Exercise performance following a carbohydrate load in chronic airflow obstruction. *J Appl Physiol (1985)*. 1985;58:1340-1346.
232. Sue DY, Chung MM, Grosvenor M, Wasserman K. Effect of altering the proportion of dietary fat and carbohydrate on exercise gas exchange in normal subjects. *Am Rev Respir Dis*. 1989;139:1430-1434.
233. Jones NL, McHardy GJR, Naimark A, Campbell EJM. Physiological dead space and alveolar-arterial gas pressure differences during exercise. *Clin Sci*. 1966;31:19-29.
234. Lamarra N, Whipp BJ, Ward SA. Physiological inferences from intra-breath measurement of pulmonary gas exchange. Paper presented at: Proceedings of the Annual International Conference of the IEEE Engineering in Medicine and Biology Society; November 4-7, 1988; New Orleans, LA.
235. Whipp BJ, Ward SA. Cardiopulmonary coupling during exercise. *J Exp Biol*. 1982;100:175-193.
236. Davis JA, Whipp BJ, Wasserman K. The relation of ventilation to metabolic rate during moderate exercise in man. *Eur J Appl Physiol Occup Physiol*.1980;44:97-108.
237. Neder JA, Berton DC, Arbex FF, et al. Physiological and clinical relevance of exercise ventilatory efficiency in COPD. *Eur Respir J*. 2017;49(3).
238. Sun XG, Hansen JE, Garatachea N, Storer TW, Wasserman K. Ventilatory efficiency during exercise in healthy subjects. *Am J Respir Crit Care Med*. 2002;166:1443-1448.

239. American Thoracic Society, American College of Chest Physicians. ATS/ACCP statement on cardiopulmonary exercise testing. *Am J Respir Crit Care Med*. 2003;167:211-277.
240. Palange P, Ward SA, Carlsen K-H, et al. Recommendations on the use of exercise testing in clinical practice. *Eur Respir J*. 2007;29:185-209.
241. Gallagher CG, Brown E, Younes M. Breathing pattern during maximal exercise and during submaximal exercise with hypercapnia. *J Appl Physiol (1987)*. 1987;63:238-244.
242. Whipp BJ, Pardy RL. Breathing during exercise. In: Macklem PT, Mead J, eds. *Handbook of Physiology, Section 3: The Respiratory System*. Washington, DC: American Physiological Society; 1986:605-629.
243. Cunningham DJC, Robbins PA, Wolff CB. Integration of respiratory responses to changes in alveolar partial pressures of CO_2 and O_2 and in arterial pH. In: Cherniack NS, Widdicombe JG, eds. *Handbook of Physiology, Section 3: The Respiratory System*. Vol 11. Bethesda, MD: American Physiological Society; 1986:475-528.
244. Dempsey JA, Adams L, Ainsworth DM, et al. Airway, lung and respiratory muscle function. In: Rowell LB, Shepherd JT, eds. *Handbook of Physiology, Section 12: Exercise: Regulation and Integration of Multiple Systems*. New York, NY: American Physiological Society; 1996:448-514.
245. Beck KC, Babb TG, Staats BA, Hyatt RE. Dynamics of breathing during exercise. In: Whipp BJ, Wasserman K, eds. *Exercise: Pulmonary Physiology and Pathophysiology*. New York, NY: Dekker; 1991:67-97.
246. Younes M. Determinants of thoracic excursions during exercise. In: Whipp BJ, Wasserman K, eds. *Exercise: Pulmonary Physiology and Pathophysiology*. New York, NY: Dekker; 1991:1-65.
247. Babb TG. Exercise ventilatory limitation: the role of expiratory flow limitation. *Exerc Sport Sci Rev*. 2013;41:11-18.
248. Sheel AW, Romer LM. Ventilation and respiratory mechanics. *Compr Physiol*. 2012;2:1093-1142.
249. Ward SA. Regulation of breathing during exercise. In: Granger DN, Granger JP, eds. *Colloquium Series on Integrated Systems Physiology: The Respiratory System*. Princeton, NJ: Morgan & Claypool Life Sciences; 2014:1-91.
250. Dempsey JA, Smith CA. Pathophysiology of human ventilatory control. *Eur Respir J*. 2014;44:495-512.
251. Whipp BJ. Control of the exercise hyperpnea: the unanswered question. *Adv Exp Med Biol*. 2008;605:16-21.
252. Duffin J. The fast exercise drive to breathe. *J Physiol*. 2014;592(pt 3):445-451.
253. Paterson DJ. Defining the neurocircuitry of exercise hyperpnoea. *J Physiol*. 2014;592:433-444.
254. Haouzi P. Tracking pulmonary gas exchange by breathing control during exercise: role of muscle blood flow. *J Physiol*. 2014;592:453-461.
255. Kaufman MP, Forster HV. Reflexes controlling circulatory, ventilatory and airway responses to exercise. In: Rowell LB, Shepherd JT, eds. *Handbook of Physiology, Section 12: Exercise: Regulation and Integration of Multiple Systems*. New York, NY: American Physiological Society; 1996:381-447.
256. Cummin ARC, Iyawe VI, Mehta N, Saunders KB. Ventilation and cardiac output during the onset of exercise, and during voluntary hyperventilation, in humans. *J Physiol* 1986;370:567-583.
257. Miyamoto Y, Hiura T, Tamura T, Nakamura T, Higuchi J, Mikami T. Dynamics of cardiac, respiratory, and metabolic function in men in response to step work load. *J Appl Physiol Respir Environ Exerc Physiol*. 1982;52:1198-1208.
258. Banner N, Guz A, Heaton R, Innes JA, Murphy K, Yacoub M. Ventilatory and circulatory responses at the onset of exercise in man following heart or heart-lung transplantation. *J Physiol*. 1988;399:437-449.
259. Theodore J, Morris AJ, Burke CM, et al. Cardiopulmonary function at maximum tolerable constant work rate exercise following human heart-lung transplantation. *Chest*. 1987;92:433-439.
260. Huszczuk A, Whipp BJ, Adams TD, et al. Ventilatory control during exercise in calves with artificial hearts. *J Appl Physiol (1985)*. 1990;68:2604-2611.
261. Parkes MJ. Reappraisal of systemic venous chemoreceptors: might they explain the matching of breathing to metabolic rate in humans? *Exp Physiol*. 2017;102:1567-1583.
262. DuBois AB, Britt AG, Fenn WO. Alveolar CO_2 during the respiratory cycle. *J Appl Physiol*. 1952;4:535-548.
263. Whipp BJ. Peripheral chemoreceptor control of exercise hyperpnea in humans. *Med Sci Sports Exerc*. 1994;26:337-347.
264. Whipp BJ, Wasserman K. Carotid bodies and ventilatory control dynamics in man. *Fed Proc*. 1980;39:2668-2673.
265. Winter B. Bilateral carotid body resection for asthma and emphysema. A new surgical approach without hypoventilation or baroreceptor dysfunction. *Int Surg*. 1972;57:458-466.
266. Paterson DJ. Potassium and ventilation in exercise. *J Appl Physiol (1985)*. 1992;72:811-820.
267. Shea SA, Andres LP, Shannon DC, Banzett RB. Ventilatory responses to exercise in humans lacking ventilatory chemosensitivity. *J Physiol*. 1993;468:623-640.
268. Adams L, Frankel H, Garlick J, Guz A, Murphy K, Semple SJ. The role of spinal cord transmission in the ventilatory response to exercise in man. *J Physiol*. 1984;355:85-97.
269. Brice AG, Forster HV, Pan LG, et al. Is the hyperpnea of muscular contractions critically dependent on spinal afferents? *J Appl Physiol (1985)*. 1988;64:226-233.
270. Brown DR, Forster HV, Pan LG, et al. Ventilatory response of spinal cord-lesioned subjects to electrically induced exercise. *J Appl Physiol (1985)*. 1990;68:2312-2321.
271. Swanson GD. Redundancy structures in respiratory control. In: Honda Y, Miyamoto Y, Konno K, Widdicombe JG, eds. *Control of Breathing and Its Modelling Perspective*. New York, NY: Plenum Press; 1992:171-177.
272. Babb TG, Wood HE, Mitchell GS. Short- and long-term modulation of the exercise ventilatory response. *Med Sci Sports Exerc*. 2010;42:1681-1687.
273. Grodins FS, Yamashiro SM. Optimization of the mammalian respiratory gas transport system. *Annu Rev Biophys Bioeng*. 1973;2:115-130.
274. Yamamoto WS. Information systems approach to integrated responses in the respiratory control system. *Ann Biomed Eng*. 1983;11:349-360.
275. Poon CS. Evolving paradigms in H^+ control of breathing: from homeostatic regulation to homeostatic competition. *Respir Physiol Neurobiol*. 2011;179:122-126.
276. Swanson GD, Robbins PA. Optimal respiratory controller structures. *IEEE Trans Biomed Eng*. 1986;33:677-680.
277. Moosavi SH, Guz A, Adams L. Repeated exercise paired with "imperceptible" dead space loading does not alter VE of subsequent exercise in humans. *J Appl Physiol*. 2002;92:1159-1168.
278. Turner DL, Sumners DP. Associative conditioning of the exercise ventilatory response in humans. *Respir Physiol Neurobiol*. 2002;132:159-168.
279. Wood HE, Fatemian M, Robbins PA. A learned component of the ventilatory response to exercise in man. *J Physiol*. 2003;553(pt 3):967-974.
280. Sutton JR, Jones NL. Control of pulmonary ventilation during exercise and mediators in the blood: CO_2 and hydrogen ion. *Med Sci Sports*. 1979;11:198–203.
281. Hagberg JM, Coyle EF, Carroll JE, Miller JM, Martin WH, Brooke MH. Exercise hyperventilation in patients with McArdle's disease. *J Appl Physiol Respir Environ Exerc Physiol*. 1982;52:991-994.
282. Scheuermann BW, Kowalchuk JM. Attenuated respiratory compensation during rapidly incremented ramp exercise. *Respir Physiol*. 1998;114:227-238.
283. Rausch SM, Whipp BJ, Wasserman K, Huszczuk A. Role of the carotid bodies in the respiratory compensation for the metabolic acidosis of exercise in humans. *J Physiol*. 1991;444:567-578.
284. Teppema LJ, Barts PWJA, Evers JAM. Effects of metabolic arterial pH changes on medullary ecf pH, csf pH and ventilation in peripherally chemodenervated cats with intact blood-brain barrier. *Respir Physiol*. 1984;58:123-136.
285. Ward SA. Control of the exercise hyperpnea. *Curr Opin Physiol*. 2019;10:166-172.
286. Stringer W, Hansen J, Wasserman K. Cardiac output estimated noninvasively from oxygen uptake during exercise. *J Appl Physiol (1985)*. 1997;82:908-912.

CHAPTER 3

Measurements During Integrative Cardiopulmonary Exercise Testing

Cardiopulmonary exercise testing (abbreviated as CPET or CPX) evaluates the ability of the cardiovascular and respiratory systems to perform their major functions during progressive or incremental exercise, that is, gas exchange between the cells and the environment.[1-3] As described in Chapter 2, exercise requires an integrative cardiopulmonary response to support the increase in muscle respiration required for exercise. Therefore, gas exchange measurements are fundamental to the understanding of the pathophysiology of exercise limitation. It is evident from the scheme shown in **Figure 1.1** that a reduction in maximal (peak) oxygen uptake ($\dot{V}O_2$max, peak $\dot{V}O_2$) can be caused by any disease process affecting skeletal muscle function or the organ systems needed to transport O_2 and CO_2 between the air and the muscle cell. Use of CPET to determine only $\dot{V}O_2$max or peak $\dot{V}O_2$, as is sometimes done, fails to employ CPET to its fullest capacity, that is, to define the pathophysiology of exercise limitation. This chapter describes measurements obtained from CPET that are useful when assessing the responses of each of the organ systems that couple external respiration (O_2 uptake [$\dot{V}O_2$] and CO_2 output [$\dot{V}CO_2$] at the airway) to cellular respiration (O_2 consumption and CO_2 production of the cells) during exercise.

Because CPET can be performed for a variety of reasons ranging, for example, from diagnosis, identification of the contributions of different organ systems to impairment, risk assessment for future complications, and determining prognosis, each CPET can be viewed as having specific clinical-physiological questions to be addressed, as shown in **Table 3.1**. In this table, the questions are paired with variables that should be helpful in answering these questions.

Conversely, **Table 3.2** links specific measurements made during CPET to physiological function or dysfunction. Fortunately, most measurements can be made noninvasively and can be performed in modern cardiology or cardiopulmonary function laboratories. In addition to the individual measured variables, many are combined as calculated variables—for example, oxygen pulse ($\dot{V}O_2$/heart rate), ventilatory equivalent for CO_2 ($\dot{V}E/\dot{V}CO_2$), physiological dead space–tidal volume ratio (V_D/V_T)—or further incorporated into more complex relationships over defined regions of the exercise test, such as the slope of $\dot{V}O_2$ versus work rate (WR) or the slope of $\dot{V}E$ versus $\dot{V}CO_2$. Finally, "patterns" of these variables provide further insight into pathophysiology, such as the identification of the anaerobic threshold (*AT*) or the determination of probable ventilatory limitation to exercise.

Valuable insights into pathophysiology and grading of severity of impairment are provided by the measurements described in this chapter, especially as these are related to the physiology of exercise (see Chapter 2), the optimal presentation of data (see Chapter 6), and the comparison to normal values (see Chapter 7). More details about methods of measurement, calculations, calibration, and assessment of accuracy are described in Chapter 5 and Appendix C.

A CPET is useful because it enables the examiner to (1) quantify the level of the individual's exercise limitation, (2) assess the adequacy of the performance of various components in the coupling of pulmonary to cellular gas exchange, (3) determine the organ system limiting exercise,

TABLE 3.1 Questions Addressed by Cardiopulmonary Exercise Testing

Question	Disorder	Markers of abnormality[a]
Is exercise capacity reduced?	Any disorder	Maximal or peak $\dot{V}O_2$ (panel 1)
Is the metabolic requirement for exercise increased?	Obesity	$\dot{V}O_2$–WR relationship (panel 1)
Is exercise limited by impaired O_2 flow?	Ischemic, myopathic, valvular, congenital heart disease	ECG; *AT*; $\Delta\dot{V}O_2/\Delta WR$; $\dot{V}O_2/HR$ (panels 1-3)
	Pulmonary vascular disease	$\Delta\dot{V}O_2/\Delta WR$; *AT*; $\dot{V}O_2/HR$; $\dot{V}E/\dot{V}CO_2$ at *AT*; $\dot{V}E$-$\dot{V}CO_2$ slope (panels 1-3, 4, 6)
	Peripheral arterial disease	BP; $\Delta\dot{V}O_2/\Delta WR$; $\Delta\dot{V}CO_2/\Delta WR$ (panels 1, 5)
	Anemia, hypoxemia, elevated COHb	$\dot{V}O_2/HR$ (panels 1-3, 7)
Is exercise limited by reduced ventilatory capacity?	Lung; chest wall	BR; ventilatory and breathing pattern response (panels 1, 4, 7, 9)
Is there an abnormal degree of $\dot{V}A/\dot{Q}$ mismatching?	Lung disease; pulmonary vascular disease; heart failure	$P(A - a)O_2$; $P(a - ET)CO_2$; VD/VT; $\dot{V}E/\dot{V}CO_2$ at *AT*; $\dot{V}E$-$\dot{V}CO_2$ slope (panels 4, 6, 7)
Is there a defect in muscle utilization of O_2 or substrate?	Muscle glycolytic or mitochondrial enzyme defect	*AT*, R, $\dot{V}CO_2$; HR versus $\dot{V}O_2$; [lactate]; [lactate]-[pyruvate] ratio (panels 1-3, 8)
Is exercise limited by a behavioral problem?	Psychogenic dyspnea; hysteria	Ventilatory and breathing pattern responses; $PETO_2$; $PETCO_2$ (panels 1, 7-9)
Is work output reduced because of poor effort?	Poor effort with secondary gain	Increased HRR; increased BR; peak R <1.0; normal *AT*, $P(A - a)O2$ and $P(a - ET)CO_2$ (panels 1-3, 8, 9)

Abbreviations: *AT*, anaerobic threshold; BP, blood pressure; BR, breathing reserve (maximum voluntary ventilation minus ventilation at maximum exercise); COHb, carboxyhemoglobin; $\Delta\dot{V}CO_2/\Delta WR$, increase in $\dot{V}CO_2$ relative to increase in work rate; $\Delta\dot{V}O_2/\Delta WR$, increase in $\dot{V}O_2$ relative to increase in work rate; ECG, electrocardiogram; HR, heart rate; HRR, heart rate reserve (predicted maximum heart rate minus maximum exercise heart rate); O_2, oxygen; $P(A - a)O_2$, alveolar-arterial PO_2 difference; $P(a - ET)CO_2$, arterial-end-tidal PCO_2 difference; peak $\dot{V}O_2$, highest O_2 uptake measured; $PETCO_2$, end-tidal PCO_2; $PETO_2$, end-tidal PO_2; R, respiratory exchange ratio ($\dot{V}CO_2/\dot{V}O_2$); VD/VT, physiological dead space-tidal volume ratio; $\dot{V}E/\dot{V}CO_2$ at *AT*, ventilatory equivalent for carbon dioxide at anaerobic threshold; $\dot{V}E$-$\dot{V}CO_2$ slope, slope of $\dot{V}E$-$\dot{V}CO_2$ relationship; $\dot{V}O_2/HR$, O_2 pulse; $\dot{V}A/\dot{Q}$, ventilation-perfusion ratio; WR, work rate.

[a]Panel numbers refer to case study plots in Chapter 10.

and (4) determine the $\dot{V}O_2$ at which exercise limitation occurs. These evaluations can be addressed during a short (approximately 10 min), progressive, nonsteady state (ie, incremental or ramp) exercise test, rather than during a more prolonged test with increments of relatively long duration. Prolonged testing is more likely to delay recovery of the patient, thereby making it more difficult for the investigator to repeat exercise testing if required. What makes CPET especially valuable is that it amplifies abnormalities in cardiopulmonary function and brings out abnormalities that are only present during exercise (eg, exercise-induced myocardial ischemia).

MEASUREMENTS

Electrocardiographic Changes With Exercise

Myocardial ischemia results from an inadequate O_2 supply to the myocardium to meet the O_2 needed in support of increased cardiac work. When the myocardium becomes anaerobic, it alters its ionic permeability. Thus, the rate of reestablishing the electrical membrane potential during repolarization is slowed in the ischemic areas of the myocardium. This causes the T wave and ST segments to change acutely when the O_2 requirement for the increased cardiac work of exercise exceeds the availability of O_2 (**Table 3.3**). Because exercise causes the heart rate (HR) to increase and the diastolic time to shorten, the time for coronary perfusion is decreased. Thus, coronary artery disease is more likely to be electrographically detected during exercise when the HR and the rate-pressure product are increasing.[4-7]

An increased frequency of ectopic beats, as the work rate increases, is also suggestive of myocardial ischemia. However, some individuals manifest occasional premature ventricular or atrial contractions at rest that disappear or become less frequent during exercise. Such ectopic beats appear to be benign and unrelated to a disturbance in the balance between myocardial O_2 availability and requirement because they are overridden by the sinus tachycardia of exercise.

In many instances, false-positive and borderline changes occur in the electrocardiogram (ECG) when one relies solely on changes in the T wave and ST segments to detect exercise-induced myocardial ischemia. When these ECG changes are accompanied by myocardial dyskinesis, $\dot{V}O_2$ may fail to increase appropriately for the increasing work rate. Thus, a reduction in the $\dot{V}O_2$–WR slope ($\Delta\dot{V}O_2/\Delta WR$) accompanied by ECG changes consistent with myocardial ischemia, with or without angina, strengthens the diagnosis of coronary artery disease involving a significant mass

TABLE 3.2 Assessing Function With Physiological Measurements

Measurements	Function
Electrocardiogram	Myocardial O_2 availability-requirement balance
$\dot{V}O_2$	Cardiac output × $C(a - \bar{v})O_2$
Peak $\dot{V}O_2$	Highest $\dot{V}O_2$ achieved during presumed maximal effort for an incremental exercise test (specific for type of exercise); may or may not equal $\dot{V}O_2max$
$\dot{V}O_2max$	Highest $\dot{V}O_2$ achievable as evidenced by failure for $\dot{V}O_2$ to increase despite increasing WR (specific for type of exercise); highest cardiac output × $C(a - \bar{v})O_2$
$\Delta\dot{V}O_2/\Delta WR$	Aerobic contribution to exercise (low value suggests high anaerobic contribution); normally 10 mL/min/W
Cardiac output	Useful when evaluating hemodynamics
Anaerobic threshold (*AT*)	Highest $\dot{V}O_2$ that can be sustained without developing a lactic acidosis; important determinant of potential for endurance work (specific for form of exercise)
O_2 pulse	Product of SV and $C(a - \bar{v})O_2$; under conditions when SV is constant, change in O_2 pulse is proportional to change in $C(a - \bar{v})O_2$
Heart rate reserve (HRR)	Difference between predicted peak and measured heart rate at peak $\dot{V}O_2$
Arterial pressure	Detecting systemic hypertension, ventricular outflow obstruction, or myocardial failure (pulsus alternans or decreasing pressure with increasing WR)
$\dot{V}E = \dot{V}A + \dot{V}D$	$\dot{V}D$ is increased due to mismatching of $\dot{V}A$ to $\dot{Q}$. $\dot{V}A$ is inversely related to $PaCO_2$, whether caused by a low $PaCO_2$ set point, metabolic acidosis, or hypoxemia.
BR = MVV − $\dot{V}E$ at max exercise, or (MVV − $\dot{V}E$ at max exercise) / MVV	Breathing reserve; theoretical additional $\dot{V}E$ available at cessation of exercise
Exercise V_D/V_T; $\dot{V}E$-$\dot{V}CO_2$ slope or $\dot{V}E/\dot{V}CO_2$ at the *AT* or VCP	Measures of mismatching of $\dot{V}A$ to $\dot{Q}$
$P(a - ET)CO_2$	Detects high $\dot{V}A/\dot{Q}$ components of lung with mismatching of $\dot{V}A/\dot{Q}$
$P(A - a)O_2$	Increased in presence of $\dot{V}A/\dot{Q}$ mismatching, diffusion defect, and/or right-to-left shunt
Expired flow pattern	Useful for indicating presence of significant airflow obstruction
V_T/IC	Fraction of the inspiratory capacity used in breathing
Immediate $\dot{V}O_2$ increase (phase I) in response to constant WR exercise	Ability to increase pulmonary blood flow at start of constant WR exercise (phase I)
$\Delta\dot{V}O_2$ (6 − 3)	Positive for constant WR exercise above *AT* and proportional to arterial [lactate] increase
Magnitude of transient decrease (nadir) in $\dot{V}E$ during abrupt switch to 100% O_2 breathing	Contribution of the carotid body chemoreflex to ventilatory drive

Abbreviations: BR, breathing reserve; $C(a - \bar{v})O_2$, arterial-mixed venous O_2 content difference; $\Delta\dot{V}O_2$ (6 − 3), difference between $\dot{V}O_2$ at 6 and 3 min during constant work rate exercise; IC, inspiratory capacity; MVV, maximal voluntary ventilation; O_2, oxygen; $PaCO_2$, arterial PCO_2; $\dot{Q}$, pulmonary perfusion; SV, stroke volume; $\dot{V}A$, alveolar ventilation; V_D, physiological dead space; $\dot{V}CO_2$, carbon dioxide output; VCP, ventilatory compensation point; $\dot{V}D$, physiological dead space ventilation; $\dot{V}E$, ventilation; $\dot{V}O_2$, oxygen uptake; $\dot{V}O_2max$, maximal oxygen uptake; V_T, tidal volume; WR, work rate.

of myocardium. The diagnosis of ischemic heart disease is further supported if systemic blood pressure decreases or HR increases disproportionately to $\dot{V}O_2$ in the presence of ECG changes characteristic of myocardial ischemia during exercise.

TABLE 3.3 Electrocardiographic Evidence of Myocardial Ischemia During Exercise

ST segment changes
T wave changes
Premature ventricular contractions that appear during exercise

Maximal and Peak Oxygen Uptake

The body clearly has an upper limit for O_2 utilization at a particular state of fitness or training and the size of the muscle group employed in the task. As discussed in Chapter 2 ("Cardiovascular Responses to Exercise" section), this is usually determined by the maximal cardiac output, the arterial O_2 content, the fractional distribution of the cardiac output to the exercising muscle, and the ability of the muscle to extract O_2. The ventilatory capacity determines the upper limit of $\dot{V}O_2$ only when ventilation ($\dot{V}E$) is insufficient to eliminate the CO_2 produced by aerobic metabolism and that resulting from bicarbonate (HCO_3^-) buffering of the metabolic (largely lactic) acidosis.[8]

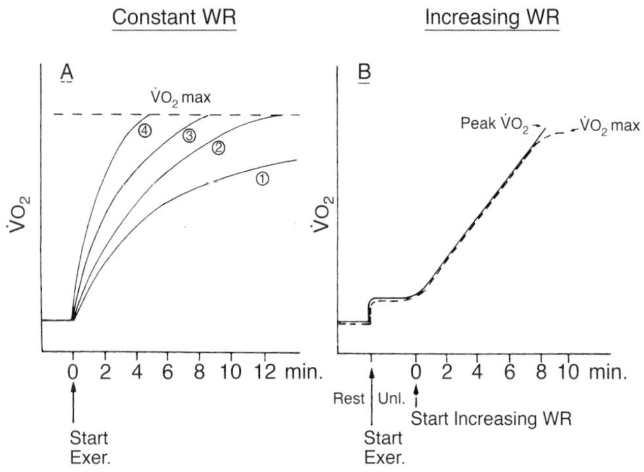

FIGURE 3.1. A: Determining the maximal oxygen uptake ($\dot{V}O_2max$) from supramaximal work rate (WR) tests. The time course of $\dot{V}O_2$ following the onset of exercise is shown for progressively higher WRs. For WR 1, the oxygen uptake ($\dot{V}O_2$) asymptote is below $\dot{V}O_2max$. The WR 2 reaches a $\dot{V}O_2$ that is the same as the highest $\dot{V}O_2$ reached by WRs 3 and 4. Because the end-exercise $\dot{V}O_2$ is the same for WRs 2, 3, and 4, this value identifies $\dot{V}O_2max$ for the modality of exercise studied. B: Distinguishing between $\dot{V}O_2max$ and peak $\dot{V}O_2$ from a maximal-effort incremental exercise test. When the subject's maximum tolerable WR results in a flattening of the $\dot{V}O_2$–WR relationship, this defines the subject's $\dot{V}O_2max$. When the rate of rise of $\dot{V}O_2$ does not slow with increasing WR despite the subject reaching his or her maximum tolerable WR, the highest $\dot{V}O_2$ attained is the peak $\dot{V}O_2$.

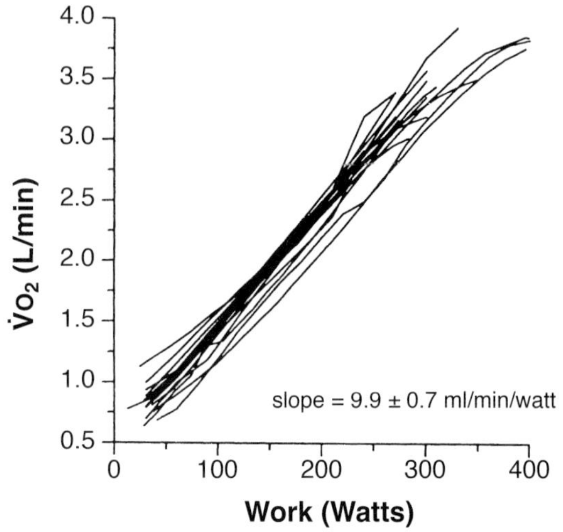

FIGURE 3.2. The relationship between oxygen uptake ($\dot{V}O_2$) and work rate during incremental cycle ergometer exercise for 17 normal individuals. The average regression slope and standard deviation are given in the equation. The slope is consistent among subjects but is displaced upward depending on body weight, as shown in Figures 2.8 and 3.6. *(Republished with permission of John Wiley & Sons, Inc. from Wasserman K, Sue DY. Coupling of external to cellular respiration. In: Wasserman K, ed.* Exercise Gas Exchange in Heart Disease. *Armonk, NY: Futura Publishing; 1996:1-15; permission conveyed through Copyright Clearance Center, Inc.)*

Maximal aerobic power (ie, maximal $\dot{V}O_2$ or $\dot{V}O_2max$) was originally measured using a series of discontinuous fatiguing constant work rate tests, each with a large increase in work rate, with intervening rest periods. It is defined as the $\dot{V}O_2$ at which performance of increasing levels of fatiguing constant work rate exercise fail to increase $\dot{V}O_2$ by 150 mL/min, despite increasing work rate.[9] This is schematized in **Figure 3.1A** and shown experimentally in **Figure 2.7**.

The advantages of determining $\dot{V}O_2max$ from discrete constant work rate tests are the following:

1. The higher intensity work rates can be selected based on the patient's responses to the lower work rate tests.
2. Timed manual bag collection of mixed expired gas for measurement of $\dot{V}O_2$ and $\dot{V}CO_2$ near the end of each test does not require rapidly responding gas analyzers.
3. The failure of $\dot{V}O_2$ to increase despite an increase in work rate provides unequivocal identification of $\dot{V}O_2max$.

The disadvantages of determining $\dot{V}O_2max$ from discrete constant work rate tests are the following:

1. The considerable time commitment required of the patient, physician, and technician
2. The tests are exhausting and may prove challenging for the patient.
3. Although such tests are often considered steady-state tests, this is not the case for work rates that exceed the *AT*.
4. The $\dot{V}O_2max$ definition has shortcomings because it is dependent on the exercise protocol and because 150 mL/min is a large fraction of the highest $\dot{V}O_2$ obtained in many patients.

The maximal $\dot{V}O_2$ may also be determined in an incremental exercise test by observing that $\dot{V}O_2$ fails to increase normally relative to the increase in work rate (<10 mL/min/W) just before the individual fatigues (**Figs. 3.1B** and **3.2**). However, flattening of the $\dot{V}O_2$–WR relationship, as peak $\dot{V}O_2$ is approached, is often not seen in incremental exercise tests (see **Fig. 3.2**). This highest $\dot{V}O_2$ is called the peak $\dot{V}O_2$ and is the terminology used to describe the highest $\dot{V}O_2$ achieved in an incremental exercise test. The highest $\dot{V}O_2$ may also be regarded as the maximal $\dot{V}O_2$ when $\dot{V}O_2$ fails to increase normally over the last 60 seconds of exercise just prior to fatigue—that is, $\dot{V}O_2$ fails to increase further despite an increase in work rate (see **Fig. 3.2**). Although the peak $\dot{V}O_2$ does not satisfy the definition of the maximal $\dot{V}O_2$ determined from repeated fatiguing constant work rate tests, it is usually equal to the actual $\dot{V}O_2max$ in normal individuals. The distinction between $\dot{V}O_2max$ and peak $\dot{V}O_2$ is diagrammed in **Figure 3.1**.

However, a strategy has been developed that allows $\dot{V}O_2peak$ to be identified as $\dot{V}O_2max$ from a standard ramp incremental (RI) test modified to include an additional subsequent verification phase, despite no plateau being evident in $\dot{V}O_2$.[10] That is, following the completion of the ramp test and a 5-minute recovery at 20 W, the subject then completes a step exercise (SE) phase to the limit of tolerance at 105% of the peak work rate achieved on the ramp test. Despite the higher work rate, $\dot{V}O_2$ rose no higher than $\dot{V}O_2peak$, thus establishing the plateau criterion (see **Fig. 3.3**). This "RISE" test has been used successfully in healthy individuals and also in heart failure patients.[11]

In summary, a similar $\dot{V}O_2$ during a series of supramaximal constant work rate tests or an incremental exercise

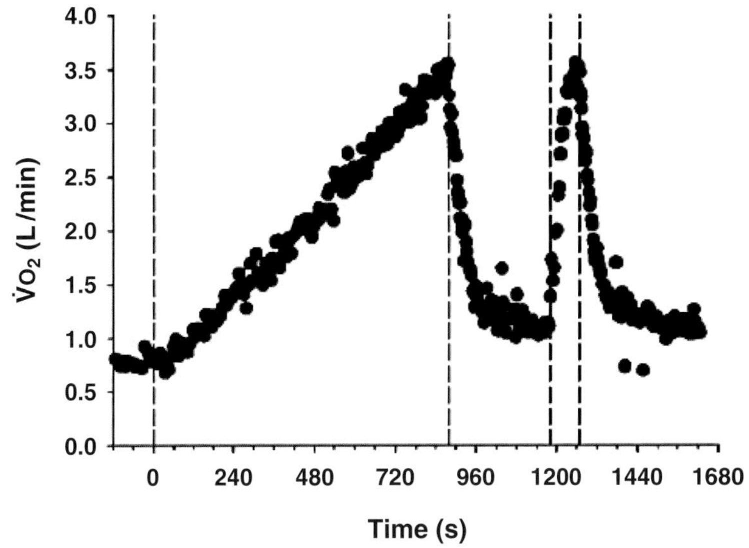

FIGURE 3.3. Oxygen uptake ($\dot{V}O_2$) profile (5-breath average) for a healthy individual during the ramp incremental (RI) and step exercise (SE) components of the RISE protocol. Dashed vertical lines show the start and end of the RI and SE components. *(Reproduced with permission from Rossiter HB, Kowalchuk JM, Whipp BJ. A test to establish maximum O_2 uptake despite no plateau in the O_2 uptake response to ramp incremental exercise. J Appl Physiol. 2006;100[3]:764-770. Copyright © 2006 American Physiological Society. All rights reserved.)*

test shows that a $\dot{V}O_2$max has, in fact, been attained. In studies on normal individuals performing incremental exercise to the limit of tolerance, only about one-third reach a plateau in $\dot{V}O_2$ (see **Fig. 3.2**). That is, after reaching their peak $\dot{V}O_2$, many individuals cannot endure the discomfort long enough to achieve a plateau in the $\dot{V}O_2$ response (see Chapter 2, "Power-Duration Curve and Critical Power" section). For normal children, the regression equations and scaling factors for those who did not reach a plateau were indistinguishable from those children who reached a plateau.[12]

A plateau in $\dot{V}O_2$ may also fail to occur during an incremental exercise test when the subject stops exercising because of leg or chest pain, shortness of breath, mechanical limitation to breathing, or lack of motivation. In these instances, the peak $\dot{V}O_2$ will not satisfy the definition of $\dot{V}O_2$max.

An incremental exercise test, as described in Chapter 5 and as illustrated in **Figures 3.1B** and **3.2**, has several advantages over high-intensity constant work rate testing:

1. The test starts out at a relatively low work rate so that it does not require the abrupt application of great muscle force with its associated sudden, large cardiorespiratory stress.
2. The $\dot{V}O_2$max or peak $\dot{V}O_2$ can be determined from a test in which the period of increasing work rate lasts only 8 to 12 minutes.
3. The subject is stressed for only a few minutes at relatively high work rates.
4. The $\dot{V}O_2$–WR relationship can be determined if the ergometer work rate can be measured, such as for the cycle.

To obtain the best data for interpreting the measured responses to an incremental exercise test, the work rate increments should be uniform in magnitude and duration, and imposed relatively rapidly. This means that the ergometer must be accurately calibrated and work rate should increase linearly with time.

The peak $\dot{V}O_2$ is the first measurement to be examined because it establishes whether the patient's physiological responses allow normal maximal aerobic function. Other measurements are then used to differentiate the cause of exercise limitation whether or not the subject reaches his or her predicted peak $\dot{V}O_2$.

Oxygen Uptake and Work Rate

Although $\dot{V}O_2$ measurements are made from respired gas measured at the mouth, the increase in $\dot{V}O_2$ reflects O_2 utilization by the muscle cells performing the work of exercise (see Chapter 2, "Oxygen Cost of Work" section). The $\dot{V}O_2$–WR relationship describes how much O_2 is used by the exercising subject in relation to the quantity of external work performed. Because this relationship gives important information concerning the coupling of external to internal (cellular) respiration, it is valuable also to graph $\dot{V}O_2$ and work rate as a function of time and to measure the ability of $\dot{V}O_2$ to track the increase in work rate. The coupling of external respiration to cellular respiration is the responsibility of the cardiovascular system. Therefore, disease of some component of the cardiovascular system will result in an abnormal pattern of $\dot{V}O_2$ in response to incremental exercise, characteristic of that component.

Normal Subjects

As described in Chapter 2 ("Oxygen Uptake Kinetics" section), following a short delay-like phase reflective of the underlying $\dot{V}O_2$ response kinetics, $\dot{V}O_2$ increases smoothly during cycle ergometry when work rate is increased relatively rapidly in a continuous ramp pattern or incrementally in equal steps of 1-minute duration (**Fig. 3.4**). This type of protocol has advantages in that work rate increments are small and therefore not readily perceptible, in contrast to when the work rate is incremented at the same rate but less frequently (eg, every 2 or 3 min) and therefore with larger (and more abrupt) changes in work rate. Because $\dot{V}O_2$

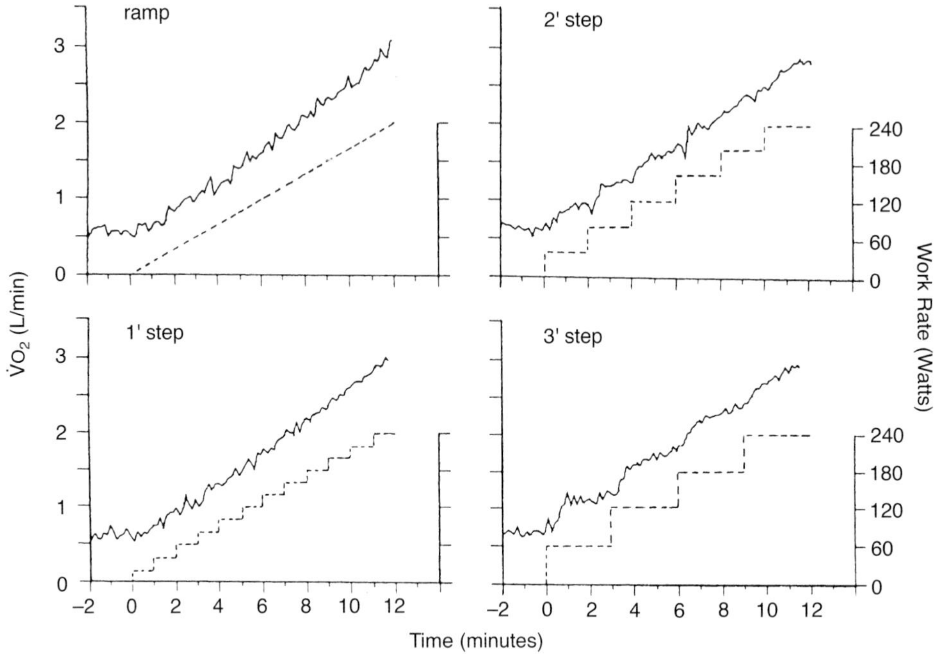

FIGURE 3.4. The oxygen uptake ($\dot{V}O_2$) response in a single individual to four different cycle ergometer protocols having the same average work rate incrementation rate with respect to time: ramp and 1-, 2-, and 3-minute increments. The dashed lines show the profile of work rate increase with time. The corresponding $\dot{V}O_2$ data are the average of 9-s periods. *(Reprinted with permission from Zhang YY, Johnson MC II, Chow N, Wasserman K. Effect of exercise testing protocol on parameters of aerobic function.* Med Sci Sports Exerc. *1991;23[5]:625-630. Copyright © 1991 The American College of Sports Medicine.)*

normally attains a steady state following imposition of a sub-*AT* constant work rate within about 3 minutes (ie, with a $\dot{V}O_2$ time constant of 35-45 s—the time to attain 63% of the final response) (see **Figs. 2.35** and **2.40**) (see Chapter 2, "Oxygen Uptake Kinetics" section), a ramp or a 1-minute incremental test will yield a smooth increase in $\dot{V}O_2$ as the work rate increases (see **Fig. 3.4**).[13] However, a stepped $\dot{V}O_2$ response profile emerges as step duration is increased (ie, there now being sufficient time on each step for $\dot{V}O_2$ to approach or even achieve its steady state value) (see **Fig. 3.4**).[13] Thus, the slope of the increase in $\dot{V}O_2$ relative to work rate ($\Delta\dot{V}O_2/\Delta WR$) can be calculated with either the ramp or 1-minute incremental exercise test[13] and, as shown in **Figure 3.2**, the normal $\Delta\dot{V}O_2/\Delta WR$ is equal to about 10 mL/min/W. Interestingly, the stepped $\dot{V}O_2$ profile characteristic of longer increment durations (eg, 3 min) becomes damped above the *AT*, reflecting the influence of the $\dot{V}O_2$ slow component, which has considerably slower kinetics than the sub-*AT* response (see **Figs. 2.35** and **2.40**) (see Chapter 2, "Oxygen Uptake Kinetics" section). This "stepped" effect is predictably less marked for endurance-fit individuals, in whom $\dot{V}O_2$ kinetics are typically more rapid (see **Fig 3.5**).[14]

Upward Displacement of $\dot{V}O_2$ as a Function of Work Rate in Obesity

The position of the $\dot{V}O_2$–WR relationship depends on body weight (**Fig. 3.6A**). For example, obese individuals require increased $\dot{V}O_2$ to do a given amount of external work (see Chapter 2, "Oxygen Cost of Work" section). This reflects the added O_2 cost to move the limbs during cycle ergometry and the cost of moving the entire body during treadmill exercise. Based on two separate studies of cycle ergometer exercise on adults, $\dot{V}O_2$ during unloaded cycling at 60 rpm was found to be displaced upward by approximately 5.8 mL/min/kg of body weight.[15,16] Although

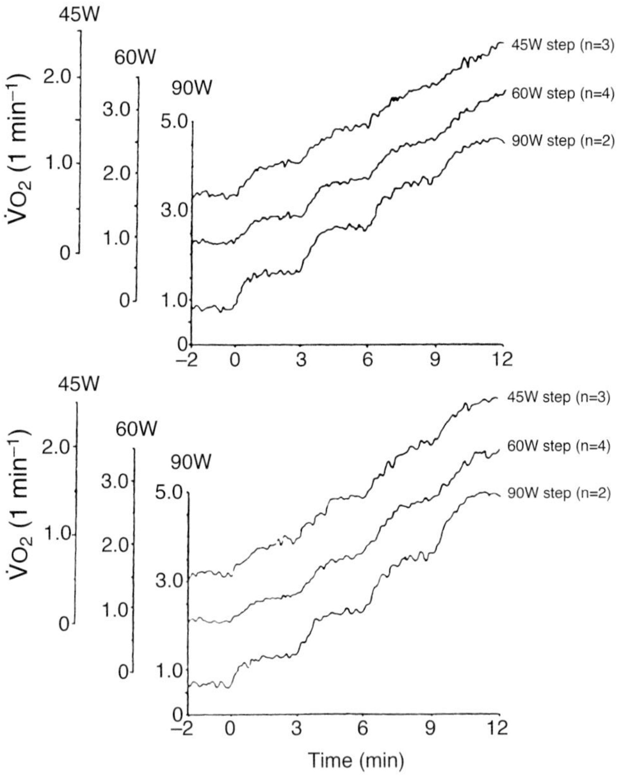

FIGURE 3.5. The average time courses of oxygen uptake ($\dot{V}O_2$) and carbon dioxide output ($\dot{V}CO_2$) for a 3-min incremental cycle ergometer exercise test in normal individuals of three different fitness levels: the fitter individuals (ie, higher $\dot{V}O_2$peak) exercised with larger work rate increments (eg, 90W vs. 45 W steps). Responses are expressed as the average over each consecutive quarter of the tolerable work rate range. At higher work rates, the $\dot{V}O_2$ responses slow and thereby appear to be more damped, although this effect is less marked in the fit individuals because their $\dot{V}O_2$ kinetics are faster. *(Reprinted by permission from Springer: Zhang YY, Johnson MC II, Chow N, Wasserman K. The role of fitness on $\dot{V}O_2$ and $\dot{V}CO_2$ kinetics in response to proportional step increases in work rate.* Eur J Appl Physiol Occup Physiol. *1991;63[2]:94-100. Copyright © 1991 Springer Nature.)*

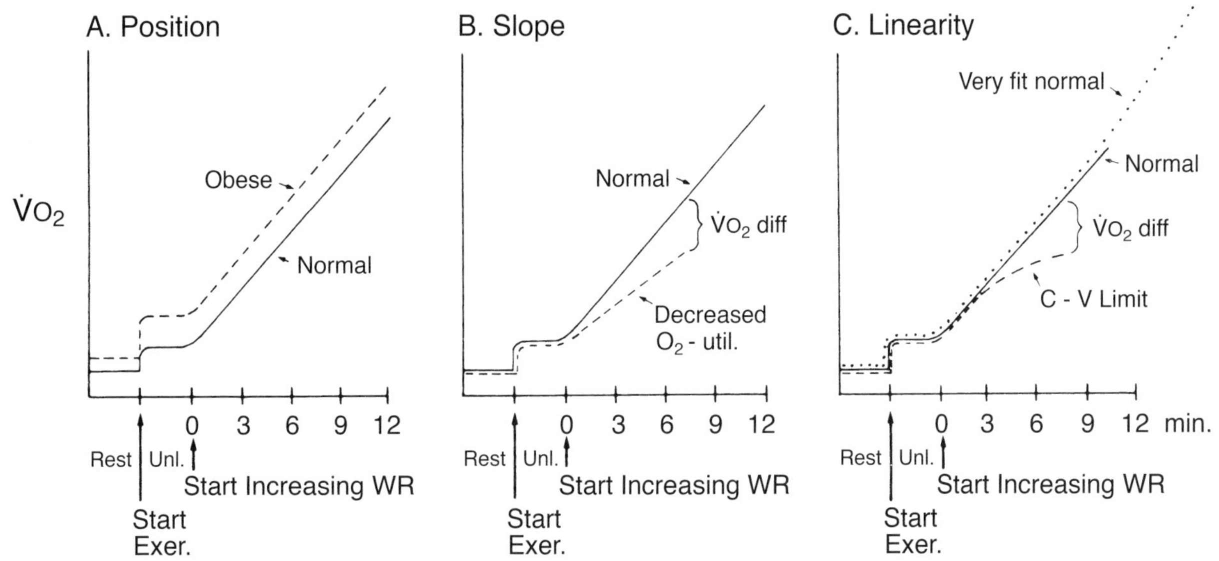

FIGURE 3.6. Position displacement (A), slope (B), and linearity (C) of the oxygen uptake ($\dot{V}O_2$)–work rate (WR) relationship for incremental exercise. Obesity displaces the $\dot{V}O_2$–work rate relationship upward, but the slope is unchanged (A). A decreased slope of the $\dot{V}O_2$–work rate relationship (B) reflects inadequate oxygen (O_2) availability to the exercising muscles, such as when peripheral blood flow is impaired. The linearity of the $\dot{V}O_2$–work rate relationship (C) can be altered in patients with cardiovascular diseases (slope becoming shallower at higher work rates) because of impaired O_2 flow to the exercising muscles or in very fit individuals (slope becoming steeper). $\dot{V}O_2$ difference ($\dot{V}O_2$ diff) is the difference between the expected $\dot{V}O_2$ and the actual $\dot{V}O_2$ at the maximum work rate.

upwardly displaced, the $\dot{V}O_2$–WR relationship in obesity often parallels that of the normal-weight individual during cycle ergometry.

For treadmill exercise, a predictable adjustment for body weight is not possible because of complex mechanical factors such as varying the subject's center of gravity as the angle of the treadmill is changed, the variable length of the stride as the speed and grade are altered, and the tendency of the subject to hold on to stationary objects for support or balance during the test. These variables make it difficult to estimate an individual's actual power output during treadmill ergometry. Pórszász et al[17] have described how to linearize a treadmill exercise protocol (see Chapter 5), which we recommend for treadmill ergometry. In addition, to avoid the temptation of holding on to the treadmill railing for balance, we advise our patients to rest the back of the hand(s) on the treadmill railing.

Slope of $\dot{V}O_2$ as a Function of Work Rate ($\Delta\dot{V}O_2/\Delta WR$)

The slope of $\dot{V}O_2$ as a function of work rate is important because it is a measure of the aerobic work efficiency (see Chapter 2, "Oxygen Cost of Work" section). The $\dot{V}O_2$-WR slope for the ramp or 1-minute incremental cycle ergometer exercise test was found to be 10.2 ± 1.0 mL/min/W for normal individuals by Hansen et al[15] and 9.9 ± 0.7 mL/min/W by Wasserman and Sue[18] (see **Fig. 3.2**). These values are similar to the value of 10.1 mL/min/W previously obtained from steady state measurements in sedentary individuals.[16] In 12 trained cyclists, Riley et al[19] obtained an average slope of 11.5 mL/min/W with a standard deviation of 0.78, suggesting that athletes may have a slightly higher $\Delta\dot{V}O_2/\Delta WR$ than nonathletes.

Linearity of $\dot{V}O_2$ as a Function of Work Rate

As discussed in Chapter 2 ("Oxygen Uptake Kinetics" section), $\dot{V}O_2$ kinetics are a more complex function of work rate than a single exponential at work rates above the *AT*. This can be reflected in a steepening of the $\dot{V}O_2$–WR relationship above the *AT* when work rate incrementation rates are slow, allowing for expression of the $\dot{V}O_2$ slow component. Also, the progressively greater increase in the work of breathing for a given increase in $\dot{V}E$ that occurs when $\dot{V}E$ achieves very high values (as in highly fit endurance athletes) or when the respiratory-mechanical impedance is abnormally increased (as in respiratory disease) could also contribute to a steepening of the $\dot{V}O_2$–WR relationship.[8,16] In addition, the use of additional muscle groups when performing heavy exercise (eg, pulling on cycle handlebars during leg cycling to brace the trunk on the ergometer as the pedals get harder to turn) can increase the oxygen cost of exercise at higher work rates.

However, the peak $\dot{V}O_2$ is not systematically affected by the work rate incrementation rate. In general, work rate increments of 15 to 25 W/min in normal men and 10 to 20 W/min in normal women give a similar rate of rise in $\dot{V}O_2$ both above and below the *AT*. A method for selecting the work rate increment for incremental exercise testing of normal individuals and patients is described in Chapter 5.

Can $\dot{V}O_2$ or METs Be Predicted From the Work Rate?

Some laboratories estimate $\dot{V}O_2$ from work rate during exercise rather than measuring $\dot{V}O_2$ directly. This practice is inaccurate and should be discouraged. A unit called a *MET* was derived from the average resting $\dot{V}O_2$ for a 70-kg, 40-year-old man. It is equal to 3.5 mL/min/kg of body weight.

By assuming a fixed relationship between the ergometer work rate and the $\dot{V}O_2$, some laboratories report an estimate of $\dot{V}O_2$ from the ergometer work rate. After obtaining this estimated $\dot{V}O_2$ and expressing it per kilogram of body weight, the $\dot{V}O_2$ per kilogram is divided by 3.5 to obtain the number of METs performed by the subject.

However, under many conditions, $\dot{V}O_2$ cannot be accurately predicted from the estimated work rate for the reasons summarized in **Table 3.4**. If $\dot{V}O_2$ does not increase linearly with increasing work rate, as is common in patients with cardiovascular diseases, $\dot{V}O_2$ cannot be estimated from work rate (see **Fig. 3.6C** and the cardiovascular cases in Chapter 10).[20] Thus, using work rate to calculate $\dot{V}O_2$ or mets will usually lead to overestimates in these patients.

In addition, work rate fails to predict $\dot{V}O_2$ if the obesity factor is not taken into account. This factor is often ignored or incorrect estimates of the effect of body weight are used. As discussed above, the $\dot{V}O_2$ to perform a given amount of external work will be higher in an obese individual than in a lean individual because of the need to expend additional energy to move a large body when effecting external work. For cycle ergometer exercise, we have found that the O_2 cost of cycling at 60 rpm on an unloaded ergometer is an additional 5.8 mL/min for each kilogram body weight.[15,16]

Appendix C and Chapter 5 should be reviewed for methods of assuring accuracy in gas exchange measurements and ergometer calibration.

Cardiac Output and Stroke Volume

Cardiac output measurement may be useful when trying to assess whether a patient's reduced peak $\dot{V}O_2$ is due to reduced O_2 transport or failure of the exercising muscles to extract O_2 for whatever cause. However, cardiac output measurement by itself, even if accurate, may not reveal whether cardiac output is adequate for the work rate performed. The major concern of exercise testing should be to determine whether the circulation is capable of providing the exercise-stressed muscles with enough oxygen. To answer this important question, measurement of the *AT* and $\Delta\dot{V}O_2/\Delta WR$ during an incremental test, as well as measurement of $\dot{V}O_2$ and $\dot{V}CO_2$ kinetics during a constant work rate test, may be more useful. Because all of these measurements are made noninvasively with CPET, they can be repeated easily.

TABLE 3.4 Conditions in Which Work Rate Fails to Predict Oxygen Update ($\dot{V}O_2$)

$\dot{V}O_2$ fails to increase linearly with work rate.
Obesity
Valvular heart disease
Coronary artery disease
Cardiomyopathy
Peripheral arterial disease
Pulmonary vascular disease
Faulty ergometer calibration

Cardiac Output Measurement

Thermodilution

Cardiac output can be determined by thermodilution. A bolus of isotonic fluid (usually 5% dextrose in water) of known volume, temperature (usually 0°C), specific heat, and specific gravity is rapidly injected into the right atrial port of a pulmonary artery catheter and the temperature change measured with a temperature sensor at the catheter tip in the pulmonary artery. The temperature change downstream reflects the volume of dilution of the bolus, and cardiac output can be calculated using an automated system. The integral of temperature over time is inversely proportional to cardiac output.[21] Stetz et al[22] reviewed several studies and concluded that values of cardiac output determined by thermodilution in catheterization laboratories and intensive care units were of comparable accuracy to those determined by Fick or dye-dilution methods. They suggested, however, that a 20% to 26% difference in cardiac output should be found before concluding that two single determinations were different. Advantages of thermodilution include safety, speed, and repeatability.

Indirect Fick Method Using $\dot{V}CO_2$ and Estimated $C\bar{v}CO_2$

Estimates of cardiac output during exercise are sometimes made with the indirect Fick method:

$$\text{Cardiac output} = \dot{V}CO_2 \,/\, C(\bar{v} - a)CO_2$$

$\dot{V}CO_2$ is measured while $C(\bar{v} - a)CO_2$ is derived from mixed venous PCO_2 ($P\bar{v}CO_2$) obtained by the CO_2 rebreathing method[23] (see Appendix C) and arterial PCO_2 ($PaCO_2$) estimated from end-tidal PCO_2 ($P_{ET}CO_2$).

This approach does have several potential errors. First, estimation of $PaCO_2$ from $P_{ET}CO_2$ measurements is unreliable, especially in patients.[24-27] $P_{ET}CO_2$ is less than $PaCO_2$ in patients with lung disease, heart failure, and pulmonary vascular disease and greater than $PaCO_2$ in normal individuals (see "Arterial–End-Tidal PCO_2 Difference" below). Second, the assumption is made that the CO_2 dissociation curve is linear, although in reality, it gets less steep the higher the PCO_2 (see **Fig. 2.32**) (see Chapter 2, "Oxyhemoglobin Dissociation" section). Third, the assumption is made that mixed venous CO_2 content ($C\bar{v}CO_2$) can be determined accurately from $P\bar{v}CO_2$ using a standard CO_2 dissociation curve that plots blood CO_2 content against blood PCO_2. However, despite $P\bar{v}CO_2$ increasing throughout incremental exercise, once the *AT* is exceeded, $C\bar{v}CO_2$ no longer continues to increase proportionately but rather falls to near resting levels as peak $\dot{V}O_2$ is approached, consequent to the developing metabolic acidosis (see Chapter 2, "Arterial and Venous PCO_2 and Carbon Dioxide Content").[28] That is, the CO_2 dissociation curve is shifted progressively downward with increasing work rates above *AT*, as HCO_3^- dissociates when it buffers the metabolic acidosis. Thus, the CO_2 rebreathing method for determining mixed venous CO_2 content, particularly above the *AT*, is not accurate—this effect cannot be estimated without direct mixed venous blood gas and pH measurements.

Direct Fick Method

This method represents the gold standard for cardiac output measurement. From the simultaneous measurement of $\dot{V}O_2$ and of arterial and mixed venous O_2 content (CaO_2, $C\bar{v}O_2$), cardiac output can be determined from the direct Fick equation:

$$\text{Cardiac output} = \dot{V}O_2 \,/\, C(a - \bar{v})O_2$$

The $C\bar{v}O_2$ and CaO_2 are determined from samples drawn from catheters in the pulmonary artery and a systemic artery, respectively. Interestingly, average cardiac outputs during incremental exercise were very similar when CO_2 was used as the test gas, compared to O_2, although the individual variability was greater.[28] This increased variability was attributed to the much lower extraction ratio for CO_2 and the greater complexity in calculation of blood CO_2 content as compared with O_2 content; raising concerns about the accuracy and precision of direct cardiac output determinations using CO_2 as the test gas.

Noninvasive Cardiac Output and Stroke Volume by the Fick Principle

Stringer et al[29] proposed that cardiac output could be estimated, noninvasively, by the Fick principle during incremental exercise with an accuracy as good as generally reported by other methods. This is based on the demonstration that $C(a - \bar{v})O_2$ is linearly related to percent $\dot{V}O_2$ peak or max for incremental exercise, achieving a value of approximately 75% to 80% at peak (**Fig. 3.7**), with a regression slope and intercept that are similar for normal individuals and patients with stable chronic heart failure regardless of severity of impairment (**Fig. 3.8**).[29-32] Agostoni et al[30] found that patients

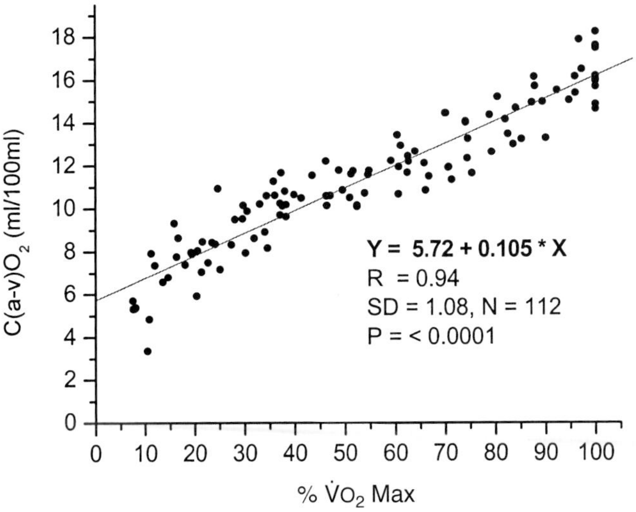

FIGURE 3.7. Arterial-mixed venous oxygen content difference $[C(a - \bar{v})O_2]$ as a function of percentage maximal oxygen uptake ($\dot{V}O_2max$) during incremental cycle ergometer exercise for 10 studies on five normal individuals. $C(a - \bar{v})O_2$ is linearly correlated with percentage $\dot{V}O_2max$: $C(a - \bar{v})O_2 = 5.72 + (0.105 \times \%\ \dot{V}O_2max)$. *(Reproduced with permission from Stringer W, Hansen J, Wasserman K. Cardiac output estimated noninvasively from oxygen uptake during exercise.* J Appl Physiol. *1997;82[3]:908-912. Copyright © 1997 American Physiological Society. All rights reserved.)*

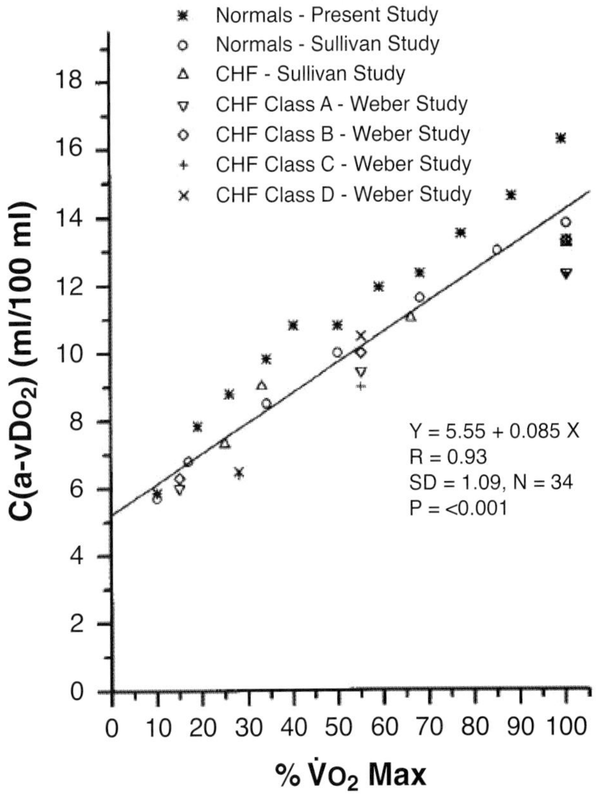

FIGURE 3.8. Arterial-mixed venous oxygen content difference $[C(a - vDO_2)]$ as a function of percentage maximal oxygen uptake ($\dot{V}O_2max$) from incremental cycle ergometer exercise studies of Stringer et al,[29] Sullivan et al,[31] and Weber and Janicki[32] in normal individuals and patients with congestive heart failure (CHF). Despite a wide variation in cardiac function, the regression slope and intercept were similar to those obtained for the normal individuals presented in Figure 3.7. *(Reproduced with permission from Stringer W, Hansen J, Wasserman K. Cardiac output estimated noninvasively from oxygen uptake during exercise.* J Appl Physiol. *1997;82[3]:908-912. Figure 6. Copyright © 1997 American Physiological Society. All rights reserved.)*

with more severe chronic heart failure, on average, had higher values for $C(a - \bar{v})O_2$ at the *AT*. However, they had similar values to normal individuals at peak $\dot{V}O_2$ (**Table 3.5**).

The resulting cardiac output values compare favorably with directly measured cardiac output using the direct Fick principle (**Fig. 3.9**). The determination of cardiac output is made from the $\dot{V}O_2$ measurement alone, at work rates at which $C(a - \bar{v})O_2$ can be estimated with relative accuracy, such as at *AT* and peak $\dot{V}O_2$.

Estimates at peak exercise for $C(a - \bar{v})O_2$ are shown in **Table 3.6**, taking into account different values for resting levels of hemoglobin (Hb). Other assumptions are hemoconcentration at peak exercise of 5%, a normal arterial O_2 saturation of 96%, an Hb-O_2 binding capacity of 1.34 mL/g Hb, a normal carboxyhemoglobin (COHb) saturation of 1%, and a mixed venous O_2 saturation at peak exercise of 24%. Allowance in the $C(a - \bar{v})O_2$ estimation can be made for factors such as [Hb], arterial O_2 saturation, [COHb], and fitness as explained in the footnote. For example, the degree of hemoconcentration varies with the peak $\dot{V}O_2$.

TABLE 3.5 Arteriovenous Oxygen (O_2) Difference and Extraction Ratio ± Standard Deviation at Rest, Anaerobic Threshold (*AT*), and Peak O_2 uptake ($\dot{V}O_2$)

	$\dot{V}O_2$ (L/min)	Arteriovenous O_2 difference (mL/dL)	Extraction ratio[a]
Normal males[b]			
Rest		6.14 ± 1.7	0.30 ± 0.09
AT	1.84 ± 0.36	11.3 ± 0.87	0.53 ± 0.04
Peak $\dot{V}O_2$	3.77 ± 0.61	16.2 ± 1.2	0.74 ± 0.07
Chronic heart failure[c]			
Rest	0.28 ± 0.07	7.8 ± 2.6	0.43 ± 0.11
AT	0.83 ± 0.25	13.0 ± 2.4	0.68 ± 0.09
Peak $\dot{V}O_2$	1.26 ± 0.39	15.0 ± 2.7	0.77 ± 0.07

[a]Extraction ratio equals fractional difference between CaO_2 and $C\bar{v}O_2$.

[b]Data from Stringer W, Hansen J, Wasserman K. Cardiac output estimated noninvasively from oxygen uptake during exercise. *J Appl Physiol (1985)*. 1997;82:908-912.

[c]Data from Agostoni PG, Wasserman K, Perego GB, et al. Non-invasive measurement of stroke volume during exercise in heart failure patients. *Clin Sci (Lond)*. 2000;98:545-551.

An initial estimate of 5% was assumed for an individual of average fitness and hemoconcentration, with an additional 5% being applied for an exceptionally fit individual and 5% being subtracted for a very unfit individual or a patient having a very low peak $\dot{V}O_2$. With regard to arterial

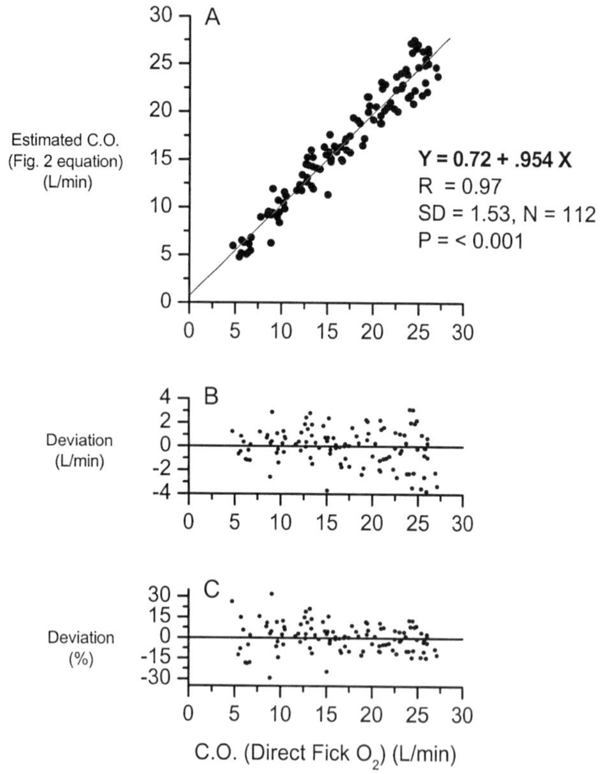

FIGURE 3.9. Estimated cardiac output (CO) from measured oxygen uptake ($\dot{V}O_2$) and estimated arterial-mixed venous oxygen content difference (using equation in Figure 3.7) compared with directly measured Fick CO during incremental cycle ergometer exercise (A). The estimated and measured values agree well (B), with a 95% confidence limit of ± 15% (C). *(Reproduced with permission from Stringer W, Hansen J, Wasserman K. Cardiac output estimated noninvasively from oxygen uptake during exercise.* J Appl Physiol. *1997;82[3]:908-912. Copyright © 1997 American Physiological Society. All rights reserved.)*

O_2 desaturation (eg, patients with lung diseases, highly fit endurance athletes at high work rates), a 1% decrease in $C(a - \bar{v})O_2$ is applied for each 1% decrease in arterial O_2 saturation below 96%. For a COHb saturation greater than 1% (eg, cigarette smokers), $C(a - \bar{v})O_2$ is decreased by COHb saturation (%) minus 1. In general, the effect on the finally derived cardiac output measurement is relatively small, especially when peak $\dot{V}O_2$ is low.

Similar adjustments to $C(a - \bar{v})O_2$ can be made for [Hb] and arterial O_2 saturation (expressed as fractional) at rest, at the *AT*, and at peak exercise. The equations for the effect of [Hb] and arterial O_2 saturation on $C(a - \bar{v})O_2$ are the following:

$$\text{At rest: } [\text{Hb}] \times 1.34 \times (\text{fractional arterial } O_2 \text{ saturation} - 0.7)$$

$$\text{At } AT\text{: } [\text{Hb}] \times 1.34 \times (\text{fractional arterial } O_2 \text{ saturation} - 0.4)$$

$$\text{At peak: } [\text{Hb}] \times 1.34 \times (\text{fractional arterial } O_2 \text{ saturation} - 0.2)$$

where 0.7, 0.4, and 0.2 are estimates of fractional mixed venous O_2 saturation.

Oxygen Pulse and Stroke Volume

The O_2 pulse, $\dot{V}O_2/HR$, equals the product of stroke volume (SV) and $C(a - \bar{v})O_2$. The O_2 pulse measured breath by breath in the transition from rest to exercise and from exercise to recovery (ie, phase I, see Chapter 2, "Oxygen Uptake Kinetics" and "Carbon Dioxide Output Kinetics" sections) is informative, as the immediate increase in O_2 pulse at the start of exercise (and decrease at exercise offset) depends primarily on stroke volume (**Fig. 3.10**). It will therefore be low in patients who cannot increase their stroke volume in response to exercise.[33] At exercise offset, the O_2 pulse often transiently increases in patients with left ventricular failure and exercise-induced myocardial ischemia. The explanation for this paradoxical response is that the afterload of the left ventricle is abruptly decreased when stopping

TABLE 3.6 Estimation of Arteriovenous Oxygen (O_2) Difference [$C(a - \bar{v})O_2$] at Peak Exercise

Hb (g/100 mL)[a]	O_2 capacity (mL/100 mL)	Arterial O_2 saturation (%)	Mixed venous O_2 saturation (%)	Arterial O_2 content (mL/100 mL)	Mixed venous O_2 content (mL/100)	$C(a - \bar{v})O_2$ (mL/100 mL)[b]
16	22.5	96	24	21.4	5.4	16.0
15	21.1	96	24	20.0	5.0	15.0
14	19.7	96	24	18.7	4.7	14.0
13	18.3	96	24	17.4	4.4	13.0
12	16.9	96	24	16.0	4.0	12.0
11	15.5	96	24	14.7	3.7	11.0
10	14.1	96	24	13.4	3.4	10.0

[a]The left column identifies the resting hemoglobin (Hb) concentration. The Hb concentration at peak exercise is considered to be 5% higher than the resting [Hb]—that is, a fitness factor of 1.05 (see text for definition). The carboxyhemoglobin concentration is assumed to be 1%.

[b]Modifications to $C(a - \bar{v})O_2$ (right column): (1) If the person is very unfit, decrease the $C(a - \bar{v})O_2$ by up to 6%; if the person is very fit, increase the $C(a - \bar{v})O_2$ by up to 6%. (2) Reduce the $C(a - \bar{v})O_2$ by 1% for each 1% increase in [carboxyhemoglobin] above 1%. (3) Reduce the $C(a - \bar{v})O_2$ by 1% for each 1% decrease in arterial oxyhemoglobin saturation below 96%.

exercise because of the immediate decrease in systemic arterial blood pressure. This allows improved ventricular ejection and increased stroke volume as the patient with the failing heart stops exercising.[34] The increase in stroke volume allows capillary blood flow to move more rapidly through the lung during the period of a heartbeat, thereby taking up more O_2.

In response to increasing work rates, the O_2 pulse normally increases with a hyperbolic profile (see **Fig. 2.28**, panel d, right; and **Fig. 3.10**), primarily because of an increasing $C(a - \bar{v})O_2$. However, if the stroke volume is reduced, the $C(a - \bar{v})O_2$ and therefore the O_2 pulse reaches maximal values at a relatively low work rate (see **Fig. 3.10**; heart disease curve).[35] The O_2 pulse is also low in individuals with anemia, high levels of COHb, marked arterial hypoxemia, and

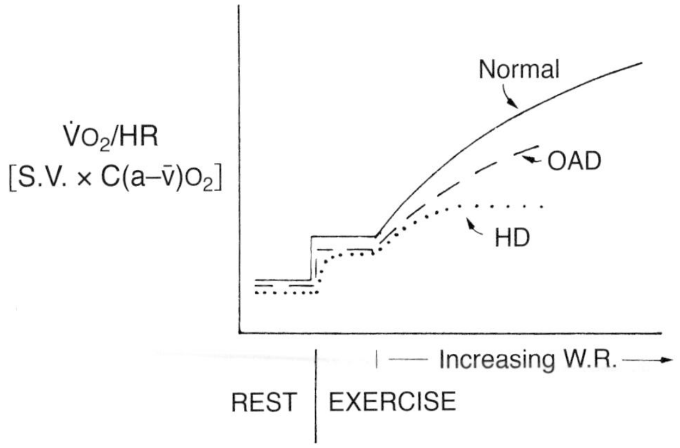

FIGURE 3.10. The oxygen (O_2) pulse, that is, oxygen uptake ($\dot{V}O_2$)/heart rate (HR) or the product of stroke volume (SV) and $C(a - \bar{v}O_2)$, response to increasing work rate (WR) imposed from a constant low-WR baseline. Patients with low stroke volumes, such as those with heart disease (HD), tend to have a lower than normal O_2 pulse trajectory that can plateau as maximal WRs are approached. In contrast, patients with obstructive airway disease (OAD) have a pattern similar to that of normal individuals, although the values are lower at each work rate, reflecting the relatively low stroke volume in these patients.

muscle mitochondrial or glycolytic enzyme defects because of a reduced $C(a - \bar{v})O_2$ at maximal exercise.

Stroke volume during exercise can be estimated from the O_2 pulse, recognizing that

$$SV = [O_2 \text{ pulse} / C(a - \bar{v})O_2] \times 100$$

where stroke volume is in milliliters per beat. For example, $C(a - \bar{v})O_2$ could be derived noninvasively from **Table 3.6**, taking account of [Hb] for example. An alternative approach is based on the recognition that the asymptotic value of the O_2 pulse during exercise is related to stroke volume, assuming that stroke volume is normally relatively invariant with increasing work rates (see Chapter 2, "Cardiac Output" section).[36]

Thus:

$$O_2 \text{ pulse} = \dot{V}O_2 / HR = (\text{cardiac output} \times CaO_2) / HR - (\text{cardiac output} \times C\bar{v}O_2) / HR$$

$$O_2 \text{ pulse} = (SV \times CaO_2) - (\text{cardiac output} \times C\bar{v}O_2) / HR$$

As it has been shown that the product of cardiac output and $C\bar{v}O_2$ is relatively constant (ie, k) over a wide range of steady state work rates:

$$O_2 \text{ pulse} = (SV \times CaO_2) - k / HR$$

Because CaO_2 is usually relatively constant in normal individuals during exercise, the O_2 pulse should change hyperbolically with respect to HR, reaching an asymptote at a value of (SV × CaO_2) at high work rates. And as this asymptotic O_2 pulse equals the slope (S) of the linear HR-$\dot{V}O_2$ relationship (see **Fig. 2.28**, panel D), exercise SV may be predicted as S/CaO_2. If CaO_2 cannot be measured, it can reasonably be assumed to equal 0.2 L/L, in which case SV = 5 × S. However, this estimator will not be valid in situations where CaO_2 is low and variable during exercise, for example, in patients with lung disease or anemia, in highly fit endurance athletes who desaturate during exercise, or at high altitude.

Anaerobic (Lactate, Lactic Acidosis) Threshold

As discussed in Chapter 2 ("Arterial Lactate Increase" section), the *AT* is defined as the level of exercise $\dot{V}O_2$ above, which aerobic energy production is supplemented by anaerobic mechanisms and is reflected by an increase in [lactate] and [lactate]–[pyruvate] (L/P) ratio in muscle and arterial blood (see **Figs. 2.2**, **2.11**, **2.12**, and **2.13**). The *AT* is thus measured as metabolic stress—that is, in units of $\dot{V}O_2$, not work rate. It is unaffected by the rate at which the work rate is incremented[37,38] or by metabolic substrate.[39-41] However, like $\dot{V}O_2$max, the *AT* is influenced by the size of the involved muscle groups.

The development of the exercise metabolic acidosis is described in Chapter 2 ("Arterial Lactate Increase" section) and illustrated by the almost equimolar increase of arterial [lactate] relative to the associated decrease of arterial [HCO_3^-] (**Fig. 3.11**). The underlying mechanism for the *AT* estimation depends on detecting the effects of the net increases in lactate and proton production (**Fig. 2.1**, pathway B). At work rates below the *AT*, the muscle and blood L/P ratios are essentially the same as at rest, and no metabolic acidosis develops. Above the *AT*, a metabolic acidosis develops. Thus, the threshold can be defined physiologically as the $\dot{V}O_2$ above which production of adenosine triphosphate (ATP) through anaerobic glycolysis supplements the aerobic ATP production (*AT*). It can also be defined in terms of changing redox state within the cell, as the $\dot{V}O_2$ at which [lactate] and L/P ratio increase (lactate threshold [*LT*]), or in terms of acid-base balance change, as the $\dot{V}O_2$ at which metabolic acidosis develops, as indicated by a decrease in standard [HCO_3^-] (lactic acidosis threshold [*LAT*]) (**Fig. 3.12**).

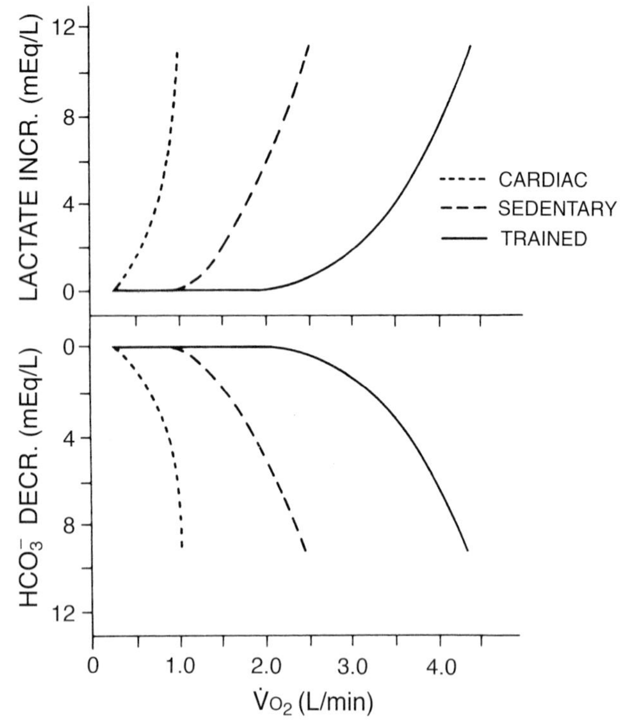

FIGURE 3.11. Arterial blood [lactate] increase and [bicarbonate] [HCO_3^-] decrease during incremental exercise in trained and sedentary normal individuals and in patients with primary cardiac disease of class II to III severity as defined by the New York Heart Association Classification. *(Republished with permission of McGraw-Hill LLC from Wasserman K. Physiological basis of exercise testing. In: Fishman AP, ed. Pulmonary Diseases and Disorders. New York, NY: McGraw-Hill; 1980:337-347; permission conveyed through Copyright Clearance Center, Inc.)*

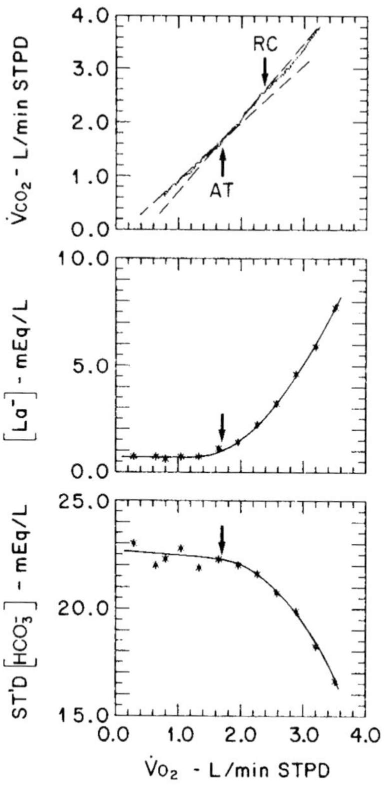

FIGURE 3.12. Responses of arterial [lactate], standard [bicarbonate] [HCO_3^-], and $\dot{V}CO_2$ as a function of $\dot{V}O_2$ during incremental cycle ergometer exercise for a single subject. Arrows indicate estimates of the anaerobic threshold (*AT*) by the plots of $\dot{V}CO_2$ versus $\dot{V}O_2$ (V-slope), and the arterial [lactate] increase and [HCO_3^-] decrease versus $\dot{V}O_2$. RC is the respiratory (ventilatory) compensation point.

Methods of Measurement

The relatively rapid incremental exercise test (ramp or 1-min steps) used in CPET can readily determine the $\dot{V}O_2$ at which metabolic acidosis first develops (ie, the *AT*) when gas exchange is measured breath by breath or as the average of several breaths. The reason gas exchange is so effective in detecting the onset of the metabolic acidosis is that the time delay between the onset of HCO_3^- buffering of the metabolic proton load and its expression in the lung gas as CO_2 is only a matter of a few seconds (see Chapter 2, "Buffering the Exercise-Induced Lactic Acidosis" section), as is the consequential $\dot{V}E$ response to this supplemental $\dot{V}CO_2$ (see Chapter 2, "Ventilatory Control" section). These two features are key to *AT* estimation. A flow diagram describing the sequence of gas exchange and $\dot{V}E$ changes in response to the developing metabolic acidosis for an incremental exercise test is shown in **Figure 3.13**.

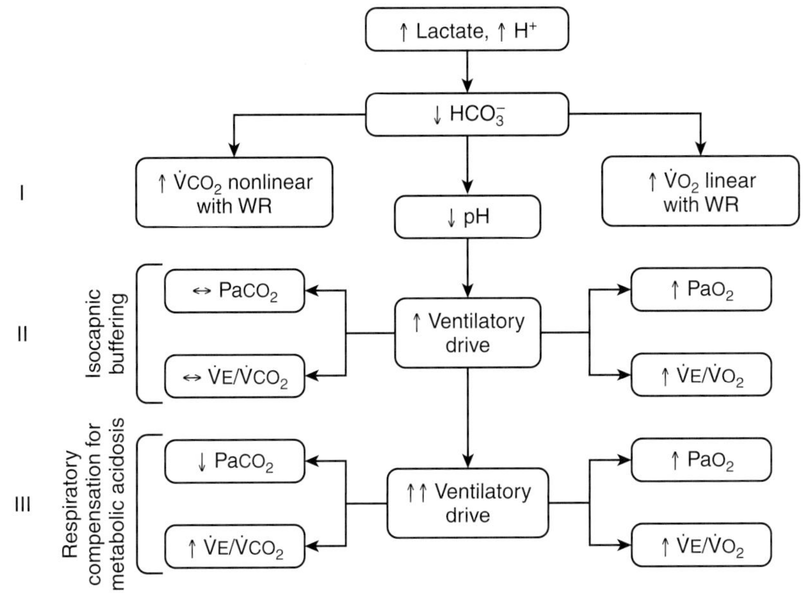

FIGURE 3.13. Effects of increasing arterial [lactate] on gas exchange (oxygen uptake [$\dot{V}O_2$], carbon dioxide output [$\dot{V}CO_2$]), ventilation ($\dot{V}E$), and arterial PO_2 and PCO_2 (PaO_2, $PaCO_2$) during an incremental exercise test. Small upward arrows indicate increases, small downward arrows indicate decreases, and horizontal arrows indicate no change. Mechanism I describes gas exchange that results solely from buffering of the metabolic acidosis (see lower left panel of Fig. 3.17). Mechanism II describes changes in arterial and end-tidal PCO_2 and PO_2 and ventilatory equivalents for oxygen (O_2) and carbon dioxide (CO_2) that result from increased ventilatory drive consequent to CO_2 generated by the buffering reaction (see right upper and lower panels of Fig. 3.17). Mechanism III describes changes caused by further increases in ventilatory drive consequent to ventilatory compensation for the metabolic acidosis (see changes to the right of anaerobic threshold lines in right upper and lower panels of Fig. 3.17). Abbreviations: HCO_3^-, bicarbonate; WR, work rate.

V-Slope Method

With the onset of a metabolic acidosis during incremental exercise, there is an obligatory increase in CO_2 production in excess of that resulting from aerobic metabolism, which represents the CO_2 generated from the HCO_3^- buffering of newly produced H^+, stoichiometrically (see **Fig. 2.2**). The point at which this supplemental $\dot{V}CO_2$ first occurs is relatively easy to as an acceleration of $\dot{V}CO_2$ relative to $\dot{V}O_2$ as work rate increases (see **Fig. 3.13**, mechanism I; see also **Figs. 2.52** and **3.14**).

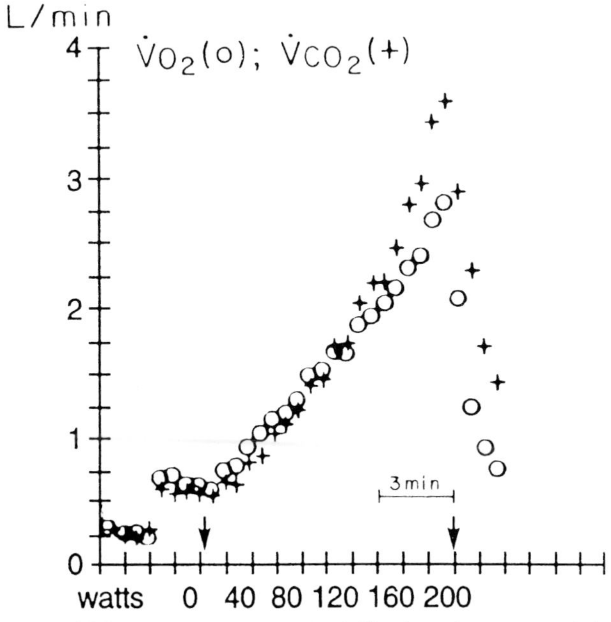

FIGURE 3.14. Carbon dioxide output ($\dot{V}CO_2$) and oxygen uptake ($\dot{V}O_2$) as functions of work rate for an incremental cycle ergometer exercise test (20 W/min). $\dot{V}CO_2$ starts to increase more steeply than $\dot{V}O_2$ in the middle work rate range, reflecting H^+ buffering above the anaerobic threshold.

Specifically, after the first minute or so of the incremental phase of the test, plotting $\dot{V}CO_2$ as a function of $\dot{V}O_2$ yields a progression of points that is commonly composed of two reasonably linear components, S_1 and S_2 (**Fig. 3.15**). The lower S_1 component has a slope slightly less than 1.0. The slope then breaks, with $\dot{V}CO_2$ increasing faster than $\dot{V}O_2$ such that the new higher S_2 slope is now clearly above 1.0. This S_1-S_2 break point is the *AT* (see **Fig. 3.15**), as confirmed with arterial standard [HCO_3^-] measurements.[42] This technique is referred to as the V-slope method because it relates the increase in $\dot{V}CO_2$ to $\dot{V}O_2$. An advantage of this approach is that it is independent of the individual's associated ventilatory response and is insensitive to irregularities in breathing. Thus, it is useful for estimating the *AT* in patients who do not develop ventilatory compensation for the exercise metabolic acidosis because of poor respiratory chemosensitivity or premature respiratory-mechanical limitation, such as in patients with severe chronic obstructive pulmonary disease (COPD) or obesity syndrome (see "Ventilatory Equivalent Method" section below).

Beaver et al[42] determined S_1 and S_2 from statistically derived regression slopes of $\dot{V}CO_2$ versus $\dot{V}O_2$ in the respective regions of interest (see **Fig. 3.15**). The break point or intersection of the two slopes can be selected by a computer program, that is, defining the $\dot{V}O_2$ above which $\dot{V}CO_2$ increases faster than $\dot{V}O_2$. Sue et al[43] simplified this method (**Fig. 3.16**). That is, as the V-slope method is predicated on the S_1 value being 1.0 or slightly less and the S_2 value greater than 1.0, the S_1-S_2 break point representing the *AT* can readily be determined as follows. A line parallel to the line of identity (ie, with a slope of 1.0 when $\dot{V}CO_2$ and $\dot{V}O_2$ are plotted on equal scales—a unitary tangent) is first placed to the right of the $\dot{V}CO_2$-$\dot{V}O_2$ profile and then moved laterally leftward (manually or by computer) until it first impacts on the $\dot{V}CO_2$-$\dot{V}O_2$ profile. The $\dot{V}O_2$ at which the data points first systematically start to lie above the unitary tangent (ie, with $\dot{V}CO_2$ starting to increase out of its previous proportion to $\dot{V}O_2$, with a

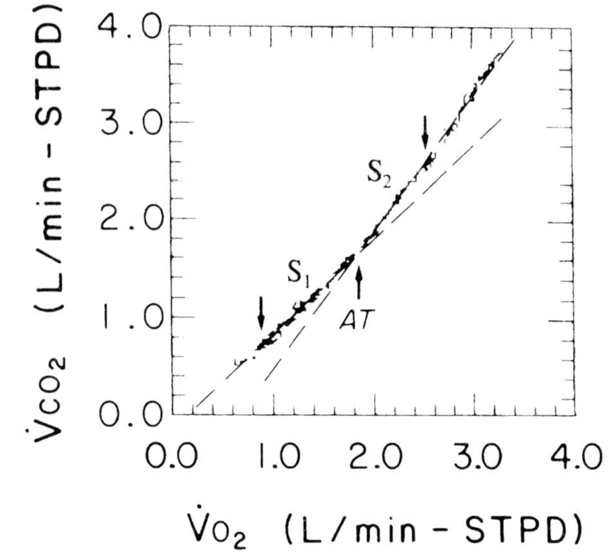

FIGURE 3.15. Example of V-slope technique. Carbon dioxide output ($\dot{V}CO_2$) as a function of oxygen uptake ($\dot{V}O_2$) during an incremental cycle ergometer exercise test (V-slope plot). The transition from aerobic metabolism, where $\dot{V}CO_2$ increases linearly relative to $\dot{V}O_2$ with a slope (S_1) slightly less than 1, to anaerobic plus aerobic metabolism, where the $\dot{V}CO_2$-$\dot{V}O_2$ slope increases to a value greater than 1 (S_2), defines the anaerobic threshold (*AT*) by gas exchange. The steeper S_2 reflects the production of additional carbon dioxide (CO_2) from bicarbonate (HCO_3^-) buffering of the metabolic acidosis over that produced by aerobic metabolism. For rapid incremental tests such as this, hyperventilation relative to CO_2 does not occur at the *AT* and therefore does not contribute to the steepening of S_2. The lower downward-directed arrow indicates where CO_2 stores are no longer increasing and calculation of S_1 starts. The upper downward-directed arrow indicates the $\dot{V}O_2$ above which hyperventilation in response to the metabolic acidosis starts. The S_1 and S_2 are calculated from the data between the two downward arrows. Abbreviation: STPD, standard temperature pressure dry. *(Modified from Beaver WL, Wasserman K, Whipp BJ. A new method for detecting anaerobic threshold by gas exchange.* J Appl Physiol. *1986;60:2020-2027.)*

$\dot{V}CO_2$-$\dot{V}O_2$ slope >1.0) is the *AT*. The assumption of the method is the recognition that the unitary tangent approximates the S_1 slope value (ie, the *ratio* of increase in $\dot{V}CO_2$ relative to increase in $\dot{V}O_2$ in the S_1 region), whose value reflects predominantly glycogen oxidation (ie, respiratory quotient ~ 1.0). The *AT* values obtained by the modified V-slope method agree closely with the directly measured *LT* and *LAT* (determined from arterial standard [HCO_3^-]).[42,43] This approach is useful when the $\dot{V}CO_2$-$\dot{V}O_2$ relationship cannot convincingly be partitioned into clearly linear S_1 and S_2 segments.

There can be instances where a patient develops a metabolic acidosis with only minimal exercise. Thus, the $\dot{V}CO_2$-$\dot{V}O_2$ plot could become steeper than 1.0 as early as the unloaded exercise phase of the test, such that the *AT* will be less than the lowest measured exercise $\dot{V}O_2$.

Ventilatory Equivalent Method

It is important to recognize that the demonstration of a break point in the $\dot{V}CO_2$-$\dot{V}O_2$ profile should not be taken, on its own, as evidence for the onset of a metabolic acidosis. For example, while hyperventilation resulting from psychogenic factors, hypoxemia or pain would be expected to introduce a break point in the $\dot{V}CO_2$-$\dot{V}O_2$ profile, it would also be accompanied by an increase in end-tidal PO_2 ($PETO_2$) and a decrease in $PETCO_2$—the latter is not normally observed at the *AT* during rapid incremental exercise (see Chapter 2, "Ventilatory Control" section). This is a reflection of the delayed ventilatory compensation for the metabolic acidosis, such that the maintained proportionality between $\dot{V}E$ and $\dot{V}CO_2$ beyond the *AT* (ie, until the ventilatory compensation point [VCP]) is reflected in $\dot{V}E/\dot{V}CO_2$ not increasing and $PETCO_2$ and $PaCO_2$ therefore not falling (ie, isocapnic buffering) (see **Fig. 3.13**, mechanism II; see also **Figs. 2.52** and **3.17**).

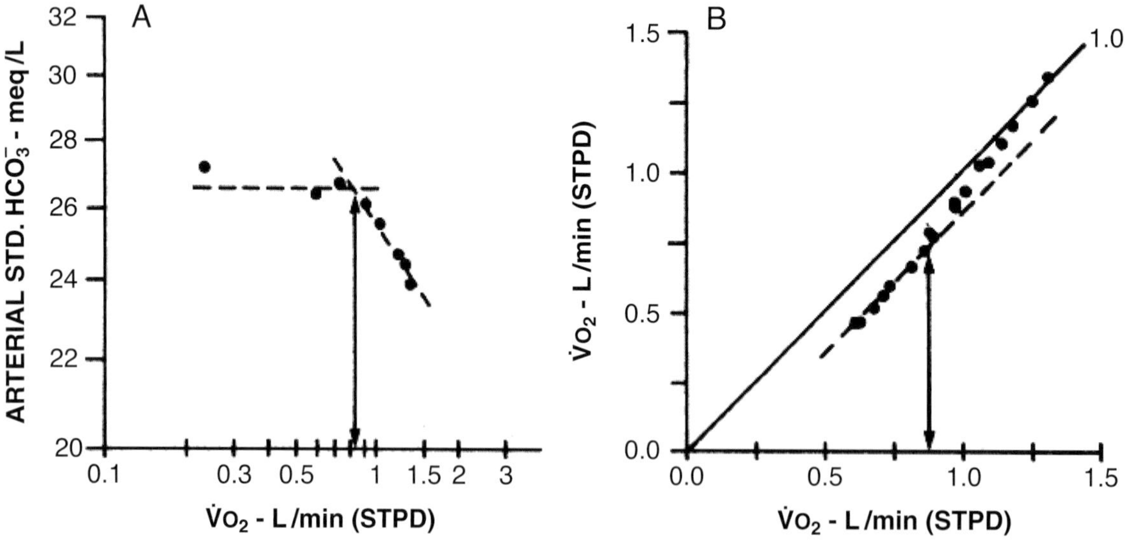

FIGURE 3.16. Example of modified V-slope technique. A: The relationship between log (standard [bicarbonate] [HCO_3^-]) and log (oxygen uptake [$\dot{V}O_2$]) during an incremental cycle ergometer exercise test. Intersection point of best-fit lines drawn to points before and after decline in log standard [HCO_3^-] is taken as the anaerobic threshold. B: The carbon dioxide output ($\dot{V}CO_2$) is plotted against $\dot{V}O_2$. Note the more rapid increase in $\dot{V}CO_2$ relative to $\dot{V}O_2$ beyond the anaerobic threshold. Abbreviation: STPD, standard temperature pressure dry. *(Reprinted from Sue DY, Wasserman K, Moricca RB, Casaburi R. Metabolic acidosis during exercise in patients with chronic obstructive pulmonary disease. Use of the V-slope method for anaerobic threshold determination.* Chest. *1988;94[5]:931-938. Figure 1. Copyright © 1988 American College of Chest Physicians. With permission.)*

However, the necessary consequence of $\dot{V}E$ continuing to increase in proportion to $\dot{V}CO_2$ in the isocapnic buffering phase is that $\dot{V}E$ has now to increase at a greater rate relative to $\dot{V}O_2$. The ventilatory equivalent for O_2 ($\dot{V}E/\dot{V}O_2$) therefore also starts to increase, as does $PETO_2$ (see **Figs. 2.52** and **3.17**). Thus, hyperventilation occurs with respect to O_2 but not CO_2 as the *AT* is exceeded.

The increase in $\dot{V}E/\dot{V}O_2$ without an increase in $\dot{V}E/\dot{V}CO_2$ can only be caused by HCO_3^- buffering of the exercise metabolic acidosis. It cannot be caused by other factors that increase $\dot{V}E$ out of proportion to $\dot{V}O_2$ (eg, hypoxemia, pain,

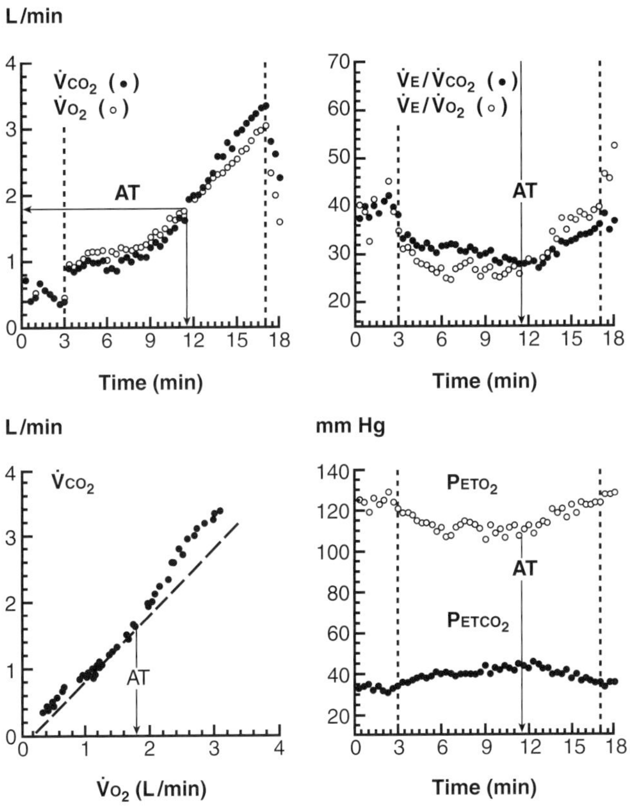

FIGURE 3.17. Ventilatory and gas exchange responses for a normal individual during an incremental cycle ergometer exercise test to illustrate the changes that take place at the anaerobic threshold (*AT*). The far-left vertical dashed line, in the three panels with time as the x-axis, indicates the start of unloading cycling. After 3 min of unloaded cycling, the work rate was increased at 25 W/min. The right vertical dashed line indicates the end of exercise. Oxygen uptake ($\dot{V}O_2$) and carbon dioxide output ($\dot{V}CO_2$) versus time (upper left panel). For the V-slope plot of $\dot{V}CO_2$ versus $\dot{V}O_2$ (lower left panel), the diagonal line is at 45° (or a slope of 1); the *AT* is where the $\dot{V}CO_2$ starts to increase faster than $\dot{V}O_2$, with the slope of the plot becoming steeper (ie, greater than 1). This is shown as the vertical arrow marked *AT*. The *AT* can also be located where the $\dot{V}E/\dot{V}O_2$ profile (right upper panel) inflects upward (vertical dashed arrow labeled *AT*). The nadir of the $\dot{V}E/\dot{V}CO_2$ profile occurs at a higher work rate and reflects the delayed start of ventilatory compensation for the metabolic acidosis characteristic of rapid incremental tests. Because of the hyperventilation with respect to O_2, end-tidal PO_2 ($PETO_2$) increases at the *AT*, whereas end-tidal PCO_2 ($PETCO_2$) does not start to decrease systematically until approximately 2 min later, coinciding with the increased ventilatory drive that serves to partially compensate for the decrease in arterial pH (right lower panel).

or anxiety) because these would cause $\dot{V}E/\dot{V}CO_2$ to increase as well as $\dot{V}E/\dot{V}O_2$. When $\dot{V}E/\dot{V}O_2$ increases without a simultaneous increase in $\dot{V}E/\dot{V}CO_2$ during an incremental exercise test, it is a specific gas exchange demonstration that the *AT* has been surpassed (see **Figs. 2.52** and **3.17**).

The primary reason for increasing work rate relatively rapidly during the CPET exercise test is that the ventilatory compensation for the exercise metabolic acidosis, most likely mediated by the carotid body chemoreceptors, develops slowly relative to the rate of work rate increase (see Chapter 2, "Ventilatory Control" section). Hence, ventilatory compensation for the metabolic acidosis does not occur when arterial pH first starts to fall (ie, at the *AT*) but at a higher $\dot{V}O_2$ (ie, at the VCP) (see **Figs. 2.52** and **3.17**). In contrast to the *AT*, the VCP is influenced by the work rate incrementation rate, being closer to the *AT* when work rates are incremented slowly and also when carotid body drive is enhanced by hypoxia increase (see Chapter 2, "Ventilatory Control" section). Beyond the VCP, the carotid chemoreceptors respond to the decreasing arterial pH and ventilatory stimulation is intensified (see **Fig. 3.13**, mechanism III; see also **Figs. 2.52** and **3.17**). This causes $PaCO_2$ to decrease, preventing pH from falling as much as would be predicted by the imposition of a lactic acidosis in a closed system. This ventilatory compensation for the metabolic acidosis is reflected in an increase in $\dot{V}E/\dot{V}CO_2$ and a decrease in $PaCO_2$ and $PETCO_2$ as well as by further increases in $\dot{V}E/\dot{V}O_2$ and $PETO_2$ (see **Figs. 2.52** and **3.17**).

A second reason for using a rapid incremental exercise test is to take advantage of the CO_2 contribution from buffering being observed only *during* the buffering process (ie, when $[HCO_3^-]$ is actually decreasing) and not after the buffering process is complete (ie, when $[HCO_3^-]$ would have stabilized at a new lower level). Thus, CO_2 generated from buffering is evident in the expired gas only when [lactate] and $[HCO_3^-]$ are *changing* but not after they have already *changed*. As a result, in contrast to tests in which work rate is incremented slowly, increasing the work rate at a relatively fast rate (as is recommended for CPET) will result in a greater rate of $[HCO_3^-]$ decrease and therefore a steeper S_2 slope, improving the discriminability of the S_1-S_2 break point and also the associated ventilatory and gas exchange indices for *AT* estimation.[39,44]

Improving Estimation of the Anaerobic Threshold

Occasionally, the *AT* cannot be reliably detected by the ventilatory equivalent method (see **Fig. 3.13**, mechanism II) by factors such as irregular breathing, an inappropriate rate of increase in work rate, suboptimal plotting scales, or a poor ventilatory response to the metabolic acidosis. To obviate these problems, one can measure arterial [lactate] or standard $[HCO_3^-]$ directly (see **Fig. 3.12**). Beaver et al[45] found that the *LT* can be most reliably identified by plotting log arterial [lactate] against log $\dot{V}O_2$. Similarly, the start of the arterial $[HCO_3^-]$ fall, indicating the onset of the developing lactic acidosis (*LAT*), can be most reliably detected from a plot of log standard arterial $[HCO_3^-]$ against log $\dot{V}O_2$ (see **Fig. 3.16**).[46] A slight difference exists in the $\dot{V}O_2$ for these thresholds. The

LT slightly precedes *LAT* because of non-HCO_3^- buffering of the initial increased proton load.[47] However, although we distinguish between *LT* and *LAT* for scientific correctness, the distinction is not of clinical significance.

When the S_1-S_2 break point (ie, $\dot{V}CO_2$ increasing faster than $\dot{V}O_2$) is not clear using the V-slope method, it is likely that the rate of CO_2 released from HCO_3^- buffering of the metabolic acidosis is slow because the rate of increase in work rate is slow relative to the subject's fitness.[48] Alternatively, a metabolic acidosis may not be elicited, such as in muscle phosphorylase deficiency (McArdle's syndrome).[49] In the former instance, the test should be repeated with a faster rate of increase in work rate. If the S_1-S_2 break point is still not observed, the possibility should be investigated that the patient is unable to raise blood lactate levels because of a muscle metabolic defect.

False Positives

There are instances, however, when a "false-positive" *AT* estimation (or pseudothreshold) can result.[44] For example, when the work rate is incremented far more rapidly than recommended (eg, 25-30 W/min), the consequently rapid rate of increase in the metabolic CO_2 production response exaggerates the normally modest transient CO_2 stores wash-in early in the test (see Chapter 2, "Substrate Utilization" and "Carbon Dioxide Output Kinetics" sections), with a smaller than normal proportion being cleared at the lungs.[50] At this time, the $\dot{V}CO_2$ response is therefore attenuated both absolutely and relative to $\dot{V}O_2$, resulting in an abnormally low $\dot{V}CO_2$-$\dot{V}O_2$ slope with respiratory exchange ratio (R) (ie, $\dot{V}CO_2/\dot{V}O_2$) falling to uncharacteristically low values (**Fig. 3.18**). The subsequent reduction in CO_2 storage rate as the test progresses leads to an increase in the $\dot{V}CO_2$ response relative to $\dot{V}O_2$, that is, an increased $\dot{V}CO_2$-$\dot{V}O_2$ slope (see **Fig. 3.18**). Furthermore, the acceleration of the $\dot{V}CO_2$ response relative to $\dot{V}O_2$ beyond the $\dot{V}CO_2$-$\dot{V}O_2$ break point triggers the cascade of ventilatory and gas exchange responses that are conventionally seen at the S_1-S_2 break point, that is, hyperventilation relative to O_2 but not CO_2 (see **Fig. 3.18**; compare with **Figs. 2.52** and **3.17**). At first sight, this response profile could reasonably be suggestive of the onset of a metabolic acidosis (see **Figs. 3.15** and **3.17**). However, the abnormally low initial $\dot{V}CO_2$-$\dot{V}O_2$ slope (ie, the "S_1" slope proxy) and falling R as the $\dot{V}CO_2$-$\dot{V}O_2$ break point is approached distinguishes it from the conventional gas exchange profile seen at the onset of the metabolic acidosis of incremental exercise, as does the lack of increase in arterial [lactate] (see **Fig. 3.18**).

A similar effect can occur when CO_2 stores are depleted prior to the test by volitional or anticipatory hyperventilation, which results in a considerable proportion of the aerobically produced CO_2 early in the exercise test being retained to replenish the stores rather than being cleared at the lungs. Again, an abnormally low initial $\dot{V}CO_2$-$\dot{V}O_2$ slope and a marked falling of R can result, together with hyperventilation relative to O_2 but not CO_2 but with no evidence of a metabolic acidosis.[51] That is, in each of these conditions, $\dot{V}CO_2$ can begin to increase at a discernibly greater rate with increasing work rate, not only simply because CO_2 begins to be produced more rapidly in the exercising muscles but also because its tissue storage rate begins to slow.

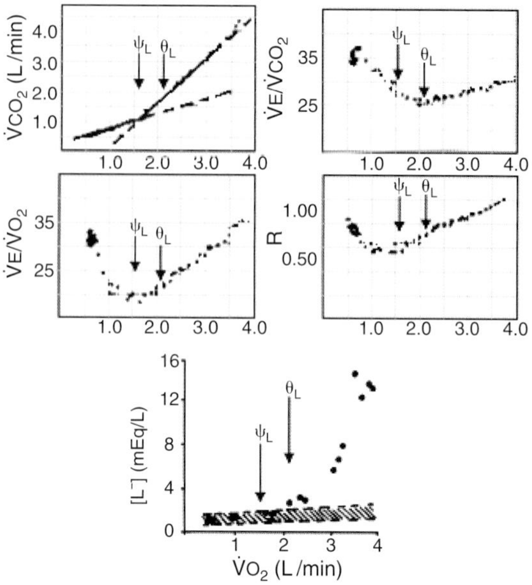

FIGURE 3.18. Response profiles of carbon dioxide output ($\dot{V}CO_2$), ventilatory equivalent for oxygen ($\dot{V}E/\dot{V}O_2$), ventilatory equivalent for carbon dioxide ($\dot{V}E/\dot{V}CO_2$), respiratory exchange ratio (R), and arterialized-venous [lactate] versus oxygen uptake ($\dot{V}O_2$) for incremental cycle ergometer exercise (25 W/min). Note that a psuedothreshold (ψ_L) was evident, occurring at a lower $\dot{V}O_2$ than the directly estimated lactate or anaerobic threshold (θ_L). *(Reprinted with permission from Springer: Ward SA, Whipp BJ. Influence of body CO_2 stores on ventilatory-metabolic coupling during exercise. In: Honda Y, Miyamoto Y, Konno K, Widdicombe JG, eds.* Control of Breathing and Its Modelling Perspective. *New York, NY: Plenum Press; 1992:425-431. Figure 5. Copyright © 1992 Springer Science+Business Media New York.)*

Heart Rate–Oxygen Uptake Relationship and Heart Rate Reserve

Heart rate normally increases linearly with $\dot{V}O_2$ during incremental exercise (**Fig. 3.19**) (see Chapter 2, "Cardiac Output" section). In heart diseases unrelated to conduction defects, HR often increases relatively steeply for the increase in $\dot{V}O_2$ because the stroke volume is reduced. In addition, $\dot{V}O_2$ commonly slows its rate of increase with work rate when the myocardium becomes ischemic, as in patients with coronary artery disease. Because HR typically continues to increase in patients whose HRs are not slowed by β-adrenergic blockade, the rate of increase in HR relative to $\dot{V}O_2$ becomes steeper, deviating from the linearity established at lower work rates (see **Fig. 3.19**). This implies that stroke volume is decreasing and that cardiac output may not be increasing in pace with the O_2 requirement. Although this curvilinear increase in the HR–$\dot{V}O_2$ relationship is not uniformly seen in patients with heart disease, it is a useful diagnostic observation and suggests a significant worsening in left ventricular function with increasing work rate.[52] Pulmonary vascular disease is also associated with a steep HR response because venous return to

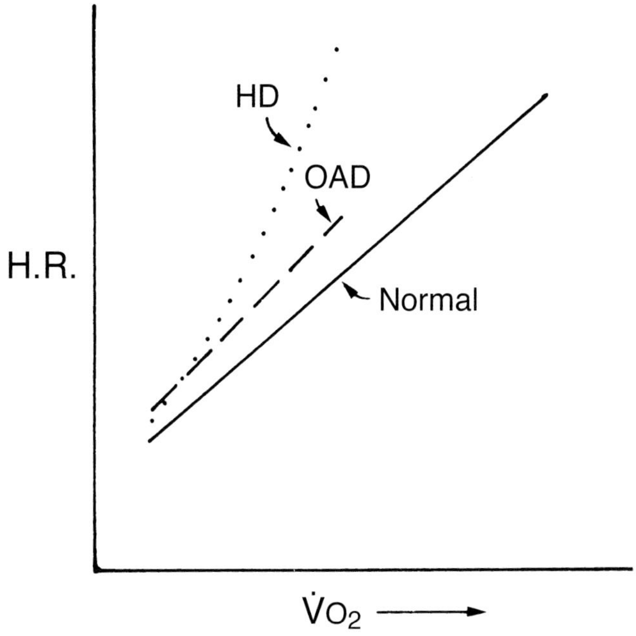

FIGURE 3.19. Characteristic changes in heart rate (HR) relative to oxygen uptake ($\dot{V}O_2$) during incremental exercise for normal individuals, patients with chronic obstructive airway disease (OAD), and those with heart disease (HD) without chronotropic incompetence. The steeper HR-$\dot{V}O_2$ relationship for the OAD patient may reflect relative unfitness or reduced stroke volume secondary to disturbed lung mechanics or pulmonary vascular occlusion. In contrast, the relatively low maximum HR reflects respiratory limitation at the peak work rate. The steepening HR-$\dot{V}O_2$ relationship seen in some HD patients reflects the failure of $\dot{V}O_2$ to increase normally in response to the increasing work rate, as illustrated in Figure 3.6C.

the left side of the heart and therefore left ventricular output are low in this disorder.[53,54]

Patients with airflow obstruction (see **Fig. 3.19**) commonly have a moderately elevated HR response at a given $\dot{V}O_2$ due to a reduced stroke volume. The latter results from a restriction in cardiac filling[55] due to high intrathoracic pressure during exhalation, or to encroachment of the lung on the cardiac fossa, or both. Heart rate increases linearly with $\dot{V}O_2$ in this disorder. However, the maximum HR in the patient with ventilatory limitation is usually below the predicted value because ventilatory limitation occurs before the cardiovascular system is maximally str essed.[35,56,57]

The estimated HR reserve is a measure of the difference between the predicted maximal HR, based on age, and the measured HR at peak $\dot{V}O_2$ (see the section on "Peak Heart Rate and Heart Rate Reserve" in Chapter 7). Although the predicted maximal HR has considerable variation, as determined from population studies, the HR reserve is still a useful concept for differential diagnosis. **Table 3.7** lists disorders in which the HR reserve may be increased. Normally, the HR reserve is relatively small (less than 15 bpm). It is also usually normal in patients with silent myocardial ischemia and valvular heart disease and in patients with disorders of the pulmonary circulation. In contrast, patients with peripheral arterial disease and patients with COPD become symptom limited before the predicted maximal HR is reached. Patients with disorders of the conducting system of the heart, or sinoatrial node, may also have a low maximum HR. Patients who take β-adrenergic blocking drugs or patients who are limited in exercise because of heart block or sick sinus syndrome have a large HR reserve. Finally, those patients who make a poor effort have an increased HR reserve because they fail to maximally stress their cardiovascular system at the time they stop exercising.

TABLE 3.7 Disorders Associated With Increased Heart Rate Reserve

Claudication limiting exercise
Angina-limiting exercise
"Sick sinus" syndrome
β-Adrenergic blockade
Lung disease with impaired ventilatory mechanics
Poor effort

Arterial Blood Pressure

Arterial pressure measurements, particularly when directly measured, are helpful for diagnostics as well as for patient safety. The normal responses of systolic, diastolic, and pulse pressures are described in Chapter 5 ("Electrocardiogram and Systemic Blood Pressure" section) and Chapter 7. Normally, the systolic pressure increases to a much greater degree than the diastolic pressure and in proportion to the work rate increase. A decrease in systolic and pulse pressures with increasing work rate suggests significant cardiac dysfunction and indicates that the exercise test should stop. The direct arterial pressure tracing (made at a fast recorder speed) showing a slow rise in arterial pressure may provide evidence for ventricular outflow obstruction, such as seen with aortic stenosis or hypertrophic cardiomyopathy.

Breathing Reserve

The breathing reserve is expressed as either the difference between the maximal voluntary ventilation (MVV) and the maximum exercise $\dot{V}E$ in absolute terms or this difference as a fraction of the MVV (**Table 3.2** and **Fig. 3.20**). Except in extremely fit endurance athletes who can attain exceptionally high metabolic rates, normal males have a breathing reserve of at least 11 L/min or 10% to 40% of the MVV (**Fig. 3.21**).[58] Female athletes might also have a low breathing reserve during exercise because, relative to height, females have a lower MVV than males. A low breathing reserve is characteristic of patients with primary lung disease who have ventilatory limitation.[1,8,16,56,57] The breathing reserve is high when cardiovascular or other diseases limit exercise performance.[1,16,32]

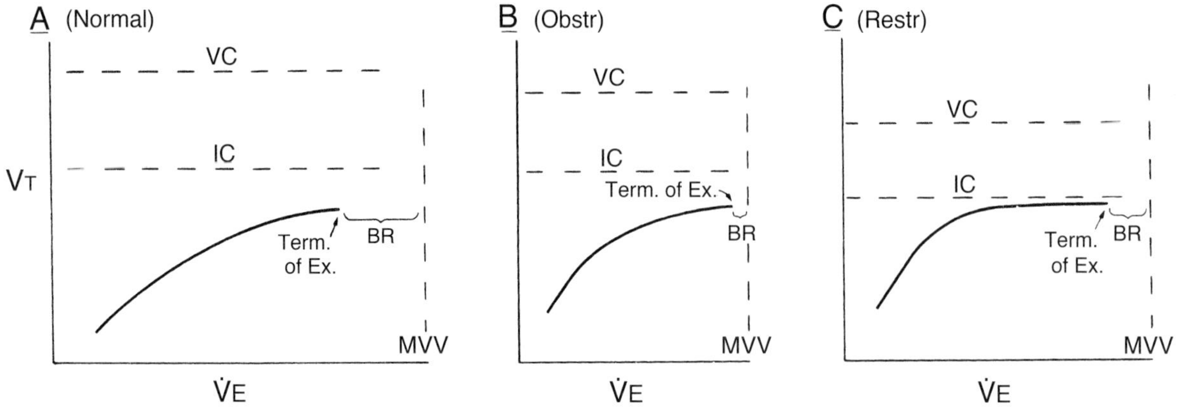

FIGURE 3.20. Characteristic examples of tidal volume (VT) response relative to ventilation (V̇E) during incremental exercise in a normal individual (A) and in patients with obstructive (B) and restrictive (C) lung diseases. The response profile ends at the individual's maximal exercise ventilation. The vertical dashed line on the x-axis indicates the individual's maximum voluntary ventilation (MVV). The horizontal dashed lines on the y-axis indicate the vital capacity (VC) and inspiratory capacity (IC). The distance on the x-axis between the V̇E at peak exercise and MVV is the individual's breathing reserve (BR). In obstructive lung disease, the BR is quite small. In restrictive lung diseases, the IC is reduced and VT closely approximates the IC near and at peak exercise.

Expiratory Flow Pattern

The expiratory flow pattern can be useful in detecting airway obstruction during exercise. The peak expiratory flow rate is near the middle of the expiratory phase of respiration in normal individuals and has an appearance of a half sine wave. In contrast, the expiratory flow pattern of the patient with obstructive airway disease has an early peak and appears trapezoidal because exhalation effort is sustained with an abrupt termination of expiration, when the next inspiration is initiated (**Fig. 3.22**). This pattern can acutely normalize in asthmatic patients after the use of inhaled bronchodilators (see **Fig. 3.22**). Although the expiratory flow pattern gives only qualitative evidence of airflow obstruction during exercise, it is obtained simply by recording expired airflow, breath by breath. Flow-volume analysis[57,59,60] can give similar information to that of the flow-time analysis.

Inspiratory Capacity

It has long been recognized that end-expiratory lung volume (EELV) increases during exercise in many patients with COPD.[8,59,60] O'Donnell et al[61] emphasized the value of the reduction in inspiratory capacity (IC) during exercise consequent to the development of hyperinflation and increase in EELV during exercise in patients with COPD. In normal individuals, the IC is maintained or slightly increases during exercise, reflecting a decrease in EELV.[8,62] In contrast, the IC decreases during exercise in COPD, reflecting hyperinflation and air trapping as the respiratory rate increases. This reduction in IC in COPD has been used to assess severity of disease. The increase in IC has been used to evaluate the therapeutic efficacy of O_2 breathing[63] and bronchodilators[61] in COPD.

Tests of Uneven V̇A/Q̇

Wasted Ventilation and Dead Space-Tidal Volume Ratio

As discussed in Chapter 2 ("Ventilatory Determinants" section), alveolar ventilation (V̇A) is the theoretical ventilation participating in pulmonary gas exchange if the ventilation–perfusion ratios of all alveolar units were the same, that is,

FIGURE 3.21. Peak exercise ventilation (V̇E peak) relative to maximum voluntary ventilation (MVV) for incremental cycle ergometer exercise in patients with chronic obstructive pulmonary disease (COPD, x) and in normal (control) individuals (•). The dashed-line isopleths indicate the percentage of breathing reserve [(MVV − V̇E peak)/MVV] × 100. The *r* values are the correlation coefficients for the control and the COPD groups. Abbreviation: BTPS, body temperature pressure saturated.

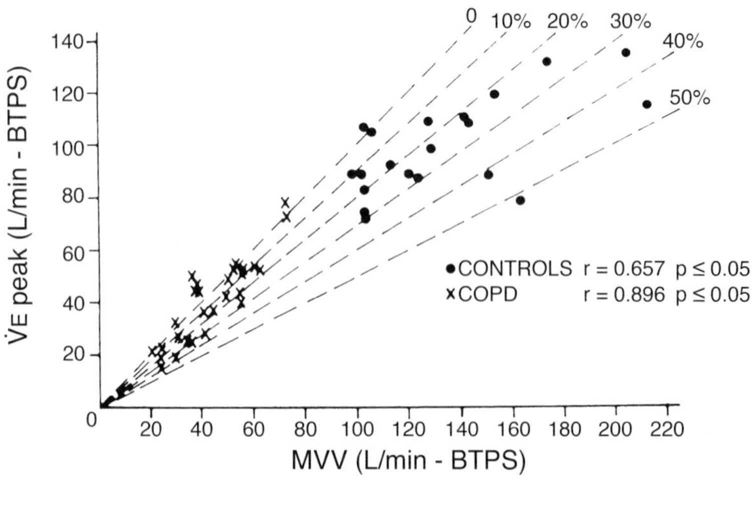

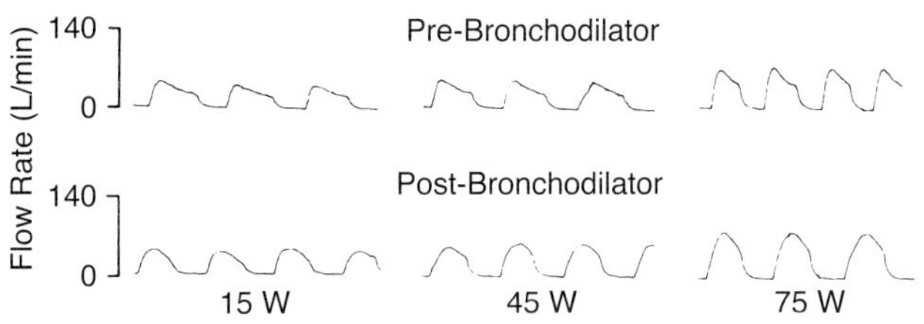

FIGURE 3.22. Expiratory flow pattern in an asthmatic patient at increasing work rates before and after acute bronchodilator therapy. *(Reprinted from Brown HV, Wasserman K, Whipp BJ. Strategies of exercise testing in chronic lung disease.* Bull Eur Physiopathol Respir. *1977;13[3]:409-423. Copyright © 1977 Elsevier. With permission.)*

the "ideal" lung. In the ideal lung, the mean alveolar P_{CO_2} is assumed to equal the arterial P_{CO_2}. However, the lung usually does not have ideal properties, and the actual ventilation (ie, $\dot{V}_E$) includes ventilation to conducting airways (ie, which do not participate in gas exchange, comprising the anatomic dead space) and alveoli that may not be ideally perfused. The difference between $\dot{V}_E$ and the ideal $\dot{V}_A$ is the physiological dead space ventilation (which includes the anatomic dead space and the alveolar dead space). A valuable estimate of the degree of mismatching of ventilation to perfusion during exercise is V_D/V_T. The V_D/V_T is lowest when alveolar ventilation relative to perfusion ($\dot{V}_A/\dot{Q}$) is uniform.

At rest, the physiological dead space volume is normally about one-third of the tidal volume. During exercise, it is reduced to about one-fifth of the tidal volume,[64] with the major decrement occurring at the lowest work rates. In patients with airway disorders, $\dot{V}_A/\dot{Q}$ relationships are uneven primarily because of nonuniform ventilation. In patients with pulmonary vascular disease, $\dot{V}_A/\dot{Q}$ relationships are uneven primarily because of nonuniform perfusion of ventilated lung. In both disorders, V_D/V_T is higher, particularly during exercise, because the V_D/V_T is increased at rest and fails to decrease during exercise.

The V_D/V_T is a valuable measurement because it is typically abnormal in patients with primary pulmonary vascular disease or pulmonary vascular disease secondary to obstructive or interstitial lung disease and patients with heart failure. This is discussed in greater detail in Chapter 4. An elevated V_D/V_T is sometimes the only gas exchange abnormality evident during exercise testing.[52] **Figure 3.23** illustrates the pattern of change in V_D/V_T as the work rate is increased in the normal individual and in patients with nonuniform $\dot{V}_A/\dot{Q}$ distributions resulting from lung or pulmonary vascular diseases. In patients with nonuniform $\dot{V}_A/\dot{Q}$, the V_D/V_T may be only slightly elevated at rest, but it remains relatively unchanged during exercise or even increases if a right-to-left shunt develops during exercise (eg, opening a foramen ovale). Thus, exercise brings out the abnormality in $\dot{V}_A/\dot{Q}$ relationships.

As discussed in Chapter 2 ("Ventilatory Determinants" section), when V_D/V_T is increased, $\dot{V}_E$ is typically abnormally high for the work rate performed. The $\dot{V}_E$ may also be high in conditions in which the Pa_{CO_2} is relatively low (low

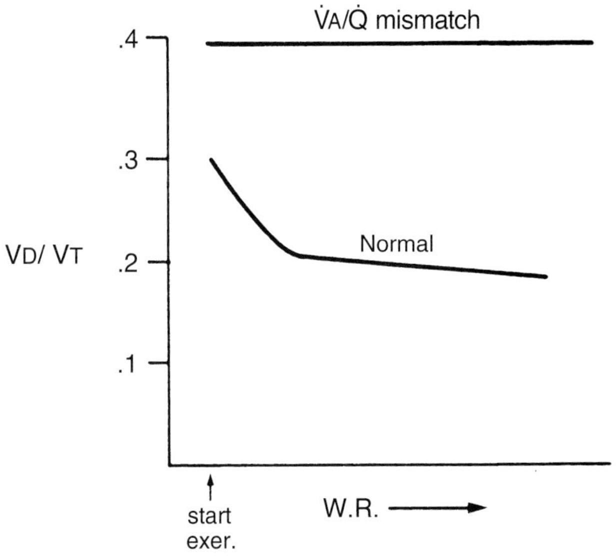

FIGURE 3.23. Characteristic examples of the ratio of physiological dead space to tidal volume (V_D/V_T) response from rest with increasing work rate (WR) for a normal individual and a patient with ventilation–perfusion ($\dot{V}_A/\dot{Q}$) mismatch.

CO_2 set point), such as with a chronic metabolic acidosis. In this setting, V_D/V_T will be normal if the lungs are normal, and arterial blood gas analysis will reveal a low Pa_{CO_2} (hyperventilation). Therefore, a high $\dot{V}_E$ at a given work rate (high $\dot{V}_E/\dot{V}_{CO_2}$) is indicative of a high V_D/V_T, hyperventilation, or both. The two pathophysiological mechanisms can be differentiated by measuring gas exchange and arterial blood gases simultaneously.

Figure 3.24 shows the $\dot{V}_E$ required for various metabolic rates ($\dot{V}_{CO_2}$) for designated values of Pa_{CO_2} and V_D/V_T. This plot is useful for demonstrating the relationships between $\dot{V}_E$, Pa_{CO_2}, $\dot{V}_{CO_2}$, and V_D/V_T. It also serves as a nomogram to determine V_D/V_T when the three other variables are known.

Arterial P_{O_2} and Alveolar–Arterial P_{O_2} Difference

Normally, Pa_{O_2} does not decrease during exercise, and the alveolar-to-arterial P_{O_2} difference $[P(A - a)_{O_2}]$ remains under 20 to 30 mm Hg, although tending to widen at higher work rates (**Fig. 3.25A**) (see Chapter 2, "Arterial P_{O_2}" section). However, in highly fit endurance athletes, $P(A - a)_{O_2}$ widens appreciably near peak exercise with a consequent fall in Pa_{O_2} (exercise-induced arterial hypoxemia). In patients with airway disease, a reduced Pa_{O_2} and an increased $P(A - a)_{O_2}$ during incremental exercise (**Fig. 3.25B**) typically result from underventilation of regions of lung relative to their perfusion—that is, lung units with low alveolar ventilation–perfusion ratios.[64,65] During exercise, when cardiac output increases, causing more desaturated blood to flow through low $\dot{V}_A/\dot{Q}$ areas of the lungs, arterial hypoxemia becomes more marked. Fortunately, the blood vessels in the poorly ventilated low $\dot{V}_A/\dot{Q}$ areas of the lung normally constrict under the influence of decreasing alveolar P_{O_2}.[66] This diversion of blood

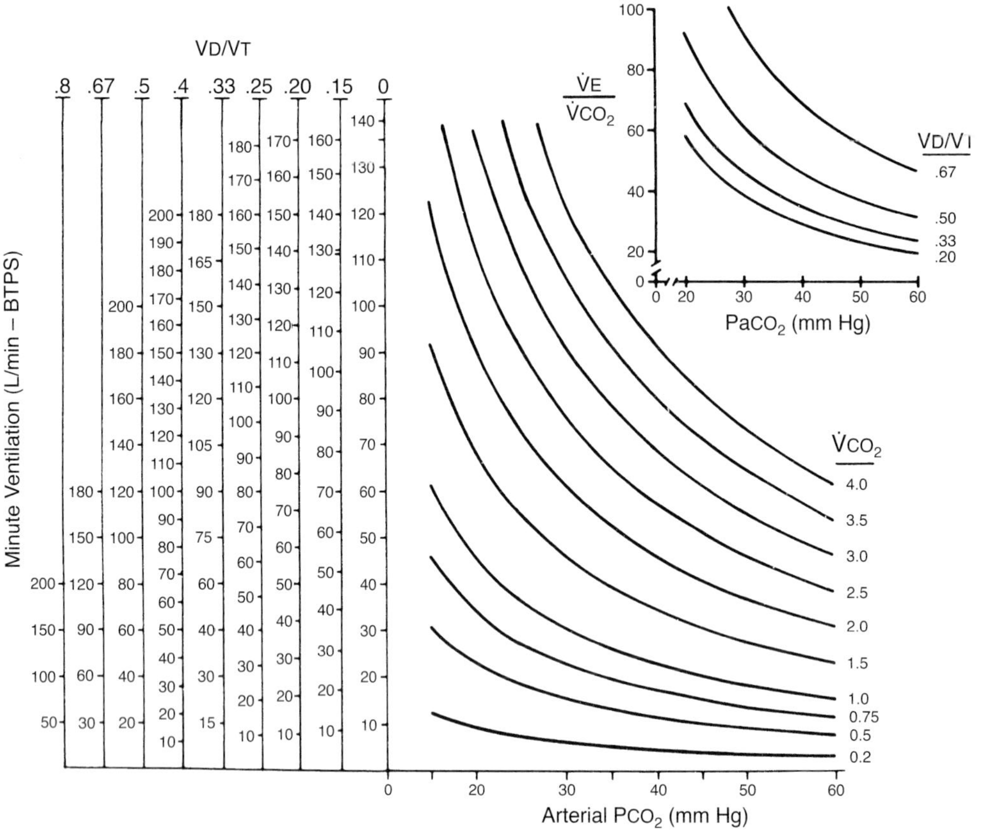

FIGURE 3.24. Main graph shows ventilation ($\dot{V}_E$) as a function of arterial P_{CO_2} (Pa_{CO_2}) for various values of carbon dioxide output ($\dot{V}_{CO_2}$) during exercise (solid curves are $\dot{V}_{CO_2}$ isopleths). The additional influence of physiological dead space–tidal volume ratio (V_D/V_T) is displayed at the left: Each vertical scale on the y-axis indicates the $\dot{V}_E$ values for a particular V_D/V_T value. If values for any three of the foregoing variables are known, the fourth can be determined. For instance, if $\dot{V}_E$, $\dot{V}_{CO_2}$, and Pa_{CO_2} are measured, then V_D/V_T can be determined from the y-axis scale that agrees with the measured $\dot{V}_E$. The inset graph (top right) shows the effect of changing Pa_{CO_2} on $\dot{V}_E/\dot{V}_{CO_2}$ during exercise at each of a range of V_D/V_T values. Abbreviation: BTPS, body temperature pressure saturated. *(Reprinted with permission of the American Thoracic Society. Copyright © 2020 American Thoracic Society. All rights reserved. Main figure from Wasserman K, Whipp BJ. Exercise physiology in health and disease.* Am Rev Respir Dis. *1975;112[2]:219-249. The American Review of Respiratory Disease* is an official journal of the American Thoracic Society. [*Now titled The American Journal of Respiratory and Critical Care Medicine])*

flow to areas of relatively good ventilation is a protective mechanism because it reduces the degree of hypoxemia that would otherwise occur. This mechanism prevents progressive hypoxemia as the work rate is increased in patients with COPD (**Fig. 3.25B**).

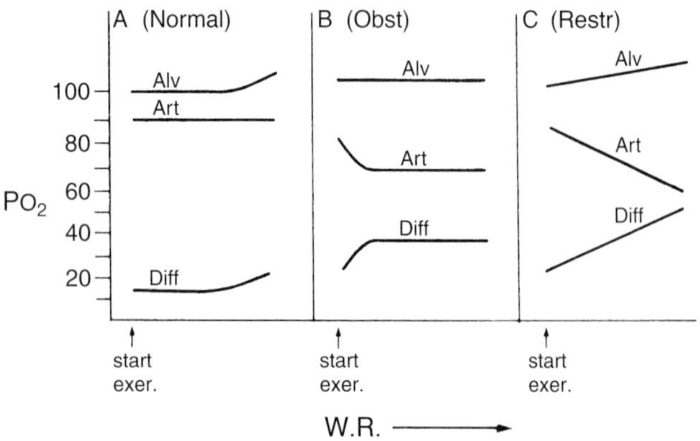

FIGURE 3.25. Characteristic pattern of arterial and alveolar P_{O_2} and alveolar-arterial P_{O_2} difference responses for incremental exercise in normal individuals (A) and in patients with obstructive (B) and restrictive (C) lung diseases. Abbreviation: WR, work rate.

Exercise hypoxemia may also develop in patients with pulmonary fibrosis or pulmonary vascular disease. Because all recruitable pulmonary blood vessels are functioning at rest in patients with a reduced pulmonary capillary bed, when cardiac output increases during exercise, no additional pulmonary capillaries are available to be recruited to accommodate the increase in pulmonary blood flow. Thus, the red cell residence or transit time must decrease at rest and further decrease during exercise, resulting in reduced time for diffusion equilibrium between alveolar P_{O_2} and red cell P_{O_2}. A pattern of decreasing Pa_{O_2} and increasing $P(A - a)_{O_2}$ with increasing work rate reflects a decrease in residence time of red cells in the pulmonary capillaries when the pulmonary capillary blood volume is critically reduced. Consequently, for disorders in which pulmonary capillary blood volume is reduced and accompanied by exercise-induced hypoxemia due to reduced time for diffusion equilibrium, hypoxemia becomes more pronounced as the work rate and pulmonary blood pressure and flow increase (**Fig. 3.25C**).

Pa_{O_2} also decreases as the work rate is increased in conditions in which the alveoli are filled with material in which

O_2 is relatively insoluble (eg, as in pulmonary alveolar proteinosis). When the perfusion increases in these lung units, O_2 in the gas space fails to equilibrate with O_2 in the red cell (alveolar capillary block), and hypoxemia becomes more marked as the blood flow increases (a diffusion defect). At rest, however, when pulmonary blood flow is relatively low, Pa_{O_2} may be normal because red cell residence time in the pulmonary capillary is long enough (>0.3 s) to reach diffusion equilibrium.

Hypoxemia will worsen in patients with lung disease when a potentially patent foramen ovale opens consequent to right atrial pressure exceeding left atrial pressure. This causes part of the venous return to shunt from right to left at the atrial level. A simple, sensitive test to diagnose a right-to-left shunt that develops during exercise uses 100% O_2 breathing. For example, when breathing 100% O_2, the Pa_{O_2} is reduced approximately 100 mm Hg below "normal" (ie, 600 mm Hg) for each 5% right-to-left shunt until the Pa_{O_2} reaches a value of about 150 mm Hg. The decrease in Pa_{O_2} is then smaller for a given shunt size.

Calculation of $P(A - a)_{O_2}$ may reveal abnormalities in blood oxygenation masked by hyperventilation. An abnormally elevated $P(A - a)_{O_2}$ is indicative of uneven $\dot{V}_A/\dot{Q}$, a diffusion defect, and/or a right-to-left shunt.

Arterial–End-Tidal P_{CO_2} Difference

Alveoli that are underperfused or unperfused have a low P_{CO_2}. The ventilation of these alveoli is wasted (alveolar dead space) because these alveoli cannot participate fully in gas exchange. Thus, in these patients, the mixed expired and end-tidal P_{CO_2} values are reduced relative to the directly measured arterial P_{CO_2}. By measuring the arterial–end-tidal P_{CO_2} difference [$P(a - ET)_{CO_2}$], we have another measurement that can be used as evidence of increased alveolar dead space or uneven $\dot{V}_A/\dot{Q}$ (**Fig. 3.26**).[24,25,64]

During exercise, P_{ETCO_2} normally increases relative to Pa_{CO_2} (**Fig. 3.26A**), provided that the functioning alveoli are relatively uniformly perfused. The mechanism for this is relatively straightforward—the consequence of an intermittent ventilation of exchanging alveoli in the face of more nearly continuous pulmonary-capillary perfusion.[67] Direct measurements of continuously measured P_{CO_2} in the respired air and arterial blood are shown in **Figure 3.27**. Thus, during exhalation, alveolar P_{CO_2} increases because of the continuing diffusion of CO_2 from pulmonary capillary blood into the alveoli, coupled with the progressive reduction of alveolar volume. The highest value alveolar P_{CO_2} attains in the respiratory cycle is equal to the P_{ETCO_2}. In the subsequent inspiration, alveolar P_{CO_2} declines progressively, reflecting the diluting action of the inhaled air. The resulting intrabreath fluctuation in alveolar P_{CO_2} (and pulmonary-capillary blood P_{CO_2}) dictates that P_{ETCO_2} will exceed the intrabreath mean alveolar P_{CO_2} and the mean arterial P_{CO_2} (when the latter is sampled over several, and ideally a unitary number of, breaths); thus, $P(a - ET)_{CO_2}$ is negative.[24,26,68,69] The intrabreath alveolar P_{O_2} shows a mirror image.

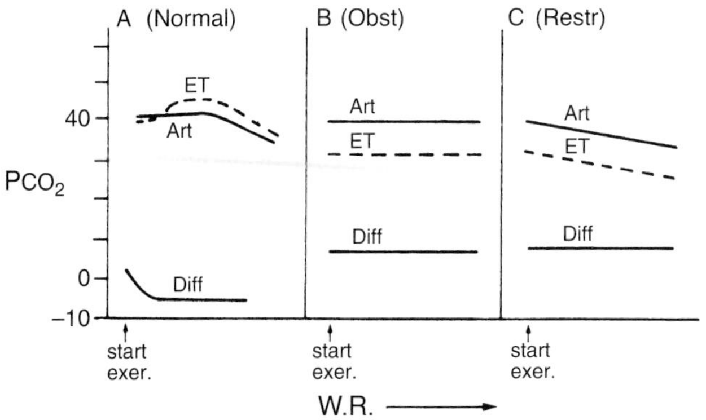

FIGURE 3.26. Characteristic pattern of arterial (Art) and end-tidal (ET) P_{CO_2} and Art-ET P_{CO_2} difference responses for incremental exercise in normal individuals (A) and in patients with obstructive (B) and restrictive (C) lung diseases. All are assumed to have normal resting Pa_{CO_2} values. Abbreviation: WR, work rate.

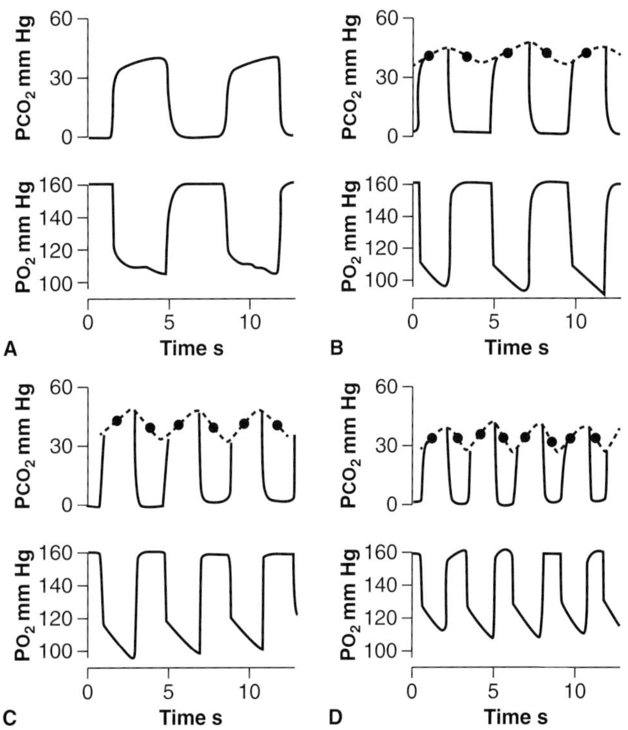

FIGURE 3.27. Intrabreath profiles of respired P_{CO_2} and P_{O_2} at rest (A), 100 W (B), 200 W (C), and 300 W (D) in a normal individual. ----, schematized time-course of alveolar (and arterial) P_{CO_2} (ie, corrected for gas-analyser transit delays); •, mean alveolar (and arterial) P_{CO_2}. *(Reprinted from Whipp BJ. The bioenergetic and gas exchange basis of exercise testing.* Clin Chest Med. *1994;15[2]:173-192. Figure 9. Copyright © 1994 Elsevier. With permission.)*

The slope of instantaneously measured exhaled P_{CO_2} during the alveolar phase of the breath increases as work rate increases, reflecting a greater driving pressure for intrapulmonary CO_2 diffusion consequent to the increasing greater mixed venous P_{CO_2}, and therefore P_{ETCO_2} rises progressively and $P(a - ET)_{CO_2}$ becomes more negative (**Fig. 3.27B,C**).[24,26,69] Further increases in P_{ETCO_2} typically become truncated at higher work rates when breathing frequency starts to increase (**Fig. 3.27D**). However, the slower the breathing rate, the closer P_{ETCO_2} would be to mixed venous P_{CO_2}, making $P(a - ET)CO_2$ even more negative.

In contrast, $P(a - ET)CO_2$ is positive in the healthy lung at rest (**Fig. 3.26A**), reflecting a small degree of regional $\dot{V}A/\dot{Q}$ inhomogeneity; Pa_{CO_2} is approximately 2 mm Hg greater than P_{ETCO_2}. If the $P(a - ET)CO_2$ remains positive during exercise, this is evidence for decreased perfusion to ventilated alveoli (uneven $\dot{V}A/\dot{Q}$ with high $\dot{V}A/\dot{Q}$ units) (**Fig. 3.26B,C**). An extreme situation may be seen when CO_2-rich venous blood is diverted to the left side of the circulation without passing through the lungs during exercise (right-to-left shunt). In this case, Pa_{CO_2} is much higher than P_{ETCO_2} because the blood perfusing the lung is subsequently hyperventilated to compensate for the CO_2 load entering the arterial circulation through the shunt.[54,70] $P(a - ET)CO_2$ is therefore markedly positive because of a decreased P_{ETCO_2}. The magnitude of the increased $P(a - ET)CO_2$ depends on the size of the right-to-left shunt.

Sue et al[25] compared the resting diffusing capacity of the lung for carbon monoxide (DLCO) with arterial blood gases during maximal exercise in 276 male shipyard workers. Fourteen of 16 individuals with a DLCO less than 70% had abnormal gas exchange during exercise, measured as an increase in $P(A - a)O_2$, VD/VT, or $P(a - ET)CO_2$. However, 88 individuals had abnormal exercise gas exchange with a normal DLCO. Increases in VD/VT and $P(a - ET)CO_2$ occurred when there was a major component of uneven, high $\dot{V}A/\dot{Q}$ lung units. Both were abnormal in the same individuals. In contrast, an increase in $P(A - a)O_2$ was abnormal when there was a major component of uneven, low $\dot{V}A/\dot{Q}$ lung units. An increased $P(a - ET)CO_2$ and VD/VT occurred more frequently than an increased $P(A - a)O_2$. When $P(A - a)O_2$ was increased, $P(a - ET)CO_2$ and VD/VT were also increased. In many instances, however, only $P(a - ET)CO_2$ and VD/VT were abnormal, without $P(A - a)O_2$ being abnormal.

Consequently, P_{ETCO_2} being equal to or less than Pa_{CO_2} during exercise is reflective of abnormal gas exchange. For these reasons, P_{ETCO_2} is not a reliable index of Pa_{CO_2} (for discussion of Pa_{CO_2} estimators).[26,27]

Ventilatory Equivalents as Indices of Uneven $\dot{V}A/\dot{Q}$

As described previously, measurements of VD/VT, $P(a - ET)CO_2$, and $P(A - a)O_2$ quantify the degree of $\dot{V}A/\dot{Q}$ mismatching and, thereby, inefficient pulmonary gas exchange. To obtain these measurements, arterial blood gas sampling is required. Because the consequence of inefficient gas exchange dictates an increased ventilatory requirement to eliminate a given amount of CO_2 from the body, two noninvasive approaches have been used to estimate $\dot{V}A/\dot{Q}$ mismatching: the slope of the $\dot{V}E$-$\dot{V}CO_2$ relationship for the work rate range below the VCP and the nadir of $\dot{V}E/\dot{V}CO_2$, which typically occurs at or between the *AT* and VCP[71-76]; generally, the values of these indices of ventilatory inefficiency are essentially identical (see Chapter 2, "Ventilatory Determinants" section). Normal values for the slope and ratio, adjusted for age and gender, are given in Chapter 7.

Figure 3.28 compares the $\dot{V}E$-$\dot{V}CO_2$ slope and the $\dot{V}E/\dot{V}CO_2$ at or between *AT* and VCP in three normal individuals. Although the difference between these two indices is small, the $\dot{V}E$-$\dot{V}CO_2$ slope, measured below the VCP, is usually slightly less than $\dot{V}E/\dot{V}CO_2$ at the *AT* or VCP, depending on the size of the positive intercept on the y-axis of the $\dot{V}E$-$\dot{V}CO_2$ plot.[76] That is, as discussed in Chapter 2 ("Ventilatory Determinants" section), the $\dot{V}E$-$\dot{V}CO_2$ relationship (over its linear range) generally has a small positive $\dot{V}E$ intercept in normal individuals. This makes the $\dot{V}E$-$\dot{V}CO_2$ slope a little less than $\dot{V}E/\dot{V}CO_2$ at the *AT* and VCP (see **Fig. 3.28**, subject 1).

A positive $\dot{V}E$ intercept implies that $\dot{V}E/\dot{V}CO_2$ will decline in a hyperbolic fashion with increasing work rate (see **Fig. 2.28**, panel A) and, if accompanied by a proportionally similar decline in VD/VT (see **Fig. 2.28**, panel B), will result in regulation of Pa_{CO_2}. However, caution is required when inferring the behavior of VD/VT and Pa_{CO_2} from the $\dot{V}E$-$\dot{V}CO_2$ slope and $\dot{V}E$ intercept or from $\dot{V}E/\dot{V}CO_2$ at or between *AT* and VCP. An increased $\dot{V}E$ intercept predictably leads to an elevated $\dot{V}E/\dot{V}CO_2$ profile with increasing work rate and an elevated $\dot{V}E/\dot{V}CO_2$ at or between *AT* and VCP (see **Fig. 3.28**, subject 2). In contrast, if the $\dot{V}E$ intercept is at or near zero, the decline in $\dot{V}E/\dot{V}CO_2$ is greatly attenuated (and, in the limit, would be flat), resulting in the $\dot{V}E$-$\dot{V}CO_2$ slope below the VCP and the $\dot{V}E/\dot{V}CO_2$ at or between *AT* and VCP being essentially equal (see **Fig. 3.28**, subject 3). This commonly occurs in pulmonary vascular disease, reflecting a high resting VD/VT that does not decline appreciably during exercise. However, it should be recognized that under conditions in which the $\dot{V}E$-$\dot{V}CO_2$ slope and the $\dot{V}E$ intercept change in opposite directions, the $\dot{V}E/\dot{V}CO_2$ nadir could potentially be relatively unaffected.[74,77]

Because the $\dot{V}E/\dot{V}CO_2$ at or between *AT* and VCP is less variable than the $\dot{V}E$-$\dot{V}CO_2$ slope below the VCP,[76] we prefer the former to the latter as an index of ventilatory inefficiency. No special calculation is required to obtain this ratio, in contrast to the regression slope through a selected range of values below the VCP for the $\dot{V}E$-$\dot{V}CO_2$ plot (see panel 6 for the cases presented in Chapter 10). $\dot{V}E/\dot{V}CO_2$ at the *AT* or VCP is read directly from panel 4 of the nine-panel plot. It is the $\dot{V}E/\dot{V}CO_2$ value least affected by anxiety hyperventilation and the H^+ stimulus to the carotid bodies caused by the exercise metabolic acidosis.

The range of normal values for the $\dot{V}E$-$\dot{V}CO_2$ slope below the VCP and the $\dot{V}E/\dot{V}CO_2$ at the *AT* or between the *AT* and VCP, as related to age and gender, is described in Chapter 7. The values are the same for cycle and treadmill exercise. Although small in most systems, the breathing valve dead space is variable from system to system and therefore should be subtracted from $\dot{V}E$ to obtain a value that could allow the measurement to be interrelated among all systems (see Appendix C). Elevated $\dot{V}E/\dot{V}CO_2$ values at the *AT* or between the *AT* and VCP (**Fig. 3.29B,C**) reflect either hyperventilation (decreased Pa_{CO_2}), an increase in VD/VT (uneven $\dot{V}A/\dot{Q}$), or a combination of both. Acute hyperventilation is

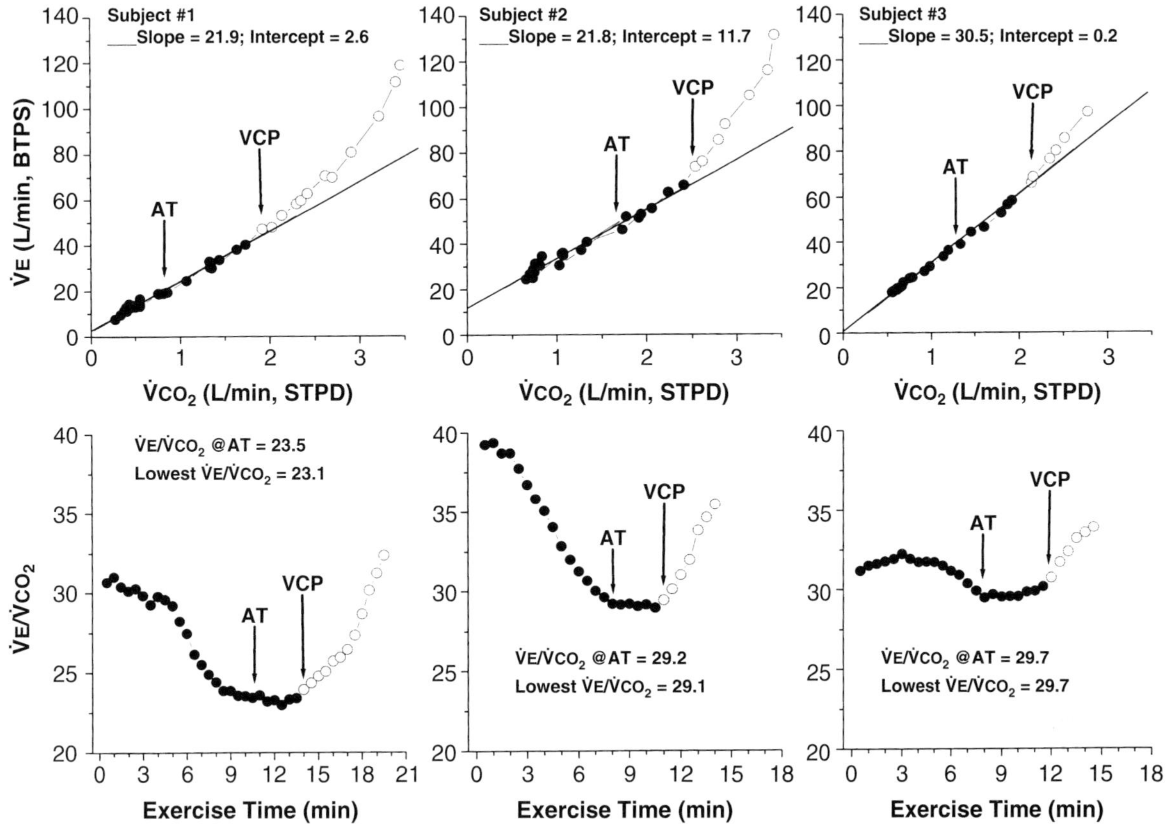

FIGURE 3.28. The ventilation ($\dot{V}_E$)-carbon dioxide output ($\dot{V}CO_2$) relationship (upper panels) and the ventilatory equivalent for carbon dioxide ($\dot{V}_E/\dot{V}CO_2$) profile as a function of time (lower panels) in three normal individuals during incremental cycle ergometer exercise. Data points are shown every 0.5 minute. The $\dot{V}_E$-$\dot{V}CO_2$ slope (straight solid lines) and $\dot{V}_E$-intercept were calculated over the linear region (upper panels), that is, points (open symbols) lying above the ventilatory compensation point (VCP) were excluded. $\dot{V}_E/\dot{V}CO_2$ profiles (lower panels) reach a nearly constant nadir between the anaerobic threshold (*AT*) and VCP. Subject 1 is typical of an average response, subject 2 has an unusually large positive $\dot{V}_E$-intercept, and subject 3 has a $\dot{V}_E$-intercept close to zero. Although the $\dot{V}_E$-$\dot{V}CO_2$ slopes for subjects 1 and 2 are similar, their differing $\dot{V}_E$-intercepts result in the $\dot{V}_E/\dot{V}CO_2$ at *AT* and VCP of subject 2 being considerably higher than for subject 1. For subjects 2 and 3, although the $\dot{V}_E/\dot{V}CO_2$ at *AT* and VCP are similar, the $\dot{V}_E$-$\dot{V}CO_2$ slopes and $\dot{V}_E$-intercepts differ appreciably. Abbreviations: BTPS, body temperature pressure saturated; STPD, standard temperature pressure dry. *(Reprinted with permission of the American Thoracic Society. Copyright © 2020 American Thoracic Society. All rights reserved. From Sun X-G, Hansen JE, Garatachea N, Storer TW, Wasserman K. Ventilatory effi ciency during exercise in healthy subjects.* Am J Respir Crit Care Med. *2002;166[11]:1443-1448. The American Journal of Respiratory and Critical Care Medicine is an official journal of the American Thoracic Society.)*

supported by an abnormally high R. At times, it might be necessary to distinguish between chronic hyperventilation and increased V_D/V_T as a cause of high $\dot{V}_E/\dot{V}CO_2$ values at the *AT* or between the *AT* and VCP. Patients with COPD (**Fig. 3.29B**), restrictive lung disease, left ventricular failure, and pulmonary vascular occlusive disease (**Fig. 3.29C**) usually have uneven $\dot{V}_A/\dot{Q}$. Therefore, $\dot{V}_E/\dot{V}CO_2$ at the *AT* or between the *AT* and VCP is often high. Because of mechanical limitation to breathing, patients with severe COPD usually do not hyperventilate or increase $\dot{V}_E/\dot{V}CO_2$ in response to metabolic acidosis, in contrast to the disorders of $\dot{V}_A/\dot{Q}$ without a breathing limitation.

FIGURE 3.29. Characteristic responses of the ventilatory equivalents for carbon dioxide ($\dot{V}_E/\dot{V}CO_2$, dashed lines) and oxygen ($\dot{V}_E/\dot{V}O_2$, solid lines) during incremental exercise for a normal individual (A) and for patients with obstructive lung disease (B) and restrictive lung disease, pulmonary vascular disease, and congestive heart failure (C). The nadir in the $\dot{V}_E/\dot{V}O_2$ response reflects the anaerobic threshold (*AT*), whereas the nadir of the $\dot{V}_E/\dot{V}CO_2$ response occurs between the *AT* and the ventilatory compensation point (VCP). Abbreviations: CHF, congestive heart failure; PVD, pulmonary vascular disease.

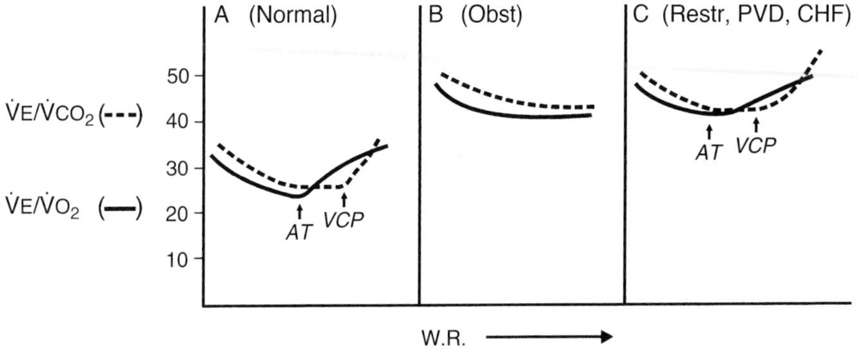

Although $\dot{V}E/\dot{V}CO_2$ normally increases from its nadir (isocapnic buffering period) to maximal exercise, with the amount depending on the magnitude of the compensatory ventilatory response to the metabolic acidosis, it fails to increase above the *AT* if the carotid chemoreceptors that detect the increased arterial $[H^+]$ are caused to be insensitive (eg, high O_2 breathing) or the work of breathing is high, such as with severe COPD or extreme obesity (**Fig. 3.29B**).

Differentiating Uneven Ventilation From Uneven Perfusion as the Cause of Uneven $\dot{V}A/\dot{Q}$

Based on the concept that end-tidal expired gas comes from the air spaces with the longest mechanical time constants for emptying and the most poorly ventilated lung acini, $PETCO_2$ would be relatively high compared to the mixed expired PCO_2 ($P\bar{E}CO_2$) in patients with uneven ventilation. In contrast, patients with uneven perfusion but uniform ventilation would have reduced end-tidal as well as mixed expired PCO_2, although the relationship between the mixed expired and end-tidal values would be normal. Thus, Hansen et al[78] studied the mixed expired and end-tidal PCO_2, as well as their ratio ($P\bar{E}CO_2/PETCO_2$), in normal individuals and patients with idiopathic pulmonary vasculopathy (idiopathic pulmonary arterial hypertension [PAH]), left ventricular failure, and COPD at rest, during unloaded cycling, and at *AT* and peak $\dot{V}O_2$. While mixed expired PCO_2 values were all comparably reduced relative to normal in all three disorders, end-tidal PCO_2 was most reduced in PAH and least reduced in COPD (**Fig. 3.30**). Despite marked reductions in mixed expired and end-tidal PCO_2 in PAH, the $P\bar{E}CO_2/PETCO_2$ ratio was normal. $P\bar{E}CO_2/PETCO_2$ was similar to normal and PAH in left ventricular failure but slightly reduced at peak exercise. In contrast, $P\bar{E}CO_2/PETCO_2$ was markedly reduced in COPD, reflecting the influence of long time-constant airways on the end-tidal gas composition (see **Fig. 3.30**).

Other Measures of Uneven $\dot{V}A/\dot{Q}$

The Fick relationship defines $\dot{V}CO_2$ as the product of $\dot{V}E$ and mixed expired CO_2 concentration (or PCO_2). Thus, $\dot{V}E$ is a hyperbolic function of mixed expired PCO_2 at a given $\dot{V}CO_2$ (see Chapter 2, "Ventilatory Determinants" section). Consequently, when $\dot{V}E$ increases in response to an exacerbated physiological dead space, mixed expired and end-tidal PCO_2 will decrease. Patients with stable left ventricular failure have an increase in physiological dead space in proportion to the severity of the disease.[79] Thus, Matsumoto et al[80] found a reduction in $PETCO_2$ during exercise in patients with left ventricular that was inversely related to the severity of disease. This is similar to the inverse $\dot{V}E/\dot{V}CO_2$-$PETCO_2$ relationship found by Yasunobu et al[81] in patients with idiopathic PAH.

Baba et al[82] reported that $\dot{V}O_2$ (y-axis) plotted as a log function of $\dot{V}E$ (x-axis) was a good correlate of cardiac function. This relationship has been referred to as the oxygen uptake efficiency slope (OUES). Apparently, $\dot{V}E$ was plotted as a log function in an attempt to provide a linear relationship that

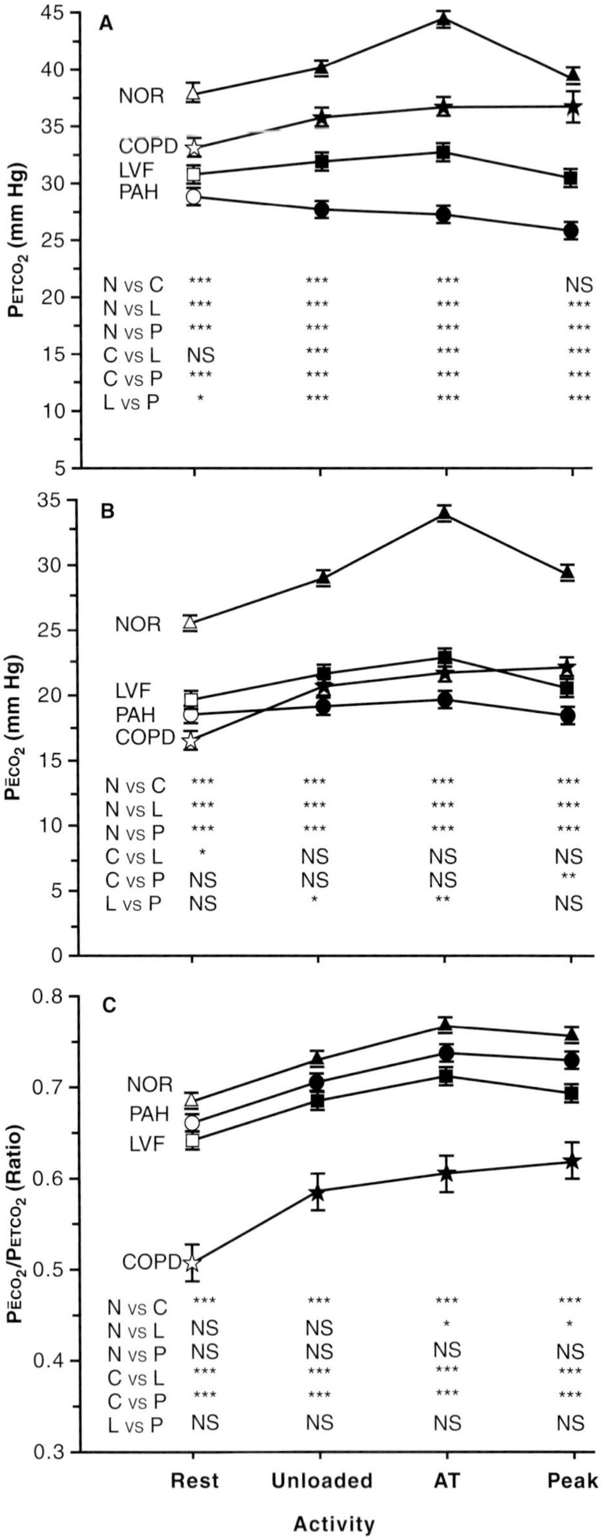

FIGURE 3.30. Values of end-tidal PCO_2 ($PETCO_2$), mixed expired PCO_2 ($P\bar{E}CO_2$), and their ratio ($P\bar{E}CO_2/PETCO_2$) for normal individuals (NOR or N), chronic obstructive pulmonary disease (COPD or C), left ventricular failure (LVF or L), and pulmonary arterial hypertension (PAH or P) during incremental cycle ergometer exercise at rest (open symbols), unloaded cycling, anaerobic threshold (*AT*), and peak exercise (closed symbols). Values are means ± standard errors of the mean. A: $PETCO_2$. B: $P\bar{E}CO_2$. C: $P\bar{E}CO_2/PETCO_2$. $^*P < .05$. $^{**}P < .01$. $^{***}P < .001$.

was readily amenable to analysis, rather than for any physiological reason. A low OUES (higher $\dot{V}_E$ relative to $\dot{V}O_2$) occurs with greater mismatching of ventilation relative to $\dot{V}O_2$, and correlated with more severe heart failure. However, Arena et al[83] found that the OUES was not as prognostically useful as the $\dot{V}_E$-$\dot{V}CO_2$ slope or $\dot{V}_E/\dot{V}CO_2$ at the *AT* or VCP for evaluating patients with left ventricular failure.

Arterial Bicarbonate and Acid-Base Response

Individuals making a maximal effort during an incremental exercise test normally develop a significant metabolic acidosis by the time the terminal work rate is reached. This is observed even for incremental protocols of relatively short duration (8-12 min) (**Fig. 3.31**; also see **Figs. 2.23** and **2.30**). The greatest increase in arterial [lactate] and reductions in arterial [HCO_3^-] and pH are noted about 2 minutes into recovery (see **Fig. 3.31**). We find that the 2-minute recovery [HCO_3^-] decreases by at least 6 mmol/L below the resting value if the effort is good and the patient is not limited by a ventilatory or mechanical disorder.

Tidal Volume/Inspiratory Capacity Ratio

Normally, V_T increases during incremental exercise, but it rarely exceeds 80% of the IC, as measured during standard resting pulmonary function tests. This ratio may become abnormal during exercise in patients with restrictive lung diseases. Such patients have a reduced IC and limited ability to increase their V_T in response to exercise (see **Fig. 3.20C**). Thus, as the work rate increases, the V_T/IC ratio reaches a value close to 1.0 at a relatively low work rate. Because a reduced V_T requires a high breathing rate to achieve the $\dot{V}_E$ needed for CO_2 elimination, we routinely relate V_T to the IC as well as to the ventilatory capacity (ie, MVV) in panel 9 of the nine-panel plot (see Chapter 8) when defining a patient's physiological response to exercise (see Chapter 10). The V_T/IC ratio is more helpful than the V_T/VC ratio because it is very unusual for V_T to exceed IC, even in severe restrictive lung disease.

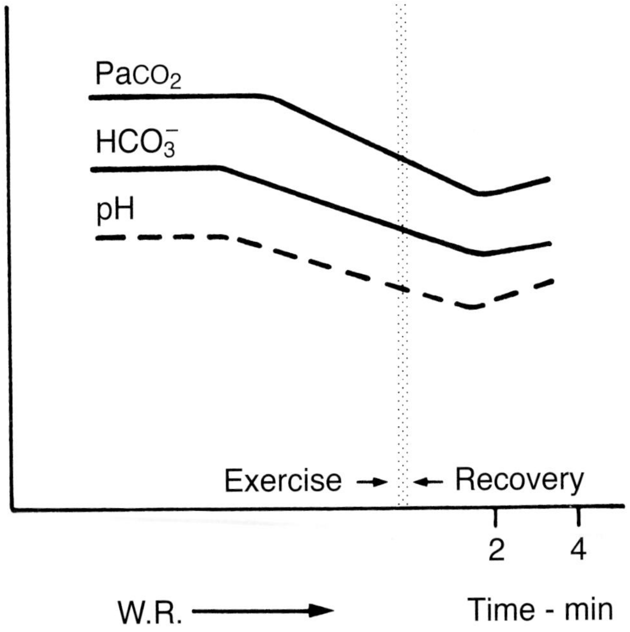

FIGURE 3.31. Normal response profiles of arterial P_{CO_2}, [bicarbonate] [HCO_3^-], and pH during incremental exercise and recovery. The stippled vertical bar indicates the point at which exercise stops. Note that the decrease in arterial P_{CO_2} is delayed relative to the decrease in [HCO_3^-] and pH (ie, the period of isocapnic buffering). The arterial P_{CO_2}, [HCO_3^-], and pH continue to decrease in the early recovery period, before starting to increase back toward normal. Abbreviation: WR, work rate.

Measurements Unique to Constant Work Rate Exercise Testing

As described in Chapter 2 ("Oxygen Uptake Kinetics" and "Carbon Dioxide Output Kinetics" sections), constant work rate tests provide a different perspective on the physiological responses of the specific organ systems that transport O_2 and CO_2, in terms of control mechanisms, speed of recruitment (kinetics), and system limitations. The following are useful measurements that can be obtained from the time course of constant work rate exercise. Adequate precision may require averaging the breath-by-breath data obtained from several constant work rate test repetitions.[84,85]

$\dot{V}O_2$ Response in Phase I

Normally, $\dot{V}O_2$ (and $\dot{V}CO_2$ and $\dot{V}_E$) abruptly increases at the start of constant work rate exercise (phase I) during upright exercise because of the immediate increase in flow of venous blood through the lungs resulting from the increased venous return (see **Fig. 2.37**) (see Chapter 2, "Oxygen Uptake Kinetics" section). The latter is enhanced at the start of exercise by increased cardiac inotropy, compression of veins by contracting muscles, and increased HR. Increased pulmonary blood flow is the predominant mechanism accounting for the increase in $\dot{V}O_2$ (and $\dot{V}CO_2$) during the first 15 to 20 seconds of exercise. Under clinical conditions in which pulmonary blood flow fails to increase abruptly at the start of exercise, the phase I increase in $\dot{V}O_2$ is also attenuated.[33,86,87] Thus, the phase I $\dot{V}O_2$ response provides a noninvasive proxy for the concomitant increase in cardiac output, whereas—as discussed earlier ("Oxygen Pulse and Stroke Volume" section)—the corresponding O_2 pulse response is an index of the stroke volume response.

$\dot{V}O_2$ Response in Phase II

During phase II, $\dot{V}O_2$ (and $\dot{V}CO_2$ and $\dot{V}_E$) increases as exponential functions when work rates lie below the *AT* (see Chapter 2, "Oxygen Uptake Kinetics" section) (see **Fig. 2.37**), that is, the speed of the response being characterized by its time constant. It has been demonstrated that the phase II $\dot{V}O_2$ kinetics are slower (ie, longer time constant) in COPD patients than for age- and gender-matched normal individuals cycling at the same relatively modest work rate (40 W) cycling (**Fig. 3.32**).[86] This resulted in an increased O_2 deficit in the COPD patients and therefore a greater reliance on anaerobic energy production from phosphocreatine

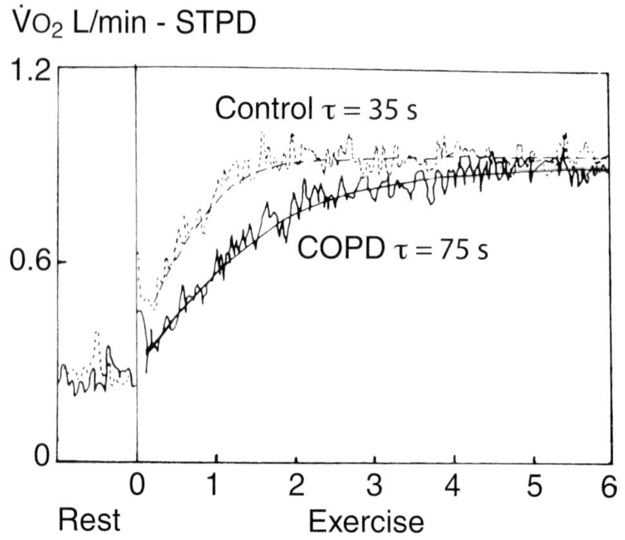

FIGURE 3.32. The $\dot{V}O_2$ response as a function of time for constant work rate cycle ergometer exercise (40 W) in a patient with chronic obstructive pulmonary disease (COPD) and an age-matched normal individual. Note that $\dot{V}O_2$ during phase I (the first 15-20 s of exercise) is less and the rate of rise of $\dot{V}O_2$ to its asymptote during phase II is slower in the COPD patient. The latter is reflected in the longer time constant (τ), compared to the normal individual. Abbreviation: STPD, standard temperature pressure dry. *(From Nery LE, Wasserman K, Andrews JD, Huntsman DJ, Hansen JE, Whipp BJ. Ventilatory and gas exchange kinetics during exercise in chronic airways obstruction.* J Appl Physiol Respir Environ Exerc Physiol. *1982;53:1594-1602.)*

hydrolysis until $\dot{V}O_2$ attained its new steady state. Thus, the phase II $\dot{V}O_2$ time constant provides a useful index of fitness and also of intramuscular mitochondrial oxidative phosphorylation recruitment (see Chapter 2, "Oxygen Uptake Kinetics" section).

$\dot{V}O_2$ Response Above the Anaerobic Threshold

As described in Chapter 2 ("Oxygen Uptake Kinetics" section), the more complex $\dot{V}O_2$ kinetics above the *AT* require characterization not only of the exponential phase II response but also the delayed $\dot{V}O_2$ slow component, which is challenging both technically and with regard to the underlying physiological assumptions. The $\dot{V}O_2$ mean response time (MRT), that is, the time taken to reach 63% of the final response amplitude, has been used as an empirical estimate of the overall supra-*AT* $\dot{V}O_2$ kinetics, that is, it collectively "captures" the phase I, phase II, and slow components as a single exponential. The $\dot{V}O_2$ MRT for supra-*AT* work rates has been demonstrated to discriminate an individual's fitness, based on incremental exercise testing—those with the highest peak $\dot{V}O_2$ per kilogram body weight having the shortest MRTs.[88] There is also the simple expedient of characterising the $\dot{V}O_2$ slow component as the magnitude of $\dot{V}O_2$ increase between 3 and 6 minutes of the exercise [$\Delta\dot{V}O_2$ (6 − 3)].[89] Thus, for sub-*AT* exercise, $\Delta\dot{V}O_2$ (6 − 3) is zero (ie, a $\dot{V}O_2$ steady state is normally attained by 3 min); however, when $\Delta\dot{V}O_2$ (6 − 3) is positive, this indicates that a $\dot{V}O_2$ slow component is evident (ie, $\dot{V}O_2$ has not stabilized within the first 6 min). The $\Delta\dot{V}O_2$ (6 − 3) can be determined by linear regression of $\dot{V}O_2$ against time between 3 and 6 minutes of exercise (**Fig. 3.33**). As $\Delta\dot{V}O_2$ (6 − 3) correlates well with the concomitant increase in arterial blood [lactate] for both normal individuals[89,90] and chronic heart failure patients[91] (see **Figs. 2.9** and **3.34**), this index is therefore useful for judging whether a particular work rate is or is not above the *AT*. This distinction can be useful in situations where the *AT* is difficult to reliably discern from incremental testing, that is, via constant work rate testing spanning the likely region of the *AT*.

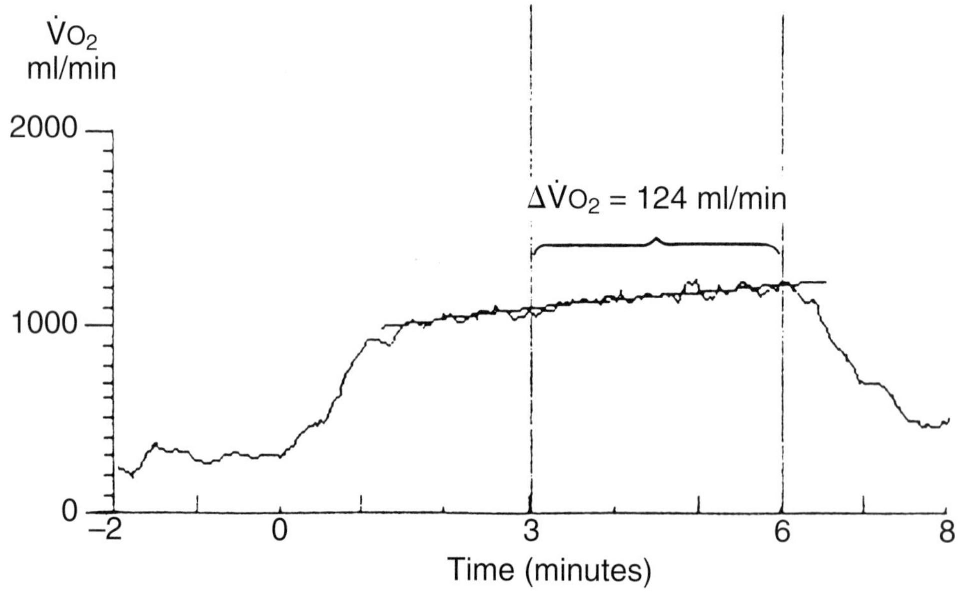

FIGURE 3.33. Method illustrating the measurement of the difference in oxygen uptake ($\dot{V}O_2$) between 3 and 6 min [$\Delta\dot{V}O_2$ (6 − 3)] for constant work rate cycle ergometer exercise (70 W) in a patient with cardiac disease. The straight line drawn on the plot between 3 and 6 min was determined by the best least-squares fit to the breath-by-breath data. The difference in $\dot{V}O_2$ at the 6- and 3-min points is calculated from the 3- and 6-min intercepts of the linear regression of the data between 3 and 6 min.

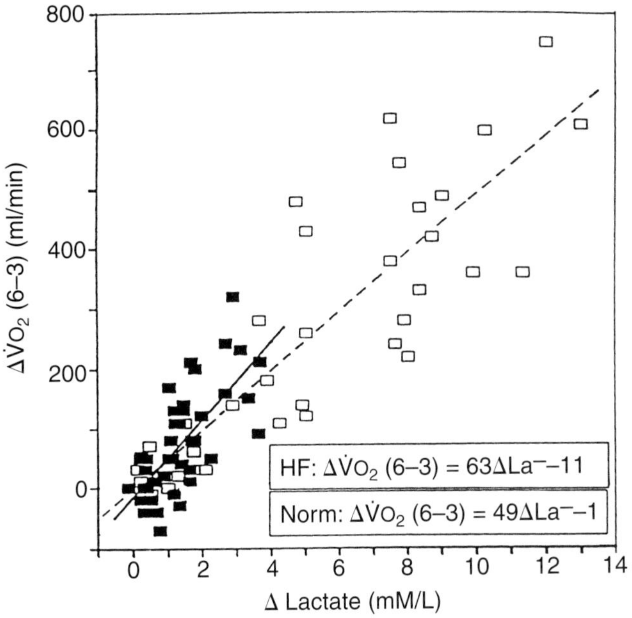

FIGURE 3.34. Degree of nonsteady state in oxygen uptake ($\dot{V}O_2$) for constant work rate cycle ergometer exercise, expressed as the increase in $\dot{V}O_2$ between 3 and 6 min [$\dot{V}O_2$ (6 − 3)], as a function of the increase in blood [lactate] above rest in normal individuals (open squares) and in patients with heart failure (solid squares). Blood was sampled from the antecubital vein at rest and at 2 min of recovery. Neither the slopes nor the intercepts of the regression equations differed significantly between the two groups. *(From Roston WL, Whipp BJ, Davis JA, Cunningham DA, Effros RM, Wasserman K. Oxygen uptake kinetics and lactate concentration during exercise in humans.* Am Rev Respir Dis. *1987;135:1080-1084; Zhang YY, Wasserman K, Sietsema KE, et al. O_2 uptake kinetics in response to exercise. A measure of tissue anaerobiosis in heart failure.* Chest. *1993;103:735-741.)*

The Power-Duration Relationship and Endurance Time

Determination of the power-duration relationship is time consuming (see Chapter 2, "Power-Duration Curve and Critical Power" section) and therefore not routinely conducted in a CPET context. However, the tolerance time (t_{lim}) for sustaining a particular supra-*AT* work rate is both readily determined and also more sensitive for CPET-based evaluation of therapeutic efficacy (eg, exercise, pharmacological therapy, supplemental O_2, heliox breathing) than indices such as peak $\dot{V}O_2$ on an incremental exercise test.[1,3,92] This results from the curvature of the power-duration relationship, which serves to translate a small improvement in peak $\dot{V}O_2$ on an incremental exercise test into an appreciable increase in t_{lim} on a high-intensity constant work rate test, especially for work rates only slightly above critical power (for higher work rates, the absolute magnitude of improvement being smaller).[93] The test can be performed on the cycle ergometer or treadmill. Target work rates typically fall in the range of 75% to 80% of peak work rate on an incremental test, with the target t_{lim} range for the preintervention test being 3 to 8 minutes. Supporting the simple measure of t_{lim} with a full complement of CPET measurements facilitates interpretation of improvements in exercise tolerance. In summary, the high-intensity constant work rate test performed to the limit of tolerance is gaining in popularity as an adjunct to incremental exercise testing.

Noninvasive Estimation of Metabolic Acidosis Buffering

Supra-*AT* constant work rate exercise tests can also be useful for estimating noninvasively the magnitude of blood [HCO_3^-] decrease or [lactate] increase. This is based on the demonstration (see Chapter 2, "Carbon Dioxide Output Kinetics" section) that $\dot{V}CO_2$ increases more rapidly than $\dot{V}O_2$ after about 1 to 2 minutes after exercise onset (see **Figs. 1.4, 2.35,** and **2.36**). This is primarily due to the buffering of newly formed protons by HCO_3^-. Thus, from the simultaneous analysis of the $\dot{V}CO_2$ and $\dot{V}O_2$ time courses, it is possible to determine whether the work rate is accompanied by a metabolic acidosis or not.

Figure 3.35 illustrates that the cumulative volume of CO_2 that is output (Cum Sum CO_2) during a 6-minute supra-*AT* constant work rate cycle ergometer test increases more rapidly and to a greater extent, than the cumulative volume of O_2 that is taken up (Cum Sum O_2), in contrast to sub-*AT* exercise.[94] The aerobic CO_2 production component of this response was calculated by multiplying $\dot{V}O_2$ by the muscle

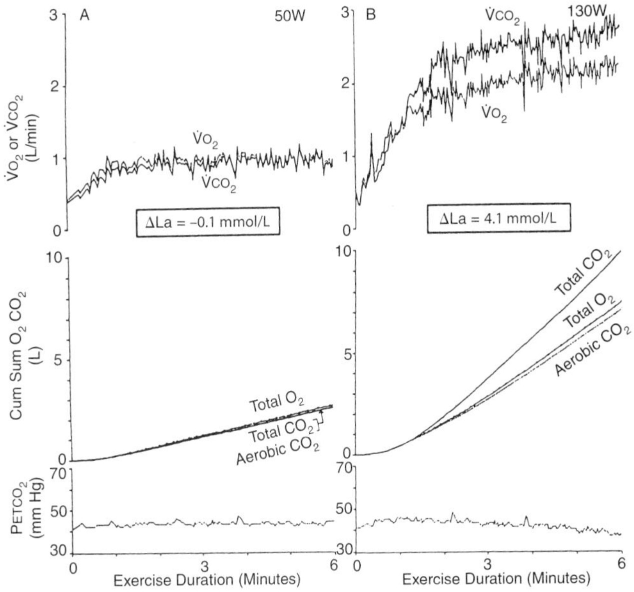

FIGURE 3.35. Breath-by-breath changes in oxygen uptake ($\dot{V}O_2$), carbon dioxide output ($\dot{V}CO_2$), total or accumulated volume of O_2 taken up (Cum Sum O_2), total or accumulated volume of CO_2 output (Cum Sum CO_2), aerobic $\dot{V}CO_2$ ($\dot{V}O_2 \times 0.95$), and end-tidal P_{CO_2} (P_{ETCO_2}) in response to 6-min constant work rate cycle ergometer exercise at 50 W (below *AT*) (A) and at 130 W (above *AT*) (B) for a normal individual. The average increase in antecubital vein [lactate] (ΔLa) at 2 min into recovery for A and B is indicated. The difference between the accumulated total volume of CO_2 output and the aerobic volume of CO_2 output is the accumulated buffer volume of CO_2 output. In A, the total and aerobic Cum Sum CO_2 curves overlap and cannot be distinguished. *(Reprinted by permission from Springer: Zhang YY, Sietsema KE, Sullivan CS, Wasserman K. A method for estimating bicarbonate buffering of lactic acid during constant work rate exercise.* Eur J Appl Physiol Occup Physiol. *1994;69:309-315. Copyright © 1994 Springer Nature.)*

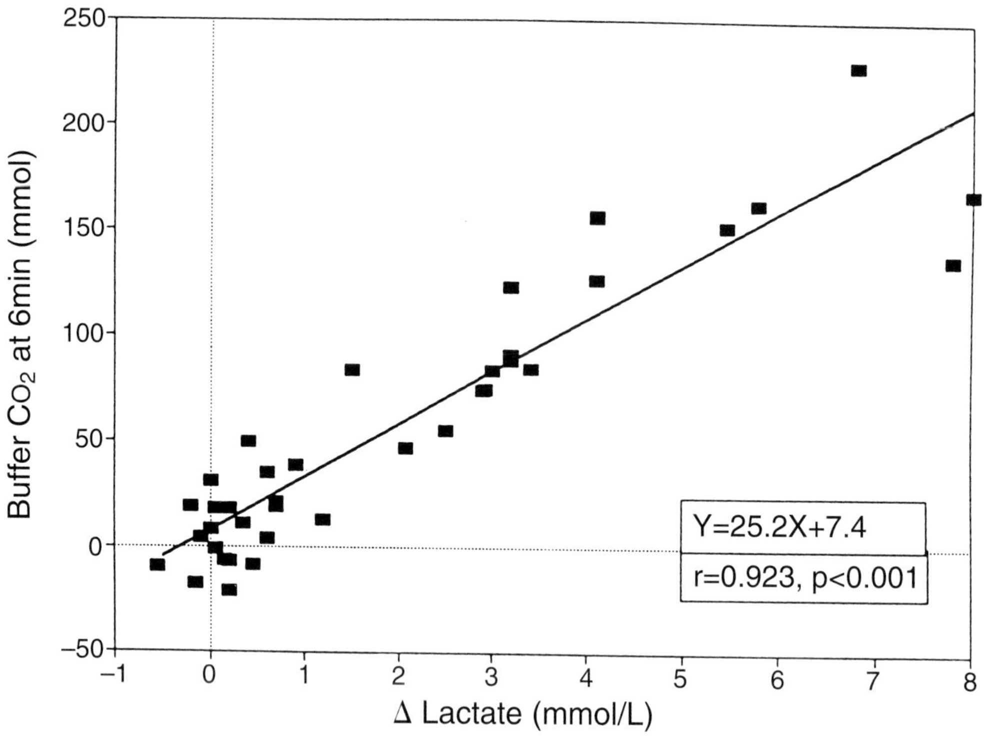

FIGURE 3.36. Buffer carbon dioxide (CO_2) (mmol) at 6 min of exercise as a function of the increase (Δ) in blood [lactate] at 2 min of recovery. The correlation coefficient, significance of the correlation, and the equation for the regression are indicated. *(Reprinted by permission from Springer: Zhang YY, Sietsema KE, Sullivan CS, Wasserman K. A method for estimating bicarbonate buffering of lactic acid during constant work rate exercise.* Eur J Appl Physiol Occup Physiol. *1994;69:309-315. Copyright © 1994 Springer Nature.)*

substrate respiratory quotient (approximately 0.95, on average), estimated as the slope of the sub-*AT* $\dot{V}CO_2$-$\dot{V}CO_2$ relationship for incremental exercise. The difference between the total volume of CO_2 output and the volume of aerobic CO_2 output over the test was taken to represent the volume of $\dot{V}CO_2$ produced from the buffering of metabolically produced protons plus, if any, the volume of CO_2 produced by the hyperventilation of respiratory compensation (see **Fig. 3.35**). The volume of CO_2 output derived from buffering at the 6-minute point correlated closely with the antecubital venous [lactate] sampled 2 minutes into recovery (**Fig. 3.36**); the slope of the regression line defining the volume of distribution of lactate (25 L, or about one-third body weight for the subject population studied). However, in those individuals who hyperventilated in response to the exercise-induced metabolic acidosis at the 6-minute point, the associated volume of CO_2 accounted for only about 6% of the excess CO_2 over that deriving from aerobic metabolism.

Carotid Body Contribution to Ventilation

Several techniques have been proposed to determine the contribution of the carotid body chemoreceptors to the exercise ventilatory response.[95,96] Of these, the Dejours oxygen test,[97] has the advantage of being short in duration, relatively unaffected by secondary influences, its applicability at work rates below or above the *AT*, and its safety (in contrast to breathing hypoxic gas mixtures to stimulate the carotid bodies),[97-100] and is applicable to patients with lung diseases. The test is designed to transiently remove the ongoing source of carotid chemoreceptor stimulation by the abrupt and surreptitious administration of 100% O_2 during the steady state of exercise (a maximal inhibitory effect is usually seen with an increase in PaO_2 to 250 mm Hg or more) (**Fig. 3.37**). This results in a decrease in $\dot{V}E$ that develops after a few breaths, the delay being consistent with the circulation time between the lungs and carotid bodies. $\dot{V}E$ reaches a nadir within about 15 to 30 seconds, and is normally about 12% to 15% of the prior control value. This $\dot{V}E$ decline has been ascribed to a silencing of the carotid chemoreceptors by the hyperoxia, and indeed it cannot be discerned in individuals who have undergone bilateral carotid body resection (**Fig. 3.37**).[99,100] $\dot{V}E$ then starts increasing back toward, but not completely to, its prior control value despite continued breathing of 100% O_2. The most likely stimulus for this rebound in $\dot{V}E$ is the increase in $PaCO_2$ caused by the abrupt decrease in $\dot{V}E$ resulting from O_2 breathing. That is, whereas hyperoxia continues to inhibit the carotid body $\dot{V}E$ drive, the increase in $PaCO_2$ resulting from this inhibition stimulates the central chemoreceptors to partially mask the carotid body silencing.

In order to define the profile of $\dot{V}E$ response with sufficient fidelity, $\dot{V}E$ must be measured breath by breath. Also, it is preferable that several repetitions of the test are undertaken, allowing an ensemble average profile to be obtained, which minimizes the influence of breath-by-breath "noise." If a pneumotachograph is used to measure $\dot{V}E$, an adjustment must be made in calculating the $\dot{V}E$ decrease to account for

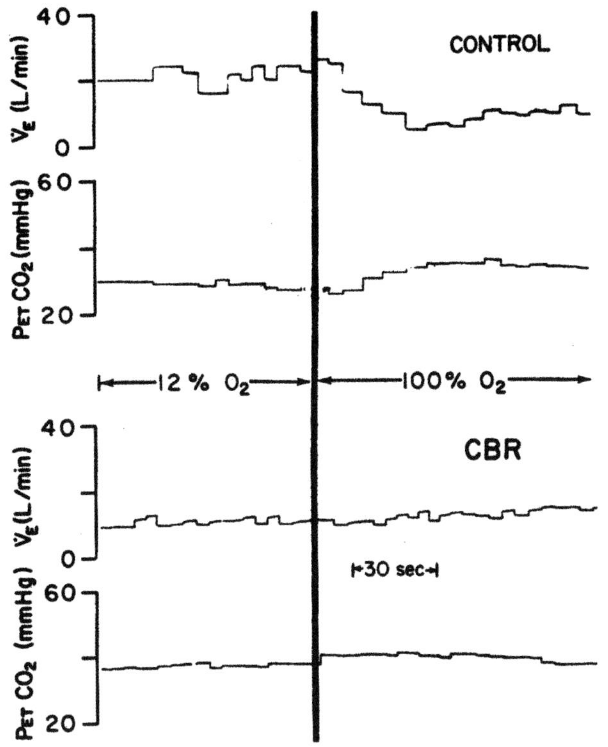

FIGURE 3.37. Breath-by-breath responses of ventilation (V̇E) and end-tidal P_{CO_2} (P_{ETCO_2}) to the abrupt inhalation of 100% oxygen (O_2) from a background of 12% O_2 in an individual who had previously undergone bilateral carotid body resection (CBR) (lower panel) and in a normal age-matched individual (CONTROL) (upper panel). Three phases are typically evident in the CONTROL V̇E response: (1) following a short delay reflecting the vascular transit delay between the lungs and carotid bodies, V̇E decreased to a nadir within approximately 15 s—reflecting the carotid bodies being maximally attenuated by the O_2—and end-tidal and arterial P_{CO_2} therefore rose; (2) in the period between approximately 15 and approximately 45 s, V̇E started to rebound toward the prior hypoxic baseline, presumably because the increased arterial P_{CO_2} stimulated the central chemoreceptors; and (3) by about 45 s, V̇E became relatively constant at a reduced value compared to the prior hypoxic baseline, and P_{ETCO_2} leveled off at an elevated value. For the CBR individual, however, no transient decline in V̇E was evident. *(From Whipp BJ, Wasserman K. Carotid bodies and ventilatory control dynamics in man.* Fed Proc. *1980;39(9):2668-2673.* Copyright *© 1980 Federation of American Societies for Experimental Biology. Reprinted by permission of John Wiley & Sons, Inc.)*

the 11% higher gas viscosity of 100% O_2 than air. The flowmeters of some commercial systems automatically correct for the difference in gas viscosity with changing O_2 concentration. This can be documented by calibrating with a known volume of air and O_2 and determining if there is a difference in recorded volume. In summary, therefore, a brief temporal window is provided, within which the effects of the carotid body chemoreceptors are effectively isolated, such that the magnitude of the V̇E decline to its nadir provides an index of the carotid body contribution to the exercise hyperpnea.

Detecting Exercise-Induced Bronchospasm

Although exercise-induced bronchospasm can often be demonstrated after standard incremental exercise testing in the afflicted individual, it may be more evident after 6 minutes of near-maximal constant work rate exercise.[101] It is necessary to obtain good baseline measurements of FEV_1 or some other index of airway obstruction immediately before exercise. Most investigators prefer the treadmill to the cycle ergometer for inducing postexercise bronchospasm, although we have used both successfully. To induce postexercise bronchospasm, it is our practice to increase the work rate to approximately 80% of the predicted maximal work rate after a 1-minute warm-up at a lower work rate. The patient inspires dry air from a bag filled from a tank of compressed air rather than room air because, according to current concepts, dry air aids in the induction of bronchospasm and reduces day-to-day variability if repeated tests are necessary.[102] After 6 minutes of heavy exercise, the mouthpiece is immediately removed. Spirometric tracings are obtained as soon as possible and at 3, 5, 10, 15, and 20 minutes after exercise. A fall of FEV_1 greater than or equal to 10% would indicate exercise-induced bronchospasm. The severity of exercise-induced bronchospasm can be graded as mild ($\geq$10% and $<$25%), moderate ($\geq$25% and $<$50%), and severe ($\geq$50%).[103]

SUMMARY

Changes in pulmonary $\dot{V}O_2$ and $\dot{V}CO_2$ reflect changes in cell respiration induced by exercise, although these relationships can become complex in nonsteady state conditions. Although the source of the increased gas exchange with exercise is the increase in cell respiration, cardiac output and ventilation modulate the gas exchange responses at the airway. Thus, diseases of the cardiovascular and ventilatory systems will affect the pulmonary gas exchange response pattern during exercise, depending on the disease pathophysiology. Measurements that assess these functions, following controlled work rate perturbations, define the physiological state of the organ systems that participate in gas transport. Defects in the coupling of external to internal respiration result in gas exchange abnormalities characteristic of the limiting organ system. For example, whereas diseases of the heart, the lungs, and the peripheral and pulmonary circulations all result in demonstrable abnormalities in gas exchange, each disorder manifests specific and relatively unique abnormalities that are amplified by exercise testing. The effects of various disease states on these measurements are described in Chapter 4.

REFERENCES

1. American Thoracic Society and American College of Chest Physicians. ATS/ACCP statement on cardiopulmonary exercise testing. *Am J Respir Crit Care Med*. 2003;167:211-277.
2. Palange P, Laveneziana P, Neder A, Ward SA, eds. *Clinical Exercise Testing*. Sheffield, United Kingdom: European Respiratory Society; 2018. European Respiratory Monograph.
3. Palange P, Ward SA, Carlsen K-H, et al. Recommendations on the use of exercise testing in clinical practice. *Eur Respir J*. 2007;28:185-209.
4. Balady GJ, Arena R, Sietsema K, et al. Clinician's guide to cardiopulmonary exercise testing in adults: a scientific statement from the American Heart Association. *Circulation*. 2010;122:191-225.
5. Belardinelli R, Lacalaprice F, Carle F, et al. Exercise-induced myocardial ischaemia detected by cardiopulmonary exercise testing. *Eur Heart J*. 2003;24:1304-1313.
6. Gibbons RJ, Balady GJ, Beasley JW, et al. ACC/AHA guidelines for exercise testing. A report of the American College of Cardiology/American Heart Association Task Force on Practice Guidelines (Committee on Exercise Testing). *J Am Coll Cardiol*. 1997;30:260-311.
7. Itoh H, Tajima A, Koike A, et al. Oxygen uptake abnormalities during exercise in coronary artery disease. In: Wasserman K, ed. *Cardiopulmonary Exercise Testing and Cardiovascular Health*. Armonk, NY: Futura Publishing; 2002:165-172.
8. Whipp BJ, Pardy RL. Breathing during exercise. In: Macklem PT, Mead J, eds. *Handbook of Physiology—The Respiratory System III*. Bethesda, MA: American Physiological Society; 1992:605-629.
9. Taylor HL, Buskirk E, Henschel A. Maximal oxygen intake as an objective measure of cardio-respiratory performance. *J Appl Physiol*. 1955;8:73-80.
10. Rossiter HB, Kowalchuk JM, Whipp BJ. A test to establish maximum O_2 uptake despite no plateau in the O_2 uptake response to ramp incremental exercise. *J Appl Physiol (1985)*. 2006;100:764-770.
11. Bowen TS, Cannon DT, Begg G, Baliga V, Witte KK, Rossiter HB. A novel cardiopulmonary exercise test protocol and criterion to determine maximal oxygen uptake in chronic heart failure. *J Appl Physiol (1985)*. 2012;113:451-458.
12. Cooper DM, Weiler-Ravell D, Whipp BJ, Wasserman K. Aerobic parameters of exercise as a function of body size during growth in children. *J Appl Physiol Environ Exerc Physiol*. 1984;56:628-634.
13. Zhang YY, Johnson MC II, Chow N, Wasserman K. Effect of exercise testing protocol on parameters of aerobic function. *Med Sci Sports Exerc*. 1991;23:625-630.
14. Zhang YY, Johnson MC II, Chow N, Wasserman K. The role of fitness on VO2 and VCO2 kinetics in response to proportional step increases in work rate. *Eur J Appl Physiol*. 1991;63:94-100.
15. Hansen JE, Sue DY, Wasserman K. Predicted values for clinical exercise testing. *Am Rev Respir Dis*. 1984;129(2, pt 2):S49-S55.
16. Wasserman K, Whipp BJ. Exercise physiology in health and disease. *Am Rev Respir Dis*. 1975;112:219-249.
17. Pórszász J, Casaburi R, Somfay A, Woodhouse LJ, Whipp BJ. A treadmill ramp protocol using simultaneous changes in speed and grade. *Med Sci Sports Exerc*. 2003;35:1596-1603.
18. Wasserman K, Sue DY. Coupling of external to cellular respiration. In: Wasserman K, ed. *Exercise Gas Exchange in Heart Disease*. Armonk, NY: Futura Publishing; 1996:1-15.
19. Riley M, Wasserman K, Fu PC, Cooper CB. Muscle substrate utilization from alveolar gas exchange in trained cyclists. *Eur J Appl Physiol Occup Physiol*. 1996;72:341-348.
20. Koike A, Hiroe M, Adachi H, et al. Anaerobic metabolism as an indicator of aerobic function during exercise in cardiac patients. *J Am Coll Cardiol*. 1992;20:120-126.
21. Weisel RD, Berger RL, Hechtman HB. Measurement of cardiac output by thermodilution. *N Engl J Med*. 1975;292:682-684.
22. Stetz CW, Miller RG, Kelly GE, Raffin TA. Reliability of the thermodilution method in the determination of cardiac output in clinical practice. *Am Rev Respir Dis*. 1982;126:1001-1004.
23. Jones NL, Campbell EJM. *Clinical Exercise Testing*. Philadelphia, PA: WB Saunders; 1982.
24. Jones NL, McHardy GJR, Naimark A, Campbell EJ. Physiological dead space and alveolar-arterial gas pressure differences during exercise. *Clin Sci*. 1966;31:19-29.
25. Sue DY, Oren A, Hansen JE, Wasserman K. Diffusing capacity for carbon monoxide as a predictor of gas exchange during exercise. *N Engl J Med*. 1987;316:1301-1306.
26. Whipp BJ, Lamarra N, Ward SA, Davis JA, Wasserman K. Estimating arterial PCO_2 from flow-weighted and time-averaged alveolar PCO_2 during exercise. In: Swanson GD, Grodins FS, eds. *Respiratory Control: Modelling Perspective*. New York, NY: Plenum Press; 1990:91-99.
27. Whipp BJ, Wagner PD, Agusti A. Determinants of the physiological systems responses to muscular exercise in healthy subjects. In: *Eur Respir Mon*. 2007;40:1-35.
28. Sun X-G, Hansen JE, Ting H, et al. Comparison of exercise cardiac output by the Fick principle using oxygen and carbon dioxide. *Chest*. 2000;118:631-640.
29. Stringer W, Hansen J, Wasserman K. Cardiac output estimated noninvasively from oxygen uptake during exercise. *J Appl Physiol (1985)*. 1997;82:908-912.
30. Agostoni PG, Wasserman K, Perego GB, et al. Non-invasive measurement of stroke volume during exercise in heart failure patients. *Clin Sci (Lond)*. 2000;98:545-551.
31. Sullivan MJ, Knight JD, Higginbotham MB, Cobb FR. Relation between central and peripheral hemodynamics during exercise in patients with chronic heart failure. Muscle blood flow is reduced with maintenance of arterial perfusion pressure. *Circulation*. 1989;80:769-781.
32. Weber KT, Janicki JS. Cardiopulmonary exercise testing for evaluation of chronic cardiac failure. *Am J Cardiol*. 1985;55:22A-31A.
33. Sietsema KE, Cooper DM, Perloff JK, et al. Dynamics of oxygen uptake during exercise in adults with cyanotic congenital heart disease. *Circulation*. 1986;73:1137-1144.
34. Koike A, Itoh H, Doi M, et al. Beat-to-beat evaluation of cardiac function during recovery from upright bicycle exercise in patients with coronary artery disease. *Am Heart J*. 1990;120:316-323.
35. Nery LE, Wasserman K, French W, Oren A, Davis JA. Contrasting cardiovascular and respiratory responses to exercise in mitral valve and chronic obstructive pulmonary diseases. *Chest*. 1983;83:446-453.
36. Whipp BJ, Higgenbotham MB, Cobb FC. Estimating exercise stroke volume from asymptotic oxygen pulse in humans. *J Appl Physiol (1985)*. 1996;81:2674-2679.
37. Buchfuhrer MJ, Hansen JE, Robinson TE, et al. Optimizing the exercise protocol for cardiopulmonary assessment. *J Appl Physiol*. 1983;55:1558-1564.
38. Davis JA, Whipp BJ, Lamarra N, Huntsman DJ, Frank MH, Wasserman K. Effect of ramp slope on determination of aerobic parameters from the ramp exercise test. *Med Sci Sports Exerc*. 1982;14:339-343.
39. Cooper CB, Beaver WL, Cooper DM, Wasserman K. Factors affecting the components of the alveolar CO2 output-O2 uptake relationship during incremental exercise in man. *Exp Physiol*. 1992;77:51-64.
40. McLellan TM, Gass GC. The relationship between the ventilation and lactate thresholds following normal, low and high carbohydrate diets. *Eur J Appl Physiol Occup Physiol*. 1989;58:568-576.
41. Yoshida T. Effect of dietary modifications on lactate threshold and onset of blood lactate accumulation during incremental exercise. *Eur J Appl Physiol Occup Physiol*. 1984;53:200-205.
42. Beaver WL, Wasserman K, Whipp BJ. A new method for detecting anaerobic threshold by gas exchange. *J Appl Physiol (1985)*. 1986;60:2020-2027.
43. Sue DY, Wasserman K, Moricca RB, Casaburi R. Metabolic acidosis during exercise in patients with chronic obstructive pulmonary disease. Use of the V-slope method for anaerobic threshold determination. *Chest*. 1988;94:931-938.
44. Whipp BJ. Physiological mechanisms dissociating pulmonary CO_2 and O_2 exchange dynamics during exercise in humans. *Exp Physiol*. 2007;92:347-355.

45. Beaver WL, Wasserman K, Whipp BJ. Improved detection of lactate threshold during exercise using a log-log transformation. *J Appl Physiol (1985)*. 1985;59:1936-1940.
46. Beaver WL, Wasserman K, Whipp BJ. Bicarbonate buffering of lactic acid generated during exercise. *J Appl Physiol (1985)*. 1986;60:472-478.
47. Stringer W, Casaburi R, Wasserman K. Acid-base regulation during exercise and recovery in humans. *J Appl Physiol (1985)*. 1992;72:954-961.
48. Wasserman K. Determinants and detection of anaerobic threshold and consequences of exercise above it. *Circulation*. 1987; 76(6, pt 2):VI29-VI39.
49. Riley M, Nicholls DP, Nugent AM, et al. Respiratory gas exchange and metabolic responses during exercise in McArdle's disease. *J Appl Physiol (1985)*. 1993;75:745-754.
50. Ward SA, Whipp BJ. Influence of body CO_2 stores on ventilatory-metabolic coupling during exercise. In: Honda Y, Miyamoto Y, Konno K, Widdicombe JG, eds. *Control of Breathing and Its Modelling Perspective*. New York, NY: Plenum Press; 1992:425-431.
51. Ozcelik O, Ward SA, Whipp BJ. Effect of altered body CO_2 stores on pulmonary gas exchange dynamics during incremental exercise in humans. *Exp Physiol*. 1999;84:999-1011.
52. Koike A, Itoh H, Taniguichi K, Hiroe M. Detecting abnormalities in left ventricular function during exercise by respiratory measurement. *Circulation*. 1989;80:1737-1746.
53. Deboeck G, Niset G, Lamotte M, Vachiéry JL, Naeije R. Exercise testing in pulmonary arterial hypertension and in chronic heart failure. *Eur Respir J*. 2004;23:747-751.
54. Sun X-G, Hansen JE, Oudiz R, Wasserman K. Gas exchange detection of exercise-induced right-to-left shunt in patients with primary pulmonary hypertension. *Circulation*. 2002;105:54-60.
55. Butler J, Schrijen F, Henriquez A, Polu JM, Albert RK. Cause of the raised wedge pressure on exercise in chronic obstructive pulmonary disease. *Am Rev Respir Dis*. 1988;138:350-354.
56. ERS Task Force on Standardization of Clinical Exercise Testing. European Respiratory Society. Clinical exercise testing with reference to lung diseases: indications, standardization and interpretation strategies. *Eur Respir J*. 1997;10:2662-2689.
57. Gallagher CG. Exercise limitation and clinical exercise testing in chronic obstructive pulmonary disease. *Clin Chest Med*. 1994;15:305-326.
58. Sue DY, Hansen JE. Normal values in adults during exercise testing. *Clin Chest Med*. 1984;5:89-98.
59. Babb TG, Rodarte JR. Exercise capacity and breathing mechanics in patients with airflow limitation. *Med Sci Sports Exerc*. 1992;24:967-974.
60. Johnson BD, Weisman IM, Zeballos RJ, Beck KC. Emerging concepts in the evaluation of ventilatory limitation during exercise: the exercise tidal flow-volume loop. *Chest*. 1999;116:488-503.
61. O'Donnell DE, Lam M, Webb KA. Spirometric correlates of improvement in exercise performance after anticholinergic therapy in chronic obstructive pulmonary disease. *Am J Respir Crit Care Med*. 1999;160:542-549.
62. Sheel AW, Romer LM. Ventilation and respiratory mechanics. *Compr Physiol*. 2012;2:1093-1142.
63. Somfay A, Pórszász J, Lee S-M, Casaburi R. Effect of hyperoxia on gas exchange and lactate kinetics following exercise onset in nonhypoxemic COPD patients. *Chest*. 2002;121:393-400.
64. Wasserman K, VanKessel A, Burton GB. Interaction of physiological mechanisms during exercise. *J Appl Physiol*. 1967;22:71-85.
65. Wagner PD, Gale GE. Ventilation-perfusion relationships. In: Whipp BJ, Wasserman K, eds. *Exercise: Pulmonary Physiology and Pathophysiology*. New York, NY: Marcel Dekker; 1991:121-142.
66. Fishman AP. Hypoxia on the pulmonary circulation. How and where it acts. *Circ Res*. 1976;38:221-231.
67. DuBois AB, Britt AG, Fenn WO. Alveolar CO_2 during the respiratory cycle. *J Appl Physiol*. 1952;4:535-548.
68. Jones NL, Robertson DG, Kane JW. Difference between end-tidal and arterial PCO2 in exercise. *J Appl Physiol Respir Environ Exerc Physiol*. 1979;47:954-960.
69. Whipp BJ, Wasserman K. Alveolar-arterial gas tension differences during graded exercise. *J Appl Physiol*. 1969;27:361-365.
70. Sietsema KE, Cooper DM, Perloff JK, et al. Control of ventilation during exercise in patients with central venous-to-systemic arterial shunts. *J Appl Physiol (1985)*. 1988;64:234-242.
71. Chua TP, Ponikowski P, Harrington D, et al. Clinical correlates and prognostic significance of the ventilatory response to exercise in chronic heart failure. *J Am Coll Cardiol*. 1997;29:1585-1590.
72. Kleber FX, Vietzke G, Wernecke KD, et al. Impairment of ventilatory efficiency in heart failure: prognostic impact. *Circulation*. 2000;101:2803-2809.
73. Metra M, Dei Cas L, Panina G, Visioli O. Exercise hyperventilation chronic congestive heart failure, and its relation to functional capacity and hemodynamics. *Am J Cardiol*. 1992;70:622-628.
74. Neder JA, Berton DC, Arbex FF, et al. Physiological and clinical relevance of exercise ventilatory efficiency in COPD. *Eur Respir J*. 2017;49(3):1602036. doi:10.1183/13993003.02036-2016.
75. Neder JA, Nery LE, Peres C, Whipp BJ. Reference values for dynamic responses to incremental cycle ergometry in males and females aged 20 to 80. *Am J Respir Crit Care Med*. 2001;164(8, pt 1):1481-1486.
76. Sun X-G, Hansen JE, Garatachea N, Storer TW, Wasserman K. Ventilatory efficiency during exercise in healthy subjects. *Am J Respir Crit Care Med*. 2002;166:1443-1448.
77. Neder JA, Arbex FF, Alencar MC, et al. Exercise ventilatory inefficiency in mild to end-stage COPD. *Eur Respir J*. 2015;45:377-387.
78. Hansen J, Ulubay G, Chow BF, Sun XG, Wasserman K. Mixed-expired and end-tidal CO_2 distinguish between ventilation and perfusion defects during exercise testing in patients with lung and heart diseases. *Chest*. 2007;132:977-983.
79. Wasserman K, Zhang YY, Gitt A, et al. Lung function and exercise gas exchange in chronic heart failure. *Circulation*. 1997;96:2221-2227.
80. Matsumoto A, Itoh H, Eto Y, et al. End-tidal CO_2 pressure decreases during exercise in cardiac patients: association with severity of heart failure and cardiac output reserve. *J Am Coll Cardiol*. 2000;36:242-249.
81. Yasunobu Y, Oudiz R, Sun X-G, Hansen JE, Wasserman K. End-tidal P_{CO_2} abnormality and exercise limitation in patients with primary pulmonary hypertension. *Chest*. 2010;127:1637-1646.
82. Baba R, Nagashima M, Goto M, et al. Oxygen uptake efficiency slope: a new index of cardiorespiratory functional reserve derived from the relation between oxygen uptake and minute ventilation during incremental exercise. *J Am Coll Cardiol*. 1996;28:1567-1572.
83. Arena R, Myers J, Hsu L, et al. The minute ventilation/carbon dioxide production slope is prognostically superior to the oxygen uptake efficiency slope. *J Card Fail*. 2007;13:462-469.
84. Whipp BJ, Rossiter HB. The kinetics of oxygen uptake: physiological inferences from the parameters. In: Jones AM, Poole DC, eds. *Oxygen Uptake Kinetics in Health and Disease*. London, United Kingdom: Routledge; 2005:64-94.
85. Whipp BJ, Ward SA, Lamarra N, Davis JA, Wasserman K. Parameters of ventilatory and gas exchange dynamics during exercise. *J Appl Physiol Respir Environ Exerc Physiol*. 1982;52:1506-1513.
86. Nery LE, Wasserman K, Andrews JD, Huntsman DJ, Hansen JE, Whipp BJ. Ventilatory and gas exchange kinetics during exercise in chronic airways obstruction. *J Appl Physiol Respir Environ Exerc Physiol*. 1982;53:1594-1602.
87. Sietsema K. Oxygen uptake kinetics in response to exercise in patients with pulmonary vascular disease. *Am Rev Respir Dis*. 1992;145:1052-1057.
88. Sietsema KE, Daly JA, Wasserman K. Early dynamics of O2 uptake and heart rate as affected by exercise work rate. *J Appl Physiol (1985)*. 1989;67:2535-2541.
89. Whipp BJ, Wasserman K. Oxygen uptake kinetics for various intensities of constant-load work. *J Appl Physiol*. 1972;33:351-356.
90. Roston WL, Whipp BJ, Davis JA, Cunningham DA, Effros RM, Wasserman K. Oxygen uptake kinetics and lactate concentration during exercise in humans. *Am Rev Respir Dis*. 1987;135:1080-1084.
91. Zhang YY, Wasserman K, Sietsema KE, et al. O_2 uptake kinetics in response to exercise. A measure of tissue anaerobiosis in heart failure. *Chest*. 1993;103:735-741.

92. Puente-Maestu L, Palange P, Casaburi R, et al. Use of exercise testing in the evaluation of interventional efficacy: an official ERS statement. *Eur Resp J*. 2016;47:429-460.
93. Whipp BJ, Ward SA. Quantifying intervention-related improvements in exercise tolerance. *Eur Respir J*. 2009;33:1254-1260.
94. Zhang YY, Sietsema KE, Sullivan S, Wasserman K. A method for estimating bicarbonate buffering of lactic acid during constant work rate exercise. *Eur J Appl Physiol Occup Physiol*. 1994;69:309-315.
95. Rebuck AS, Slutsky AS. Measurement of ventilatory responses to hypercapnia and hypoxia. In: Hornbein TF, ed. *Regulation of Breathing*. New York, NY: Marcel Dekker; 1991:745-772.
96. Severinghaus JW. Proposed standard determination of ventilatory responses to hypoxia and hypercapnia in man. *Chest*. 1976;70(suppl 1): 129-131.
97. Dejours P. Chemoreflexes in breathing. *Physiol Rev*. 1962;42:335-358.
98. Ward SA. Assessment of peripheral chemoreflex contributions to exercise hyperpnea in humans. *Med Sci Sports Exerc*. 1994;26:303-310.
99. Whipp BJ. Peripheral chemoreceptor control of exercise hyperpnea in humans. *Med Sci Sports Exerc*. 1994;26:337-347.
100. Whipp BJ, Wasserman K. Carotid bodies and ventilatory control dynamics in man. *Fed Proc*. 1980;39:2668-2673.
101. Cropp GJ. The exercise bronchoprovocation test: standardization of procedures and evaluation of response. *J Allergy Clin Immunol*. 1979;64(6, pt 2):627-633.
102. Deal EC Jr, McFadden ER Jr, Ingram RH Jr, Strauss RH, Jaeger JJ. Role of respiratory heat exchange in production of exercise-induced asthma. *J Appl Physiol Environ Exerc Physiol*. 1979;46:467-475.
103. Parsons JP, Hallstrand TS, Mastronarde JG, et al. An official American Thoracic Society clinical practice guideline: exercise-induced bronchoconstriction. *Am J Respir Crit Care Med*. 2013;187(9):1016-1027.

CHAPTER 4

Pathophysiology of Disorders Limiting Exercise

The coupling of external to cellular respiration to perform exercise involves many organ systems. **Figure 4.1** illustrates that the blood, the peripheral circulation, the heart, the pulmonary circulation, the lungs, the chest wall, respiratory control, and metabolic pathways in bioenergetics all influence the normal coupling of external to cellular respiration. Thus, defects of any might limit exercise performance. The objective of this chapter is to describe the changes in external respiration that may characterize the pathophysiology brought about by diseases of some of the major organ systems that are required for the support of the exercise bioenergetic mechanisms. Common categories of disorders are listed in **Table 4.1**, accompanied by descriptions of major pathophysiology and physiological limitations and how these are reflected in measurements made during cardiopulmonary exercise testing (CPET). Individually or in combination, these disorders limit exercise by causing symptoms of dyspnea, fatigue, and/or pain.

OBESITY

Although the obese individual has some increase in resting metabolic rate (resting oxygen uptake [$\dot{V}O_2$]) relative to the nonobese individual, the increase is more marked during dynamic exercise (see **Figs. 2.8** and **3.6**). Additional energy is needed to move a larger body mass while ambulating and often even to lift heavier legs in cycling exercise.[1] This adds to the O_2 needed to perform external work in proportion to the excess body weight (**Fig. 4.2**).[2] Because the metabolic rate is increased to perform the external work, obese people require an increased cardiorespiratory response to perform the same amount of exercise. However, the heart, blood

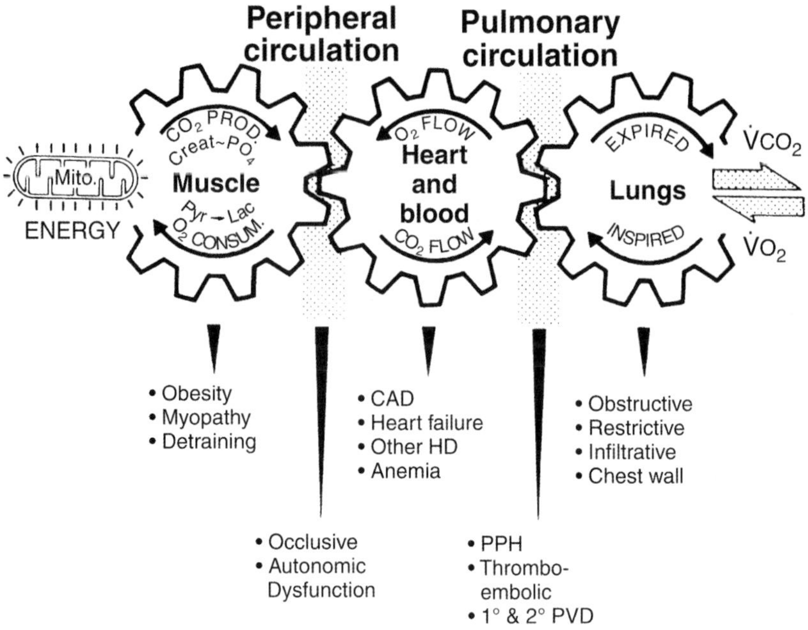

FIGURE 4.1. Sites of interference in the metabolic-cardiovascular-ventilatory coupling caused by some common disease states. Abbreviations: CAD, coronary artery disease; HD, heart disease; Mito, mitochondrion; PPH, primary pulmonary hypertension; PVD, pulmonary vascular disease; $\dot{V}CO_2$, carbon dioxide output; $\dot{V}O_2$, oxygen uptake.

vessels, lungs, and muscles do not usually increase in size commensurate with the individual's added weight. Consequently, for the obese individual to do any amount of physical work, there must be greater than normal cardiovascular and ventilatory responses. Because more O_2 transport than normal is needed to support body movement itself, less O_2 transport is available for effective external work in obesity.

Constraints are imposed on the maximal exercise performance because of altered cardiovascular and ventilatory mechanics in obesity, especially in the extremely obese individual. Because of the large mass, there is already some increase in the resting cardiac output per kilogram of lean body weight. Thus, the cardiac output reserve available to support the increased muscle O_2 requirement for exercise is reduced. Furthermore, the added mass on the chest wall and the increased pressure in the abdomen cause an increase in ventilatory work. In very obese subjects, the increased abdominal pressure may constrain diaphragmatic descent during inspiration, reducing the inspiratory capacity and tidal volume. Both the increased abdominal pressure and the added weight to the chest wall effectively "straps the chest" of the obese individual[3] causing the resting end-expiratory lung volume (functional residual capacity, FRC) to be reduced (in extreme cases, close to the residual volume).[4] This can lead to atelectasis of peripheral lung units and hypoxemia at rest. In addition, pulmonary vascular resistance may be increased, primarily as a result of pulmonary insufficiency, especially if there is associated sleep-disordered breathing or obesity hypoventilation syndrome. In extreme cases, over time, cor pulmonale may develop with hypoxemia, secondary erythrocytosis, hepatomegaly, peripheral edema, and right ventricular hypertrophy and/or failure.

The average increase in O_2 cost for performing mechanical work associated with obesity is predictable and well worked out for cycle ergometry.[1,2,5] The $\dot{V}O_2$–work rate relationship is displaced upward, depending on the degree of obesity, by an average of 5.8 mL/min/kg (see **Fig. 4.2**). However, obesity causes no discernible change in the slope of the $\dot{V}O_2$–work rate relationship ($\Delta\dot{V}O_2/\Delta WR$).[2,5] The effect of adipose tissue distribution in the body (ie, legs or trunk) on $\dot{V}O_2$ has had limited study,[6] but, as expected, a high waist-hip circumference ratio identifying women with "abdominal" obesity compared to lower body obesity had higher $\dot{V}O_2$ during progressive exercise and displayed a shallower and more rapid breathing pattern. Some of the increase observed in $\dot{V}O_2$ is likely due to increased work of breathing.[7]

The peak $\dot{V}O_2$ and anaerobic threshold (*AT*) are low when related to actual body weight but usually normal or high when related to height[2] or to predicted weight or lean body mass. Because of the high metabolic cost of doing even modest levels of exercise, an active, otherwise healthy, obese individual may have good cardiovascular fitness but reduced work capacity. Thus, the actual peak $\dot{V}O_2$ may be greater than that predicted for a normal sedentary subject based on height or lean body weight.

The hypoxemia commonly present at rest in obesity results from atelectasis of peripheral lung units. When this is the case, it usually improves during exercise because the increase in tidal volume reexpands atelectatic lung units. It is the only pulmonary condition in which arterial oxygenation improves during exercise. Because ventilation–perfusion relationships usually normalize during exercise in the patient with uncomplicated obesity, dead space/tidal volume ratio (V_D/V_T), alveolar-arterial partial pressure of O_2 difference [$P(A - a)O_2$], and arterial minus end-tidal partial pressure CO_2 difference [$P(a - ET)CO_2$] values are usually within the normal range during exercise, although small differences have been shown in comparison to healthy, nonobese individuals.[8] However, ventilatory compensation for the lactic acidosis of exercise may be less than normal at peak $\dot{V}O_2$ because of the increased work of breathing in the obese individual[9]; reduced maximum inspiratory and expiratory pressure may play a role.[8]

TABLE 4.1 Selected Categories of Disorders Limiting Work Tolerance and Associated Pathophysiology and CPET Findings

Disorder	Limitation	Pathophysiology	Characteristic findings on CPET
Obesity	Decreased capacity for "external work" due to metabolic cost of supporting or moving body weight	Increased metabolic requirements relative to increase in WR	• $\Delta\dot{V}O_2/\Delta WR$ normal but shifted upward so higher $\dot{V}O_2$ required for a given WR • Low $\dot{V}O_2$/kg body weight
		Respiratory (chest wall) restriction	• Low breathing reserve • Tidal volume low relative to IC
		Increased work of breathing and/or reduced response to chemical stimulation	• Sometimes reduced or no respiratory compensation for metabolic acidosis • If associated with obesity hypoventilation syndrome, there may be hypercapnia, low $\dot{V}E/\dot{V}CO_2$, and sometimes hypoxemia.
Cardiovascular disorders	Limited capacity for transport of O_2 to exercising muscles	Impaired increase in systemic cardiac output due to limited stroke volume and/or HR	In most cardiovascular disorders: • Low peak $\dot{V}O_2$, *AT*, and O_2 pulse • Steep slope of HR versus $\dot{V}O_2$ Exceptions: With chronotropic insufficiency: • Low peak HR and shallow slope of HR versus $\dot{V}O_2$ • High O_2 pulse if stroke volume can be augmented via Starling mechanism
	Lag in $\dot{V}O_2$ responses and resulting increase in O_2 deficit	Slow rate of adaptation (kinetics) of metabolic responses to exercise or of circulatory responses to metabolic changes	Abnormal $\Delta\dot{V}O_2/\Delta WR$ during incremental exercise: • With heart failure, PAD, PVD: $\Delta\dot{V}O_2/\Delta WR$ slope may be abnormal across entire test, but $\Delta\dot{V}CO_2/\Delta WR$ increases normally. • With CAD: $\Delta\dot{V}O_2/\Delta WR$ slope initially normal but decreases when ischemia causes impaired contractility or diastolic filling; $\dot{V}CO_2$ increases normally • With PAD: With severe occlusive disease, both $\Delta\dot{V}O_2/\Delta WR$ and $\Delta\dot{V}CO_2/\Delta WR$ may be shallow above the *AT*. Slow recovery of $\dot{V}O_2$ and HR after exercise
	Uneven distribution of pulmonary blood flow	Areas of high and/or low pulmonary $\dot{V}A/\dot{Q}$ relationships	With heart failure: • High $\dot{V}E/\dot{V}CO_2$ at *AT*; steep slope of $\dot{V}E$ versus $\dot{V}CO_2$ With PVD: • High $\dot{V}E/\dot{V}CO_2$ at *AT*; steep slope of $\dot{V}E$ versus $\dot{V}CO_2$; often decreased arterial O_2 saturation
Distinctive patterns in certain cardiovascular conditions	Right to left shunt (eg, through septal defect or patent foramen ovale), present before or developing during exercise	New or increased admixture of venous blood into systemic arterial circulation during exercise	• Onset or worsening of systemic arterial desaturation • Augmentation of $\dot{V}E$ to compensate for shunting of CO_2 with (usually) abrupt decrease in P_{ETCO_2} and simultaneous increases in P_{ETO_2}, R, and ventilatory equivalents
	Oscillatory breathing in heart failure	Altered ventilatory control due to changes in circulation time, blood flow dynamics, or other factors	• Regular waxing and waning of $\dot{V}E$ and other gas exchange variables with a periodicity of 45-90 s at rest and early exercise

(Continued)

TABLE 4.1 Selected Categories of Disorders Limiting Work Tolerance and Associated Pathophysiology and CPET Findings *(Continued)*

Disorder	Limitation	Pathophysiology	Characteristic findings on CPET
Pulmonary disorders	Airflow obstruction	Reduced breathing capacity	• Low breathing reserve
		Increased and heterogeneous airway resistance causing abnormal $\dot{V}_A/\dot{Q}$	• Elevated $\dot{V}_E/\dot{V}_{CO_2}$ at *AT* and elevated V_D/V_T • Arterial hypoxemia
		Air trapping	• Dynamic hyperinflation detectable by increasing IC; sometimes decreasing V_T
		Increased work of breathing; increased demand for blood flow to respiratory muscles	• Reduced peak $\dot{V}_E$
		Limited capacity to increase pulmonary blood flow due to loss of capillary volume and/or increased intrathoracic pressure impairing systemic venous return	Features of cardiovascular impairment including: • Shallow $\Delta\dot{V}_{O_2}/\Delta WR$ • Low peak O_2 pulse and steep HR versus $\dot{V}_{O_2}$ slope
	Interstitial lung disease	Reduced breathing capacity	• Low breathing reserve
		Limited capacity for pulmonary blood flow due to loss of capillary volume	Features of cardiovascular disorders may be prominent including: • Shallow $\Delta\dot{V}_{O_2}/\Delta WR$ • Low peak O_2 pulse and steep HR versus $\dot{V}_{O_2}$ slope
		Pulmonary $\dot{V}_A/\dot{Q}$ mismatch	• Elevated $\dot{V}_E/\dot{V}_{CO_2}$ at *AT* and elevated V_D/V_T • Systemic arterial hypoxemia
	Extrapulmonary restriction (eg, by chest wall abnormalities)	Reduced breathing capacity	• Low breathing reserve but normal pulmonary gas exchange
Defects in hemoglobin content and quality	Anemia	Reduced blood O_2 content; limited capacity to widen $C(a - \bar{v})O_2$	• Low peak $\dot{V}_{O_2}$, *AT*, and O_2 pulse
	Increased carboxyhemoglobin	Reduced blood O_2 content; limited capacity to widen $C(a - \bar{v})O_2$; increased affinity of hemoglobin for O_2	• Low peak $\dot{V}_{O_2}$, *AT*, and peak O_2 pulse
	Hemoglobinopathy with high P_{50}	Increased O_2 affinity for hemoglobin (left-shifted HbO_2 dissociation curve) and impaired diffusive O_2 delivery	• Low peak $\dot{V}_{O_2}$, *AT*, and peak O_2 pulse
Metabolic acidosis	Chronic low pH with low HCO_3^-	Increased ventilatory requirement to maintain normal pH	• High $\dot{V}_E/\dot{V}_{CO_2}$ at *AT* • Low Pa_{CO_2} and PET_{CO_2}
Muscle metabolic disorders	Glycolytic enzyme defect	Deficiency in utilization of carbohydrate substrate; dependence on fatty acid metabolism; inability to regenerate ATP by anaerobic pathways	• Low peak $\dot{V}_{O_2}$ • Absence of lactic acidosis or discernible *AT* • Low steady state R values
	Lipid metabolism defect	Limited energy sources for long duration exercise; fatigue or muscle symptoms during sustained or fasting exercise	• Often no abnormalities
	Electron transport defect	Metabolic acidosis at low work rate Hyperdynamic circulatory response to exercise	• Low *AT* or lactic acidosis at rest • Low peak $\dot{V}_{O_2}$ and O_2 pulse • Shallow $\Delta\dot{V}_{O_2}/\Delta WR$ • Steep HR versus $\dot{V}_{O_2}$ slope • Steep cardiac output versus $\dot{V}_{O_2}$ slope

TABLE 4.1 Selected Categories of Disorders Limiting Work Tolerance and Associated Pathophysiology and CPET Findings *(Continued)*

Disorder	Limitation	Pathophysiology	Characteristic findings on CPET
Noncardiorespiratory limitations	Anxiety or idiopathic hyperventilation	Unknown	• High $\dot{V}_E$, often with deep regular breathing pattern • Low Pa_{CO_2} and $P_{ET}CO_2$ • Although $\dot{V}_E/\dot{V}CO_2$ at *AT* may be high, V_D/V_T is normal. • Lightheadedness, paresthesia if severe
	Volitional low performance	Secondary gain	• Chaotic or atypical breathing pattern • Exercise ending prior to clear cardiovascular limits
	Incomplete effort	Exercise limited by noncardiorespiratory factors, fear of discomfort or complications, submaximal motivation	• Low peak $\dot{V}O_2$, low peak HR with normal *AT*

Abbreviations: *AT*, anaerobic threshold; ATP, adenosine triphosphate; CAD, coronary artery disease; CO_2, carbon dioxide; CPET, cardiopulmonary exercise testing; HCO_3^-, bicarbonate; HR, heart rate; IC, inspiratory capacity; O_2, oxygen; P_{50}, partial pressure of PO_2 in blood associated with 50% oxyhemoglobin saturation; Pa_{CO_2}, arterial P_{CO_2}; PAD, peripheral arterial disease; $P_{ET}CO_2$, end-tidal P_{CO_2}; $P_{ET}O_2$, end-tidal P_{O_2}; PVD, pulmonary vascular disease; R, respiratory exchange ratio; $\dot{V}_A/\dot{Q}$, alveolar ventilation/perfusion ratio; $\dot{V}CO_2$, CO_2 output; V_D/V_T, dead space/tidal volume ratio; $\dot{V}_E$, minute ventilation; $\dot{V}_E/\dot{V}CO_2$, ventilatory equivalent for CO_2; $\dot{V}O_2$, oxygen uptake; WR, work rate.

The $\dot{V}_E$ versus CO_2 output ($\dot{V}CO_2$) slope appears to be normal in mild-to-moderate obesity, likely because it is not effort dependent and does not require reaching maximum exercise. In one study of heart failure patients, the slope maintained its prognostic value regardless of body mass index.[10]

PATTERNS OF EXERCISE GAS EXCHANGE COMMON TO CARDIOVASCULAR DISEASES

The cardiovascular system has a major role in exercise by subserving the delivery of oxygen to exercising muscle and carbon dioxide to the lung. As a result, many cardiovascular conditions can affect the $\dot{V}O_2$ response to exercise, including the peak $\dot{V}O_2$, *AT*, and peak O_2 pulse (see **Table 4.1**). These findings are typical of any condition limiting maximal cardiac output whether due to limitation of left or right ventricular function or of the pulmonary or the peripheral circulations. The underlying bioenergetic relationship between oxygen consumption, adenosine triphosphate (ATP) production, and muscular work is not altered by impairment in oxygen delivery, but the rate of adaptation of oxygen delivery and/or utilization can be slower in patients with cardiovascular disease, and under the nonsteady state of an incremental exercise test, there may therefore be marked lag in the rate of $\dot{V}O_2$ increase relative to changing work rate ($\Delta\dot{V}O_2/\Delta WR$) in the submaximal range of exercise.[11]

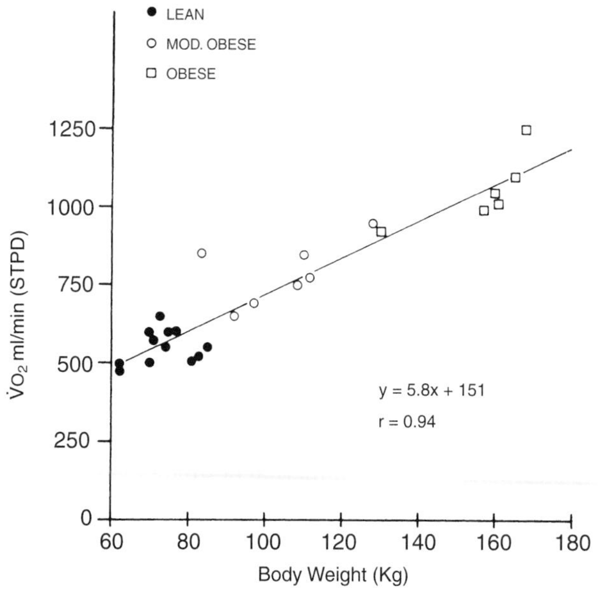

FIGURE 4.2. The O_2 cost of performing unloaded cycling as related to body weight. Abbreviation: STPD, standard temperature and pressure dry. *(Reprinted with permission of the American Thoracic Society. Copyright © 2020 American Society. All rights reserved. From Wasserman K, Whipp BJ. Exercise physiology in health and disease.* Am Rev Respir Dis. *1975;112[2]:219-249. The American Review of Respiratory Disease* is an official journal of the American Thoracic Society. [*Now titled The American Journal of Respiratory and Critical Care Medicine])*

$\dot{V}O_2$ Response to Increasing Work Rate ($\Delta\dot{V}O_2/\Delta WR$) in Patients With Cardiovascular Abnormalities

An example of a normal $\Delta\dot{V}O_2/\Delta WR$ (10 mL/min/W) is illustrated in **Figure 4.3A**. If the circulatory coupling of external respiration to cellular respiration is inadequate to keep pace with the changing O_2 requirement, the rate of increase of $\dot{V}O_2$ relative to changing work rate may be shallower than normal (**Fig. 4.3B-E**). The pattern of alteration in $\Delta\dot{V}O_2/\Delta WR$ slope often differs depending on the cardiovascular pathophysiology limiting exercise (see **Fig. 4.3**). In left ventricular failure, the linearity of the $\dot{V}O_2$–work rate relationship is commonly abnormal and the $\Delta\dot{V}O_2/\Delta WR$ slope is reduced to a different extent depending on the rate at which work rate is increased.[12] The $\dot{V}O_2$ may increase normally as the work rate is increased at low levels, but the rate of increase becomes progressively less as the peak $\dot{V}O_2$ is approached.[5] In contrast, in patients with coronary disease, the $\Delta\dot{V}O_2/\Delta WR$ slope may be normal during the early portion of exercise.

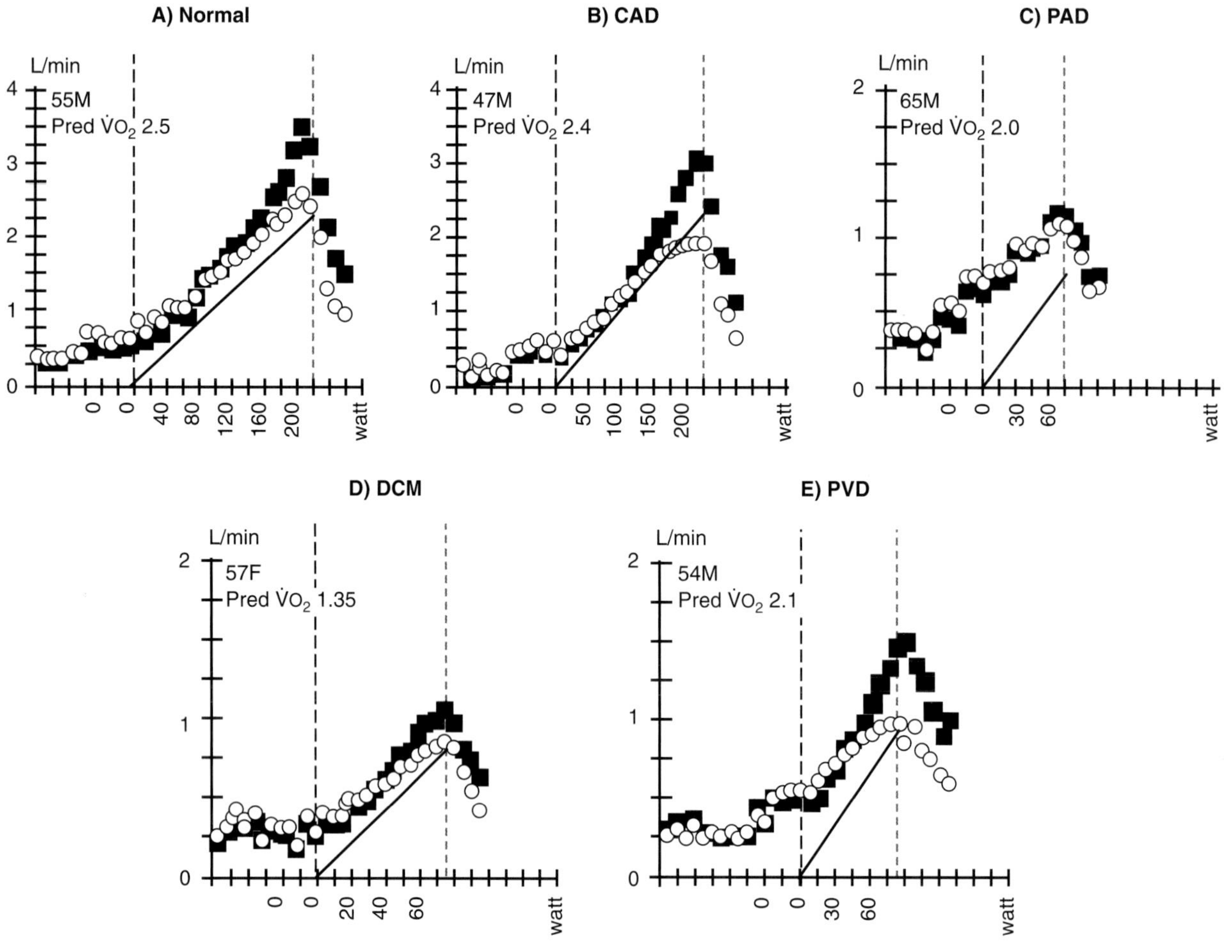

FIGURE 4.3. The pattern of increase in oxygen uptake ($\dot{V}O_2$) (open circles) and carbon dioxide output ($\dot{V}CO_2$) (solid boxes) as related to increasing work rate (WR) (diagonal line) in four individuals with different cardiovascular pathophysiologies (B-E) compared to a normal individual (A). The diagonal line shows the theoretical normal increase in $\dot{V}O_2$ relative to increase in WR of 10 mL/min/W. A: A 55-year-old man whose peak $\dot{V}O_2$ and $\Delta\dot{V}CO_2/\Delta WR$ are normal. B: A 47-year-old man with coronary artery disease (CAD) with reduced peak $\dot{V}O_2$ and myocardial dyskinesis demonstrable starting at about 150 W. C: A 65-year-old man with claudication-limited exercise due to peripheral artery disease (PAD) with reduced peak $\dot{V}O_2$, reduced $\Delta\dot{V}O_2/\Delta WR$, and reduced $\Delta\dot{V}CO_2/\Delta WR$ starting from unloaded cycling. D: A 57-year-old woman with dilated cardiomyopathy (DCM) and reduced ejection fraction heart failure with reduced peak $\dot{V}O_2$, decreasing $\Delta\dot{V}O_2/\Delta WR$, and normally increasing $\Delta\dot{V}CO_2/\Delta WR$ starting from unloaded cycling. E: A 54-year-old man with an idiopathic pulmonary hypertension (PVD) with reduced peak $\dot{V}O_2$, reduced $\Delta\dot{V}O_2/\Delta WR$, and normally increasing $\Delta\dot{V}CO_2/\Delta WR$ starting from unloaded cycling.

When the myocardial O_2 demand exceeds the myocardial O_2 supply due to myocardial ischemia, however, exercise-induced myocardial dyskinesis may be evident at the work rate and rate-pressure product at which the ischemia occurs.[13] The break in the $\Delta\dot{V}O_2/\Delta WR$ slope appears to occur before the electrocardiographic evidence of myocardial ischemia becomes evident or even without electrocardiogram (ECG) changes.[14] Patients with primary and secondary pulmonary vasculopathies have abnormally high pulmonary vascular resistance that prevents the normal recruitment of pulmonary vascular bed and appropriate increase in pulmonary blood flow in response to exercise. The limitation to right-sided cardiac output has the same effect on the pattern of $\dot{V}O_2$ relative to work rate as is seen in left-sided heart failure (see **Fig. 4.3E**). Additional differences in these conditions include the frequent occurrence of arterial hypoxemia in patients with pulmonary vasculopathy, with or without a right-to-left shunt through a patent foramen ovale,[15] whereas patients with stable chronic left ventricular failure rarely develop hypoxemia during exercise.[16] In each of these conditions, the slope of $\dot{V}CO_2$ relative to work rate increase ($\Delta\dot{V}CO_2/\Delta WR$ slope) continues to rise relatively steeply (see **Fig. 4.3B**, **D**, and **E**). The increasing difference between the rise in $\dot{V}CO_2$ relative to that of $\dot{V}O_2$ reflects the CO_2 released from the bicarbonate (HCO_3^-) buffering of simultaneously generated lactic acid. In occlusive peripheral arterial disease, fixed atherosclerotic stenoses limit the normal increase in blood flow to exercising muscles. Therefore, with lower extremity exercise, $\dot{V}O_2$ may increase linearly but relatively shallowly, as shown for the patient in **Figure 4.3C**. In this case, and in contrast to other cardiovascular disorders, the $\Delta\dot{V}CO_2/\Delta WR$ may also be relatively shallow, which may result from diffuse vascular obstruction and correspondingly low fraction of the cardiac output flowing through the ischemic muscle.

Why Do Cardiovascular Disorders Impair Gas Transport?

Because gas transport is the major and most immediate function of the cardiovascular system, cardiac dysfunction of most types of heart disease (ie, heart rate [HR] impairment, coronary artery disease, cardiomyopathy, and structural defects) will cause changes in the pattern of minute ventilation ($\dot{V}E$), $\dot{V}O_2$, $\dot{V}CO_2$, end-tidal partial pressures of CO_2 ($PETCO_2$), end-tidal partial pressures of O_2 ($PETO_2$), HR, and blood pressure responses to exercise and their relationships.

In nearly all heart defects (in the absence of intrinsic or pharmacologic impairment in HR), the increase in HR as a function of $\dot{V}O_2$ is steeper than normal. This reflects the increased dependence on HR and arteriovenous O_2 extraction to increase O_2 transport, which is essential for exercise.

Because of the relatively low cardiac output response, mixed venous oxygen reaches its lowest value and the arterial–mixed venous oxygen difference [$C(a - \bar{v})O_2$] its highest value at a low work rate.[17] Consequently, the O_2 pulse [$C(a - \bar{v})O_2 \times SV$, where SV = stroke volume] reaches a constant value that is abnormally low and occurs at an unusually low work rate compared to normal (**Fig. 4.4**). The increase in $\dot{V}O_2$ as WR increases commonly becomes smaller near the maximum work rate (see **Fig. 4.3**), reflecting a lower proportion of energy from aerobic metabolism compared to normal, presumably because of impaired O_2 transport[18] or utilization.[19]

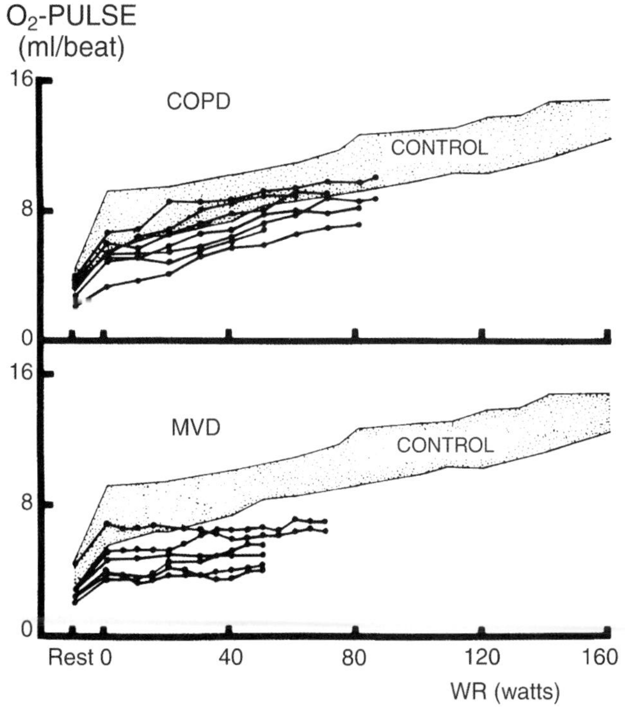

FIGURE 4.4. The O_2-pulse response to incremental exercise in patients with chronic obstructive pulmonary disease (COPD) (upper panel) and mitral valve disease (MVD) (lower panel) compared with the range of values of a control group (stippled area). *(Modified from Nery LE, Wasserman K, French W, Oren A, Davis JA. Contrasting cardiovascular and respiratory responses to exercise in mitral valve and chronic obstructive pulmonary diseases.* Chest. *1983;83[3]:446-453. Copyright © 1983 American College of Chest Physicians. With permission.)*

A number of studies have shown that patients with chronic left ventricular failure have high effective V_D/V_T, reflecting mismatching of ventilation relative to pulmonary perfusion of the high alveolar ventilation/perfusion ratio ($\dot{V}A/\dot{Q}$) type. This results in a further increase in the breathing requirement to maintain blood pH homeostasis.[16,20-23] The need to maintain pH homeostasis in the presence of the increase in V_D/V_T is the major factor, along with the increase in $\dot{V}CO_2$ in response to developing lactic acidosis, accounting for the increased ventilatory response to exercise,[24] and likely contributes to the symptom of dyspnea in patients with chronic left ventricular failure.

Constant work rate tests may be helpful for evaluating the cardiovascular response to specific levels of exercise in heart diseases.[25,26] If the work rate is above the lactic acidosis threshold, $\dot{V}O_2$ will not reach a steady state by 3 minutes. The magnitude of the increase in $\dot{V}O_2$ between 3 and 6 minutes [$\Delta\dot{V}O_2$ (6 − 3)] is correlated with the exercise lactic acidosis.

HEART DISEASES

Coronary Artery Disease

Although mild coronary artery disease may be difficult to detect, simultaneous gas exchange measurements with the ECG improve the diagnostic capabilities of an exercise stress test. Coronary artery disease will often cause the peak $\dot{V}O_2$ to be reduced. Patients with coronary artery disease may or may not experience chest pain with exercise. When the exercise-induced increase in myocardial oxygen requirement is not met by the myocardial oxygen supply, myocardial ischemia may result with characteristic ECG changes. These might be preceded by the characteristic $\dot{V}O_2$ changes of exercise-induced myocardial ischemia (see **Fig. 4.3B**).

The $\dot{V}O_2/\Delta WR$ slope is normal at low work rates of an incremental exercise test but abruptly decreases when myocardial ischemia fails to generate sufficient ATP to maintain myocardial contraction and stroke volume (myocardial dyskinesis). The ECG usually becomes abnormal, whether or not chest pain develops, when or after $\Delta\dot{V}O_2/\Delta WR$ starts to decrease.[13,27-29] Despite a decrease in $\Delta\dot{V}O_2/\Delta WR$ because of myocardial dyskinesis, $\dot{V}CO_2$ continues to increase steeply, creating a large disparity between the increases in $\dot{V}CO_2$ and $\dot{V}O_2$. With myocardial ischemia, HR usually increases more steeply as a function of $\dot{V}O_2$, developing a curvilinear HR versus $\dot{V}O_2$ relationship rather than the normal linear relationship.

The O_2 pulse fails to increase to its normal predicted value when myocardial ischemia develops, often becoming flat or decreasing despite increasing work rate. The decreased O_2 pulse is likely due to a decrease in stroke volume secondary to myocardial dyskinesis while $C(a - \bar{v})O_2$ is simultaneously increasing. These simultaneous changes often maintain a constant, albeit reduced, O_2 pulse during increasing work rate in patients with heart failure (see **Fig. 4.4**) and coronary artery disease.

In normal persons, the O_2 pulse decreases immediately after exercise. However, a paradoxical increase in O_2 pulse sometimes occurs in patients who develop myocardial ischemia during exercise or who have heart failure. This paradoxical increase in O_2 pulse may be due to an immediate increase in stroke volume because of the abrupt decrease in left ventricular afterload when exercise stops.[30]

Metabolic acidosis usually develops because of impaired O_2 transport resulting from the failure to increase cardiac output commensurate with the increasing work rate when a significant portion of the left ventricle stops contracting normally. How much metabolic acidosis develops depends on duration that exercise is maintained after ischemia develops.

In patients with coronary artery disease, the breathing reserve is normal or high because the individual is forced to stop exercise from symptoms at a relatively low metabolic rate. The ventilatory equivalents are normal, reflecting relatively uniform ventilation–perfusion relationships, in contrast to the nonuniform ventilation–perfusion relationships observed in patients with chronic stable heart failure.

Myopathic Heart Disease (Heart Failure)

Patients with heart failure, whether ischemic or idiopathic, and with reduced or preserved left ventricular ejection fraction, have difficulty in transporting oxygen to the skeletal muscles during exercise. As a result, the increase in $\dot{V}O_2$ relative to the increase in work rate is slower than normal. This slowing, however, is not abrupt in onset, in contrast to that seen in patients who develop acute myocardial ischemia during exercise. The failure to transport O_2 at the rate needed to regenerate the ATP needed for muscular contraction makes it impossible to sustain muscular contraction; consequently, muscles fatigue and the individual must stop.

The peak $\dot{V}O_2$ is reduced consequent to the reduced peak cardiac output response to exercise. The *AT* is also commonly reduced.[31] The peak O_2 pulse is low because of the reduced stroke volume. The HR increase is commonly steep relative to the increase in $\dot{V}O_2$, except when on β-adrenergic blocking or other negative chronotropic drugs. The maximal HR and rate of change in HR relative to $\dot{V}O_2$ may be reduced in patients with heart failure when cardiomyopathy is accompanied by chronotropic incompetence, β-adrenergic blockade, or early exercise fatigue. Consequently, the O_2 pulse, $[C(a - \bar{v})O_2] \times SV$, reaches a constant value that is low and that occurs at an unusually low work rate compared with normal (see **Fig. 4.4**).

Patients with heart failure have a high ventilatory requirement relative to the metabolic rate.[20,22,31,32] In fact, the ventilatory requirement relative to $\dot{V}CO_2$ is recognized as a prognosticator of survival.[20,32,33] A number of factors can contribute to the higher ventilatory requirement.[34] Most importantly, the effective V_D/V_T is increased reflecting mismatching of ventilation relative to pulmonary perfusion, particularly of the high $\dot{V}_A/\dot{Q}$ type. Constraints on the increase in tidal volumes due to pulmonary congestion may also contribute to an elevated exercise V_D/V_T. The degree of ventilatory inefficiency correlates with the degree of functional impairment in exercise performance (**Fig. 4.5**). This reduced gas exchange efficiency is a major factor accounting for the increased ventilatory output in heart failure. In addition, a metabolic acidosis occurs at lower work rates

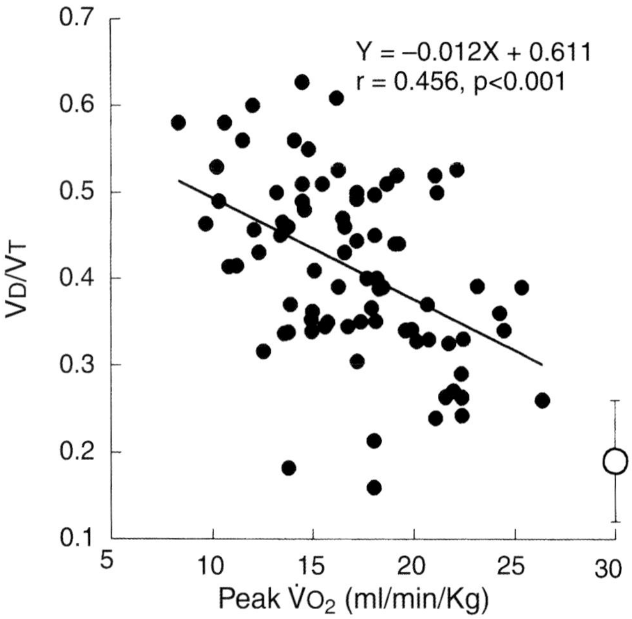

FIGURE 4.5. Ratio of physiological dead space to tidal volume (V_D/V_T) as a function of peak oxygen uptake ($\dot{V}O_2$) on a cycle ergometer in 78 patients with chronic stable heart failure. The open circle on the right is the mean V_D/V_T ± standard deviation for normal subjects. *(Reprinted with permission from Wasserman K, Zhang YY, Gitt A, et al. Lung function and exercise gas exchange in chronic heart failure.* Circulation. *1997;96[7]:2221-2227. Copyright © 1997 by American Heart Association.)*

in patients with heart failure compared with normal.[24,35,36] The increase in CO_2 produced at low work rates, because of the buffering of lactic acid by HCO_3^-, increases the acid load to the ventilatory system. These factors combine to increase the breathing requirement to maintain arterial H^+ homeostasis in response to exercise[24] and likely contribute to exertional dyspnea.

A regular oscillatory pattern of breathing in which $\dot{V}O_2$, $\dot{V}CO_2$, $\dot{V}_E$, and related variables wax and wane with a period of approximately 45 to 90 seconds is observed in some patients with more severe heart failure. Up to one-third of patients with either heart failure with reduced ejection fraction or heart failure with preserved ejection fraction will have oscillatory breathing.[37-39] This oscillatory pattern in gas exchange is most marked at rest and at lower work rates and tends to diminish and even to disappear as maximum exercise is approached. During oscillatory breathing, the phasic changes in $\dot{V}O_2$ lead $\dot{V}CO_2$ and, more particularly, $\dot{V}_E$.[40] This suggests that flow through the pulmonary circulation is oscillating such that oscillatory changes in arterial blood gases (P_{O_2}, P_{CO_2}) and pH could be inducing the gas exchange patterns. The mechanism(s) of oscillatory changes in ventilation and gas exchange in the presence of heart failure remain controversial. Potential mechanisms include effects of heart failure on features of the ventilatory control mechanisms, such as enhanced gain of the carotid bodies, reduction in system damping, and instability in ventilatory controller feedback. Other postulated mechanisms relate to the behavior of the failing heart and include cyclic changes in left ventricular afterload originating from the vasomotor center (Traube-Hering waves), increased circulatory time, and variations in cerebral blood flow sensed in the medulla.[37,41,42] Cyclic breathing patterns are occasionally seen in individuals without heart failure, so this finding is not completely unique to cardiovascular disease. Among patients with heart failure, however, the presence of oscillatory or periodic breathing during exercise is associated with a poor prognosis.[43]

Finally, about 20% of heart failure patients have chronic atrial fibrillation, and the presence of atrial fibrillation is also associated with a lower exercise performance and lower peak $\dot{V}O_2$.[44]

Valvular Heart Disease

Exercise pathophysiology in these conditions is dependent on the valve involved and the type of valve disease. Common clinically important valvular diseases include mitral regurgitation, valvular aortic stenosis (AS), and aortic regurgitation or insufficiency; mitral stenosis is less commonly seen, and right-sided valvular lesions are less clinically significant, including commonly seen mild tricuspid regurgitation. In regurgitant valvular lesions, ventricular stroke volume may be increased, as blood leaves the ventricle in the retrograde direction (mitral regurgitation, tricuspid regurgitation), but "forward" stroke volume may be reduced. In significant valvular stenosis, especially AS, stroke volume may be impaired because of central circulatory obstruction and cannot be made up by increased contractility. When stroke volume is reduced, the increase in $\dot{V}O_2$ relative to increase in work rate is usually reduced (ie, low $\Delta\dot{V}O_2/\Delta WR$). Both the *AT* and the peak $\dot{V}O_2$ are typically reduced, and the O_2 pulse is reduced and reaches a plateau value at a relatively low work rate (see **Fig. 4.4**). The HR generally increases steeply relative to $\dot{V}O_2$, with the maximal HR achieved at a relatively low work rate, as the increase in cardiac output is increasingly dependent on increased HR with low stroke volume. Inability to increase stroke volume and cardiac output in AS makes CPET contraindicated in patients who are symptomatic.

Congenital Heart Disease

Pathophysiology of exercise in the various forms of congenital heart disease depends highly on the underlying anatomy; duration of disease; compensatory changes; and presence, timing, and type of surgical repair. Nevertheless, among adults with congenital heart disease, Mantegazza et al[45] have suggested that findings commonly include reduced peak $\dot{V}O_2$, early *AT* (low $\dot{V}O_2$ at the *AT*), a blunted HR response, reduced increase in tidal volume, and increased $\dot{V}E/\dot{V}CO_2$. Not surprisingly, exercise impairment tends to be least for simple disorders and greatest for patients with more complex anatomic lesions. Patients with simple valve lesions or surgically repaired lesions may have exercise capacity within the normal range. Despite this, the range of exercise capacity varies widely even within a given anatomic diagnosis.[46] The CPET is an important tool for objectively assessing functional capacity in adults with congenital lesions due to the difficulty of accurate assessment by clinical history and patient report alone.[47] In addition to providing an objective assessment of cardiorespiratory capacity, CPET also provides information on prognosis in this population. Both peak $\dot{V}O_2$ and ventilatory efficiency have been identified as prognostic in congenital lesions. Dimopoulos et al[48] reported that increased $\dot{V}E/\dot{V}CO_2$ slope was the most powerful predictor among noncyanotic patients, although was not predictive among cyanotic patients, for whom the slope was particularly high due to the effect of right to left shunt on ventilation as described in the following text.

Studies of constant work rate exercise tests have been of particular value in understanding responses to exercise in patients with complex congenital heart disease. Because the increases in $\dot{V}O_2$ and $\dot{V}CO_2$ are determined by the increase in flow of O_2-desaturated, CO_2-rich blood through the pulmonary circulation, the pattern of increase in blood flow through the lungs can be appreciated from the $\dot{V}O_2$ and $\dot{V}CO_2$ kinetics. Thus, patients with pulmonary valve obstruction or obliterative pulmonary vascular disease may fail to demonstrate a normal increase in blood flow at the start of exercise, resulting in a reduced or absent phase I increase in $\dot{V}O_2$ and $\dot{V}CO_2$.[49] The inability to augment pulmonary blood flow can result in most or all of the increased venous return being directed through the central circulatory shunt (eg, septal defect), if present, with marked arterial desaturation as a consequence. Phase II kinetics are also inappropriately slow, and the magnitude of phase II becomes a relatively large portion of the total O_2 requirement at low work rates.[50] A slowly rising $\dot{V}O_2$ is also evident at relatively low work rates during phase III. As in other cardiovascular disorders, the peak $\dot{V}O_2$ and *AT* are reduced.

A markedly elevated ventilatory response is also noted at the start of exercise in patients with cyanotic congenital heart disease and variable right to left intracardiac shunt.[51] In these disorders, the blood flowing through the lungs is hyperventilated to compensate for the blood that bypasses the lungs and enters the left side of the circulation through the shunt. An increase in right to left shunt at the start of exercise is marked by hyperventilation of the blood passing through the lungs. This results in an immediate decrease in P_{ETCO_2}, an increase in P_{ETO_2}, an increase in the respiratory exchange ratio (R), and usually an increase in $\dot{V}E/\dot{V}O_2$ and $\dot{V}E/\dot{V}CO_2$; these changes are usually sustained until the start of recovery. The arterial P_{CO_2} (Pa_{CO_2}) and pH remain relatively unchanged during modest levels of exercise in patients with a right-to-left shunt, whereas the arterial P_{O_2} (Pa_{O_2}) decreases.[49] The relatively unchanged acid-base status suggests that the respiratory control mechanism is sensitive to the regulation of arterial $[H^+]$ and is not greatly influenced by the high pulmonary artery pressures in this population of patients. In congenital heart diseases accompanied by a left-to-right shunt—for example, a patent ductus arteriosus—or in dialysis patients with a systemic arteriovenous fistula, peak $\dot{V}O_2$ and *AT* may be reduced because of the diversion of a sizable part of the systemic cardiac output through the low-resistance shunt.

PULMONARY VASCULAR DISEASES

Causes of Increased Ventilation

Patients with disorders of the pulmonary circulation, such as pulmonary arterial hypertension (idiopathic or familial), chronic pulmonary emboli, and other causes of pulmonary vasculopathy,[52] experience hypoperfusion to ventilated alveoli, particularly during exercise. Consequently, other lung units must accept a greater than normal perfusion and must be ventilated to a proportionately greater degree than normal to remove the metabolic CO_2 and maintain Pa_{CO_2}, Pa_{O_2}, and pH at appropriate levels. Ventilation of the poorly perfused alveoli is wasted and in combination with high ventilation of better perfused alveoli contributes to the elevated calculated dead space (ie, high $\dot{V}_A/\dot{Q}$). Because of this increase in physiological dead space ventilation, minute ventilation is increased in patients with pulmonary vascular diseases at rest and to a greater degree during exercise. The increased dead space ventilation is manifested as a high V_D/V_T, low P_{ETCO_2}, and a persistently positive $P(a - ET)CO_2$ during exercise. A low P_{ETCO_2} is found in pulmonary hypertension for two reasons: (1) hypoperfusion of ventilated lung regions and, in some, (2) opening of the foramen ovale, causing a right-to-left shunt during exercise that may not be present at rest. If a right-to-left shunt develops during exercise, the calculated V_D/V_T and $P(a - ET)CO_2$ will increase further as the size of the shunt increases because overall alveolar ventilation must increase to counter the increased delivery of venous blood to the arterial side through the right-to-left shunt.

Exercise Arterial Hypoxemia

An additional cause of increased ventilatory drive during exercise in many patients with pulmonary vascular occlusive disease is arterial hypoxemia, which gets worse during exercise. The decrease in Pa_{O_2} stimulates the carotid bodies, which are the chemoreceptors that stimulate ventilation in the presence of arterial hypoxemia.

The Pa_{O_2} may be near normal at rest, but there may be striking arterial oxyhemoglobin desaturation during exercise. Several mechanisms may play a role. First, the time available for diffusion equilibrium of O_2, already shortened at rest by the reduced size of the functional capillary bed, is further shortened by the exercise-induced increase in pulmonary blood flow. Red cell residence time remains above 0.3 second (the time required for O_2 equilibration between capillary and alveolar space in a normal acinus) in the normal individual despite increasing cardiac output as much as fourfold at maximal exercise because of recruitment of pulmonary capillaries (approximately doubling the resting capillary blood volume). However, in the presence of pulmonary vascular occlusive disease, the functional capillary bed is reduced and any capillary bed that should be available for recruitment during exercise is already perfused at rest. Thus, red cell transit times through the pulmonary capillaries are shortened during exercise. Consequently, the desaturated red cell arriving from the systemic venous circulation may not remain in the pulmonary capillary bed long enough for diffusion equilibrium of O_2 between the alveolar gas and red cell to occur, especially in response to exercise. High $\dot{V}_A/\dot{Q}$ lung units predominate in chronic pulmonary vascular occlusive disease in patients without airway disease.

Another cause of hypoxemia during exercise in patients with increased pulmonary vascular resistance is the development of a right-to-left shunt resulting from the opening of a potentially patent foramen ovale. An estimated 35% of the normal population is thought to have an "unsealed" foramen ovale. In the healthy individuals, this is usually of no consequence because left atrial pressure is normally higher than right atrial pressure and blood does not shunt in either direction. However, if pulmonary vascular resistance is increased so that the right ventricle cannot pump the venous return into the pulmonary circulation as fast as it is delivered (right ventricular failure), right ventricular end-diastolic pressure and, therefore, right atrial pressure will increase. If the right atrial pressure exceeds that of the left atrium, some of the right atrial flow will pass through the unsealed foramen ovale, constituting a right-to-left shunt. This can cause marked hypoxemia and may be only evident during exercise.[15] The development of a right-to-left shunt is reflected in an abrupt increase in P_{ETO_2}, abrupt decrease in P_{ETCO_2}, and a sustained increase in R, accompanied by increases in $\dot{V}_E/\dot{V}_{O_2}$ and $\dot{V}_E/\dot{V}_{CO_2}$ at the start of exercise. Repeating the exercise test while the subject breathes 100% oxygen can confirm and quantify a right-to-left shunt. If the shunt develops during O_2 breathing, the increase in Pa_{O_2} value should be well below that predicted for normal subjects (>550 mm Hg), and for every 3% to 5% of cardiac output passing through the right-to-left shunt, the Pa_{O_2} while breathing 100% O_2 will be approximately 100 mm Hg less than expected.

In both pulmonary arterial hypertension and chronic left ventricular failure, the V_D/V_T and $\dot{V}_E/\dot{V}_{CO_2}$ at the *AT* and the $\dot{V}_E$ versus $\dot{V}_{CO_2}$ slope are increased. However, the finding of arterial oxyhemoglobin desaturation may help distinguish the two. Oxygenation is normal in patients with uncomplicated left ventricular failure, presumably because of the slow flow through the pulmonary capillary bed. In contrast, systemic arterial blood is often desaturated in patients with pulmonary vascular occlusive disease. As described earlier, the pulmonary capillary blood volume is reduced in the latter condition.

Effect on Systemic Hemodynamics

Pulmonary vascular occlusive diseases cause a hemodynamic stenosis in the central circulation, making it difficult for the right ventricle to deliver blood to the left atrium at a rate sufficient to meet the increased systemic cardiac output needed for exercise. Because the cardiac output (O_2 delivery) increase in response to exercise is reduced, the *AT* and peak $\dot{V}_{O_2}$ and O_2 pulse are reduced in patients with pulmonary vascular disease, similar to that seen in patients with left heart failure.

The clinical spectrum of patients with pulmonary vascular disease is, of course, very wide. Care should be taken in distinguishing the pathophysiology of those with pulmonary hypertension primarily due to vasoconstriction or occlusion of the pulmonary arteries from those whose primarily defect is elevated pulmonary venous pressures. These include, for example, left ventricular failure, mitral stenosis, and pulmonary veno-occlusive disease. The pathophysiology in those with elevated pulmonary arterial pressure due to impaired left ventricular systolic function may have different gas exchange findings during exercise compared to those with pulmonary arterial hypertension (previously called idiopathic or primary pulmonary hypertension) and may have gas exchange responses more like patients with chronic heart failure.

PERIPHERAL ARTERIAL DISEASES

Because of atherosclerotic changes that reduce the internal diameter of the conducting arteries to the limbs, peripheral arterial diseases prevent the increase in blood flow needed to meet the increased metabolic demand of exercise. Thus, O_2 flow to muscles fails to increase sufficiently to satisfy the O_2 requirement for performing exercise. The inability to supply sufficient O_2 to the exercising muscles to meet the O_2 requirement is reflected in a reduced $\Delta\dot{V}O_2/\Delta WR$ ratio at low work levels (see **Fig. 4.3C**). Although a compensatory increase in mitochondrial number in the ischemic muscle may occur with time, the improved O_2 extraction that this mechanism portends is inadequate to make up for the deficiency in O_2 flow.[53] Consequently, the ischemic muscles produce lactic acid at relatively low work rates, with subsequent leg pain, heaviness, or fatigue. With diffuse disease, and slow blood flow through the ischemic leg, the wash out of lactic acid and the CO_2 from HCO_3^- buffering may be delayed, such that $\Delta\dot{V}CO_2/\Delta WR$ may, like $\Delta\dot{V}O_2/\Delta WR$, be relatively shallow. The maximum $\dot{V}O_2$ and the lactic acidosis threshold are reduced, although the latter may be difficult to detect.

Systemic arterial hypertension is a risk factor for peripheral arterial disease, so it is not uncommon for blood pressure response at low work rates to be excessive. Airways disease or additional forms of cardiovascular disease are also common due to shared risk factors. The HR at maximum exercise is usually relatively low because the patient stops exercise from symptoms of claudication at a work rate too low to provide maximal HR stimulation.

VENTILATORY DISORDERS

Obstructive Lung Diseases

Patients with chronic obstructive pulmonary diseases (COPD), including emphysema, chronic bronchitis, asthma, and mixtures of these disease entities, are usually limited during exercise by dyspnea or fatigue. Dyspnea generally results from difficulty in achieving the ventilation and, possibly, the O_2 cost of ventilation needed to eliminate the additional CO_2 generated during exercise at the level of $PaCO_2$ regulated by the patient (the patient's PCO_2 set point). Complicating matters, some of these patients are highly sedentary due to avoidance of exertional dyspnea and therefore develop a lactic acidosis at a relatively low work rate (**Table 4.2**). The added CO_2 load resulting from the HCO_3^- buffering of lactic acid and the H^+ provide additional chemical stimuli to breathe but to an inefficient gas-exchanging lung.

Ventilatory Capacity-Ventilatory Requirement Imbalance

Figure 4.6 conceptualizes the pathophysiological features leading to dyspnea in patients with COPD. The two major contributing factors are the decreased ventilatory capacity and the increased ventilatory requirement. In emphysema, the decreased ventilatory capacity is due to increased airflow obstruction combined with reduced lung elastic recoil, whereas in chronic bronchitis and asthma, the decreased ventilatory capacity is due to increased airway resistance.

The increased ventilatory requirement in patients with COPD is primarily due to inefficient ventilation of the lungs consequent to the regional mismatching of ventilation to perfusion; that is, certain regions of the lungs are hypoventilated, whereas others are hyperventilated. This has the effect of increasing the fraction of the breath that is

TABLE 4.2 Effect of Airway Obstruction Due to Emphysema on Average Blood Lactate Concentration, Minute Ventilation, and Work Rate at an O_2 Consumption of Approximately 1.0 L/min

FEV_1 (L)	$\dot{V}O_2$ (L/min, STPD)	WR (W)	$\dot{V}E$ (L/min, BTPS)	$\dot{V}E/\dot{V}O_2$	La^- (mmol/L)	$La^-/\dot{V}O_2$
1.02	0.90	35	35	39	3.03	3.37[a]
1.80	1.05	34	36	34	2.95	2.80[b]
Normal	~1.0	50	25	25	<1.0	1.0[c]

Abbreviations: BTPS, body temperature pressure saturated; FEV_1, forced expiratory volume in 1 second; La^-, blood lactate concentration; STPD, standard temperature and pressure dry; $\dot{V}E$, minute ventilation; $\dot{V}E/\dot{V}O_2$, ventilatory equivalent for O_2; $\dot{V}O_2$, O_2 uptake; WR, work rate.

[a]Mean data from Cooper CB, Daly JA, Burns MR, et al. Lactic acidosis contributes to the production of dyspnea in chronic obstructive pulmonary disease. *Am Rev Respir Dis*. 1991;143:A80.

[b]Mean data from Casaburi R, Patessio A, Ioli F, Zanaboni S, Donner CF, Wasserman K. Reductions in exercise lactic acidosis and ventilation as a result of exercise training in patients with obstructive lung disease. *Am Rev Respir Dis*. 1991;143:9-18.

[c]Mean data from Chapter 2.

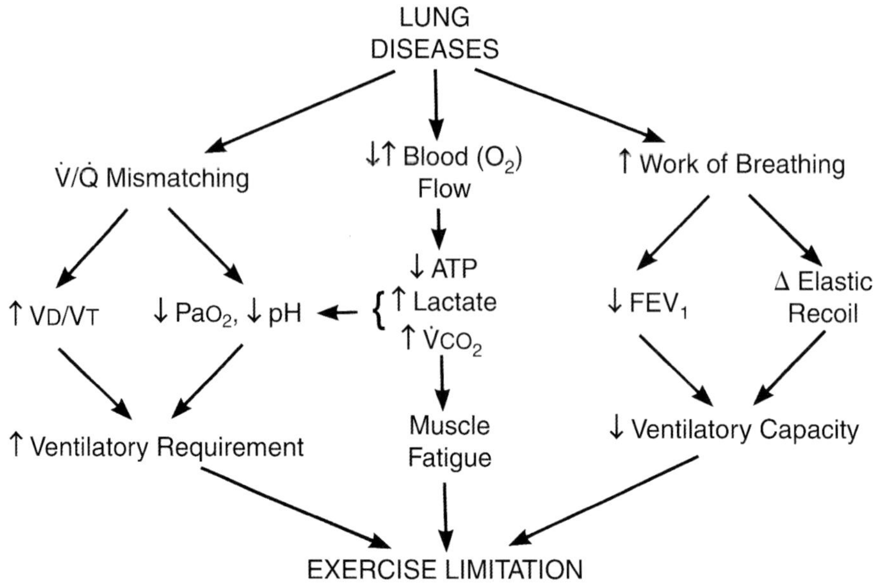

FIGURE 4.6. Factors that play a role in exercise limitation and dyspnea in patients with chronic obstructive pulmonary disease. These patients have both an increase in ventilatory requirement to perform exercise and a reduction in ventilatory capacity. See text for a detailed discussion of each of the factors shown. ATP, adenosine triphosphate; FEV_1, forced expiratory volume in 1 second; Abbreviations: VD/VT, dead space–tidal volume ratio; V̇/Q̇, ventilation-perfusion ratio.

wasted (increased VD/VT), thereby requiring an increased ventilation to eliminate the CO_2 produced by the patient to maintain the $Paco_2$ at its apparent set point.

As shown in **Figure 4.7**, ambulatory patients with stable obstructive lung disease regulate $Paco_2$ at a reasonably constant level despite increasing work rates. However, ventilatory compensation for the exercise-induced lactic acidosis may not occur in these patients. With severe airway obstruction, $Paco_2$ may increase during exercise because of the increased work of breathing, thereby worsening the exercise acidosis.[54] Hypoxemia in COPD results from underventilation of perfused lung units. Despite increasing ventilatory drive through the carotid body chemoreceptors, the hypoxic stimulus is insufficient to induce an increased respiratory drive that decreases $Paco_2$ in patients with COPD. Although regulation of Pao_2 is less precise than $Paco_2$ in these patients (**Fig. 4.8**), Pao_2 typically does not fall to extremely low levels, even at the patient's maximum work rate.

The P(A − a)O_2 is usually increased as a consequence of the perfusion of relatively poorly ventilated airspaces. The increase in P(A − a)O_2 is usually not progressive with increasing work rate, as is common in patients with primary pulmonary vascular diseases or pulmonary fibrosis. The P(a − ET)CO_2 is also increased, reflecting overventilation relative to perfusion. Thus, P(a − ET)CO_2 remains relatively constant and elevated as work rate is increased, rather than decreasing and becoming negative as in normal subjects. Because patients with COPD ventilate the fast time constant lung units predominantly, the mixed expired CO_2 is low relative to the end-tidal CO_2, which is derived predominantly from the slow, low V̇A/Q̇ lung units. Thus, the ratio of mixed expired Pco_2 to P_{ETCO_2} has been shown to distinguish between uneven V̇A/Q̇ due to uneven perfusion from uneven ventilation.[55]

Although one may predict that the O_2 cost of breathing will be increased in patients with COPD, this is difficult to measure directly. That these patients do have an increased metabolic cost is evident, however, when one examines the external work that can be performed for a given $\dot{V}o_2$. This is illustrated by data in **Table 4.2** showing that work rate was reduced at a $\dot{V}o_2$ of 1 L/min in patients with COPD compared to healthy controls. Moreover, patients with COPD

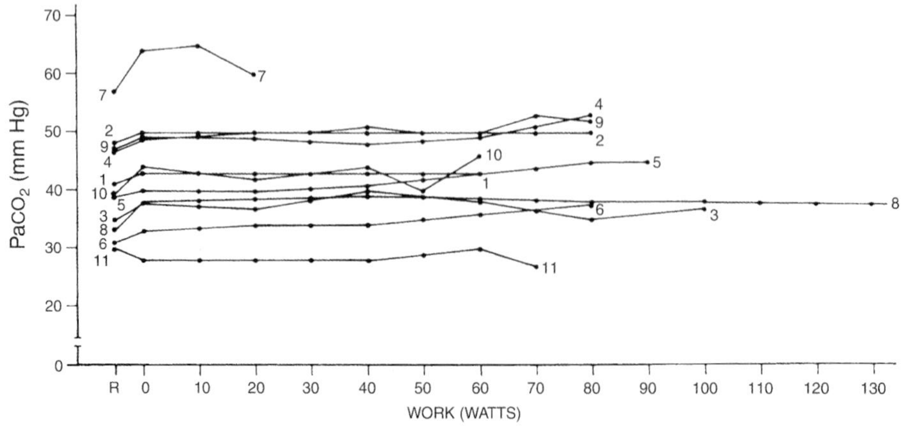

FIGURE 4.7. The arterial Pco_2 ($Paco_2$) as related to work rate in 11 patients with stable chronic airflow obstruction (each point is a different work rate). The numbers on each curve identify the patient.

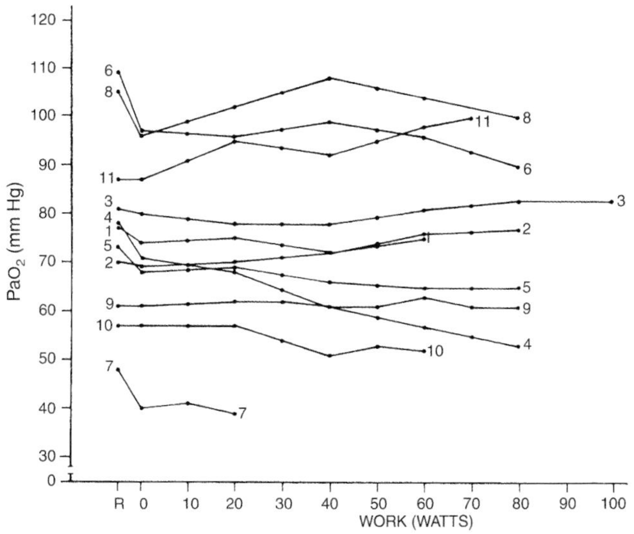

FIGURE 4.8. The arterial P_{O_2} (Pa_{O_2}) as related to increase in work rate for the same 11 patients shown in Figure 4.7 (each point is a different work rate). The numbers on each curve identify the patient and allow cross correlation with each patient's arterial P_{CO_2} (Pa_{CO_2}), shown in Figure 4.7.

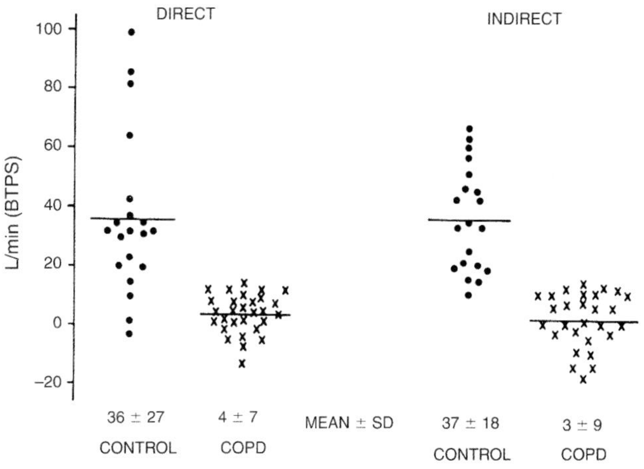

FIGURE 4.9. Breathing reserve (maximal voluntary ventilation [MVV] − max $\dot{V}_E$) for a group of normal subjects and a group of patients with stable chronic obstructive pulmonary disease (COPD). The values under each column show the mean ± standard deviation. Measurements are made using the directly measured MVV and the indirectly measured MVV calculated by multiplying forced expiratory volume in 1 second (FEV_1) by 40. Note that the breathing reserve in patients with COPD is small and the standard deviation is narrow, reflecting the importance of airflow limitation in determining exercise intolerance. Abbreviation: BTPS, body temperature pressure saturated.

may develop a lactic acidosis at a relatively low work rate.[56] This may result from sedentary lifestyle and/or systemic effects of chronic disease on the structure and function of skeletal muscle. Exercise training can be effective in reducing the lactate level for a given work rate and therefore the ventilatory requirement for a given level of exercise.

Dyspnea can result from an imbalance between how much air *must* be breathed to keep pace with metabolism and how much *can* be breathed. Patients with COPD, because of their increase in V_D/V_T, low work rate lactic acidosis, and hypoxemia, must breathe more to maintain blood gases and pH, but peak ventilation is less than normal. Although many approaches have been taken to determine if patients with COPD are ventilatory limited, the breathing reserve is the most obvious. The maximal voluntary ventilation (MVV) measured at rest or calculated from the forced expiratory volume in 1 second (FEV_1) is a reasonable estimate of the patient's ventilatory capacity. Work tasks requiring ventilation rates in excess of this value cannot be sustained. Thus, the breathing reserve, defined as the difference between the MVV and $\dot{V}_E$ at the maximum level of exercise that the subject could perform, is decreased to values close to zero in patients with COPD (**Fig. 4.9**). This contrasts with the large ventilatory reserve at the end of exercise found in most normal individuals and, particularly, in patients with heart disease.

Examining the expiratory flow pattern can be useful in documenting airflow limitation. Typically, as shown in **Fig. 3.21**, the pattern has an early expiratory peak and then a sustained expiratory flow until the point of inhalation, giving a trapezoidal appearance to the recorded pattern. No apneic pause occurs at the end of exhalation, in contrast to the finding in normal subjects when work rate is not excessively high. After effective bronchodilatation, the expiratory flow pattern normalizes, with the peak flow moving to the middle of the expiratory phase of respiration (see **Fig. 3.21**).

With exercise, as breathing frequency rises, air trapping may increase, albeit not homogenously. When patients develop air trapping with exercise, the FRC increases, as evidenced by a reduction in the inspiratory capacity. The inspiratory capacity can be measured during exercise by instructing the patient to take a maximum breath after a normal exhalation. This requires some practice to get reliable measurements in patients with obstructive lung disease and normal subjects. In contrast to the decrease in inspiratory capacity in patients with airflow obstruction, normal subjects typically have an increase in inspiratory capacity, suggesting that their FRC had decreased during exercise. Further evidence of air trapping in COPD can sometimes be evidenced by a decrease in tidal volume as exercise work rate is increased. The increase in alveolar pressure with airway closure in COPD increases intrathoracic pressure and therefore the left ventricular transmural pressure. These pressure changes can impair venous return to the heart and increase the external work of the heart, respectively.

Whereas the peak $\dot{V}O_2$ is reduced in patients with uncomplicated obstructive lung disease, the $\dot{V}O_2$ usually does not decrease its rate of rise as work rate is increased in response to a progressively increasing work rate test, in contrast to this frequent finding in patients with circulatory limitation. This is because ambulatory patients with stable obstructive lung disease are usually more limited in their ability to eliminate CO_2 (ventilatory limitation) than in their ability to make O_2 available to the mitochondria.

Often, patients with COPD develop a lactic acidosis at relatively low work rates (see **Table 4.2**). Other patients with very severe airflow obstruction may not be able to exercise sufficiently to reach their *AT*. Those who do develop a significant lactic acidosis should benefit most from skeletal muscle training because they have the potential to decrease the lactic acidosis stimulus to ventilatory drive.

The HR at maximum work rate is generally low (high HR reserve; **Fig. 4.10**), but maximum HR can be increased if the patient's maximum work rate can be improved through O_2 breathing or bronchodilatation. In contrast to cardiac disorders, O_2 pulse continues to increase normally with increasing work rate, although the final absolute values are usually reduced at peak exercise.

Oxygen Transport–Oxygen Requirement Imbalance

To sustain exercise, ATP must be regenerated aerobically. Failure of the left and right ventricular outputs to keep pace with the muscle O_2 demand will force the patient to stop exercise due to muscular fatigue. An inadequate transport of O_2 to muscles relative to its requirement will be reflected in a decreased peak $\dot{V}O_2$ and a reduced rate of increase in $\dot{V}O_2$ as work rate increases. Secondary effects of COPD on cardiovascular function can contribute to failure to meet the O_2 requirement of a progressively increasing work rate test:

1. Positive intrathoracic pressure. Positive pressures develop in the chest during exhalation in patients with poor lung elastic recoil and hyperinflation (patients with emphysema). Thus, intrathoracic pressure increases during exhalation, limiting diastolic (atrial) filling and stroke volume. This process becomes more marked as breathing rate increases to maintain arterial blood gas homeostasis with associated decrease in exhalation time. The impediment to venous return to the heart can account for the relatively low cardiac output and stroke volume observed in emphysema patients during exercise.
2. Increased pulmonary vascular resistance. Increased pulmonary vascular resistance might also cause right and left ventricular outputs to be inadequate during exercise. Many patients with emphysema have significantly elevated pulmonary vascular resistance due to loss of cross-sectional area and recruitability of the pulmonary microcirculation, which, although not limiting at rest, might prevent increasing pulmonary blood flow at the rate needed to meet the muscle O_2 requirement during exercise.
3. Coexistent factors, such as primary heart disease and reduced arterial oxygen content. Patients with lung diseases might also have coincident heart disease that independently limits the circulatory response to exercise. Other mechanisms that contribute to the impairment of O_2 flow to the muscles, such as reduced arterial O_2 content due to reduced PaO_2, anemia, and carboxyhemoglobinemia, when combined with the pathophysiology of COPD, might worsen symptoms of fatigue and/or dyspnea beyond that expected from the degree of the underlying pathophysiology.

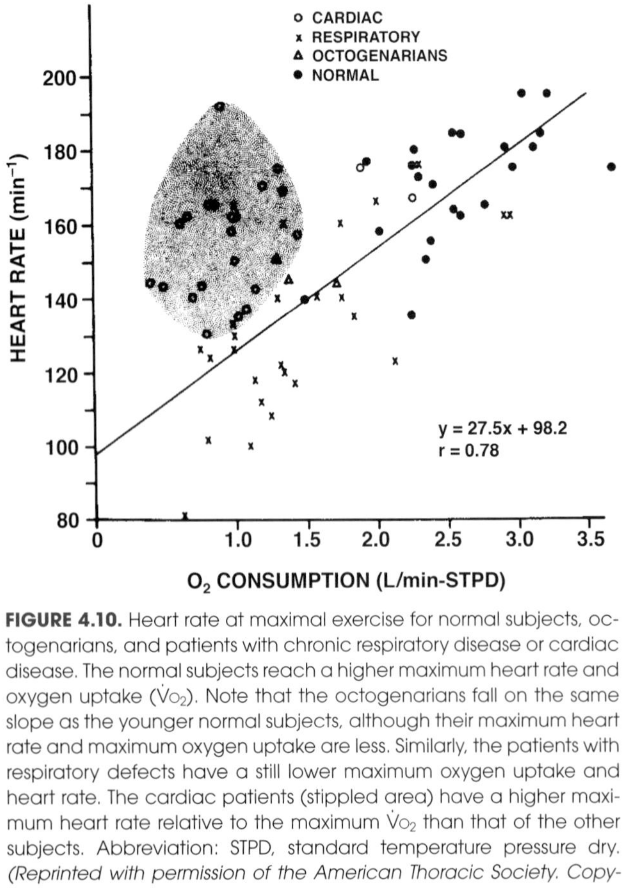

FIGURE 4.10. Heart rate at maximal exercise for normal subjects, octogenarians, and patients with chronic respiratory disease or cardiac disease. The normal subjects reach a higher maximum heart rate and oxygen uptake ($\dot{V}O_2$). Note that the octogenarians fall on the same slope as the younger normal subjects, although their maximum heart rate and maximum oxygen uptake are less. Similarly, the patients with respiratory defects have a still lower maximum oxygen uptake and heart rate. The cardiac patients (stippled area) have a higher maximum heart rate relative to the maximum $\dot{V}O_2$ than that of the other subjects. Abbreviation: STPD, standard temperature pressure dry. *(Reprinted with permission of the American Thoracic Society. Copyright © 2020 American Thoracic Society. All rights reserved. From Wasserman K, Whipp BJ. Exercise physiology in health and disease.* Am Rev Respir Dis. *1975;112[2]:219-249. The American Review of Respiratory Disease* is an official journal of the American Thoracic Society. [*Now titled The American Journal of Respiratory and Critical Care Medicine])*

Physiological Markers of Inadequate Oxygen Transport

Although respiratory mechanics are significantly impaired in patients with COPD, it is imperative to evaluate exercise gas exchange in these patients in order to determine if reduced O_2 transport is caused by impaired ventilatory mechanics or by metabolic changes with increased ventilatory drive characteristic of heart failure. The increased ventilatory drive in these patients results from the increased H^+ accompanying the increased lactate as well as the CO_2 released by the increased rate of buffering lactic acid. Thus, in the presence of reduced O_2 transport, the *AT*, $\Delta\dot{V}O_2/\Delta WR$, as well as the peak $\dot{V}O_2$ are likely to be reduced.

Restrictive Lung Diseases

Patients with restrictive lung mechanics due to interstitial lung disease tend to be exercise limited because of dyspnea or fatigue or both. These patients have both disturbed lung mechanics and a reduction in the functional pulmonary capillary bed (**Fig. 4.11**). Hansen and Wasserman,[57] in a study of a population of patients with interstitial lung diseases of mixed etiology, found that many of the patients were also limited by their inability to increase pulmonary blood flow appropriately in response to exercise (see **Fig. 4.11**). Not only did their patients have a reduced peak $\dot{V}O_2$, but the *AT* was also usually reduced. In contrast to patients with

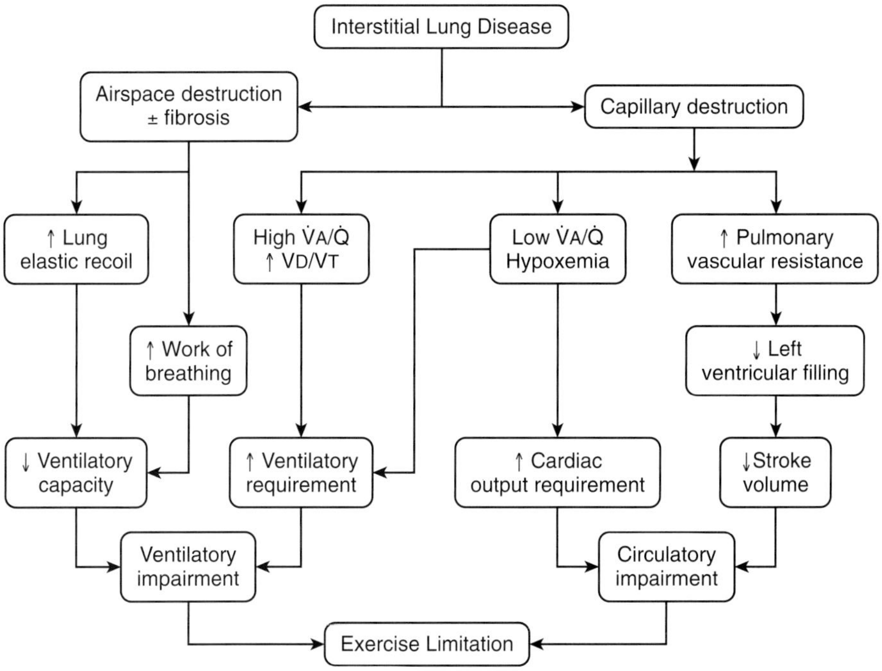

FIGURE 4.11. Pathophysiology of exercise limitation in patients with interstitial lung disease and idiopathic pulmonary fibrosis. Abbreviations: $\dot{V}A/\dot{Q}$, ratio of alveolar ventilation/perfusion; VD/VT, dead space–tidal volume ratio.

COPD, $\Delta\dot{V}O_2/\Delta WR$ was reduced, with the slope of the relationship becoming shallower as peak $\dot{V}O_2$ was approached.

An example of restrictive lung disease is idiopathic pulmonary fibrosis. This disorder has features resembling those resulting from chronic lung inflammation[58] but likely results from a progressive fibrotic process. Pathologic features are usually nonuniform, so some acini, including their blood supply, are completely replaced by scar tissue. In contrast, neighboring units that are less involved or uninvolved may undergo compensatory hyperinflation. From the point of view of lung mechanics, the net effect of the pathophysiology of idiopathic pulmonary fibrosis is a reduction in the total number of functioning acini and, consequently, a relatively poorly compliant small lung. Both total lung capacity and its subcompartments are reduced, predominantly that of the inspiratory capacity. Thus, the extent to which the tidal volume can increase with exercise is limited, and the patient must increase breathing frequency to a value higher than normal to meet the ventilatory requirement for exercise. Consequently, during exercise, the tidal volume/inspiratory capacity ratio (VC/IC) is high and approaches 1. The breathing frequency at maximum exercise often exceeds 50 breaths per minute. Such high breathing frequencies are unusual in patients with COPD because of the detrimental effect of worsening hyperinflation. Ventilation at the maximum work rate may approach the MVV if the patient is not limited by the inability to increase cardiac output earlier because of the restricted pulmonary capillary bed. However, often, the pathophysiology reflects both a failure to increase $\dot{V}O_2$ appropriately for the work rate performed and an increased ventilatory response due to exercise lactic acidosis, hypoxemia, and ventilation–perfusion mismatching (increased VD/VT).

In interstitial lung diseases, the pulmonary capillary bed is functionally reduced and normal recruitment of additional capillary bed in response to exercise may fail to occur. This restricted capillary bed results in a shortened red cell transit time in the pulmonary capillaries as the exercise work rate is increased. The progressive reduction of the red cell residence time in the pulmonary capillary as work rate and cardiac output increase results in a systematic decrease in PaO_2 as $\dot{V}O_2$ increases, similar to that seen in pulmonary vascular occlusive disease. This systematic decrease in PaO_2 is usually not seen if pulmonary blood flow fails to increase normally with exercise (as reflected in the $\dot{V}O_2$ response). Low $\dot{V}A/\dot{Q}$ regions of the lung might also contribute to the hypoxemia in patients with interstitial lung disease.

The ventilatory response of patients with interstitial lung disease is often steep, sometimes because of a reduced $PaCO_2$ set point in some patients, but mainly because of an increased VD/VT. Also contributing are worsening hypoxemia as work rate is increased, elevated dead space ventilation caused by uneven ventilation–perfusion ratios, and increased lactic acidosis from impaired O_2 transport. These along with reduced ability to increase tidal volume leading to rapid shallow breathing contribute to dyspnea in these patients. In addition, exercise fatigue might be brought about by the inability to provide O_2 to the skeletal muscles at a rate sufficient for the exercise work rate to be performed aerobically.

A relatively rare cause of restrictive disease, pulmonary alveolar proteinosis, is manifest by exercise hypoxemia that is likely primarily due to impaired diffusion of oxygen. This disease results from alveolar filling by a semisolid proteinaceous material rather than a primary interstitial process. Frequently, vital capacity and total lung capacity are only slightly reduced, and FEV_1/forced vital capacity is normal.

Because the mean path length from lung gas to lung capillaries is increased in this disorder by a medium unfavorable for O_2 diffusion, mass flow of O_2 into the pulmonary capillaries is impaired. During exercise, when red cell transit time in the capillary bed is reduced and its residence time shortened, less time is available for diffusion equilibrium. Thus, the major findings in this disorder are a systematic decrease in Pa_{O_2} and an increase in $P(A - a)_{O_2}$ with increasing work rate.

Chest Wall (Respiratory Pump) Disorders

Disorders of the respiratory pump include muscle weakness, chest deformities, rigidity of the thoracic cage (as in ankylosing spondylitis), muscle and motor nerve disorders, and extreme obesity. Patients with these disorders have a limited ability to increase tidal volume. Although their lungs are essentially normal, the intrapleural pressure necessary to expand the lungs is requires a higher than normal work of breathing. The increase in tidal volume as work rate is increased is thus often lower than average, and to increase $\dot{V}_E$ required for exercise, these patients must increase breathing frequency predominantly.

The reduced peak $\dot{V}_{O_2}$ defines the degree of exercise limitation. The $\dot{V}_{O_2}$ increases normally with increasing work rate. Because the lung parenchyma is essentially normal, Pa_{O_2} is usually normal and does not decrease as the work rate is increased. The breathing reserve is low when symptom-limited exercise is reached (usually due to dyspnea). Because of impaired ventilatory mechanics, these patients may not develop normal ventilatory compensation for the lactic acidosis of exercise. In some cases, exercise hypercapnia may actually occur. The HR reserve is high at maximal exercise because maximum exercise is limited by low breathing capacity.

DEFECTS IN HEMOGLOBIN CONTENT AND QUALITY

A considerable increase in O_2 flow from the atmosphere to the mitochondria is essential for the normal exercise response. This function is critically dependent on convective transport by the circulation of O_2 from the lungs to the exercising muscles. Therefore, it is appropriate to consider how changes in the properties of blood might impair O_2 delivery to the mitochondria and thereby reduce exercise capacity.

Oxygen delivery is the product of cardiac output and the amount of O_2 carried by the blood (arterial O_2 content). In order to meet the increased O_2 demand of exercise in patients with reduced blood O_2 content, cardiac output must increase (increased HR and stroke volume) to make up the difference. The stroke volume is normal or even increased in anemic patients, in contrast to patients with cardiac diseases and disorders of the pulmonary circulation, and there is relative tachycardia. Because the arterial O_2 content is low, the ability to increase arterial-venous O_2 difference in response to exercise is reduced. Consequently, the maximum O_2 pulse (product of stroke volume and $C[a - \bar{v}]_{O_2}$) is reduced. As in other disorders of reduced maximal O_2 flow, peak $\dot{V}_{O_2}$ and *AT* are also reduced. **Table 3.6** describes the reduction in maximal $C(a - \bar{v})_{O_2}$ resulting from reduced hemoglobin concentration. From this and peak $\dot{V}_{O_2}$, the cardiac output and stroke volume can be estimated at peak exercise. Specific mechanisms of reduced arterial O_2 content include low O_2 saturation due to hypoxemia, of course, but also anemia, hemoglobinopathies that decrease O_2 carrying capacity, and carboxyhemoglobinemia (decreased O_2 carrying capacity and left-shifted oxyhemoglobin curve).

Anemia

Because anemia results in a proportionally reduced blood O_2 carrying capacity, it compromises O_2 delivery to the mitochondria (see **Fig. 4.1**). With anemia, the exercising muscle capillary P_{O_2} falls more rapidly than normal during the transit of blood from artery to vein (see **Fig. 2.15**). Thus, the diffusion gradient of O_2 from the blood to the mitochondria decreases more rapidly than in nonanemic conditions. Consequently, a critically low capillary P_{O_2} may be reached at a lower $\dot{V}_{O_2}$ than normal, necessitating additional anaerobic mechanisms for ATP regeneration, with earlier and increasing lactate concentrations and metabolic acidosis.

Subjects with anemia commonly experience breathlessness during exercise. Although the arterial O_2 content is low, the Pa_{O_2} is not reduced. Because the carotid bodies respond to Pa_{O_2} and not O_2 content, the reduced O_2 content is not itself the cause of the increased ventilatory drive and, therefore, is unlikely to account for the symptom of breathlessness. More likely, the breathlessness and increased ventilatory drive with exercise in the anemic patient are due to the metabolic acidosis that accompanies the patient's low *AT*. The acidemia results in an increased ventilatory drive (also mediated by the carotid bodies) and a relatively high minute ventilation at a low maximum work rate.

The role of anemia in the reduction of peak $\dot{V}_{O_2}$ can be estimated when the subject is normoxic. Indeed, because each gram of hemoglobin binds 1.34 mL of O_2 and because, at peak exercise, O_2 extraction is approximately 75%, each gram of hemoglobin delivers about 1 mL of O_2. Thus, for example, if cardiac output is 10 L/min, each 1 g/dL of hemoglobin accounts for 100 mL/min of $\dot{V}_{O_2}$.

Left-Shifted Oxyhemoglobin Dissociation Curve

Conditions that cause a leftward shift in the oxyhemoglobin dissociation curve (reduced P_{50}), such as some hemoglobinopathies, a decrease in 2,3-diphosphoglycerate due to a defect in red cell metabolism, an increase in carboxyhemoglobin, or increased glycosylated hemoglobin found in poorly controlled diabetic patients, should cause the capillary blood P_{O_2} to decrease more rapidly than normal. Thus, the P_{O_2} difference between capillary and mitochondrion may reach a critical value at a reduced work rate. Consequently, O_2 flow through the exercising muscle may not provide the O_2

needed by the mitochondria to support ATP regeneration at the individual's predicted *AT*. Thus, anaerobic regeneration of ATP would be needed to support the energy requirement at a relatively lower work rate. Exercise studies on patients with a left-shifted hemoglobinopathy support the concept that these disorders lead to anaerobic glycolysis and increased net lactate production at reduced work rates.[59]

Carboxyhemoglobinemia and Cigarette Smoking

Carboxyhemoglobinemia from exposure to carbon monoxide results in a reduced O_2-carrying capacity. When the carboxyhemoglobin level is increased, arterial oxygen content is reduced, and, in addition, there is a leftward shift in the oxyhemoglobin dissociation curve. This reduces the peak $\dot{V}O_2$ and *AT*.[60,61]

Cigarette smoking adversely affects exercise tolerance by its effects on the blood carboxyhemoglobin, the cardiovascular system, and the lungs. The HR, blood pressure, and the rate-pressure product (HR times systolic blood pressure) are increased when one performs exercise immediately after smoking.[60] Ventilation–perfusion relationships also become abnormal, as evident from the increased $P(a - ET)CO_2$ during exercise. Although short-term cigarette smoking did not have an immediate effect on airway resistance in a study of young men, it was observed to cause acute cardiovascular changes and changes consistent with worsened $\dot{V}A/\dot{Q}$ mismatch.[60]

CHRONIC METABOLIC ACIDOSIS

Chronic metabolic acidosis with a reduced blood $[HCO_3^-]$ can result from poorly controlled diabetes, chronic kidney disease, primary renal tubular acidosis, or secondary to treatment with a carbonic anhydrase inhibitor such as acetazolamide. To restore normal arterial pH due to the decrease in arterial $[HCO_3^-]$, ventilation is stimulated, presumably by H^+, until $PaCO_2$ reaches a new lower PCO_2 set point, bringing pH closer to 7.4.[62,63] The magnitude of the increase in ventilation is approximately proportional to the reduction in $[HCO_3^-]$ and $PaCO_2$. To maintain the reduced $PaCO_2$ during exercise, ventilation must increase proportionally to the increase in $\dot{V}CO_2$. The higher the work rate, the higher the additional ventilation. The increased ventilatory requirement needed to maintain the arterial pH, when arterial $[HCO_3^-]$ is reduced, leads to an apparent increase in "sensitivity" of the respiratory control mechanism.

The presence of a chronic metabolic acidosis before exercise begins is evident from the resting arterial blood gases. The $[HCO_3^-]$ and $PaCO_2$ are reduced, and pH is only slightly reduced or normal. During exercise, $\dot{V}E$ increases proportionally with the increase in CO_2 production (see **Fig. 2.48**). Because the slope of the $\dot{V}E$–$\dot{V}CO_2$ relationship is steeper, the lower the $PaCO_2$, the effect of the metabolic acidosis is to amplify the ventilatory response as work rate is increased (see **Figs. 2.49** and **3.26**). Without measuring arterial blood gases, a relatively steep slope relationship between $\dot{V}E$ and $\dot{V}CO_2$ during exercise, with R in the normal range, signifies either chronic hyperventilation or increased VD/VT. Arterial blood gas and pH measurements differentiate these two potential causes of a high ventilatory response.

By itself, chronic metabolic acidosis is not a prominent cause of dyspnea. However, in conjunction with other disorders, such as obstructive airways disease, it may lower the CO_2 set point to such a marked degree that the ventilatory requirement to perform a given work rate represents a disproportionately high fraction of the individual's MVV and result in the sensation of dyspnea. Correction of the metabolic acidosis might reduce the ventilatory requirement below the individual's MVV and relieve the sensation of dyspnea.

METABOLIC MUSCLE DISORDERS

There is a wide range of primary muscle diseases, including genetic, inflammatory, autoimmune, and infectious processes, that impair motor function and exercise capacity. Many are characterized by muscle-specific symptoms of weakness or pain, directing evaluation to the muscle and neuromuscular apparatus. There is a subset of primary muscle diseases, however, that result from disorders in the pathways of muscle energy metabolism. These may manifest primarily with symptoms of dyspnea or general exercise intolerance and may therefore be referred for exercise testing for diagnostic evaluation.[64] These metabolic myopathies can be broadly divided into three categories: disorders of carbohydrate metabolism, disorders of lipid metabolism, and disorders of the mitochondrial electron transport chain.[65]

Disorders of Carbohydrate Metabolism

Disorders of carbohydrate metabolism are the basis for the glycogen storage diseases. The most common and well studied of these is McArdle syndrome, or glycogen storage disease type V, which results from a defect in the muscle form of phosphorylase.[66] Without myophosphorylase, patients with McArdle disease are unable to mobilize glucose from muscle glycogen stores so are dependent predominantly on lipid oxidation for regenerating ATP during exercise. Their capacity for anaerobic energy production is extremely limited due to the inability or limited ability to use muscle glycogen as substrate for glycolysis and the very limited extent to which use of circulating glucose can compensate for this. As a result, they are unable to exercise to work levels that normally require anaerobic mechanisms and demonstrate little or no lactate response to exercise. These patients typically experience severe muscle pain and may have the release of myoglobin and creatine kinase from muscle when attempting to exercise at levels that would normally induce a lactic acidosis. The maximum work capacity of these patients is thus limited to work rates near the *AT* of normal healthy individuals. The $\dot{V}O_2$–work rate relationship appears to be normal for work rates below the level that induces pain.[67] Their ventilatory response to exercise is generally normal,[67] although it has also been reported to be high.[68] The HR and cardiac output responses of these patients are inordinately high for the metabolic rate, and the arterial-venous O_2 difference at maximal work rate is low[69] because of limited extraction of O_2 from the peripheral capillary blood. This is attributable to limited capacity for utilization of oxygen through pathways of lipid metabolism and/or the absence of lactic acidosis to induce rightward shift in the oxyhemoglobin dissociation curve for the unloading of O_2 from hemoglobin (Bohr effect). The Bohr effect is needed for the normal maximal O_2 extraction from blood during exercise.[70] Patients with McArdle disease are limited in their ability to perform high levels of exercise, and demonstrate low peak $\dot{V}O_2$. Constant work rate exercise testing at a level of work within their capability is useful for demonstrating a "second wind" phenomenon, unique to McArdle disease, in which perceived exertion and HR both decrease to lower levels at around 8 to 10 minutes into the exercise.[71] Other defects involving enzymes in the glycolytic pathways are also associated with exercise impairment and have other distinct clinical features depending on the specific enzyme defect.

Disorders of Lipid Metabolism

Disorders in lipid metabolism include defects in the proteins responsible for mobilizing and transporting fatty acids into the mitochondria and for their beta oxidation.[65] Because muscle energy metabolism transitions from carbohydrate to lipid substrate when moderate exercise is sustained for prolonged periods, these disorders typically cause intolerance for prolonged exercise. Symptoms are especially likely if exercise is associated with fasting, heat or other stress, and may include episodes of rhabdomyolysis. Because pathways for carbohydrate metabolism are intact, and carbohydrates are the primary substrate for energy production during short durations of exercise, patients with disorders of lipid metabolism often have entirely normal responses to incremental CPET.

Disorders of Mitochondrial Electron Transport Chain

Patients with defects in the mitochondrial electron transport chain can develop lactic acidosis at exceptionally low work rates or may have elevated lactate at rest.[72,73] Mitochondrial disorders can result from mutations in either nuclear or mitochondrial DNA and may have different phenotypic features even within a family with the same genetic defect. Nonuniform distribution of mitochondria during embryonic development and subsequent replication within tissues also results in heterogeneity of expression of mitochondrial dysfunction between and within organs of a given affected individual. Multiple organ systems, for example, central nervous, hepatic, or endocrine system, may be affected by mitochondrial dysfunction, so these disorders are often syndromic and identified early in life. There are nevertheless some patients whose symptoms do not develop until later in life and are predominantly or solely manifest as exercise intolerance. The impairment in exercise capacity and peak $\dot{V}O_2$ in patients with mitochondrial myopathy is directly related to the proportion of muscle mitochondria that are abnormal.[74] The *AT* may be low, or, because there may be elevated lactate at rest, there may not be a discrete *AT* identified on incremental CPET. Indeed, stimulation of ventilation due to pervasive or early exercise metabolic acidosis accounts for at least a substantial component of the high exercise ventilation observed in patients with mitochondrial defects.[75] A hyperdynamic circulation with greater than normal cardiac output versus $\dot{V}O_2$ is characteristic of mitochondrial myopathy[74] and is reflected in a steep increase in HR relative to $\dot{V}O_2$. The O_2 pulse is usually low due to failure of $C(a - \bar{v})O_2$ to widen, reflecting reduced capacity of the muscle for consuming oxygen. Myocardial involvement may further complicate the findings.

Toxin- or Drug-Induced Muscle Impairment

A variety of toxins and drugs can affect skeletal muscle function and impair exercise capacity. Because of their widespread use, HMG-CoA reductase inhibitors, or statins, used for reduction of blood cholesterol levels, are of particular interest. This class of agents is associated with major decreases in primary and secondary complications of atherosclerotic cardiovascular disease. However, they are also associated with a 15% to 25% risk of muscle disorders ranging from asymptomatic elevation of creatine phosphokinase in the blood to muscle pain, weakness, and rhabdomyolysis, with risk factors possibly including genetics, age, gender, renal function, and others.[76] In a small study of symptomatic and asymptomatic statin users and normal controls, peak $\dot{V}O_2$, maximal work rate, and ventilatory efficiency were not different, whereas the $\dot{V}O_2$ at the *AT* (expressed as percent of predicted peak $\dot{V}O_2$) was significantly lower for symptomatic statin users and statin users in general.[77] The apparent earlier onset of anaerobic metabolism was supported in this study by evidence of decreased mitochondria content and oxidative enzyme activity.

Endocrine Disorders

The endocrine system participates in many aspects of the normal exercise response, but while untreated disorders of thyroid, sex steroids, or the adrenal cortical axis could have profound effects on CPET, there would be little reason to perform exercise testing in the setting of a severe endocrinopathy endocrinopathy. Some endocrine disorders or hormonal states may significantly impact exercise function even when treated, however, the most common consideration being diabetes. Diabetes mellitus affects large arteries (atherosclerosis), small blood vessels, and capillaries. When the disease is poorly controlled, patients with diabetes also have a leftward shift in the oxyhemoglobin dissociation curve (glycosylated hemoglobin). Any and all of these abnormalities could cause a reduction in *AT* and peak $\dot{V}O_2$.[78] Studies in children with diabetes suggest that the *AT* and peak $\dot{V}O_2$ are reduced even when the patient's diabetes is under good control.

Patients with poorly regulated diabetes increase their use of fatty acids for energy. During short duration exercise, use of fatty acids by muscle, in contrast to the normally preferred carbohydrate, should make the patients with poorly controlled diabetes require slightly more O_2 for the same energy production. **Figure 2.4** illustrates the effect of the proportion of carbohydrate to fatty acid in the metabolic substrate mix on metabolic efficiency with respect to O_2 consumption to energy yield during exercise.

The ventilatory response to exercise has been demonstrated to be increased and the Pa_{CO_2} reduced in women during the luteal phase of the menstrual cycle. The effect of this increased ventilatory drive on maximal exercise performance in women is unknown. In a study of a small group of women performing exercise during the follicular and luteal phases of the menstrual cycle, work rate, peak $\dot{V}O_2$, HR, and R; and blood lactate measured at rest, at end of exercise, and at the *AT* were not different between phases.[79] However, they observed higher $\dot{V}E/\dot{V}O_2$, $\dot{V}E/\dot{V}CO_2$, and $\dot{V}E$ at each point, suggesting higher ventilatory drive during the luteal phase, possibly related to higher progesterone levels.

NONMETABOLIC CAUSES OF EXERCISE LIMITATION AND DYSPNEA

Anxiety Reactions

Anxiety reactions occasionally cause dyspnea during exercise. One manifestation of anxiety is intense hyperventilation with development of acute respiratory alkalosis. The hyperventilation pattern is unique in that the breathing frequency is high and often quite regular. In addition, the tachypnea starts abruptly, as though switched on, rather than gradually, as is normally seen during progressive exercise. Hyperventilation might actually start at rest, in anticipation of the exercise. Psychogenic dyspnea might also be evident as rapid and unusually shallow breathing. Usually, $P_{ET}CO_2$ is very low and $P_{ET}O_2$ is high in the early phase of exercise in someone who is hyperventilating. If the individual is unable to maintain the high exercise ventilation, with exceptionally low $P_{ET}CO_2$ and high $P_{ET}O_2$, these values may gradually change in the normal direction toward the end of exercise. In such a case, the R ($\dot{V}CO_2/\dot{V}O_2$) may be elevated at the beginning of exercise and decrease as the patient approaches symptom limited maximum work rate.

Poor Effort and Manipulated Exercise Performance

It is important to distinguish manipulated exercise performance from organic disorders, although this can sometimes be challenging. An exercise test in which both HR reserve and breathing reserve are high and the *AT* is not reached strongly suggests poor effort. However, inadequate effort may also be evident when the *AT* is normal, accompanied by a high HR reserve and breathing reserve without the normal increase in R expected during a progressively increasing work rate test.

A chaotic breathing pattern may be a sign of volitional abnormalities in the exercise test. Normally, ventilation, tidal volume, and breathing frequency increase in a distinct systematic pattern, increasing tidal volume primarily with increasing $\dot{V}E$ below the *AT* and then increasing breathing frequency above the *AT*. A chaotic breathing pattern and psychogenic dyspnea are most readily diagnosed during exercise when gas exchange is monitored breath by breath. Variable and inconsistent changes in breath-by-breath measurements of $P_{ET}CO_2$ and $P_{ET}O_2$ provide evidence for manipulated exercise performance.

Before stating that a claimant for disability is not impaired on a pulmonary basis, it may be necessary to sample arterial blood sequentially for measurement of lactate increase, as well as to confirm a normal $P(A - a)O_2$, $P(a - ET)CO_2$, and V_D/V_T during exercise. Arterial blood gas and pH measurements are alternatively valuable if they identify subtle abnormalities of gas exchange that may reflect early pulmonary or pulmonary vascular disease, which may not be evident on resting lung function measurements.[80]

COMBINATIONS OF DEFECTS

A patient's symptoms may be more marked than expected from the nonexercise assessment of the severity of their disease. This might be noted particularly when the primary disease is combined with a complicating problem, such as cigarette smoking, obesity, or medications. Thus, patients with coronary artery disease who smoke and have hypertension might be less symptomatic and have better exercise tolerance if their blood pressure were under adequate control and they abstained from smoking. Similarly, patients with obstructive lung disease complicated by deconditioning due to inactivity, coexisting cardiovascular disease, or anemia may approach ventilatory limits early due to early onset of lactic acidosis. Thus, the combined defects may interact causing the patient to be more symptomatic with less exercise than expected for the severity of the primary condition alone. When more than one disease is present that can cause the same symptom(s) during exercise, a cardiopulmonary exercise test is particularly useful for identifying how the multiple processes contribute to the patient's symptoms.

SUMMARY

The major function of the cardiovascular and ventilatory systems is gas exchange between the cells and the atmosphere. Therefore, impairments in cardiovascular and respiratory function are most apparent during exercise because cell respiration is stimulated and defects are amplified. Because each component of the gas transport system that couples external to internal respiration has a different role, the pattern of the gas exchange abnormality differs according to the pathophysiology. Recognition of these differences allows the examiner to evaluate which organ system most likely accounts for the patient's exercise limitation.

REFERENCES

1. Neder JA, Nery LE, Andreoni S, Sachs A, Whipp BJ. Oxygen cost for cycling as related to leg mass in males and females, aged 20 to 80. *Int J Sports Med.* 2000;21:263-269.
2. Hansen JE, Sue DY, Wasserman K. Predicted values for clinical exercise testing. *Am Rev Respir Dis.* 1984;129(2, pt 2):S49-S55.
3. Gilbert R, Sipple JH, Auchincloss JH Jr. Respiratory control and work of breathing in obese subjects. *J Appl Physiol.* 1961;16:21-26.
4. Ray CS, Sue DY, Bray G, Hansen JE, Wasserman K. Effects of obesity on respiratory function. *Am Rev Respir Dis.* 1983;128:501-506.
5. Wasserman K, Whipp BJ. Exercise physiology in health and disease. *Am Rev Respir Dis.* 1975;112:219-249.
6. Li J, Li S, Feuers RJ, Buffington CK, Cowan GS. Influence of body fat distribution on oxygen uptake and pulmonary performance in morbidly obese females during exercise. *Respirology.* 2001;6:9-13.
7. Babb TG, Ranasinghe KG, Comeau LA, Semon TL, Schwartz B. Dyspnea on exertion in obese women: association with an increased oxygen cost of breathing. *Am J Respir Crit Care Med.* 2008;178:116-123.
8. Gläser S, Ittermann T, Koch B, et al. Influence of smoking and obesity on alveolar-arterial gas pressure differences and dead space ventilation at rest and peak exercise in healthy men and women. *Respir Med.* 2013;107:919-926.
9. Zavorsky GS, Murias JM, Kim DJ, Gow J, Christou NV. Poor compensatory hyperventilation in morbidly obese women at peak exercise. *Respir Physiol Neurobiol.* 2007;159:187-195.
10. Chase P, Arena R, Myers J, et al. Relation of the prognostic value of ventilatory efficiency to body mass index in patients with heart failure. *Am J Cardiol.* 2008;101:348-352.
11. Hansen JE, Sue DY, Oren A, Wasserman K. Relation of oxygen uptake to work rate in normal men and men with circulatory disorders. *Am J Cardiol.* 1987;59:669-674.
12. Agostoni P, Bianchi M, Moraschi A, et al. Work-rate affects cardiopulmonary exercise test results in heart failure. *Eur J Heart Fail.* 2005;7:498-504.
13. Belardinelli R, Lacalaprice F, Carle F, et al. Exercise-induced myocardial ischaemia detected by cardiopulmonary exercise testing. *Eur Heart J.* 2003;24:1304-1313.
14. Chaudhry S, Arena R, Hansen J, et al. The utility of cardiopulmonary exercise testing to detect and track early-stage ischemic heart disease. *Mayo Clin Proc.* 2010;85:928-932.
15. Sun XG, Hansen JE, Oudiz RJ, Wasserman K. Gas exchange detection of exercise-induced right-to-left shunt in patients with primary pulmonary hypertension. *Circulation.* 2002;105:54-60.
16. Wasserman K, Zhang YY, Gitt A, et al. Lung function and exercise gas exchange in chronic heart failure. *Circulation.* 1997;96:2221-2227.
17. Perego GB, Marenzi GC, Guazzi M, et al. Contribution of PO2, P50, and Hb to changes in arteriovenous O2 content during exercise in heart failure. *J Appl Physiol (1985).* 1996;80:623-631.
18. Wasserman K, Stringer W. Critical capillary PO2, net lactate production, and oxyhemoglobin dissociation: effects on exercise gas exchange. In: Wasserman K, ed. *Exercise Gas Exchange in Heart Disease.* Armonk, NY: Futura Publishing; 1996:157-181.
19. Sullivan MJ, Green HJ, Cobb FR. Altered skeletal muscle metabolic response to exercise in chronic heart failure. Relation to skeletal muscle aerobic enzyme activity. *Circulation.* 1991;84:1597-1607.
20. Kleber FX, Vietzke G, Wernecke KD, et al. Impairment of ventilatory efficiency in heart failure: prognostic impact. *Circulation.* 2000;101:2803-2809.
21. Kobayashi T, Itoh H, Kato K. The role of increased dead space in the augmented ventilation of cardiac patients. In: Wasserman K, ed. *Exercise Gas Exchange in Heart Disease.* Armonk, NY: Futura Publishing; 1996:145-156.
22. Metra M, Raccagni D, Carini G, et al. Ventilatory and arterial blood gas changes during exercise in heart failure. In: Wasserman K, ed. *Exercise Gas Exchange in Heart Disease.* Armonk, NY: Futura Publishing; 1996:125-143.
23. Sun XG, Hansen JE, Beshai JF, Wasserman K. Oscillatory breathing and exercise gas exchange abnormalities prognosticate early mortality and morbidity in heart failure. *J Am Coll Cardiol.* 2010;55:1814-1823.
24. Wasserman K. New concepts in assessing cardiovascular function. The Dickinson W. Richards lecture. *Circulation.* 1988;78:1060-1071.
25. Koike A, Hiroe M, Adachi H, et al. Oxygen uptake kinetics are determined by cardiac function at onset of exercise rather than peak exercise in patients with prior myocardial infarction. *Circulation.* 1994;90:2324-2332.
26. Koike A, Yajima T, Adachi H, et al. Evaluation of exercise capacity using submaximal exercise at a constant work rate in patients with cardiovascular disease. *Circulation.* 1995;91:1719-1724.
27. Bussotti M, Apostolo A, Andreini D, Palermo P, Contini M, Agostoni P. Cardiopulmonary evidence of exercise-induced silent ischaemia. *Eur J Cardiovasc Prev Rehabil.* 2006;13:249-253.
28. Itoh H, Tajima A, Koike A, et al. Oxygen uptake abnormalities during exercise in coronary artery disease. In: Wasserman K, ed. *Cardiopulmonary Exercise Testing and Cardiovascular Health.* Armonk, NY: Futura Publishing; 2002:165-172.
29. Tajima A, Itoh H, Osada N, et al. Oxygen uptake kinetics during and after exercise are useful markers of coronary artery disease in patients with exercise electrocardiography suggesting myocardial ischemia. *Circ J.* 2009;73:1864-1870.
30. Koike A, Itoh H, Doi M, et al. Beat-to-beat evaluation of cardiac function during recovery from upright bicycle exercise in patients with coronary artery disease. *Am Heart J.* 1990;120:316-323.
31. Gitt AK, Wasserman K, Kilkowski C, et al. Exercise anaerobic threshold and ventilatory efficiency identify heart failure patients for high risk of early death. *Circulation.* 2002;106:3079-3084.
32. Chua TP, Ponikowski P, Harrington D, et al. Clinical correlates and prognostic significance of the ventilatory response to exercise in chronic heart failure. *J Am Coll Cardiol.* 1997;29:1585-1590.
33. Koike A, Itoh H, Kato M, et al. Prognostic power of ventilatory responses during submaximal exercise in patients with chronic heart disease. *Chest.* 2002;121:1581-1588.
34. Sue DY. Excess ventilation during exercise and prognosis in chronic heart failure. *Am J Respir Crit Care Med.* 2011;183:1302-1310.
35. Sullivan MJ, Duscha B, Slentz CA. Peripheral determinants of exercise intolerance in patients with chronic heart failure. In: Wasserman K, ed. *Exercise Gas Exchange in Heart Disease.* Armonk, NY: Futura Publishing; 1996:209-227.
36. Wilson JR, Martin JL, Schwartz D, Ferraro N. Exercise intolerance in patients with chronic heart failure: role of impaired nutritive flow to skeletal muscle. *Circulation.* 1984;69:1079-1087.
37. Agostoni P, Apostolo A, Albert RK. Mechanisms of periodic breathing during exercise in patients with chronic heart failure. *Chest.* 2008;133:197-203.
38. Guazzi M, Myers J, Peberdy MA, Bensimhon D, Chase P, Arena R. Exercise oscillatory breathing in diastolic heart failure: prevalence and prognostic insights. *Eur Heart J.* 2008;29:2751-2759.
39. Koike A, Shimizu N, Tajima A, et al. Relation between oscillatory ventilation at rest before cardiopulmonary exercise testing and prognosis in patients with left ventricular dysfunction. *Chest.* 2003;123:372-379.
40. Ben-Dov I, Sietsema KE, Casaburi R, Wasserman K. Evidence that circulatory oscillations accompany ventilatory oscillations during exercise in patients with heart failure. *Am Rev Respir Dis.* 1992;145(4, pt 1):776-781.
41. Murphy RM, Shah RV, Malhotra R, et al. Exercise oscillatory ventilation in systolic heart failure: an indicator of impaired hemodynamic response to exercise. *Circulation.* 2011;124:1442-1451.
42. Yajima T, Koike A, Sugimoto K, Miyahara Y, Marumo F, Hiroe M. Mechanism of periodic breathing in patients with cardiovascular disease. *Chest.* 1994;106:142-146.

43. Corrà U, Pistono M, Mezzani A, et al. Sleep and exertional periodic breathing in chronic heart failure: prognostic importance and interdependence. *Circulation*. 2006;113:44-50.
44. Agostini PG, Emdin M, Corrà U, et al. Permanent atrial fibrillation affects exercise capacity in chronic heart failure patients. *Eur Heart J*. 2008;29:2367-2372.
45. Mantegazza V, Apostolo A, Hager A. Cardiopulmonary exercise testing in adult congenital heart disease. *Ann Am Thorac Soc*. 2017;14(suppl 1):S93-S101.
46. Inuzuka R, Diller GP, Borgia F, et al. Comprehensive use of cardiopulmonary exercise testing identifies adults with congenital heart disease at increased mortality risk in the medium term. *Circulation*. 2012;125:250-259.
47. Warnes CA, Williams RG, Bashore TM, et al. ACC/AHA 2008 guidelines for the management of adults with congenital heart disease: a report of the American College of Cardiology/American Heart Association Task Force on Practice Guidelines (Writing Committee to Develop Guidelines on the Management of Adults with Congenital Heart Disease). Developed in Collaboration with the American Society of Echocardiography, Heart Rhythm Society, International Society for Adult Congenital Heart Disease, Society for Cardiovascular Angiography and Interventions, and Society of Thoracic Surgeons. *J Am Coll Cardiol*. 2008;52(23):e143-e263.
48. Dimopoulos K, Okonko DO, Diller GP, et al. Abnormal ventilatory response to exercise in adults with congenital heart disease relates to cyanosis and predicts survival. *Circulation*. 2006;113:2796-2802.
49. Sietsema KE, Cooper DM, Perloff JK, et al. Dynamics of oxygen uptake during exercise in adults with cyanotic congenital heart disease. *Circulation*. 1986;73:1137-1144.
50. Sietsema K. Oxygen uptake kinetics in response to exercise in patients with pulmonary vascular disease. *Am Rev Respir Dis*. 1992;145:1052-1057.
51. Sietsema KE, Cooper DM, Perloff JK, et al. Control of ventilation during exercise in patients with central venous-to-systemic arterial shunts. *J Appl Physiol (1985)*. 1988;64:234-242.
52. Oudiz RJ, Roveran G, Hansen J, Sun XG, Wasserman K. Effect of sildenafil on ventilatory efficiency and exercise tolerance in pulmonary hypertension. *Eur J Heart Fail*. 2007;9:917-921.
53. Bylund-Fellenius AC, Walker PM, Elander A, Holm S, Holm J, Scherstén T. Energy metabolism in relation to oxygen partial pressure in human skeletal muscle during exercise. *Biochem J*. 1981;200:247-255.
54. Nery LE, Wasserman K, French W, Oren A, Davis JA. Contrasting cardiovascular and respiratory responses to exercise in mitral valve and chronic obstructive pulmonary diseases. *Chest*. 1983;83:446-453.
55. Hansen J, Ulubay G, Chow BF, Sun XG, Wasserman K. Mixed-expired and end-tidal CO2 distinguish between ventilation and perfusion defects during exercise testing in patients with lung and heart diseases. *Chest*. 2007;132:977-983.
56. Casaburi R, Patessio A, Ioli F, Zanaboni S, Donner CF, Wasserman K. Reductions in exercise lactic acidosis and ventilation as a result of exercise training in patients with obstructive lung disease. *Am Rev Respir Dis*. 1991;143:9-18.
57. Hansen JE, Wasserman K. Pathophysiology of activity limitation in patients with interstitial lung disease. *Chest*. 1996;109:1566-1576.
58. Lederer DJ, Martinez FJ. Idiopathic pulmonary fibrosis. *N Engl J Med*. 2018;378:1811-1823.
59. Butler WM, Spratling LS, Kark JA, Schoomaker EB. Hemoglobin Osler: report of a new family with exercise studies before and after phlebotomy. *Am J Hematol*. 1982;13:293-301.
60. Hirsch GL, Sue DY, Wasserman K, Robinson TE, Hansen JE. Immediate effects of cigarette smoking on cardiorespiratory responses to exercise. *J Appl Physiol (1985)*. 1985;58:1975-1981.
61. Koike A, Wasserman K, Taniguichi K, Hiroe M, Marumo F. Critical capillary oxygen partial pressure and lactate threshold in patients with cardiovascular disease. *J Am Coll Cardiol*. 1994;23:1644-1650.
62. Jones NL, Sutton JR, Taylor R, Toews CJ. Effect of pH on cardiorespiratory and metabolic responses to exercise. *J Appl Physiol Respir Environ Exerc Physiol*. 1977;43:959-964.
63. Oren A, Wasserman K, Davis JA, Whipp BJ. Effect of CO2 set point on ventilatory response to exercise. *J Appl Physiol Respir Environ Exerc Physiol*. 1981;51:185-189.
64. Riley MS, Nicholls DP, Cooper CB. Cardiopulmonary exercise testing and metabolic myopathies. *Ann Am Thorac Soc*. 2017;14(suppl 1):S129-S139.
65. Berardo A, DiMauro S, Hirano M. A diagnostic algorithm for metabolic myopathies. *Curr Neurol Neurosci Rep*. 2010;10:118-126.
66. McArdle B. Myopathy due to a defect in muscle glycogen breakdown. *Clin Sci*. 1951;10:13-35.
67. Riley M, Nugent A, Steele IC, et al. Gas exchange during exercise in McArdle's disease. *J Appl Physiol*. 1993;75:745-754.
68. Haller RG, Lewis SF. Abnormal ventilation during exercise in McArdle's syndrome: modulation by substrate availability. *Neurology*. 1986;36:716-719.
69. Lewis SF, Haller RG. The pathophysiology of McArdle's disease: clues to regulation in exercise and fatigue. *J Appl Physiol (1985)*. 1986;61:391-401.
70. Wasserman K, Hansen JE, Sue DY. Facilitation of oxygen consumption by lactic acidosis during exercise. *Physiology*. 1991;6:29-34.
71. Vissing J, Haller RG. A diagnostic cycle test for McArdle's disease. *Ann Neurol*. 2003;54(4):539-542.
72. Bogaard JM, Scholte HR, Busch FM, Stam H, Versprille A. Anaerobic threshold as detected from ventilatory and metabolic exercise responses in patients with mitochondrial respiratory chain defect. In: Tavassi L, DiPrampero PE, eds. *Advances in Cardiology. The Anaerobic Threshold: Physiological and Clinical Significance*. Basel, Switzerland: Karger; 1986:135-145.
73. Haller RG, Lewis SF, Estabrook RW, DiMauro S, Servidei S, Foster DW. Exercise intolerance, lactic acidosis, and abnormal cardiopulmonary regulation in exercise associated with adult skeletal muscle cytochrome C oxidase deficiency. *J Clin Invest*. 1989;84:155-161.
74. Taivassalo T, Jensen TD, Kennaway N, DiMauro S, Vissing J, Haller RG. The spectrum of exercise tolerance in mitochondrial myopathies: a study of 40 patients. *Brain*. 2003;126(pt 2):413-423.
75. Heinicke K, Taivassalo T, Wyrick P, Wood H, Babb TG, Haller RG. Exertional dyspnea in mitochondrial myopathy: clinical features and physiological mechanisms. *Am J Physiol Regul Integr Comp Physiol*. 2011;301:R873-R884.
76. Nguyen KA, Li L, Lu D, et al. A comprehensive review and meta-analysis of risk factors for statin-induced myopathy. *Eur J Clin Pharmacol*. 2018;74:1099-1109.
77. Allard NAE, Schirris TJJ, Verheggen RJ, et al. Statins affect skeletal muscle performance: evidence for disturbances in energy metabolism. *J Clin Endocrinol Metab*. 2018;103:75-84.
78. Lau AC, Lo MK, Leung GT, Choi FP, Yam LY, Wasserman K. Altered exercise gas exchange as related to microalbuminuria in type 2 diabetic patients. *Chest*. 2004;125:1292-1298.
79. Smekal G, von Duvillard SP, Frigo P, et al. Menstrual cycle: no effect on exercise cardiorespiratory variables or blood lactate concentration. *Med Sci Sports Exerc*. 2007;39:1098-1106.
80. Agostoni P, Smith DD, Schoene RGB, Robertson HT, Butler J. Evaluation of breathlessness in asbestos workers. Results of exercise testing. *Am Rev Respir Dis*. 1987;135:812-816.

CHAPTER 5

Performance of Clinical Cardiopulmonary Exercise Testing

EXERCISE LABORATORY AND EQUIPMENT

General Laboratory Environment

The proper interpretation of cardiopulmonary exercise test (CPET) data depends on accurate data collection and correct calculations. Useful exercise testing can be performed with minimal equipment; for instance, a measured course, stairway, or hallway can provide a reproducible and functional exercise stress. After review of symptoms and physical examination, information collected from such testing might include heart and breathing rates and blood pressure at the conclusion of exercise; however, real-time data for pulse oximeter O_2 saturation and heart rate (HR) are usually not available without the addition of a portable device. To obtain more complete real-time data, a properly equipped CPET laboratory provides serial gas exchange measurements, coupled with blood pressure, oximeter, blood drawing, and electrocardiographic capabilities. The patient can be relatively stationary on the ergometer during a controlled and reproducible exercise stress while measurements are continuously made, and blood may be sampled. **Figure 5.1** diagrams the devices and primary and derived measurements that are generally available in a modern exercise laboratory.

The laboratory should be climate controlled and regulated at a comfortable temperature and humidity. The patient's view should be pleasant and not cluttered with tubing, wires, or a bulletin board with distracting papers. Ideally, data displays of the monitoring devices and timers or clocks should not be positioned in the patient's view. If blood is to be sampled, the syringes should be prepared and placed in a convenient location to avoid confusion or extra motion during the time of the study. Extraneous sounds should be kept to a minimum. Soft background music may help to dampen noise without interfering with communication between the patient, examiner, and laboratory personnel. The number of people in the laboratory should be limited to the minimum required for obtaining the measurements and patient safety. It is generally favored that a physician be present in the room during testing to continually asses patient safety and provide immediate intervention if complications occur. A mobile gurney is optimal to allow a light-headed patient to lie down, and the laboratory should have an immediately available

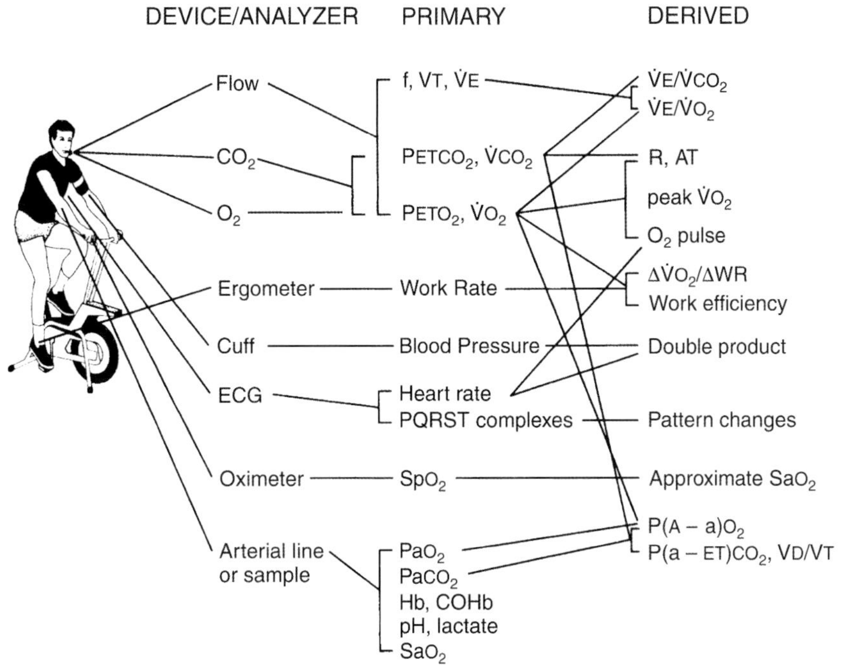

FIGURE 5.1. Devices and analyzers used to measure variables during exercise on a cycle ergometer. Devices and analyzers individually or collectively may measure a single or several primary variables. The variables in the right-hand column are usually calculated from two or more primary variables. Abbreviations: *AT*, anaerobic threshold; CO_2, carbon dioxide; COHb, carboxyhemoglobin; $\Delta\dot{V}O_2/\Delta WR$, change in $\dot{V}O_2$/change in work rate; ECG, electrocardiogram; f, frequency; Hb, hemoglobin; O_2, oxygen; $P(A - a)O_2$, alveolar-arterial PO_2 difference; $P(a - ET)CO_2$, arterial-end-tidal PCO_2 difference; $PETCO_2$, end-tidal PCO_2; $PETO_2$, end-tidal PO_2; R, respiratory exchange ratio; SaO_2, arterial O_2 saturation; SpO_2, O_2 saturation as measured by pulse oximetry; $\dot{V}CO_2$, CO_2 output; V_D/V_T, physiological dead space-tidal volume ratio; $\dot{V}_E$, minute ventilation; $\dot{V}_E/\dot{V}CO_2$, ventilatory equivalent for CO_2; $\dot{V}_E/\dot{V}O_2$, ventilatory equivalent for O_2; $\dot{V}O_2$, O_2 uptake; V_T, tidal volume.

crash cart. Furthermore, a definite plan for summoning help and responding to urgent or emergent situations should be part of the laboratory's standard operating procedures, especially if the facility is not within a hospital environment. In summary, a comfortable, professional, safe environment for exercise testing is needed to obtain the maximum confidence and therefore optimal performance by the patient. Additional expert consensus on standards of practice for exercise testing relevant to particular clinical contexts and patient populations can be found in statements and guidelines updated periodically by professional societies.[1-5]

Gas Exchange Measurement

Although exercise testing can be performed with little or no equipment, the more sophisticated and potentially useful analysis of cardiopulmonary function during exercise necessitates gas exchange measurement. A variety of systems, measuring devices, algorithms, recorders, and other equipment have been put together for these purposes. There are excellent commercial systems that determine gas exchange using either a gas-mixing chamber or, more commonly, breath-by-breath analysis of respired gas.[1,2,6-12]

Mixing Chambers

In systems using a mixing chamber, expired ventilation (minute ventilation [$\dot{V}_E$]) is determined using a flow or volume measurement device while expired gas is passed into a fixed or variable-sized mixing chamber from which gas is sampled and analyzed for O_2 and CO_2 concentrations. With proper mixing of expired gas from each breath, differences in O_2 and CO_2 concentration from the beginning to the end of each breath are minimized, and the resultant O_2 and CO_2 concentrations are equal to the volume-weighted average or "mixed expired" fractional concentrations ($F\bar{E}O_2$, $F\bar{E}CO_2$). These are equivalent to the O_2 and CO_2 concentrations that would have been obtained by collecting all of the expired gas in a Douglas bag.

An ideal mixing chamber would be of sufficient size for complete mixing of each whole breath. It would provide a gas composition identical to that of the mixed expired gas for the series of whole breaths corresponding to the time of expired flow measurement. A large gas flow (or $\dot{V}_E$) or a mixing chamber of small size has a short time constant. Under these conditions, this chamber would respond rapidly to a change in gas concentration; however, the small volume means that an individual with a large tidal volume will produce marked fluctuations in gas concentrations in the chamber. Thus, the size of the mixing chamber relative to the size of the tidal volume is important. Too large a mixing chamber volume compared with tidal volume results in an impracticably long time to reach any new equilibrium, making the mixing chamber poorly responsive to rapid changes in gas concentration. A fixed-volume mixing chamber may be satisfactory during exercise when $\dot{V}_E$, $F\bar{E}O_2$, and $F\bar{E}CO_2$ change slowly, but may be unsatisfactory when rapid changes are expected. If $\dot{V}_E$ is continuously measured, a time or volume adjustment must be made to match the correct mixed expired gas concentrations with the correct $\dot{V}E$ value.

Breath-by-Breath Systems

Our laboratories use breath-by-breath systems for both research applications and for patient evaluations. A breath-by-breath, real-time system measures airflow or volume continuously throughout the breath and simultaneously determines instantaneous expired CO_2 and O_2 concentrations. After time alignment of O_2 and CO_2 concentrations with the instantaneous flow, the O_2 uptake ($\dot{V}O_2$) and CO_2 output ($\dot{V}CO_2$) for each breath are calculated, as first described by Beaver et al.[13] The $\dot{V}O_2$ and $\dot{V}CO_2$ are calculated for the respective breath by cross-multiplying volume (integrated flow), usually every 0.01 second, by the time-corrected gas concentration. To make accurate measurements, flow and gas concentrations must be measured as near to continuously as possible. To enhance the characterization of the $\dot{V}E$, $\dot{V}O_2$, and $\dot{V}CO_2$ (and associated) responses to rapid changes in work rate, their typical breath-by-breath variability can be greatly reduced by interpolating the breath-by-breath responses (eg, second by second) and averaging these over a longer period (eg, 10 s). If necessary for further time resolution of measured responses, replicate studies with time-averaging of the second-by-second values can be performed.[14,15]

Measurement of Volume, Flow Rate, and Ventilation

Several methods of measuring respired gas volume and flow rates during exercise are used during CPET.[1,6,11,12] Although expired flow is usually measured with a flow sensor and integrated into volume, physiological variables can also be calculated from inspired volume or flow with the appropriate mathematical adjustment to convert to expired volume. Alternatively, systems that use both inspiratory and expiratory flow to separately determine the inspired and expired volumes accurately could be developed; however, these are presently not widely available on the market. Since devices for measuring volume or flows are typically part of the breathing circuit, then flow resistance, linearity, and frequency response are important considerations. Commercially used flow devices include pneumotachographs, pitot tubes, turbines, and hot-wire anemometers. Volume can alternatively be measured directly using a gas meter, spirometer, or volume transducer. The technical considerations relevant to measuring ventilated volumes are dependent on the particular devise that is used in the gas exchange measurement system.

Pneumotachographs measure flow as the pressure drop across a low-resistive element (typically an assembly of small parallel tubes) designed to constrain the flow to laminar, according to Poiseuille law, and are thus sensitive to gas viscosity. When flow becomes nonlaminar or turbulent, the relationship between flow and pressure becomes nonlinear. Fleisch-type pneumotachographs come in different sizes to accommodate the expected flow rates; in adult patients, a size no. 3 Fleisch pneumotachograph is appropriate. Compensation for nonlinearities in the pressure-flow relationship can be made by altering the output of the differential pressure transducer either electrically or mathematically using a computer. In commercial systems, empirical calibration curves may be used to optimize pneumotachograph performance.

Because expired gas is usually warmer and contains more water vapor than ambient air, contact of warm expired gas with an ambient-temperature pneumotachograph could result in condensation and obstruction of the pneumotachograph resistance elements. Pneumotachographs are therefore often equipped with an electric heater to warm the device to a temperature slightly above that of expired gas. However, a heated pneumotachograph not only warms and increases the volume of the inspired gas but also warms it by a variable amount depending on the flow. Although theoretical methods can be used to estimate the degree of warming, two practical methods may eliminate the problem. In the first method, the expired gas is kept warm, and the temperature of the pneumotachograph is only slightly warmer (approximately 0.5°C) than the temperature of the gas passing through it. Another way is to distance the pneumotachograph from the mouth so that it can be allowed to cool to ambient temperature before flow is measured.

Pitot tubes measure flow as the difference in pressure between an opening placed directly facing the flow stream and an opening perpendicular to the flow stream, according to Bernoulli law. Thus, the velocity of flow movement is proportional to the square root of the pressure difference; from the cross-sectional area of the device, the flow can be calculated. The pitot tube has the advantage of being nonresistive and dependent on turbulent flow rather than on laminar flow conditions. For exercise applications, two differential pressure transducers are required to assure linearity over more than one order of magnitude (ie, to cover flow rates from <0.5 L/s to over 10 L/s): one linearized to the lower flow-rate range and the second linearized to the higher flow-rate range. The linearization algorithms incorporate corrections for gas density and temperature. The electronics and software reconstruct the two flow signals to one continuous composite signal. Advantages of such a device include low resistance, lack of a requirement for laminar flow, and minimal problems with heating or cooling of inspired or expired gas.

Mass flow meters (hot-wire anemometers) measure the mass flow of gas by determining the change in electrical current, compared with baseline, needed to maintain a constant temperature of a wire placed in the air stream. The wire material is selected, so the wire resistance is strongly influenced by the wire temperature. The rate of mass movement of gas and its thermal capacity relate to the current change; by using an appropriate model, the flow of gas can be calculated. Although this method is inherently nonlinear, digital computer algorithms can correct this nonlinearity.

Turbine flow sensors measure volume rather than flow, each rotation of a low-resistance vane being directly proportional to the gas volume in the flow stream. They have the advantage of being relatively unaffected by changes in gas viscosity and density.

Breathing Valves, Mouthpieces, and Masks

Some gas exchange measurement systems require the use of a breathing valve to separate inspired from expired gas flows so that expired gas can be collected and analyzed. This is a necessity, for example, if the inspired gas is something other than room air, such as when supplemental oxygen is being provided during the test. The ideal valve prevents contamination of either inspired or expired gas flow by the other, has no resistance to breathing, has low rebreathed volume (low valve dead space), is of minimal weight and size, is easily cleaned and sterilized, is low cost, does not generate turbulence, and operates silently.

Dead space for the valve plus attached mouthpiece can be determined by measuring the volume of water it can hold. Valve resistance can be determined during constant airflow using a pressure transducer and flow sensor. Valves may develop back leaks, especially when subjected to high flows and pressures during heavy exercise. These leaks should be suspected for any valve but especially after prolonged use, excessive secretions, or damage to component parts. Errors in ventilation or gas exchange measurements may be important clues to a leaking breathing valve. If a leak is suspected, simultaneous recording of inspiratory and expiratory flow during exercise may reveal the presence and location of the leak.

Traditionally, patients have used nose clips so that all inspired and expired gases are routed through rubber, soft plastic, or silicone mouthpieces. However, it is now common to employ comfortable face masks of differing sizes and shapes to cover the patient's nose and mouth. The dead space represented by the mask is usually only slightly more than with a mouthpiece and nose clip.

Gas Analyzers

For gas exchange measurements, the concentration of O_2 and CO_2 in the respired gas can be determined by several devices. Mass spectrometers convert sampled gases to positively charged ions with an electron beam. Then, in a near vacuum, the ions are accelerated by an electric field and are then subjected to a magnetic field. The direction that the ions take in the magnetic field is dependent on their mass-to-charge ratios. The different ions representing different gases are detected by appropriately located detectors that each produces a voltage output proportional to the number of ions that strike the collector per unit time. Because the total voltage is dependent on the sum of the individual detector voltages, any gas for which there is no detector does not contribute to the total. For respiratory mass spectrometry, detectors for O_2, CO_2, and nitrogen (N_2) are typically used; however, there are no detectors for water vapor, argon, or other inert gases present in trace amounts in air. Thus, the O_2, CO_2, and N_2 concentrations given by a mass spectrometer are concentrations relative to a dry gas whether or not water vapor was a component of the originally sampled gas. Commercially available CPET systems commonly contain discrete gas analyzers, one for O_2 and one for CO_2, rather than interfacing with a mass spectrometer.

Carbon dioxide analyzers measure absorption by CO_2 of appropriate wavelengths of infrared light. Infrared light is passed through a cell containing the gas to be measured, and the amount of light transmitted is compared with a reference value. Absorption is proportional to the fractional CO_2 concentration. The measurement cell must be kept clean and free of water condensation.

Oxygen analyzers use several different principles. The paramagnetic analyzer measures the change in a magnetic field introduced by differences in oxygen concentration. Other respiratory gases have little paramagnetic susceptibility and do not affect the magnetic field. Alternatively, electrochemical O_2 analyzer depends on chemical reactions between O_2 and a substrate that generates a small electrical current. This current is proportional to the rate of O_2 molecules reacting with the substrate and thus to the concentration of O_2.

Carbon dioxide and oxygen analyzers measure gas concentration that the software converts to partial pressure. These calculations are affected by water vapor, resistances in the sampling systems, changes in barometric pressure, and altitude. Thus, for a given fractional concentration of gas, changes in any of these conditions at the sensor location will erroneously result in different measured gas fractions. Updating these factors is therefore an essential component of calibration prior to a test. Because the sample flow rate delivering gas to the analyzer is held constant, a change in sampling site pressure may result from changes in resistance of the delivery tubing. Using a high-pressure suction pump and a large resistance in the connection between the analyzer and the pump minimizes this effect. Care must be taken to ensure that sample tube resistance is identical during calibration and patient measurement and that water condensation, saliva, or foreign bodies are not trapped in the delivery tubing.

Both carbon dioxide and oxygen analyzers report the fraction of CO_2 or O_2 in the total gas volume, including any water vapor present. This is especially important to consider during calibration because ambient air contains water vapor. Expired gas is saturated with water vapor at the lowest temperature that it reaches before reaching the gas analyzers. Because temperature determines the partial pressure of water in a saturated gas, this temperature must be accurately known or estimated if expired P_{CO_2} and P_{O_2} are to be accurately determined. This requirement can be circumvented by using sampling tubing that contains Nafion, a sulfonated tetrafluoroethylene-based fluoropolymer-copolymer that is selectively and highly permeable to water.

The rapid serial binding of water to sulfonic acid moieties transports water molecules from the internal surface of the tubing along its pressure gradient to the exterior (with first-order kinetics). Thus, the water vapor pressure in the sampled gas rapidly equilibrates with that of ambient air, resulting in the sampled gas containing relatively little water vapor on arrival at the analyser. Additional discussion of the significance of water vapor can be found in Appendix C.

Elevated Inspired Fractional Oxygen Concentration

Commercially available systems make it possible to determine gas exchange rapidly and accurately under many conditions, including the inhalation of elevated O_2 inspirates (high fraction of inspired O_2 [High F_{IO_2}]). This can be valuable when testing individuals who are dependent on supplemental O_2 and in whom it is desired to maintain arterial oxygenation levels during testing either for safety reasons or to allow assessment of exercise capacity exclusive of the confounding effects of hypoxemia. For this, the inspiratory arm of the breathing circuit can be connected via a low-resistance valve to a reservoir balloon containing a humidified gas mixture with the desired oxygen concentration and the gas being replenished as needed during exercise from a gas tank or using an anesthesia gas blender. It must be noted that the use of higher oxygen concentrations raises special considerations for calculation of $\dot{V}O_2$. Conventionally, calculating $\dot{V}O_2$ from analysis of exhaled breath has used the Haldane transformation to calculate the unmeasured inspired volumes, but this becomes inaccurate under conditions of high F_{IO_2}. As a result, CPET has not generally been considered to be accurate when the F_{IO_2} exceeds 0.5.[6] A recent new approach replaces the Haldane transformation with what has been termed the Eschenbacher transformation when calculating $\dot{V}O_2$ at elevated F_{IO_2} effectively eliminating the calculation error associated with the Haldane transformation.[16] The use of gases that differ from room air in oxygen concentration, density, or viscosity may also require special calibration procedures depending on the range over which the analyzers are calibrated and the type of flow transducer used. Procedures needed to prepare for testing patients on elevated F_{IO_2} therefore depend on the specifications and software of the particular equipment in use. It is recommended that validation of the ability of the system to accurately measure gas exchange on elevated F_{IO_2} be done using healthy volunteers performing a series of steady-state constant work rate tests to verify that metabolic measurements made when breathing the higher F_{IO_2} are comparable to those made for the same work rate when breathing air (see "Quality Control, Validation, and Maintenance" section).

Ergometers: Treadmills and Cycles

Although many different ergometers can be used in exercise testing, by far, the most common are treadmill and stationary cycle ergometer. Details of these have been described comprehensively.[1,2,6]

Treadmill

Treadmills allow individuals to walk, jog, or run at measured speeds and grades of incline. A variety of protocols for increasing work rate have been designed, and both low and high work rates may be imposed. Treadmills have some advantages over cycle ergometers. An individual exercising on a treadmill generally has a higher peak $\dot{V}O_2$ than on a cycle ergometer, with the differences usually reported in the range of 5% to 10%.[17] Because walking is a nearly universal component of daily activity, treadmill exercise may also extrapolate more directly to functional capacity than cycling. On the other hand, treadmills have some disadvantages, including a greater likelihood of movement artifacts in measurement of ventilation, pulmonary gas exchange, blood pressure, and electrocardiogram (ECG).

Of greatest importance is the fact that if the individual being tested holds on to any part of the treadmill (eg, a hand railing or the arm of a technician or physician), the amount of work performed is reduced, thus interfering with the accurate determination of the $\dot{V}O_2$-WR relationship and work efficiency. It is therefore important to have the patient practice to achieve a quasi-normal walking pattern on the treadmill, with the handrail being used only for balance purposes.

If a normal, unaided, and unencumbered walk is achieved, the work rate (WR) on treadmill is determined by the subject's weight (m, kg), walking speed (v, m/s), and the grade of treadmill inclination (α) (Equation 1):

$$WR = m \cdot g \cdot v \cdot \sin(\alpha) \quad (1)$$

where g is the gravitational constant (9.81 m/s^2) and α is arctangent (% grade/100). It has been shown that although there are differences in physiological responses to incremental exercise on cycle and treadmill, the $\dot{V}O_2$-WR response is linear and essentially the same.[6,18] Whereas treadmill walking is not identical to free-range walking, repeated experience on the treadmill may lead to some increase in the efficiency of walking.

Changes in length of stride as speed or grade is changed, shift of center of gravity, and change from walking to jogging can each affect the patient's metabolic requirement. A treadmill protocol has been developed that uses only walking (from as low as 0.7 mph to a reasonable 3.3 mph), without having the patient switch to jogging or running, resulting in a linear increase in the metabolic rate.[19] More recently, this has been further modified to linearize the metabolic rate across a wider range of speeds from below 1 mph up to about 12 mph, assuming that the metabolic rate is proportional to kinetic energy (using the square function of walking speed).[20] As a result, very similar profiles of incremental exercise can be achieved with either treadmills or cycle ergometers.

Cycle Ergometer

Cycle ergometers enable a precise estimation of the work rate. Leg cycling may be performed sitting or supine. Advantages of the cycle ergometer include the ability to vary the work rate in step, incremental, or ramp fashion without changes in ergonomic efficiency due to factors such as gait and stride length; the ability to determine work efficiency; potentially enhanced patient comfort and/or safety because the patient is supported at all times; and less movement artifact in measurements. However, some patients may not be able to cycle because of lack of coordination or experience, and some may be intolerant of seat discomfort during a long study. Additional considerations that could limit cycle use in some circumstances include weight capacity of the apparatus and pedal spacing, which may create limitations for individuals with extreme obesity, and the range of heights that can be accommodated.

When the patient is seated in the upright position, seat height should be adjusted so that the leg is almost completely extended at the lowest point of the crank. It is useful to record the seat height in the patient's records so that future studies may be done identically. Subjects should be asked to wear shoes suitable for the types of pedals on the cycle. Toe clips or straps may be used as desired. Because subjects should cycle at a relatively constant rate, a metronome or cadence tachometer should be used to assist cycling frequency.

Two types of cycle ergometers are in general use. For mechanical cycle ergometers, the breaking force is applied to a flywheel by adjusting the tension of the breaking belt on the flywheel. The breaking force is dependent on the tension of the belt and is independent of the cycling frequency. The work rate is the product of the torque and the cycling frequency.

An electrically braked cycle ergometer uses a variable electromagnetic field to produce a resistance to pedaling that changes hyperbolically with the flywheel speed, thus achieving work rates that are independent of the cycling frequency. However, because the internal (metabolic) work is proportional to the cycling frequency, it is advisable to maintain the cycling frequency within a narrow range in order to avoid sudden changes in metabolic rate during the test. The desired work rate may be controlled from a remote controller, or it may be adjusted on the built-in controller unit of the cycle ergometer.

When an individual pedals on the cycle with no resistance added (ie, "unloaded" or "zero watt"), some work is done on the weight of the legs and the small frictional force on the flywheel. This "internal work rate" depends on the frictional forces and also on cycling frequency and accounts for approximately 5 to 15 W. The low associated O_2 cost may nevertheless exceed the maximal capacity of some severely limited patients. Manufacturer's specifications may provide information on the work rate of unloaded cycling, but users should make this determination for themselves.

We have in the past used a special protocol (see "Selecting the Rate of Work Rate Increase" later in this chapter) that uses an accessory motor attached to the cycle flywheel to start the flywheel rotating and to maintain it at the desired speed, thus removing the inertial energy needed by the subject to start cycling while simultaneously minimizing the "unloaded" work rate (virtually zero watts above the power output needed for moving the legs at the assigned cycling frequency). Many cycle ergometers now have this capacity built in. This facility is particularly helpful for testing patients with limited strength in their legs.

Cycle Versus Treadmill

Whether the treadmill or the cycle ergometer is the preferable mode of exercise for CPET has been a subject of considerable debate (**Table 5.1**). The treadmill has been in common use in the United States and elsewhere for decades. It allows one to exercise most ambulatory patients except those who are severely dyspneic, uncoordinated, or confused or those who have significant lower extremity musculoskeletal disease. As noted before, in most healthy individuals and patients, peak $\dot{V}O_2$, peak O_2 pulse, and anaerobic threshold (*AT*) values are generally higher on the treadmill than cycle.[17,18] Also, for some applications, the bulk of data published regarding the significance of CPET variables has been derived from treadmill testing, making it reasonable to perform treadmill testing when characterizing responses of patients studied for the same indication.

TABLE 5.1 Comparison of Treadmill and Cycle Ergometers for Exercise Testing

Features	Treadmill	Cycle
Highest peak $\dot{V}O_2$ and peak O_2 pulse	+	
Highest peak heart rate and peak $\dot{V}E$	+	+
Familiarity of exercise	++	+
Patient stability	+/−	++
Quantitation of external work	+/−	++
Freedom from artifacts in ECG, airflow, and blood pressure signals	−	+
Ease of sampling blood	− −	++
Eliciting heart rate response by rate-adaptive pacemakers	+	−
Eliciting hemoglobin desaturation in patients with chronic lung disease	++	+/−

Abbreviations: ECG, electrocardiogram; O_2, oxygen; $\dot{V}E$, minute ventilation; $\dot{V}O_2$, oxygen uptake; +, ++, potential advantage or strength of testing mode; −, − −, potential disadvantage or weakness of testing mode; +/−, variable advantage or disadvantage of testing mode depending on patient factors.

Whereas suffering injury during treadmill testing is extremely rare, cycle exercise is generally viewed as safer for those patients who are less coordinated or who are particularly frail and may be more prone to fall. Even the most athletic of patients may require several minutes of practice prior to testing to be able to safely start and end treadmill exercise. Because patients can lose their balance on the moving belts, it is wise to have additional help immediately available on the sideboard of the treadmill, particularly for elderly patients. Ending a cycle exercise test may be less intimidating than ending a treadmill test because a patient can stop exercise independently, whereas with the treadmill, he or she must generally signal the examiner, who then turns off the treadmill. Thus, stopping the exercise is dependent not only on the patient but also on the reaction time of the examiner controlling the device and the subsequent slowing of the belt. Treadmills used in CPET are commonly equipped with an emergency stop button that facilitates stopping the belt quickly, should this be necessary.

Lesser patient movement during cycle ergometry compared to treadmill exercise can reduce artifact in signals and also make it easier to obtain blood samples if indicated. Other ancillary measures such as cardiac imaging may be more readily accomplished as well. Seat discomfort can be a problem with longer and repeated testing on a cycle but is rarely limiting with the short protocols typically used in CPET.

As identified above, probably, the greatest limitation to the widespread use of treadmills in CPET has been the uncertainty of accurately quantifying work rate for treadmill exercise so that it can be related to metabolic rate. Although the linearized work rate protocol described above[19] overcomes this, to date, this protocol has not been built into commercially available systems. Therefore, users need to enter the individualized protocol into their systems. Independent of the profile of the imposed work rate, however, holding the railings of the treadmill or anything else (eg, blood pressure measuring devices or steadying hands) can significantly reduce the patient's actual work rate. Therefore, for treadmill exercise, it is recommended to allow patients to touch the handrail only for balance purposes and to minimize the stabilizing effect of holding the patient's arm when taking blood pressure measurements. When safety considerations do dictate use of the handrails, the test interpreter should not presume accuracy of the estimated work rate.

There are two important clinical situations in which treadmill testing is uniquely advantageous. Patients who are dependent on rate-adaptive pacemakers for increases in HR and cardiac output are more likely to experience an appropriate increase in HR during treadmill exercise than during cycle ergometer exercise. This is because with cycling, there may not be sufficient rhythmic change in the center of gravity to be sensed by the pacemaker accelerometer. Therefore, during incremental exercise on a cycle, the pacemaker may fail to accelerate HR above the resting rate constraining the increase in cardiac output. Treadmill exercise is more frequently effective in eliciting a change in HR under these circumstances, presumably because of the walking-related shoulder and torso movement. The other situation favoring the use of treadmill testing relates to identifying and quantifying the degree of oxyhemoglobin desaturation that may occur during exercise in patients with significant chronic obstructive pulmonary disease (COPD). Hsia et al[18] compared the cycle to the treadmill using linear protocols increasing work rate at similar rates in 16 patients with COPD. With the treadmill, they found similar exercise times, peak work rates, and peak $\dot{V}E$ but significantly higher peak $\dot{V}O_2$, peak $\dot{V}CO_2$, *AT* (absolute and percentage peak $\dot{V}O_2$), and peak P_{ETCO_2} with significantly lower peak respiratory exchange ratio (R), peak end-tidal PO_2 (P_{ETO_2}), and peak ventilatory equivalent for CO_2 ($\dot{V}E/\dot{V}CO_2$). Importantly, oxygen saturation as measured by pulse oximetry (SpO_2) was approximately 5% to 8% lower on the treadmill than the cycle ergometer at equivalent $\dot{V}O_2$. Because the *AT* occurs at a lower $\dot{V}O_2$ on the cycle ergometer, $\dot{V}E$ at a given supra-*AT* $\dot{V}O_2$ is greater than on the treadmill. This results in a higher PaO_2, effectively preventing or constraining desaturation. Thus, when testing for the severity of arterial desaturation in COPD patients, treadmill exercise appears to be more sensitive than cycle ergometry.

In agreement with Åstrand,[21] we prefer the cycle to the treadmill for routine clinical testing because we may be able to quantify external work rate more frequently and thereby establish the patient's $\dot{V}O_2$-WR relationship, a valuable construct in assessing cardiovascular function. For individuals with good walking form, however, a reasonably linear $\dot{V}O_2$-WR relationship can be achieved on treadmill.[19] For a significant proportion of patients, therefore, either type of ergometer can be used for CPET and the choice for a given laboratory determined by factors that include characteristics of the clinical populations served, indications for testing, and the frequency of need for ancillary measures.

Work and Work Rate (Power)

In basic physical units, force ($kg\text{-}m/s^2$ or N) equals the product of mass (kg) and acceleration (m/s^2). When this force is applied over a distance, work is performed. Thus, work ($kg\text{-}m^2/s^2$ or N-m or J) equals the product of force ($kg\text{-}m/s^2$ or N) and distance (m). However, we are most often interested in the rate of work or power, which equals work ($kg\text{-}m^2/s^2$ or N-m or J) per second. The unit of power or work rate is the watt (W), and 1 W is defined as $1\ J/s = 1\ N\text{-}m/s = 1\ kg\text{-}m^2/s^3$.

During exercise against the resistance of a cycle ergometer, the work rate is the distance traveled by a point on the circumference of the wheel × the rotational frequency of the flywheel × the restraining force, that is, torque. The torque can be expressed as newtons or, commonly, as kiloponds (kp), where $1\ kp = 1\ kg \times 9.81\ m/s^2$. In practice, cycle ergometer work rate is expressed as W or kp-m/min. To convert from kp-m/min to W, divide the former by 6.12. For example, a work rate of 612 kp-m/min equals 100 W.

Electrocardiogram and Systemic Blood Pressure

Exercise Electrocardiogram

Silver or silver chloride ECG electrodes with circumferential adhesive provide good electrical contact and minimize movement artifacts. These are similar to those used in the intensive care unit for ECG monitoring. The skin is shaved if necessary and is rubbed with alcohol before the patches are applied on areas of the body that will not be subject to great motion during exercise. A net vest may reduce artifacts due to movement.

We use 12-lead ECGs for all patients to monitor HR and document rhythm and any abnormalities in repolarization. Precordial leads are placed in the same standard position as used for resting ECG, but the limb leads are moved to the torso to minimize motion artifacts during exercise.[22] Leads normally placed on the arms (LA and RA) are placed in the infraclavicular space or over the distal capita of the clavicle since there is only a small underlying muscle mass and the tissue is relatively motion free during exercise (thus minimizing measurement artifacts). Leg leads are recommended to be placed on the lower anterolateral torso, midway between the lower margin of the ribs and the iliac crests in the midclavicular line. It may be necessary to modify this placement based on individual patients' body habitus, especially for cycle testing, to avoid artifact due to "bounce" of underlying soft tissue during exercise. Nonstandard placement of the limb leads and upright posture can alter the axis and QRS and repolarization morphology relative to the standard supine ECG, but rate and rhythm determination are not affected. Commercial systems developed for recording exercise ECG usually have a built-in filter (usually 100 Hz) that can be activated should the ECG signal be disturbed by motion artifacts. As a general rule, the exercise should be stopped and the electrode placement be corrected if the signal is noisy to an extent that it prevents adequate monitoring.

Systemic Blood Pressure

Arterial blood pressure should be measured frequently during exercise to be aware of extreme hypertension or to detect impending hypotension. Blood pressure can be measured and recorded using several commercial devices: mechanically controlled or automated inflatable cuffs and auscultation or pressure transducers placed over the radial or brachial artery. Commercial devices that use the ECG to synchronize the pressure measurement are usually more reliable and are preferred. Noninvasive blood pressure measurement devices should be cross-validated against sphygmomanometer measurements. Indwelling arterial catheters are less frequently used but allow nearly continuous direct measurement of arterial blood pressure. The pressure transducer of such systems should be located at the level of the left atrium and the transducer carefully calibrated. More commonly, blood pressure is measured with an aneroid manometer, inflatable arm cuff, and auscultation. During treadmill exercise, it is important that the arm is released from the handrail and relaxed in order to assure a relatively noise-free condition for optimal auscultation, whether automatic or manual measurement is the chosen procedure.

Oximetry, Blood Sampling, and Arterial Catheters

Valid measurements of Pa_{O_2}, P_{CO_2} (Pa_{CO_2}), or pH from direct arterial blood samples for calculation or measurement of arterial oxygen saturation (Sa_{O_2}), alveolar-arterial P_{O_2} difference [$P(A - a)_{O_2}$], arterial–end-tidal P_{CO_2} difference [$P(a - ET)_{CO_2}$], or the physiological dead space fraction of the breath (physiological dead space–tidal volume ratio [V_D/V_T]) are useful for CPET interpretation. However, on many occasions, correct diagnoses and interpretations can be made using noninvasive measurements.

Pulse Oximetry

Pulse oximetry estimates Sa_{O_2} using pulsatile changes in light absorption. Since the late 1970s, the principle of pulse oximetry has been widely used.[23,24] This technique estimates arterial S_{O_2} from a combination of spectrophotometry and pulse plethysmography. These devices use two wavelengths of light produced by light-emitting diodes, one in the red and one in the infrared spectrum, and a detector that measures transmitted or reflected light from the ear lobe, fingertip, or forehead. Differential absorption of light at these two wavelengths provides information to determine the ratio of oxyhemoglobin to total hemoglobin, assuming that all the pulsatile change is due to the effects of arterial blood. Pulse oximetry is theoretically independent of skin pigmentation and the thickness of the ear lobe or finger; however, some studies have shown that dark skin pigmentation may affect results.[25,26]

Some newer pulse oximeters use eight wavelengths for analysis and detection and thus can now accurately distinguish carboxyhemoglobin and methemoglobin as well as reduced and oxyhemoglobin.[27] In general, pulse oximetry becomes less accurate when arterial S_{O_2} is less than 75%.[23,28]

During exercise, movement artifact and stray incidental light may interfere with pulse oximeter accuracy. Although some studies have found acceptable accuracy of pulse oximeters during exercise,[26,28,29] Hansen and Casaburi[30] have shown that overestimation and underestimation of arterial S_{O_2} may occur near the patient's maximum work rate. Reasons for this may include dependence of the pulse oximeter on sufficient blood flow to the vascular bed measured, a change in the shape of the arterial pulse waveform, a change in empirically determined calibration factors, or movement artifacts. Newer generation pulse oximeters have improved algorithms that allow the devices to cope better with motion artifacts, reduced perfusion, and changes in pulsatile waveforms. These have been tested in critically ill patients and to a lesser extent in the exercise laboratory.[31,32] Fewer motion artifacts may be encountered if a reflectance oximeter probe is placed on the forehead or other less vigorously moving parts of the body.

The major disadvantage of pulse oximetry is that Sa_{O_2} rather than Pa_{O_2} is measured. Thus, although the correlation between arterial SO_2 measured directly and by indirectly pulse oximetry (SpO_2) is good, it is not perfect and significant decreases in PaO_2 when above 60 mm Hg result in only small decreases in arterial SO_2. On occasions, when a more modest abnormality of oxygenation requires documentation or a determination regarding O_2 prescription is needed, direct PaO_2 measurements may be necessary. In patients with left heart disease, declines in SpO_2 may sometimes occur near end-exercise. If such a decline is accompanied by declining blood pressure, light-headedness, or premature plateaus in $\dot{V}O_2$ or O_2 pulse, the decline in SpO_2 can usually be attributed to poor tissue perfusion under the oximeter. On some occasions, direct blood gas measurements will be necessary for accurate diagnoses.

Newer devices can also accurately measure arterialized capillary PCO_2 transcutaneously, using a Severinghaus electrode. This electrode is essentially a pH electrode that is calibrated to report PCO_2. The electrode is heated to facilitate vasodilation and diffusion through the skin of the earlobe or the skin on the upper torso or forehead. The device reliably records arterialized capillary PCO_2 that can be used in the calculation of dead space ventilation, as illustrated in **Figure 5.2.**[6,34-37] The simultaneous transcutaneous measurement of PO_2 and PCO_2 has recently gained a role in CPET. This technology has been shown to be reasonably accurate as measured against direct arterial blood gas sampling and has been used in clinical applications in cardiovascular and pulmonary disease.

Single Samples of Arterial Blood by Puncture

Arterial blood samples allow direct measurement of SaO_2, PaO_2, $PaCO_2$, pH, and lactate and calculation of $P(A - a)O_2$, V_D/V_T, and $P(a - ET)CO_2$. Often, a single sample of arterial blood is obtained by puncture during the middle or late portion of an exercise test to assess the adequacy of blood gases. If this is done, the sample must be obtained before the end of the exercise because rapid changes occur in PaO_2 and

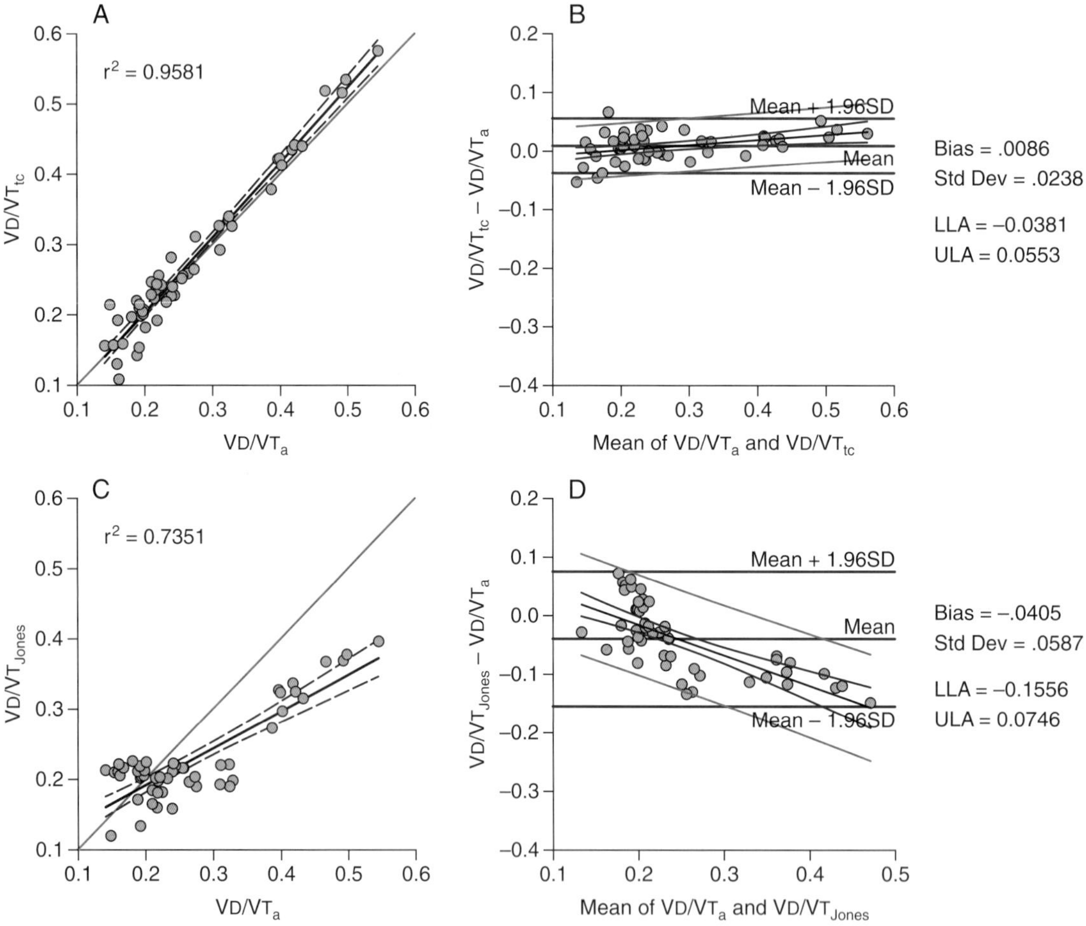

FIGURE 5.2. Physiological dead space–tidal volume ratio (V_D/V_T) values at rest and exercise for patients with chronic obstructive lung disease based on PCO_2 values measured by arterial blood gas analysis (V_D/V_{Ta}), transcutaneous electrode (V_D/V_{Ttc}), and extrapolation of end-tidal PCO_2 measurement as described by Jones et al[33](V_D/V_{TJones}). Panels A and C show correlations of V_D/V_{Ttc} (upper) and V_D/V_{TJones} (lower), against V_D/V_{Ta}. Panels B and D are the corresponding Bland Altman plots. The V_D/V_T values derived from $P_{tc}CO_2$ were highly correlated with those derived from $PaCO_2$, whereas values derived from end-tidal PCO_2 analysis tended to overestimate low values and overestimate high values. *(Reprinted with permission from Orogian A, Corey SM, Calmelat R, et al. Validation of transcutaneous PCO₂ to estimate deadspace ventilation [VD/VT] during exercise in patients with COPD.* Am J Crit Care Med. *2018;197:A4326.)*

Pa_{CO_2} early into recovery from exercise.[38-40] Optimally, the sample should be drawn over an integral number of breaths spanning an interval of approximately 10 to 20 seconds, so the result can be matched with concurrent breath-by-breath gas exchange measurements averaged over the same time period. The radial artery is the more common site for a single sample; local anesthesia to that site administered before exercise reduces patient discomfort.

Multiple Samples of Arterial Blood by Catheterization

An indwelling arterial catheter makes repeated sampling of arterial blood for blood gases simple and fast and can also provide continuous monitoring of arterial blood pressure. The most common insertion sites are the radial and brachial arteries, and the same kinds of small-bore catheters used in intensive care unit for arterial catheterization can be used. With meticulous care, we have never had a serious complication of either brachial or radial artery catheterization in several thousand insertions. However, the radial artery site has the advantage that the ulnar artery can supply blood to the hand if the radial artery is injured, whereas the brachial artery is the sole blood supply of the lower arm. A disadvantage of the radial artery site is that it may interfere with gripping of the cycle ergometer handlebars; in addition, referring direct blood pressure measurements to the left atrial level may be more difficult. Potential complications of arterial punctures and catheterization include bleeding, arterial spasm, distal arterial thromboembolism, thrombosis, infection, and local pain or discomfort. Arterial catheters should be used with special care or avoided in patients with known peripheral arterial disease and in patients with clotting or bleeding disorders.

Free-Flowing Ear Capillary Blood

Some investigators and clinicians use free-flowing ear capillary blood as a substitute for arterial blood.[41] When such blood is used, it is important that the blood be free-flowing into the receiving capillary tube. The differences between concurrently collected ear capillary and arterial blood are both technique and exercise-intensity dependent. Therefore, it would be desirable for sites that use ear capillary blood to make some simultaneous capillary and arterial blood measures during rest and exercise to determine the pH, P_{CO_2}, and P_{O_2} differences between these sites. In optimal circumstances, there are trivial differences in pH values (<0.01 units), minor differences in P_{CO_2} values (1-2 mm Hg higher in capillary samples), but considerable differences in P_{O_2} values (5-10 mm Hg lower in capillary samples with Sa_{O_2} >90%). Thus, capillary values should be used cautiously in calculating and interpreting values of $P(a - ET)CO_2$, V_D/V_T, and $P(A - a)O_2$.

Invasive Cardiopulmonary Exercise Testing With Pulmonary Artery Catheter

For some patients, an invasive CPET with a pulmonary artery (PA) catheter and other simultaneous invasive and noninvasive testing (eg, echocardiography) may add valuable diagnostic information.[42,43] For example, it may be useful to measure central vascular pressures during exercise in selected patients with suspected primary or secondary pulmonary hypertension in whom resting PA pressures are not overtly elevated. The failure to recruit pulmonary capillary bed during exercise in patients with pulmonary vasculopathy can result in the PA pressure increasing strikingly even with a relatively small exercise-induced increase in blood flow. Similarly, in patients with impaired left ventricular relaxation, there could be significant increase in pulmonary capillary wedge pressure during exercise despite normal values at rest. The PA catheter also allows for sampling of mixed venous blood to quantify peripheral oxygen extraction and to calculate cardiac output.

The PA catheter is balloon tipped and flow directed and can be passed through a large vein in the arm through the right atrium, right ventricle, and into the PA, generally with fluoroscopic guidance in the catheterization laboratory prior to exercise testing. Because of the potential for arrhythmias and heart block during placement, insertion should be done with ECG monitoring and availability of appropriate resuscitation equipment and medications. For pressure measurements, a calibrated transducer and recorder are used. During exercise, especially with patients with lung disease, large swings in intrathoracic pressure with respiration may be transmitted to the PA and wedge pressures, and pressure measurements may therefore be subject to large variation with breathing. Intravascular pressures at end exhalation are selected by convention and are usually most relevant. Blood samples can be drawn from the PA distal port to be analyzed for mixed venous P_{O_2} and O_2 content needed for the calculation of cardiac output using the Fick equation (see Chapter 3) or calculation of venous admixture.

Cardiac output can also be determined by thermodilution (see Chapter 3), that is, by rapidly injecting a bolus of isotonic fluid (usually 5% dextrose in water) of known volume, temperature (usually 0°C), specific heat, and specific gravity into the right atrial port of the PA catheter and measuring the temperature change with a thermistor or temperature sensor at the catheter tip in the PA. The temperature change downstream reflects the volume of dilution of the bolus, and cardiac output can be calculated using an automated system. The integral of temperature over time is inversely proportional to cardiac output. Stetz et al[44] reviewed several studies and concluded that values of cardiac output determined by thermodilution in catheterization laboratories and ICUs were of comparable accuracy to those determined by Fick or dye-dilution methods. These authors suggested, however, that a 20% to 26% difference in cardiac output should be found before concluding that two single determinations were different. Advantages of thermodilution include safety, speed, and repeatability.

The use of invasive hemodynamic measurements increases the risks, costs, and preparation time of CPET. Although uncommon, complications can include arrhythmia, heart block, bleeding, perforation of the access vein or of the right ventricle or PA, and infections. Under specific circumstances, however, measuring of central circulatory pressures, quantifying changes in stroke volume or peripheral oxygen extraction, or determining the slope of cardiac output relative to $\dot{V}O_2$ over the course of progressive exercise provides critical diagnostic information otherwise not available from noninvasive testing alone. In such cases, the benefits gained can outweigh the risks of the procedures.

Data Sampling and Computation

Automated exercise gas exchange systems make use of computers for data collection, calculations, and data storage and display. The speed and capability of computerized calculations can correct data from nonlinear analyzers and make adjustments for different environmental or subject characteristics. Ergometer protocols can also be computer controlled allowing for near continuous changes in work rate. Typically, data sampled from a flow sensor, gas analyzer, pulse oximeter, HR monitor, or other device undergo analog-to-digital conversion under computer control. Accurate calculations require a sufficiently high sampling rate, which for most gas exchange systems is 100 Hz.

Many commercial CPET systems come with a variety of options for data display and can compile tables and graphs summarizing the results of CPETs in customizable formats (see Chapters 6 and 10). These tools facilitate data management and reporting and have the potential to be interfaced with electronic health records or other databases.

Quality Control, Validation, and Maintenance

Assessment and assurance of data quality in the CPET laboratory are extensively covered in the references.[1,6,8,11,12,45,46] Flow sensor validation is essential for confidence in the ability of the device to measure respired volumes accurately and reproducibly under testing conditions. Large volume syringes of 1 to 4 L that can deliver known inspiratory and expiratory volumes at very slow to very rapid flow rates are commonly used to calibrate flow devices. If the flow signals are further processed by analog or digital means, the results will be subject to the response characteristics and calculation methods of these instruments. Accurate flow integration is documented by constant volumes over the range of gas flows expected to be encountered. The accuracy of flow and volume can also be determined using a calibrated oscillating pump.

Gas analyzers should be checked for accuracy and linearity within the range of needed values. This can be done by using gases of known concentration of O_2 and CO_2. The Scholander and Haldane methods for gas analysis are accurate, but they are also time-consuming, tedious, and now uncommonly used.[47] They may be useful for initial calibration of gas analyzers and primary analysis of stored gases used for calibration purposes. Alternatively, gas having O_2 and CO_2 concentrations of acceptable precision can be obtained from a reliable gas supplier. Such high-precision gases are expensive, but such a tank may be kept for years and used only periodically to assay less expensive gases used for day-to-day calibration. After long storage, it is best to roll tanks to avoid gas stratification.

If an analyzer is nonlinear, a calibration curve can be constructed by observing the analyzer output at several gas concentrations. The analyzers should be warmed up for sufficient time to ensure against electrical drift. Once linearity has been established, a two-point calibration can be used. Room air is often used as one calibration point, assuming an O_2 concentration of 20.93% and CO_2 concentration of 0.04%. A calibration gas of approximately 15% O_2, 5% CO_2, and balance N_2 (but whose actual values are accurately known) is appropriate for the second point because these concentrations are near the expected expired gas concentrations.

For the breath-by-breath calculation of $\dot{V}O_2$ and $\dot{V}CO_2$, the gas transport delay time and the response time of each analyzer to the detection of a new gas concentration are important to know. How these play a role in the calculation is further addressed in Appendix C.

Treadmill speed and grade should be routinely checked for accuracy and reproducibility. Grade may be determined by using a plumb line and tape measure. Speed can be accurately determined by using a stopwatch to time the movement of a mark made on the treadmill belt.

Cycle calibration is highly desirable both during initial setup of the laboratory and periodically thereafter. Manufacturers' specifications and calibration procedures should be followed. Commercially available or specially built devices that generate known amounts of power can act as standards for calibration and verification

In the past, systems of analyzers and computers for determination of gas exchange during exercise were developed and assembled in individual laboratories. The first of these to report the requirements for a breath-by-breath system was Beaver et al.[13] This was later modified to a true alveolar breath-by-breath gas exchange system to correct for changes in alveolar volume and gas concentrations.[48] Many good exercise systems are now commercially available, although any system requires initial and ongoing validation and monitoring for accuracy and reproducibility of results.

Validation can be performed by simultaneous collection of mixed expired gas while the exercise system is collecting data. For mixing chamber and breath-by-breath systems, extremes of tidal volume and flow are particularly challenging. It is easiest to collect expired gas during the steady state of constant work rate exercise, but such validation may not provide evidence of accurate measurement during rapidly changing exercise protocols or when the focus is on short-term changes in gas exchange.

A particularly useful device is an automated metabolic calibrator that simulates gas exchange at a known and reproducible rate. One type of calibrator uses a pump of known volume and measurable frequency to provide an accurate "expired minute ventilation."[49] Gas exchange rates

($\dot{V}O_2$ and $\dot{V}CO_2$) with an R value of approximately 1 are simulated by the introduction of a gas mixture containing 21% CO_2 and balance N_2 into a reservoir bag where it mixes with room air (or the "inspirate") to yield the "expirate," which is then drawn into the gas exchange measurement system by the calibrator pump. The $\dot{V}O_2$ and $\dot{V}CO_2$ measured by the system should be equal to 0.21 × the flow rate of the 21% CO_2 in N_2 mixture flowing into the reservoir bag. The R is somewhat higher than 1.0 because the CO_2 concentration (21.00%) is slightly higher than the O_2 concentration in room air (20.93%). An adjustment of the exercise system algorithms may be necessary to accommodate the nearly dry room-temperature gas delivered by the calibrator to the gas exchange measuring device that is set up to measure under body temperature, saturated conditions. This metabolic calibrator has been demonstrated to provide an accurate simulation of gas exchange that can be used for validation and for detection of the source of instrument or algorithm errors when an erroneous value is detected. In addition, the device is useful for routine periodic checks of reproducibility. If an error (or change) in measured $\dot{V}E$, $\dot{V}O_2$, or $\dot{V}CO_2$ is found, analysis of the differences in the measurements may also suggest the nature of the problem. Commercial providers may be able to offer this service for a charge if requested.

However, "biological" calibration provides an inexpensive and relatively simple way to test the validity of the entire system, including the ergometer.[46,50] This requires a healthy individual (typically a member of the laboratory personnel) to cycle at two or three constant sub-*AT* work rates, for example, 20 and 70 W, for 6 minutes each. On such tests, the $\dot{V}O_2$ after 3 minutes should be in a steady state, and the $\dot{V}O_2$ difference for this 50 W increment should be approximately 500 mL/min (ie, corresponding to 10 mL/min/W) and within 5% to 10% of previously measured values (approximately 0.7 L/min for an individual of average size exercising at 20 W and 1.2 L/min at 70 W, with a difference of 0.5 ± 0.05 L/min). Values significantly deviant from prior tests suggest errors in flow, gas analyzer, or delay measurements or errors in ergometer calibration. If the tested individual can control his or her breathing frequency appropriately, there should be less than 5% difference in $\dot{V}O_2$ whether breathing at a frequency of 15, 30, or 60 breaths/min. Although this can be challenging to perform, it is an excellent test of the validity of gas analyzer transit delay times and the rapidity of gas analyzer responses: greater variation in $\dot{V}O_2$ values at higher breathing frequencies suggesting errors in analyzer delay and/or response time.

The accuracy and precision of the gas exchange measurement system assessed by "biological" calibration can be evaluated using the combined *z* score method.[46] The combined *z* score assigns 0.5 of the *z* score to $\dot{V}O_2$ at 70 W and 0.5 to the $\dot{V}O_2$-WR slope. The quality control results of a larger clinical trial employing treadmill exercise demonstrated that if the combined *z* score is <0.7, both the accuracy and the precision are acceptable. With a combined *z* score between 0.7 and 0.9, the accuracy is still acceptable, and the coefficient of variation, due to nonnormal distribution of the sample, is greater than desired but still <10%.[46] Systematic biological quality control is needed in multicenter clinical trials in order to assure the accuracy and precision of all sites' CPET systems. Keeping the standard deviation consistently low will benefit the power analysis and the final results of the study.

Many commercial systems have an option to print a listing of the current status of environmental conditions, gas analyzers, calibration gas concentrations, temperature, and other important system variables, including historical values. These validation and reproducibility data should be regularly reviewed and kept for future reference and evidence of change, since this information can be helpful in identifying and resolving problems.

PREPARING FOR THE EXERCISE TEST

The objective of CPET should be to learn the maximum about the extent and/or cause of a patient's exercise limitation with the greatest accuracy, with the least required stress to the patient, and in the shortest period of time. The optimal examination allows the simultaneous evaluation of the adequacy of the muscles, heart, the peripheral and pulmonary circulations, and the lungs to meet the gas exchange requirements of exercise. The exercise test should enable the investigator to distinguish disorders in these systems from inadequate effort, obesity, anxiety, or deconditioning.

For the differential diagnosis of exercise limitation caused by cardiovascular or respiratory disease and also to extract indices relevant to judgments on interventional change and prognostication, relatively complete gas exchange measurements should be made. Exercise with large muscle groups is needed to stimulate internal respiration sufficiently to stress the cardiovascular and pulmonary systems. Therefore, either a cycle ergometer or a treadmill should be used. Isometric exercise is of limited value because it is largely anaerobic, providing little information about the ability of the cardiovascular and respiratory systems to support the energy requirements of sustained exercise. The protocol selected for exercise testing depends on the purpose of the test (see "Performing the Exercise Test" in the following text).

Requesting the Test and Notifying the Patient

We request relevant demographic and clinical information in advance of the test from the patient's referring clinician including the following:

- Patient's name and contact information
- Patient's weight, height, gender, and age
- Known or tentative medical diagnoses and current medications
- The indication or reason for the study
- Type of test requested and special requirements

In the case of testing for diagnostic purposes, results of prior diagnostic tests, laboratory measures, and imaging studies are extremely useful. The referring clinician may not be familiar with CPET procedures or know what information is most relevant to provide. Optimally, therefore, a direct discussion with the referring clinician should occur so that the purpose of the test is clear beforehand. This helps the laboratory decide several issues regarding the protocol, specifically whether the cycle or treadmill is the preferable form of ergometry, whether an arterial or even a PA catheter is desired, whether measurements should be included to assess for exercise-induced bronchospasm or dynamic hyperinflation, and whether supplemental O_2 is needed during the exercise test (see Chapter 3).

At the time the exercise test is scheduled, the patient is advised to wear comfortable nonbinding clothing and low-heeled or athletic shoes, eat no more than a light meal 2 or more hours before arrival, avoid cigarettes and coffee for at least 2 hours prior to testing, and take his or her usual scheduled medications. The only exception to the latter is when testing is performed to assess for exercise-induced bronchoconstriction, for which medications modifying this response should be suspended. The patient is also provided a brief description of the exercise test, including how long it will take and what to expect.

The Patient in the Exercise Laboratory

Preliminary Tests

Because spirometric data are used in the final report, the vital capacity, inspiratory capacity, forced expiratory volume in 1 second (FEV_1), and maximum voluntary ventilation (MVV) should be obtained when the patient arrives at the exercise laboratory according to published standards.[51] The direct MVV can be calculated from a 12-second maneuver of rapid and deep breathing or the indirect MVV by multiplying the FEV_1 by 40. The MVV values are needed for determination of the exercise breathing reserve (see Chapter 3). In patients with conditions that constrain deep rapid breathing, such as inspiratory obstruction, neuromuscular disorders, or severe obesity, the direct MVV should be used even if it is considerably less than the indirect MVV. In other patients with poor spirometric efforts, the indirect MVV is usually a more reliable measure of ventilatory capacity.

Recent hemoglobin and, ideally, current carboxyhemoglobin levels, should be known or measured as well as the resting diffusing capacity of the lung for carbon monoxide (D_{LCO}) in those patients with lung disease or dyspnea. An accurate shoeless height and weight should be obtained the day of testing.

Physician Evaluation

The physician should obtain relevant clinical information directly from the patient and available medical records, with particular emphasis on medications, tobacco and recreational drug use, accustomed activity level, the presence of angina or other exercise-induced symptoms, or conditions that could represent contraindications to testing. A focused examination should be performed on the day of testing with particular attention to the heart, lungs, peripheral pulses, and musculoskeletal system. If this examination reveals findings such as decompensated heart or lung disease, or inadequately controlled blood pressure, testing should usually be deferred until these are medically optimized. The physician determines the type of exercise test and protocol on the basis of the exercise request, the clinical evaluation, review of the current ECG and other preliminary tests, and any other special considerations.

Informed consent for the exercise test is needed. The patient should be told what to expect and that he or she will be asked to make a maximal effort (for most studies) but also advised that exercise can be stopped at any time. The patient is advised that, if the laboratory staff note any patient safety issues (eg, arrhythmias, ischemia, marked desaturation), the test will be stopped. The patient is advised of potential discomfort and risks associated with the procedure, the kinds of information that will be obtained, and how this may benefit him or her. Finally, the patient is encouraged to ask questions about the testing before giving consent. Because patients may be apprehensive about performing exercise, it is helpful to explicitly identify that the test is designed to begin at an easy level and increase in difficulty gradually, is individualized to their capabilities, and can be stopped at any time.

Equipment Familiarization

We find it particularly useful to familiarize the patient with the exercise testing equipment before starting the actual test. If the treadmill is used, time is provided for practice trials so the patient can get on and off the moving treadmill belt with confidence. If the cycle is used, the position of the handlebars is adjusted, and the seat height is adjusted so the legs are nearly completely extended when the pedals are at their lowest point and the cadence is checked to ensure the patient can cycle effectively. These settings should be noted for future reference.

The mask or mouthpiece and nose clip are demonstrated before the actual test. The patient is advised that it is acceptable to swallow with the mouthpiece in place, moisten the inside of the mouth with the tongue, or cough but to refrain from talking as it affects the data quality. We also explain the importance of having a good seal of the lips around the mouthpiece or the mask about the face.

Ending the Exercise

We advise patients that they can stop exercise if they feel distressed. Alternatively, we stop the exercise if we note important abnormalities. Because a mouthpiece or mask interferes with the ability of the patient to communicate verbally in response to questions regarding symptoms, the patient is encouraged to use the signal "thumbs up" if everything is satisfactory and "thumbs down" if he or she is experiencing any difficulty but does not wish to stop. The patient is advised to point to the site of discomfort (eg, chest or leg), and the technician or physician will explore the details of the discomfort.

Arterial Blood Sampling and Use of Catheter

If the study requires repeated arterial blood sampling, a catheter is inserted into a peripheral artery. To avoid spurious dilution of the blood specimen with heparin-containing solution, the dead space of the catheter tubing (usually about 0.5 mL of fluid) is discarded before collecting each arterial blood sample. Each sample is collected over 10 to 20 seconds so that the measured gas partial pressures are minimally influenced by respiratory variations and are therefore representative of mean arterial values. The catheter lumen is flushed with heparinized saline between samples. We usually sample blood at rest, at the end of 3 minutes of unloaded cycling or lowest level treadmill exercise, every 2 minutes during the period of increasing work rate, and at 2 minutes of recovery, but the number and frequency of samples is dependent on the purpose of the test.

After use, the arterial catheter is removed with the same precautions applicable to other medical contexts, including keeping direct pressure over the puncture site for at least 5 to 10 minutes to minimize hematoma formation. The site is then inspected carefully for evidence of bleeding, and pressure is continued for additional time if needed. A light dressing covered with a firm elastic bandage is then applied over the puncture site, and the peripheral pulses are checked. The patient is advised to remove the dressing after 4 to 6 hours and to not use that arm for heavy exercise for the next 24 hours

After an exercise test with blood sampling, it is advisable to review the blood gas results before discarding any remaining blood in the sampling syringes. This makes it possible to reanalyze samples for which the results are questionable.

PERFORMING THE EXERCISE TEST

The following sections describe several different protocols that are used for addressing various clinical questions. Most often, we use a maximum (symptom-limited) incremental exercise test on a cycle ergometer; this protocol is described in detail here. It addresses most clinical and fitness issues. However, if the patient is being evaluated for detection of exercise-induced bronchospasm, value of oxygen supplementation in exercise, or other reasons, other protocols may be more appropriate.

Incremental Exercise Test to Symptom-Limited Maximum

In this protocol, the patient exercises on a cycle ergometer (or a treadmill) while measurements of gas exchange are made (ideally breath by breath) at rest, during 3 minutes of unloaded cycling (or level grade walking for treadmill), and throughout the incremental phase where the work rate is increased each minute (incremental) or continuously (ramp pattern). In general, the patient should be encouraged to continue as long as he or she feels able. This encouragement is usually sufficient for most patients to go to their reproducible peak $\dot{V}O_2$. In some contexts, particularly if there is history of exertional syncope or other concerning symptoms, we do not coax patients to maximal exertion but advise them to stop exercise at a level that they would normally do so in their daily activities.

Selecting the Rate of Work Rate Increase

We select the rate of work rate increase after considering the patient's history (especially the amount and intensity of his or her daily activity), physical examination (notably, obesity and evidence of cardiac or respiratory disease), and pulmonary function evaluation (particularly, the FEV_1 and MVV). If we expect the patient to reach a near-normal work rate, we estimate the $\dot{V}O_2$ at unloaded pedaling from the patient's body weight and estimate the peak $\dot{V}O_2$ from the patient's age and height. We then calculate the work rate increment necessary to reach the patient's estimated peak $\dot{V}O_2$ in 10 minutes. The steps that we use to approximate the correct increment for the cycle are as follows:

1. $\dot{V}O_2$ unloaded in milliliters per minute = 150 + (6 × weight in kilograms)
2. Peak $\dot{V}O_2$ in milliliters per minute = (height in centimeters − age in years) multiplied by 20 for sedentary men or by 14 for sedentary women (or calculated from normal reference equations, as discussed in Chapter 7)
3. Work rate increment per minute in W = (peak $\dot{V}O_2$ in milliliters per minute − $\dot{V}O_2$ unloaded in milliliters per minute) / 100

For example, given an apparently healthy sedentary man 180 cm in height, 100 kg in weight, and 50 years of age, his anticipated $\dot{V}O_2$ unloaded in milliliters per minute = 150 + 6 × 100 kg = 750 mL/min; and his anticipated peak $\dot{V}O_2$ = (180 − 50) × 20 = 2600 mL/min. To achieve an incremental test duration of 10 minutes, we would therefore use a work rate increment of (2600 − 750) / 100 = 18.5 W/min. Practically, we would select an increment of 20 W/min and expect the test duration to be slightly less than 10 minutes.

If the patient has history or symptoms suggestive of chronic disease that will limit exercise capacity, the expected peak $\dot{V}O_2$ in step 2 is reduced the amount being judged by our preexercise assessment of impairment. Ideally, we reduce the size of the work rate increment in an attempt to keep the total incremental exercise time at about 10 minutes. In some patients, their disease is so severe that they cannot tolerate incremental exercise for more than a few minutes. With too large an increment, the test will be too brief, although the patient will recover quickly, which is an advantage if retesting is necessary. With too small an increment, however, the patient may stop for ambiguous reasons and may feel too fatigued for retesting. It is important to stress that we do not concern ourselves with attaining an exercise duration of exactly 10 minutes. We prefer it to be shorter rather than longer than the 10-minute target because we are likely to get a more reproducible and therefore easier test for interpretation (eg, for *AT* estimation, see Chapter 3). Exercise tests as short as 5 minutes can often be satisfactorily interpreted.

When the patient has severe cardiovascular or pulmonary disease or extreme obesity (with extreme obesity, leg cycling at 60 rpm without an added load may require a $\dot{V}O_2$ of as much as 1.0 L/min), a modified protocol can be useful, in which, after the rest period, the work rate is incremented less rapidly than usual and with an extended lower work rate range. For this, the 3-minute unloaded pedaling phase (with an accessory motor engaged: see "Cycle Ergometer" above) occurs at a pedaling rate of 20 rpm. The incremental phase then starts with the patient still cycling with no added load but at an increased pedaling rate of 40 rpm for a minute, followed by a pedaling rate of 60 rpm for the next minute. With the patient continuing to pedal at 60 rpm, the work rate is then increased by 5 to 10 W/min for the remainder of the test. This protocol allows the accumulation of more data at a tolerable metabolic rate and frequently allows delineation of very low *AT* values that are otherwise unmeasurable because they were exceeded during the first phase of the test.

Resting Measures

A 12-lead ECG may be obtained with the patient in the supine position and again when in the upright exercise position. If an arterial catheter is placed, resting blood samples are obtained in the supine and sitting positions, before the patient breathes through the mouthpiece. After the patient is positioned on the cycle or treadmill and is made comfortable, the breathing apparatus is attached, either mouthpiece and nose clip, or face mask, and checked for leaks.

The HR, breathing frequency or tidal volume, $\dot{V}E$, $\dot{V}O_2$, $\dot{V}CO_2$, $\dot{V}E/\dot{V}CO_2$, ventilatory equivalent for O_2, R, $PETO_2$, $PETCO_2$, and SpO_2 can be displayed or graphed in real-time on a monitor. Although these are measured breath by breath, it is most useful to monitor values averaged over several breathes or time periods of 10 seconds or so as the data are collected. The ECG tracings should also be visible. The measured and calculated variables are plotted after the test, as shown in Chapters 6 and 10. With an arterial catheter, arterial blood pressure can be recorded continuously and arterial blood is sampled for blood gases, pH, lactate, co-oximetry, and hemoglobin values at rest and during exercise. If an arterial catheter is not used, blood pressure is obtained with a pressure cuff. Inspiratory capacity maneuvers, if desired, should be obtained initially at rest on the cycle or treadmill and then every 2 minutes throughout the exercise test to minimize the effect on data collection.

Unloaded Exercise and Cycling Rate

To overcome the inertia of the cycle flywheel with an electromagnetically braked cycle, an accessory motor can be used to rotate the flywheel at a rate of slightly over 60 rpm while the patient's feet are motionless on the pedals (see "Cycle Ergometer" above). At a verbal signal, the patient begins 3 minutes of unloaded pedaling. An rpm meter or metronome may be used to assist the patient in maintaining a cadence of 60 rpm. After the patient has established the cycling rhythm, the motor controlling the flywheel speed is turned off so that the patient controls the speed of the unloaded flywheel. A 12-lead ECG, blood pressure measurement, and, if the patient has an arterial catheter, a blood sample are obtained near the end of the 3 minutes of unloaded pedaling. During this initial period of exercise, a new baseline of metabolic rate and cardiorespiratory output is established in the moderate (below *AT*) domain of exercise, prior to beginning the linear increase in work rate. Omitting this initial stage of the test can complicate interpretation of the exercise data since the dynamic responses to the step-up in metabolic rate at the start of exercise, and responses to progressively increasing work rate, are superimposed.

Incremental Exercise

Measurements are continued while the work rate is increased continuously (ramp test)[52] or by a uniform amount each minute (incremental test) until the patient is limited by symptoms or the examiner believes that exercise cannot be continued safely (**Fig. 5.3**). A 12-lead ECG is monitored continuously for arrhythmias and ischemic signs and recorded every 1 or 2 minutes. Arterial blood samples for blood gas and pH measurement are ordinarily obtained every 2 minutes if the patient has an indwelling arterial catheter. The technician and physician work cooperatively in observing the patient's facial expression, monitoring blood pressure and ECG signals for untoward changes and arrhythmias, looking for nose or mouthpiece leaks, observing for signals of distress from the patient, and quietly encouraging the patient to maximize his or her performance. This is done by commenting on the satisfactory nature of the study as well as encouraging patients to do their best but to stop when they feel that they must. The resistance of the cycle is removed for evidence of patient distress, a consistent fall in systolic or mean blood pressure greater than 20 mm Hg, significant arrhythmia, or ST segment depression of 3 mm or greater with symptoms of angina, or if the patient stops on his or her own volition. The exercise is also terminated if the patient is unable to consistently maintain the cycling frequency above 40 to 45 rpm or to keep pace with the belt on the treadmill without use of handrail support. The test should not be stopped for arbitrary endpoints, such as an HR $>85\%$, $\dot{V}E/MVV >85\%$, an R value above 1.1 or 1.15, etc.

Recovery

We ask the patient to continue to breathe through the mouthpiece during 2 to 3 minutes of recovery, unless there

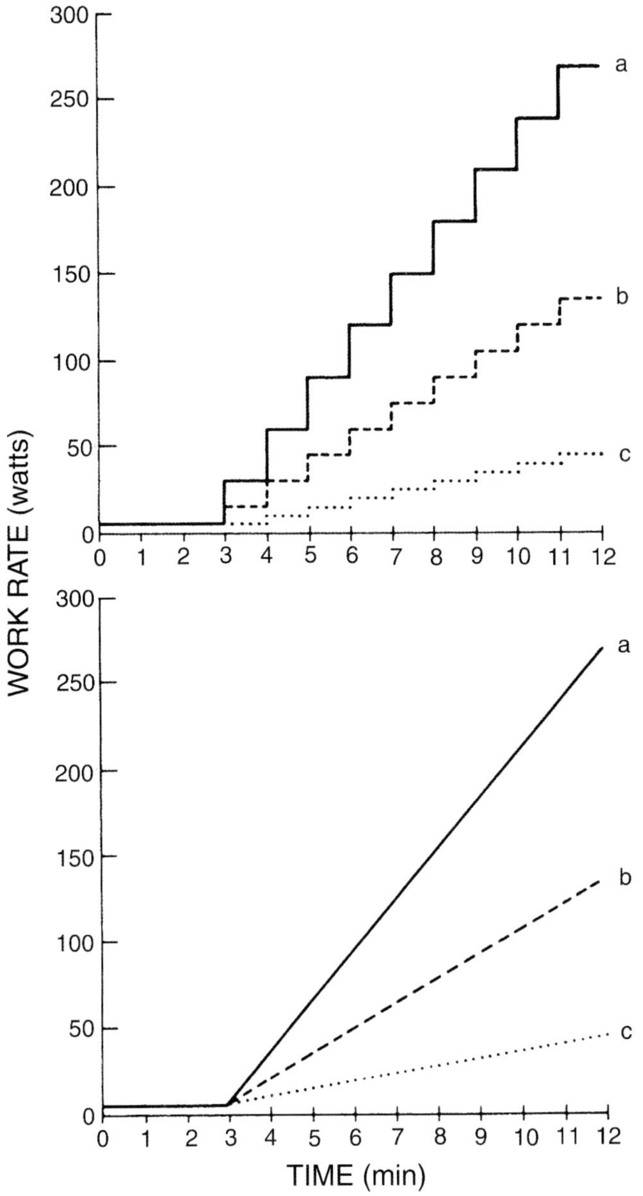

FIGURE 5.3. One-minute incremental (upper) and ramp incremental (lower) protocols for cycle ergometry. In both cases, the subject initially cycles for 3 min of unloaded pedaling. In the example shown, the work rate is incremented 30 W (a), 15 W (b), or 5 W (c) per minute depending on the height, age, gender, and health of the subject. The increment is added at the start of each minute for the 1-min test, whereas for the ramp test the work rate is increased continuously (eg, second by second) with the increment value being attained at the end of each minute. Larger or intermediate increments can also be used. The load is returned to the unloaded setting when the cycling frequency cannot be maintained over 40 rpm or when the physician or subject decides to terminate the exercise.

are safety concerns dictating otherwise. In the immediate postexercise period, the patient is advised to continue to pedal at a slow frequency without a load on the ergometer or to walk at a slow pace at zero grade on the treadmill. This leg movement tends to minimize the precipitous fall in blood pressure and light-headedness that may be experienced with the abrupt decrease in venous return due to lower extremity vasodilatation. Attention to the patient and the monitoring devices continue during recovery as exercise-induced arrhythmias or hypoxemia may persist or worsen in the first few minutes after exercise ends. If blood is being sampled via a catheter, a final sample is obtained at 2 minutes of recovery, since this is when lactate concentrations peak and pH values reach their nadir.

Postexercise Questioning and Review

At the conclusion of the test and soon after removal of the mouthpiece, the examiner should question the patient in a nonleading fashion about what caused him or her to stop exercise. A series of questions may be required to assess just what the patient means by his or her limiting symptoms, for example, "Did your lungs or your legs limit your exercise?" It is important to differentiate calf from thigh pain and to determine the exact character of any chest discomfort and when it occurred during exercise or recovery. In particular, it is always worthwhile to find out if the symptoms reproduce the complaints of exertional dyspnea, chest pain, or other discomfort experienced by the patient outside the laboratory.

If, on review of the data, it appears that a symptom-limited test was terminated prematurely because of suboptimal patient effort, a repeat test after a recovery period of 30 to 45 minutes may be indicated. For instance, if the patient made an insufficient effort, as suggested by the combination of high breathing and HR reserves, a low R, and only a slight fall in arterial [bicarbonate] (if measured), the test bears repeating with greater encouragement from the examiner. In these repeat tests, the reproducibility of the patient's performance should be examined. We believe having a physician in the room helps with both safety and encouragement in obtaining a maximal effort.

Incremental Tests

A number of exercise protocols have been described using consistent increases in work rate at regular intervals. Balke and colleagues[53,54] introduced the use of 1-minute incremental treadmill tests for the study of fitness in military personnel, using a constant treadmill speed and either a 1% or 2% increment in grade per minute. Others, including Consolazio et al,[55] Jones,[56] and Spiro,[57] used the cycle ergometer with the work rate incremented an equal amount every minute or half minute.[58] We introduced the use of a continuously incrementing (ramp-pattern) exercise protocol in 1981 and have used it extensively since then in adults and children.[52]

As discussed in Chapter 3, when comparing the ramp test with 1-, 2-, and 3-minute incremental tests at the same overall average work rate increase, there are no significant differences in peak $\dot{V}O_2$, *AT*, peak $\dot{V}E$, peak HR, $\dot{V}O_2$-WR slope, or exercise duration in healthy individuals. Step patterns in some measures could be seen in the 2- and 3-minute incremental protocols, however (see **Fig. 3.3**). Thus, although any of these protocols might be used, either the ramp or the

1-minute incremental test seems most practical and preferable for patients because they do not feel sudden increases in work rate.

A number of observations support the desirability of adjusting the work rate increment according to the patient's cardiorespiratory status. Tests that are too brief (ie, with the work rate increased too rapidly) may not allow a sufficient quantity of data to be accumulated. Tests that are too long (ie, with too small a work rate increase) are likely to be terminated prematurely because of boredom or "seat discomfort." We found that tests in which the incremental part of the protocol is completed between 6 and 12 minutes give the highest peak $\dot{V}O_2$ in healthy individuals.[59] Longer or shorter tests are likely to give slightly lower values. We know of no similar study in patients with heart or lung disease but assume that the findings would be similar. Therefore, we attempt to select a work rate increment that will result in termination of the incremental part of the exercise test in 8 to 10 minutes, but tests as short as 5 minutes are acceptable.

It can be asked whether the peak $\dot{V}O_2$ is as high in continuous incremental protocols as in discontinuous protocols and, therefore, whether the highest $\dot{V}O_2$ reached (peak $\dot{V}O_2$) should be identified as the $\dot{V}O_2$max. As discussed in Chapters 2 and 3, Taylor et al[60] defined the $\dot{V}O_2$max from a series of progressively fatiguing constant work rate tests as the $\dot{V}O_2$ at which further increases in work rate resulted in an increase of $\dot{V}O_2$ of less than 150 mL/min. This criterion is appropriate for tests in fit individuals using large work rate increments, such as a 2.5% grade change at a treadmill speed of 7 mph. In tests featuring a 15 W/min increase in work rate, however, the normal rate of increase in $\dot{V}O_2$ is only 150 mL/min. Therefore, at increments of 15 W/min or less, the criterion of Taylor et al[60] is not relevant to discerning whether the peak $\dot{V}O_2$ is indeed the $\dot{V}O_2$max.

A single study[61] reported an approximately 10% lower peak $\dot{V}O_2$ using a continuous rather than a discontinuous graded work rate treadmill test, although the long duration (20-30 min) of the continuous tests in this analysis could have accounted for this. In contrast, others[62,63] found no systematic difference in peak $\dot{V}O_2$ measured in continuous incremental treadmill tests compared with discontinuous constant work rate tests. Pollock and colleagues[64] found a plateau in $\dot{V}O_2$ in 59% to 69% of the continuous incremental treadmill tests they administered. We found a similar peak $\dot{V}O_2$ in healthy males for ramp-incremental cycle ergometer tests, whether the increase was 20, 30, or 50 W/min.[65] Thus, we believe that the $\dot{V}O_2$max can be approximated with continuous incremental protocols of the proper duration and that peak $\dot{V}O_2$ is the appropriate term for the oxygen uptake value at the end of the test, if it was considered to be maximal patient effort.

As described in Chapter 3, a modified CPET protocol has been proposed for verifying whether the peak $\dot{V}O_2$ measured on an incremental test is a valid approximation of maximal $\dot{V}O_2$.[66] For this, a brief period of cycling to tolerance at an effectively supramaximal work rate follows shortly after completing the incremental test (see **Fig. 3.1**). Although this approach has not had wide use in clinical testing, it is reported to be well tolerated even by patients with chronic heart failure. Using the ramp exercise test, we also found that the *AT*, the $\dot{V}O_2$ time constant, work efficiency, peak $\dot{V}E$, and peak HR were comparable to values found with constant work rate tests.[52,65] Because we were concerned that the non–steady-state incremental exercise test might give different values for $\dot{V}E$, $\dot{V}O_2$, $\dot{V}CO_2$, $P(A - a)O_2$, $P(a - ET)CO_2$, and HR as compared to steady-state sub-*AT* constant work rate exercise at the same $\dot{V}O_2$, we studied 23 men (11 normal and 12 with chronic lung disease) using both test formats (**Table 5.2**).[67] We found that $\dot{V}CO_2$, $\dot{V}E$, PaO_2, and R were slightly lower during incremental exercise than constant work rate exercise at the same $\dot{V}O_2$. These differences were consistent with the influence of the response kinetics of $\dot{V}CO_2$ and $\dot{V}E$ throughout the non–steady-state incremental test. However, the $P(A - a)O_2$, $P(a - ET)CO_2$, $PaCO_2$, $\dot{V}E/\dot{V}CO_2$, and VD/VT values were in close agreement in both protocols for both the normal individuals and the patients. This was important in

TABLE 5.2 Effect of Protocol on Measurements of PaO_2, $P(A - a)O_2$, and VD/VT During Cycling at the Same Mean $\dot{V}O_2$ (0.92 ± 0.03 L/min)[a]

		PaO_2, mm Hg		$P(A - a)O_2$, mm Hg		VD/VT	
	N	Incremental[b]	Constant[c]	Incremental	Constant	Incremental	Constant
Normal	11	89	94	14	13	0.26	0.25
Restrictive lung disease	3	87	89	18	21	0.21	0.19
Obstructive lung disease	9	79	83	25	22	0.32	0.32
All subjects	23	85[d]	89	19	17	0.27	0.28

Abbreviations: $P(A - a)O_2$, alveolar-arterial PO_2 difference; VD/VT, physiological dead space–tidal volume ratio; $\dot{V}O_2$, oxygen uptake.

[a]Data from Furuike AN, Sue DY, Hansen JE, Wasserman K. Comparison of physiologic dead space/tidal volume ratio and alveolar-arterial PO_2 difference during incremental and constant work exercise. *Am Rev Respir Dis.* 1982;126:579-583.

[b]One-minute incremental exercise protocol.

[c]Constant moderate-intensity work rate protocol; measurements were made at 6 min.

[d]Indicates significant difference between 1-min incremental and constant work rate test at $P < .05$ by paired *t* test; other differences are not significantly different.

demonstrating that it is possible to make measurements of gas exchange and ventilation-perfusion matching equally well during incremental as during moderate steady-state exercise.

Constant Work Rate Exercise Tests

As discussed in Chapters 2 and 3, exercise tests performed with individuals exercising at a constant work rate may be useful in particular situations. The design of such tests requires the patient to have previously completed a standard incremental exercise test. The selection of the appropriate work rate depends on the question being addressed and the number of different work rates that are chosen. For example, sub-*AT* tests are useful in determining ventilatory and gas exchange kinetics, with supplemental supra-*AT* tests allowing the influence of the $\dot{V}O_2$ "slow component" to be quantitated. Sub-*AT* tests are also the basis for the biological quality control processes described earlier in this chapter. High-intensity, supra-*AT*, tests performed to the limit of tolerance allow $\dot{V}O_2max$ to be determined. Also, the tolerable duration of such tests (t_{lim}) has proved to be a more sensitive index of therapeutic efficacy (eg, exercise, pharmacological therapy, supplemental O_2, heliox breathing) than indices such as peak $\dot{V}O_2$ on an incremental exercise test. This has proven to be an extremely effective way of assessing efficacy of interventions in clinical trials directed at improving exercise tolerance. In situations where the *AT* cannot be convincingly estimated from an incremental exercise test, constant work rate tests spanning the likely region of the *AT* can be useful. The contribution of the carotid bodies to the exercise hyperpnea during exercise can be judged from the magnitude of transient $\dot{V}E$ decline in response to the surreptitious imposition of brief episodes of hyperoxia. Finally, near-maximal constant work rate tests are the preferred protocol for the diagnosis of exercise-induced bronchospasm.

Treadmill Test for Detecting Myocardial Ischemia

Incremental treadmill exercise protocols have long been used for provoking and detecting ECG changes consistent with myocardial ischemia, some of which are illustrated in **Figure 5.4**.

Notably, Bruce[68] developed a protocol that begins with 3-minute stages of walking at 1.7 mph at 0%, 5%, or 10% grade (**Fig. 5.4C**). The 0% and 5% grades are omitted in fitter individuals. Thereafter, the grade is incremented 2% every 3 minutes and the speed is incremented 0.8 mph every 3 minutes until the treadmill reaches 18% grade and 5 mph. After this, the speed is increased by 0.5 mph every 3 minutes. The Ellestad[69] protocol uses seven periods, each of 2 or 3 minutes' duration, at progressively increasing speeds of 1.7, 3, 4, 5, 6, 7, and 8 mph (**Fig. 5.4E**). The grade is 10% for the first four periods, with durations of 3, 2, 2, and 3 minutes, respectively, and 15% grade for the last three periods, each of 2 minutes' duration. Patterson et al[70] used 10 exercise periods of 3 minutes' duration, each separated by rest periods of 3 minutes (**Fig. 5.4A**). The grade and speed of each period were 0% and 1 mph, 0% and 1.5 mph, 0% and 2 mph, 3.5% and 2 mph, 7% and 2 mph, 5% and 3 mph, 7.5% and 3 mph, 10% and 3 mph, 12.5% and 3 mph, and 15% and 3 mph.

In each of these treadmill protocols, blood pressure is measured and a multiple-lead ECG is recorded at each work rate and during recovery. From this, the rate pressure product (systolic blood pressure multiplied by HR) can be calculated as an index of cardiac oxygen requirement. Tests are terminated at the physician's discretion (eg, for decline in blood pressure, significant arrhythmia, progressive ST segment changes, or attainment of a given HR) or by the patient's symptoms.

Itoh et al[71] and Belardinelli et al[72] advanced the application of the exercise ECG in diagnosing myocardial ischemia by combining it with gas exchange measurements. They found that accompanying changes in the ECG, the $\dot{V}O_2$-WR relationship becomes more shallow, providing evidence of myocardial dyskinesis.

Comment

These treadmill protocols have had extensive clinical use, and experience with them has provided important information on the safety of incremental exercise in individuals with suspected heart disease. A survey in 1977 concluded that the complication rate for such exercise stress testing was 3.6 myocardial infarctions, 4.8 serious arrhythmias, and 0.5 deaths per 10 000 tests.[73] In this survey, the treadmill was the ergometer used most often (71%), and the most common protocol was that of Bruce (65%). Recent safety data indicates a 2 to 5 per 100 000 mortality in a population undergoing evaluation for lung and heart transplantation.[1,74]

The peak $\dot{V}O_2$ is generally 5% to 11% higher with treadmill as compared with cycle ergometer testing, whereas peak HR is similar. Bruce et al[75] showed a high correlation between peak $\dot{V}O_2$ and the duration of treadmill exercise in their normal population. The $\dot{V}O_2$-WR relationship can be distorted by cardiovascular disease, however, so using the duration of exercise as a measure of peak $\dot{V}O_2$ in patients suspected of having cardiovascular disease is not reliable, or is peak HR given the variability in peak HR and wide use of β-adrenergic blocking drugs. The $\dot{V}E$, breathing pattern, and gas exchange have not routinely been measured in testing using these protocols, so information on gas exchange and pulmonary system function is not available. The unequal duration of increment and variability in increment size are disadvantages of these tests, since it makes it difficult to compare results of one protocol to another, especially when interpretation is not based on measurements of $\dot{V}O_2$.

Treadmill Tests With Even Increments in Work Rate

In contrast to the above protocols, Jones[56] and Buchfuhrer et al[59] proposed using a constant treadmill speed and incrementing the grade by a constant amount each minute for the entire study, similar to the Balke protocol. After 3 minutes of warm-up at zero grade at a comfortable walking speed

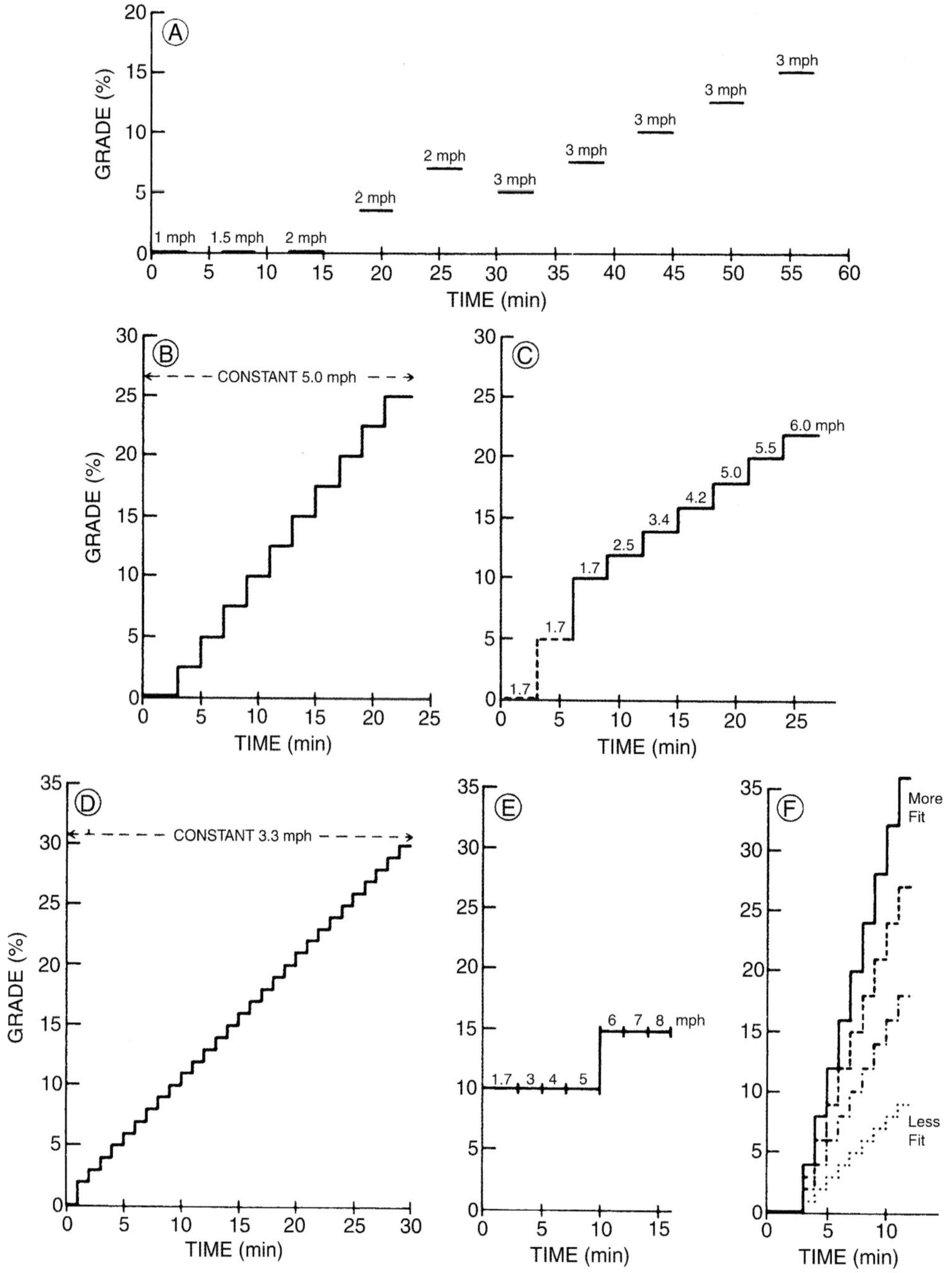

FIGURE 5.4. Profiles of several widely used treadmill protocols. A: Naughton protocol. Three-minute exercise periods of increasing work rate alternate with 3-min rest periods. The exercise periods vary in grade and speed. B: Åstrand protocol. The speed is constant at 5 mph. After 3 min at 0% grade, the grade is increased 2.5% every 2 min. C: Bruce protocol. Grade and speed are changed every 3 min. The 0% and 5% grades are omitted in healthier individuals. D: Balke protocol. After 1 min at 0% grade and 1 min at 2% grade, the grade is increased 1% per minute, all at a speed of 3.3 mph. E: Ellestad protocol. The initial grade is 10% and the later grade is 15% while the speed is increased every 2 or 3 min. F: Modified Balke protocol. After 3 min of walking at a comfortable speed, the grade is increased at a constant preselected amount each minute—1%, 2%, or 3%—so that the subject reaches his or her peak oxygen uptake in approximately 10 min.

(which may range from 0.8 to 4.5 mph, depending on the examiner's assessment of the patient's fitness), we use an even grade increment of 1%, 2%, or 3% each minute, also based on estimated capacity, to the patient's maximum tolerance. Speed and grade are selected with the goal of there being approximately 10 minutes of incremental exercise (**Fig. 5.4F**).

We have also successfully used the more recently developed treadmill protocol of Porszasz et al[19] (see "Ergometers: Treadmills and Cycles") that produces a linear increase in work rate illustrated in **Figure 5.5**. This protocol uses a slower speed and a low grade for the 3 minutes of warm-up, followed by a linear increase in speed and a curvilinear increase in grade so as the estimated work rate is increasing

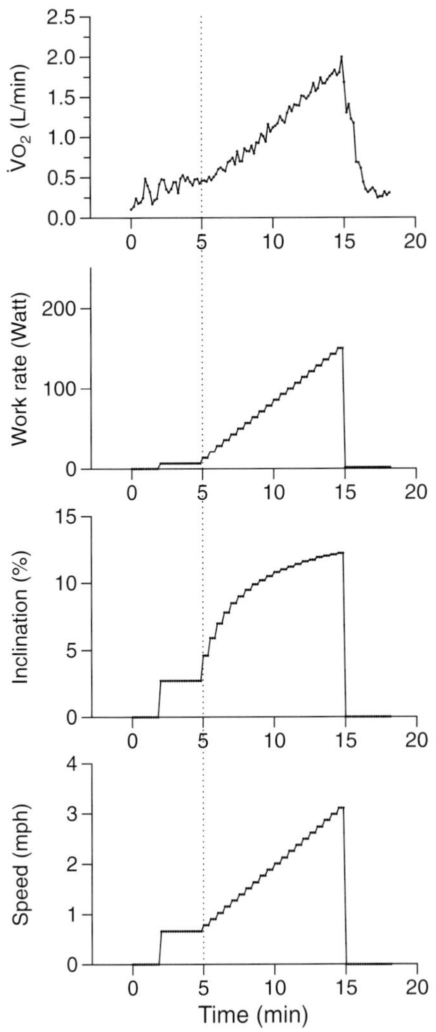

FIGURE 5.5. Linearized treadmill protocol. Speed, inclination, the estimated work rate (Watt), and the metabolic response, oxygen uptake ($\dot{V}O_2$), are shown as a function of time. The vertical dotted line marks the start of the ramp after a slow walking speed of about 0.7 mph. Of note, the slow walking speed is in an increase of $\dot{V}O_2$ of less than 0.5 L/min, which is commensurable that of the unloaded cycling on the cycle ergometer. After this, the simultaneous linear increase in walking speed and the estimated work rate elicits a linear increase in metabolic rate.

linearly. This protocol can be set up as either a stepwise or a ramp profile to maximal tolerance and, of course, gas exchange is measured breath by breath throughout ($\dot{V}O_2$, $\dot{V}CO_2$, and $\dot{V}E$). The low initial speed avoids the large step-up in $\dot{V}O_2$ at the start of testing that sometimes occurs with other protocols. The $\dot{V}O_2$ response to this protocol is essentially identical to that of the cycle ergometer ramp protocol. However, there are well-defined and expected differences in other physiological variables as discussed earlier.[6]

Arm Ergometry

Arm exercise protocols similar to those for lower extremity exercise are usually done because of dysfunction of the lower extremities. The usual technique is to use a converted cycle ergometer with the axle placed at or below the level of the shoulders while the subject sits or stands and moves the pedals so the arms are alternately fully extended; commercial arm ergometers are also available, however. The most common frequency is 50 rpm. Occasionally, upper extremity exercise is performed using wheelchair wheels coupled to a cycle ergometer or by rowing, paddling, or swimming. These modes may be particularly useful for paraplegics and for competitive rowers, kayakers, and swimmers. However, to obtain maximal cardiovascular and respiratory stress, arm cycling must be done concurrently with lower extremity exercise.

If the person performing the test is healthy and has not undergone specific upper extremity training, the peak $\dot{V}O_2$ for arm cycling will approximate 50% to 70% of that for leg cycling.[76] The *AT* for arm cycling for most healthy individuals is also lower than that of leg cycling. Peak $\dot{V}E$ is similarly reduced, whereas peak HR is only 2% to 12% less than with leg cycle exercise. Thus, the peak O_2 pulse is less with arm than with leg cycling.

Critique

Although arm cycling exercise has occasional uses, for most individuals, it does not stress the cardiovascular and respiratory systems as much as leg cycling or treadmill exercise and also requires a specialized arm ergometer. As such, it is a poor substitute when one assesses the cardiovascular and respiratory systems, except when lower extremity exercise is impossible.

Other Tests Suitable for Fitness or Serial Evaluations

A variety of tests have been used to evaluate individuals or groups without attempting to ascertain whether a particular system (eg, cardiovascular, respiratory, musculoskeletal) or the motivation of the performer is limiting exercise. Some such tests are likely to be used for children, young adults, military personnel, or workers exposed to environmental stress or exposures (**Fig. 5.5B,D**). These tests are often considered measures of cardiovascular fitness and may allow division of the population studied into several levels of fitness, but they can also be used to serially evaluate patients with known disorders. Formerly, these tests could be repeated frequently only with simple equipment. Now, with wearable telemetry devices, gas exchange measurements are possible. A few of these tests are briefly described in the following text.

Harvard Step Test and Modifications

The original Harvard step test consisted of having the subject step up and down at a uniform rate of 30 steps up per minute onto a platform 20 inches high for a period of 5 minutes, if possible, with HR measurements for 30 seconds after 1 minute of recovery.[47] Multiple modifications to this have been introduced including the following:

1. The addition of backpacks that add approximately one-third to the subject's weight
2. Reduction in the duration of the test to 3 minutes
3. Reduction in the step height to 17 inches for women

4. Measurement of HR during exercise
5. Change in the time of measurement of recovery HR
6. Change in test scoring
7. Use of a gradational step in which the height of the platform can be raised 2 cm every minute or 4.5 cm every 2 minutes

600-Yard Run-Walk

The 600-yard run-walk requires that the subject cover a 600-yard level distance in the shortest possible time.[77] He or she may intersperse running with walking but must try to finish as quickly as possible. A properly marked track or football field is suitable. For 87 male university staff and faculty members, time for completion showed a moderately good correlation ($r = 0.644$) with peak $\dot{V}O_2$ measured by an incremental cycle ergometer test (ranging from 25 to 50 mL/min/kg).

12-Minute Field Test

In the 12-minute field performance test, the subjects—dressed in exercise attire—cover as much distance as possible by running or walking. The distance covered was shown to correlate well ($r = 0.897$) with $\dot{V}O_2max$ measured during an intermittent incremental treadmill test in 115 military personnel ($\dot{V}O_2max$ range of 30-60 mL/min/kg).[78]

12-Minute Walk Test

The distance covered in 12 minutes of walking[79-82] has been used for assessing disability. The patient is instructed to cover as much distance as possible on foot in 12 minutes, walking over a marked course, for example, in a hospital corridor. The patient is told to try to keep going but not to be concerned if he or she has to slow down or stop to rest. The aim is for the patient to feel that at the end of the test, he or she could not have covered more ground in the time given. A physician or therapist accompanies the patient, acting as timekeeper and giving encouragement as necessary.

Some learning effect has been described on a 12-minute test repeated on consecutive days. In 35 patients with lung disease, the distance correlated significantly with peak $\dot{V}O_2$ ($r = 0.52$), peak $\dot{V}E$ ($r = 0.53$), and forced vital capacity ($r = 0.406$), but not with FEV_1 ($r = 0.283$).[83]

6-Minute Walk Test

The 6-minute walk test evolved in the 1980s as a less strenuous test than the 12-minute walk test, suitable for patients with symptomatic heart and lung disorders.[79-82,84,85] It is a relatively simple self-paced test useful for measuring the response to interventions in patients with known disease. It requires a flat, hard surface, such as a long indoor hallway with a path of 100 feet (30 m) in length, over which the patient travels back and forth as rapidly as he or she can with standardized encouragement by a monitor. Testing should be performed only where a rapid response to an emergency is possible. Patients with unstable angina or recent myocardial infarctions should not be tested.

The distance covered correlates reasonably well with peak $\dot{V}O_2$ measured during incremental tests in impaired populations. When conducted on 2 consecutive days, the distance covered on the second day is systematically higher, indicating a significant learning effect. The test does not discriminate between the different organ systems that may limit activity and is therefore should not be viewed as a diagnostic test. Several standards have been proposed as a clinically significant increase in walking distance on this test: 54 ± 17 m,[86] 35 ± 6 m,[87] and 31 ± 13 m.[88] This test has been successfully used in evaluating patients with lung resection, pulmonary rehabilitation, heart failure, pulmonary hypertension, cystic fibrosis, peripheral vascular disease, and obstructive lung disease.

It must be emphasized that the 6-minute walk test does not measure exercise tolerance but, at best, exercise performance. It is a self-paced test, with walk distance best correlated with habitual activity rather than maximal exercise tolerance. Because of a well-recognized "ceiling effect," it is not discriminatory of fitness levels among relatively young healthy persons. It is also not consistently sensitive to therapeutic interventions in populations of impaired patients. For example, it has been very effective in detecting changes in function in therapeutic trials for patients with isolated pulmonary arterial hypertension but has been variably effective in studies involving more complex populations with end-stage renal disease or chronic heart failure.

Incremental Shuttle Walk Test and Endurance Shuttle Walk Tests

Shuttle walk tests[79-82] count the number of times an individual can ambulate back and forth between marked end points on a defined course. For incremental shuttle walk tests, the walking pace is dictated by a metronome or other signal and increases on successive laps. In this way, the test simulates the profile of an incremental treadmill or cycle test and is intended to elicit a maximal effort without the need for an exercise ergometer.

SUMMARY

Numerous exercise devices, protocols, and physiological measuring systems are available for the safe and economical evaluation of normal individuals, athletes, and patients suspected of having (or known to have) respiratory, cardiovascular, or neuromuscular disease. The specific exercise performed can be tailored to the diagnostic or therapeutic questions being asked and the facilities and technical and professional expertise available. Ordinarily, a maximum amount of information can be obtained by making ventilatory, gas exchange, ECG, blood pressure, and blood gas measurements during a cycle or treadmill test that includes measurements sitting or standing at rest, followed by unloaded cycling or treadmill walking for 3 minutes, further followed by ramp or 1-minute incremental exercise with an increment size enabling the subject to reach his or her maximally tolerated work rate in about 10 minutes, and finally ending in a 2- to 3-minute recovery period. Less frequently, constant work rate tests, arm ergometry, or walking tests measuring time or distance may be useful.

REFERENCES

1. American Thoracic Society, American College of Chest Physicians. ATS/ACCP statement on cardiopulmonary exercise testing. *Am J Respir Crit Care Med*. 2003;167(2):211-277.
2. American College of Sports Medicine. *ACSM's Resource Manual for Guidelines for Exercise Testing and Prescription*. 10th ed. Philadelphia, PA: Wolters Kluwer; 2017.
3. Balady GJ, Arena R, Sietsema K, et al; and American Heart Association Exercise, Cardiac Rehabilitation, and Prevention Committee of the Council on Clinical Cardiology; Council on Epidemiology and Prevention; Council on Peripheral Vascular Disease; Interdisciplinary Council on Quality of Care and Outcomes Research. Clinician's guide to cardiopulmonary exercise testing in adults: a scientific statement from the American Heart Association. *Circulation*. 2010;122: 191-225.
4. Myers J, Arena R, Franklin B, et al; for American Heart Association Committee on Exercise, Cardiac Rehabilitation, and Prevention of the Council on Clinical Cardiology, the Council on Nutrition, Physical Activity, and Metabolism, and the Council on Cardiovascular Nursing. Recommendations for clinical exercise laboratories: a scientific statement from the American Heart Association. *Circulation*. 2009;119(24):3144-3161.
5. Arena R, Myers J, Williams MA, et al. Assessment of functional capacity in clinical and research settings: a scientific statement from the American Heart Association Committee on Exercise, Rehabilitation, and Prevention of the Council on Clinical Cardiology and the Council on Cardiovascular Nursing. *Circulation*. 2007;116(3):329-343.
6. Porszasz J, Stringer W, Casaburi R. Equipment, measurements and quality control. In: Palange P, Laveneziana P, Neder JA, Ward S, eds. *Clinical Exercise Testing*. Sheffield, United Kingdom: European Respiratory Society; 2018:59-81. *European Respiratory Society Monograph*; vol 80.
7. Davis JA. Direct determination of aerobic power. In: Maude PJ, Foster C, eds. *Physiological Assessment of Human Fitness*. Champaign, IL: Human Kinetics; 1995:9-17.
8. Lamarra N, Whipp BJ. Measurement of pulmonary gas exchange. In: Maud PJ, Foster C, eds. *Physiological Assessment of Human Fitness*. Champaign, IL: Human Kinetics; 1995:19-35.
9. Macfarlane DJ. Automated metabolic gas analysis systems: a review. *Sports Med*. 2001;31:841-861.
10. Macfarlane DJ. Open-circuit respirometry: a historical review of portable gas analysis systems. *Eur J Appl Physiol*. 2017;117:2369-2386.
11. Porszasz J, Stringer W, Casaburi R. Equipment, measurements and quality control in clinical exercise testing. In: Ward SA, Palange P, eds. *Clinical Exercise Testing*. Sheffield, United Kingdom: European Respiratory Society Journals; 2007:108-128. *European Respiratory Society Monograph*; vol 40.
12. Ward SA. Open-circuit respirometry: real-time, laboratory-based systems. *Eur J Appl Physiol*. 2018;118:875-898.
13. Beaver WL, Wasserman K, Whipp BJ. On-line computer analysis and breath-by-breath graphical display of exercise function tests. *J Appl Physiol*. 1973;34(1):128-132.
14. Whipp BJ, Ward SA, Lamarra N, Davis JA, Wasserman K. Parameters of ventilatory and gas exchange dynamics during exercise. *J Appl Physiol Respir Environ Exerc Physiol*. 1982;52:1506-1513.
15. Sietsema KE, Cooper DM, Perloff JK, et al. Dynamics of oxygen uptake during exercise in adults with cyanotic congenital heart disease. *Circulation*. 1986;73(6):1137-1144.
16. Lang S, Herold R, Kraft A, Harth V, Preisser AM. Spiroergometric measurements under increased inspiratory oxygen concentration (F_{IO_2})—putting the Haldane transformation to the test. *PLoS One*. 2018;13(12):e0207648.
17. Hansen JE. Exercise instruments, schemes, and protocols for evaluating the dyspneic patient. *Am Rev Respir Dis*. 1984;129(2, pt 2):S25-S27.
18. Hsia D, Casaburi R, Pradhan A, Torres E, Porszasz J. Physiological responses to linear treadmill and cycle ergometer exercise in COPD. *Eur Respir J*. 2009;34(3):605-615.
19. Porszasz J, Casaburi R, Somfay A, Woodhouse LJ, Whipp BJ. A treadmill ramp protocol using simultaneous changes in speed and grade. *Med Sci Sports Exerc*. 2003;35(9):1596-1603.
20. Bar-Yoseph R, Porszasz J, Radom-Aizik S, Stehli A, Law P, Cooper DM. The effect of test modality on dynamic exercise biomarkers in children, adolescents, and young adults. *Physiol Rep*. 2019;7(14):e14178.
21. Åstrand I. Aerobic work capacity in men and women with special reference to age. *Acta Physiol Scand Suppl*. 1960;49(169):1-92.
22. Kligfield P, Gettes LS, Bailey JJ, et al. Recommendations for the standardization and interpretation of the electrocardiogram: part I: the electrocardiogram and its technology: a scientific statement from the American Heart Association Electrocardiography and Arrhythmias Committee, Council on Clinical Cardiology; the American College of Cardiology Foundation; and the Heart Rhythm Society: endorsed by the International Society for Computerized Electrocardiology. *Circulation*. 2007;115:1306-1324.
23. Clark JS, Votteri B, Ariagno RL, et al. Noninvasive assessment of blood gases. *Am Rev Respir Dis*. 1992;145(1):220-232.
24. Jubran A. Pulse oximetry. *Crit Care*. 2015;19:272.
25. Smyth RJ, D'Urzo AD, Slutsky AS, Galko BM, Rebuck AS. Ear oximetry during combined hypoxia and exercise. *J Appl Physiol (1985)*. 1986;60(2):716-719.
26. Zeballos RJ, Weisman IM. Reliability of noninvasive oximetry in black subjects during exercise and hypoxia. *Am Rev Respir Dis*. 1991;144(6):1240-1244.
27. Barker SJ, Curry J, Redford D, Morgan S. Measurement of carboxyhemoglobin and methemoglobin by pulse oximetry: a human volunteer study. *Anesthesiology*. 2006;105(5):892-897.
28. Ries AL, Farrow JT, Clausen JL. Accuracy of two ear oximeters at rest and during exercise in pulmonary patients. *Am Rev Respir Dis*. 1985;132(3):685-689.
29. Powers SK, Dodd S, Freeman J, Ayers GD, Samson H, McKnight T. Accuracy of pulse oximetry to estimate HbO_2 fraction of total Hb during exercise. *J Appl Physiol (1985)*. 1989;67(1):300-304.
30. Hansen JE, Casaburi R. Validity of ear oximetry in clinical exercise testing. *Chest*. 1987;91(3):333-337.
31. Gehring H, Hornberger C, Matz H, Konecny E, Schmucker P. The effects of motion artifact and low perfusion on the performance of a new generation of pulse oximeters in volunteers undergoing hypoxemia. *Respir Care*. 2002;47(1):48-60.
32. Yamaya Y, Bogaard HJ, Wagner PD, Niizeki K, Hopkins SR. Validity of pulse oximetry during maximal exercise in normoxia, hypoxia, and hyperoxia. *J Appl Physiol (1985)*. 2002;92(1):162-168.
33. Jones NL, McHardy GJR, Naimark A, Campbell EJM. Physiological dead space and alveolar-arterial gas pressure differences during exercise. *Clin Sci*. 1966;31:19-29.
34. Carter R, Banham SW. Use of transcutaneous oxygen and carbon dioxide tensions for assessing indices of gas exchange during exercise testing. *Respir Med*. 2000;94(4):350-355.
35. Stege G, van den Elshout FJ, Heijdra YF, et al. Accuracy of transcutaneous carbon dioxide tension measurements during cardiopulmonary exercise testing. *Respiration*. 2009;78(2):147-153.
36. Sridhar MK, Carter R, Moran F, Banham SW. Use of a combined oxygen and carbon dioxide transcutaneous electrode in the estimation of gas exchange during exercise. *Thorax*. 1993;48(6):643-647.
37. Orogian A, Corey SM, Calmelat R, et al. Validation of transcutaneous P_{CO_2} to estimate deadspace ventilation (V_D/V_T) during exercise in patients with COPD. *Am J Crit Care Med*. 2018;197:A4326.
38. Frye M, DiBenedetto R, Lain D, et al. Single arterial puncture vs arterial cannula for arterial gas analysis after exercise. Change in arterial oxygen tension over time. *Chest*. 1988;93:294-299.
39. O'Neill AV, Johnson DC. Transition from exercise to rest. Ventilatory and arterial blood gas responses. *Chest*. 1991;99:1145-1150.
40. Ries AL, Fedullo PF, Clausen JL. Rapid changes in arterial blood gas levels after exercise in pulmonary patients. *Chest*. 1983;83:454-456.
41. Mollard P, Bourdillon N, Letournel M, et al. Validity of arterialized earlobe blood gases at rest and exercise in normoxia and hypoxia. *Respir Physiol Neurobiol*. 2010;172:179-183.
42. Maron BA, Cockrill BA, Waxman AB, Systrom DM. The invasive cardiopulmonary exercise test. *Circulation*. 2013;127:1157-1164.
43. Huang W, Resch S, Oliveira RK, Cockrill BA, Systrom DM, Waxman AB. Invasive cardiopulmonary exercise testing in the evaluation of

unexplained dyspnea: insights from a multidisciplinary dyspnea center. *Eur J Prev Cardiol*. 2017;24(11):1190-1199.
44. Stetz CW, Miller RG, Kelly GE, Raffin TA. Reliability of the thermodilution method in the determination of cardiac output in clinical practice. *Am Rev Respir Dis*. 1982;126:1001-1004.
45. Sue DY, Hansen JE, Blais M, Wasserman K. Measurement and analysis of gas exchange during exercise using a programmable calculator. *J Appl Physiol Respir Environ Exerc Physiol*. 1980;49(3):456-461.
46. Porszasz J, Blonshine S, Cao R, Paden HA, Casaburi R, Rossiter HB. Biological quality control for cardiopulmonary exercise testing in multicenter clinical trials. *BMC Pulm Med*. 2016;16:13.
47. Consolazio CF, Johnson RE, Pecora LI. *Physiological Measurements of Metabolic Function in Man*. New York, NY: McGraw-Hill; 1963.
48. Beaver WL, Lamarra N, Wasserman K. Breath-by-breath measurement of true alveolar gas exchange. *J Appl Physiol Respir Environ Exerc Physiol*. 1981;51:1662-1675.
49. Huszczuk A, Whipp BJ, Wasserman K. A respiratory gas exchange simulator for routine calibration in metabolic studies. *Eur Respir J*. 1990;3:465-468.
50. Revill SM, Morgan MD. Biological quality control for exercise testing. *Thorax*. 2000;55:63-66.
51. Graham BL, Steenbruggen I, Miller MR, et al. Standardization of spirometry 2019 update. An official American Thoracic Society and European Respiratory Society technical statement. *Am J Respir Crit Care Med*. 2019;200(8):e70-e88.
52. Whipp BJ, Davis JA, Torres F, Wasserman K. A test to determine parameters of aerobic function during exercise. *J Appl Physiol Respir Environ Exerc Physiol*. 1981;50:217-221.
53. Balke B. *Correlation of Static and Physical Endurance. 1. A Test of Physical Performance Based on the Cardiovascular and Respiratory Response to Gradually Increased Work*. San Antonio, TX: United States Air Force School of Aviation Medicine; 1952. Project No. 21-32-004, Report No. 1.
54. Balke B, Ware RW. An experimental study of physical fitness of Air Force personnel. *U S Armed Forces Med J*. 1959;10:675-688.
55. Consolazio CF, Nelson RA, Matoush LO, Hansen JE. Energy metabolism at high altitude (3,475 m). *J Appl Physiol*. 1966;21:1732-1740.
56. Jones NL. *Clinical Exercise Testing*. Philadelphia, PA: WB Saunders; 1988.
57. Spiro SG. Exercise testing in clinical medicine. *Br J Dis Chest*. 1977;71:145-172.
58. Fairshter RD, Walters J, Salvess K, et al. Comparison of incremental exercise test during cycle and treadmill ergometry. *Am Rev Respir Dis*. 1982;125(suppl):254.
59. Buchfuhrer MJ, Hansen JE, Robinson TE, Sue DY, Wasserman K, Whipp BJ. Optimizing the exercise protocol for cardiopulmonary assessment. *J Appl Physiol Respir Environ Exerc Physiol*. 1983;55:1558-1564.
60. Taylor HL, Buskirk E, Henschel A. Maximal oxygen intake as an objective measure of cardio-respiratory performance. *J Appl Physiol*. 1955;8:73-80.
61. Froelicher VF Jr, Brammell H, Davis GD, Noguera I, Stewart A, Lancaster MC. A comparison of three maximal treadmill exercise protocols. *J Appl Physiol*. 1974;36:720-725.
62. Maksud MG, Coutts KD. Comparison of a continuous and discontinuous graded treadmill test for maximal oxygen uptake. *Med Sci Sports*. 1971;3:63-65.
63. McArdle WD, Katch FI, Pechar GS. Comparison of continuous and discontinuous treadmill and bicycle tests for max $\dot{V}O_2$. *Med Sci Sports*. 1973;5:156-160.
64. Pollock ML, Bohannon RL, Cooper KM, et al. A comparative analysis of four protocols for maximal treadmill stress testing. *Am Heart J*. 1976;92:39-46.
65. Davis JA, Whipp BJ, Lamarra N, Huntsman DJ, Frank MH, Wasserman K. Effect of ramp slope on determination of aerobic parameters from the ramp exercise test. *Med Sci Sports Exerc*. 1982;14:339-343.
66. Rossiter HB, Kowalchuk JM, Whipp BJ. A test to establish maximum O_2 uptake despite no plateau in the O_2 uptake response to ramp incremental exercise. *J Appl Physiol (1985)*. 2006;100(3):764-770.
67. Furuike AN, Sue DY, Hansen JE, Wasserman K. Comparison of physiologic dead space/tidal volume ratio and alveolar-arterial P_{O_2} difference during incremental and constant work exercise. *Am Rev Respir Dis*. 1982;126:579-583.
68. Bruce RA. Exercise testing of patients with coronary heart disease. Principles and normal standards for evaluation. *Ann Clin Res*. 1971;3:323-332.
69. Ellestad MH. *Stress Testing*. Philadelphia, PA: FA Davis; 1980.
70. Patterson JA, Naughton J, Pietras RJ, et al. Treadmill exercise in assessment of the functional capacity of patients with cardiac disease. *Am J Cardiol*. 1972;30:757-762.
71. Itoh H, Tajima A, Koike A, et al. Oxygen uptake abnormalities during exercise in coronary artery disease. In: Wasserman K, ed. *Cardiopulmonary Exercise Testing and Cardiovascular Health*. Armonk, NY: Futura Publishing; 2002:165-172.
72. Belardinelli R, Lacalaprice F, Carle F, et al. Exercise-induced myocardial ischaemia detected by cardiopulmonary exercise testing. *Eur Heart J*. 2003;24:1304-1313.
73. Stuart RJ Jr, Ellestad MH. National survey of exercise stress testing facilities. *Chest*. 1980;77:94-97.
74. Myers J, Voodi L, Umann T, Froelicher VF. A survey of exercise testing: methods, utilization, interpretation, and safety in the VAHCS. *J Cardiopulm Rehabil*. 2000;20(4):251-258.
75. Bruce RA, Kusumi F, Hosmer D. Maximal oxygen intake and nomographic assessment of functional aerobic impairment in cardiovascular disease. *Am Heart J*. 1973;85:546-562.
76. Larsen RT, Christensen J, Tang LH, et al. A systematic review and meta-analysis comparing cardiopulmonary exercise test values obtained from the arm cycle and the leg cycle respectively in healthy adults. *Int J Sports Phys Ther*. 2016;11(7):1006-1039.
77. Fleishman EA. *The Structure and Measurement of Physical Fitness*. Englewood Cliffs, NJ: Prentice-Hall; 1964.
78. Cooper KM. A means of assessing maximal oxygen intake. Correlation between field and treadmill testing. *JAMA*. 1968;203:201-204.
79. Singh SJ, Puhan MA, Andrianopoulos V, et al. An official systematic review of the European Respiratory Society/American Thoracic Society: measurement properties of field walking tests in chronic respiratory disease. *Eur Respir J*. 2014;44:1447-1478.
80. Garvey C, Boylan AM, Miller DL, et al; for American Thoracic Society Implementation Task Force. Field walking tests in chronic respiratory disease. *Ann Am Thorac Soc*. 2015;12(3):446-447.
81. Puente-Maestu L, Palange P, Casaburi R, et al. Use of exercise testing in the evaluation of interventional efficacy: an official ERS statement. *Eur Respir J*. 2016;47:429-460.
82. Holland AE, Spruit MA, Troosters T, et al. An official European Respiratory Society/American Thoracic Society technical standard: field walking tests in chronic respiratory disease. *Eur Respir J*. 2014;44:1428-1446.
83. McGavin CR, Gupta SP, McHardy GJR. Twelve-minute walking test for assessing disability in chronic bronchitis. *Br Med J*. 1976;1:822-823.
84. ATS Committee on Proficiency Standards for Clinical Pulmonary Function Laboratories. ATS statement: guidelines for the six-minute walk test. *Am J Respir Crit Care Med*. 2002;166(1):111-117.
85. Salzman SH. The 6-min walk test: clinical and research role, technique, coding, and reimbursement. *Chest*. 2009;135(5):1345-1352.
86. Redelmeier DA, Bayoumi AM, Goldstein RS, Guyatt GH. Interpreting small differences in functional status: the six minute walk test in chronic lung disease patients. *Am J Respir Crit Care Med*. 1997;155:1278-1282.
87. Puhan MA, Mador MJ, Held U, Goldstein R, Guyatt GH, Schünemann HJ. Interpretation of treatment changes in 6-minute walk distance in patients with COPD. *Eur Respir J*. 2008;32:637-643.
88. Sciurba FC, Slivka WA. Six-minute walk testing. *Semin Respir Crit Care Med*. 1998;19:383-392.

CHAPTER 6

Approaches to Data Summary and Interpretation

Reporting results of a cardiopulmonary exercise test (CPET) entails first distilling a large amount of data into a discrete set of variables that characterize the individual's exercise capacity or performance in standardized terms. Interpretation of the test attaches meaning to the results by comparison with appropriately selected reference values and identifying their significance in the context of the clinical indication for which the test was conducted.

The processes of summarizing and interpreting data are both greatly aided by use of graphical displays of measurements across the period of testing. This allows the interpreter to verify that the discrete values reported in the summary are reasonable representations of the data as a whole and sometimes also to identify meaningful aspects of the test responses that are not reflected in the summary values. The approach to analysis of incremental CPET presented here includes a systematic review of an array of nine panels of graphs (see **Fig. 6.1**), which is the same format used for presenting data of the case examples later in this book. Users may choose alternative formats for data display that include additional measurements or relationships important to particular applications, but the approach to reviewing and summarizing data can be applied independent of the details of formatting.

CONSIDERATIONS IN FORMATTING AND SUMMARIZING DATA

Averaging Breath-by-Breath Data

Many systems for measuring pulmonary gas exchange calculate values on a breath-by-breath basis. Variations in tidal volume (V_T) and end-expiratory lung volumes can add "noise" to the individual measurements from exhaled

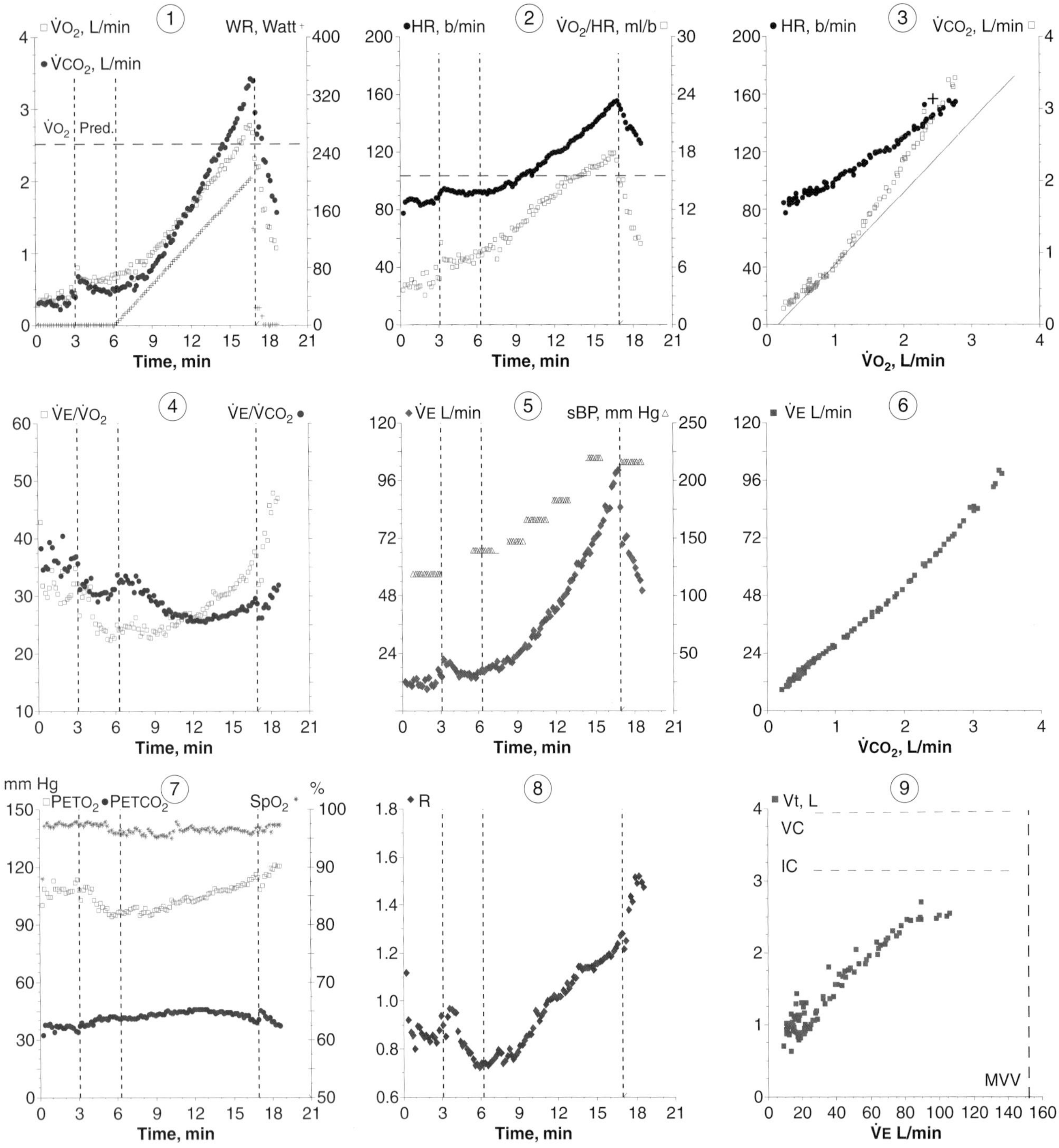

FIGURE 6.1. Example of a nine-panel array of data from an incremental exercise test on a cycle ergometer. The patient was a 58-year-old man with hypertension treated with an angiotensin-converting enzyme inhibitor. Testing was performed as he was resuming exercise after a period of inactivity due to an orthopedic injury. Data are displayed as 10-second averages of breath-by-breath measurements made over 3 minutes of rest, 3 minutes of unloaded cycling, and progressive increase in work rate of 20 W/min to symptom limitation, followed by 2 minutes of recovery. The patient terminated exercise with symptoms of leg fatigue. In the first two columns, time is on the x-axis and vertical dashed lines mark the onsets of unloaded cycling, incremental phase, and recovery. Horizontal dashed lines indicate the normal reference values chosen for comparison: panel 1, peak $\dot{V}O_2$; panel 2, peak O_2-pulse; panel 3, peak HR. In panel 3 a diagonal line indicates a slope of 1 for changes in $\dot{V}CO_2$ relative to $\dot{V}O_2$, and the predicted peak values for $\dot{V}O_2$ and HR are indicated by a cross mark. In panel 9, dashed lines show values for vital capacity (VC), inspiratory capacity (IC), and maximum voluntary ventilation (MVV) measured prior to exercise. For other abbreviations see text.

breaths compared to the simultaneous rates of carbon dioxide (CO_2) production and oxygen (O_2) consumption by the body. Averaging breath-by-breath data over a number of breaths or over set periods of time is widely used for reducing random noise and also condenses the data set to a more manageable size. Obviously, the longer the period of averaging, the more extraneous noise is dampened, but so too is the true magnitude of any rapid changes occurring during that period. The latter is important to consider for commonly used incremental test protocols in which measurements progress from rest to maximal exercise levels over a relatively short period of time.

Formatting Data for Viewing During and After Testing

A rolling, or moving, average of values measured over a set number of successive breaths is a convenient format for viewing measures in real time. With this format, the time interval represented by each data point varies with breathing frequency, and any abrupt changes in measured values are dampened by preceding measurements. Once data collection is complete, the breath-by-breath data can be converted to a time-based format and then averaged over a set interval. In most cases, averages over 10 to 20 seconds work well for purposes of graphing. Thirty-second averages may be more appropriate for longer tests and are convenient for tabular summaries. Sometimes, the averaging strategy obscures an underlying pattern that is of interest. This is the case for oscillatory variations in ventilation and gas exchange that are characteristic of some patients with chronic heart failure, which is often most clearly demonstrated on a rolling average of breath-by-breath data.

Quantifying Peak Values

The highest measures at the end of an incremental test are termed peak values, acknowledging that these may or may not correspond to true maximal responses. By convention, averages of the last 30 seconds of measurements at peak exercise are used as a reasonable balance between avoiding spurious values resulting from breath-to-breath noise and underestimating peak values by inclusion of too much submaximal data. Even though some variables, heart rate (HR) in particular, may not be subject to breath-related noise, when used to calculate composite variables such as the O_2 pulse, it is appropriate to use the same averaging interval as for the gas exchange variables.

Characterizing Submaximal Exercise Patterns

Measurements characterizing exercise responses in the submaximal range include linear and nonlinear relationships between variables, which are best appreciated from graphical displays. These often have the advantage of being independent of maximal effort so may be more repeatable than peak values. Software may facilitate manipulation of data on screen, for example, to superimpose multiple variables in one graph, select appropriate ranges of data, and calculate slopes of linear relationships.

ORGANIZING DATA: APPROACH TO REVIEW OF A NINE-PANEL GRAPHICAL DISPLAY

A consistent approach to displaying data and systematic approach to their review facilitates interpretation and helps ensure that no important finding is overlooked. For this, the data shown in **Figure 6.1** can be divided into sets representing three aspects of the physiologic responses to exercise (**Table 6.1**).

- Graphs representing O_2 uptake ($\dot{V}O_2$) and its relation to other variables (panels 1, 2, 3, and 8). Because $\dot{V}O_2$ depends on oxygen transport and utilization, these can be broadly considered to reflect the cardiovascular and metabolic responses to exercise.
- Graphs depicting minute ventilation ($\dot{V}E$) and its components (panels 5 and 9), which reflect the scale and mechanics of breathing during exercise
- Graphs reflecting efficiency of pulmonary gas exchange (panels 4, 6, and 7). These include the proportionality between ventilation and gas exchange and the partial pressures of gases in exhaled breath, blood, and/or tissue.

These three sets of data and the processes they reflect are clearly interdependent and also include measurements not represented in the graphs. While this breakdown is therefore simplistic, it provides a useful framework for organizing the exercise data for review and also for generating an interpretation for the test report.

Data Reflecting Cardiovascular and Metabolic Responses

Panels 1, 2, 3, (**Fig. 6.2**) and 8 (see **Fig. 6.3**) show data most directly related to the processes of oxygen delivery and utilization.

Panel 1: $\dot{V}O_2$, CO_2 output ($\dot{V}CO_2$), and work rate versus time. Predicted peak $\dot{V}O_2$ is shown for reference as a dashed horizontal line.

$\dot{V}O_2$ and $\dot{V}CO_2$. Peak $\dot{V}O_2$ is a global measure of exercise capacity or performance and a primary finding of CPET. How the subject's peak $\dot{V}O_2$ compares to the reference value selected for comparison is readily appreciated from its relation to the horizontal dashed line. The validity of the peak $\dot{V}O_2$ as an estimate of the subject's true maximal $\dot{V}O_2$ depends on effort, so an assessment of this will need to be incorporated into its interpretation. One of the factors in this assessment is whether the subject exercised substantially beyond his or her lactate threshold, and because $\dot{V}CO_2$ reflects the gas exchange consequence of lactic acidosis, the relative positions of $\dot{V}CO_2$ and $\dot{V}O_2$ in this graph at end exercise provides an initial impression of whether a lactic acidosis was achieved during the test. The relationship between $\dot{V}O_2$ and $\dot{V}CO_2$ will be analyzed further in panels 3 and 8.

Work rate slope ($\Delta\dot{V}O_2/\Delta WR$). With the onset of incremental work, after a short time lag, $\dot{V}O_2$ increases progressively to the end of exercise. In the figure, the increases in

TABLE 6.1 Three Aspects of the Cardiopulmonary Response to Exercise as Reflected in CPET Variables[a]

Aspect of exercise response	Panels (see Fig. 6.1)	Variables	Potential abnormalities	Representative conditions
Cardiovascular and metabolic	1, 3	$\Delta\dot{V}O_2/\Delta WR$ *AT*	Low	• Any disease limiting oxygen delivery or utilization, including heart failure, myocardial ischemia, peripheral vascular disease, pulmonary vascular disease, metabolic myopathy
	1, 2, 3	Peak $\dot{V}O_2$ Peak $\dot{V}O_2$/HR	Low	• Any of the conditions above • Any condition terminating the test prior to maximal cardiovascular stress
	2, 3	$\Delta HR/\Delta\dot{V}O_2$ slope Peak $\dot{V}O_2$/HR	Shallow High	• Chronotropic impairment
		ECG	ST segment displacement Ectopy, arrhythmia	• Ischemic heart disease • Arrhythmia • Conduction system defect
		Blood pressure increase	Excessive	• Hypertensive cardiovascular disease
			Reduced	• Severe cardiovascular impairment • Autonomic insufficiency
	Additional measures related to cardiovascular and metabolic responses			
		ΔCardiac output/$\Delta\dot{V}O_2$	Low (<5)	• Cardiovascular impairment
			High (>6)	• Muscle oxidative defect • Autonomic dysfunction
Ventilatory	5, 9	Breathing reserve	Low (<15 L/min or 20% of MVV)	• Chronic obstructive lung disease • Interstitial lung disease • Extrapulmonary restriction
	9	Inspiratory capacity and inspiratory reserve volume	Reduced from rest to exercise	• Obstructive airways disease with dynamic hyperinflation
	5, 9	Breathing pattern	Chaotic	• Volitional hyperventilation • Anxiety
			Oscillatory	• Heart failure
	Additional measures related to ventilatory response			
		post exercise spirometry	flow rate or volume changes	• Exercise induced broncho-constriction • Upper airway dysfunction
Efficiency of pulmonary gas exchange	4, 6	$\dot{V}E/\dot{V}CO_2$ V_D/V_T	High	• Heart failure • Lung disease: obstructive or interstitial • Pulmonary vascular disease
	7	SpO_2, SaO_2, PaO_2 $P(A-a)O_2$	Low High	• Pulmonary vascular disease • Lung disease: obstructive or interstitial • Right to left shunt

Abbreviations: *AT*, anaerobic threshold; ECG, electrocardiogram; HR, heart rate; IC, inspiratory capacity; MVV, maximum voluntary ventilation; V_D/V_T, dead space–tidal volume ratio; $\dot{V}E/\dot{V}CO_2$, ventilatory equivalent for CO_2; $\dot{V}O_2$, O_2 uptake; WR, work rate.

[a]The first column shows the aspects of the responses: cardiovascular and metabolic, ventilatory, and efficiency of pulmonary gas exchange. The second column indicates where the data are located in the graph in Figure 6.1, if relevant, and the third column indicates the specific variables. The two right-hand columns show possible abnormalities in the variables and examples of clinical conditions in which they would typically be seen.

$\dot{V}O_2$ and work rate appear parallel because the two y-axes were intentionally scaled with the range of $\dot{V}O_2$ (in mL/min) 10 times the range of work rate (in W). As a result, the two variables will be plotted as parallel if $\dot{V}O_2$ increased at the expected rate of 10 mL/min/W. The slope can usually be quantified by fitting a straight line to the data, excluding the first 1 to 2 minute of incremental work during which there is a relative lag in the increase of $\dot{V}O_2$ due to inherent kinetics of the response. Although this slope typically reflects normal skeletal muscle bioenergetics, an abnormally shallow $\Delta\dot{V}O_2/\Delta WR$ slope does not imply unusually high metabolic efficiency but instead suggests failure of oxygen delivery (cardiovascular function)[1] or utilization (muscle oxidative capacity)[2,3] to keep pace with rapid changes in

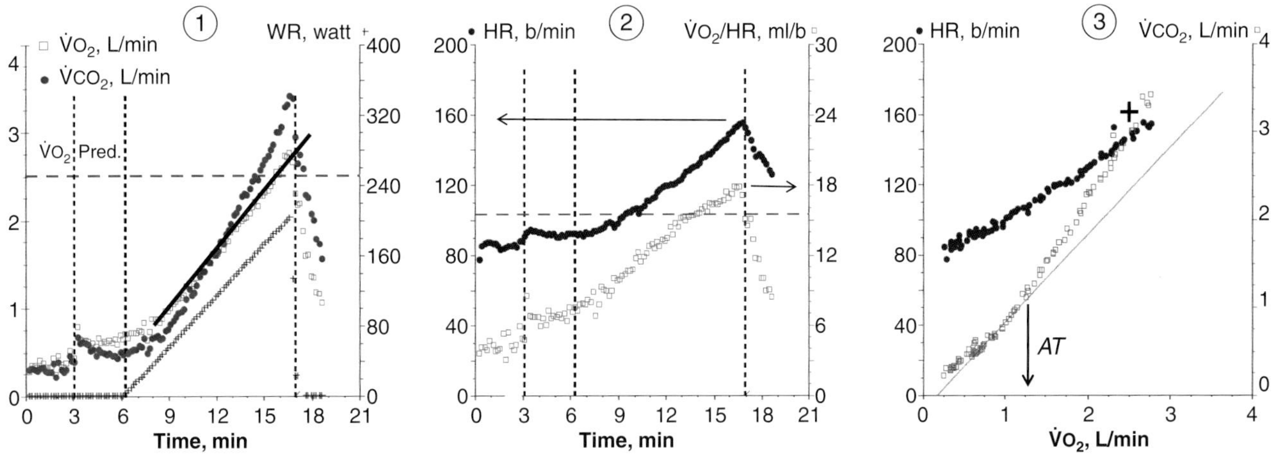

FIGURE 6.2. Graphs used to quantify variables related to $\dot{V}O_2$ reflecting cardiovascular and metabolic responses to exercise. From panel 1, peak $\dot{V}O_2$ and its relationship to the reference value and the $\Delta\dot{V}O_2/\Delta WR$ slope can be identified. Panel 2 shows peak heart rate (HR) and peak O_2 pulse ($\dot{V}O_2$/HR) as well as the pattern of change in these over the range of work. Panel 3 shows the slope of HR relative to $\dot{V}O_2$ and the relationship of these to their peak reference values. The HR reserve is the vertical difference between the predicted peak HR and the actual peak HR. The V-slope ($\dot{V}CO_2$ versus $\dot{V}O_2$) for identifying the anaerobic threshold (*AT*) is shown along with a diagonal line referencing a slope of 1.0 for these variables.

metabolic demand as work rate increases. In some cases, a decrease in an initially normal slope may develop during exercise due to development of, for example, exercise-induced myocardial dysfunction due to ischemic heart disease.[4-6] Care should be taken in reporting the $\Delta\dot{V}O_2/\Delta WR$ slope. For cycle ergometry, precision of work rate is uncertain in the range of less than around 15 W, and work rate is difficult to quantify accurately for treadmill exercise in any range. Although formulae are available to estimate work rate from treadmill grade and speed, the calculations are based on individuals with good treadmill walking economy and not using side rails or other support that alters the external work.[7] The reporting of $\Delta\dot{V}O_2/\Delta WR$ therefore should generally be reserved for tests on a well-calibrated cycle in which there are a least several minutes of exercise above 15 W.

Pattern of $\dot{V}O_2$ in transitions between rest and exercise. In **Figure 6.1**, it can be seen that $\dot{V}O_2$ approximately doubled during unloaded cycling relative to rest. This is typical for a normally proportioned person, although for one with heavy legs due to obesity or with inefficient pedaling ergonomics due to body habitus, or neurologic or orthopedic issues, this increment may be larger. For treadmill exercise, the initial increase in $\dot{V}O_2$ may be even more dependent on the individual's weight and ergonomics because of the added work of supporting body weight. In this example, $\dot{V}O_2$ reached a new steady state within the 3-minute period, which is typical for a work rate in the moderate-intensity domain. Ideally, the exercise protocol should be designed so that this initial period of exercise is moderate intensity, that is, below the individual's anaerobic threshold (*AT*). At the start of recovery, $\dot{V}O_2$ normally begins to drop exponentially back toward resting levels. If an abnormal energy deficit accumulated during exercise, however, recovery of $\dot{V}O_2$ can be delayed. $\dot{V}O_2$ recovery times are thus a corollary of the $\Delta\dot{V}O_2/\Delta WR$ slope. The recovery speed correlates with peak $\dot{V}O_2$ and might substitute for the $\Delta\dot{V}O_2/\Delta WR$ assessment in situations in which work rate is not readily known. Methods and quantitative reference values for characterizing $\dot{V}O_2$ recovery are not as well standardized as for other variables discussed here.[8,9]

Panel 2: Heart rate and O_2 pulse versus time

Heart rate. Heart rate is usually derived from the RR interval of the electrocardiogram (ECG) over several cardiac cycles. There is typically an acute increase in heart rate immediately at the start of exercise from rest, attributable to a reflex withdrawal of parasympathetic tone. Later in exercise, progressive sympathetic stimulation further stimulates heart rate. The decrease in heart rate from peak value over the first minute of recovery has long been used as an index of cardiovascular fitness with prognostic significance.[10] Variations in heart rate pattern may result from cardiovascular disease, medications, conditions affecting autonomic function, or pretest anticipation.

Peak heart rate and heart rate reserve. A peak heart rate near the predicted maximal value is useful in supporting the impression of adequate effort on an incremental test. The range of normal maximal heart rate is wide, however, even in healthy unmedicated persons, so the presence of a heart rate reserve (predicted maximum HR − peak HR) does not necessarily indicate poor effort. Peak heart rate can be reduced by medications or by intrinsic chronotropic impairment.

Oxygen pulse. $\dot{V}O_2$/HR or O_2 pulse is equal to the product of stroke volume and $C(a - \bar{v})O_2$. Both of these factors are expected to increase during exercise, with most of the increment in stroke volume occurring early in exercise and $C(a - \bar{v})O_2$ increasing progressively from rest until maximal

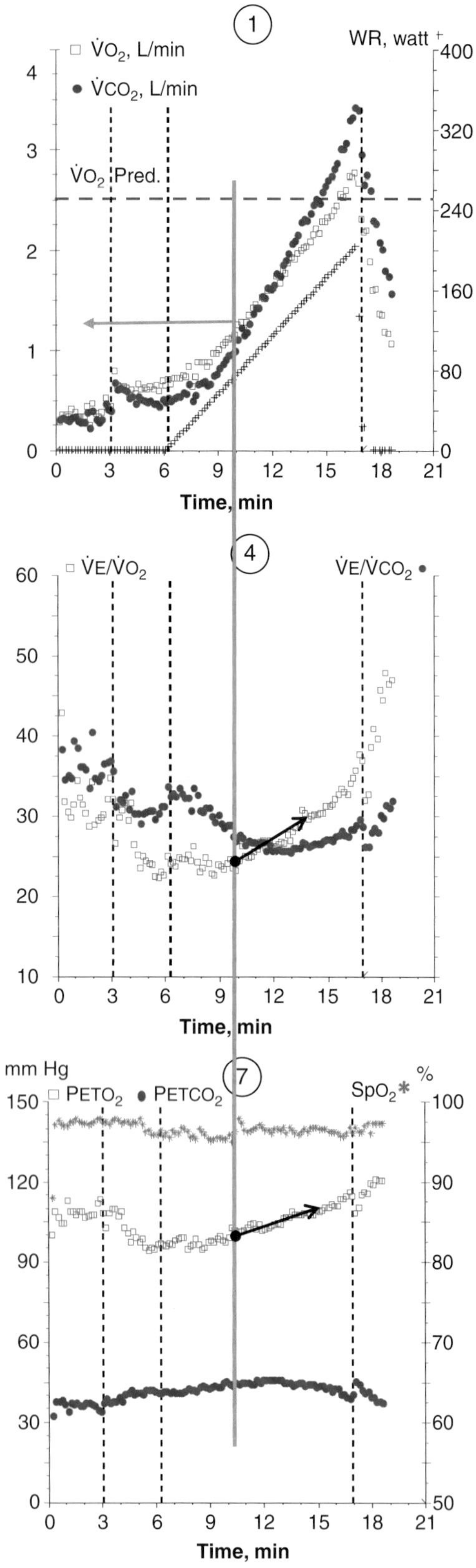

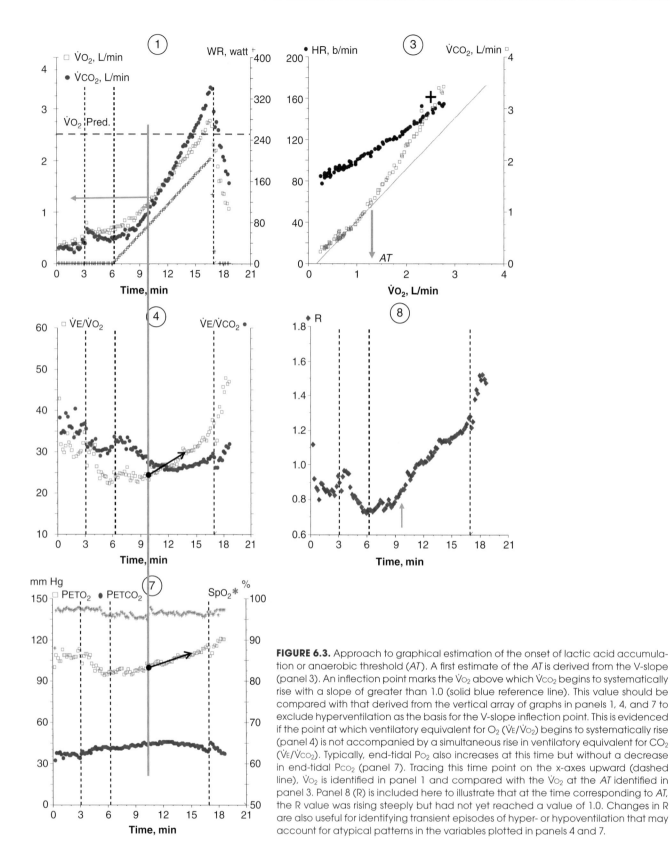

FIGURE 6.3. Approach to graphical estimation of the onset of lactic acid accumulation or anaerobic threshold (*AT*). A first estimate of the *AT* is derived from the V-slope (panel 3). An inflection point marks the $\dot{V}O_2$ above which $\dot{V}CO_2$ begins to systematically rise with a slope of greater than 1.0 (solid blue reference line). This value should be compared with that derived from the vertical array of graphs in panels 1, 4, and 7 to exclude hyperventilation as the basis for the V-slope inflection point. This is evidenced if the point at which ventilatory equivalent for O_2 ($\dot{V}E/\dot{V}O_2$) begins to systematically rise (panel 4) is not accompanied by a simultaneous rise in ventilatory equivalent for CO_2 ($\dot{V}E/\dot{V}CO_2$). Typically, end-tidal PO_2 also increases at this time but without a decrease in end-tidal PCO_2 (panel 7). Tracing this time point on the x-axes upward (dashed line), $\dot{V}O_2$ is identified in panel 1 and compared with the $\dot{V}O_2$ at the *AT* identified in panel 3. Panel 8 (R) is included here to illustrate that at the time corresponding to *AT*, the R value was rising steeply but had not yet reached a value of 1.0. Changes in R are also useful for identifying transient episodes of hyper- or hypoventilation that may account for atypical patterns in the variables plotted in panels 4 and 7.

effort. If the O_2 pulse plateaus at a stable value that does not increase with progressive rise in work rate, the peak value can be interpreted as maximal. A lower than expected maximal O_2 pulse could result from numerous factors, including low exercise stroke volume, reduction in arterial oxygen content, or, less commonly, limitation of maximal oxygen extraction due to failure to distribute blood flow to the muscle or a defect in muscle oxidative capacity. When the O_2 pulse does not clearly reach a plateau, a low peak value could simply reflect premature ending of the test prior to attainment of maximal oxygen extraction. Higher than average values for O_2 pulse, on the other hand, usually reflect high exercise stroke volume. Increased stroke volume is characteristic of endurance-trained individuals but can also result in nonathletes from impairment of heart rate by medication or disease.

Rate-pressure product. A variable not explicitly shown in **Figure 6.2** is the product of heart rate and systolic blood pressure (shown in **Figure 6.1**, panel 5). The rate pressure product is an estimate of myocardial oxygen consumption and frequently used to judge the adequacy of an exercise stress for precipitation or exclusion of exercise-induced myocardial ischemia due to coronary disease.

Panel 3: $\dot{V}CO_2$ and heart rate as functions of $\dot{V}O_2$

HR to $\dot{V}O_2$ slope ($\Delta HR/\Delta\dot{V}O_2$). The change in heart rate relative to $\dot{V}O_2$ over incremental testing is normally quite linear, with a shallower slope for persons who are fit compared to those who are less fit. When peak heart rate is low, this panel can be helpful in distinguishing between a generalized impairment in heart rate response versus submaximal effort.[11] An upward inflection in the $\Delta HR/\Delta\dot{V}O_2$ in this panel corresponds to plateauing of O_2 pulse in panel 2.

V-slope estimate of onset of lactic acidosis. The graph of $\dot{V}CO_2$ as a function of $\dot{V}O_2$ or "V-slope,"[12] demonstrates the point at which $\dot{V}CO_2$ accelerates relative to $\dot{V}O_2$ due to excess CO_2 being evolved from the buffering of lactic acid by bicarbonate. Analysis of this graph is the most useful first step to identifying the *AT*. There are a number of factors that can affect the appearance and interpretation of this graph. The earliest portion of the data reflects the different dynamics of $\dot{V}O_2$ and $\dot{V}CO_2$ as they increase at the start of exercise; because $\dot{V}O_2$ has a faster time course, in a nonhyperventilating subject, the earliest points on this plot will increase with a slope of less than 1. Beyond this early dynamic phase, $\dot{V}O_2$ and $\dot{V}CO_2$ increase in a ratio close to 1:1, reflecting the metabolism of carbohydrate as the primary substrate used by muscle during short-duration, moderate-intensity exercise. At the onset of lactate accumulation, the slope exceeds a value of 1 as $\dot{V}CO_2$ accelerates relative to $\dot{V}O_2$. In **Figure 6.2**, the length and scaling of the $\dot{V}O_2$ and $\dot{V}CO_2$ axes are identical so that the slope of the data just prior to *AT* increase at a 45° angle. A 45° angled ruler or electronic equivalent can be aligned with these data to aid in visual identification of the inflection point. Note that if the initial phase of exercise requires a $\dot{V}O_2$ at or above the subject's lactate threshold, the *AT* cannot be discretely identified. In addition, hyperventilation alone can cause an apparent inflection point in the V-slope because excess ventilation can wash CO_2 out of the pulmonary capillary blood with little effect on the intake of oxygen. Additional graphs (particularly the ventilatory equivalents in panel 4 and end-tidal gas tensions in panel 7) should be examined to exclude nonphysiologic hyperventilation as cause of a breakpoint in the V-slope. Variables used for identifying the *AT* from gas exchange are shown together in **Figure 6.3**.

Panel 8: R

R ($\dot{V}CO_2/\dot{V}O_2$). The relationship between $\dot{V}CO_2$ and $\dot{V}O_2$ has already been considered in the graphs in panels 1 and 3. Here, their ratio, R (or RER, respiratory exchange ratio), is shown as a function of time. Under resting steady state conditions, R is equivalent to the RQ (respiratory quotient) and reflects the mix of substrate undergoing oxidative metabolism in all tissues of the body. However, during an incremental exercise test, conditions are not in a steady state and R has a complex pattern reflecting the aggregate effects of changes in the overall mix of substrate metabolized by the body, discordant dynamics of $\dot{V}O_2$ and $\dot{V}CO_2$ in response to work, the development of an additional nonmetabolic source of CO_2 from lactic acid buffering, and any superimposed effects of hyper- or hypoventilation. Prior to exercise, with a mix of fat and carbohydrate metabolism, R is usually around 0.8. With exercise, the *increases* in $\dot{V}O_2$ and $\dot{V}CO_2$ reflect the increment in metabolism of the exercising muscles, which, for short duration exercise, is fueled predominantly by carbohydrate. As a result, the R tends to increase toward 1.0 during moderate-intensity exercise as pulmonary gas exchange reflects increasing contributions from muscle metabolism. The R increases further above the lactate threshold although R typically does not exceed a value of 1.0 until some time after the onset of lactate accumulation. End-exercise R values are usually greater than 1 due to the effect of additional CO_2 evolving from buffering. However, the *rate* of production of CO_2 from buffering varies with the rate of work rate increase. The more gradual the work rate is incremented, the more gradual the rate of lactate accumulation and buffering, and the lower the peak R. Peak R may also be low when exercise is limited by noncardiovascular factors such as breathing mechanics or, alternatively, may be misleadingly high in the setting of nonphysiologic hyperventilation. At the onset of recovery, R values normally increase above the peak value, reflecting the faster time course of recovery for $\dot{V}O_2$ relative to $\dot{V}CO_2$. If oxygen delivery and utilization during exercise are severely impaired, and recovery of $\dot{V}O_2$ is significantly delayed, R may instead decrease in early recovery.

Cardiovascular and Metabolic Variables: Summary

To summarize cardiovascular and metabolic responses on a CPET, begin with panels 1 and 3 to identify peak $\dot{V}O_2$ and the *AT*, reflecting overall exercise capacity and the upper limit of the domain of moderate exercise, respectively. Cross-validate the inflection point in the V-slope as the *AT* by reviewing other variables to exclude hyperventilation as its basis. Identify peak heart rate in panel 2 and evaluate its linearity with $\dot{V}O_2$ in panel 3. Identify the peak value of O_2 pulse in panel 2 as a reflection of the composite changes in stroke volume and oxygen extraction and note whether the pattern suggests it was a maximal response. Review ECG tracings for abnormalities of rhythm, conduction, or repolarization, along with changes in blood pressure. Note findings that are abnormal and consider whether the abnormalities may be limiting to overall function.

Data Reflecting Ventilation Responses to Exercise

Panels 5 and 9 (**Fig. 6.4**) show the scale and pattern of breathing during exercise, which can be supplemented with additional spirometry to assess the role of ventilation as a limitation to exercise.

Panel 5: $\dot{V}E$ as a function of time

Peak $\dot{V}E$ needs to be considered in the context of breathing capacity. The latter is most often estimated by the maximum voluntary ventilation (MVV), which can be plotted on the $\dot{V}E$ axis of panel 5 and/or panel 9. Breathing reserve is expressed either as difference between MVV and peak $\dot{V}E$ in L/min or as percent of MVV. The MVV can be measured directly, but many prefer to calculate it as 40 or 35 times the measured forced expiratory volume in the first second of expiration. A small or absent breathing reserve strongly suggests that an individual's exercise capacity is subject to constraint by breathing mechanics. This can occur at an abnormally low level of exercise either due to a reduced breathing capacity or due to exaggerated breathing requirements due to inefficiency of pulmonary gas exchange. Well-conditioned individuals may also approach or reach the limits of breathing capacity even with normal lung function, by virtue of the ability to attain very high levels of $\dot{V}O_2$ and $\dot{V}CO_2$, which require corresponding high levels of ventilation. Whereas a small or absent breathing reserve is evidence of limitation to exercise due to lung mechanics, the presence of a breathing reserve does not necessarily exclude exercise limitation due to pulmonary factors causing dyspnea.

Panel 9: VT as a function of ventilation

Exercise breathing patterns vary but most commonly increases in VT predominate early in exercise and increases in breathing frequency predominate later. In panel 9, resting inspiratory capacity (IC) and vital capacity are shown as dashed horizontal lines to provide reference for the spontaneous VTs. Spontaneous inhalations generally remain below a maximal lung inflation, that is, VT remains below IC. Operational lung volumes may shift during exercise, however, normally by a modest decrease in end-expiratory lung volume and reciprocal increase in IC. The opposite, that is, an increase of end-expiratory volume and therefore decrease of IC, may occur due to "breath stacking" in patients with obstructive lung disease, resulting in dynamic hyperinflation and dyspnea.[13] Detection of dynamic hyperinflation requires reassessment of lung volumes during the exercise, most commonly by periodic measures of IC that can then be graphed in panel 9 to show the actual relationship of exercise VT with IC. Other breathing patterns that may be noted during testing include an oscillatory pattern in $\dot{V}E$ and gas exchange variables that is characteristic of some patients with severe heart disease. It is not unique to this condition but when present is a marker of disease severity. A chaotic breathing pattern of variable VT and frequency is sometimes present in patients with hyperventilation syndromes.

Ventilatory Variables: Summary

These variables are used primarily to assess whether breathing mechanics are limiting to maximal exercise. Compare peak $\dot{V}E$ in panel 5 or 9 with MVV after review of the source and validity of the MVV value. More subtle limitation related to breathing mechanics may take the form of dyspnea related to high work of breathing due for example to dynamic hyperinflation or to pulmonary or extrapulmonary restriction to breathing. The breathing pattern in panel 9, tidal flow–volume relationships, and reported symptoms are all potentially helpful.

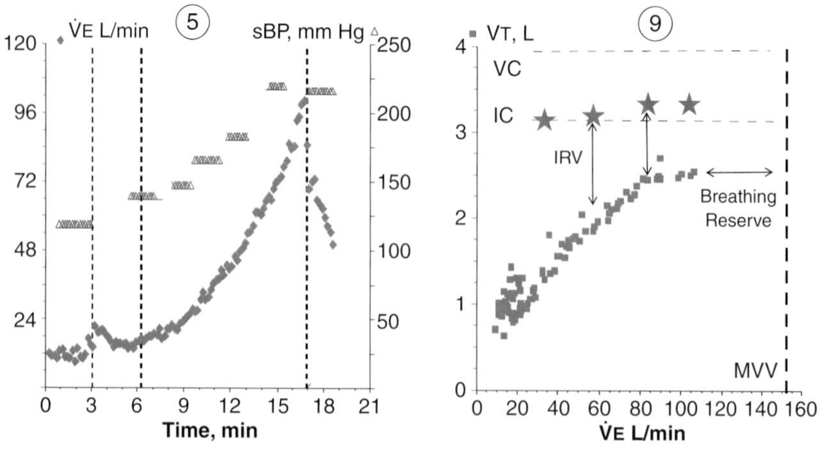

FIGURE 6.4. Graphs showing variables reflecting the ventilatory response to exercise. Peak minute ventilation ($\dot{V}E$) is identified in either panel 5 or 9 and compared with the maximum voluntary ventilation (MVV) to determine the breathing reserve. Changes in tidal volume are shown in panel 9 in comparison with resting inspiratory capacity (IC) or IC measured during exercise to identify changes in operational lung volumes such as dynamic hyperinflation. Abbreviation: IRV, inspiratory reserve volume.

Data Reflecting Efficiency of Pulmonary Gas Exchange

Close matching of regional ventilation and perfusion ($\dot{V}/\dot{Q}$) in the lung results in nearly full oxygenation of the arterial blood and sufficient clearance of CO_2 to maintain acid-base balance with optimal efficiency with respect to ventilation and work of breathing. Regional overperfusion or underventilation (low $\dot{V}/\dot{Q}$) results in impaired oxygenation, whereas regional overventilation or underperfusion (high $\dot{V}/\dot{Q}$) effectively waste ventilation. The net effects of $\dot{V}/\dot{Q}$ matching or mismatching are reflected in **Figure 6.5** including panels 4 and 6, which show the relationship between ventilation and gas exchange, and panel 7, which shows gas tensions in body tissues and exhaled breath resulting from these relationships.

Panel 4: $\dot{V}_E/\dot{V}_{CO_2}$ and $\dot{V}_E/\dot{V}_{O_2}$

Ventilatory equivalents for $\dot{V}_{CO_2}$ and $\dot{V}_{O_2}$ both typically decrease from rest to midexercise and then increase later in the test. The initial decrease reflects an improved ventilatory efficiency due to reduction in the effective V_D/V_T. This can be attributed in part to the increase in V_T, which is greater than any corresponding increase in anatomic dead space, and in part to reduction of high $\dot{V}/\dot{Q}$ regions in the lung due to recruitment of pulmonary capillaries that were underperfused at rest in the upright position. Later in exercise, there is often an increase in $\dot{V}_E/\dot{V}_{CO_2}$ due to the disproportionate increase in $\dot{V}_E$ relative to $\dot{V}_{CO_2}$ at and after the onset of respiratory compensation for metabolic acidosis. This respiratory compensation point occurs sometime after the *AT* and may not occur prior to the end of the incremental test, so it is not always evident.

An increase in $\dot{V}_E/\dot{V}_{O_2}$, usually in midexercise, marks the *AT*, as it results from $\dot{V}_E$ tracking $\dot{V}_{CO_2}$ as it increases disproportionate to $\dot{V}_{O_2}$. Because of the delay between this and the respiratory compensation point, there is a period of "isocapnic buffering." The stability of $\dot{V}_E/\dot{V}_{CO_2}$ during this time is taken as evidence that the increase in $\dot{V}_E/\dot{V}_{O_2}$ is not simply the result of nonphysiologic hyperventilation.

Panel 6: $\dot{V}_E$ vs. $\dot{V}_{CO_2}$ slope

The slope of $\dot{V}_E$ relative to $\dot{V}_{CO_2}$ is essentially linear over most of the range of exercise, with an upward inflection usually occurring at the high end of the range, corresponding to the onset of respiratory compensation for metabolic acidosis. The $\dot{V}_E$ vs. $\dot{V}_{CO_2}$ slope (or $\Delta\dot{V}_E/\Delta\dot{V}_{CO_2}$) is best determined over the early linear range, exclusive of data above the respiratory compensation point. Omitting the latter phase from calculation of the slope makes the slope independent of the duration of the test and of the individual's effort and response to metabolic acid. This reduces variability of the slope, which is particularly valuable when used in serial

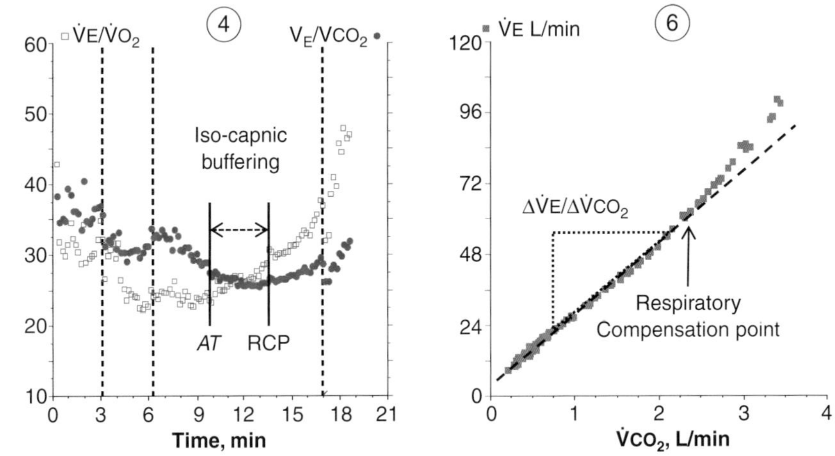

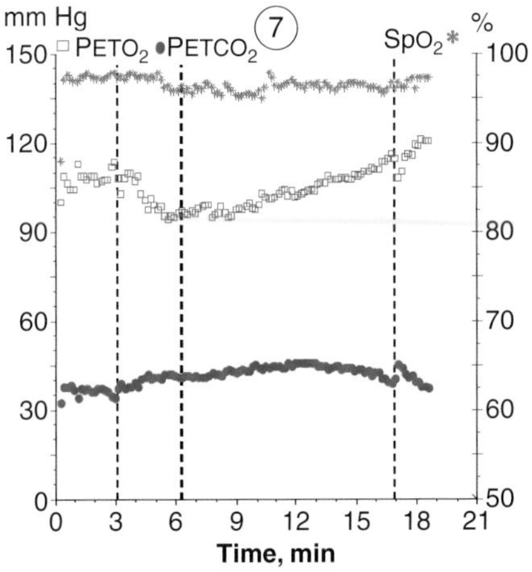

FIGURE 6.5. Primary graphs demonstrating variables related to the efficiency of pulmonary gas exchange. Panel 6 shows the near-linear increase in minute ventilation ($\dot{V}_E$) relative to carbon dioxide (CO_2) output ($\dot{V}_{CO_2}$) in early exercise, which is characterized as a slope ($\Delta\dot{V}_E/\Delta\dot{V}_{CO_2}$) over the region below respiratory compensation point. In panel 4, the related value of the ventilatory equivalent for CO_2 ($\dot{V}_E/\dot{V}_{CO_2}$) is identified at its nadir, which is usually at or shortly after the anaerobic threshold (*AT*). The pattern of change in $\dot{V}_E/\dot{V}_{CO_2}$ over the course of the test reflects decreasing values associated with decreasing V_D/V_T, stabilization during the isocapnic buffering period following *AT*, and increase with the onset of respiratory compensation for metabolic acidosis. Partial pressures of gases at the end of each breath (end-tidal) and pulse oximeter estimates of arterial oxygenation are shown in panel 7. Additional gas tensions from arterial blood or other sensors may also be displayed here.

assessments of a given patient. The $\dot{V}E$ vs. $\dot{V}CO_2$ slope demonstrated in panel 6 is closely related to the nadir value of $\dot{V}E/\dot{V}CO_2$ in panel 4 but typically lower by a few units reflecting the positive y-intercept of the slope.

An abnormally high $\dot{V}E$ vs. $\dot{V}CO_2$ slope or $\dot{V}E/\dot{V}CO_2$ have emerged as independent prognostic variables in certain clinical conditions, including chronic heart failure. This is also seen in other cardiac, pulmonary, or pulmonary vascular diseases that result in elevated effective V_D/V_T. The $\dot{V}E/\dot{V}CO_2$ may also be elevated in the presence of low arterial PCO_2, so a finding of elevated $\dot{V}E/\dot{V}CO_2$ cannot be attributed to V_D/V_T abnormalities without analysis of arterial PCO_2.

Panel 7: partial pressures of CO_2 and O_2 and SpO_2

Panel 7 shows partial pressures of gases, including at a minimum end-tidal values of PCO_2 and PO_2 in exhaled breath. Also plotted when available are pulse oximeter derived estimates of arterial O_2 saturation, transcutaneous estimates of arterial PCO_2, and arterial PCO_2 and PO_2. Arterial PO_2 and PCO_2 and the $P(A - a)O_2$ and V_D/V_T values calculated from them, are the most direct and sensitive measures of the normalcy of pulmonary gas exchange. End-tidal gas tensions are easy to measure but can be very difficult to interpret. An upward deflection of end-tidal PO_2 ($PETO_2$) is helpful in identification of the *AT*. End-tidal PCO_2 ($PETCO_2$) is typically low when V_D/V_T is high. However, $PETCO_2$ is also low when arterial PCO_2 is low, so identifying the cause of a low $PETCO_2$ requires determining arterial values.

Pulse oximeter estimates of arterial saturation are useful but may also be subject to error due to motion artifact, suboptimal perfusion, or ambient light. Small inaccuracies in the estimate of saturation can correspond to large differences in the corresponding partial pressure. Transcutaneous PCO_2 analyzers can provide close estimates of arterial values but their response times make them insensitive to rapid changes.

Pulmonary Gas Exchange Efficiency: Summary

Adequacy of oxygenation can usually be determined from pulse oximeter data, although if precise assessment of PO_2 is needed, arterial blood must be sampled. The efficiency of ventilation for clearing CO_2 and the pattern typical of a falling V_D/V_T in the transition from rest to exercise are demonstrated in panels 4 and 6. If noninvasive estimates of gas exchange efficiency are unexpectedly abnormal, blood gas assessment with calculation of $P(A - a)O_2$ and V_D/V_T can confirm and quantify abnormalities.

Graphing Strategies to Facilitate Data Analysis

The figures in this chapter and in Chapter 10 case presentations were plotted using some conventions that assist in visual analysis. This includes in panel 1 scaling $\dot{V}O_2$ and work rate values in a 10:1 ratio so that these data appear as parallel lines if the $\dot{V}O_2$ is increasing by the expected 10 mL/min/W. In panel 3, using axes of equal length and equal scaling for $\dot{V}O_2$ and $\dot{V}CO_2$ in the V-slope makes it easy to identify a breakpoint by aligning the angle of a 45° ruler along the early portion of the data. The same instrument can be used to quickly assess whether the slope of $\dot{V}E/\dot{V}CO_2$ in panel 6 is above or below a slope of 30, roughly demarcating abnormal and normal, by scaling the $\dot{V}E$ and $\dot{V}CO_2$ axes in a ratio of 30:1. Finally, the vertical array of the left hand column of graphs allows one to use a straightedge to align typical patterns for the *AT* occurring in ventilatory equivalents (panel 4) and end-tidal gas tensions (panel 7) with $\dot{V}O_2$ in panel 1. For the graphs not using time on the x-axis, recovery data are omitted from the graphs or plotted with different symbols to avoid confusion with the exercise responses.

Summarizing Key Variables

The key variables used to characterize exercise performance discussed earlier can be summarized in tabular format such as shown in **Table 6.2**, with reference values listed alongside. Software often support the creation of a summary table of the values, which should always be cross-checked during the process of reviewing the original study data to ensure accuracy.

EXAMPLES OF FINDINGS IN THE NINE-PANEL DISPLAY IN SELECTED CARDIORESPIRATORY DISORDERS

In **Figures 6.6** through **6.14** each of the nine panels in the montage discussed earlier are shown for eight patients with different clinical disorders in comparison with a normal individual. The findings illustrated are not invariant among all patients with the diseases represented, but they serve to demonstrate the potential for the underlying disorder to constrain or distort some of the normal exercise responses in patterns that are useful for diagnostic assessment.

In **Figures 6.6** through **6.14**, data for a particular panel are shown for (A) 55-year-old man who is apparently healthy, (B) a 47-year-old man with coronary artery disease (CAD), (C) a 65-year-old man with intermittent claudication due to peripheral arterial disease (PAD), (D) a 57-year-old woman with reduced ejection fraction heart failure due to nonischemic cardiomyopathy (DCM), (E) a 54-year-old man with idiopathic pulmonary arterial hypertension (PVD), (F) a 37-year-old man with uncomplicated obesity, (G) a 50-year-old man with chronic obstructive pulmonary disease (COPD), (H) a 29-year-old man with interstitial and pulmonary vascular disease due to sarcoidosis, and (I) a 20-year-old man with severe interstitial pulmonary fibrosis (IPF).

Panel 1: $\dot{V}O_2$, $\dot{V}CO_2$, and Work Rate as Related to Time

The first panel of the nine-panel array for nine different individuals is shown in **Figure 6.6**. The parallel increases in plotted values for $\dot{V}O_2$ and work rate, as shown for the normal individual A, indicate that $\Delta\dot{V}O_2/\Delta WR$ is the expected 10 mL/min/W, because work rate is plotted on a scale one-tenth of the $\dot{V}O_2$ scale. A shallower slope (less than

TABLE 6.2 Key Variables Summarizing Data From a Cardiopulmonary Exercise Test and Their Standard Formats

Variable	Formats
Cardiovascular/metabolic	
Peak $\dot{V}O_2$	mL/min, mL/min/kg % of predicted
Anaerobic threshold $\dot{V}O_2$	mL/min % of predicted peak $\dot{V}O_2$
$\Delta\dot{V}O_2/\Delta WR$	mL/min O_2/W
Peak $\dot{V}O_2$/HR	(mL/min O_2)/heart beat
Peak HR	beats/min
Heart rate reserve	beats/min
Blood pressure	mm Hg at rest, peak exercise
Peak work rate	Watts (cycle), speed and grade (treadmill)
Ventilation	
Peak $\dot{V}E$	L/min
Breathing reserve	L/min
Peak respiratory rate	breaths/min
Delta IC	mL
Gas exchange efficiency	
$\dot{V}E/\dot{V}CO_2$	Slope of linear domain $\Delta\dot{V}E/\Delta\dot{V}CO_2$ or nadir $\dot{V}E/\dot{V}CO_2$ value at or shortly after *AT*
SpO_2	%: rest, peak exercise; mm Hg: rest, peak exercise
Additional gas exchange efficiency variables when arterial blood gas data are available	
PaO_2	mmHg: rest, peak exercise
$P(A - a)O_2$	mmHg: rest, peak exercise
V_D/V_T	Rest, peak exercise

Abbreviations: *AT*, anaerobic threshold; HR, heart rate; IC, inspiratory capacity; V_D/V_T, dead space–tidal volume ratio; $\dot{V}E$, minute ventilation; $\dot{V}E/\dot{V}CO_2$, ventilatory equivalent for CO_2; $\dot{V}O_2$, O_2 uptake; WR, work rate.

approximately 8.5) suggests a condition impairing delivery and/or utilization of O_2, which is most commonly due to a cardiovascular impairment. This is illustrated by data from several patients in **Figure 6.6**, including C, D, E, H, and I with PAD, DCM, PVD, pulmonary sarcoidosis, and IPF, respectively. Of note, patient B, with CAD, initially demonstrates a normal $\Delta\dot{V}O_2/\Delta WR$ slope, but this became abnormal coincident with the development of ischemic changes on ECG, consistent with disruption of the normal cardiac output response to increasing work rate due to myocardial ischemia. For each of the patients with abnormal $\Delta\dot{V}O_2/\Delta WR$ slope, the peak $\dot{V}O_2$ was also lower than predicted, also consistent with lower than normal capacity for oxygen delivery and/or utilization. Note that patient F was tested on a treadmill, and because variations in walking economy make it difficult to know work rate precisely, $\Delta\dot{V}O_2/\Delta WR$ slope was not calculated. For patient G, with COPD, the $\Delta\dot{V}O_2/\Delta WR$ was normal up to the level of work attained. Failure of oxygen delivery and utilization to keep pace with requirements of increasing work rate results in accumulation of an "oxygen deficit" during the exercise. As a consequence, the return of $\dot{V}O_2$ back to resting levels is prolonged as additional O_2 uptake is needed to replete oxygen stores and regenerate depleted high-energy phosphate stores. This is best illustrated in **Figure 6.6** by the data for patient H, for whom $\dot{V}O_2$ remained elevated close to peak values over the first 2 minutes of recovery. Less dramatic is the slow $\dot{V}O_2$ recovery pattern for patients E and I, when compared with that for the healthy individual A. The time course of $\dot{V}O_2$ recovery after exercise can thus provide indirect evidence of abnormal $\dot{V}O_2$ increase during the test, even for tests in which the work rate cannot be precisely quantified.

Panel 3: Heart Rate and Carbon Dioxide Output as a Function of Oxygen Uptake

In **Figure 6.7**, data for individual A demonstrate the normal linear increase of heart rate relative to $\dot{V}O_2$ toward their respective predicted maximum values, marked by the *X* in the figure. The heart rate:VO_2 slope is often steeper than normal, and may become nonlinear, in patients with cardiac disease, such as patients B and D, or pulmonary vascular disease, illustrated by patients E, H, and I. Not illustrated among these examples is a shallow slope of heart rate relative to $\dot{V}O_2$ and low peak heart rate, which would be characteristic of treatment with β-adrenergic blocking agents or intrinsic impairment of chronotropic function. A shallow slope is also characteristic of cardiorespiratory fitness; however, in that case, the peak heart rate would be in the normal range and peak $\dot{V}O_2$ would likely be above the average expected for sedentary individuals. On the same graph in **Figure 6.7** is the "V-slope" relationship showing $\dot{V}CO_2$ as a function of $\dot{V}O_2$ for identifying the *AT*. The *AT* is often reduced in cardiovascular disease as illustrated by patients D, E, H, and I.

Panel 2: Heart Rate and Oxygen Pulse as a Function of Time

Panel 2 of the nine-panel array is shown in **Figure 6.8**. The abrupt increase in heart rate at the start of unloaded cycling, due to reflex withdrawal of parasympathetic tone, with subsequent progressive rise with increasing work rate, is illustrated by data for the normal individual A. Low peak heart rate is seen in patients with chronotropic incompetence or β-blocker therapy, such as in patient D with DCM, or when the exercise ends because of conditions or symptoms limiting exercise prior to maximal cardiac stress, such as for patient C with PAD, and patient G with COPD.

Also graphed in this panel is the O_2 pulse, or $\dot{V}O_2$/HR, which equals the product of stroke volume and $C(a - \bar{v})O_2$. Although this variable often reaches an asymptote in

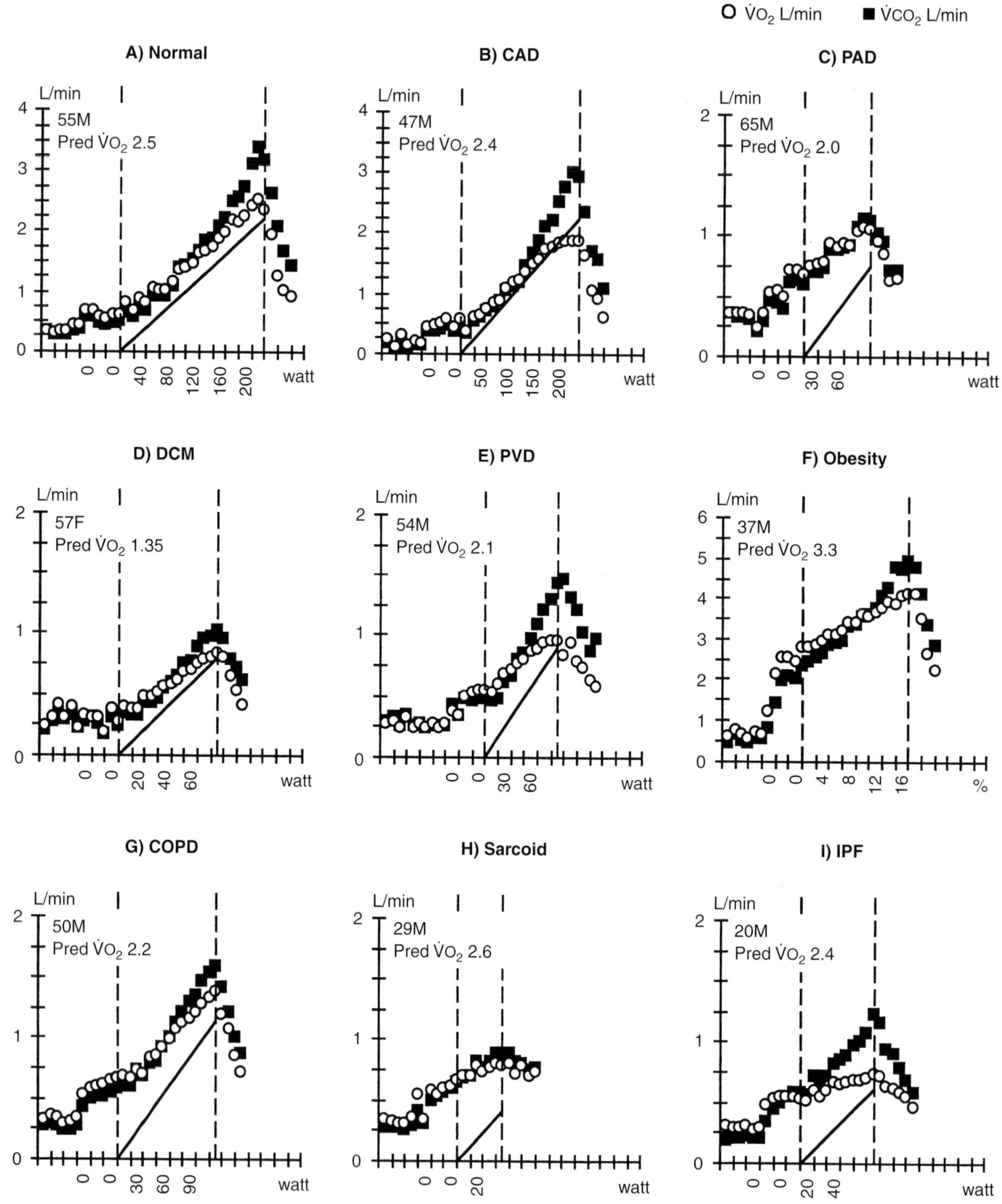

FIGURE 6.6. Plots of $\dot{V}O_2$ (open circles) and $\dot{V}CO_2$ (filled squares) as functions of time and work rate (watts) and time and work rate (1 min between tick marks on x-axis) for nine individuals, including one with normal exercise performance (A), and for patients with diagnoses of coronary artery disease (CAD) (B), peripheral arterial disease (PAD) (C), dilated cardiomyopathy (DCM) (D), pulmonary vascular disease (PVD) (E), obesity (abscissa is percentage treadmill grade) (F), chronic obstructive pulmonary disease (COPD) (G), sarcoidosis (H), and interstitial pulmonary fibrosis (IPF) (I). The data to the left of the first 0 are from the rest period. Zero work rate is unloaded cycling. The period of increasing work rate starts at the left vertical dashed line and ends at the right vertical dashed line as indicated by the solid diagonal line. The predicted peak $\dot{V}O_2$ is shown in the upper left of each panel along with the age and sex of the patient. Abbreviations: CAD, coronary artery disease; COPD, chronic obstructive pulmonary disease; DCM, dilated cardiomyopathy; IPF, interstitial pulmonary fibrosis; PAD, peripheral arterial disease; PVD, pulmonary vascular disease.

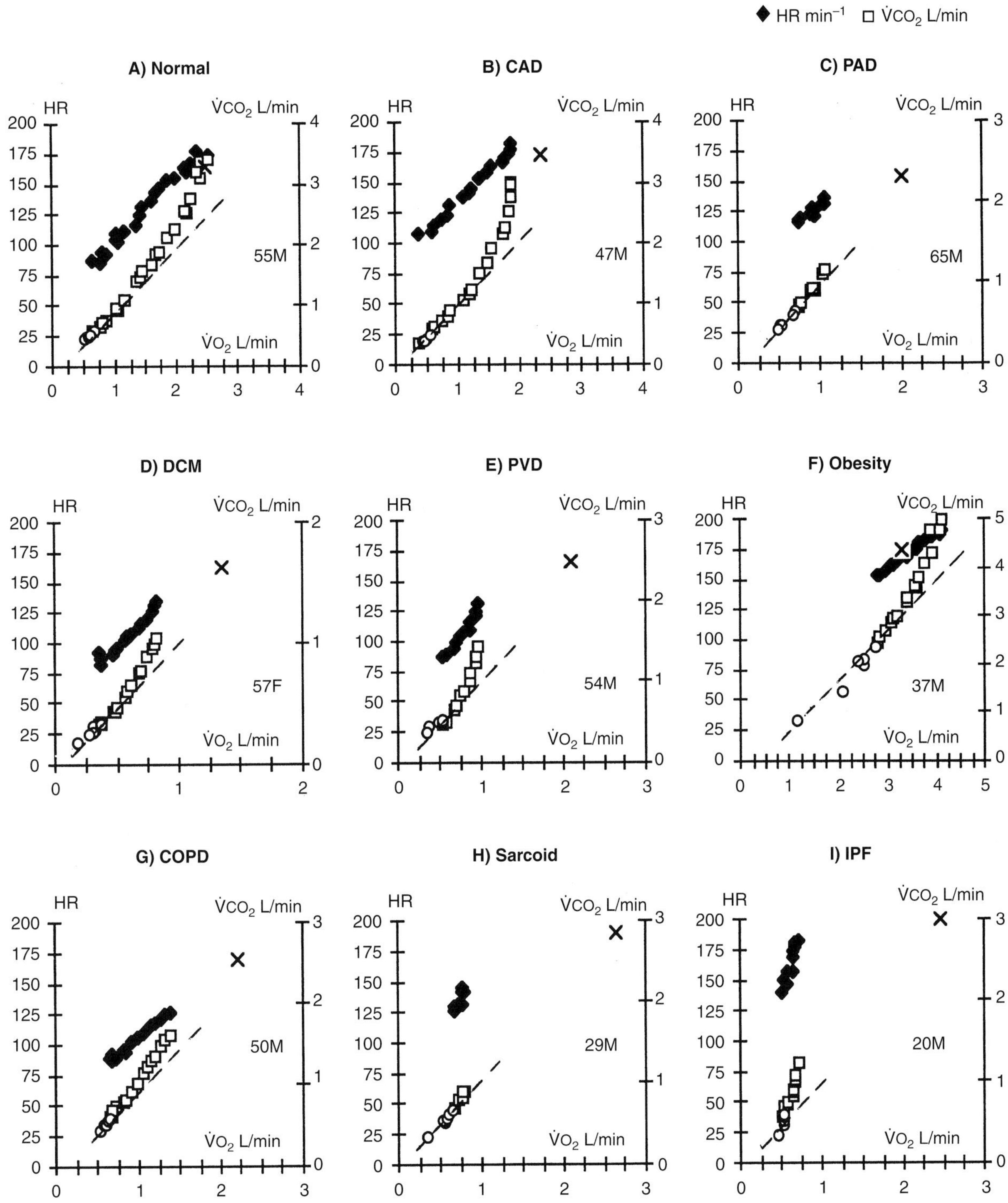

FIGURE 6.7. Plots of heart rate (HR) (filled squares) and $\dot{V}CO_2$ (open circles), both as functions of $\dot{V}O_2$ at rest and exercise; recovery data are omitted. An X marks the predicted peak values for HR and peak $\dot{V}O_2$. The scaling on the $\dot{V}O_2$ and $\dot{V}CO_2$ axes are identical, so the diagonal dashed line shows a slope of 1.0 for $\dot{V}CO_2$ relative to $\dot{V}O_2$. The test protocols and tested individuals are the same as for Figure 6.6.

healthy individuals as peak exercise is approached, a flattening of the response at a lower than expected value implies that both stroke volume and $C(a - \bar{v})O_2$ reached their limits and that one or both was lower than normal. This is frequently the case for patients with impaired cardiac stroke volume, as illustrated for patient D with DCM. Early flattening of the O_2 pulse in patients E, H, and I, similarly, likely reflects constraint on stroke volume of the right ventricle, although there is additional limitation on $C(a - \bar{v})O_2$ due to exercise-induced hypoxemia (shown in **Fig. 6.12**). Anemia could also limit the maximal $C(a - \bar{v})O_2$ due to reduced arterial oxygen content. For patient B with CAD,

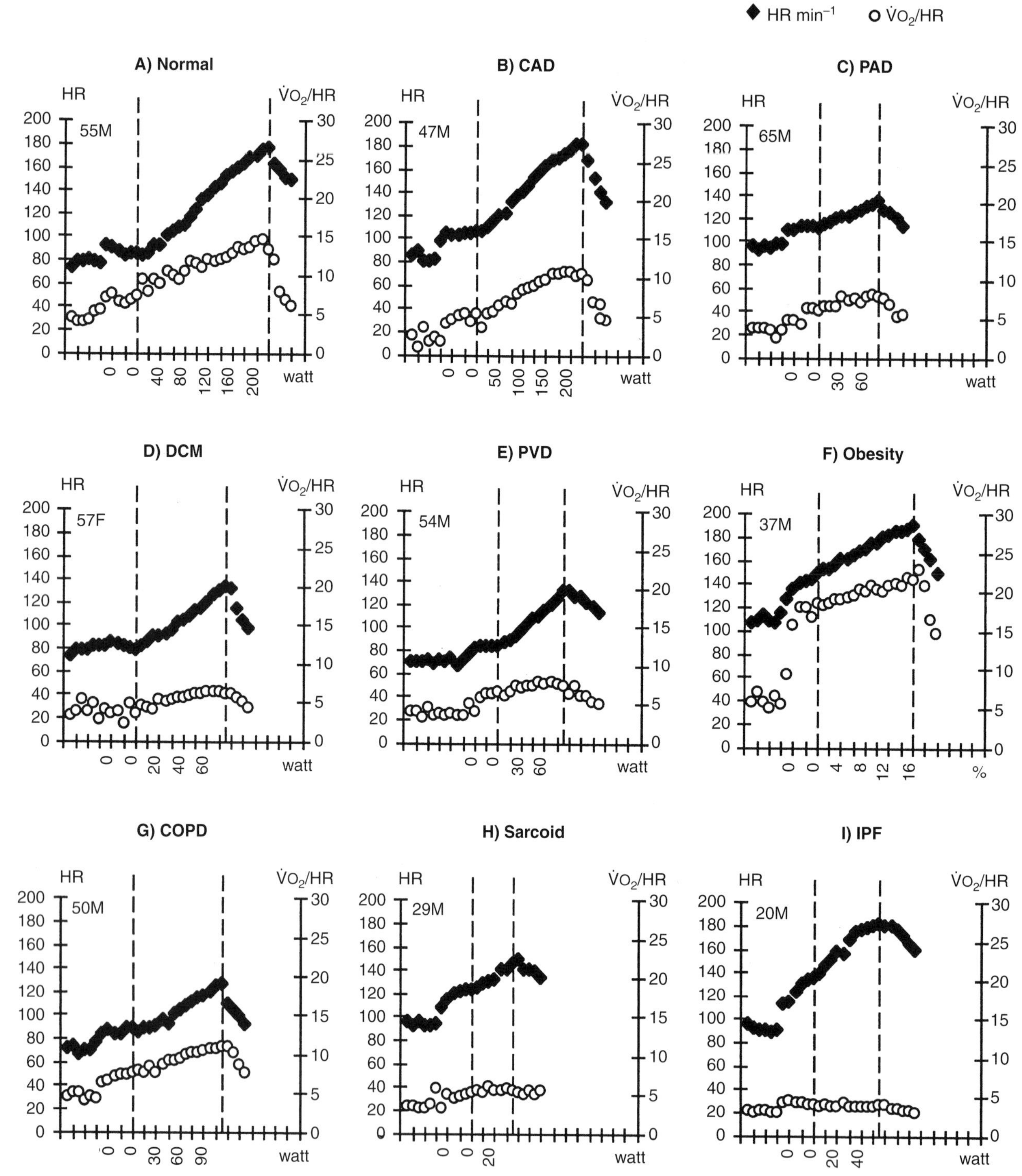

FIGURE 6.8. Plot of heart rate (HR) (filled squares) and O_2 pulse (open circles) as functions of work rate and time at rest, exercise, and recovery. The test protocols and tested individuals are the same as for Figure 6.6.

the initial increase in O_2 pulse appeared normal but it leveled off at the time ischemic changes developed on ECG, consistent with an ischemia-induced reduction in exercise stroke volume. In patients with impairment of heart rate but otherwise intact cardiac function, a higher than average O_2 pulse is typically seen due to partial compensation for the reduced heart rate by increased stroke volume.

Panel 9: Tidal Volume as a Function of Exercise Minute Ventilation

The VT is plotted as a function of V̇E in panel 9 of the nine-panel array and shown in **Figure 6.9**. As illustrated for individual A, there is usually a breathing reserve at end exercise, and VT usually remains below the IC throughout exercise. Changes in end-expiratory lung volume during

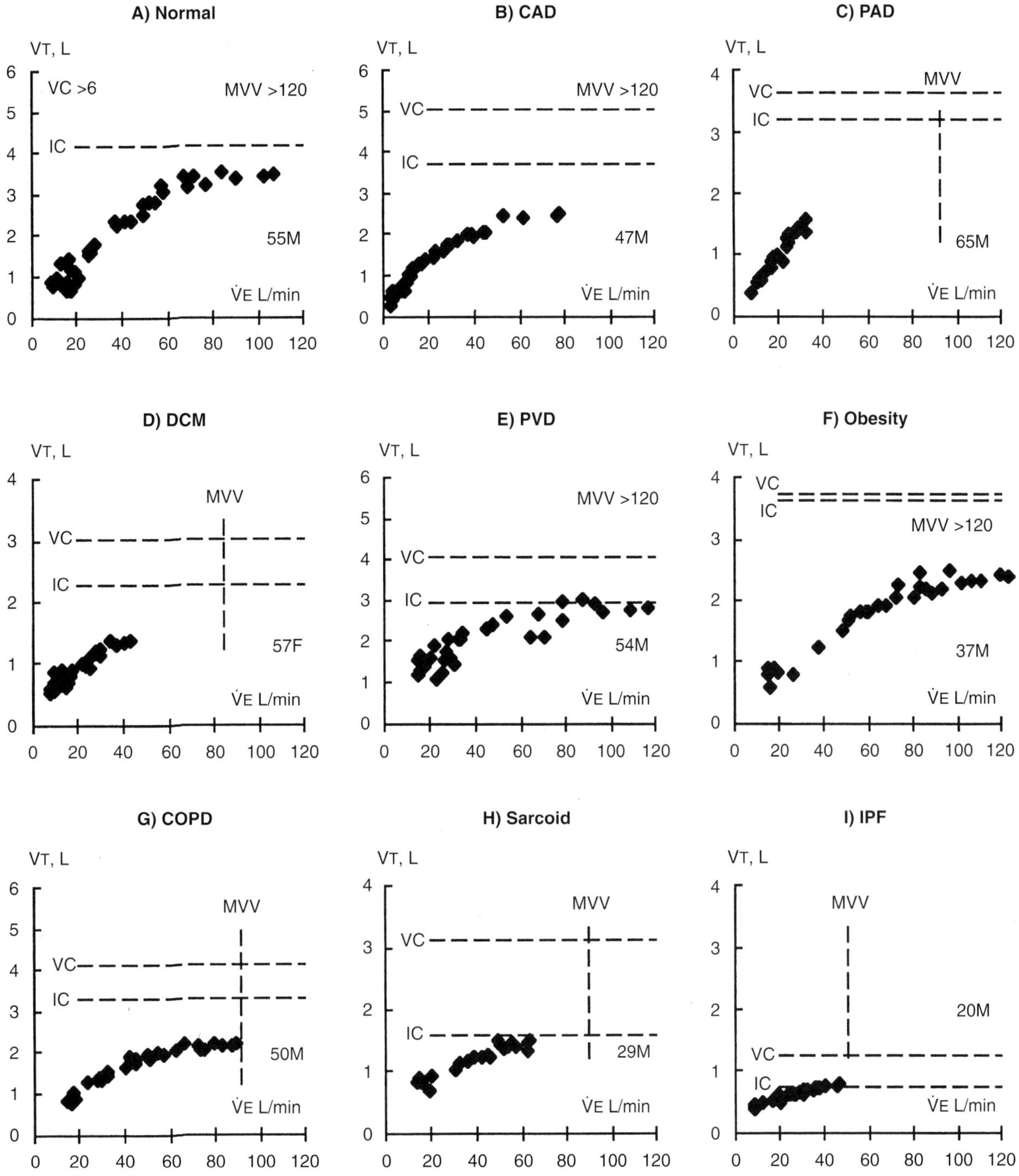

FIGURE 6.9. Plot of tidal volume (VT) as a function of exercise minute ventilation (V̇E) during rest and exercise. Also shown are the individuals' maximum voluntary ventilations (MVV) on the abscissa (vertical dashed lines) and the subject's resting inspiratory capacity (IC) and vital capacity (VC) on the ordinate (horizontal dashed lines) unless above scale. The test protocols and tested individuals are the same as for Figure 6.6.

exercise may shift IC to higher or lower levels than measured at rest, however. Although hyperinflation (increased end-expiratory lung volume) may sometimes be evidenced by a reduction in VT, at high levels of V̇E, this is not as sensitive as demonstrating the reciprocal decrease in IC on serial measures during exercise. In patients with restrictive lung disease, VT may reach or even exceed the resting IC as illustrated by patients H and I with pulmonary sarcoidosis and IPF, respectively, likely reflecting a decrease in end-expiratory lung volume during exercise. The lack of breathing reserve for patients G and I with COPD and IPF, respectively, is evidence of exercise limitation due to breathing mechanics.

Breathing pattern is rarely diagnostic of a specific disorder in and of itself. Exceptions to this include identification of dynamic hyperinflation as a driver of dyspnea in obstructive lung disease or the finding of an erratic breathing pattern with evidence for acute hyperventilation reproducing the presenting symptom of dyspnea. Patients with laryngeal dysfunction may have lower than expected VTs due to functional obstruction of the upper airway during inspiration, with or without audible stridor, but this diagnosis is best established by laryngoscopic visualization of the airways during symptoms.[14]

Panel 6: Exercise Minute Ventilation as a Function of Carbon Dioxide Output

$\dot{V}E$ is plotted as a function of $\dot{V}CO_2$ in panel 6 of the nine-panel array and shown in **Figure 6.10**. This slope may be steeper than normal in a wide range of conditions for which there are high ventilation to perfusion ($\dot{V}/\dot{Q}$) relationships in the lung, that is, high effective VD/VT. A steeper than normal slope is typical of heart failure as

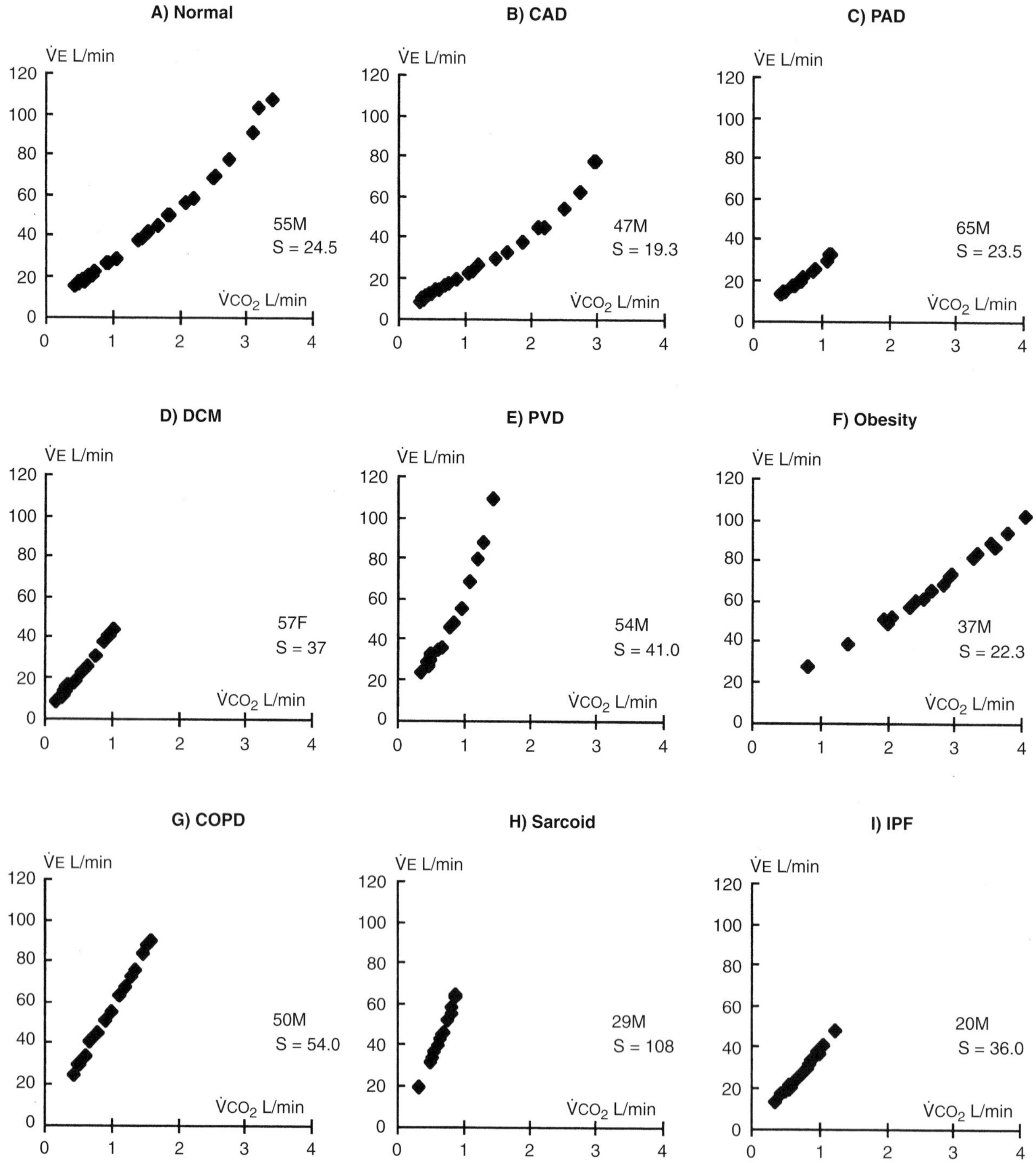

FIGURE 6.10. Plot of minute ventilation ($\dot{V}E$) as a function of $\dot{V}CO_2$ at rest and exercise; recovery data are omitted. Scaling for each reflects a ratio of 30:1 for $\dot{V}E$ relative to $\dot{V}CO_2$ such that a 45° slope corresponds to a $\dot{V}E/\dot{V}CO_2$ slope of 30. The test protocols and tested individuals are the same as for Figure 6.6.

illustrated by patient D with DCM and also of primary or secondary pulmonary vascular disease as illustrated by patients E, G, H, and I. Although each of these cases is likely associated with $\dot{V}/\dot{Q}$ abnormalities, a steep slope may also result from acute or chronic respiratory alkalosis, resulting, for example, from acute hyperventilation or respiratory compensation for chronic metabolic acidosis. The slope is typically not affected by conditions of CAD without heart failure, PAD, or obesity, as illustrated by patients B, C, and F.

Panel 4: Ventilatory Equivalents for Oxygen and Carbon Dioxide Versus Time

The ventilatory equivalents are shown in panel 4 of the nine-panel array and in **Figure 6.11**. The same factors affecting the slope of $\dot{V}E/\dot{V}CO_2$ shown in **Figure 6.10** determine

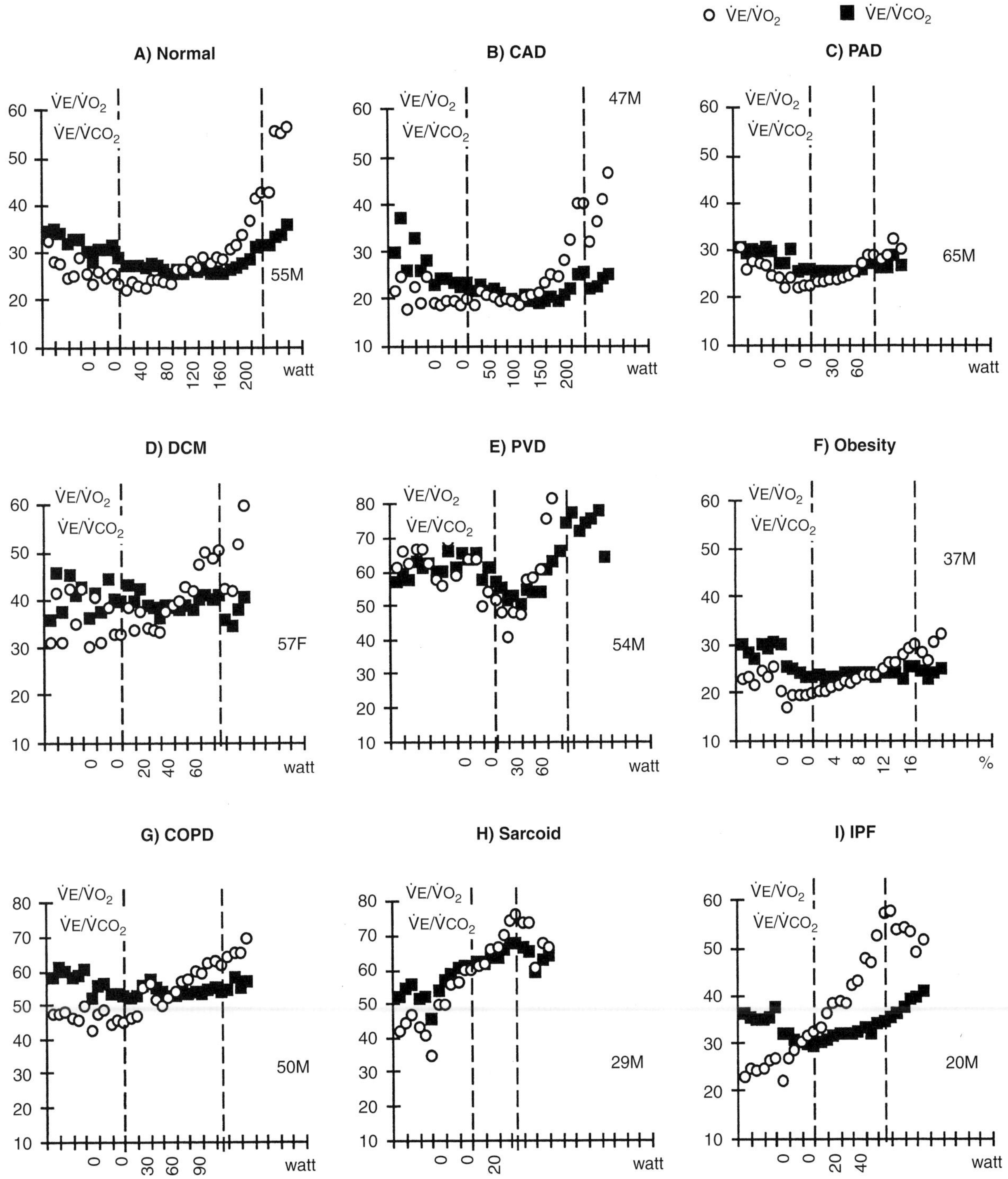

FIGURE 6.11. Plot of ventilatory equivalent for O_2 ($\dot{V}E/\dot{V}O_2$) (open circles) and CO_2 ($\dot{V}E/\dot{V}CO_2$) (closed squares) as functions of work rate and time at rest, exercise, and recovery. The test protocols and tested individuals are the same as for Figure 6.6.

the value of the $\dot{V}E/\dot{V}CO_2$ ratio. Failure of $\dot{V}E/\dot{V}CO_2$ to decrease in the transition from rest to moderate exercise implies a failure of V_D/V_T to decrease normally. This is typical of conditions in which there are no recruitable pulmonary capillaries to accept the increased venous return at the start of exercise due to congestive (eg, patient D) or obliterative (eg, patients G and H) pulmonary vascular conditions. $\dot{V}E/\dot{V}CO_2$ decreases to a nadir between the *AT* and ventilatory compensation point at values that are usually in the 20s, as shown in for individual A and patients B, C, and F. Values remain higher in patients with abnormal slopes of $\dot{V}E/\dot{V}CO_2$ as identified earlier. The pattern of $\dot{V}E/\dot{V}O_2$ relative to $\dot{V}E/\dot{V}CO_2$ is also useful in the determination or confirmation of *AT*. The typical finding on this panel of stable $\dot{V}E/\dot{V}CO_2$ at the point where $\dot{V}E/\dot{V}O_2$ begins to increase provides supporting evidence that the inflection of $\dot{V}CO_2$ identified on the V-slope of panel 3 was driven by buffering of lactate, rather than by primary hyperventilation. In contrast, a simultaneous increase in both ratios suggests a hyperventilation event. For patient H with advanced sarcoidosis, both ventilatory equivalents increase together at the start of pedaling; however, review of data in panel 3 (see **Fig. 6.8**) and panel 7 (see **Fig. 6.12**) are not indicative of hyperventilation and suggest instead that this resulted from his having exceeded his *AT* soon after the start of exercise.

Panel 7: End-Tidal Oxygen and Carbon Dioxide Tensions Versus Time

P_{ETO_2} and P_{ETCO_2}—and, when available, Pa_{O_2} and Pa_{CO_2}—are plotted in panel 7 of the nine-panel array and are shown in **Figure 6.12**. Other measures of respiratory gases, including oxyhemoglobin saturation from pulse oximetry, or transcutaneous measures of P_{CO_2} can also be displayed. Note that although the P_{ETO_2} and P_{ETCO_2} values for the normal individual, A, appear quite similar to the corresponding arterial blood values, in the presence of diseases affecting pulmonary $\dot{V}/\dot{Q}$ matching, such as patients E, H, and I, the P_{ETCO_2} were lower than arterial values. Furthermore, in healthy individuals, P_{ETCO_2} usually exceeds Pa_{CO_2} during heavy exercise. Thus, low P_{ETCO_2} can indicate low Pa_{CO_2}, high V_D/V_T, or both, and high P_{ETCO_2} may or may not reflect arterial hypercapnia.

When evaluating patients with diseases known to alter the efficiency of gas exchange, there is often no need to confirm the abnormalities with arterial blood gases. When clinically necessary, however, the most precise way to identify and quantify gas exchange abnormalities is to measure arterial blood gases and calculate the $P(A - a)O_2$ and V_D/V_T; formulae are found in Appendix C. The $P(A - a)O_2$ may be abnormally wide even without definitive desaturation by oximetry in patients with early lung or pulmonary vascular disease. Elevation of V_D/V_T with or without abnormal oxygenation may indicate a primary or secondary pulmonary vascular process. Chronic metabolic acidosis may result in exercise intolerance due to augmented ventilation associated with the associated respiratory compensation.

Panel 5: Minute Ventilation as a Function of Time

The $\dot{V}E$ is plotted as a function of time in panel 5 of the nine-panel array shown in **Figure 6.13**. The normal pattern is illustrated by individual A: a linear increase of $\dot{V}E$ relative to work rate during moderate exercise, acceleration at the *AT*, and further acceleration at the ventilatory compensation point. Respiratory compensation for metabolic acidosis may not occur prior to the end of exercise or may be attenuated in patients with constraints on breathing pattern due to body habitus, as seen for patient F with obesity, or severe lung disease, as for patients H and I with interstitial lung diseases. Although not shown in **Figure 6.13**, intermittent measures of systolic blood pressure are also plotted on this panel in the case examples in Chapter 10.

Panel 8: Respiratory Exchange Ratio at Rest, Increasing Work Rate Exercise, and Recovery

The R as a function of time is shown in panel 8 of the nine-panel array and in **Figure 6.14**. The normal pattern of R from rest through peak exercise is described earlier and illustrated for the normal individual A. The R values may be elevated at rest if there is transient hyperventilation when first breathing through the mouthpiece or mask used for testing. Although usually self-limited, hyperventilation, and relative hypoventilation occurring once hyperventilation resolves, can alter typical values of R and other CPET variables. A progressive rise of R during exercise to values exceeding 1.0 is expected for patients able to exercise beyond *AT*, but this may not occur if exercise is limited by symptoms, poor motivation, or other factors prior to development of lactic acidosis. Immediately postexercise, R normally increases further because recovery of $\dot{V}O_2$ toward baseline values is more rapid than the corresponding fall in $\dot{V}CO_2$. In some patients with substantial limitation in oxygen delivery and/or utilization, R may decrease, rather than increase, at the start of recovery due to delayed recovery of $\dot{V}O_2$, as illustrated by patients H and I in **Figure 6.14**.

Summary of Sample Response Patterns

Abnormalities in individual variables and graphs described here are usually not unique to a specific clinical condition. Any one finding is best interpreted in light of all other findings on the examination and additional information from the patient's clinical history. Similarly, not all patients with a particular clinical condition will have identical limitations in their exercise responses. Indeed, CPET is uniquely valuable in demonstrating how impairments of function in an organ system, which may or may not be apparent at rest, affect a particular individual during exercise, and how the effects of multiple impairments interact in determining overall function.

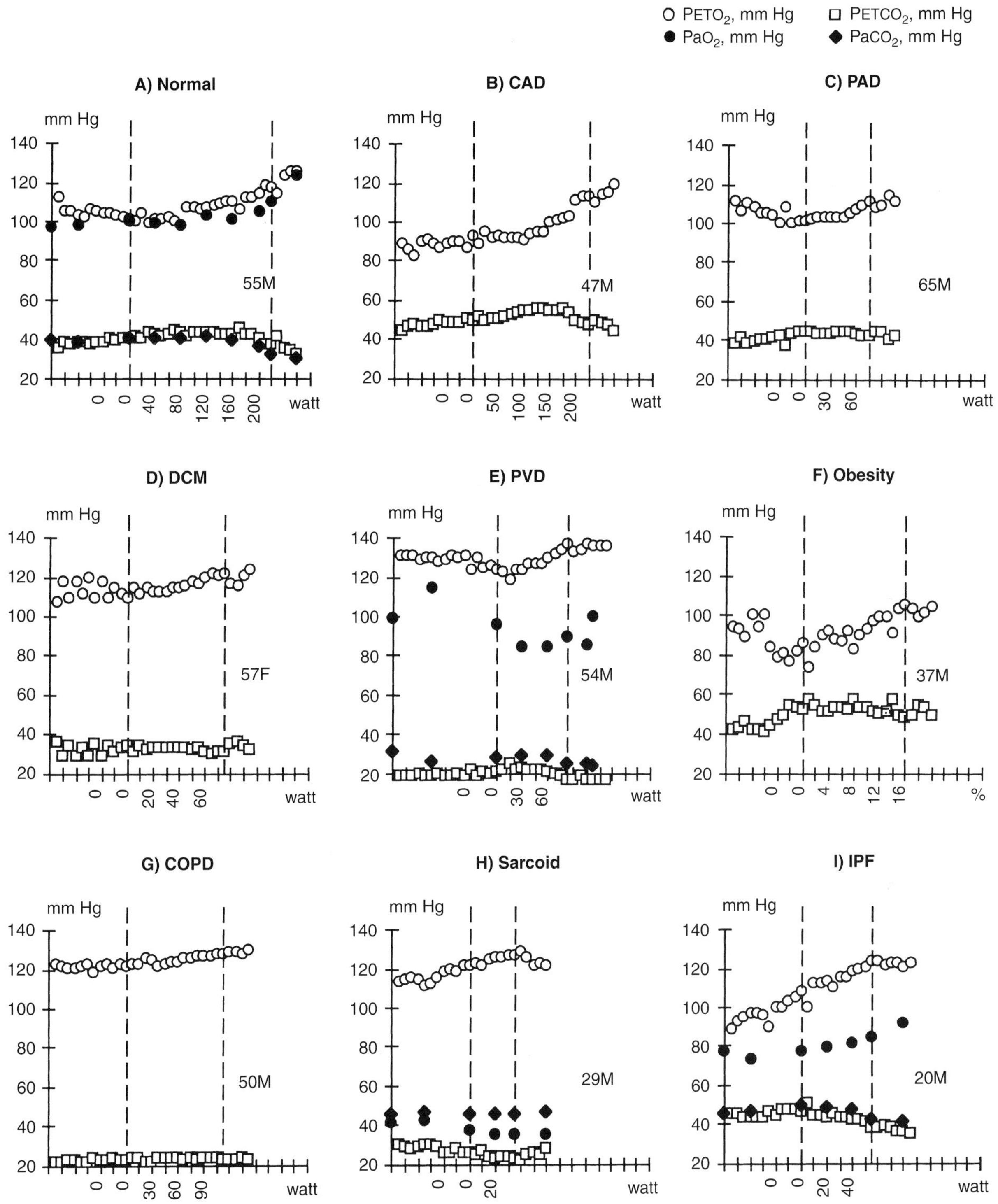

FIGURE 6.12. Plot of end-tidal gas tensions, P_{ETCO_2} (open circles) and P_{ETO_2} (open squares), and, in four cases, the corresponding arterial values (filled circles and squares) as functions of work rate and time at rest, exercise, and recovery. The test protocols and tested individuals are the same as for Figure 6.6.

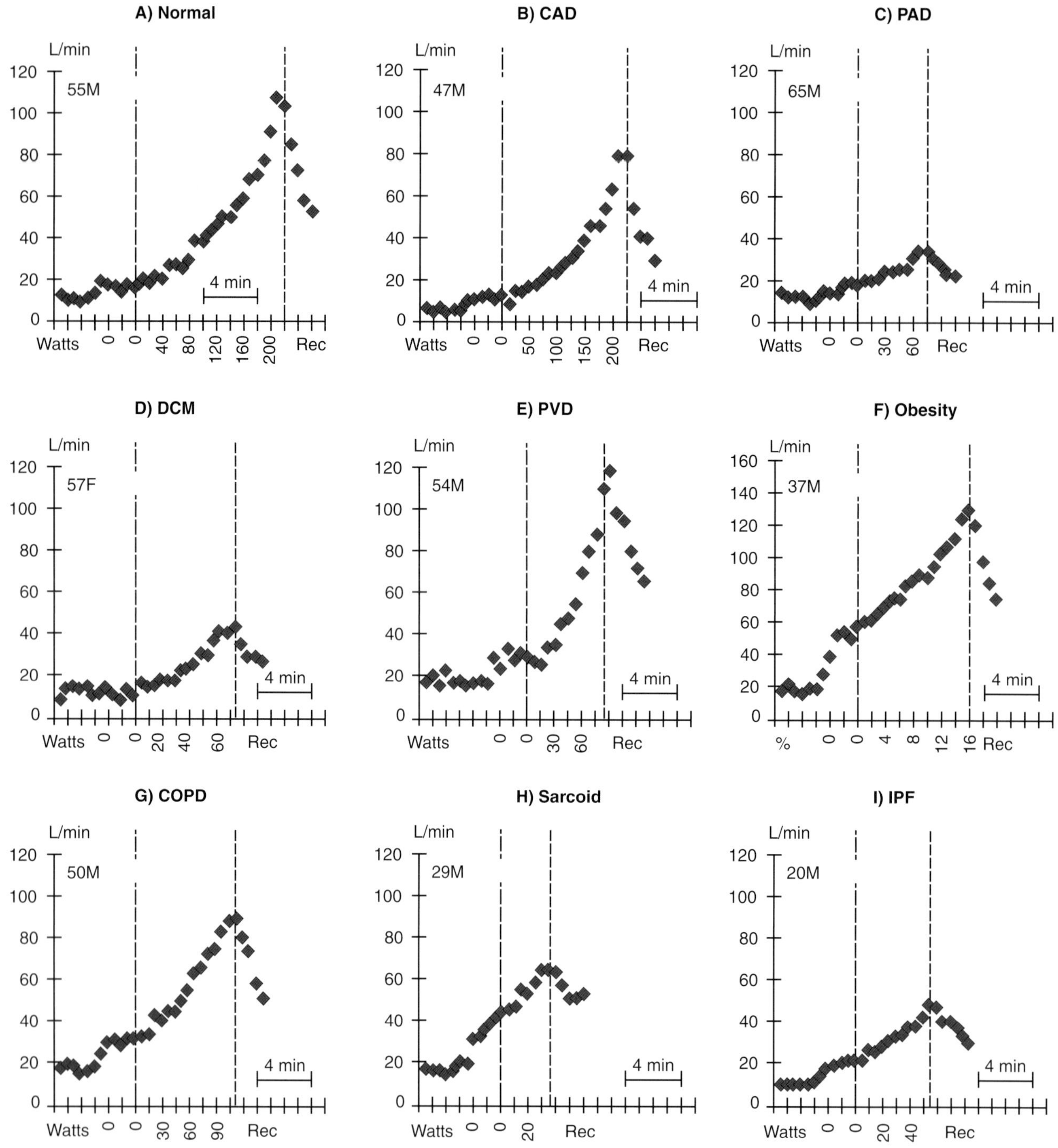

FIGURE 6.13. Plot of minute ventilation ($\dot{V}_E$) at rest, exercise, and recovery as a function of work rate and time during rest, exercise, and recovery. The test protocols and tested individuals are the same as for Figure 6.6.

WRITING AN EXERCISE TEST REPORT

Elements of the Report

Elements of a CPET report are summarized in **Table 6.3**. These include identification of the individual tested, the indication for the test, details of the exercise protocol, and any unexpected findings or complications as well as the resulting data. Test data should be reported in quantitative terms using standard units and formats as discussed elsewhere in this text. The interpretation should be in terms understandable to the intended reader but, regardless of the intended end user, should contain sufficient data and information for an independent reviewer with expertise in exercise testing to formulate his or her own interpretation. The context of

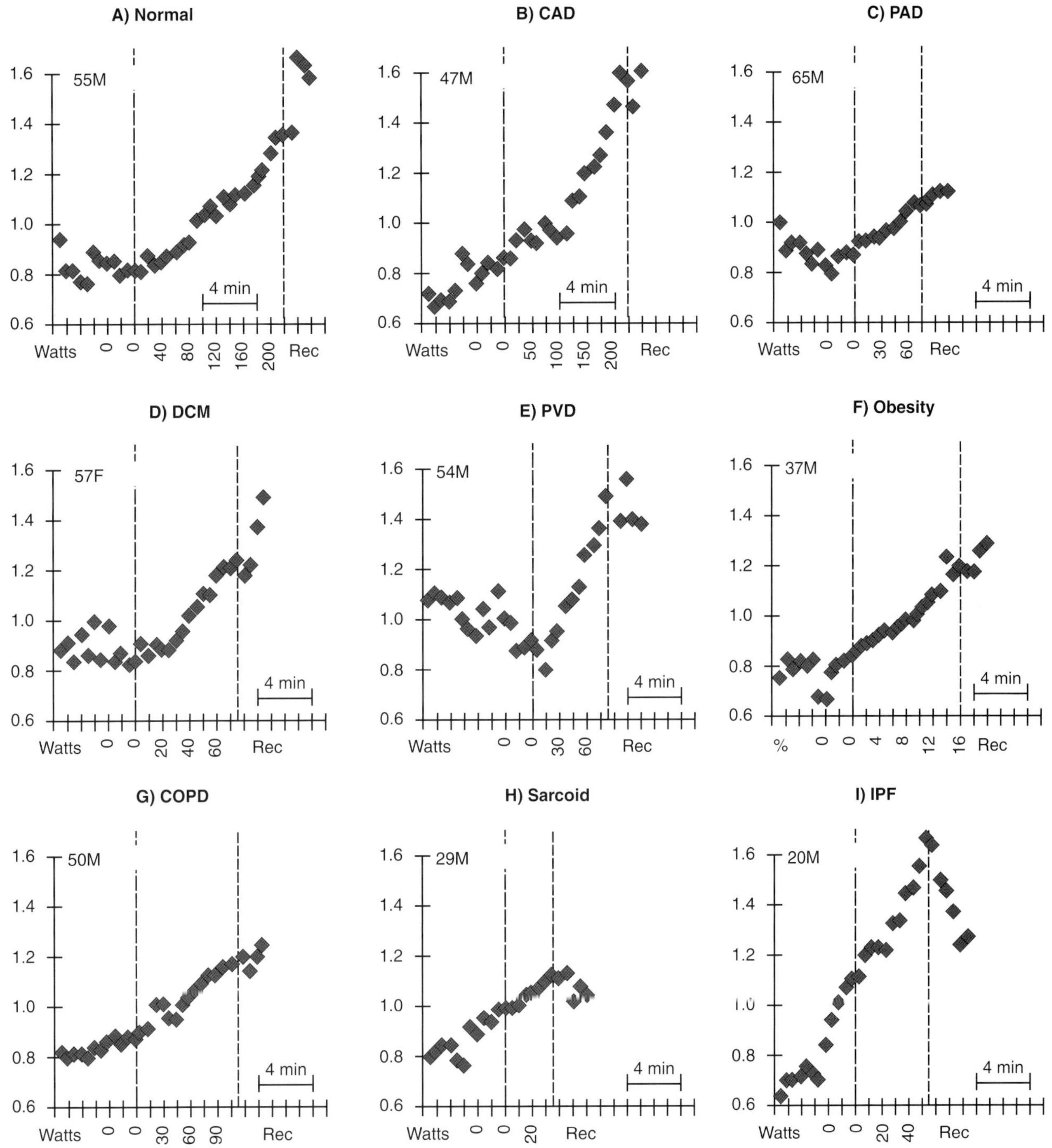

FIGURE 6.14. Plot of the respiratory gas exchange ratio (R, $\dot{V}CO_2/\dot{V}O_2$) as a function of work rate and time at rest, exercise, and recovery. The test protocols and tested individuals are the same as for Figure 6.6.

the test may dictate additional elements required to support appropriate clinical coding or exportation to clinical or research databases.

Interpretation

Interpretation begins with assessment of how measures for a patient compare with the selected reference values, that is, whether they are above or below average or frankly abnormal. Knowledge of the source and nature of the reference values will enter into interpretation if there are differences in demographics, habitual exercise, or other features of the patient compared to those of subjects represented in the normal reference data set. The remainder of the interpretation is an assessment of the significance of the test results in the clinical context of the test.

TABLE 6.3 Outline of Major Elements Included in a Comprehensive Report of a Cardiopulmonary Exercise Test

Element		Examples or relevant information
Identifiers and patient information	Identity of subject	Name, medical record number, and/or other identifiers
	Reason for the test	For example: • Assessing severity of known disease • Prognosis assessment • Preoperative risk stratification • Diagnostic evaluation for unexplained symptoms • Exercise training prescription
	Referral source	
	Relevant clinical history	In particular: • History of conditions affecting exercise function or indicating a modification of test protocol • Clinical stability at the time of testing • Exercise habits and tolerance in daily life • Exercise symptoms, particularly dyspnea, chest pain, syncope
	Medications	Especially important to record are medications modifying heart rate or treating conditions likely to affect exercise function.
Methods	Type of ergometer	Cycle, treadmill, other
	Test protocol	Profile of work rate increase and rest and recovery periods
	Equipment and measurements	Gas exchange equipment, variables measured, monitoring, frequency of blood pressure, etc
	Ancillary measurements, if any	Imaging, postexercise spirometry, etc
Results	Reason for ending the test	Examples: • Predetermined end point • Subject symptoms or inability to maintain work rate • Safety concerns
	Limiting symptoms	Also note, if relevant, whether the test reproduced the symptoms being investigated.
	Peak exercise settings	Work rate or treadmill settings at end exercise
	Unexpected or adverse events	Abnormal blood pressure, ECG, oximetry findings, or health threatening event, with interventions and outcome
	Results of safety monitoring	Indicate whether ECG, blood pressure, and oximetry findings were normal or identify abnormalities.
	Test data	• Table of values for key variables and corresponding reference values • Summary of ECG findings and representative tracings • Graphical data • Spirometry or other ancillary measures
Interpretation	Statement of overall exercise capacity or performance	Quantify as peak $\dot{V}O_2$ in, mL/min, mL/min/kg, Percentage of reference value Identify if there is reason to regard the peak value to be submaximal. Identify as normal, reduced, above or below average, etc.
	Summarize responses: • Cardiovascular/metabolic • Ventilatory • Gas exchange efficiency	• Identify whether findings were normal or abnormal. • Identify evidence of abnormal limitation to maximal function. • Detail of each based on relevance
	Conclude: Identify results most relevant to test indication in format appropriate to the referring provider.	For example: • Values of variables measured for prognosis in a particular condition • Findings of specific pathologies • Findings indicating need for further diagnostic evaluation • Values used for planning exercise prescription
Explanatory information	Source of reference values	
	Glossary and abbreviations	

Abbreviation: ECG, electrocardiogram.

Interpretation of Tests Conducted for Determination of Selected Variables

Some CPETs are conducted with specific goal of determining the value of a variable having known utility in a particular clinical condition. In healthy persons, this might be determination of peak $\dot{V}O_2$ and *AT* to characterize fitness or design a training regimen. For clinical populations, this might be for assessing severity of known disease or for judging prognosis. For example, a patient with lung cancer might be tested to determine if the peak $\dot{V}O_2$ is in a range predicting sufficient cardiorespiratory reserve to tolerate lung resection surgery. Test interpretations in these cases should explicitly include assessment of whether the key variables measured were technically accurate and valid for use in the intended decision making. In any case, the core variables described here should also be reported as standard components of the CPET.

Interpretation of CPETs Conducted for Diagnostic Purposes

In the case of patients referred for CPET as part of a diagnostic evaluation of unexplained symptoms, interpretation may be more complex. The implicit strategy is to identify the pattern of findings for the patient's test and attempt to match it to the pattern of a known clinical condition which could explain the symptoms. A CPET can lead to a specific diagnosis in some such cases when the exercise reproduces the patient's symptoms together with a specific and corresponding pathologic finding such as exercise-induced arrhythmia or stridor. Exercise intolerance can arise from a myriad of conditions[14,15] that do not all have unique findings on CPET, however. Furthermore, many patients with exercise intolerance have multiple chronic conditions each of which can affect CPET responses.[16] As a result, the contribution of CPET to diagnosis of unexplained symptoms often consists of narrowing a broad differential diagnosis, rather than of establishing a single diagnosis.[17]

Proposed approaches to interpreting CPET for diagnostic purposes take a number of forms. A stepwise flow chart to guide diagnostic thinking is presented in Chapter 9. The framework presented in **Table 6.1** and discussed earlier for summarizing findings can also be used in a more iterative fashion for formulating a diagnostic interpretation. For this, abnormal and/or limiting findings can be sought within each of the three aspects of exercise function (cardiovascular and metabolic, ventilatory, and gas exchange efficiency) as discussed previously in this chapter. The range of clinical conditions that could be associated with abnormalities in each of the categories is then considered in the light of the others and all available clinical information. Normal or abnormal findings in one category can limit the differential diagnosis represented by findings in another area, and elements from the clinical history may independently restrict potential diagnoses. Although specific diagnoses may not be definitively established, distinction can often be made between limitation due to pulmonary versus cardiovascular disorders, or particular pretest concerns may be excluded by test results, all of which are useful for directing further targeted diagnostics.[15,18] As an example, abnormalities in $\dot{V}O_2$-related variables are common to a wide range of conditions, particularly cardiac but also peripheral vascular, pulmonary vascular, and skeletal muscle disorders. A concomitant finding of high $\dot{V}E/\dot{V}CO_2$ would implicate disruption of normal pulmonary $\dot{V}/\dot{Q}$ matching, which is typical of heart failure, pulmonary, and pulmonary vascular conditions. If there is also abnormal oxygenation, however, this is unlikely attributable to heart failure alone, so diseases of the pulmonary parenchyma or vasculature become most likely. The CPET results can thus inform the choice of targeted testing to confirm or exclude potential diagnoses. Examples of tests conducted for diagnostic purposes and approaches to their interpretation are included in Chapter 10.

Tests demonstrating low or low-normal exercise capacity but without specific pathologic findings are not uncommon. These may represent early cardiopulmonary disease, deconditioning, suboptimal effort, or other conditions causing dyspnea or effort intolerance by unclear mechanisms. In these cases, clinical context should determine whether to monitor conservatively or pursue more invasive diagnostic studies. Adding hemodynamic measurements to CPET sometimes brings unique diagnostic findings to these cases.[19,20] For example, the addition of cardiac output measurement in patients with reduced exercise capacity can identify whether the cardiac output response to exercise is hypo- or hyperdynamic relative to the normal 5 to 6 L/min increase expected for each liter increase in $\dot{V}O_2$. Hyperdynamic responses are characteristic of metabolic myopathy or autonomic dysfunction. Hypodynamic responses most commonly result from intrinsic cardiac dysfunction.

Direct measurement of central circulatory pressures requires an invasive procedure but may be needed to confirm exercise-induced changes in pulmonary vascular or cardiac filling pressures that are not detectable at rest. This may be useful for identifying exercise-induced pulmonary arterial hypertension due to early pulmonary vascular disease or pulmonary venous hypertension due to left ventricular diastolic dysfunction. Low cardiac filling pressures, in contrast, may identify deficits in blood volume regulation or impairment in venous return resulting in reduced cardiac preload limiting the cardiac output response.

Confounding Factors

The presence of comorbid conditions can clearly confound the appearance of typical exercise response patterns. Although this may complicate diagnostic algorithms, CPET is sometimes performed explicitly to help clarify which of multiple known conditions is the proximal cause of limitation. In addition to chronic cardiovascular and pulmonary conditions, a number of other factors can impact exercise function and affect the responses measured on CPET. Some which should be readily recognized and identified prior to testing include obesity, anemia, and acid-base disorders.

Obesity obligates a disproportionate amount of metabolic capacity to support of the body weight so that less external work can be accomplished for a given $\dot{V}O_2$ while the relationship between changes in $\dot{V}O_2$ and work rate (ie, the $\Delta\dot{V}O_2/\Delta WR$ slope) remains unaffected. Anemia limits arterial oxygen carrying capacity and therefore oxygen delivery and peak $\dot{V}O_2$. Carboxyhemoglobin may be less obvious but also reduces oxygen carrying capacity and may be significantly elevated in smokers or others exposed to products of incomplete combustion. Either of these can affect the $\dot{V}O_2$ responses and may represent modifiable factors affecting exercise tolerance. Acid-base disorders alter ventilatory set point and therefore $\dot{V}E/\dot{V}CO_2$ relationships. In the case of chronic metabolic acidosis with respiratory compensation, maintaining a lower arterial PCO_2 will necessitate higher $\dot{V}E$ for a given metabolic rate. Conversely, patients with a chronic respiratory acidosis, resulting, for example, from obesity-hypoventilation syndrome, will have lower $\dot{V}E$ requirements for a given $\dot{V}CO_2$ due to arterial $PaCO_2$ being regulated at a higher level. Knowledge of basic laboratory findings is thus important in the interpretation of CPET performed for clinical indications.

REFERENCES

1. Hansen JE, Sue DY, Oren A, Wasserman K. Relation of oxygen uptake to work rate in normal men and men with circulatory disorders. *Am J Cardiol*. 1987;59:669-674.
2. Gimenes AC, Neder JA, Dal Corso S, et al. Relationship between work rate and oxygen uptake in mitochondrial myopathy during ramp-incremental exercise. *Braz J Med Biol Res*. 2011;44:354-360.
3. Taivassalo T, Jensen TD, Kennaway N, DiMauro S, Vissing J, Haller RG. The spectrum of exercise tolerance in mitochondrial myopathies: a study of 40 patients. *Brain*. 2003;126(pt 2):413-423.
4. Belardinelli R, Lacalaprice F, Tiano L, Muçai A, Perna GP. Cardiopulmonary exercise testing is more accurate than ECG-stress testing in diagnosing myocardial ischemia in subjects with chest pain. *Int J Cardiol*. 2014;174:337-342.
5. Belardinelli R, Lacalaprice F, Carle F, et al. Exercise-induced myocardial ischaemia detected by cardiopulmonary exercise testing. *Eur Heart J*. 2003;24:1304-1313.
6. Koike A, Hiroe M, Adachi H, et al. Cardiac output-O_2 uptake relation during incremental exercise in patients with previous myocardial infarction. *Circulation*. 1992;85:1713-1739.
7. Berling J, Foster C, Gibson M, Doberstein S, Porcari J. The effect of handrail support on oxygen uptake during steady-state treadmill exercise. *J Cardiopulm Rehabil*. 2006;26:391-394.
8. Cohen-Solal A, Laperche T, Morvan D, Geneves M, Caviezel B, Gourgon R. Prolonged kinetics of recovery of oxygen consumption after maximal graded exercise in patients with chronic heart failure. Analysis with gas exchange measurements and NMR spectroscopy. *Circulation*. 1995;91:2924-2932.
9. Mitchell SH, Steele NP, Leclerc KM, Sullivan M, Levy WC. Oxygen cost of exercise is increased in heart failure after accounting for recovery costs. *Chest*. 2003;124:572-579.
10. Cole CR, Blackstone EH, Pashkow FJ, Snader CE, Lauer MS. Heart-rate recovery immediately after exercise as a predictor of mortality. *N Engl J Med*. 1999;341:1351-1357.
11. Neder JA, Nery LE, Peres C, Whipp BJ. Reference values for dynamic responses to incremental cycle ergometry in males and females aged 20 to 80. *Am J Respir Crit Care Med*. 2001;164(8 pt 1):1481-1486.
12. Beaver WL, Wasserman K, Whipp BJ. A new method for detecting anaerobic threshold by gas exchange. *J Appl Physiol (1985)*. 1986;60:2020-2027.
13. O'Donnell DE, Revill SM, Webb KA. Dynamic hyperinflation and exercise intolerance in chronic obstructive pulmonary disease. *Am J Respir Crit Care Med*. 2001;164:770-777.
14. Olin JT, Clary MS, Fan EM, et al. Continuous laryngoscopy quantitates laryngeal behaviour in exercise and recovery. *Eur Respir J*. 2016; 48(4):1192-1200.
15. Martinez FJ, Stanopoulos I, Acero R, Becker FS, Pickering R, Beamis JF. Graded comprehensive cardiopulmonary exercise testing in the evaluation of dyspnea unexplained by routine evaluation. *Chest*. 1994;105:168-174.
16. Waraich S, Sietsema KE. Clinical cardiopulmonary exercise testing: patient and referral characteristics. *J Cardiopulm Rehabil Prev*. 2007;27:400-406.
17. Palange P, Ward SA, Carlsen KH, et al; for ERS Task Force. Recommendations on the use of exercise testing in clinical practice. *Eur Respir J*. 2007; 29:185-209.
18. Pratter MR, Abouzgheib W, Akers S, Kass J, Bartter T. An algorithmic approach to chronic dyspnea. *Respir Med*. 2011;105:1014-1021.
19. Huang W, Resch S, Oliveira RK, Cockrill BA, Systrom DM, Waxman AB. Invasive cardiopulmonary exercise testing in the evaluation of unexplained dyspnea: insights from a multidisciplinary dyspnea center. *Eur J Prev Cardiol*. 2017;24:1190-1199.
20. Maron BA, Cockrill BA, Waxman AB, Systrom DM. The invasive cardiopulmonary exercise test. *Circulation*. 2013;127(10):1157-1164.

CHAPTER 7

Normal Values

Interpretation of the results of exercise tests requires knowledge of the normal responses. This chapter presents values for important physiological variables that we think represent the best predictive data available for sedentary normal adults and children during exercise. In some instances, several sets of normal values for the same measurement are included. When doing so, we have made recommendations as to which to use.

POTENTIAL LIMITATIONS OF PUBLISHED REFERENCE VALUES FOR CARDIOPULMONARY EXERCISE TESTING

In 2001, the American Thoracic Society (ATS)/American College of Chest Physicians (ACCP) statement on cardiopulmonary exercise testing (CPET) included a review of available published normal or reference values for a number of variables during exercise.[1] Reported studies were critiqued based on several concepts, some of which are included in **Table 7.1**. For example, including only a small number of subjects meant that few individuals contributed to the distribution around the derived normal or reference values and would decrease confidence in the reported value. Optimally, subjects would be from a community-based sample instead of from a hospital or medical facility to minimize the likelihood of disease, even in those who have no medical diagnosis. When using a community-based population, care should have been taken to avoid "volunteers," who may bias the sample with those who are more physically active or competitive. Thus, a randomized sample from the whole population is more likely to be representative.

Often, a single regression equation is reported for each individual variable, for example, exercise peak oxygen uptake (peak $\dot{V}O_2$), with independent variables being size (height or weight), age, gender, and type of exercise. Because of large

The contributions of Dr. James E. Hansen, an original author of this chapter and source of much insight regarding reference data in our laboratories, are gratefully acknowledged.

TABLE 7.1 Potential Criticisms of Studies Reporting Normal or References Values for Cardiopulmonary Exercise Testing[a]

- Small number of subjects studied
- Retrospective study
- Lack of randomization
- Inclusion of smokers in the sample studied
- Exclusion of different racial groups
- Level of physical activity not reported
- Lack of quality control
- Lack of definition of confidence limits for individual or specified characteristics
- Mixing of subjects with likely differences in exercise performance
- Inclusion of data from different methodology
- Lack of a validation cohort to compare reference values from a derivation sample
- Not all relevant variables measured in same subject sample

[a]Modified from American Thoracic Society, American College of Chest Physicians. ATS/ACCP statement on cardiopulmonary exercise testing. *Am J Respir Crit Care Med.* 2003;167:211-277.

differences in peak $\dot{V}O_2$ between genders, separate equations will generally offer less variability, despite being derived from a smaller sample. This would also be true for developing separate equations for other factors, such as has been done for age (pediatric versus adult population), size (obese versus nonobese), race, and other factors. At some point, however, the convenience of a single or a few equations is generally accepted rather than multiple separate equations.

Methodology is a major consideration when deriving reference values, including the separate reporting of subjects using different ergometers, different exercise protocols, different methods for gas exchange measurements, and other factors. Efforts to ensure consistent methodology, calibration, and protocol should be reported. Finally, all variables of interest would ideally be measured in the same sample of subjects; this would be especially important for measurements that are subsequently combined, such as oxygen (O_2) pulse, ventilatory equivalent for carbon dioxide ($\dot{V}E/\dot{V}CO_2$), and $\dot{V}O_2$ at the anaerobic threshold (*AT*) compared with peak $\dot{V}O_2$. A validation cohort demonstrating comparable results to the cohort of subjects used for derivation is highly desirable.

Paap and Takken,[2] in their systematic review of 35 studies in 2014, again recommended that in the absence of ideal reference values, individual laboratories select those that best match their patient populations and methodology. In recent years, greater attention to these criteria have led to several larger, better defined, and more detailed potential normal reference values for exercise testing taken from randomized sampling. These include larger and more comprehensive references for children,[3] systematic studies of adults from several different countries, and data obtained from large randomly selected samples of adults.

PREDICTED VALUES FOR ADULTS

Peak Oxygen Uptake

The selection of peak $\dot{V}O_2$ predicted values (both mean and at the 95% confidence level) is a challenging problem, especially because the geographic area, body sizes, and activity levels of a specific clinical population may differ from those of reference populations. Peak $\dot{V}O_2$ in normal subjects during exercise varies with age, gender, body size, lean body mass, level of ordinary activity, and type of exercise. When comparing the peak $\dot{V}O_2$ of an individual to the predicted peak $\dot{V}O_2$, a predicted value generated or modified for the same form of exercise should be used. It is preferable if the population from which the predicting equations were obtained included a large number of individuals with similar characteristics to the patient being tested.

Astrand and Rodahl[4] pointed out that peak $\dot{V}O_2$ expressed as (mL/min) $\times$ kg^{-1} is higher in smaller compared with larger elite athletes, even when obesity is not a factor. However, when expressed as (mL/min) $\times$ $kg^{-2/3}$, peak $\dot{V}O_2$ differs minimally between smaller and larger athletes. They argued against the practice of using weight as a primary variable in predicting peak $\dot{V}O_2$. Despite their rational explanation and the obvious bias introduced by obesity on peak values when expressed as (mL/min) $\times$ kg^{-1}, many exercise physiologists and clinicians continue to estimate cardiovascular function by comparing actual values to values predicted from age, gender, and weight, even in obese individuals. However, this practice will frequently predict too high a peak $\dot{V}O_2$ in obese individuals. We believe that sufficient evidence exists to assert that, even though peak $\dot{V}O_2$ values may still be expressed as (mL/min) $\times$ kg^{-1} in many publications, this practice is not optimal for the clinical evaluation of the cardiorespiratory function of patients.[5-7]

Age and Gender

Many investigators have reported that peak $\dot{V}O_2$ declines with age and is smaller for women than men.[8] Although cross-sectional studies of change in peak $\dot{V}O_2$ with age are easier to perform than longitudinal studies, they may be misleading on account of selection bias. Older subjects included in a cross-sectional study are more likely to be active, relative to their peers, than their younger counterparts; hence, the peak $\dot{V}O_2$ values in older subjects in cross-sectional studies tend to decrease more slowly than peak $\dot{V}O_2$ values in longitudinal studies. In a longitudinal study, Astrand et al[9] measured $\dot{V}O_2max$ during cycling exercise (highest level of $\dot{V}O_2$ despite further increase in work rate) in 66 well-trained, physically active men and women aged 20 to 33 years and studied them again 21 years later. The mean decrease in $\dot{V}O_2max$ was 22% for the 35 women and 20% for the 31 men.

Bruce et al[10] used stepwise multiple regression analysis to identify whether gender, age, physical activity, weight, height, or smoking aided in the prediction of $\dot{V}O_2max$ during treadmill exercise in adults. They found that gender and age were the two most important factors. The $\dot{V}O_2max$ values of women were approximately 77% of the $\dot{V}O_2$max of men when adjusted for body weight and activity. Astrand[11] reported 17% lower $\dot{V}O_2$max for 18 women students compared with 17 male students of comparable size.

Activity Level

Investigators generally agree that values obtained from athletes, physical education teachers, servicemen, or participants in organized exercise groups are not representative as reference values for a clinical population. Drinkwater et al[8] found that the peak $\dot{V}O_2$ of extremely active women did not decline over two decades despite a gradual increase in body weight. The decline in peak $\dot{V}O_2$ with age is more rapid in habitually inactive men, even allowing for greater weight gain in the inactive group. Importantly, even brief periods of physical training can increase peak $\dot{V}O_2$ by 15% to 25% or more.[12]

Matching Predicting or Reference Equations to Body Size

The diagnosis of cardiovascular and other diseases depends not only on pattern analysis but also on comparing actual with predicted peak exercise values. As can be seen in **Figure 7.1**, the population that is referred to us for clinical exercise testing at our institution includes a great many very obese individuals. It is very likely that this situation occurs at many other locations as well. Therefore, it is essential to have predicting equations that are valid for overweight, obese, and morbidly obese patients. As illustrated in **Figures 7.2** and **7.3**, there are relatively small differences in predicted peak $\dot{V}O_2$ values for individuals of average height (men of 170-180 cm and women of 160 cm) who are not obese (body mass index [BMI] <22 kg/m^2). However, the differences in predicted peak $\dot{V}O_2$ values become significantly more diverse when the subjects (or patients) are shorter, taller, or obese.[13-18] Because the differences are markedly exaggerated with increasing obesity, it is important and necessary to compare predicted peak $\dot{V}O_2$ values of otherwise healthy men and women at different heights, ages, and BMI levels.

Tables 7.2 and **7.3** give the equations for reference values for peak $\dot{V}O_2$ in the several series displayed in **Figures 7.4** and **7.5**. Part of the differences between series relate to subject selection and their activity and fitness level at each site:

1. The Inbar et al[15] equations of peak $\dot{V}O_2$ treadmill values for Israeli men, which included 20% to 27% smokers, are reduced by 10% to estimate cycle peak $\dot{V}O_2$ values. The small changes dependent on rural versus urban residence and activity level are not given nor plotted.
2. The Itoh et al[16] equations are from a relatively small sample (72 men and 27 women) of leaner Japanese men and women and depend on age and gender.
3. Two equations derived from 100 Canadian men and women during cycle ergometer exercise published by Jones et al[17] are compared. *Jones 1* equations use height but not weight as variables; *Jones 2* equations use both height and weight.
4. The equations by Neder et al[18] were derived from 10 randomly selected sedentary Brazilian subjects of each gender from six decades from a population of more than 8000 subjects. The authors derived several equations for peak $\dot{V}O_2$; the ones reported here use age, weight, and height and do not include physical activity score or lean body mass because these did not improve prediction. Ethnicity of subjects and history of light smoking were not significant variables.
5. The Study of Health in Pomerania (SHIP) equations[14] were derived from a normal large northeast German population, with 577 men and 626 women completing CPET out of a randomly selected sample. These included a significant portion of healthy obese subjects (24% with BMI >30 kg/m^2) and about 26% current smokers. In addition, equations could be used to get reference values for current smokers (or not) and for those on moderate doses of β-blockers. These equations were published in the previous edition of this book. Of interest, SHIP investigators had earlier published equations[20] based on 534 subjects that excluded those with BMI >30 kg/m^2 as

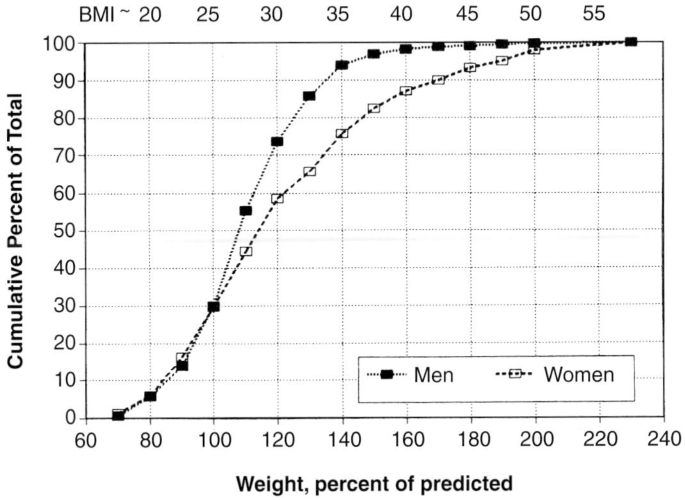

FIGURE 7.1. Cumulative percentage of the total number of patients (approximately 1000) evaluated for symptoms requiring cardiopulmonary exercise testing at Harbor-UCLA Medical Center, as related to actual body mass index (BMI; top x-axis) and percentage of predicted body weight (bottom x-axis). Normal (predicted) weight for men in kilograms = 0.79 × height in centimeters − 60.7 and for women in kilograms = 0.65 × height in centimeters − 42.8. Our patient population can be seen to include a high proportion of overweight, obese, and morbidly obese individuals. *(Data and formulas from Bruce RA, Kusumi F, Hosmer D. Maximal oxygen intake and nomographic assessment of functional aerobic impairment in cardiovascular disease.* Am Heart J. *1973;85:546-562.)*

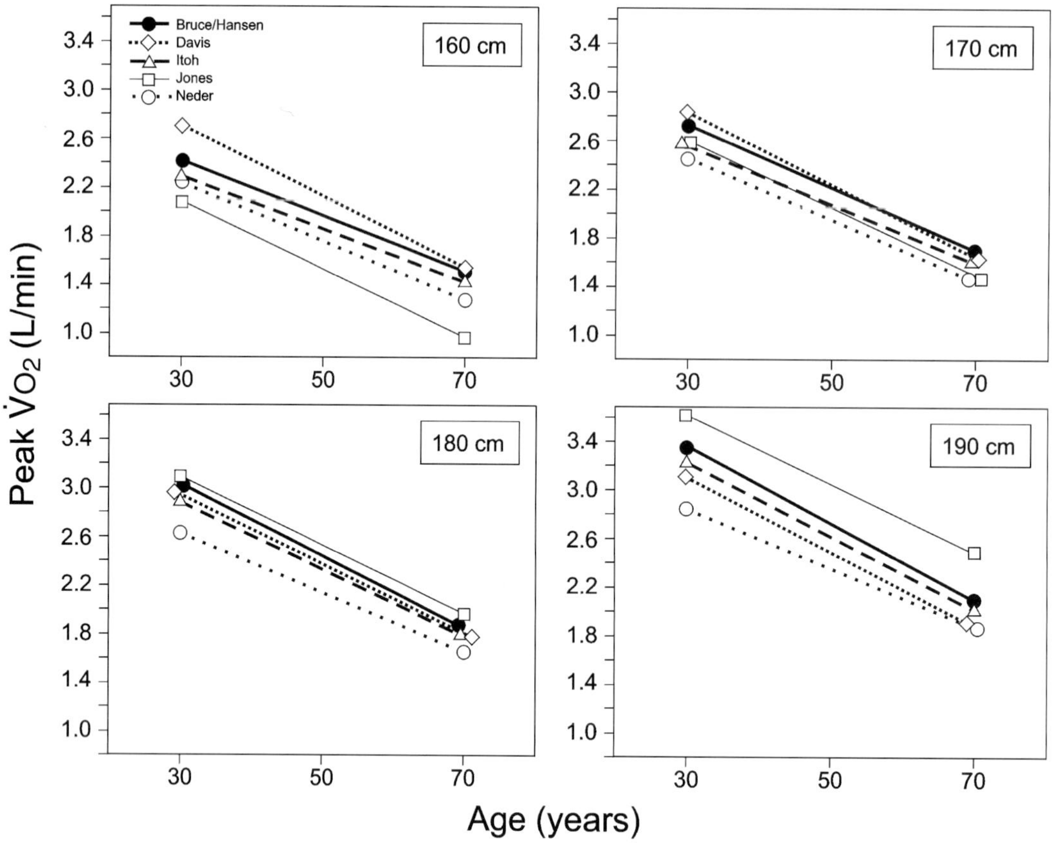

FIGURE 7.2. Comparison of predicted peak oxygen uptake ($\dot{V}O_2$) for cycle ergometry of sedentary men with body mass index of 22 calculated from five reference series for ages 30 to 70 for four different heights and weights: 160 cm and 56 kg, 170 cm and 64 kg, 180 cm and 71 kg, and 190 cm and 80 kg. *(Data are from Bruce RA, Kusumi F, Hosmer D. Maximal oxygen intake and nomographic assessment of functional aerobic impairment in cardiovascular disease.* Am Heart J. *1973;85:546-562; Jones NL, Makrides L, Hitchcock C, Chypchar T, McCartney N. Normal standards for an incremental progressive cycle ergometer test.* Am Rev Respir Dis. *1985;131:700-708; as modified by Hansen JE, Sue DY, Wasserman K. Predicted values for clinical exercise testing.* Am Rev Respir Dis. *1984;129[2, pt 2]:S49-S55; Itoh H, Taniguchi K, Koike A, Doi M. Evaluation of severity of heart failure using ventilatory gas analysis.* Circulation. *1990;81[1 suppl]:II31-II37; Davis JA, Storer TW, Caiozzo VJ, Pham PH. Lower reference limit for maximal oxygen uptake in men and women.* Clin Physiol Funct Imaging. *2002;22:332-338; Neder JA, Nery LE, Castello A, et al. Prediction of metabolic and cardiopulmonary responses to maximum cycle ergometry: a randomised study.* Eur Respir J. *1999;14:1304-1313.)*

well as current smokers. These equations are presented as SHIP 2009 for comparison.

6. The Hansen/Wasserman equations from **Tables 7.2** and **7.3** (compatible with Bruce/Hansen in earlier editions) are based on a large Seattle population[10] and our experience with a Southern California population of healthy asbestos-exposed men including many who were smokers or obese.[5,7] Gender, age, height, and predicted ideal weight are primary factors with secondary adjustments dependent on differences between actual and ideal weight.
7. Recently, the Fitness Registry and the Importance of Exercise National Database (FRIEND registry) provided data to develop equations for peak $\dot{V}O_2$ for treadmill exercise.[21] A generalized equation suitable for treadmill or cycle ergometer in men and women was published recently.[19] The derivation cohort included 7617 subjects, 68% men, with 64% exercising on a treadmill. Results from these equations are included in the tables and figures on succeeding pages.
8. Schneider[22] used a different approach by performing regression analysis on 18 studies of healthy adults over 40 years and then weighting these regression equations to arrive at relatively simple equations for peak $\dot{V}O_2$ and other variables. These are notable because only gender and age were included, without height or weight as independent variables but are somewhat surprisingly rather consistent with other equations despite the primary data collected over many years and from different populations. There are wide differences shown, however, between individual regression equations.

Figures 7.4 and **7.5** show the variability in predicted peak $\dot{V}O_2$ between series as BMI values increase from 20 to 30 to 40. Comparing the reference values for men with BMI of 20 at all heights, the Jones 1 equations yield reference peak $\dot{V}O_2$ values well above average because they do not include weight as a variable. The Jones 2 equations, which have weight as a variable, give high reference peak $\dot{V}O_2$ values at 185 cm and 35 years but the lowest values at

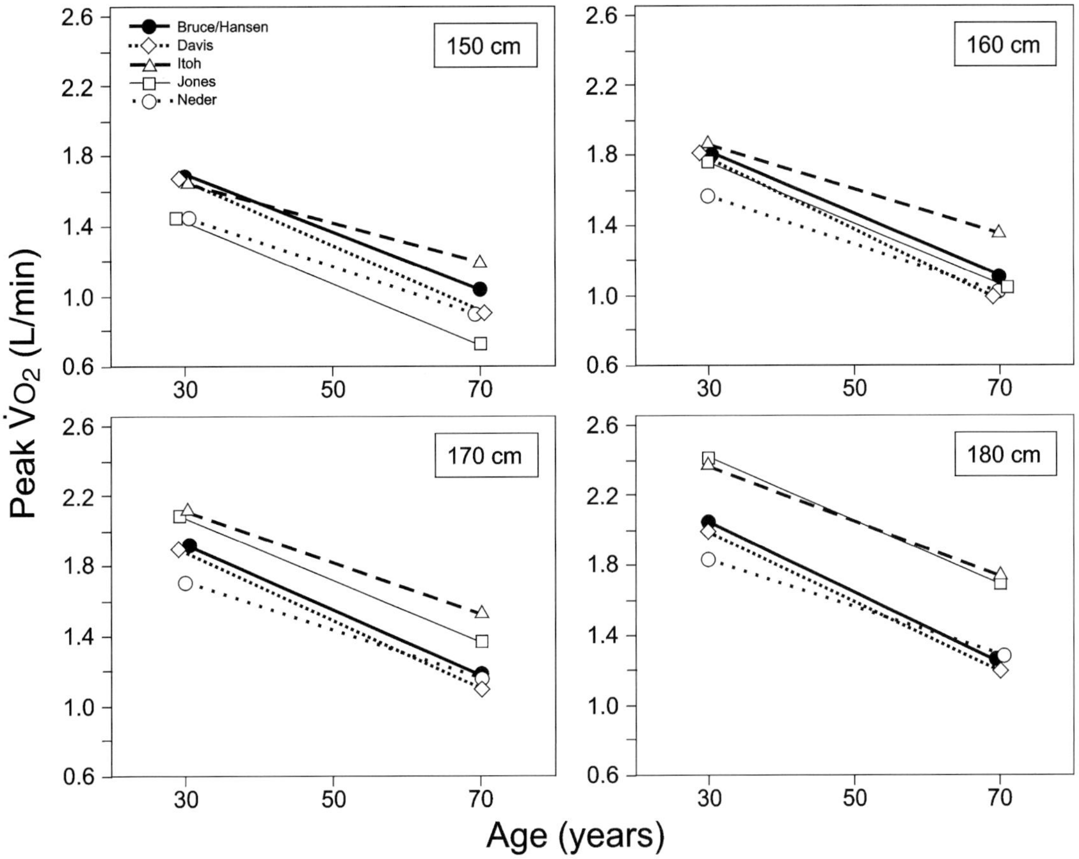

FIGURE 7.3. Comparison of predicted peak oxygen uptake ($\dot{V}O_2$) for cycle ergometry of sedentary women with body mass index of 22 calculated from five reference series for ages 30 to 70 for four different heights and weights: 150 cm and 50 kg, 160 cm and 56 kg, 170 cm and 64 kg, and 180 cm and 71 kg. *(Data are from Bruce RA, Kusumi F, Hosmer D. Maximal oxygen intake and nomographic assessment of functional aerobic impairment in cardiovascular disease.* Am Heart J. *1973;85:546-562; Jones NL, Makrides L, Hitchcock C, Chypchar T, McCartney N. Normal standards for an incremental progressive cycle ergometer test.* Am Rev Respir Dis. *1985;131:700-708; as modified by Hansen JE, Sue DY, Wasserman K. Predicted values for clinical exercise testing.* Am Rev Respir Dis. *1984;129[2, pt 2]:S49-S55; Itoh H, Taniguchi K, Koike A, Doi M. Evaluation of severity of heart failure using ventilatory gas analysis.* Circulation. *1990;81[1 suppl]:II31-II37; Davis JA, Storer TW, Caiozzo VJ, Pham PH. Lower reference limit for maximal oxygen uptake in men and women.* Clin Physiol Funct Imaging. *2002;22:332-338; Neder JA, Nery LE, Castello A, et al. Prediction of metabolic and cardiopulmonary responses to maximum cycle ergometry: a randomised study.* Eur Respir J. *1999;14:1304-1313.)*

160 cm and 70 years. The Inbar and Neder reference values are slightly below average. The predicted values of peak $\dot{V}O_2$ for SHIP 2009 and SHIP 2010 were very close and similar to others.

At BMI values of 30, typical for many of our patients, Itoh's reference values are highest at 35 years, whereas the Jones 2 reference values are highest at 185 cm and lowest and 160 cm at 70 years. At BMIs of 40, Itoh and Jones 2 reference values are uniformly high. Note that the Itoh equations do not include height as a variable because the population tested was likely uniformly nonobese, typical of the Japanese people. The Hansen/Wasserman, SHIP 2010, Neder, and Inbar equations yield relatively similar predicted values. The SHIP 2009 equations are somewhat higher at BMI of 40, possibly because they excluded overweight subjects in their sample. The values generated by Schneider's composite regression equation are relatively low with obesity; neither weight nor height is included in these equations.

Reference peak $\dot{V}O_2$ values for women at three differing BMI levels, are usually with more variability than for men. The Itoh and Jones 1 reference values, which do not include weight as a factor, are similar for thin, overweight, and very obese individuals and thus vary considerably from the overall averages. At BMI of 20, Jones 1 has the highest reference values at 175 cm but very low values at 150 cm at 70 years. Itoh and Jones 2 reference values are next highest for 175 cm at 35 years and next lowest for 150 cm at 70 years. At BMIs of 30 and 40, Itoh reference values for men are lower than all others. At BMI of 30, Jones 2 reference values are high for age 70 and low for age 35 years. At BMI of 40, Jones 1 reference values are again low for 150-cm subjects regardless of age and Jones 2 reference values are high for 175-cm subjects, whereas the Neder, SHIP 2010, and Hansen/Wasserman reference values are all reasonably similar. For women with higher BMI, the SHIP 2009 values appear higher, again likely because overweight patients were excluded.

TABLE 7.2 Equations for Adult Men for Prediction of Peak $\dot{V}O_2$ in L/min for Cycle[a]

Reference	Country	Equation for peak $\dot{V}O_2$
Inbar et al[15]	Israel	Peak $\dot{V}O_2$ = 0.9 × [0.183 + 0.0114 × height + 0.0172 × weight − 0.0227 × age]
Itoh et al[16]	Japan	Peak $\dot{V}O_2$ = 0.9 × weight × [0.0521 − 0.00038 × age]
Jones et al[17] (Jones 1 equations)	Canada	Peak $\dot{V}O_2$ = −4.31 + 0.046 × height − 0.021 × age
Jones et al[17] (Jones 2 equations)	Canada	Peak $\dot{V}O_2$ = −3.76 + 0.034 × height + 0.022 × weight − 0.028 × age
Neder et al[18]	Brazil	Peak $\dot{V}O_2$ = 0.702 + 0.0098 × height + 0.0125 × weight − 0.0246 × age
Gläser et al[14] (SHIP 2010)	Germany	Peak $\dot{V}O_2$ = −0.069 + 0.01402 × height + 0.00744 × weight + 0.00148 × age − 0.0002256 × age × age
Hansen[b] (Hansen/Wasserman)	United States	Ideal weight (kg) = 0.79 × height (cm) − 60.7 If actual weight equals or exceeds ideal weight: Peak $\dot{V}O_2$ = 0.0337 × height − 0.000165 × age × height − 1.963 + 0.006 × weight (actual − ideal) If actual weight is less than ideal weight: Peak $\dot{V}O_2$ = 0.0337 × height − 0.000165 × age × height − 1.963 + 0.014 × weight (actual − ideal) (Use age of 30 y for adults younger than 30 y.)
de Souza E Silva[19] (FRIEND registry)	United States	Peak $\dot{V}O_2$ = 33.38 − 0.35 × age − 0.33 × weight + 0.2677 × height

Abbreviations: FRIEND, Fitness Registry and the Importance of Exercise National Database; SHIP, Study of Health in Pomerania; $\dot{V}O_2$, oxygen uptake.
[a]Units of measure: peak $\dot{V}O_2$, L/min; height, cm; weight, kg; age, years.
[b]J. E. Hansen, Written, 2001.

Table 7.4 summarizes and quantifies the differences between reference peak $\dot{V}O_2$ values from several of these series. It is apparent that there are major differences in peak $\dot{V}O_2$ between the Jones 1 and 2 equations as well as the SHIP and Hansen/Wasserman equations. Jones 1 and the Hansen/Wasserman reference equations were recommended as acceptable by the ATS/ACCP committee in 2001.[1] It is also apparent that the Hansen/Wasserman and SHIP 2010 reference values are the most similar of the values considered, whereas the Neder and Inbar reference values show only small differences from the SHIP 2010 and Hansen/Wasserman reference values. Similarity does not necessarily indicate accuracy, but the large population size, careful exclusion of disease states, meticulous measurements, and

TABLE 7.3 Equations for Adult Women for Prediction of Peak $\dot{V}O_2$ in L/min for Cycle[a]

Reference	Country	Equation for peak $\dot{V}O_2$
Itoh et al[16]	Japan	Peak $\dot{V}O_2$ = 0.9 × weight × [0.0404 − 0.00023 × age]
Jones et al[17] (Jones 1 equations)	Canada	Peak $\dot{V}O_2$ = −4.93 + 0.046 × height − 0.021 × age
Jones et al[17] (Jones 2 equations)	Canada	Peak $\dot{V}O_2$ = −2.26 + 0.025 × height + 0.01 × weight − 0.018 × age
Neder et al[18]	Brazil	Peak $\dot{V}O_2$ = 0.372 + 0.0074 × height + 0.0075 × weight − 0.0137 × age
Gläser et al[14] (SHIP 2010)	Germany	−0.588 + 0.00913 × height + 0.02688 × weight − 0.01133 × age − 0.00012 × weight × weight
Hansen et al[b] (Hansen/Wasserman)	United States	Ideal weight (kg) = 0.65 × height (cm) − 42.8 Peak $\dot{V}O_2$ = 0.001 × height × (14.783 − 0.11 × age) + 0.006 × weight (actual − ideal) (Use age of 30 y for adults younger than 30 y)
de Souza E Silva et al[19] (FRIEND registry)	United States	Peak $\dot{V}O_2$ = 22.48 − 0.35 × age − 0.033 × weight + 0.2677 × height

Abbreviations: FRIEND, Fitness Registry and the Importance of Exercise National Database; SHIP, Study of Health in Pomerania; $\dot{V}O_2$, oxygen uptake.
[a]Units of measure: peak $\dot{V}O_2$, L/min; height, cm; weight, kg; age, years.
[b]J. E. Hansen, Written, 2001.

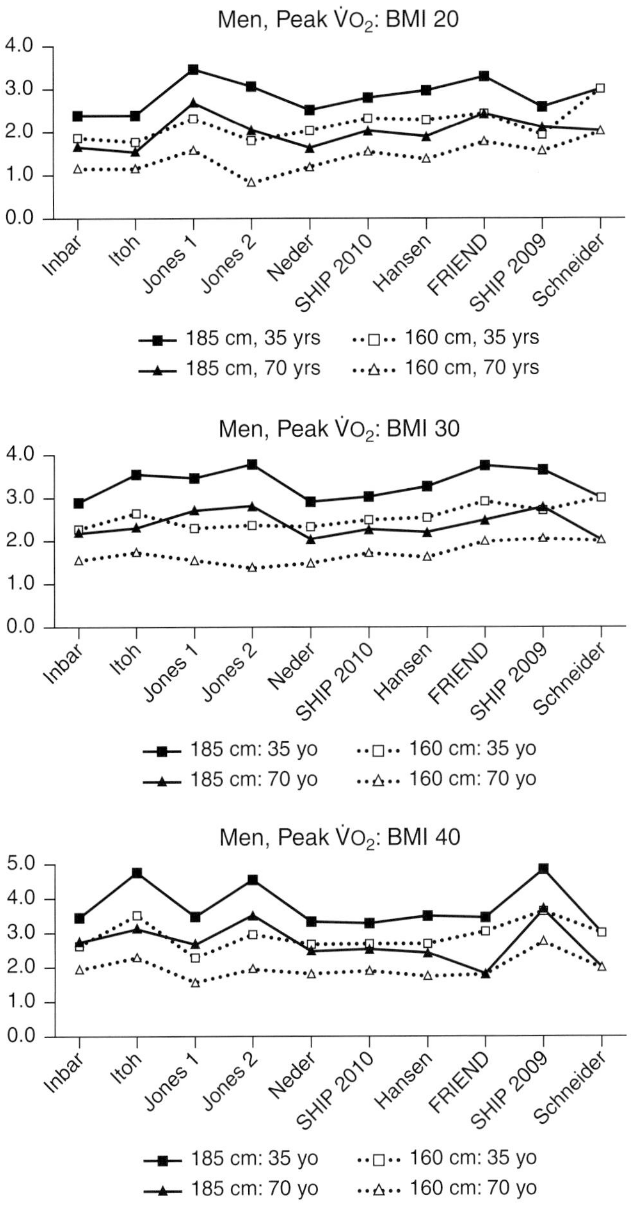

FIGURE 7.4. Comparison of predicted peak oxygen uptake ($\dot{V}O_2$) values for men of two ages (35 and 70 years), two heights (160 and 185 cm), and three nutritional states (body mass index [BMI] of 20, 30, and 40) for seven series. The similarities and differences are discussed in the text. Abbreviations: FRIEND, Fitness Registry and the Importance of Exercise National Database; SHIP, Study of Health in Pomerania. *(Data and predictive equations are from Inbar O, Oren A, Scheinowitz M, Rotstein A, Dlin R, Casaburi R. Normal cardiopulmonary responses during incremental exercise in 20- to 70-yr-old men.* Med Sci Sports Exerc. *1994;26:538-546; Itoh H, Taniguchi K, Koike A, Doi M. Evaluation of severity of heart failure using ventilatory gas analysis.* Circulation. *1990;81[1 suppl]:II31-II37; Jones NL, Makrides L, Hitchcock C, Chypchar T, McCartney N. Normal standards for an incremental progressive cycle ergometer test.* Am Rev Respir Dis. *1985;131:700-708; Neder JA, Nery LE, Castello A, et al. Prediction of metabolic and cardiopulmonary responses to maximum cycle ergometry: a randomised study.* Eur Respir J. *1999;14:1304-1313; Gläser S, Koch B, Itterman T, et al. Influence of age, sex, body size, smoking, and beta blockade on key gas exchange exercise parameters in an adult population.* Eur J Cardiovasc Prev Rehabil. *2010;17:469-476; Hansen JE, Sue DY, Wasserman K. Predicted values for clinical exercise testing.* Am Rev Respir Dis. *1984;129[2, pt 2]:S49-S55; de Souza E Silva CG, Kaminsky LA, Arena R, et al. A reference equation for maximal aerobic power for treadmill and cycle ergometer exercise testing: analysis from the FRIEND registry.* Eur J Prev Cardiol. *2018;25:742-750; Koch B, Schäper C, Ittermann T, et al. Reference values for cardiopulmonary exercise testing in healthy volunteers: the SHIP study.* Eur Respir J. *2009;33:389-397; Schneider J. Age dependency of oxygen uptake and related parameters in exercise testing: an expert opinion on reference values suitable for adults.* Lung. *2013;191:449-458.)*

well-analyzed data of the SHIP 2010 series should give some confidence that the SHIP 2010 equations and the Hansen/Wasserman, Neder, and Inbar reference values for peak $\dot{V}O_2$ are all likely to be reasonable, especially considering the diversity of values about the mean in each series.

The selection of reference equations is of importance in ascertaining whether a patient's peak $\dot{V}O_2$ and related variables (*AT* and peak O_2 pulse) are within normal limits or reduced. Over a broad age, height, and weight span, the SHIP and Hansen/Wasserman equations (see **Tables 7.2** and **7.3**) give the most similar reference values (see **Table 7.4**). The SHIP equations are derived from a well-selected, very large German population and differ minimally from the Hansen/Wasserman predicted values. The Inbar and Neder equations values give reference peak $\dot{V}O_2$ values, which are usually similar or only slightly lower than those of SHIP and Hansen/Wasserman equations.

Exercise Mode

The type of exercise is an important determinant of peak $\dot{V}O_2$. Peak $\dot{V}O_2$ during arm-cranking ergometer exercise (which is inappropriate to use in evaluating most patients) is about 70% of that of leg cycling exercise because of the smaller mass of muscle and lower maximum work rate achievable. The peak $\dot{V}O_2$ of leg cycling is approximately 89% to 95% of the maximal values achieved with treadmill exercise.[23] Thus, the form of ergometry and muscle groups involved must be considered when predicting peak $\dot{V}O_2$.

Recommendations

- Reported peak $\dot{V}O_2$ values should preferably be based on the average of 20 or 30 seconds of data at peak exercise. It should not be based on a single breath or less than 10 seconds of data. Peak $\dot{V}O_2$ values can include data obtained

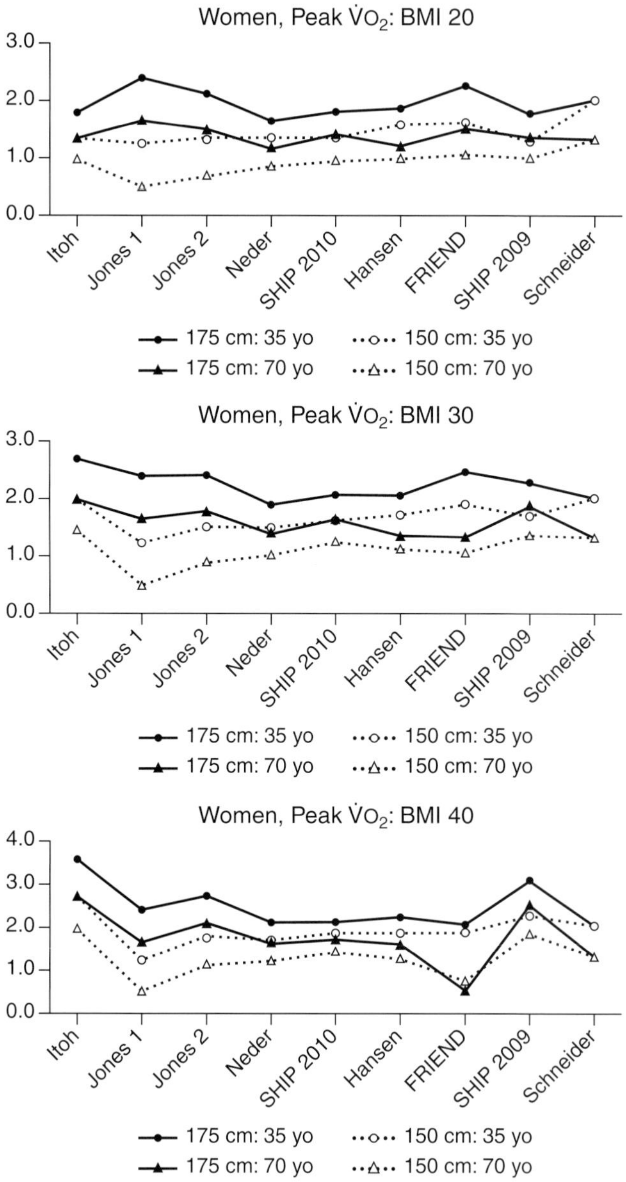

FIGURE 7.5. Comparison of predicted peak oxygen uptake ($\dot{V}O_2$) values for women of two ages (35 and 70 years), two heights (150 and 175 cm), and three nutritional states (body mass index [BMI] of 20, 30, and 40) for six series. The similarities and differences are discussed in the text. Abbreviations: FRIEND, Fitness Registry and the Importance of Exercise National Database; SHIP, Study of Health in Pomerania. *(Data and predictive equations are from Itoh H, Taniguchi K, Koike A, Doi M. Evaluation of severity of heart failure using ventilatory gas analysis.* Circulation. *1990;81[1 suppl]:II31-II37; Jones NL, Makrides L, Hitchcock C, Chypchar T, McCartney N. Normal standards for an incremental progressive cycle ergometer test.* Am Rev Respir Dis. *1985;131:700-708; Neder JA, Nery LE, Castello A, et al. Prediction of metabolic and cardiopulmonary responses to maximum cycle ergometry: a randomised study.* Eur Respir J. *1999;14:1304-1313; Gläser S, Koch B, Itterman T, et al. Influence of age, sex, body size, smoking, and beta blockade on key gas exchange exercise parameters in an adult population.* Eur J Cardiovasc Prev Rehabil. *2010;17:469-476; Hansen JE, Sue DY, Wasserman K. Predicted values for clinical exercise testing.* Am Rev Respir Dis. *1984;129[2, pt 2]:S49-S55; de Souza E Silva CG, Kaminsky LA, Arena R, et al. A reference equation for maximal aerobic power for treadmill and cycle ergometer exercise testing: analysis from the FRIEND registry.* Eur J Prev Cardiol. *2018;25:742-750; Koch B, Schäper C, Ittermann T, et al. Reference values for cardiopulmonary exercise testing in healthy volunteers: the SHIP study.* Eur Respir J. *2009;33:389-397; Schneider J. Age dependency of oxygen uptake and related parameters in exercise testing: an expert opinion on reference values suitable for adults.* Lung. *2013;191:449-458.)*

one or two breaths after cessation of peak exercise, if it increases the peak value.

- Reference values for patients aged 18 to 29 years should generally be the same as for age 30 years. Therefore, for subjects of this age group, use age 30 in reference equations for peak $\dot{V}O_2$ derived for adults rather than actual age.
- The reference values given are for relatively sedentary men and women. Higher values should be expected in athletes or those who vigorously exercise during work or play. Relatively short periods (2 wk) of extreme inactivity will reduce peak $\dot{V}O_2$ values in most individuals.
- For societies with higher levels of physical activity, the recommended predicted values may be too low. There is no good evidence that ethnicity, per se, modifies predicted values.
- For societies with very low levels of physical activity, the reference values given here may be somewhat too high.
- In sedentary populations, values of peak $\dot{V}O_2$ at 1600 m (1 mile) elevation above sea level will be mildly (5%) reduced; at 3200 m, values will be reduced by 15% to 20%.
- Medications given to relatively healthy individuals may reduce peak $\dot{V}O_2$ values. β-Adrenergic blocking drugs, especially in higher dosages, are likely to do so.
- It is wise to compare reference values from two or more series, as given in **Tables 7.2** and **7.3**, especially for subjects at extremes of age, height, or weight. Considering the wide variability in the populations studied and the variability among reference mean values in multiple series, the lower limit of normal values should approximate 75% of the selected mean reference value.
- The SHIP 2010 or Hansen/Wasserman equations listed in **Tables 7.2** and **7.3** are recommended for predicting reference values for peak $\dot{V}O_2$ in Western societies. The Inbar and Neder values may also be useful in this case.

TABLE 7.4 Average Absolute Differences of Peak Oxygen Uptake in L/min Between Several Reference Equations for Men and Women of Two Ages, Three Body Mass Indexes, and Two Heights, in Order of Descending Differences[a]

Series compared[b]	Men	Women	Combined
Jones 1 versus Jones 2[b]	0.493	0.403	0.448
Jones 2 versus Hansen/Wasserman[c]	0.453	0.297	0.375
Jones 1 versus Hansen/Wasserman	0.307	0.437	0.372
Jones 1 versus SHIP[d]	0.307	0.400	0.353
Jones 2 versus SHIP	0.487	0.210	0.348
Inbar[e] versus SHIP	0.203	—	—
Inbar versus Hansen/Wasserman	0.187	—	—
Inbar versus Neder	0.160	—	—
Neder[f] versus SHIP	0.187	0.153	0.170
Neder versus Hansen/Wasserman	0.186	0.127	0.157
SHIP versus Hansen/Wasserman	0.110	0.127	0.119

Abbreviation: SHIP, Study of Health in Pomerania.

[a]Ages are 35 and 70 y; Body mass indexes are 20, 30, and 40 kg/m^2; heights are 160 and 185 cm for men and 150 and 175 cm for women.

[b]Jones 1 and 2 equations are from Jones NL, Makrides L, Hitchcock C, Chypchar T, McCartney N. Normal standards for an incremental progressive cycle ergometer test. *Am Rev Respir Dis.* 1985;131:700-708.

[c]Hansen/Wasserman equations are from Hansen JE, Sue DY, Wasserman K. Predicted values for clinical exercise testing. *Am Rev Respir Dis.* 1984;129(2, pt 2):S49-S55.

[d]SHIP equations are from Gläser S, Koch B, Itterman T, et al. Influence of age, sex, body size, smoking, and beta blockade on key gas exchange exercise parameters in an adult population. *Eur J Cardiovasc Prev Rehabil.* 2010;17:469-476.

[e]Inbar equations are from Inbar O, Oren A, Scheinowitz M, Rotstein A, Dlin R, Casaburi R. Normal cardiopulmonary responses during incremental exercise in 20- to 70-yr-old men. *Med Sci Sports Exerc.* 1994;26:538-546.

[f]Neder equations are from Neder JA, Nery LE, Castello A, et al. Prediction of metabolic and cardiopulmonary responses to maximum cycle ergometry: a randomised study. *Eur Respir J.* 1999;14:1304-1313.

Peak Heart Rate and Heart Rate Reserve

The maximum or peak heart rate (HR) achieved declines with age in all studies. Previously, only small differences have been found between men and women or among the types of exercise used (eg, leg cycling, stepping, inclined treadmill, walking, running).

The two most common formulas for predicting peak HR in adults are as follows: 220 − age (years) and 210 − 0.65 × age (years).[24] The standard deviation (SD) for each formula is 10 beats/min. As reported by Sheffield et al[25] and Astrand and Rodahl,[4] the peak HRs derived from fit individuals approximate either formula reasonably well. Our finding that the peak HR was reduced in obese men is consistent with the suggestion that a sedentary existence may reduce peak HR even in well-motivated subjects.[5]

The expected peak HR = 220 − age (years) for all subjects has been challenged in recent years, partly because of the limited number and characteristics of subjects used to develop this formula but largely because of new data from large clinical trials. Sydó and colleagues[26] reported on a large number of subjects performing treadmill exercise tests and, after exclusion of those suspected of reasons for different peak HR, men closely followed the 220 − age (years) regression line, peak HR = 220 − 0.95 × age (years). However, for women, the best-fit peak HR = 210 − 0.79 × age (years). Arena et al,[27] Tanaka et al,[28] Gellish et al,[29] and the HUNT study[30] found that regression equations resulted in somewhat higher peak HRs in older subjects and lower peak HRs in young subjects. In the SHIP database, increased BMI had a significant effect by lowering peak exercise HR. A comparison of predicted peak HR with age is shown in **Figure 7.6**, including 220 − age (years). It is not clear that the higher predicted peak HR in the regression formulas that did not include weight or BMI had many overweight subjects in their samples. It can be seen that while peak HR = 220 − age (years) does fit within the range of other regression formulas, the rate of fall with age appears to be slightly more marked compared to the more recent studies.

The concept of heart rate reserve (HRR) can be useful for estimating the relative stress of the cardiovascular system during exercise, but it should be used with caution. A normal HRR is zero, but the SD for predicted peak HR is wide, and the mean predicted peak HR may not be reached because of normal population variability, poor motivation, medications such as β-adrenergic blockers, or because of heart, peripheral vascular, lung, endocrine, or musculoskeletal diseases. Caution is emphasized in using peak HR and HRR compared to predicted, as the sole judge of the subject or patient's effort during the test.

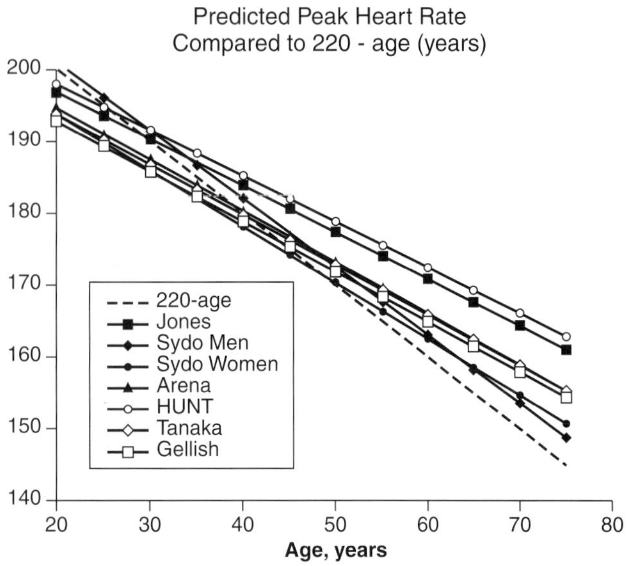

FIGURE 7.6. Mean predicted peak exercise heart rate for "traditional" formula (peak HR = 220 − age [years]) compared with several other prediction equations versus age. Several studies show a trend of less steep fall in peak heart rate with age. *(Data are from Sydó N, Abdelmoneim SS, Mulvagh SL, Merkely B, Gulati M, Allison TG. Relationship between exercise heart rate and age in men vs women.* Mayo Clin Proc. *2014;89:1664-1672; Arena R, Myers J, Kaminsky LA. Revisiting age-predicted maximal heart rate: can it be used as a valid measure of effort?* Am Heart J. *2016;173:49-56; Tanaka H, Monahan KD, Seals DR. Age-predicted maximal heart rate revisited.* J Am Coll Cardiol. *2001;37:153-156; Gellish RL, Goslin BR, Olson RE, McDonald A, Russi GD, Moudgil VK. Longitudinal modeling of the relationship between age and maximal heart rate.* Med Sci Sports Exerc. *2007;39:822-829; Nes BM, Janszky I, Wisløff U, Støylen A, Karlsen T. Age-predicted maximal heart rate in healthy subjects: the HUNT fitness study.* Scand J Med Sci Sports. *2013;23:697-704.)*

Recommendations

Peak HR values should be measured and averaged at the same time as the peak $\dot{V}O_2$ values. The following equations can be used to estimate the predicted peak HR and the HRR for adults and children:

- Maximum HR (beats/min) = 220 − age (years), although some recent studies have challenged use of this equation for both men and women and with increased BMI.
- HRR = predicted peak HR − observed peak HR

Relationship of Oxygen Uptake and Heart Rate: Peak Oxygen Pulse

In a given individual, a consistent relationship exists between $\dot{V}O_2$ and HR during exercise. The quotient of the $\dot{V}O_2$ and HR is the O_2 pulse, in turn equal to the product of stroke volume and the difference between the arterial and mixed venous blood O_2 content. The arteriovenous O_2 difference is dependent on the hemoglobin, arterial blood oxygenation, and peripheral oxygen extraction. Although much emphasis is placed on the O_2 pulse at peak exercise (peak $\dot{V}O_2$/HR), this value must be interpreted in conjunction with the pattern of rise of $\dot{V}O_2$ and HR prior to peak exercise.

Examples of normal and abnormal $\dot{V}O_2$ versus HR responses and O_2 pulse responses are shown in **Figure 7.7A** (note that the O_2 pulse at any given point is the "inverse" of the slope of a line drawn from the origin to each point). The normal relationship of HR with $\dot{V}O_2$ (patients 1 and 2)

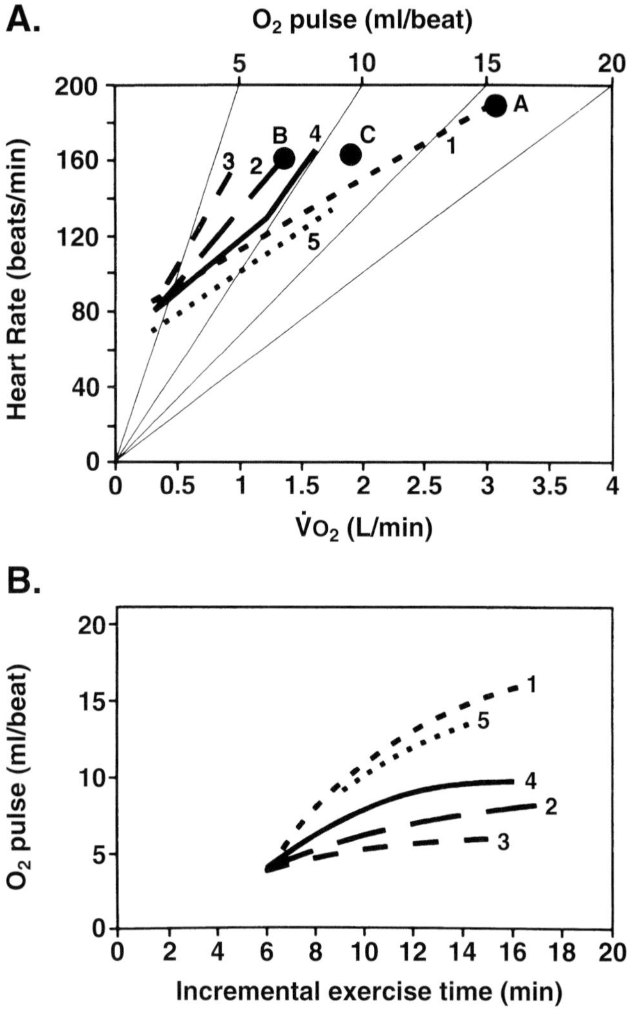

FIGURE 7.7. Values of $\dot{V}O_2$, heart rate, and oxygen pulse (O_2 pulse) for five individuals during incremental cycle ergometer tests. For clarity, the resting, unloaded pedaling, and recovery data are not shown. **A:** Isopleths for O_2 pulse at 5, 10, 15, and 20 mL per beat. The three large solid circles are maximal exercise target values (each of which depends on each patient's age, gender, size, activity level, and exercise mode) and are labeled *A* for patients 1 and 5, *B* for patients 2 and 3, and *C* for patient 4. The responses for patients 1 and 2 are normal. Patient 3 had decreased cardiovascular function throughout the test and would not have reached target values even if able to exercise longer. Patient 4 manifested decreased cardiovascular function about 2 minutes before the cessation of exercise. Patient 5 stopped exercise prematurely for other than cardiovascular causes. **B:** Plots of the same O_2 pulse data against time for the five patients. Patients 1 and 2 reach their target values, whereas patients 3, 4, and 5 do not. The plateau in O_2 pulse seen for patient 4 is abnormal.

is linear throughout a ramp exercise test, with a positive intercept on the HR axis. Although sedentary patients 1 and 2 differ considerably in their predicted peak values (because they differ in age and gender or size), both have normal responses. An exercise response with a higher $\dot{V}O_2$/HR than predicted indicates better than average cardiorespiratory function, whereas a response with a lower $\dot{V}O_2$/HR indicates poorer cardiorespiratory function (patient 3). In our clinical population, this latter response is most commonly due to low stroke volume, but it could be due to anemia or carboxyhemoglobinemia, poor blood oxygenation in the lung, right-to-left shunt, or (rarely) low peripheral oxygen extraction. In patient 4, the increasing slope of the HR versus $\dot{V}O_2$ relationship for the last several minutes of exercise is abnormal, indicating that the rise in HR is disproportionately faster than $\dot{V}O_2$, as work rate increases. In patient 5, the rate of rise of the HR versus $\dot{V}O_2$ is normal, but exercise ends at a relatively low work rate. If the cessation of incremental exercise is due to pain, musculoskeletal disease, ventilatory insufficiency, or volition, these factors (rather than circulatory disease) may be the cause of an abnormally low maximum O_2 pulse.

Figure 7.7B shows O_2 pulse versus time for the same responses. Normally, the rate of increase in O_2 pulse declines gradually as the O_2 pulse approaches maximum values. This is a necessary consequence of a linear $\dot{V}O_2$ versus HR response with a positive intercept on the HR axis. This curvilinear response of the O_2 pulse during incremental exercise is clearly demonstrated in **Figure 7.7B**. Thus, both the peak values and the patterns of change of $\dot{V}O_2$, HR, and O_2 pulse may vary importantly in various diseases.

The predicted peak O_2 pulse at any given work rate is strongly dependent on the individual's body size, gender, age, degree of fitness, and hemoglobin concentration. Normal values for the predicted peak O_2 pulse on the cycle ergometer range from approximately 5 mL per beat in a 7-year-old child to 8 mL per beat in a 150-cm, 70-year-old woman, or to 17 mL per beat in a 190-cm, 30-year-old man. The actual peak O_2 pulse may be considerably higher than predicted in the cardiovascularly fit person. β-Adrenergic blocking drugs might also increase the O_2 pulse. Most commonly, predicted peak O_2 pulse is determined by dividing the predicted peak $\dot{V}O_2$ by the predicted peak HR, but as noted earlier, there are several reference equations for both variables that can be chosen. Therefore, some authors have included regression equations based on peak O_2 pulse itself, such as the SHIP study,[14] which may be better suited for certain populations or have decreased variance.

Recommendations

- Predicted peak O_2 pulse (mL/beat) = predicted peak $\dot{V}O_2$ (mL/min)/predicted peak HR (beats/min)
- Both the pattern of change as well as the absolute values of O_2 pulse should be considered when interpreting a clinical study.

Relationship of Heart Rate and $\dot{V}O_2$: $\Delta HR/\Delta \dot{V}O_2$

A graph of HR versus $\dot{V}O_2$ during a progressive exercise test has an intercept on the HR axis (resting HR) and a slope that reflects overall "fitness" of the individual. A steep response indicates that the increase in $\dot{V}O_2$ is achieved by larger increases in HR, rather than increasing stroke volume and increasing O_2 extraction. In well-randomized normal subjects during cycle exercise reported by Neder et al,[31] the slope was related to gender and age as well as weight.

$$\text{Men: } \Delta HR/\Delta \dot{V}O_2 = 0.42 \times \text{age (years)} - 0.53 \times \text{weight (kg)} + 73.5 \text{ (SEE 11.2)}$$

$$\text{Women: } \Delta HR/\Delta \dot{V}O_2 = 0.42 \times \text{age, (years)} - 0.28 \times \text{weight (kg)} + 78.1 \text{ (SEE 12.1)}$$

Systemic Blood Pressure

Blood pressure can be measured by auscultation during exercise by skilled technicians or physicians, but assessing the fourth Korotkoff phase diastolic pressure (muffling of sound) and the fifth Korotkoff phase diastolic pressure (disappearance of sound) may be difficult because of the background noise of the ergometer. An American Heart Association statement[32] addressed the problems related to the measurement of blood pressure by sphygmomanometry. However, intra-arterial pressures can be accurately and continuously measured by means of a pressure transducer attached to an indwelling radial or brachial arterial catheter whenever arterial blood specimens are not being drawn through the catheter. Accurate intra-arterial blood pressure values are more difficult to obtain during treadmill ergometry because of movement artifacts. When the subject is using the cycle, the hand on the handlebar stabilizes the arm and transducer, but tight gripping should be avoided to minimize the hypertensive effect of isometric exercise. The blood pressure measurements recorded in **Table 7.5** are from a small sample of predominantly cigarette-smoking, sedentary men.[5,33] Values may be lower in nonsmoking, more active individuals. Noteworthy are the striking rise in systolic (by both cuff and direct intra-arterial recording) and mean pressures, the considerable rise in intra-arterial diastolic pressures, the modest rise in fourth-phase cuff diastolic pressures, and the gradual decline in fifth-phase cuff diastolic pressures during incremental exercise. Although resting pressures are higher in older men, the mean maximum exercise systolic and diastolic pressures are similar in both groups. Note that the true mean arterial pressure closely approximates the diastolic pressure plus half the pulse pressure, rather than one-third the pulse pressure during exercise when using a cuff.[33]

From larger more recent cohorts including women, **Figure 7.8** show systolic and diastolic blood pressures at peak exercise as mean values[34] from the FRIEND registry or from regression equations from the SHIP cohort[35]

TABLE 7.5 Blood Pressure During 1-min Incremental Cycle Exercise Measured Directly From Catheter in Brachial Artery and in Opposite Arm by Cuff[a,b]

	Prior examination at rest	Rest on cycle	Exercise near anaerobic threshold	Exercise near maximum
Sedentary, nonhypertensive men, ages 34 to 74				
Systolic intra-arterial	—	142 ± 18	182 ± 23	207 ± 27
Systolic cuff	124 ± 11	131	171	200
Diastolic intra-arterial	—	86 ± 10	92 ± 11	99 ± 12
Diastolic fourth phase	79 ± 7	84	86	88
Diastolic fifth phase	—	81	80	77
Mean intra-arterial	—	107	128	142
Sedentary, nonhypertensive men, ages 19 to 24				
Systolic intra-arterial	—	129	—	203
Diastolic intra-arterial	—	78	—	106
Mean intra-arterial	—	96	—	141

[a]Values are mean or mean ± standard deviation in mm Hg.

[b]Data are from Hansen JE, Sue DY, Wasserman K. Predicted values for clinical exercise testing. *Am Rev Respir Dis.* 1984;129(2, pt 2):S49-S55; Robinson TR, Sue DY, Huszczuk A, Weiler-Ravell D, Hansen JE. Intra-arterial and cuff blood pressure responses during incremental cycle ergometry. *Med Sci Sports Exerc.* 1988;20:142-149.

for men and women. Both obtained blood pressures at peak exercise by standardized auscultation methods. In agreement with other studies, systolic and diastolic blood pressures rise on average to peak exercise. The SHIP participants had higher blood pressures than the FRIEND registry subjects, but comparable to other studies, the SHIP investigators found a significant relationship of higher blood pressure with larger BMI. Notably, the FRIEND cohort, on average, had a relatively lower mean BMI, but systolic and diastolic blood pressures were considerably lower in both genders.

Recommendations

The brachial artery blood pressure values of nonhypertensive men, measured directly (intra-arterially) or by cuff and sphygmomanometer during 1-minute incremental exercise, are given in **Table 7.5**, but the range of expected peak systolic and diastolic blood pressures may be wide, different by gender, and related to BMI.

Anaerobic Threshold

The *AT* is expressed in milliliters or liters of $\dot{V}O_2$ per minute. The $\dot{V}O_2$ at which the blood lactate level begins to rise (lactate threshold) has been used to define the *AT* in normal subjects.[36,37] A noninvasive measurement using the V-slope method[38-40] determines the lactic acidosis threshold, the $\dot{V}O_2$ of which is systematically slightly higher than the lactate threshold for the reasons described in Chapter 3. In these studies, the lowest values of *AT* in a number of studies of normal subjects is about 40% of predicted peak $\dot{V}O_2$, approximately the O_2 cost of walking at a moderate pace.[5,14,17,41] The ratio of predicted *AT* to predicted peak $\dot{V}O_2$ tends to rise with increasing age, approaching peak $\dot{V}O_2$ in the most elderly.

Reference equations for *AT* were also derived from 616 healthy subjects, including 333 women, for the SHIP cohort[42] from northeastern Germany, with separate equations for men and women:

Men: $\dot{V}O_2$ at *AT* (mL/min) = −329.082 − 4.9426 × age (years) + 4.3686 × height (cm) + 5.4209 × weight (kg). Lower 95% confidence limit for $\dot{V}O_2$ at *AT* (mL/min) = 29.509 − 0.5930 × age (years) + 3.1446 × height (cm) + 3.9946 × weight (kg)

Women: $\dot{V}O_2$ at *AT* (mL/min) = 298.823 − 1.5512 × age (years) + 2.3848 × height (cm) + 4.7977 × weight (kg). Lower 95% confidence limit for $\dot{V}O_2$ at *AT* (mL/min) = 913.901 − 0.7278 × age (years) − 2.9840 × height (cm) + 4.3668 × weight (kg)

Similar to older studies with smaller numbers of subjects, mean *AT* as a percentage of predicted peak $\dot{V}O_2$ ranged from 44% to 57% in men and 47% to 59%, with the percentage increasing with age. The lower 95% confidence limits were similar but somewhat lower than **Table 7.6**: men 27% to 41% and women 33% to 42%. These data are shown in **Figures 7.9A** and **7.9B**, and these values are comparable to the values shown in **Table 7.6**. The mode of exercise affects the value of *AT* in normal subjects. Davis et al[43] studied 39 healthy college-aged men. Mean $\dot{V}O_2$ at the *AT* was 46% ± 9% of peak $\dot{V}O_2$ for arm cycling, 64% ± 9% of peak $\dot{V}O_2$ for leg cycling, and 59% ± 6% of peak $\dot{V}O_2$ for treadmill exercise. A substantial difference was noted between the *AT* during arm cycling and either form of leg exercise, but

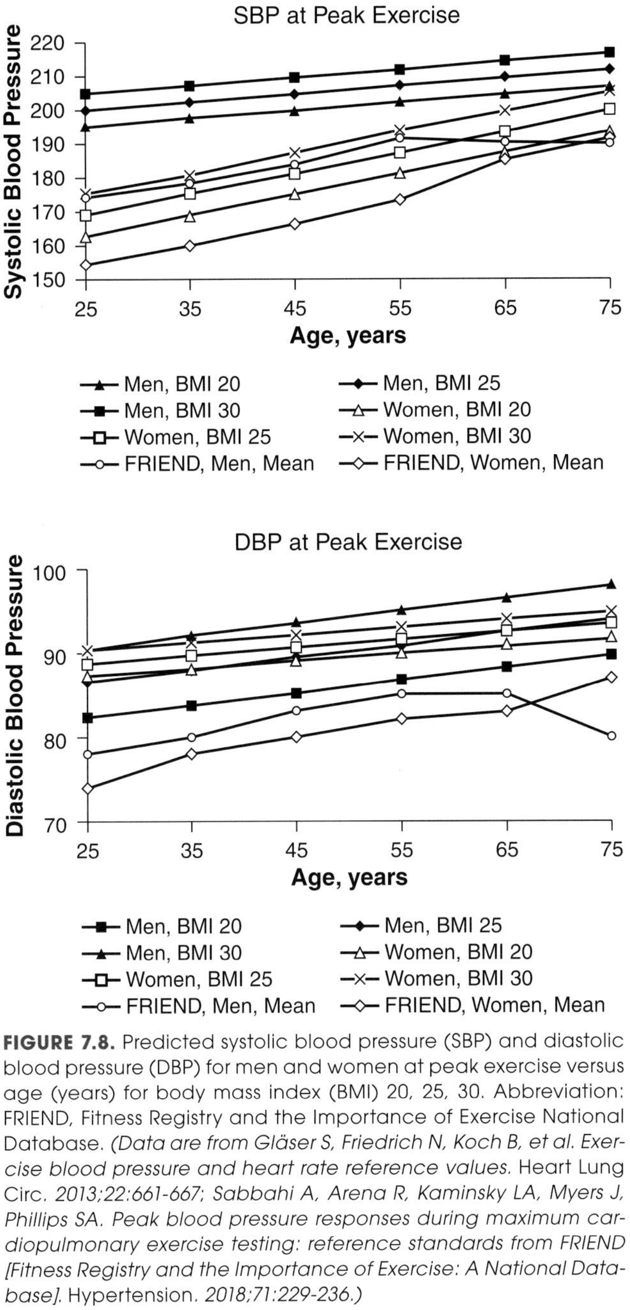

FIGURE 7.8. Predicted systolic blood pressure (SBP) and diastolic blood pressure (DBP) for men and women at peak exercise versus age (years) for body mass index (BMI) 20, 25, 30. Abbreviation: FRIEND, Fitness Registry and the Importance of Exercise National Database. *(Data are from Gläser S, Friedrich N, Koch B, et al. Exercise blood pressure and heart rate reference values.* Heart Lung Circ. *2013;22:661-667; Sabbahi A, Arena R, Kaminsky LA, Myers J, Phillips SA. Peak blood pressure responses during maximum cardiopulmonary exercise testing: reference standards from FRIEND [Fitness Registry and the Importance of Exercise: A National Database].* Hypertension. *2018;71:229-236.)*

no significant difference existed between the *AT* obtained from cycle exercise and that obtained from treadmill exercise. Buchfuhrer et al[44] found similar ratios of *AT* to peak $\dot{V}O_2$ for treadmill and for cycle exercise: 50% ± 9% and 47% ± 11%, respectively. Withers et al,[45] however, comparing highly trained cyclists and runners, found a higher *AT* for the total group on the treadmill (mean 76% of peak $\dot{V}O_2$) than on the cycle (mean 64% of peak $\dot{V}O_2$), with the cyclists reaching higher *AT* and *AT*/peak $\dot{V}O_2$ on the cycle and runners reaching higher *AT* and *AT*/peak $\dot{V}O_2$ on the treadmill.

TABLE 7.6 Mean and Lower 95% Confidence Limits for Ratio of Predicted Anaerobic Threshold to Predicted Peak Oxygen Uptake in Adults, as a Percentage[a]

	Men		Women	
Age (y)	Mean	Lower 95% limit	Mean	Lower 95% limit
25	50	40	53	40
35	52	42	55	42
45	54	44	57	44
55	56	46	59	46
65	58	48	61	48
75	60	50	63	50

[a]Data are from Jones NL, Makrides L, Hitchcock C, Chypchar T, McCartney N. Normal standards for an incremental progressive cycle ergometer test. *Am Rev Respir Dis.* 1985;131:700-708; Davis JA, Storer TW, Caiozzo VJ. Prediction of normal values for lactate threshold estimated by gas exchange in men and women. *Eur J Appl Physiol Occup Physiol.* 1997;76:157-164; Gläser S, Koch B, Itterman T, et al. Influence of age, sex, body size, smoking, and beta blockade on key gas exchange exercise parameters in an adult population. *Eur J Cardiovasc Prev Rehabil.* 2010;17:469-476; Hansen JE, Sue DY, Wasserman K. Predicted values for clinical exercise testing. *Am Rev Respir Dis.* 1984;129(2, pt 2):S49-S55.

Recommendations

Reference values for mean and lower limit of normal *AT* values for sedentary nonathletes, as related to reference values for peak $\dot{V}O_2$, are given in the text and **Table 7.6**.

Oxygen Uptake-Work Rate Relationship

When a progressively increasing work rate test is initiated, a delay occurs before $\dot{V}O_2$ begins to increase in a linear fashion. This delay must be considered in the calculation of the overall value of the $\dot{V}O_2$–work rate relationship ($\Delta\dot{V}O_2/\Delta WR$). This kinetic delay is equal to the time constant of $\dot{V}O_2$ following a stepwise increase, is accounted for by the kinetics of muscle O_2 utilization, and is normally between one-half and three-quarters of a minute. Thus, the formula used to calculate $\Delta\dot{V}O_2/\Delta WR$ for cycle exercise is:

$$\Delta\dot{V}O_2/\Delta WR = (\text{peak } \dot{V}O_2 - \text{unloaded } \dot{V}O_2) / [(T - 0.75) \times S]$$

where $\dot{V}O_2$ is measured in milliliters per minute, *T* is the time of incremental exercise, and *S* is the slope of work rate increment in watts per minute.[46] The $\Delta\dot{V}O_2/\Delta WR$ relationship can be calculated by linear regression during the entire incremental exercise test or during specific portions of the test. It is also convenient simply to measure the slope of $\dot{V}O_2$ plotted against work rate, using only points after the early delay in increase in $\dot{V}O_2$.

The overall $\Delta\dot{V}O_2/\Delta WR$ during incremental cycle ergometer exercise varies modestly with the slope of work rate increase, the cardiovascular fitness of the individual, and the duration of the test.[46-48] In 10 normal young men, tests of

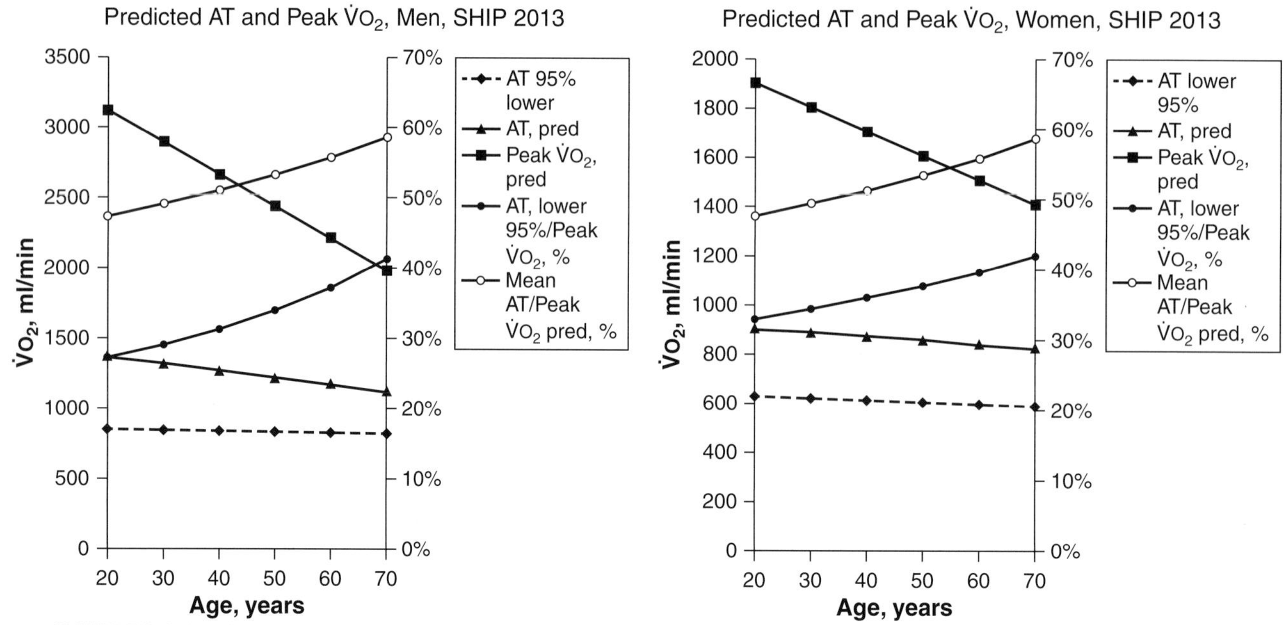

FIGURE 7.9. A: Predicted mean peak anaerobic threshold (*AT*) for men, expressed as oxygen uptake ($\dot{V}O_2$), mL/min, and as percentage of predicted peak $\dot{V}O_2$ along with lower 95% confidence limit, expressed in the same way. Note that while peak $\dot{V}O_2$ and $\dot{V}O_2$ at the *AT* are both declining with age, $\dot{V}O_2$ at the *AT* declines more slowly, so the ratio of $\dot{V}O_2$ at the *AT*/peak $\dot{V}O_2$ increases with age. *(Data are from Gläser S, Koch B, Itterman T, et al. Influence of age, sex, body size, smoking, and beta blockade on key gas exchange exercise parameters in an adult population.* Eur J Cardiovasc Prev Rehabil. *2010;17:469-476.)* **B:** Predicted mean peak *AT* for women, expressed as $\dot{V}O_2$, mL/min, and as percentage of predicted peak $\dot{V}O_2$ along with lower 95% confidence limit, expressed in the same way. Note that while peak $\dot{V}O_2$ and $\dot{V}O_2$ at the *AT* are both declining with age, $\dot{V}O_2$ at the *AT* declines more slowly, so the ratio of $\dot{V}O_2$ at the *AT*/peak $\dot{V}O_2$ increases with age. *(Data are from Gläser S, Koch B, Itterman T, et al. Influence of age, sex, body size, smoking, and beta blockade on key gas exchange exercise parameters in an adult population.* Eur J Cardiovasc Prev Rehabil. *2010;17:469–476.)*

approximately 15 minutes' duration (15-W/min increment) gave higher $\Delta\dot{V}O_2/\Delta WR$ values (11.2 ± 0.15 mL/min/W) than tests of approximately 5 minutes' duration (60-W/min increment) (8.8 ± 0.15 mL/min/W). The change in $\Delta\dot{V}O_2/\Delta WR$ occurred primarily above the *AT*. The $\Delta\dot{V}O_2/\Delta WR$ below the *AT* was not significantly affected by the rate of work rate increase. In tests of long duration (slowly increasing work rate tests), a higher fraction of the total energy cost of the work above the *AT* is supported by oxygen transport relative to anaerobic sources (eg, lactate production). In contrast, a lower fraction of the total energy cost of work is derived from oxygen extracted from the inspired air above the *AT* in the rapidly increasing work rate test. Thus, $\Delta\dot{V}O_2/\Delta WR$ is slightly greater for the slower increasing work rate test.

The reverse allocation of energy support occurs in maximal tests of short duration. In tests of intermediate duration, however, the mean ± standard error of $\Delta\dot{V}O_2/\Delta WR$ found in 10 normal young men[48] was 10.2 ± 0.16 mL/min/W, and in 54 older sedentary normal men,[46] the mean ± SD was 10.3 ± 1.0 mL/min/W. The mean ± SD of 17 normal men was 9.9 ± 0.7 mL/min/W. Jones et al[17] also found a $\Delta\dot{V}O_2/\Delta WR$ of 10.3 mL/min/W in 100 healthy adult men and women. This range is small enough that the $\Delta\dot{V}O_2/\Delta WR$ is potentially clinically useful in identifying patients with circulatory disorders.

Most patients with circulatory disorders have a significantly reduced $\Delta\dot{V}O_2/\Delta WR$,[46,48,49] notably above their *AT*. The most obvious reason is that O_2 transport is inadequate to perform the work. Thus, anaerobic metabolism (anaerobic glycolysis with lactate as the byproduct) contributes a larger proportion of the total energy requirement than normal.

We have seen that athletes may have a higher than average $\Delta\dot{V}O_2/\Delta WR$ (in the range of 11-12 mL/min/W) when cycling, perhaps due to their tendency to involve arm, chest, abdominal, and back musculature more than nonathletes.

Recommendations

For incremental cycle ergometry exercise of 6 to 12 minutes' duration, the $\Delta\dot{V}O_2/\Delta WR$ for sedentary adults is 10.0 mL/min/W, with an SD of 1.0 mL/min/W and a lower limit of normal at the 95% confidence level of 8.4 mL/min/W.

Ventilatory Limitation During Exercise

Exercise Ventilation and Breathing Reserve

Maximum exercise minute ventilation ($\dot{V}E$), even in normal subjects, is dependent on multiple factors, including peak $\dot{V}O_2$, the respiratory exchange ratio at end-exercise, the set-point for $PaCO_2$, and the subjects dead space/tidal volume ratio (V_D/V_T). It is not surprising, therefore, that there are relatively few reference values for maximum $\dot{V}E$ but rather more estimates based on maximum voluntary ventilation (MVV).

The maximum $\dot{V}E$ is similar for leg cycling, treadmill walking, and running[44] but is less for arm cycling[43] because the maximal metabolic rate is lower when smaller muscle groups are used. The breathing reserve relates the ventilatory response during maximum exercise to the maximum ability to breathe. Because normal, untrained subjects do not ordinarily have ventilatory limitations in their ability to perform work,[1] some ability to increase ventilation further is usually present during maximal exercise. This potential increase in ventilation is generally estimated from the MVV, a test performed at rest over 12 to 15 seconds but highly dependent on the subject's motivation and effort. The difference between the measured MVV and the maximum $\dot{V}_E$ during exercise is used as a measure of the ventilatory or breathing reserve. A low breathing reserve suggests that a patient's exercise capacity may be limited by his or her ventilatory capacity. The breathing reserve is usually reduced in patients with moderate to severe restrictive or obstructive lung disease (see **Fig. 4.9**).

Many investigators have examined the normal relationship between the MVV and the maximum exercise $\dot{V}_E$. Maximum exercise $\dot{V}_E$ averages 50% to 80% of the 12- or 15-second MVV, indicating a breathing reserve of 20% to 50% of the MVV. Because the MVV is dependent on the subject's cooperation, effort, and technique of performance, the MVV is sometimes indirectly estimated from the forced expired volume in 1 second (FEV_1) or $FEV_{0.75}$. Gandevia and Hugh-Jones[50] suggested that this "indirect" MVV could be estimated as $FEV_1 \times 35$, whereas Cotes[51] suggested $FEV_{0.75} \times 40$ or $(36.8 \times FEV_1 - 2.8)$. Our data[5] indicate that $FEV_1 \times 40$ provides an optimal estimate of the measured MVV both in normal subjects and in patients with obstructive lung disease. If the directly measured MVV is less than the indirectly measured MVV ($FEV_1 \times 40$), poor cooperation or understanding in the performance of the maneuver, extreme obesity, neurologic disorders, or inspiratory obstruction may be possible causes. If one is uncertain regarding a discrepancy between the direct MVV and the indirect MVV, or if the patient has variable obstruction, it may be necessary to have the patient repeat the direct MVV measurement or to accept the $FEV_1 \times 40$, which should be a more reproducible measurement. In the case of patients with interstitial lung disease, it is common for them to have direct MVV values that are 50 or 60 times the FEV_1. This is likely due to the fact that they have strong ventilatory muscles, have increased elastic recoil so that their airways do not tend to collapse during forced exhalations, and their breathing frequencies during the MVV tests are very high, sometimes as high as 100 to 120 breaths/min. Because such high breathing frequencies are rarely achieved during CPET, and their direct MVV values can markedly exceed $FEV_1 \times 40$, we now recommend that the indirect MVV ($FEV_1 \times 40$) be used in calculating breathing reserve.

In 77 normal middle-aged subjects participating in an incremental cycle ergometer exercise test clinical study,[5,7] the mean direct MVV was 131 ± 23.6 L/min (range 81-203 L/min). The mean maximum exercise $\dot{V}_E$/MVV was 71.5% ± 14.6%; only 13 subjects had a value greater than 80%. When we used $FEV_1 \times 40$ as an indirect estimate of the MVV, the mean maximum exercise $\dot{V}_E$/indirect MVV was 71.5% ± 15.3%, the same percentage as for the directly measured MVV. By expressing breathing reserve as MVV minus maximum exercise $\dot{V}_E$, we obtained an average of 38.1 ± 22.0 L/min using the directly measured MVV and 38.0 ± 21.5 L/min using the indirect MVV. We consider it likely that a patient is ventilatory limited when the breathing reserve is less than 11 L/min.

Recently, Kaminsky et al,[52] using 5232 US subjects from the FRIEND registry, looked at both treadmill peak $\dot{V}_E$ and its relationship with FEV_1 (in 3434) and MVV ($FEV_1 \times 40$ and $FEV_1 \times 35$). The excluded those with chronic obstructive pulmonary disease (COPD) and with peak respiratory exchange ratio <1.0 but did not exclude those with some other chronic diseases. They derived a regression equation for peak $\dot{V}_E$ based on size and gender as well as a regression equation for peak $\dot{V}_E$ compared to FEV_1.

$$\text{Peak } \dot{V}_E = 17.32 - 28.33 \times \text{sex (men} = 0, \text{ women} = 1) - 0.79 \times \text{age (years)} + 0.728 \times \text{height (cm)}$$

$$\text{Peak } \dot{V}_E = 5.51 + 26.79 \times FEV_1$$

Peak $\dot{V}_E$ as generally expected was lower in women compared to men and in shorter subjects and declines with age. These regression equations result in predicted peak $\dot{V}_E$ somewhat smaller than predicted from other studies; notably, peak $\dot{V}_E = 5.51 + 26.79 \times FEV_1$ is smaller than 35 or $40 \times FEV_1$.

Tidal Volume and Breathing Frequency

We consider that patients are likely to have ventilatory limitation if the exercise tidal volume (V_T) reaches the resting inspiratory capacity (IC), particularly early during a progressively increasing work rate test, or if the breathing frequency (*f*) exceeds 50 breaths/min. The expected maximum exercise V_T, like vital capacity (VC) and other resting pulmonary function measurements, depends on the subject's height, age, and gender. In addition, the dead space or rebreathed volume of the breathing apparatus influences ventilation. A V_T can be related to $\dot{V}_E$ to analyze the breathing pattern, such as is shown in **Figure 3.20**. At low exercise intensity, the increase in $\dot{V}_E$ is accomplished primarily by an increase in V_T. After the V_T reaches approximately 50% to 60% of the VC, further increases in $\dot{V}_E$ are accomplished primarily by increasing *f*.[51] Thus, *f* is a curvilinear function of $\dot{V}_E$. In contrast, Cotes[51] suggested that maximum V_T is about 50% of VC for VC values between 2.0 and 5.0 L in normal men and women of European descent. Astrand and Rodahl[4] found that, at maximal exercise, the V_T averaged between 1.9 and 2.0 L, or 52% to 58% of the VC, whereas *f* at maximal exercise ranged between 34 and 46 breaths/min. Little difference in V_T/VC was noted among age groups, but *f* was lower in the older subjects studied.

Wasserman and Whipp[53] compared exercise V_T to IC. They found that V_T does not usually exceed approximately 70% of the IC during exercise, but it increases to a value approaching 100% in patients with restrictive lung disease, suggesting that the IC may limit the increase in V_T (see **Fig. 3.20**). In a series of 77 healthy middle-aged men, the mean resting V_T of 0.71 ± 0.26 L increased to 1.44 ± 0.43 L at the *AT* and 2.28 ± 0.43 L at maximum exercise.[5,7] Maximum *f* was 41.6 ± 9.6 breaths/min. Maximum V_T averaged 70.0% ± 10.7% of the IC and 55.0% ± 8.7% of the VC. No one had a maximum exercise V_T greater than his or her resting IC, and only 3 had a maximal exercise *f* greater than 60 breaths/min.

Partitioning the ventilatory cycle duration (T_{TOT}) into inspiratory (T_I) and expiratory (T_E) times may also prove useful. However, this measurement is not commonplace in clinical exercise testing. The T_I/T_{TOT} should increase during exercise due to shortening of T_E.

Recommendations

- Use indirect MVV ($FEV_1 \times 40$) rather than direct MVV unless there are compelling circumstances (eg, inspiratory obstruction or severe neuromuscular disorder) to do otherwise.
- Use the direct MVV to test for respiratory muscle fatigue or weakness (eg, myasthenia gravis).
- Breathing reserve = MVV − highest $\dot{V}_E$ during exercise averaged during a 20- to 30-second period.
- Breathing reserve <10% of indirect MVV or <11 L/min is likely abnormal, suggesting ventilatory limitation to exercise.
- The *f* uncommonly exceeds 55/min except in athletes and interstitial lung disease.
- Exercise V_T uncommonly reach more than 85% to 90% of resting IC volumes. Higher percentages often occur with interstitial lung disease.

Gas Exchange Relationships and Ventilatory Efficiency: $\dot{V}_E$ and $\dot{V}CO_2$

Because ventilation is more closely linked to carbon dioxide output ($\dot{V}CO_2$) than $\dot{V}O_2$, ventilatory efficiency is best defined by the relationship of the liters of ventilation required to eliminate a liter of CO_2. Mathematically, this relationship can be expressed either as a ratio ($\dot{V}_E/\dot{V}CO_2$) or a slope ($\dot{V}_E$ versus $\dot{V}CO_2$) (see **Fig. 3.28**), with the only factors being V_D/V_T, $PaCO_2$, and a constant ($k = 863$) to adjust for gases at standard temperature pressure dry (STPD) and body temperature pressure saturated (BTPS), and to convert fractional concentrations to pressures:

$$\dot{V}_E/\dot{V}CO_2 = k \;/\; [PaCO_2 \times (1 - V_D/V_T)]$$

Practically, the efficiency or inefficiency of elimination of CO_2 is measured as $\dot{V}_E/\dot{V}CO_2$ at a level of ventilation that appears to be the least variable in the region of the *AT* or the ventilatory compensation point (VCP) or the slope of $\dot{V}_E$ compared with $\dot{V}CO_2$ from the start of exercise to just below the *AT*. Because both $\dot{V}_E/\dot{V}CO_2$ and the slope are strongly affected by changes in lung gas exchange caused by both lung and heart diseases, the measurement of $\dot{V}_E/\dot{V}CO_2$ at the *AT* or VCP and the slope of $\dot{V}_E$ versus $\dot{V}CO_2$ are clinically very useful. An increase above normal for either variable indicates either lower $PaCO_2$ (hyperventilation) or greater inefficiency of ventilation. Despite the mathematical similarity between $\dot{V}_E/\dot{V}CO_2$ and the slope of $\dot{V}_E$ versus $\dot{V}CO_2$, any single measurement of $\dot{V}_E/\dot{V}CO_2$ may not be equal to the slope; this is because the graph of $\dot{V}_E$ versus $\dot{V}CO_2$ has a positive intercept on the $\dot{V}_E$ axis.

Slope of $\dot{V}_E$ (BTPS) versus $\dot{V}CO_2$ (STPD)

The slope of $\dot{V}_E$ (BTPS) versus $\dot{V}CO_2$ (STPD) has been characterized in patients[54-58] and normal subjects[14,15,18,51,56,59,60] to evaluate their relationship. We compared the variability between several large series of normal subjects that measured slopes only below the VCP to assess similarities and dissimilarities. For women, we compared the formulas of Kleber et al,[56] Neder et al,[18] the SHIP investigators,[14] and Sun et al[59] at ages 30 and 70 years with normal heights and BMIs. We added the formula of Inbar et al[15] for men. The formulas of Sun et al,[59] Neder et al,[18] and Kleber et al[56] showed the least variability from the overall means, with absolute differences of 0.8, 1.0, and 1.6 units, respectively.

Formulas for $\dot{V}_E$ versus $\dot{V}CO_2$ slope are

Sun et al[59] = 34.4 − 0.0723 cm + 0.082 years (SD 3.0) for both genders

Neder et al[18] = 21.0 + 0.12 years (SD 2.5) for men
= 25.2 + 0.08 years (SD 2.8) for women

Kleber et al[56] = 19.9 + 0.13 years (SD 4.0) for men
= 24.4 + 0.12 years (SD 4.0) for women

Gläser et al[14] = 20.9 + 0.139 × age (years) − 0.043 × height (cm) + 0.044 × weight (kg) + 1.45 × current smoker (no = 0, yes = 1) for men
= 26.7 + 0.046 × age (years) − 0.039 × height (cm) + 0.030 × weight (kg) for women

$\dot{V}_E/\dot{V}CO_2$ Near the *AT*

To evaluate ventilatory efficiency or inefficiency for gas exchange at the lungs, Sun et al[59] measured $\dot{V}_E/\dot{V}CO_2$ ratios at the *AT* and also at their lowest level. They were virtually identical and had less variability than the slope of $\dot{V}_E$ versus $\dot{V}CO_2$, which normally has an intercept on the $\dot{V}_E$ axis. Advantages to the using the lowest $\dot{V}_E/\dot{V}CO_2$ formula of Sun et al[59] are (1) the SD around the mean is smaller than the value at the *AT* and (2) it is not necessary to identify the *AT* to use the lowest $\dot{V}_E/\dot{V}CO_2$ ratios. The regression formulas for $\dot{V}_E/\dot{V}CO_2$ at the *AT* published by the Gläser et al[14] (SHIP) were similar to Sun et al[59] measured at the *AT*, although somewhat lower in younger men and older women.

To evaluate ventilatory inefficiency, we recommend lowest $\dot{V}_E/\dot{V}CO_2$ ratios or the $\dot{V}_E/\dot{V}CO_2$ at the *AT*, described by Sun et al[59] (**Table 7.7**):

$\dot{V}_E/\dot{V}CO_2$ at *AT* = 28.2 + 0.105 years − 0.0375 cm + 1.0 for women (SD 2.39)

$\dot{V}_E/\dot{V}CO_2$ at lowest level = 27.9 + 0.106 years − 0.0376 cm + 1.0 for women (SD 2.43)

TABLE 7.7 Ventilatory Efficiency During Exercise for Men[a,b]

Age (y)	N	$\dot{V}_E$ versus $\dot{V}CO_2$ slope	Lowest $\dot{V}_E/\dot{V}CO_2$
<20	46	22.9 ± 2.8	23.5 ± 2.0
21-30	90	23.6 ± 2.8	23.9 ± 2.1
31-40	49	23.9 ± 3.1	25.0 ± 2.7
41-50	37	25.2 ± 2.9	26.1 ± 2.2
51-60	54	27.2 ± 3.0	28.0 ± 2.9
>60	34	27.5 ± 3.1	29.4 ± 2.3

[a]To determine values for women, add 1 to the values shown for men.

[b]Data from Sun XG, Hansen JE, Garatachea N, Storer TW, Wasserman K. Ventilatory efficiency during exercise in healthy subjects. *Am J Respir Crit Care Med.* 2002;166(11):1443-1448.

Recommendations

- $\dot{V}CO_2$ (STPD), $\dot{V}O_2$ (STPD), and $\dot{V}_E$ (BTPS) should be measured and calculated synchronously over the same period(s) of time.
- In all calculations, mouthpiece mechanical dead space ventilation (V_D) (usually approximating 50-60 mL per breath) should be subtracted from overall $\dot{V}_E$.
- $\dot{V}_E$ versus $\dot{V}CO_2$ slope should be calculated from rest or onset of exercise to VCP by linear regression or by estimation from the graph. Reference value for $\dot{V}_E$ versus $\dot{V}CO_2$ slope = 34.4 − 0.0723 × height (cm) + 0.082 × age (years). For both genders, SD = 3.0 and upper limit of normal (ULN) = mean predicted + 4.9.
- Lowest $\dot{V}_E/\dot{V}CO_2$ or $\dot{V}_E/\dot{V}CO_2$ at *AT* for men = 27.9 + 0.106 × age (years) − 0.0376 × height (cm). Add 1.0 for women. For both genders, SD = 2.43 and ULN = mean predicted + 4.0.

Oxygen Uptake Efficiency Slope: $\dot{V}_E$ and $\dot{V}O_2$

A variable somewhat recently introduced is the oxygen uptake efficiency slope (OUES) that may be useful in assessment of heart failure prognosis and response to therapy. It is expressed as the slope of $\dot{V}O_2$ versus log $\dot{V}_E$ and is relatively linear throughout a progressive exercise test. Thus, the slope measured during submaximal exercise is similar to the slope measured throughout exercise to maximum. A higher slope suggests that $\dot{V}O_2$ is more efficient relative to $\dot{V}_E$; a lower slope, less efficient. As heart failure is potentially associated with a smaller rise in $\dot{V}O_2$ with progressive exercise and because $\dot{V}O_2 = \dot{V}CO_2 \times R$, a low OUES would also seem to have similar meaning as a lower $\Delta\dot{V}O_2/\Delta WR$ in addition to high $\dot{V}_E/\dot{V}CO_2$ ratio or high $\dot{V}_E$ versus $\dot{V}CO_2$ slope. These may be reasons for the potential usefulness of OUES.

Sun et al[61] published reference equations for OUES derived from 417 normal adult men and women:

$$\text{OUES, adult men} = -0.610 - 0.032 \times \text{age (years)} + 0.023 \times \text{height (cm)} + 0.008 \times \text{weight (kg)}$$

$$\text{OUES, adult women} = -1.178 - 0.032 \times \text{age (years)} + 0.008 \times \text{weight (kg)}$$

Physiological Dead Space–Tidal Volume Ratio

The physiological V_D is dependent on anatomic and physiological factors, whereas the physiological V_D/V_T is also dependent on the pattern of breathing. At rest, the V_D/V_T may be elevated because of rapid shallow breathing or anxiety. Physiological control mechanisms usually stabilize V_D/V_T at a lower, more efficient breathing pattern soon after the onset of exercise (**Fig. 7.10**) in normal subjects. Calculation of the V_D and V_D/V_T must be carefully performed, making an adjustment for the apparatus dead space (see Appendix C). In addition, gas exchange measurements must be synchronous with arterial blood sampling for measuring $PaCO_2$.

All studies have shown a fall in V_D/V_T during exercise in normal subjects. Thus, although mean V_D/V_T at rest ranged from 0.28 to 0.35 in several studies of normal subjects, mean V_D/V_T decreases to approximately 0.20 soon after exercise starts (see **Fig. 7.10**). It remains at about this level to the end of exercise, regardless of the level of work.[5,60,62]

Figure 7.10 shows the effect of exercise on V_D/V_T at various levels of cycle exercise in normal young men. As can be seen, the V_D/V_T stabilizes at a new low value soon after exercise starts and is slightly lower at higher work rates. Cotes[51] suggested that V_D (mL) equals 140 + 0.07 V_T (mL) with an SD of 90 mL in young men during exercise. Recently, the SHIP investigators reported regression equations for V_D/V_T based on age, sex, height, weight, and smoking status.[63] Compared to the recommendations below, although similar, resting V_D/V_T values were somewhat lower for younger subjects and peak V_D/V_T had a wider range based on age (**Figure 7.11**).

As a reminder, the practice of substituting end-tidal PCO_2 ($P_{ET}CO_2$) for $PaCO_2$ to determine a "noninvasive V_D/V_T" is invalid, largely because an abnormal V_D/V_T is closely associated with increased difference between $P_{ET}CO_2$ and $PaCO_2$ (increased P[a − ET]).

Recommendations

Normal values for V_D/V_T at rest and during upright exercise after allowance for valve dead space are as follows:

- **For men under age 40:**
  V_D/V_T (mean ± SD) = 0.29 ± 0.06 at rest
  = 0.17 ± 0.05 at the *AT*
  = 0.16 ± 0.04 at maximum exercise
- **For men over age 40:**
  V_D/V_T (mean ± SD) = 0.30 ± 0.08 at rest
  = 0.20 ± 0.07 at the *AT*
  = 0.19 ± 0.07 at maximum exercise[5]
- **Upper 95% confidence limits for men over 40:**
  V_D/V_T = 0.45 at rest
  = 0.33 at the *AT*
  = 0.30 at maximum exercise[5]
- For a suitable patient population with features similar to the SHIP cohort,[63] an alternative for peak exercise V_D/V_T = −0.251 + 0.0026 × age (years) + 0.0013 ×

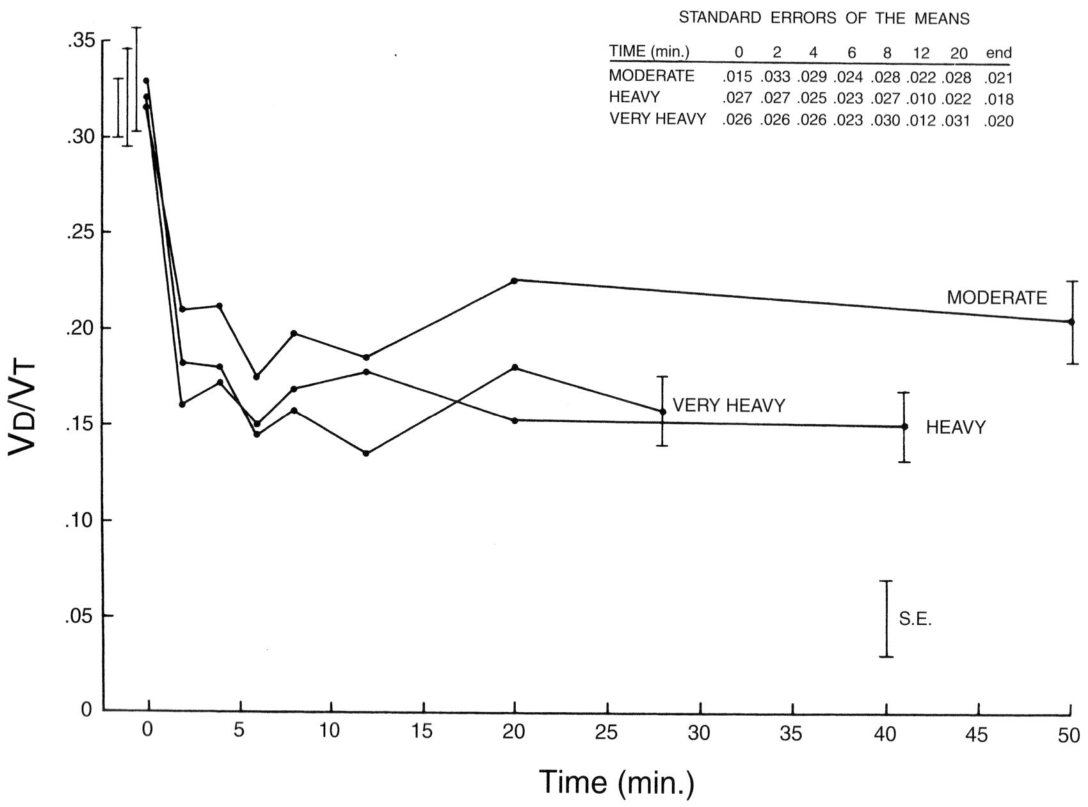

FIGURE 7.10. The physiological dead space–tidal volume ratio (VD/VT) in 10 normal young men at rest and during three intensities of cycle ergometer exercise as related to exercise time. The standard errors of the means are given in the table inset. *(Reproduced with permission from Wasserman K, Van Kessel A, Burton GG. Interaction of physiological mechanisms during exercise.* J Appl Physiol. *1967;22[1]:71-85. Copyright © 1967 American Physiological Society. All rights reserved.)*

height (cm) + 0.0001 × weight (kg) + 0.029 × (men = 1, women = 2). They reported an upper 95% percentile = 0.414 + 0.0025 × age (years) − 0.0013 × height (cm) + 0.0002 × weight (kg) − 0.03 × (men = 1, women = 2).

Arterial, End-Tidal, and Mixed-Expired Carbon Dioxide Pressures

Resting P_{ETCO_2} and Pa_{CO_2} values are dependent on the degree of apprehension, anxiety, and experience of the subject. Some anxious individuals have a tendency to hyperventilate, especially while breathing through a mouthpiece and awaiting the signal to begin exercise (**Fig. 7.12**). Once exercise starts, however, the blood gases and pH are not discernibly different whether the individual is performing the work while breathing through a low resistance breathing valve or breathing normally without a mouthpiece.[53] In more apprehensive individuals, the Pa_{CO_2} values may rise from rest to moderate exercise, because physiological control mechanisms suppress psychogenic hyperventilation. In the relaxed individual, Pa_{CO_2} values remain relatively stable at rest and during mild and moderate exercise. The Pa_{CO_2} values cannot be predicted accurately from P_{ETCO_2} values in an individual, particularly in a patient with lung or heart disease.

Wasserman and Whipp[53] found that the difference between Pa_{CO_2} and P_{ETCO_2} (P[a − ET]CO_2) changed from approximately +2.5 mm Hg at rest to −4 mm Hg during heavy work in 10 normal men (**Fig. 7.13**). In 77 asbestos-exposed but healthy men,[5,7] P(a − ET)CO_2 at rest was 0.3 ± 2.9 mm Hg (mean ± SD) and decreased to −4.1 ± 3.2 mm Hg at maximum exercise.[5] At the peak of exercise, a positive value for P(a − ET)CO_2 was rare. Gläser et al,[63] in 190 women and 286 men without disease but including smokers and obesity, found that P(a − ET)CO_2 was related to age, height, weight, and gender, with predicted values at rest ranging from +2.7 to +4.2 mm Hg for a 170-cm, 70-kg man. At peak exercise, predicted values ranged from −5.4 to −1 mm Hg, with the less negative values anticipated in older individuals.

Hansen et al[64] studied the absolute values and relationships between mixed expired P_{CO_2} ($P\bar{E}_{CO_2}$) and P_{ETCO_2} during CPET in 100 individuals, including 25 normal, 25 with COPD, 25 with pulmonary arterial hypertension, and 25 with left ventricular heart failure. Their findings are summarized in **Figure 7.14**, which shows the successive mean changes in each group, from resting successively to end of unloaded cycling to *AT* to peak exercise. At all stages of rest and exercise, absolute values of $P\bar{E}_{CO_2}$ and P_{ETCO_2} are highest in normal subjects (indicating good perfusion of the lung).

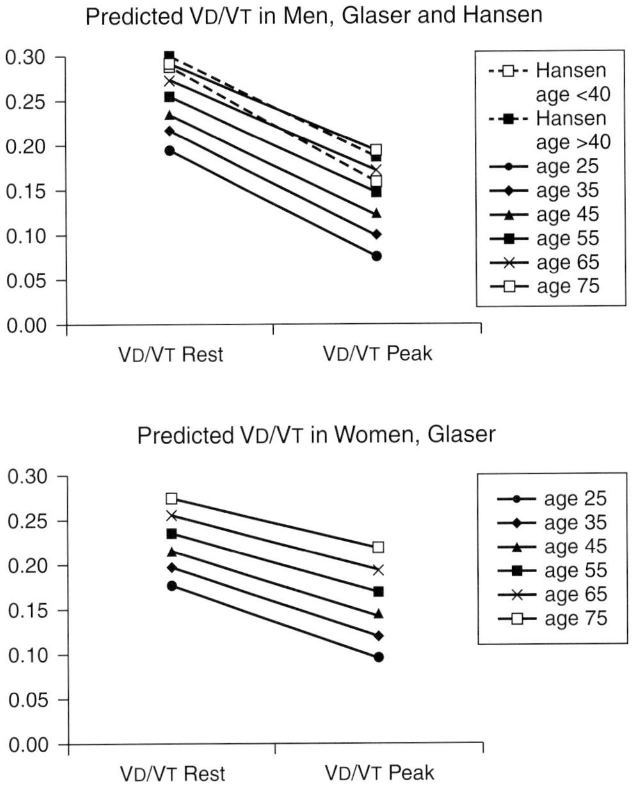

FIGURE 7.11. Predicted dead space–tidal volume ratio (V_D/V_T) for men at rest and peak exercise for ages 25 to 75 based on reference formula from Hansen et al,[5] and for men and women, Gläser et al.[63]

Recommendations

Normal values at sea level during upright exercise in adult men are as follows:

- **Pa_{CO_2}**: resting value = 36 to 42 mm Hg; stable or increasing slightly during mild and moderate exercise, decreasing with heavy exercise
- **P_{ETCO_2}**: resting value = 36 to 42 mm Hg; increases normally by 3 to 8 mm Hg during mild and moderate exercise (depending on breathing pattern), and decreases with heavy exercise
- $P(a - ET)CO_2$ (mean ± SD) at rest is close to 0, at the *AT* = −3 ± 3 mm Hg. At maximum exercise, the $P(a - ET)CO_2$ = −4 ± 3 mm Hg and is negative (P_{ETCO_2} exceeds Pa_{CO_2}) in more than 95% of normal men.
- For a population similar to the SHIP cohort,[63] another estimate is peak $P(a - ET)CO_2$ = −16.0 + 0.11 × age (years) + 0.04 × height (cm) − 0.010 × weight (kg) + 2.3 × (men = 1, women = 2), with the 95th percentile estimated = 7.5 + 0.11 × age (years) − 0.03 × height (cm) − 0.019 × weight (kg) − 0.5 × (men = 1, women = 2).

Arterial, Alveolar, and End-Tidal Oxygen Tensions and Arterial Oxyhemoglobin Saturation

The normal resting Pa_{O_2} is dependent on age, body position, and nutritional status, decreasing with age, obesity, fasting, and the supine position. Nevertheless, sea-level Pa_{O_2} values less than 80 mm Hg are not seen in normal persons younger

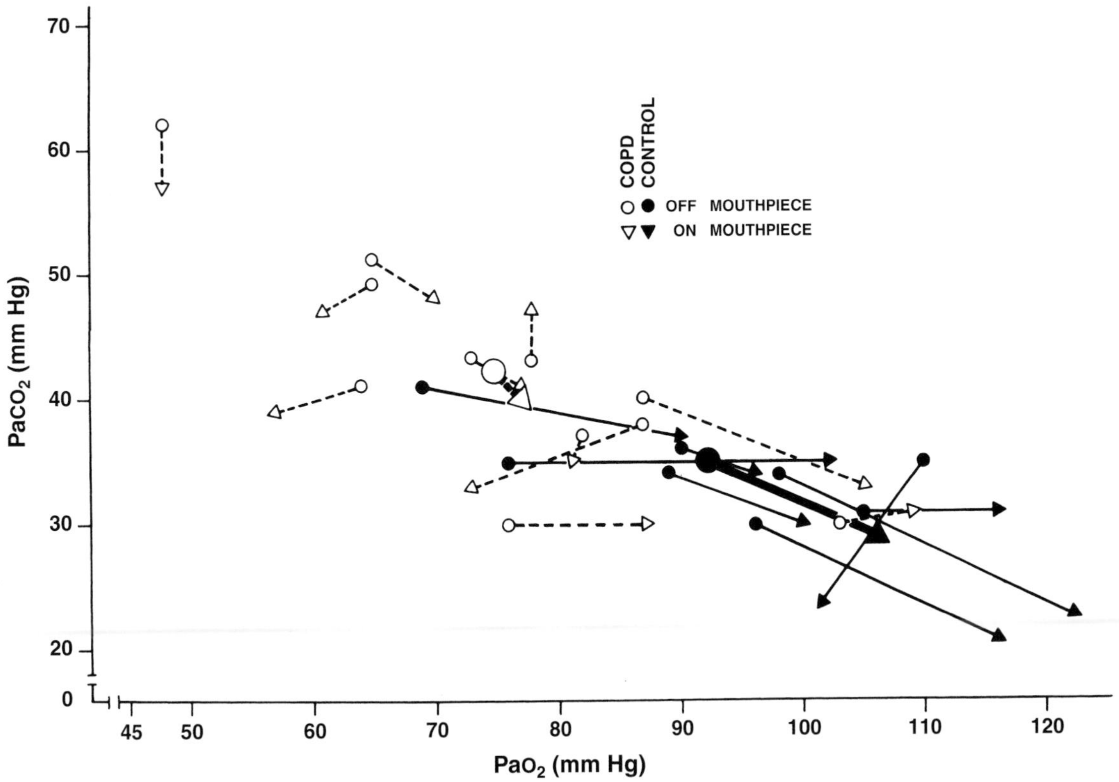

FIGURE 7.12. Resting Pa_{CO_2} and Pa_{O_2} in normal control subjects and in patients with chronic obstructive pulmonary disease (COPD) off and acutely on the mouthpiece while awaiting the signal to start cycle ergometer exercise. Small arrows show individual values, and large arrows show mean values. Note the small mean decline in Pa_{CO_2} and the increase in Pa_{O_2} in the patients with COPD while breathing on the mouthpiece. In contrast, the controls show a larger decline in Pa_{CO_2} and a much larger rise in Pa_{O_2} with the same mouthpiece at rest. *(Courtesy of J.D. Andrews, MD.)*

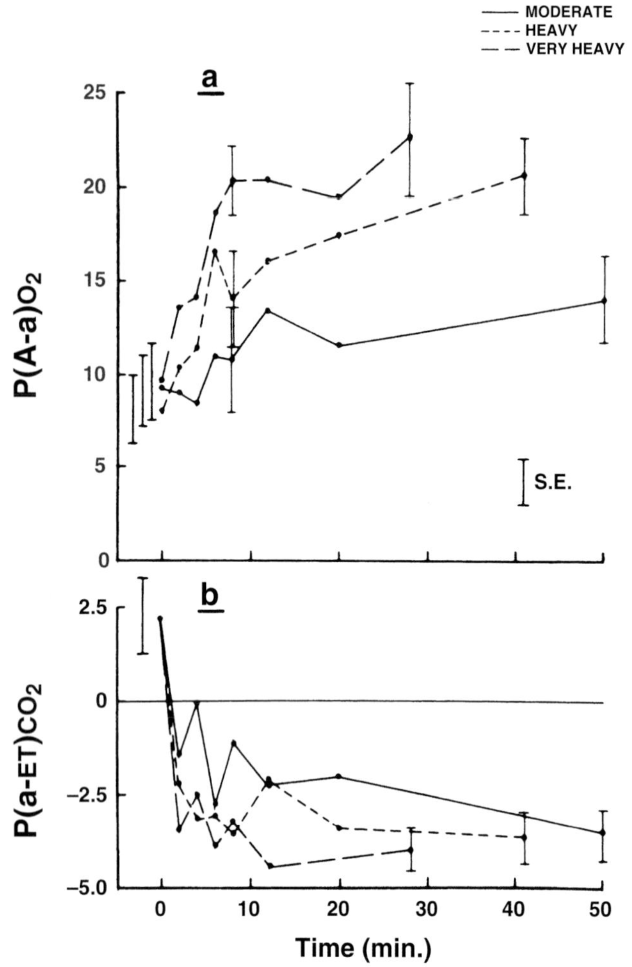

FIGURE 7.13. The P(A − a)O_2 and P(a − ET)CO_2 values in 10 normal young men at rest and during three intensities of cycle ergometer exercise as related to exercise duration. The mean and standard error of the mean are depicted. *(Reproduced with permission from Wasserman K, Van Kessel A, Burton GG. Interaction of physiological mechanisms during exercise.* J Appl Physiol. *1967;22[1]:71-85. Copyright © 1967 American Physiological Society. All rights reserved.)*

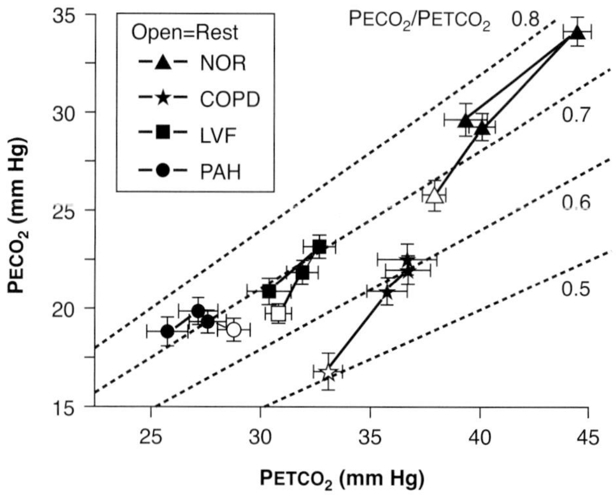

FIGURE 7.14. Mean and standard error of the mean values of mixed expired P_{CO_2} ($P\bar{E}_{CO_2}$), end-tidal P_{CO_2} (P_{ETCO_2}), in mm Hg are shown for four groups: normal (NOR), chronic obstructive pulmonary disease (COPD), left ventricular failure (LVF), and pulmonary arterial hypertension (PAH). The open symbols are resting values; the solid symbols represent a progression at end of warmup period, at *AT*, and at end of exercise. The dashed diagonal lines indicate the $P\bar{E}_{CO_2}/P_{ETCO_2}$ ratios from 0.5 to 0.8. See text for further interpretation. *(Reprinted from Hansen JE, Ulubay G, Chow BF, Sun XG, Wasserman K. Mixed-expired and end-tidal CO₂ distinguish between ventilation and perfusion defects during exercise testing in patients with lung and heart diseases.* Chest. *2007;132[3]:977-983. Copyright © 2007 American College of Chest Physicians. With permission.)*

than 70 years in the sitting position except in those who are quite obese. The end-tidal partial pressure of O_2 (P_{ETO_2}) and alveolar partial pressure of O_2 (P_{AO_2}) (the latter calculated from the alveolar gas equation; see Appendix C) are normally similar, but they may differ by 10 or more mm Hg in patients with severe maldistribution of ventilation. The P_{AO_2} and Pa_{O_2} decrease transiently soon after the start of exercise (because the rise in $\dot{V}E$ is slower than the rise in $\dot{V}O_2$, that is, respiratory exchange ratio [R] decreases) and then increase back to approximately resting values.

The arterial oxyhemoglobin saturation (Sa_{O_2}) normally changes less than 2% from rest to maximal exercise. In highly motivated athletes, the Sa_{O_2} has been reported to fall below resting values.[65-67]

The P_{ETO_2} normally increases 10 to 30 mm Hg for exercise above the *AT* because of metabolic acidosis–induced hyperventilation, rising R and high ratio ventilation-perfusion mismatching at maximal exercise.

Reports show that the P(A − a)O_2 increases during heavy exercise in normal subjects. In five healthy young men, Whipp and Wasserman[62] found a P(A − a)O_2 of 7.4 ± 4.2 mm Hg (mean ± SD) at rest and 10.8 ± 3.6 mm Hg at heavy exercise.

Similar results were obtained by Wasserman and Whipp[53] in 10 healthy young men; values are shown at rest and at three work intensities as related to time in **Figure 7.13**. In 77 normal older men (aged 34-74 years), we found P(A − a)O_2 values (mean ± SD) of 12.8 ± 7.4 mm Hg at rest and 19.0 ± 8.8 mm Hg at maximum exercise.[5,7] At maximum exercise, P(A − a)O_2 was greater than 35 mm Hg in only 3 of these 77 men. Gläser et al[63] found a somewhat higher predicted P(A − a)O_2 of 19 mm Hg at rest, increasing to 22 mm Hg at peak exercise for a 180 cm 40-year-old man weighing 80 kg. Their regression equation for P(A − a)O_2 at rest and peak exercise included age, height, weight, smoking status, and gender, with a somewhat large variance around the mean. The 95% confidence limits from this cohort ranged up to the mid- to high 30s. Of note is that the regression equations for P(A − a)O_2 predict higher values at rest with smaller or no increase at peak exercise. The authors noted a significant effect of increased BMI on predicted peak exercise P(A − a)O_2 but not on resting P(A − a)O_2; this could be because basilar lung atelectasis is diminished during exercise and lung gas exchange improves.

Recommendations

The normal arterial blood and P_{ETO_2} values at sea level during upright exercise in adult men are as follows:

- Free-flowing capillary blood P_{O_2} values are usually 5 to 10 mm Hg less than concurrently measured Pa_{O_2}, but the differences are variable and technique dependent.
- Pa_{O_2} at rest and peak exercise = 80 mm Hg or greater; usually increases slightly with heavy exercise
- Sa_{O_2} at rest = 95% or greater; no decrease with exercise
- P_{ETO_2} at rest = 90 mm Hg or greater; increases with heavy exercise
- $P(A - a)O_2$ (mean ± SD) for ages 20 to 39 years: at rest = 8 mm Hg, at the *AT* = 11 mm Hg, and at maximum exercise = 15 mm Hg
- $P(A - a)O_2$ (mean ± SD) for ages 40 to 69 years: at rest = 13 ± 7 mm Hg, at the *AT* = 17 ± 7 mm Hg, and at maximum exercise = 19 ± 9 mm Hg. The ULN (95% confidence level) at the *AT* = 28 mm Hg and at maximum exercise = 35 mm Hg
- For a patient population similar to that in the SHIP cohort,[63] a suitable estimate for peak exercise $P(A - a)O_2 = -1.0 + 0.05 \times$ age (years) $+ 0.07 \times$ height (cm) $+ 0.14 \times$ weight (kg) $- 1.2 \times$ (men = 1, women = 2). The 95th percentile is estimated at $21.9 + 0.09 \times$ age (years) $- 0.01 \times$ height (cm) $+ 0.16 \times$ weight (kg) $- 2.5 \times$ (men = 1, women = 2).

Femoral and Mixed Venous Values and Estimation of Cardiac Output

Muscle blood flow and oxygen extraction both increase strikingly with exercise. At near-maximum leg exercise, femoral vein values in normal subjects reach the following mean ± SE values: P_{O_2} = 20 ± 2 mm Hg, S_{O_2} = 17% ± 3%, pH = 7.00 ± 0.04, P_{CO_2} = 80 ± 5 mm Hg, and lactate = 10 ± 1 mmol/L. In patients with heart disease, minimum mean femoral vein values are similar: P_{O_2} = 18 mm Hg and S_{O_2} = 18% to 21%. Concurrent mixed venous values in the same patients are 2 mm Hg and 4% higher, respectively.

The usual values found for mixed venous O_2 saturation ($S\bar{v}_{O_2}$) at peak treadmill or cycle exercise approximate 25%. In normal subjects, as well as in patients with heart failure, $S\bar{v}_{O_2}$, mixed venous O_2 content ($C\bar{v}_{O_2}$), arterial-mixed venous O_2 content difference ($C[a - \bar{v}]O_2$), and O_2 extraction ratio $[C(a - \bar{v})O_2/Ca_{O_2}]$ change in relatively linear fashion as $\dot{V}_{O_2}$ changes from rest to peak values. In five normal men, the $C(a - \bar{v})O_2$ values (in mL/100 mL blood) were $5.72 + 0.1 \times$ % peak $\dot{V}_{O_2}$, with an SD of 1.08 mL/100 mL, $r = 0.94$. Combining the data from three studies involving normal subjects and patients with congestive heart failure,[68-70] the $C(a - \bar{v})O_2$ values (in mL/100 mL blood) were $5.55 + 0.085 \times$ % peak $\dot{V}_{O_2}$, with an SD of 1.09, $r = 0.97$. Absolute Ca_{O_2} values are dependent on the hemoglobin concentration, which usually rises 5% to 8% at peak exercise in healthy individuals.

Recommendations

- In the normal person and the patient with heart disease, femoral vein mean ± standard error values are P_{O_2} = 19 ± 3 mm Hg and S_{O_2} = 19% ± 3% at maximum leg exercise, when such exercise is not limited by other than cardiovascular factors.
- Concurrent mixed venous values are P_{O_2} = 21 ± 3 mm Hg and S_{O_2} = 23% ± 3%. In such individuals, the $S\bar{v}_{O_2}$, $C\bar{v}_{O_2}$, $C(a - \bar{v})O_2$, and O_2 extraction ratio change in near linear fashion from rest to maximum exercise.
- In the absence of anemia, hypoxemia, or significant carboxyhemoglobinemia, $C(a - \bar{v})O_2$ in mL/100 mL of blood is $5.55 + 0.085 \times$ % peak $\dot{V}_{O_2}$ with an SD = 1.1 mL/100 mL blood. These values can be used to estimate cardiac output and stroke volume, especially at maximum exercise.[71]

Acid-Base Balance

In the normal individual, an intense metabolic acidosis is induced by heavy exercise. Measurement of the acid-base status at the termination of an incremental exercise test is valuable in deciding whether the subject has made a good effort and performed near maximum exercise. Resting venous and arterial lactate values are normally less than 1 mmol/L and typically rise substantially before the termination of maximal exercise. During exercise, venous lactate values can be dependent on the site of lactate production and the sampling site,[70] whereas arterial or mixed venous lactate values give a better indication of the total body lactate burden.

The rise in blood lactate during exercise is accompanied by a nearly equimolar decline in bicarbonate (HCO_3^-) as HCO_3^- is converted to CO_2 and a decrease in pH. The extra CO_2 generated by HCO_3^- buffering of lactic acid is reflected by an increase in R. The arterial lactate and R reach their peak and the pH and HCO_3^- reach their nadir at about 2 minutes into recovery (**Table 7.8**). The magnitudes of the lactate and HCO_3^- changes indicate the severity of exercise-induced metabolic acidosis.

Normal values for younger[72] and older[5] men for incremental cycle exercise tests are given in **Table 7.8**. Small changes signify a mild degree of exercise stress secondary to low motivation or disorders that preclude the performance of exercise at a significant level above the *AT*.

Recommendations

- Mean R values (± SD) in normal older men at end of exercise are 1.21 ± 0.12 and are 1.59 ± 0.19 at 2 minutes of recovery. However, the value of R depends on the rate at which lactate increases and HCO_3^- decreases, not on the work rate per se.
- Decline in HCO_3^- and increase in lactate (both in mmol/L) at end of exercise are approximately 6 ± 2 in younger men and 4 ± 2.5 in older men; at 2 minutes of recovery, these are approximately 8.4 ± 2.5 in all men.

TABLE 7.8 Metabolic Acidosis at the End of and During Recovery From Maximum Incremental Cycle Ergometer Exercise in Normal Sedentary Men[a]

	At end of exercise		2 min into recovery	
Age (y)	18-24	34-74	18-24	34-74
Number studied	10	77	10	77
Average exercise duration (min)	18	9	18	9
Arterial lactate increase (mmol/L)[b]	6.6 ± 1.4	—	7.6 ± 1.8	—
Arterial HCO_3^- decrease from rest (mmol/L)[b]	6.2 ± 2.3	4.0 ± 2.5	8.7 ± 2.6	8.5 ± 2.9
Arterial pH[b]	7.31 ± 0.04	7.37 ± 0.04	7.29 ± 0.04	7.33 ± 0.03
Respiratory exchange ratio (R)[b]	—	1.21 ± 0.12	—	1.59 ± 0.19

Abbreviation: HCO_3^-, bicarbonate.

[a]Data are from Hansen JE, Sue DY, Wasserman K. Predicted values for clinical exercise testing. *Am Rev Respir Dis.* 1984;129(2, pt 2):S49-S55; Beaver WL, Wasserman K, Whipp BJ. Bicarbonate buffering of lactic acid generated during exercise. *J Appl Physiol (1985).* 1986;60:472-478.

[b]Values are means ± standard deviations.

PREDICTED VALUES FOR CHILDREN

Cardiopulmonary exercise tests in children present several particular problems. A major one is the establishment of reference values in subjects who likely require considerable adjustment for changes in body size and especially for the effects of growth, muscle mass, and other factors related to puberty. In contrast to adult reference values, simple age is unlikely to be the key variable because the range of pediatric ages is small. In their review of 34 papers presenting pediatric reference values for CPET through 2014, Blais et al[73] concluded that only a few studies were of most usefulness, based on methodology, number of subjects, and validation for either cycle or treadmill exercise, and many of these were performed several years ago. Recently, Blanchard and colleagues[3] published a set of reference values based on 228 healthy "non-athletic" children from Quebec City and Sherbrooke, Quebec, Canada, aged 12 to 17 performing ramp cycle exercise. Of note, the authors devoted considerable effort to adjusting their model for overweight, including fat free mass, BMI for age, and corrected body mass. The children were self-reported to be 87.7% Caucasian. In addition to variables described here, **Tables 7.9** and **7.10**, taken from Blanchard et al[3] permit calculation of predicted

TABLE 7.9 Predicted Values for Boys During Cardiopulmonary Exercise Testing[a,b]

	Predicted mean					Predicted SD	
	a	*b*	*c*	*d*	*e*	*f*	*g*
Peak $\dot{V}O_2$, mL/min	−0.297	105.9	36.6	0	−8660	6.45	−717.1
Peak O_2 pulse	−0.00131	0.459	0.214	0	−37.48	0.0277	−2.67
Peak work rate, W	0.0182	−5.324	2.824	4.170	378.9	0.220	−7.62
Peak $\dot{V}E$, L/min	0.00228	−0.419	0.981	3.168	2.704	0.405	−52.54
Peak HR, beats/min	−0.00053	0.313	−0.259	0	169.5	0.0966	−7.47
Peak RER	0	0.00142	−0.00098	0.0155	0.786	−0.00016	0.0935
OUES	−0.171	57.8	39.1	0	−4247	8.61	−1043
OUES, below *AT*	0.0923	−30.4	32.7	0	3181	7.27	−783.6
$\dot{V}E/\dot{V}CO_2$ slope	0	−0.0407	0	0	35.1	−0.00559	4.48
$\dot{V}E/\dot{V}CO_2$ slope, below *AT*	−0.00092	0.319	−0.0466	−0.599	7.87	−0.0527	11.04
$\dot{V}E/\dot{V}CO_2$ at *AT*	0.00128	−0.434	−0.0924	0	68.39	−0.0289	7.28
$\dot{V}O_2$ at *AT*, mL/min	−0.146	56.3	18.0	−48.3	−3898	3.11	−90.9
$\dot{V}O_2$/work rate slope, mL/min/W	0	−0.00871	0	0	12.4	0.0121	−0.995

Abbreviations: *AT*, anaerobic threshold; HR, heart rate; O_2, oxygen; OUES, oxygen uptake efficiency slope; RER, respiratory exchange ratio; $\dot{V}CO_2$, carbon dioxide output; $\dot{V}E$, minute ventilation; $\dot{V}O_2$, oxygen uptake.

[a]Mean predicted value for each variable = *a* × height, cm^2 + *b* × height, cm + *c* × corrected body mass, kg (see text) + *d* × age, years + *e*. Standard deviation (SD) = *f* × height, cm + *g*.

[b]Data are selected from Blanchard J, Blais S, Chetaille P, et al. New reference values for cardiopulmonary exercise testing in children. *Med Sci Sports Exerc.* 2018;50:1125-1133.

TABLE 7.10 Predicted Values for Girls During Cardiopulmonary Exercise Testing[a,b]

	Predicted mean					Predicted SD	
	a	*b*	*c*	*d*	*e*	*f*	*g*
Peak $\dot{V}O_2$, mL/min	−0.244	86.80	14.7	0	−6424	2.12	−45.9
Peak O_2 pulse	−0.00019	0.075	0.1007	0	−1.83	−0.00320	2.17
Peak work rate, W	−0.06025	20.57	0.741	0	−1622	0.284	−24.41
Peak $\dot{V}E$, L/min	−0.00697	2.56	0.528	1.14	−202.86	0.0681	3.72
Peak HR, beats/min	−0.0213	7.198	−0.193	−0.809	−391.1	−0.121	28.41
Peak RER	0	0.00122	−0.00195	0.0143	0.906	−0.00109	0.251
OUES	−0.251	91.4	13.8	0	−6768	4.48	−406.1
OUES, below *AT*	−0.0333	12.8	15.9	0	35.6	5.13	−476
$\dot{V}E/\dot{V}CO_2$ slope	0.000191	−0.112	0.0697	0	37.9	−0.0103	5.37
$\dot{V}E/\dot{V}CO_2$ slope, below *AT*	−0.00558	1.83	0.0191	−0.2901	−120.7	0.00481	1.98
$\dot{V}E/\dot{V}CO_2$ at *AT*	−0.00548	1.81	−0.0232	0	−119.1	0.0181	−0.00423
$\dot{V}O_2$ at *AT*, mL/min	−0.00407	−2.14	15.9	−26.7	1282	0.454	215.3
$\dot{V}O_2$/work rate slope, mL/min/W	0.00145	−0.500	0.0152	0	52.17	−0.00247	1.58

Abbreviations: *AT*, anaerobic threshold; HR, heart rate; O_2, oxygen; OUES, oxygen uptake efficiency slope; RER, respiratory exchange ratio; $\dot{V}CO_2$, carbon dioxide output; $\dot{V}E$, minute ventilation; $\dot{V}O_2$, oxygen uptake.

[a]Mean predicted value for each variable = *a* × height, cm^2 + *b* × height, cm + *c* × corrected body mass, kg (see text) + *d* × age, years + *e*. Standard deviation (SD) = *f* × height, cm + *g*.

[b]Data are selected from Blanchard J, Blais S, Chetaille P, et al. New reference values for cardiopulmonary exercise testing in children. *Med Sci Sports Exerc*. 2018;50:1125-1133.

values and *z* scores from this sample. Using the values in the columns under the letters in italics from these table, the formulas are presented in the form:

$$\text{Predicted value} = a \times \text{height}^2\ (\text{cm}) + b \times \text{height}\ (\text{cm}) + c \times \text{corrected body mass} + d \times \text{age}\ (\text{years}) + e$$

$$z = [a \times \text{height}^2\ (\text{cm}) + b \times \text{height}\ (\text{cm}) + c \times \text{corrected body mass} + d \times \text{age}\ (\text{years}) + e]\ /\ [f \times \text{height}\ (\text{cm}) + g]$$

To determine corrected body mass, calculate the subject's BMI and then compare to 85th percentile of BMI for age (World Health Organization [WHO]). For ages 12 to 18, 85th percentile of BMI (kg/m^2) for age can be estimated for boys as (age 12, 19.9; age 13, 20.8; age 14, 21.8; age 15, 22.7; age 16, 23.5: age 17, 24.3, age 18, 24.9) and for girls as (age 12, 20.8; age 13, 21.8; age 14, 22.7; age 15, 23.5; age 16, 24.1; age 17, 24.5; age 18, 24.9). If the subject's BMI is less than the 85th percentile BMI for age, use actual mass in kg. If the subject's BMI exceeds the 85th percentile BMI for age, multiply the 85th percentile BMI by (measured height)^2 and use that value as the corrected body mass.

Peak $\dot{V}O_2$ in Children

Although sustained heavy exercise rarely occurs in children, traditional exercise testing focuses largely on the peak or maximal oxygen uptake ($\dot{V}O_2$max), which can only be measured from sustained exercise precisely in the high-intensity range. The $\dot{V}O_2$max probably occurs only in the confines of the exercise laboratory, and a "true" $\dot{V}O_2$max (ie, a plateau in $\dot{V}O_2$ while the work rate continues to increase) is observed in only about 28% of children and adolescents.[74] Because of this, CPET in children includes a growing variety of less effort dependent and less quantitative protocols, like physical work capacity (PWC) at a specified HR. In the PWC testing paradigm,[75,76] the subject performs a progressive exercise test in which the main variable is the work rate achieved at a specified submaximal HR (usually around 150-170 beats/min). The PWC has been used in a number of studies of exercise and pediatric lung diseases such as asthma and cystic fibrosis.[77,78] Other submaximal approaches to exercise testing that are more amenable to field studies, such as the 20-m shuttle run and the 6-minute walk per run test, have also been used to assess fitness in children with a variety of lung diseases and pulmonary hypertension.[79-82]

A reduction in physical activity has become apparent worldwide over the past several decades,[83] which is a worrisome trend. Here, we present measurements of aerobic function for children in our environment. Ideally, each laboratory should compare a sample of local, healthy children to help choose an appropriate set of normal values relative to those presented here. Some relatively large-sample normative values for children are included in the references.[84-87]

Cooper et al[74,88] reported peak $\dot{V}O_2$ for 109 children, aged 6 to 17 years, who performed cycle ergometry using a continuously increasing work rate protocol. Because these subjects were not obese, peak $\dot{V}O_2$ correlated similarly with

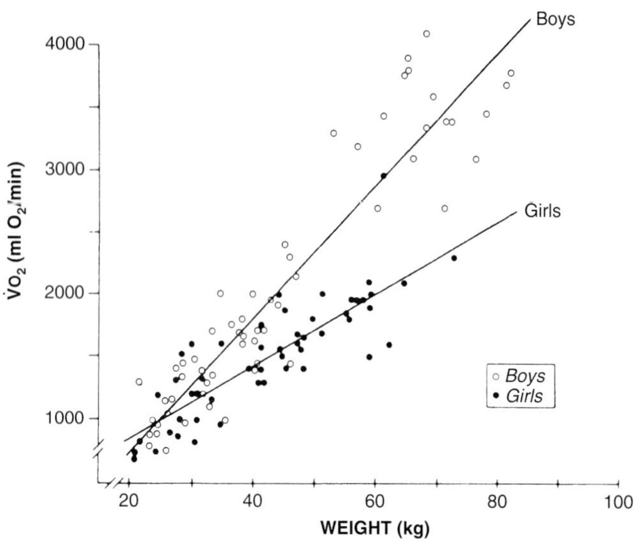

FIGURE 7.15. Peak oxygen uptake ($\dot{V}O_2$) of 109 normal North American boys and girls for leg cycling. Regression equations for peak $\dot{V}O_2$ (mL/min) as function of body weight (kg) were as follows: for boys, $\dot{V}O_2 = 52.8 \times$ weight $- 303$ ($r = 0.94$); for girls, $\dot{V}O_2 = 28.5 \times$ weight $+ 288$ ($r = 0.84$). *(Reproduced with permission from Cooper DM, Weiler-Ravell D, Whipp BJ, Wasserman K. Aerobic parameters of exercise as a function of body size during growth in children. J Appl Physiol Respir Environ Exerc Physiol. 1984;56[3]:628-634. Copyright © 1984 American Physiological Society. All rights reserved.)*

either weight or height (**Fig. 7.15**). The prediction equations are as follows:

For normal boys: Peak $\dot{V}O_2$ (mL/min) = $52.8 \times$ weight (kg) $- 303.4$
$r = 0.94$

For normal girls: Peak $\dot{V}O_2$ (mL/min) = $28.5 \times$ weight (kg) $+ 288.2$
$r = 0.84$

The study by Blanchard et al[3] showed that values for peak $\dot{V}O_2$ depended on height, corrected body mass, and age, with separate equations for girls and boys. The authors estimated "corrected body mass" as the subject's body mass (kg) from which mass in excess of the 85th percentile limit of BMI for age (WHO) is subtracted, if the subject is overweight. In addition, they presented *z* scores based on these variables that allow prediction of, for example, the lower 95% or 98% percentile. Because the peak $\dot{V}O_2$ regression equation includes height (cm) as a major factor along with weight, it is somewhat difficult to compare these examples with Cooper et al.[88] However, we find that for reasonably expected height for weight in nonobese children, the mean peak $\dot{V}O_2$ derived from Blanchard et al[3] are extremely close for boys and very slightly higher for girls.

For normal boys: Peak $\dot{V}O_2$ (mL/min) = $-0.297 \times$ height^2 (cm) $+ 105.9 \times$ height (cm) $+ 36.6 \times$ corrected body mass (kg) $- 8600$

For normal girls: Peak $\dot{V}O_2$ (mL/min) = $-0.244 \times$ height^2 (cm) $+ 86.8 \times$ height (cm) $+ 14.7 \times$ corrected body mass (kg) $- 6424$

Recommendations

- Recommended mean values for peak $\dot{V}O_2$ for children of average activity levels performing cycle ergometry are

For normal boys: Peak $\dot{V}O_2$ (mL/min) = $52.8 \times$ weight $- 303.4$
$r = 0.94$

For normal girls: Peak $\dot{V}O_2$ (mL/min) = $28.5 \times$ weight $+ 288.2$
$r = 0.84$

The data and correlations for predicted peak $\dot{V}O_2$ for leg cycling for children are shown in **Figure 7.15**. For overweight children, increase the predicted peak $\dot{V}O_2$ by 6 mL/min for each kilogram of weight above normal (predicted) weight.

- Regression equations for peak $\dot{V}O_2$ given by Blanchard et al[3] above appear to be very close to those of Cooper et al[88] for nonobese children. Because their formulas use "corrected body mass" in obesity, this requires an additional calculation if subjects are obese (defined as BMI >85th percentile).

Peak Heart Rate and Heart Rate Reserve

The maximum or peak HR achieved generally declines with age, but it should be noted that the age range in pediatric studies is quite small, and an average range for all children studied is practical. No consistent differences have been found between boys and girls or among the types of exercise used (eg, leg cycling, stepping, inclined treadmill, walking, running). Scandinavian children were found to have an average peak HR of 205 beats/min,[4] whereas North American children aged 8 to 18 years had an average peak HR of 187 beats/min, with a lower 95% confidence limit of 160.[86] In healthy Canadian children with a mean age of 15 years, Blanchard et al[3] found no statistical change with age in their multivariate analysis for boys and only a small change with age in girls, although there were small changes related to height and weight. For children of average size, predicted peak HR were somewhat lower than 220 − age (years).

Scandinavian children were found to have an average peak HR of 205 beats/min,[4] whereas North American children aged 8 to 18 years had an average peak HR of 187 beats/min, with a lower 95% confidence limit of 160.[74]

The concept of HRR can be useful for estimating the relative stress of the cardiovascular system during exercise, but it should be used with caution. A normal HRR is zero. The mean predicted peak HR may not be reached because of normal population variability; poor motivation; medications such as β-adrenergic blockers; or because of heart, peripheral vascular, lung, endocrine, or musculoskeletal diseases.

Recommendations

Peak HR values should be measured and averaged at the same time as the peak $\dot{V}O_2$ values. The following equations can be used to estimate the predicted peak HR and the HRR for adults and children:

- Predicted peak HR (beats/min) = 220 − age (years)
- HRR = predicted peak HR − observed peak HR

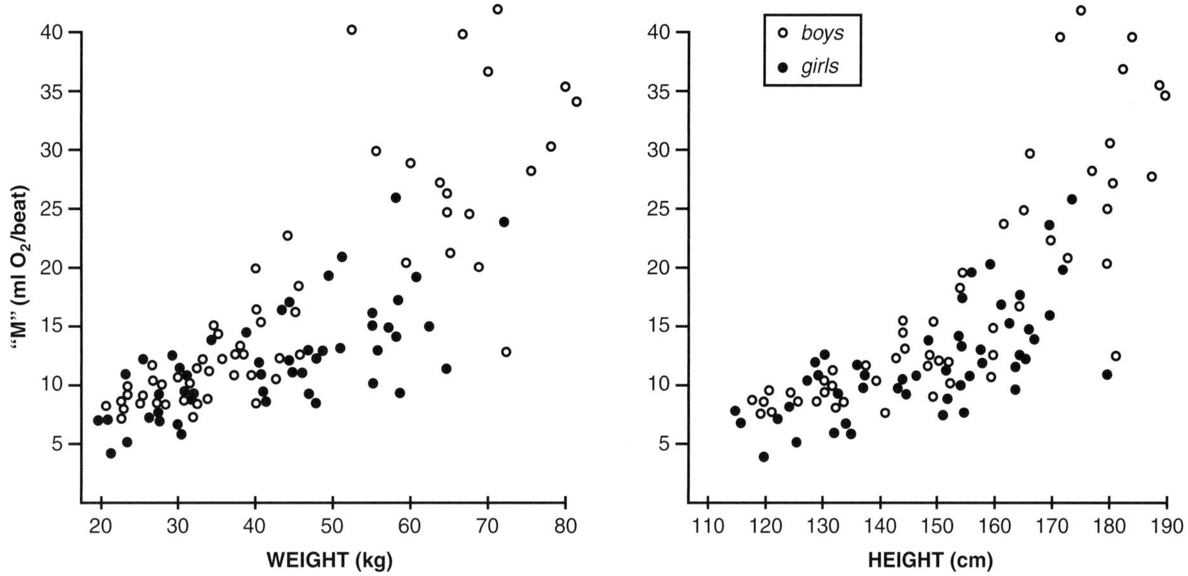

FIGURE 7.16. The slope *M* of the oxygen uptake–heart rate ($\dot{V}O_2$-HR) relationship as a function of body weight (left panel) and height (right panel) in the study population. The slope increased systematically with increasing body size but more rapidly in boys than in girls. Using height, the linear regression equation was $M = 0.32\ (Ht) - 33.9$, $r = 076$, for the whole study population. *(Reprinted by permission from Springer: Cooper DM, Weiler-Ravell D, Whipp BJ, Wasserman K. Growth-related changes in oxygen uptake and heart rate during progressive exercise in children.* Pediatr Res. *1984;18(9):845-851. Copyright © 1984 Springer Nature.)*

- However, as noted, there is very little practical change in predicted peak HR with age in the pediatric age range. For example, using 220 − age (years), the difference in peak HR from age 12 to 18 is only 6 beats/min.

Relationship of Oxygen Uptake and Heart Rate: The Peak Oxygen Pulse

Cooper et al[74] related the slope of the $\dot{V}O_2$ to HR to weight and height for boys and girls (**Fig. 7.16**). The slope gets steeper with growth. When normalized to weight, there is no systematic change in slope of $\dot{V}O_2$ versus HR with aging (**Fig. 7.17**). However, past puberty, the slope of $\dot{V}O_2$ versus HR for boys is steeper than that for girls. The peak O_2 pulse for boys and girls as related to size is shown in **Figure 7.18**. From the data of Blanchard et al,[3] derived regression equations for predicted peak O_2 pulse did not find that age was a significant for either boys or girls, although size was significant.

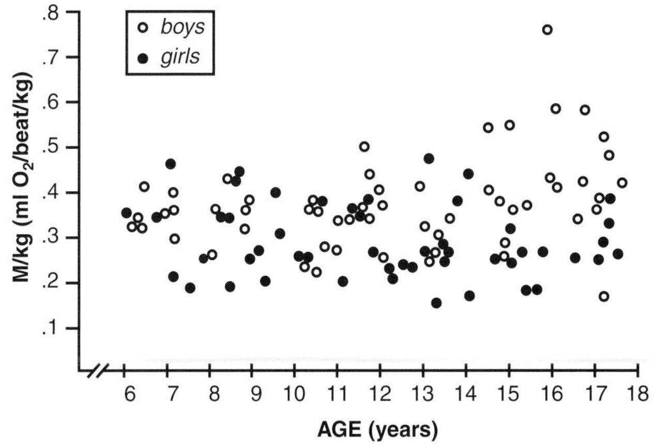

FIGURE 7.17. The slope *M* of the oxygen uptake–heart rate ($\dot{V}O_2$-HR) relationship normalized for body weight: (*M*/kg) as a function of age. There was no systemic change for *M*/kg in the population as a whole, but values for boys were significantly higher than for girls. *(Reprinted by permission from Springer: Cooper DM, Weiler-Ravell D, Whipp BJ, Wasserman K. Growth-related changes in oxygen uptake and heart rate during progressive exercise in children.* Pediatr Res. *1984;18(9):845-851. Copyright © 1984 Springer Nature.)*

Recommendations

See **Figures 7.16** and **7.17** and Cooper et al[74] for slope of $\dot{V}O_2$-HR relationship. See **Figure 7.18** for predicted peak O_2 pulse and Blanchard et al[3] for addition reference equations.

Alternatively, the regression equations of predicted peak O_2 pulse from Blanchard et al[3] for Canadian children are based on height, gender, and weight:

$$\text{Predicted peak } O_2 \text{ pulse (boys)} = -0.00131 \times \text{height}^2\ (\text{cm}) + 0.459 \times \text{height (cm)} + 0.214 \times \text{corrected body mass (kg)} - 37.48$$

$$\text{Predicted peak } O_2 \text{ pulse (girls)} = -0.00019 \times \text{height}^2\ (\text{cm}) + 0.075 \times \text{height (cm)} + 0.1007 \times \text{corrected body mass (kg)} - 1.83$$

Anaerobic Threshold

Cooper and Weiler-Ravell[89] tested 51 girls and 58 boys between the ages of 6 and 17 years. The subjects were healthy and not obese but did not participate in vigorous sports. Mean *AT* was 58% of peak $\dot{V}O_2$, and the lower limit of normal for this sample of normal children was 44% of peak $\dot{V}O_2$ (**Fig. 7.19**). From the data of Blanchard et al,[3] mean values for $\dot{V}O_2$ at *AT*/predicted peak $\dot{V}O_2$, % ranged from 65% to 75% in those 12 years old, and 61% to 70% in boys and girls age 15. The lower 95% confidence limits were between roughly 37% to 45% at age 12 and 35% to 42% at age 15.

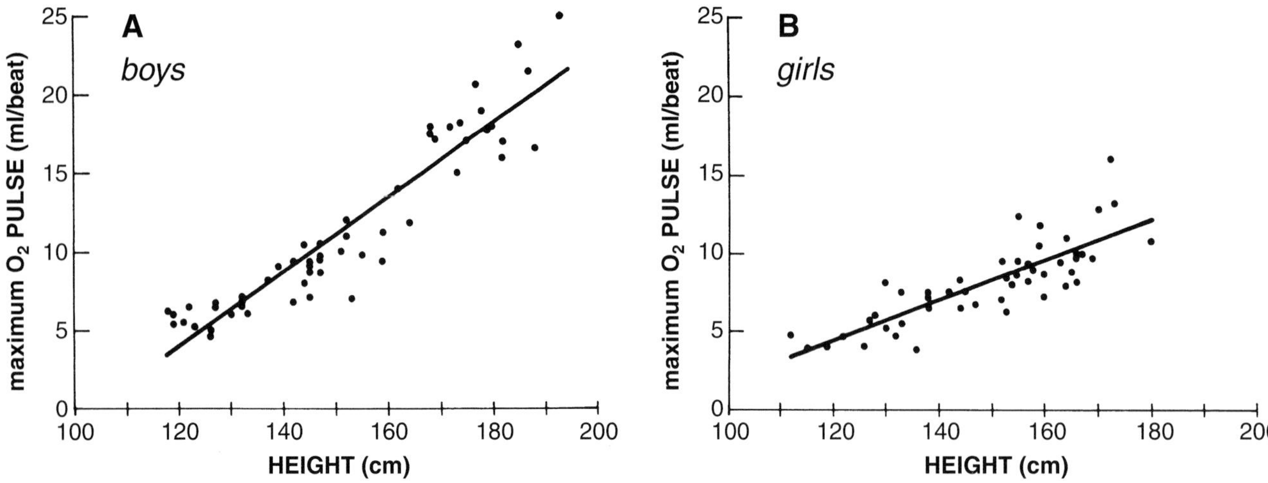

FIGURE 7.18. Maximum oxygen (O_2) pulse for normal North American boys (A) and girls (B). For boys, the best-fit regression line is O_2 pulse (mL/beat) = 0.23 × height (cm) − 24.4. The lower 95% confidence limit is 3.8 mL/beat below the regression line. For girls, the equation is O_2 pulse (mL/beat) = 0.128 × height (cm) − 10.9 with a lower 95% confidence limit of 3.0 mL/beat below the regression line. *(Modified by permission from Springer: Cooper DM, Weiler-Ravell D, Whipp BJ, Wasserman K. Growth-related changes in oxygen uptake and heart rate during progressive exercise in children.* Pediatr Res. *1984;18[9]:845-851. Copyright © 1984 Springer Nature.)*

Comparative values for *AT* in children with a variety of disease states, such as cerebral palsy[90] and congenital heart disease,[91] are also available.

Recommendations

The mean values and confidence limits for the predicted *AT* in normal children are given in **Table 7.11**, with the ratios of predicted *AT* to predicted peak $\dot{V}O_2$ in **Figure 7.19.** It can be seen in the latter that the lower 95% confidence limit for the ratio of predicted *AT* to predicted peak $\dot{V}O_2$ is about 44%. Also, consider using the prediction formula by Blanchard et al,[3] if suitable.

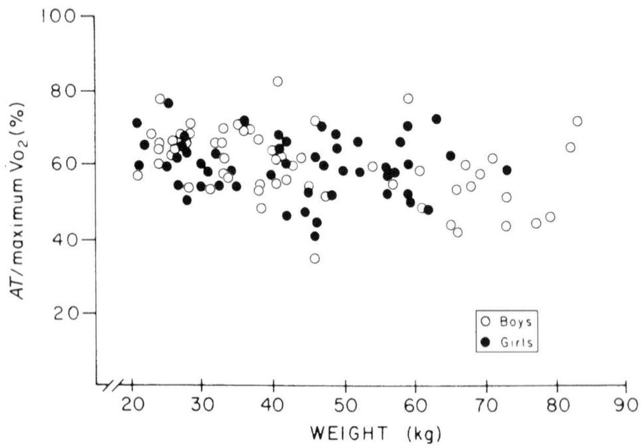

FIGURE 7.19. The ratio of anaerobic threshold to peak oxygen uptake (*AT*/peak $\dot{V}O_2$), as a percentage, for 109 normal North American boys and girls. *(Reproduced with permission from Cooper DM, Weiler-Ravell D, Whipp BJ, Wasserman K. Aerobic parameters of exercise as a function of body size during growth in children.* J Appl Physiol Respir Environ Exerc Physiol. *1984;56[3]:628-634. Copyright © 1984 American Physiological Society. All rights reserved.)*

Oxygen Uptake–Work Rate Relationship

Recommendations

Blanchard et al[3] reported regression equations for $\Delta\dot{V}O_2/\Delta WR$ for boys and girls.

$$\Delta\dot{V}O_2/\Delta WR\text{ (boys), mL/min/watt} = -0.00871 \times \text{height (cm)} + 12.4$$

$$\Delta\dot{V}O_2/\Delta WR\text{ (girls), mL/min/watt} = 52.17 + 0.00145 \times \text{height}^2\text{ (cm)} - 0.5 \times \text{height (cm)} + 0.0152 \times \text{corrected mass (kg)}$$

We note that there is only small variation in $\Delta\dot{V}O_2/\Delta WR$ with size or age. Values are in the range of 10 to 11 mL/min/W with an SD of about 1.0 to 1.2 mL/min/W.

Ventilatory Efficiency

There is a linear relationship between $\dot{V}E$ and $\dot{V}CO_2$ for most of the progressively increasing work rate test.[92] Normal values have now been established for slope of the relationship ($\Delta\dot{V}E/\Delta\dot{V}CO_2$).[93-95] The $\Delta\dot{V}E/\Delta\dot{V}CO_2$ decreases with increasing size among children and teenagers (**Fig. 7.20**).

Younger children need to breathe more than adults for a given increase in metabolic rate (ie, $\Delta\dot{V}CO_2$). Whether this results from a lower $PaCO_2$ or a higher VD/VT with lower body size has not been determined.[96,97] However, the range of $\Delta\dot{V}E/\Delta\dot{V}CO_2$ values average 26 for a 20-kg child and 20 for an 80-kg child.

Additional data demonstrate substantial differences between children and adults in the $\dot{V}E$ and $\dot{V}CO_2$ responses to and recovery from 1 minute of high-intensity exercise. We used these short exercise protocols because they more closely mimic patterns of activity actually observed in real life in children. Adults took longer than did children to recover from exercise, and $\tau\dot{V}CO_2$ (τ is the recovery time constant; the time required

TABLE 7.11 Predicted Peak oxygen uptake ($\dot{V}O_2$) and Anaerobic Threshold in Normal Children for Cycle Ergometry[a]

	Boys		Girls	
Age	≤13 y	>13 y	≤11 y	>11 y
Number studied	37	21	24	27
Peak $\dot{V}O_2$, mL/min/kg (mean ± SD)	42 ± 6	50 ± 8	38 ± 7	34 ± 4
Lower 95% confidence limit	32	37	26	27
Anaerobic threshold, mL/min/kg (mean ± SD)	26 ± 5	27 ± 6	23 ± 4	19 ± 3
Lower 95% confidence limit	18	17	16	14

Abbreviation: SD, standard deviation.

[a]Data from Cooper DM, Weiler-Ravell D, Whipp BJ, Wasserman K. Aerobic parameters of exercise as a function of body size during growth in children. *J Appl Physiol Respir Environ Exerc Physiol.* 1984;56(3):628-634.

to reach 63% of the end-exercise to preexercise steady-state values) and τ$\dot{V}E$ increased with work intensity in adults but not in children. These results are consistent with the hypothesis of a reduced anaerobic capability in children (see following text). If high-intensity exercise in children results in a smaller increase in lactic acid concentrations, then less CO_2 will be produced from HCO_3^- buffering of hydrogen ion.

The $PaCO_2$ seems to be controlled at lower levels in children compared with adults.[98] These observations were corroborated indirectly by the measurements of $PETCO_2$ made in our 1-minute exercise studies showing that preexercise and peak exercise values were significantly lower in children compared with adults, and more directly in a study of arterial $PaCO_2$ in children by Ohuchi et al.[97] A lower CO_2 set point may also explain, in part, the greater slopes of the $\dot{V}E$-$\dot{V}CO_2$ relationship that were observed in progressive exercise tests;[99] if alveolar PCO_2 is lower, then more $\dot{V}E$ is needed to excrete a given amount of CO_2.

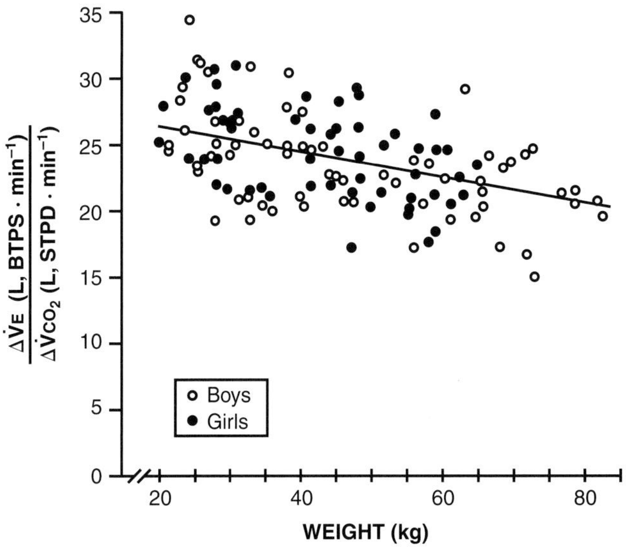

FIGURE 7.20. Slope of the minute ventilation-carbon dioxide output ($\dot{V}E$-$\dot{V}CO_2$) relationship as a function of body weight in 128 normal subjects ranging in age from 6 to 18 years. Boys are represented by open circles; girls by closed circles. There was a small but significant negative correlation between the slope and body weight. Abbreviations: BTPS, body temperature pressure saturated; STPD, standard temperature pressure dry. *(Reprinted by permission from Springer: Cooper DM, Kaplan MR, Baumgarten L, Weiler-Ravell D, Whipp BJ, Wasserman K. Coupling of ventilation and CO_2 production during exercise in children.* Pediatr Res. *1987;21(6):568-572. Copyright © 1987 Springer Nature.)*

The coupling of $\dot{V}CO_2$ and $\dot{V}E$ is closer in children than in adults. The rise in $PETCO_2$ with exercise seen in both children and adults indicates that $\dot{V}CO_2$ increased more rapidly than $\dot{V}E$, but the exercise-induced increase in $PETCO_2$ was much smaller in children (from 37.8 ± 0.4 to 40.1 ± 0.3 mm Hg) compared to adults (from 40.5 ± 0.2 to 49.9 ± 0.4), suggesting that $\dot{V}E$ kept pace with $\dot{V}CO_2$ better in children than in adults during exercise and early in recovery. Ratel et al[100] explored the implications of this close coupling on acid-base balance during exercise in children. Although recovery τ$\dot{V}E$ was significantly longer than τ$\dot{V}CO_2$ in adults following 1 minute of high-intensity exercise, the recovery times for $\dot{V}E$ and $\dot{V}CO_2$ were indistinguishable in the children.

Recommendations

Normal values for $\dot{V}E/\dot{V}CO_2$ and $\dot{V}E$ versus $\dot{V}CO_2$ below the respiratory compensation point (with $\dot{V}E$ expressed as L/min BTPS and $\dot{V}CO_2$ as L/min STPD) for cycle or treadmill ergometry are given in **Figure 7.20** and Cooper et al.[92]

Also, if comparing to a suitable population, Blanchard et al[3] provided normal values for $\dot{V}E/\dot{V}CO_2$ at the *AT* and $\dot{V}E$ versus $\dot{V}CO_2$ below the *AT* (similar to below the respiratory compensation point).

$$\dot{V}E/\dot{V}CO_2 \text{ at the } AT \text{ (boys)} = 68.39 + 0.00128 \times \text{height}^2\text{ (cm)} - 0.434 \times \text{height (cm)} - 0.0924 \times \text{corrected body mass (kg)}$$

$$\dot{V}E/\dot{V}CO_2 \text{ at the } AT \text{ (girls)} = -119.1 - 0.00548 \times \text{height}^2\text{ (cm)} + 1.81 \times \text{height (cm)} - 0.0232 \times \text{corrected body mass (kg)}$$

$$\dot{V}E \text{ versus } \dot{V}CO_2 \text{ below the } AT \text{ (boys)} = 7.87 - 0.00092 \times \text{height}^2\text{ (cm)} + 0.319 \times \text{height (cm)} - 0.0466 \times \text{corrected body mass (kg)} - 0.599 \times \text{age (years)}$$

$$\dot{V}E \text{ versus } \dot{V}CO_2 \text{ below the } AT \text{ (girls)} = -120.73 - 0.00558 \times \text{height}^2\text{ (cm)} + 1.83 \times \text{height (cm)} - 0.2901 \times \text{corrected body mass (kg)}$$

SUMMARY

This chapter presented and critiqued absolute values and patterns of change during CPET from rest to peak exercise and through recovery for a number of variables, including $\dot{V}O_2$, $\dot{V}CO_2$, $\dot{V}E$, HR, blood pressure, end-tidal CO_2 and O_2, as well as arterial blood O_2, CO_2, and $[H^+]$ values. Also considered were the *AT*, O_2 pulse, $\Delta\dot{V}O_2/\Delta WR$, $\Delta\dot{V}O_2/\Delta HR$, V_D/V_T, $\dot{V}CO_2$, and $\dot{V}O_2$ values in adults and children.

REFERENCES

1. American Thoracic Society, American College of Chest Physicians. ATS/ACCP statement on cardiopulmonary exercise testing. *Am J Respir Crit Care Med*. 2003;167:211-277.
2. Paap D, Takken T. Reference values for cardiopulmonary exercise testing in healthy adults: a systematic review. *Expert Rev Cardiovasc Ther*. 2014;12:1439-1453.
3. Blanchard J, Blais S, Chetaille P, et al. New reference values for cardiopulmonary exercise testing in children. *Med Sci Sports Exerc*. 2018;50:1125-1133.
4. Astrand PO, Rodahl K. *Textbook of Work Physiology*. 3rd ed. New York, NY: McGraw-Hill; 1986.
5. Hansen JE, Sue DY, Wasserman K. Predicted values for clinical exercise testing. *Am Rev Respir Dis*. 1984;129(2, pt 2):S49-S55.
6. Jones NL, Summers E, Killian KJ. Influence of age and stature on exercise capacity during incremental cycle ergometry in men and women. *Am Rev Respir Dis*. 1989;140:1373-1380.
7. Sue DY, Hansen JE. Normal values in adults during exercise testing. *Clin Chest Med*. 1984;5:89-98.
8. Drinkwater BL, Horvath SM, Wells CL. Aerobic power of females, ages 10 to 68. *J Gerontol*. 1975;30:385-394.
9. Astrand I, Astrand PO, Hallbäck I, Kilbom A. Reduction in maximal oxygen uptake with age. *J Appl Physiol*. 1973;35:649-654.
10. Bruce RA, Kusumi F, Hosmer D. Maximal oxygen intake and nomographic assessment of functional aerobic impairment in cardiovascular disease. *Am Heart J*. 1973;85:546-562.
11. Astrand PO. Human physical fitness with special reference to sex and age. *Physiol Rev*. 1956;36:307-335.
12. Davis JA, Frank MH, Whipp BJ, Wasserman K. Anaerobic threshold alterations caused by endurance training in middle-aged men. *J Appl Physiol Respir Environ Exerc Physiol*. 1979;46:1039-1046.
13. Davis JA, Storer TW, Caiozzo VJ, Pham PH. Lower reference limit for maximal oxygen uptake in men and women. *Clin Physiol Funct Imaging*. 2002;22:332-338.
14. Gläser S, Koch B, Itterman T, et al. Influence of age, sex, body size, smoking, and beta blockade on key gas exchange exercise parameters in an adult population. *Eur J Cardiovasc Prev Rehabil*. 2010;17:469-476.
15. Inbar O, Oren A, Scheinowitz M, Rotstein A, Dlin R, Casaburi R. Normal cardiopulmonary responses during incremental exercise in 20- to 70-yr-old men. *Med Sci Sports Exerc*. 1994;26:538-546.
16. Itoh H, Taniguchi K, Koike A, Doi M. Evaluation of severity of heart failure using ventilatory gas analysis. *Circulation*. 1990;81(1 suppl): II31-II37.
17. Jones NL, Makrides L, Hitchcock C, Chypchar T, McCartney N. Normal standards for an incremental progressive cycle ergometer test. *Am Rev Respir Dis*. 1985;131:700-708.
18. Neder JA, Nery LE, Castello A, et al. Prediction of metabolic and cardiopulmonary responses to maximum cycle ergometry: a randomised study. *Eur Respir J*. 1999;14:1304-1313.
19. de Souza E Silva CG, Kaminsky LA, Arena R, et al. A reference equation for maximal aerobic power for treadmill and cycle ergometer exercise testing: analysis from the FRIEND registry. *Eur J Prev Cardiol*. 2018;25:742-750.
20. Koch B, Schäper C, Ittermann T, et al. Reference values for cardiopulmonary exercise testing in healthy volunteers: the SHIP study. *Eur Respir J*. 2009;33:389-397.
21. Myers J, Kaminsky LA, Lima R, Christle JW, Ashley E, Arena R. A reference equation for normal standards for VO_2 max: analysis from the Fitness Registry and the Importance of Exercise National Database (FRIEND registry). *Prog Cardiovasc Dis*. 2017;60:21-29.
22. Schneider J. Age dependency of oxygen uptake and related parameters in exercise testing: an expert opinion on reference values suitable for adults. *Lung*. 2013;191:449-458.
23. Faulkner JA, Roberts DE, Elk RL, Conway J. Cardiovascular responses to submaximum and maximum effort cycling and running. *J Appl Physiol*. 1971;30:457-461.
24. Jones NL. *Clinical Exercise Testing*. Philadelphia, PA: WB Saunders; 1988.
25. Sheffield LT, Maloof JA, Sawyer JA, Roitman D. Maximal heart rate and treadmill performance of healthy women in relation to age. *Circulation*. 1978;57:79-84.
26. Sydó N, Abdelmoneim SS, Mulvagh SL, Merkely B, Gulati M, Allison TG. Relationship between exercise heart rate and age in men vs women. *Mayo Clin Proc*. 2014;89:1664-1672.
27. Arena R, Myers J, Kaminsky LA. Revisiting age-predicted maximal heart rate: can it be used as a valid measure of effort? *Am Heart J*. 2016;173:49-56.
28. Tanaka H, Monahan KD, Seals DR. Age-predicted maximal heart rate revisited. *J Am Coll Cardiol*. 2001;37:153-156.
29. Gellish RL, Goslin BR, Olson RE, McDonald A, Russi GD, Moudgil VK. Longitudinal modeling of the relationship between age and maximal heart rate. *Med Sci Sports Exerc*. 2007;39:822-829.
30. Nes BM, Janszky I, Wisløff U, Støylen A, Karlsen T. Age-predicted maximal heart rate in healthy subjects: the HUNT fitness study. *Scand J Med Sci Sports*. 2013;23:697-704.
31. Neder JA, Nery LE, Peres C, Whipp BJ. Reference values for dynamic responses to incremental cycle ergometry in males and females aged 20 to 80. *Am J Respir Crit Care Med*. 2001;164(8, pt 1):1481-1486.
32. Perloff D, Grim C, Flack J, et al; for American Heart Association. Human blood pressure determination by sphygmomanometry. *Circulation*. 1993;88:2460-2470.
33. Robinson TR, Sue DY, Huszczuk A, Weiler-Ravell D, Hansen JE. Intra-arterial and cuff blood pressure responses during incremental cycle ergometry. *Med Sci Sports Exerc*. 1988;20:142-149.
34. Sabbahi A, Arena R, Kaminsky LA, Myers J, Phillips SA. Peak blood pressure responses during maximum cardiopulmonary exercise testing: reference standards from FRIEND (Fitness Registry and the Importance of Exercise: A National Database). *Hypertension*. 2018;71: 229-236.
35. Gläser S, Friedrich N, Koch B, et al. Exercise blood pressure and heart rate reference values. *Heart Lung Circ*. 2013;22:661-667.
36. Wasserman K, McIlroy MB. Detecting the threshold of anaerobic metabolism in cardiac patients during exercise. *Am J Cardiol*. 1964;14:844-852.
37. Wasserman K. The anaerobic threshold measurement to evaluate exercise performance. *Am Rev Respir Dis*. 1984;129(2, pt 2):S35-S40.
38. Beaver WL, Wasserman K, Whipp BJ. A new method for detecting the anaerobic threshold by gas exchange. *J Appl Physiol (1985)*. 1986;60:2020-2027.
39. Sue DY, Wasserman K, Morrica RB, Casaburi R. Metabolic acidosis during exercise in patients with chronic obstructive pulmonary disease. Use of the V-slope method for anaerobic threshold determination. *Chest*. 1988;94:931-938.
40. Wasserman K, Beaver WL, Whipp BJ. Gas exchange theory and the lactic acidosis (anaerobic) threshold. *Circulation*. 1990;81(1 suppl): II14-II30.
41. Davis JA, Storer TW, Caiozzo VJ. Prediction of normal values for lactate threshold estimated by gas exchange in men and women. *Eur J Appl Physiol Occup Physiol*. 1997;76:157-164.
42. Gläser S, Ittermann T, Schäper C, et al. The Study of Health in Pomerania (SHIP) reference values for cardiopulmonary exercise testing [in German]. *Pneumologie*. 2013;67:58-63.
43. Davis JA, Vodak P, Wilmore JH, Vodak J, Kurtz P. Anaerobic threshold and maximal aerobic power for three modes of exercise. *J Appl Physiol*. 1976;41:544-550.

44. Buchfuhrer MJ, Hansen JE, Robinson TE, Sue DY, Wasserman K, Whipp BJ. Optimizing the exercise protocol for cardiopulmonary assessment. *J Appl Physiol Respir Environ Exerc Physiol*. 1983;55:1558-1564.
45. Withers RT, Sherman WM, Miller JM, Costill DL. Specificity of the anaerobic threshold in endurance trained cyclists and runners. *Eur J Appl Physiol Occup Physiol*. 1981;47:93-104.
46. Hansen JE, Sue DY, Oren A, Wasserman K. Relation of oxygen uptake to work rate in normal men and men with circulatory disorders. *Am J Cardiol*. 1987;59:669-674.
47. Boone J, Koppo K, Bouckaert J. The VO2 response to submaximal ramp cycle exercise: influence of ramp slope and training status. *Respir Physiol Neurobiol*. 2008;161:291-297.
48. Hansen JE, Casaburi R, Cooper DM, Wasserman K. Oxygen uptake as related to work rate increment during cycle ergometer exercise. *Eur J Appl Physiol Occup Physiol*. 1988;57:140-145.
49. Sietsema KE, Cooper DM, Rosove MH, et al. Dynamics of oxygen uptake during exercise in adults with cyanotic congenital heart disease. *Circulation*. 1986;73:1137-1144.
50. Gandevia B, Hugh-Jones P. Terminology for measurements of ventilatory capacity; a report to the Thoracic Society. *Thorax*. 1957;12:290-293.
51. Cotes JE. *Lung Function: Assessment and Application in Medicine*. Oxford, United Kingdom: Blackwell Scientific Publications; 1975.
52. Kaminsky LA, Harber MP, Imboden MT, Arena R, Myers J. Peak ventilation reference standards from exercise testing: from the FRIEND registry. *Med Sci Sports Exerc*. 2018;50:2603-2608.
53. Wasserman K, Whipp BJ. Exercise physiology in health and disease. *Am Rev Respir Dis*. 1975;112:219-249.
54. Chua TP, Ponikowski P, Harrington D, et al. Clinical correlates and prognostic significance of the ventilatory response to exercise in chronic heart failure. *J Am Coll Cardiol*. 1997;29:1585-1590.
55. Gitt AK, Wasserman K, Kilkowski C, et al. Exercise anaerobic threshold and ventilatory efficiency identify heart failure patients for high risk of early death. *Circulation*. 2002;106:3079-3084.
56. Kleber FX, Vietzke G, Wernecke KD, et al. Impairment of ventilatory efficiency in heart failure: prognostic impact. *Circulation*. 2000;101:2803-2809.
57. Metra M, Raccagni D, Carini G, et al. Ventilatory and arterial blood gas changes during exercise in heart failure. In: Wasserman K, ed. *Exercise Gas Exchange in Heart Disease*. Armonk, NY: Futura Publishing; 1996.
58. Wasserman K, Zhang YY, Gitt A, et al. Lung function and exercise gas exchange in chronic heart failure. *Circulation*. 1997;96:2221-2227.
59. Sun XG, Hansen JE, Garatachea N, Storer TW, Wasserman K. Ventilatory efficiency during exercise in healthy subjects. *Am J Respir Crit Care Med*. 2002;166:1443-1448.
60. Wasserman K, Van Kessel A, Burton GB. Interaction of physiological mechanisms during exercise. *J Appl Physiol*. 1967;22:71-85.
61. Sun XG, Hansen JE, Stringer WW. Oxygen uptake efficiency plateau: physiology and reference values. *Eur J Appl Physiol*. 2012;112:919-928.
62. Whipp BJ, Wasserman K. Alveolar-arterial gas tension differences during graded exercise. *J Appl Physiol*. 1969;27:361-365.
63. Gläser S, Ittermann T, Koch B, et al. Influence of smoking and obesity on alveolar-arterial gas pressure differences and dead space ventilation at rest and peak exercise in healthy men and women. *Respir Med*. 2013;107:919-926.
64. Hansen J, Ulubay G, Chow BF, Sun XG, Wasserman K. Mixed-expired and end-tidal CO2 distinguish between ventilation and perfusion defects during exercise testing in patients with lung and heart diseases. *Chest*. 2007;132:977-983.
65. Dempsey JA, Hanson P, Henderson K. Exercise-induced arterial hypoxaemia in healthy humans at sea level. *J Physiol*. 1984;355:161-175.
66. Dominelli PB, Foster GE, Dominelli GS, et al. Exercise-induced arterial hypoxaemia and the mechanics of breathing in healthy young women. *J Physiol*. 2013;591:3017-3034.
67. Gaston AF, Durand F, Roca E, Doucende G, Hapkova I, Subirats E. Exercise-induced hypoxaemia developed at sea-level influences responses to exercise at moderate altitude. *PLoS One*. 2016;11:e0161819.
68. Stringer W, Hansen J, Wasserman K. Cardiac output estimated noninvasively from oxygen uptake during exercise. *J Appl Physiol (1985)*. 1997;82:908-912.
69. Sullivan MJ, Knight JD, Higginbotham MB, Cobb FR. Relation between central and peripheral hemodynamics during exercise in patients with chronic heart failure. Muscle blood flow is reduced with maintenance of arterial perfusion pressure. *Circulation*. 1989;80:769-781.
70. Weber KT, Janicki JS. Cardiopulmonary exercise testing for evaluation of chronic cardiac failure. *Am J Cardiol*. 1985;55:22A-31A.
71. Agostoni PG, Wasserman K, Perego GB, et al. Oxygen transport to muscle during exercise in chronic congestive heart failure secondary to idiopathic dilated cardiomyopathy. *Am J Cardiol*. 1997;79:1120-1124.
72. Beaver WL, Wasserman K, Whipp BJ. Bicarbonate buffering of lactic acid generated during exercise. *J Appl Physiol (1985)*. 1986;60:472-478.
73. Blais S, Berbari J, Counil FP, Dallaire F. A systematic review of reference values in pediatric cardiopulmonary exercise testing. *Pediatr Cardiol*. 2015;36:1553-1564.
74. Cooper DM, Weiler-Ravell D, Whipp BJ, Wasserman K. Growth-related changes in oxygen uptake and heart rate during progressive exercise in children. *Pediatr Res*. 1984;18:845-851.
75. Eisenmann JC, Katzmarzyk PT, Thériault G, Song TM, Malina RM, Bouchard C. Cardiac dimensions, physical activity, and submaximal working capacity in youth of the Québec Family Study. *Eur J Appl Physiol*. 2000;81:40-46.
76. Trudeau F, Laurencelle L, Shephard RJ. Tracking of physical activity from childhood to adulthood. *Med Sci Sports Exerc*. 2004;36:1937-1943.
77. Basaran S, Guler-Uysal F, Ergen N, Seydaoglu G, Bingol-Karakoç G, Ufuk Altintas D. Effects of physical exercise on quality of life, exercise capacity and pulmonary function in children with asthma. *J Rehabil Med*. 2006;38:130-135.
78. Orenstein DM, Hovell MF, Mulvihill M, et al. Strength vs aerobic training in children with cystic fibrosis: a randomized controlled trial. *Chest*. 2004;126:1204-1214.
79. Gabriele C, Pijnenburg MW, Monti F, Hop W, Bakker ME, de Jongste JC. The effect of spirometry and exercise on exhaled nitric oxide in asthmatic children. *Pediatr Allergy Immunol*. 2005;16:243-247.
80. Lammers AE, Diller GP, Odendaal D, Tailor S, Derrick G, Haworth SG. Comparison of 6-min walk test distance and cardiopulmonary exercise test performance in children with pulmonary hypertension. *Arch Dis Child*. 2011;96:141-147.
81. Lesser DJ, Fleming MM, Maher CA, et al. Does the 6-min walk test correlate with the exercise stress test in children? *Pediatr Pulmonol*. 2010;45:135-140.
82. Liem RI, Nevin MA, Prestridge A, Young LT, Thompson AA. Functional capacity in children and young adults with sickle cell disease undergoing evaluation for cardiopulmonary disease. *Am J Hematol*. 2009;84:645-649.
83. Tomkinson GR, Léger LA, Olds TS, Cazorla G. Secular trends in the performance of children and adolescents (1980–2000): an analysis of 55 studies of the 20m shuttle run test in 11 countries. *Sports Med*. 2003;33:285-300.
84. Lobelo F, Pate RR, Dowda M, Liese AD, Ruiz JR. Validity of cardiorespiratory fitness criterion-referenced standards for adolescents. *Med Sci Sports Exerc*. 2009;41:1222-1229.
85. Priesnitz CV, Rodrigues GH, Stumpf CS, et al. Reference values for the 6-min walk test in healthy children aged 6–12 years. *Pediatr Pulmonol*. 2009;44:1174-1179.
86. Ten Harkel AD, Takken T, Van Osch-Gevers M, Helbing WA. Normal values for cardiopulmonary exercise testing in children. *Eur J Cardiovasc Prev Rehabil*. 2011;18:48-54.
87. van der Cammen-van Zijp MH, Ijsselstijn H, Takken T, et al. Exercise testing of pre-school children using the Bruce treadmill protocol: new reference values. *Eur J Appl Physiol*. 2010;108:393-399.
88. Cooper DM, Weiler-Ravell D, Whipp BJ, Wasserman K. Aerobic parameters of exercise as a function of body size during growth in children. *J Appl Physiol Respir Environ Exerc Physiol*. 1984;56:628-634.
89. Cooper DM, Weiler-Ravell D. Gas exchange response to exercise in children. *Am Rev Respir Dis*. 1984;129(2, pt 2):S47-S48.

90. Verschuren O, Bloemen M, Kruitwagen C, Takken T. Reference values for anaerobic performance and agility in ambulatory children and adolescents with cerebral palsy. *Dev Med Child Neurol*. 2010;52:e222-e228.
91. Reybrouck T, Boshoff D, Vanhees L, Defoor J, Gewillig M. Ventilatory response to exercise in patients after correction of cyanotic congenital heart disease: relation with clinical outcome after surgery. *Heart*. 2004;90:215 216.
92. Cooper DM, Kaplan MR, Baumgarten L, Weiler-Ravell D, Whipp BJ, Wasserman K. Coupling of ventilation and CO_2 production during exercise in children. *Pediatr Res*. 1987;21:568-572.
93. Guerrero L, Naranjo J, Carranza MD. Influence of gender on ventilatory efficiency during exercise in young children. *J Sports Sci*. 2008;26:1455-1457.
94. Marinov B, Kostianev S, Turnovska T. Ventilatory response to exercise and rating of perceived exertion in two pediatric age groups. *Acta Physiol Pharmacol Bulg*. 2000;25:93-98.
95. Marinov B, Kostianev S, Turnovska T. Ventilatory efficiency and rate of perceived exertion in obese and non-obese children performing standardized exercise. *Clin Physiol Funct Imaging*. 2002;22:254-260.
96. Barstow TJ, Cooper DM, Sobel E, Landaw EM, Epstein S. Influence of increased metabolic rate on [13C]bicarbonate washout kinetics. *Am J Physiol*. 1990;259:R163-R171.
97. Ohuchi H, Kato Y, Tasato H, et al. Ventilatory response and arterial blood gases during exercise in children. *Pediatr Res*. 1999;45:389-396.
98. Springer C, Cooper DM, Wasserman K. Evidence that maturation of the peripheral chemoreceptors is not complete in childhood. *Respirat Physiol*. 1988;74:55-64.
99. Nagano Y, Baba R, Kuraishi K, et al. Ventilatory control during exercise in normal children. *Pediatr Res*. 1998;43:704-707.
100. Ratel S, Duche P, Hennegrave A, Van Praagh E, Bedu M. Acid-base balance during repeated cycling sprints in boys and men. *J Appl Physiol*. 2002;92:479-485.

CHAPTER 8

Clinical Applications of Cardiopulmonary Exercise Testing

The increasing number of applications for which cardiopulmonary exercise testing (CPET) is currently employed attests to the growing recognition of its importance in medicine. This chapter describes current applications of CPET. In some instances, these applications are well established, as described in a number of reviews.[1-9] In others, the applications are underappreciated or evolving. The applications of CPET are of great value in patient care and have the potential to reduce health care costs by streamlining diagnosis and facilitating treatment decisions.

CARDIOPULMONARY EXERCISE TESTING IN THE DIAGNOSTIC EVALUATION OF EXERCISE INTOLERANCE

Exertional symptoms, particularly shortness of breath or fatigue, are common complaints that can arise from a wide range of underlying disorders. For most patients with these complaints, a diagnosis is readily established through common assessment tools of history, physical examination, and basic laboratory tests and diagnostics available in the office or clinic. However, there will remain some such patients whose symptoms are not readily explained. A CPET, using a rapid incremental or ramp-type exercise test on a cycle ergometer or a treadmill, is particularly suited to evaluation of these patients because it simulates the condition which induces the symptoms, and provides the clinician with measurements that reflect the integrated responses of cardiovascular, ventilatory, and pulmonary gas exchange systems linking internal (cellular) to external (airway) respiration.

Because defects at different stages of the coupling of cellular to external respiration affect these measurements in different ways, the responses to CPET can often reveal which aspects of the exercise response—cardiac, ventilatory, or gas exchange—are abnormal. This, together with the clinical history, can narrow a broad differential diagnosis to focus on one or another of the key systems involved. Typical effects on the responses to CPET of a number of common conditions limiting exercise are illustrated and discussed in detail in Chapter 4. The organization and interpretation of data from CPET for this purpose is further described in Chapter 6.

There are certain conditions which result in unique findings during CPET that point to a specific process or diagnosis. These include exercise-induced myocardial ischemia, arrhythmias, or chronotropic incompetence limiting the cardiac output response; exercise-induced bronchoconstriction; and upper airway dysfunction resulting in stridor and dyspnea. There are additionally a number of conditions that result in distinctive, if not entirely unique, findings on CPET, which can serve to confirm or direct the clinical assessment. These include diastolic dysfunction, the development of a right-to-left shunt during exercise, pulmonary vascular disease, some disorders of skeletal muscle that impair muscle bioenergetics, and nonphysiological hyperventilation syndromes. A CPET may also be valuable in confirming normal findings that make significant disease unlikely and may thus allow for conservative follow-up with deferral of additional more invasive testing.

Disorders With Unique or Distinctive Findings During Cardiopulmonary Exercise Testing

Myocardial Dyskinesis Secondary to Myocardial Ischemia During Exercise

The normal contraction of the myocardium depends on the ability of the myofibrils of the heart muscle to contract synchronously in response to the electrical depolarization set off by the sinoatrial pacemaker. As is the case for skeletal muscle, adenosine triphosphate (ATP) is consumed by the heart, primarily during systole, and regenerated in diastole when the myocardium is resupplied with oxygenated blood. For normal regeneration of ATP, the myocardial oxygen (O_2) supply must be adequate. When the diastolic period shortens as heart rate increases, there is less time to resupply O_2 to the myocardium. Thus, exercise may precipitate myocardial ischemia in regions of the heart that have impaired ability to resupply O_2 commensurate with the increased myocardial O_2 demand. The latter is dictated by the increase in cardiac work during exercise, which is proportional to the pressure-pulse rate product (systolic blood pressure × heart rate).

Asynchronous contraction of the myocardium (myocardial dyskinesis) or impaired diastolic relaxation, can result from ischemia causing reduction in stroke volume and potentially a decreased amount of oxygen per heart beat to be delivered to the exercising muscle in response to increased work rate. Thus, O_2 uptake ($\dot{V}O_2$) may fail to increase in proportion to the increase in work rate, as illustrated in the examples shown in **Figure 4.3** of Chapter 4 and **Figure 6.6** of Chapter 6. The slowing or failure of $\dot{V}O_2$ to increase with increasing work rate suggests that cardiac output is not increasing appropriately.

In patients with pathological electrocardiogram (ECG) changes consistent with myocardial ischemia, with or without chest pain, simultaneous reduction in the slope of the $\dot{V}O_2$-WR relationship ($\Delta\dot{V}O_2/\Delta WR$) and flattening of the O_2 pulse with increasing work rate and heart rate, strongly suggest functional changes in cardiac output and stroke volume associated with the ECG findings. The ECG changes without chest pain and without corresponding changes in gas exchange suggesting myocardial dyskinesis, on the other hand, make the diagnosis of myocardial ischemia less certain. By measuring gas exchange, therefore, the physician can be more confident in interpretation of the stress ECG.[10]

This was illustrated by the study by Belardinelli et al[11] of 1265 consecutive patients with chest pain who underwent CPET with incremental cycle ergometry. Diagnosis of myocardial ischemia during CPET was made by an inflection in the normally linear $\dot{V}O_2$-WR relationship along with flattening of the O_2 pulse. A diagnosis of ischemia was excluded if there was absence of inflection in the $\dot{V}O_2$-WR relationship or a flattened O_2 pulse profile, and peak $\dot{V}O_2$ was >90% of predicted. Seventy-three subjects with a positive CPET and 71 of 1192 with a negative CPET by these criteria underwent single-photon emission computerized tomography imaging and coronary angiography with an average follow-up of 4 years. Sensitivity for coronary artery disease (CAD) was 88% with 98% specificity, 88% positive predictive value, and 99% negative predictive value. In terms of specificity, there was no evidence of CAD in any patient with both peak $\dot{V}O_2$ >91% of predicted and no related signs of myocardial ischemia.

Chaudhry et al[12] also emphasized that CPET variables could serve as surrogate markers of cardiac output and stroke volume. They noted that, specifically in a subset of patients with nonobstructive CAD or microvascular ischemia, conventional testing (stress ECG with and without imaging) was less sensitive and specific; therefore, CPET may offer clinical advantages for these patients.

Chronic Heart Failure With Preserved Left Ventricular Ejection Fraction

Heart failure with reduced left ventricular (LV) ejection fraction (HFrEF) is usually easily confirmed in a patient with fatigue, exertional dyspnea, and pulmonary and peripheral edema by the finding of a low ejection fraction by echocardiography or other imaging. On the other hand, it is clear that around half of patients with heart failure have normal or only slightly reduced LV ejection fraction, that is, heart failure with preserved ejection fraction (HFpEF), in which the underlying problem is impaired diastolic relaxation. These patients, with normal ejection fraction and normal systolic LV wall contraction, frequently are women and elderly, and have hypertension (hypertension alone has about 60% sensitivity and specificity for HFpEF), atrial fibrillation, and anemia more often than those with HFrEF.[13] Indeed, a composite score incorporating obesity, atrial fibrillation, age older than 60 years, treatment with two or more antihypertensives, an echocardiographic E/e' ratio >9, and echocardiographic pulmonary artery systolic pressure <35 mm Hg demonstrated high predictive value for HFpEF.[14]

Confounding the diagnosis of HFpEF, however, are the high prevalence of risk factors and the likelihood that patients presenting with dyspnea and fatigue, especially those who are older and hypertensive, may have other contributing diagnoses.[15] A CPET may be helpful in these patients. Obokata and colleagues[16] tested 50 patients with proven HFpEF during cardiac catheterization at rest and CPET with supine cycle ergometry and found reduced peak $\dot{V}O_2$, elevated $\dot{V}E$-$\dot{V}CO_2$ slope, elevated dead space–tidal volume ratio (VD/VT), and decreased breathing reserve. These features are quite similar to findings in those with HFrEF. In a direct comparison of a small number of patients with HFrEF (n = 32) and HFpEF (n = 27), Van Iterson et al[17] showed that both groups had high $\dot{V}E$-$\dot{V}CO_2$ slopes, and, although both had elevated VD/VT and low $PaCO_2$, the relative contributions of each appeared different with a greater role of increased VD/VT in HFpEF. Prognosis in HFpEF is also similarly related to peak $\dot{V}O_2$ and $\dot{V}E$-$\dot{V}CO_2$ slope in univariate analyses, as in HFrEF[18]; in this study, $\dot{V}E$-$\dot{V}CO_2$ slope was more predictive of a combined end point of death and hospitalization. Nadruz et al[19] also found that peak $\dot{V}O_2$ and $\dot{V}E$-$\dot{V}CO_2$ slope have prognostic value in heart failure and, in fact, provide greater risk information in HFpEF compared with HFrEF. Exercise function thus appears to be similarly valuable for grading the severity of heart failure whether it is associated with reduced or preserved ejection fraction.

Pulmonary Vascular Occlusive Disease and Clinical Pulmonary Arterial Hypertension (Pulmonary Vasculopathy)

Most patients limited in exercise because of pulmonary vascular disease have exertional dyspnea well before they have signs of pulmonary hypertension. Once signs of pulmonary hypertension are present, there is usually considerable structural change in the pulmonary circulation and a reduction in capacity to recruit pulmonary blood vessels normally available for recruitment during exercise. By this time, the opportunity to intervene at an early stage of the disease, for example with specific pulmonary hypertension therapy or other treatment, may be lost. There are a number of distinct clinical entities represented by pulmonary hypertension. Although the classification scheme has varied over time, it is based on purported etiology (or lack of a defined cause), association with other disorders, especially heart, lung, rheumatological, and chronic thromboembolic disease, and central hemodynamics.[20] Regardless of the classification or cause, pulmonary vascular disease results in certain characteristic findings reflecting inability to increase pulmonary blood flow normally during exercise, such that CPET has the potential to identify patients early when findings at rest may be absent or only mild.

In patients with pulmonary vascular diseases, $\dot{V}O_2$ often does not continue to increase with the normal slope of 10 mL/min/W during ramp-type incremental exercise tests. Rather, the rate of rise gradually decreases (see **Fig. 6.6E**) up to the point where continuation of exercise becomes intolerable, usually because of dyspnea or fatigue or both. This likely reflects abnormally low O_2 delivery for the level of exercise being performed. The $\dot{V}E$-$\dot{V}CO_2$ slope and $\dot{V}E/\dot{V}CO_2$ at the *AT* or at its nadir (indices of ventilatory inefficiency) are characteristically quite elevated in patients with pulmonary vascular disease (see **Figs. 6.11E** and **6.12E**) because of increased VD/VT.

In pulmonary vascular disease, reductions in the peak $\dot{V}O_2$ (see **Fig. 6.6E**) and *AT*, increase in $\dot{V}E/\dot{V}CO_2$ at the *AT* or at its nadir and $\dot{V}E$-$\dot{V}CO_2$ slope (see **Figs. 6.10E** and **6.11E**), and decrease in end-tidal partial pressure of CO_2 ($PETCO_2$) at the *AT* (see **Fig. 6.12E**) quantifies disease severity[21,22] and, when the patient is followed serially, reflects worsening related to disease progression or improvement related to effective therapies. A steep heart rate rise and low peak O_2 pulse (likely reflecting a low stroke volume) will be evident in panels 2 and 3 of the nine-panel array (see **Figs. 6.7E** and **6.8E**). The $\dot{V}E$-$\dot{V}CO_2$ slope (panel 6), which is normally about 25, will be much higher in patients with pulmonary vascular disease (see **Fig. 6.10E**). This increase depends primarily on the increase in VD/VT and also on the development of exercise hypoxemia with attendant ventilatory stimulation. This effect is amplified if the hypoxemia is due to exercise-induced right-to-left shunt as discussed next.[23,24]

Development of a Right-to-Left Shunt During Exercise

Intracardiac right-to-left (central venous to systemic arterial) shunt may develop, or existing shunt fraction may increase, during exercise in patients with cyanotic congenital heart diseases. Ventilation during exercise in these conditions often appears excessive. However, when arterial blood gases have been measured, $PaCO_2$ is generally maintained at preexercise resting levels, at least for modest exercise.[25,26] That is, the marked exercise $\dot{V}E$ typical of these conditions is appropriate for maintaining $PaCO_2$, rather than being hyperventilatory due to the associated hypoxemia. Part of the reason for unusually high $\dot{V}E$ requirements in these patients may be the presence of high $\dot{V}A/\dot{Q}$ regions in the lung resulting from obliterative pulmonary vascular changes, but, whether or not this is the case, higher levels of $\dot{V}E$ result from the need to compensate for intracardiac shunting of venous carbon dioxide (CO_2) into the arterial circuit, which increases with exercise. Indeed, the augmentation of $\dot{V}E$ required to compensate for increased shunting of CO_2 may be so great that some patients fail to compensate and actually have an increase in $PaCO_2$ during incremental exercise despite abnormally steep increases in $\dot{V}E$.[25]

Even in the absence of structural heart disease, some 25% of the population have a potentially patent foramen ovale in the interatrial septum,[27] but this is functionally unimportant unless right atrial pressure exceeds left atrial pressure. However, a rise in right atrial pressure sufficient to open a patent foramen ovale may develop during exercise in patients with elevated pulmonary vascular resistance due to primary or secondary pulmonary vascular disease. Thus, a right-to-left shunt, absent at rest, may develop in these patients during exercise. This is most frequently evident at the start of exercise when there is an acute increase in venous return to the right heart.

An opened patent foramen ovale allows some amount of systemic venous blood to flow from the right to the left atrium when right atrial exceeds left atrial pressure. The desaturated venous blood mixed with oxygenated blood in the left atrium will result in a rapid decrease in Pa_{O_2} and increased Pa_{CO_2} and $[H^+]$ that will quickly stimulate arterial and subsequently central chemoreceptors to increase $\dot{V}E$. These phenomena can occur despite a normal or near-normal arterial oxyhemoglobin saturation at rest. A CPET with 100% O_2 breathing allows estimation of the size of a right-to-left shunt developing during exercise, based on arterial P_{O_2} measurement.

The diagnosis of a right-to-left shunt developing during exercise can be suspected from characteristic changes in gas exchange,[28] including an abrupt decrease in P_{ETCO_2} and increase in P_{ETO_2} (panel 7) of the nine panel graph, along with simultaneous abrupt increases in R (panel 8), and $\dot{V}E/\dot{V}O_2$ and $\dot{V}E/\dot{V}CO_2$ (panel 4). These findings are to be expected because stimulation of $\dot{V}E$ to maintain homeostasis of Pa_{CO_2} and pHa results in increased alveolar ventilation while blood flow to the lungs fails to increase as much as normal because some blood is diverted through the foramen ovale. Thus, the true pulmonary blood is essentially "hyperventilated," decreasing alveolar P_{CO_2} and increasing alveolar P_{O_2} while increasing $\dot{V}E/\dot{V}O_2$ and $\dot{V}E/\dot{V}CO_2$. Although all of the ventilatory and gas exchange findings described here (except the associated arterial desaturation) could result from simple hyperventilation at the start of exercise, when observed in a patient with established diagnosis of pulmonary hypertension, there is high concordance with demonstration of a patent foramen ovale by contrast echocardiography.[28] Arterial O_2 desaturation resulting from the shunt can usually be documented with a pulse oximeter (panel 7), although this may appear to develop more slowly than the $\dot{V}E$ responses due to the response time of the instrument.

An example of gas exchange abnormalities revealing the intermittent development of a right-to-left shunt during exercise in a patient with pulmonary arterial hypertension (PAH) is shown in **Figure 8.1** in a series of studies at 4-month intervals over a 16-month period during treatment with continuous intravenous epoprostenol. In test 1, when blood begins to shunt from right to left during exercise, $\dot{V}E$ abruptly increases, with an increase in $\dot{V}E/\dot{V}CO_2$ (lowest panel) rather than the usual decrease seen in normal individuals following exercise onset. The $\dot{V}E/\dot{V}CO_2$ sharply increases at the work rate at which the blood starts to shunt right to left ($\dot{V}E/\dot{V}CO_2$ versus time in test 1 of **Fig. 8.1**). The reason $\dot{V}E$ increases so steeply when the shunt develops is that Pa_{CO_2} and pHa (primary ventilatory stimulants) are normally closely regulated. Because shunting of high CO_2 and H^+ blood from the venous system into the left side of the circulation bypasses the lungs,[29] the shunted blood reaches the arterial and subsequently the central chemoreceptors, stimulating $\dot{V}E$ in proportion to the shunted CO_2 and H^+ loads.

In test 2 (see **Fig. 8.1**), the shunt is not evident early in exercise, likely because of a treatment-related reduction in right atrial pressure. However, it did develop later in exercise. This abrupt ventilatory stimulus presumably prompted the patient to stop exercise soon after the development of the right-to-left shunt. By test 3 (after 8 months of treatment), the pulmonary hypertension was much reduced, peak $\dot{V}O_2$ and peak O_2 pulse had increased, and the evidence for an exercise-induced right-to-left shunt had disappeared. Then, and in the remaining two tests, $\dot{V}E/\dot{V}CO_2$ (third panel down) remained relatively constant, although abnormally elevated. This implies that V_D/V_T remained elevated, although shunting of venous blood into the arterial circulation was no longer evident. The patient was removed from the lung transplantation list and was subsequently studied over an additional 12 years of CPET-guided therapy. Of note is that this information about the patient's pathophysiology and change with treatment over time was obtained noninvasively, and testing could thereby be repeated relatively easily as often as clinically needed.

Pulmonary Vascular Disease Limiting Exercise in Chronic Obstructive Pulmonary Disease

Although patients with chronic obstructive pulmonary disease (COPD) usually are exercise limited because of abnormal lung mechanics, as reflected by a low exercise breathing reserve, some are limited primarily by a reduced pulmonary capillary bed, which limits the increase in pulmonary blood flow and cardiac output in response to exercise. This distinction can be important in guiding treatment decisions. For example, lung reduction surgery might improve lung mechanics but not improve exercise tolerance if pulmonary blood flow cannot increase beyond that achieved before surgery. A CPET can be done before lung reduction surgery to confirm whether impaired function is attributable to limitation of CO_2 elimination and pH due to impaired lung mechanics or is instead attributable to limitation of systemic blood flow and O_2 transport due to loss of pulmonary vascularity.

Neder et al[30] published an extensive review of studies focused specifically on ventilatory efficiency in COPD patients, beginning with the notion that as COPD patients have a limited ability to increase $\dot{V}E$ because of abnormal airway mechanics and the effects of hyperinflation, these patients should be primarily ventilatory limited during exercise. In addition, the authors noted that abnormally decreased ventilatory efficiency has been largely assessed in disease states not consistently associated with ventilatory limitation, such as chronic heart failure. Thus, they suggest an important role for looking at ventilatory efficiency in COPD, potentially to address comorbidities as well as opportunities for understanding pathophysiology and treatment options. Their review summarized data from multiple studies looking at the $\dot{V}E$-$\dot{V}CO_2$ slope or $\dot{V}E/\dot{V}CO_2$ at the *AT* or at its nadir and found associations between higher values and degree of breathlessness (especially out of proportion to forced expiratory volume in 1 second [FEV_1]), comorbidities such as heart failure and pulmonary hypertension, poorer

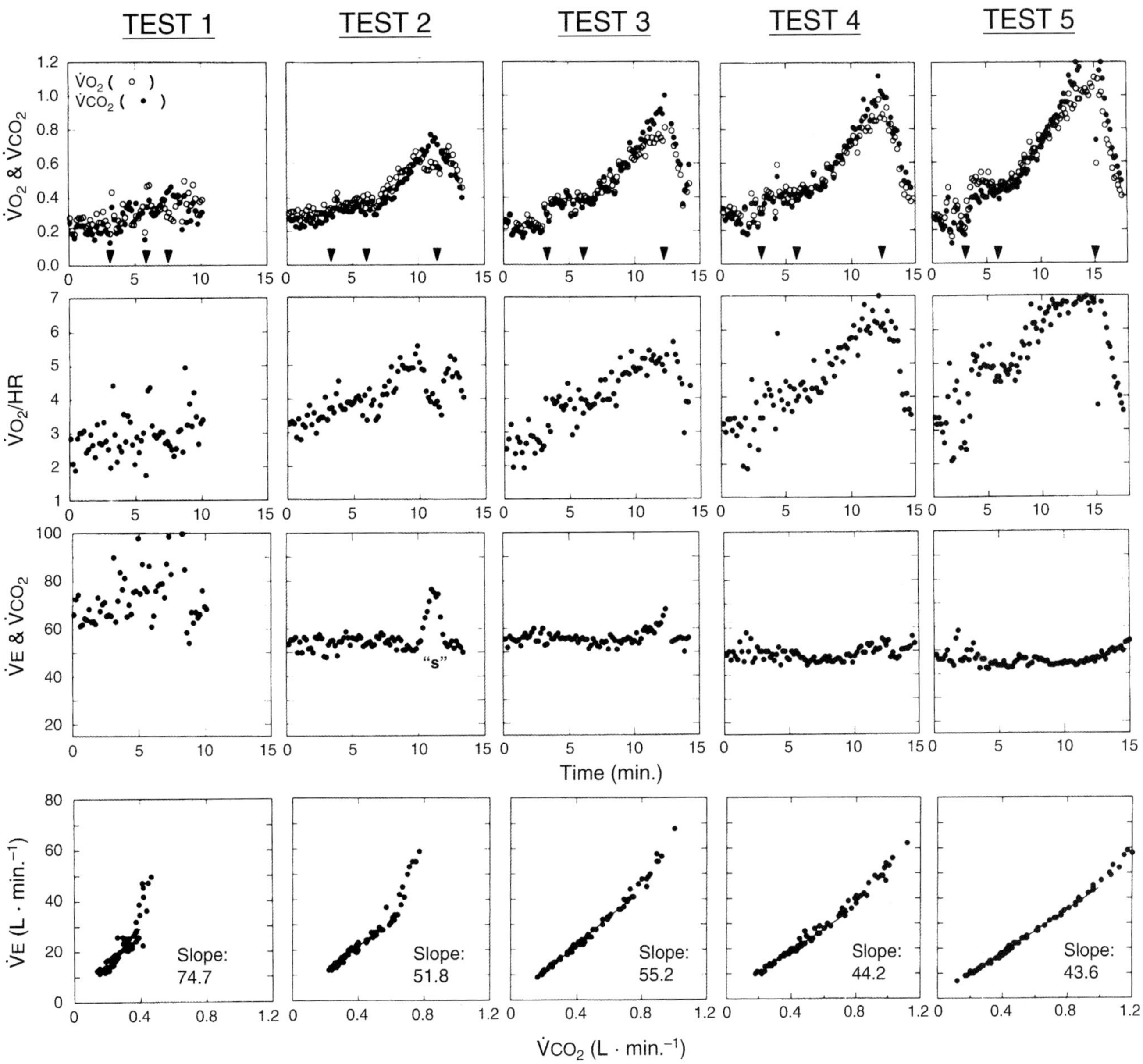

FIGURE 8.1. Five incremental exercise tests in a patient with primary pulmonary hypertension, each done at 4-month intervals. Test 1 was done as a control before the start of continuous intravenous epoprostenol, a preparation of prostacyclin. Test 2 was done after 4 months of treatment, and test 3 was done 4 months later, and so on, for a total of 16 months. Although the full nine-panel plots were obtained, for ease of comparing the physiological changes with time, only four panels of data are shown for each test. The top panel contains plots of oxygen (O_2) uptake ($\dot{V}O_2$) and carbon dioxide (CO_2) output ($\dot{V}CO_2$) against time. On the abscissa of this plot are three arrows, the left indicating the transition from rest to unloaded cycling, the middle arrow indicating the start of the increasing exercise period, and the arrow on the right indicating the end of exercise. As is evident from this panel in test 1, the patient could perform very little exercise. At that time, her O_2 pulse (mL/beat) (second panel down) could not increase in response to exercise, indicating that the product of the stroke volume and arteriovenous O_2 difference was at its maximum. The ventilatory equivalents for CO_2 (third panel down) are very high at rest (first 3 minutes) and increase further after exercise starts presumably due to the opening of a right-to-left shunt through the foramen ovale. This is reflected in a large change in the $\dot{V}E$-$\dot{V}CO_2$ slope in the fourth panel down. The slope value shown in this panel is that for the lower slope before the diverting of blood through the right-to-left shunt. The slope value of 74.7 is very high (normal being about 25; see Chapter 7). This steep slope primarily reflects the poor perfusion to ventilated lung (increased dead space–tidal volume ratio). The abrupt steepening of this slope reflects an increase in right-to-left shunt. The repeat study 4 months after the start of treatment (test 2) shows a significant increase in peak $\dot{V}O_2$ and O_2 pulse and a reduced ventilatory response as evident from the decrease in $\dot{V}E/\dot{V}CO_2$ and in the lower $\dot{V}E$-$\dot{V}CO_2$ slope (51.8 versus 74.7). The latter two values indicate that perfusion to ventilated lung had become more uniform, although still quite abnormal. Just before the end of exercise, a right-to-left shunt is evident, reflected in the abrupt decrease in $\dot{V}O_2$ and O_2 pulse and the increase in $\dot{V}E$-$\dot{V}CO_2$ slope, designated by *S* in the third panel down, and the abrupt steepening of the $\dot{V}E$-$\dot{V}CO_2$ slope in the fourth panel down. The next three tests show improvement in all measurements, reaching a plateau response by the fifth test. Additional tests were done over the next 4 years and are not shown because there was no significant change from test 5. Thus, the patient improved and stabilized but still had significant inability to increase cardiac output, as reflected by a reduced peak $\dot{V}O_2$ and O_2 pulse (60% and 70% of predicted, respectively) and an elevated $\dot{V}E$-$\dot{V}CO_2$ slope and $\dot{V}E/\dot{V}CO_2$ at the *AT*.

outcomes in lung resection surgery, and improvement in some patients with lung transplantation or lung resection.

Similarly, Boerrigter et al[31] found that COPD patients at similar stages divided into no, moderate, and severe pulmonary hypertension had lower mixed venous O_2 saturation with more severe pulmonary hypertension. Higher mean pulmonary artery pressure was also associated in several studies with higher $\dot{V}E/\dot{V}CO_2$ nadir values and $\dot{V}E$-$\dot{V}CO_2$ slope.[32,33]

Impaired Muscle Bioenergetics

As discussed in Chapter 4, skeletal muscle enzyme defects affect exercise gas exchange, with the gas exchange abnormality depending on the muscle enzyme defect. Thus, a patient with a myopathy that affects myophosphorylase or one of the glycolytic enzymes (eg, phosphofructokinase) would have a reduced maximum exercise tolerance because of the inability to develop a lactic acidosis and thereby benefit from the Bohr effect facilitating oxygen unloading (see Chapter 2, "Oxygen Supply and Critical Capillary PO_2" section). This will be reflected in exercise gas exchange,[34] not only by a reduced peak $\dot{V}O_2$ but also by failure to produce extra CO_2 from buffering of the lactic acidosis, as described by Riley et al.[35] In contrast, enzyme defects in the mitochondrial electron transport chain cause a lactic acidosis at a very low work rate,[36] with accompanying gas exchange abnormalities similar to those observed in patients with heart failure, but without the changes due to $\dot{V}A/\dot{Q}$ mismatch.[37,38] A CPET is a good screening technique for detecting or characterizing muscle enzyme defects affecting bioenergetics, and may be useful for directing the histo-chemical evaluation of a muscle sample or objectively assessing therapeutic interventions.

Exercise-Induced Airflow Obstruction

Exercise provocation is an established tool in the identification of exercise-induced bronchoconstriction.[39] The unique findings in these assessments are postexercise changes in the FEV_1. The profile of exercise stress most effective for inducing bronchoconstriction in susceptible individuals differs from the incremental protocols commonly used for CPET, because the goal is to quickly impose a work rate in the high-intensity range and maintain high levels of $\dot{V}E$ for a number of minutes to induce cooling and dehydration of the airways. Although bronchoprovocation testing does not rely on measurement of pulmonary gas exchange, using the CPET system for testing is useful for measuring $\dot{V}E$ and heart rate to standardize the exercise provocation. The American Thoracic Society guideline[39] recommends for acceptable reproducibility and sensitivity that the subject breathe dry air during a rapid increase in exercise intensity over 2 to 4 minutes, enough to raise heart rate to 80% to 90% of predicted or raise $\dot{V}E$ to 17.5 to 21 times FEV_1 and, then continue for 4 to 6 minutes.

Upper airway dysfunction—the development of airflow obstruction due to inappropriate narrowing of laryngeal or supralaryngeal structures during inspiration—is another cause of dyspnea and exercise intolerance that can be provoked with CPET. Many patients with upper airway dysfunction are initially diagnosed as having exercise-induced asthma and treated empirically with asthma medications. The development of audible inspiratory stridor distinguishes this clinically from exercise-induced bronchoconstriction, which is typically expiratory obstruction. Although there may not be distinctive gas exchange findings related to exercise-induced upper airway dysfunction, there is potential for identifying the functional obstruction from analysis of inspiratory flow rates on spontaneous flow volume loops or inferring it from reduction in volitional inspiratory capacity maneuvers during high-intensity exercise. The sensitivity of these findings has not been systematically described. Laryngoscopic examination at the time of symptoms is the gold standard for identifying upper airway dysfunction and defines the structures involved. The feasibility of doing this evaluation during CPET has been demonstrated, although it requires a specialized set of instruments and patient preparation as well as a pretest suspicion of the disorder.[40]

Psychogenic Dyspnea and Behavioral Causes of Exercise Intolerance

How do physicians diagnose psychogenic dyspnea or behavioral causes (volitional or nonvolitional) of exertional intolerance? It is difficult to make these determinations reliably, but the evaluation is enhanced by observing the patient at rest and during CPET.

These patients often undergo extensive diagnostic assessments, at great expense, that indirectly evaluate the cause of exercise intolerance. Without the diagnostic benefits of CPET, the physician may prescribe an irrelevant therapy that only adds to the patient's problem. Obviously, to diagnose the cause(s) of exercise intolerance, the patient should be studied during exercise, and the essential variables that evaluate cellular and external respiration should be measured. Logically, CPET should be done before the patient undergoes expensive imaging studies and/or an extensive invasive workup that searches, in a state of rest, for an abnormality that takes place during exercise. There are individuals with exercise intolerance for whom no clear findings of organic disease are evident, and responses to CPET are also normal. From the patient's perspective, symptoms are real whether or not their physicians can name the cause, and the designation of symptoms as "psychogenic" may be interpreted as dismissive. On the other hand, recognizing that symptoms can arise from processes that do not represent cardiorespiratory disease may prompt focusing attention on previously unidentified social or psychological stressors that are amenable to intervention. In many cases, patients may be reassured by acknowledgment that, although their symptoms are indeed unexplained, they have normal cardiovascular, respiratory, and metabolic responses to acute exercise stress. Also, volitional behavioral causes of exercise intolerance may be unmasked by findings of nonphysiological breathing responses on CPET and lack of true pathological findings.

GRADING SEVERITY OF HEART FAILURE

Symptoms had been the primary method by which physicians graded severity of heart failure before the useful development of CPET. The New York Heart Association (NYHA) classification of severity of heart failure, based on symptoms, has been almost universally used for almost six decades.[41] It has four classifications (classes I to IV) based on the perceived activity level of the patient. Matsumura et al[42] found that the NYHA classification correlated reasonably well with the *AT* and peak $\dot{V}O_2$, showing that symptoms and the ability to transport O_2 were correlated. However, the peak $\dot{V}O_2$ and *AT* had a relatively large range of values within a given NYHA class. This is thought to be due to differences in how patients perceive their own symptoms and differences in how physicians interpret their description of those symptoms.

Because of this subjectivity, Weber and Janicki[43] sought a more objective assessment based on peak $\dot{V}O_2$ and *AT*. They established an A through D classification for progressive severity as a function of the decline in peak $\dot{V}O_2$/kg (**Table 8.1**). They found that this classification corresponded to the degree of hemodynamic impairment and was an objective means of assessing cardiac dysfunction. This approach to objectively grading severity of heart failure was incorporated into a consensus statement[44] on prioritizing patients with heart failure for heart transplantation in 1993 and has remained a component of professional society guidelines related to heart failure since that time. Importantly, the physiological assessment (using peak $\dot{V}O_2$/kg) has been determined to be a more reliable independent predictor of survival than the NYHA symptom classification or measurements of resting ejection fraction.[45-48]

There are some studies that find that measures of exercise cardiac output and stroke volume may have independent prognostic, clinical, or confirmatory value in the evaluation of heart failure.[49-52] Exercise $\dot{V}O_2$ is clearly related to the cardiac output response, and therefore, estimation of cardiac output and stroke volume from noninvasive CPET data is physiologically plausible using the Fick relationship, together with informed estimates of the $C(a - \bar{v})O_2$. Note that there are multiple factors that can affect the actual $C(a - \bar{v})O_2$ including hemoglobin concentration, arterial saturation, and degree of conditioning (**Table 8.2** and **Figure 8.2**). Furthermore, there are limited data to identify how direct or indirect assessments of hemodynamic variables should be used clinically to assess disease severity or to provide prognostic information for a given patient. This is because there are relatively few studies that include cardiac output or stroke volume as a marker of prognosis while in the last 30 years, surrogate markers of cardiac performance, such as peak $\dot{V}O_2$, ventilatory inefficiency, and the *AT* have demonstrated robust clinical decision-making assistance.

TABLE 8.1 Weber's Exercise Functional Classification Based on Maximal Oxygen Uptake and Anaerobic Threshold[a]

Class	$\dot{V}O_2$max (mL/min/kg)	*AT* (mL/min/kg)	CImax (L/min/m²)
A	>20	>14	>8
B	16-20	11-14	6-8
C	10-15	8-11	4-6
D	<10	<8	<4

Abbreviations: *AT*, anaerobic threshold; CImax, maximal exercise cardiac index (cardiac output per square meter of body surface area); $\dot{V}O_2$max, maximal or peak $\dot{V}O_2$.

[a]Republished with permission of John Wiley & Sons, Inc. from Weber KT. Cardiopulmonary exercise testing and the evaluation of systolic dysfunction. In: Wasserman K, ed. *Exercise Gas Exchange in Heart Disease*. Armonk, NY: Futura Publishing; 1996:55-62, permission conveyed through Copyright Clearance Center, Inc.

TABLE 8.2 Estimation of Arteriovenous Oxygen Difference [$C(a - \bar{v})O_2$] at Peak Exercise

Hb (g/100 mL)[a]	O_2 capacity (mL/100 mL)	Arterial O_2 saturation (%)	Mixed venous O_2 saturation (%)	Arterial O_2 concentration (mL/100 mL)	Mixed venous O_2 concentration (mL/100)	$C(a - \bar{v})O_2$ (mL/100 mL)[b]
16	22.5	96	24	21.4	5.4	16.0
15	21.1	96	24	20.0	5.0	15.0
14	19.7	96	24	18.7	4.7	14.0
13	18.3	96	24	17.4	4.4	13.0
12	16.9	96	24	16.0	4.0	12.0
11	15.5	96	24	14.7	3.7	11.0
10	14.1	96	24	13.4	3.4	10.0

Abbreviation: Hb, hemoglobin; O_2, oxygen.

[a]The left column identifies the resting hemoglobin concentration. The hemoglobin concentration at peak exercise is assumed to be 5% higher than the resting hemoglobin. The carboxyhemoglobin concentration is assumed to be 1%.

[b]Modifications: (1) If the individual is very unfit, the $C(a - \bar{v})O_2$ (right column) may be decreased by up to 6%; if the person is very fit, the $C(a - \bar{v})O_2$ may be increased by up to 6%. (2) If carboxyhemoglobin is higher than 1%, reduce the $C(a - \bar{v})O_2$ by 1% for each 1% increase. (3) If arterial oxyhemoglobin saturation is less than 96%, reduce the $C(a - \bar{v})O_2$ by 1% for each 1% decrease below 96%.

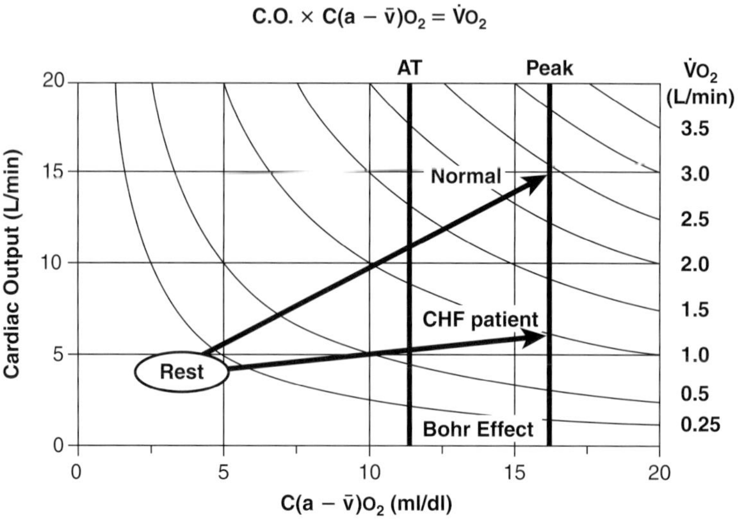

FIGURE 8.2. Oxygen uptake ($\dot{V}O_2$)-based estimations of cardiac output during exercise. Each $\dot{V}O_2$ isopleth is a product of cardiac output and arterial-mixed venous O_2 difference [$C(a - \bar{v})O_2$]. If $C(a - \bar{v})O_2$ can be estimated, such as at peak $\dot{V}O_2$ or at the anaerobic threshold (*AT*), cardiac output can be estimated at those points. The arrows illustrate how the values of $\dot{V}O_2$ at the *AT* and peak exercise can be used to estimate an individual's cardiac output noninvasively. This graph also illustrates that the *AT* becomes a larger fraction of the peak $\dot{V}O_2$ the lower the peak $\dot{V}O_2$. CHF, cardiac heart failure.

The most reliable work rate domain for cardiac output estimation from $\dot{V}O_2$ appears to be during exercise near the *AT*. Accordingly, in the first analysis of clinical data using cardiac output estimated from $\dot{V}O_2$, Bigi et al[53] used this range in a study of patients after anterior myocardial infarction. The study included 39 male and 7 female patients aged 55 ± 8 years (mean ± SD) with an ejection fraction of 39 ± 7%. Each individual underwent CPET and coronary angiography following hospital discharge. The estimated cardiac output was calculated using the linear regression of $C(a - \bar{v})O_2$ against percentage $\dot{V}O_2max$ (see **Fig. 3.6**).[54] In this study, cardiac output at the *AT* of less than 7.3 L/min was the best cutoff value for identifying multivessel CAD (relative risk = 3.1). Angiographic scores were significantly higher in patients with a cardiac output at the *AT* of less than 7.3 L/min and were inversely and significantly correlated to cardiac output at the *AT*. Moreover, cardiac output at the *AT* of less than 7.3 L/min was associated with an increased risk of further cardiac events (odds ratio, 5; 95% confidence interval, 1.4-17) and was a significant discriminator of survival for the combined end point of cardiac death, reinfarction, and clinically driven revascularization. Cardiac output at the *AT* thus appears to be a safe and useful measurement for providing additional diagnostic and prognostic information in patients with CAD.

CPET FOR EVALUATING PROGNOSIS IN HEART AND LUNG DISEASES

Because measurement of gas exchange during exercise can reflect the functions of the heart, lungs, and systemic and pulmonary circulations, CPET would be anticipated to provide prognostic information for diseases of these organs, especially because of the likely confounding effects of comorbid conditions or development of complications from the primary disorder. Indeed, exercise capacity is so global a measure of health it is found to be predictive of survival in many different populations, including apparently healthy persons and those with a variety of chronic diseases. Interestingly, prognostication using CPET has been most extensively and convincingly used in chronic heart failure with somewhat fewer studies of PAH and chronic lung diseases.[55] In the next sections, selected examples of studies relating gas exchange variables to outcome in patients with heart or lung disease are presented.

Prognosis in Heart Failure

Cardiopulmonary exercise testing makes a variety of contributions to the understanding of exercise impairment and exertional dyspnea in chronic heart failure.[56] A number of investigators have found that measurements of cardiac function at rest, both invasive and noninvasive, are poorly predictive of patients' symptoms, exercise capacity, prognosis, and/or need for heart transplantation. Concurrently, CPET has emerged as the most important method for assessing severity in chronic heart failure, including identification of patients with the poorest prognosis who are likely the best candidates for advanced therapy such as heart transplantation and LV assist devices. Currently, the most important prognostic variables measured during CPET include (1) reduced maximum exercise capacity, expressed as low peak $\dot{V}O_2$; (2) low *AT*; (3) abnormally increased $\dot{V}E$ relative to $\dot{V}CO_2$, expressed as an increased $\dot{V}E$-$\dot{V}CO_2$ slope and an increased $\dot{V}E/\dot{V}CO_2$ at the *AT* or at its nadir (ie, ventilatory inefficiency); and (4) a pattern of oscillatory $\dot{V}E$ during exercise. Other variables have also proved useful, including the trajectory of $\dot{V}O_2$ increase and the relationship of $\dot{V}E$ to $\dot{V}O_2$ during submaximal exercise. Because CPET has been used for prognostication over the last 30 years, concomitant advances in therapy leading to better outcomes in chronic heart failure require ongoing recalibration of the prognostic significance of CPET values.[57]

Peak $\dot{V}O_2$, Anaerobic Threshold, and Prognosis in Chronic Heart Failure

Weber[58] compared resting cardiac function with exercise capacity in patients with heart failure and found that variables such as cardiac index, left ventricular ejection fraction (LVEF), wedge pressure, and radiographic heart size correlated poorly with peak $\dot{V}O_2$. Also, neither resting nor exercise pulmonary capillary wedge pressure correlated significantly with peak $\dot{V}O_2$. However, peak $\dot{V}O_2$ did correlate with maximum cardiac output during exercise, as should be expected. Matsumura et al[42] and Itoh et al[59] showed that peak $\dot{V}O_2$ and *AT* correlated with symptom scores as measured by NYHA class. Mean *AT* was 90% ± 15%, 77% ± 14%, and 60% ± 12% of the predicted values for NYHA class I, class II, and class III, respectively, in the study of Itoh et al[59] In contrast, *AT* correlated only weakly with resting LVEF measured by echocardiogram or angiography.

Weber[58] introduced the classification of heart failure based on peak $\dot{V}O_2$ and *AT*, as shown in **Table 8.1**. Koike et al[60] similarly linked exercise capacity to symptom score. In the latter analysis, peak $\dot{V}O_2$, *AT*, $\Delta\dot{V}O_2/\Delta WR$, and maximum WR decreased as NYHA symptom scores worsened. The NYHA class III patients had a peak $\dot{V}O_2$ averaging 17 ± 3 mL/min/kg, *AT* of 11 ± 2 mL/min/kg, $\Delta\dot{V}O_2/\Delta WR$ equal to 6.2 ± 2 mL/min/W, and maximum work rate of 98 ± 22 W.

A number of clinical trials beginning in the 1990s confirmed the value of CPET, especially peak $\dot{V}O_2$, for providing critical criteria in predicting survival and subsequently in prioritizing patients for cardiac transplantation.[61-65] The well-known prospective study by Mancini et al[46] analyzed patients referred for heart transplantation according to the following groups: those with peak $\dot{V}O_2$ greater than 14 mL/kg/min who were considered too well for transplantation, those with peak $\dot{V}O_2$ less than 14 mL/kg/min who were listed for transplantation, and those with peak $\dot{V}O_2$ less than 14 mL/kg/min who were not accepted for surgery for noncardiac reasons. For those with peak $\dot{V}O_2$ greater than 14 mL/kg/min, the 1-year survival was 94%, which was not different from the 1-year survival of patients following cardiac transplantation at that center. In contrast, those patients with peak $\dot{V}O_2$ below 14 mL/min/kg had a 70% 1-year survival with medical management alone. This study was important not only in confirming the prognostic significance of peak $\dot{V}O_2$ in the setting of heart failure but also in demonstrating the principle that CPET values measured in these seriously ill patients could be used effectively in clinical decision making. Osada et al[66] reported that exercise blood pressure response also contributed to prognosis in heart failure. Of 500 consecutive patients referred for cardiac transplantation, they identified 154 with a peak $\dot{V}O_2$ equal to or less than 14 mL/min/kg. Among these, the 3-year survival rate was reduced from 83% to 55% in those patients unable to reach a systolic blood pressure of 120 mm Hg during exercise. Stevenson et al[67] further demonstrated that serial CPET assessment could be used to identify meaningful improvement in clinical condition of patients with severe heart failure. They identified 68 heart transplantation candidates with peak $\dot{V}O_2$ less than 14 mL/min/kg who had repeat CPETs at a mean 6 ± 5 months after the initial evaluation following a period of intensified medical therapy. On repeat testing, 30 were without "major" improvement, but 38 had an increase in peak $\dot{V}O_2$ of more than 2 mL/min/kg to a value greater than 12 mL/kg/min. Of these, 7 patients reported no clinical improvement, but 31 were clinically improved. The improvement group also had increased *AT*, peak O_2 pulse, and exercise heart rate reserve, and a decrease in resting heart rate. In the 31 patients removed from the heart transplantation waiting list based on these findings, the actuarial survival rate was 100%.

Myers et al[47] reported the results of studies on 644 patients with chronic heart failure over a 10-year period. They found that peak $\dot{V}O_2$ outperformed right heart catheterization data, exercise time, and the usual clinical variables used to assess heart failure patients in predicting outcome. They concluded that direct measurement of $\dot{V}O_2$ should be made when clinical or surgical decisions need to be made in patients referred for evaluation of heart failure or for consideration of heart transplantation.

The means of expressing values of peak $\dot{V}O_2$ in the preceding assessments warrants comment. Although most of these studies normalized the peak $\dot{V}O_2$ to body weight and ignored the variables of age and sex, Stelken et al[48] compared the sensitivity of percentage of predicted peak $\dot{V}O_2$ based on weight, age, and gender using the predicted values described in Chapter 7. In 181 ambulatory patients with NYHA class II to III symptoms, peak $\dot{V}O_2$, percentage predicted peak $\dot{V}O_2$, and *AT* were significantly different for survivors and nonsurvivors when compared at 12 and 24 months. A total of 89 patients with a peak $\dot{V}O_2$ of less than 50% predicted had 1- and 2-year survival rates of 74% and 43%, respectively, compared with 98% and 90% for the 92 patients who had a peak $\dot{V}O_2$ greater than 50% predicted. Although this study found the percentage predicted value to be a better predictor of survival than that of $\dot{V}O_2$/kg, Gitt et al,[68] making the same comparison, found that normalizing to body weight was a better predictor. The difference might be due to the relative obesity factor in the two populations and its effect on the $\dot{V}O_2$/kg index. Obesity is an increasingly common comorbid condition in clinical populations, and there are limited data addressing whether to use a patient's actual weight or ideal weight in the expression of peak $\dot{V}O_2$/kg in this context. Clearly, however, if a low peak $\dot{V}O_2$/kg is attributable to a significant degree to the weight in the denominator, one can question whether this value, or the patient's prognosis, would be improved by a transplantation.

In many early studies of exercise capacity in heart failure, the study cohorts did not include sufficient numbers of female subjects to evaluate the differential effects of sex on prognostic value of CPET variables. This was examined by Elmariah et al[69] in a study of 594 patients with heart failure, 28% of whom were women. This study found that although peak $\dot{V}O_2$/kg was lower for the women than for the men, survival was better among the women and proposed that distinct thresholds for men and women be used in prognostic assessments.

Although peak $\dot{V}O_2$ has consistently been found to be a robust prognostic variable, it might be underestimated due to reduced patient effort as well as by premature termination of exercise by the examiner. It is therefore desirable to identify variables in the submaximal range during incremental exercise that have prognostic value. Gitt et al[68] and Sun et al[70] studied the submaximal criteria of *AT* and $\dot{V}E$-$\dot{V}CO_2$ slope below the ventilatory compensation point (VCP) compared with peak $\dot{V}O_2$, normalized to both body weight and percentage predicted, as measures of heart failure severity based on survival.

The *AT* reflects the maximal sustainable aerobic $\dot{V}O_2$ and is an objective parameter of exercise capacity. It can be derived from submaximal exercise testing and therefore does not require maximal patient effort. Gitt et al[68] compared the peak $\dot{V}O_2$ and the submaximal parameters as predictors of 6-month and 24-month patient survival rate in a cohort of 223 patients. Stratifying peak $\dot{V}O_2$ at 14 mL/min/kg, *AT* at 11 mL/min/kg, and $\dot{V}E$-$\dot{V}CO_2$ slope below the VCP at 35, they found that each of these parameters separated the high-risk from the low-risk patients (**Fig. 8.3**).

Figure 8.4 shows the odds ratio of early death when these parameters are in the high-risk range. The combination of *AT* and $\dot{V}E$-$\dot{V}CO_2$ below the VCP was found to be the best predictor of early death (within 6 months) in patients with LV failure, using the threshold criteria selected in this study. Because both *AT* and $\dot{V}E$-$\dot{V}CO_2$ slope below the VCP are determined at submaximal work rates and are not effort dependent, these are exceptionally valuable measurements. Sun et al[70] confirmed the 6-month findings

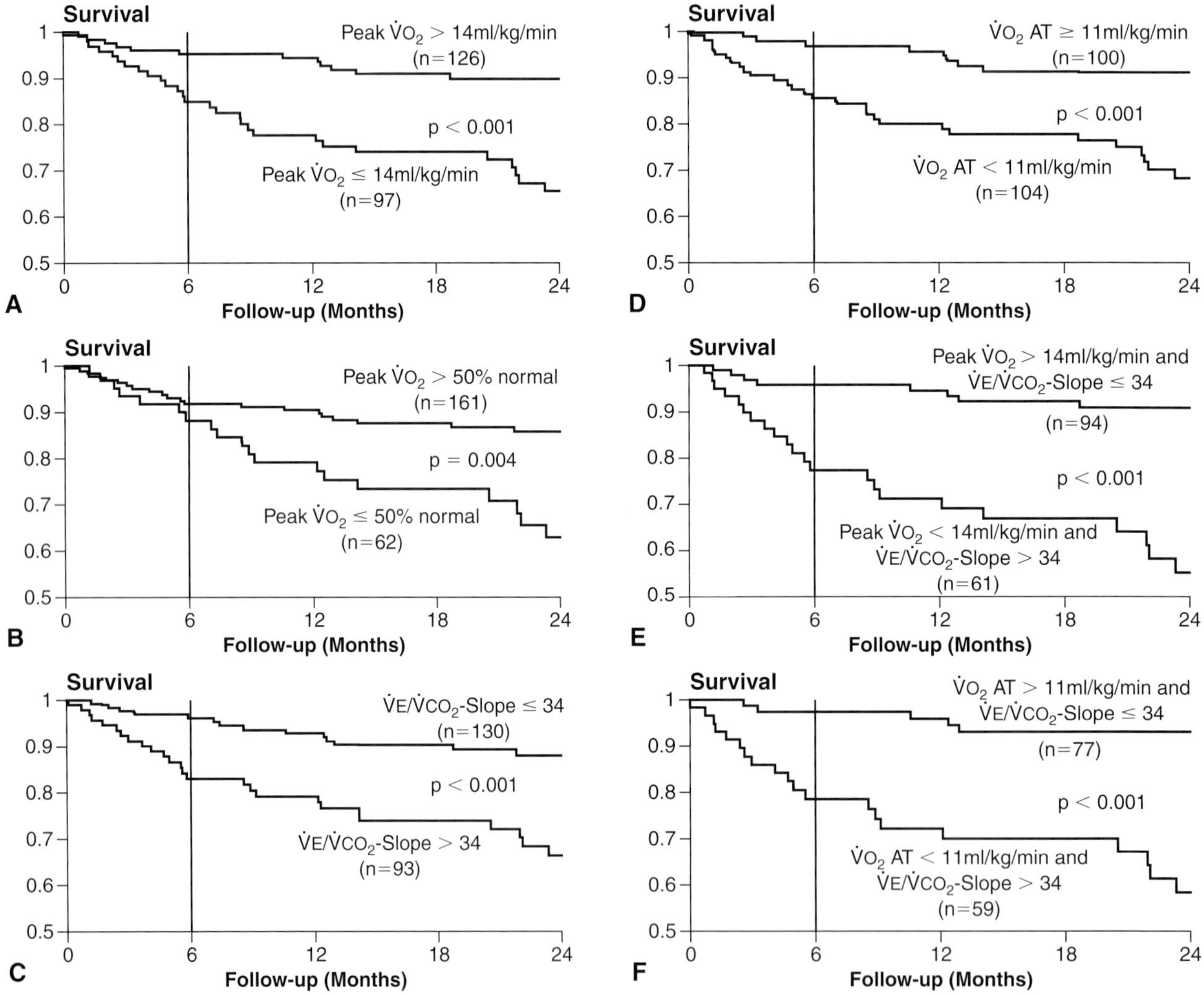

FIGURE 8.3. Kaplan–Meier survival curves using peak oxygen uptake ($\dot{V}O_2$) ≤14 (A), peak $\dot{V}O_2$ <50% predicted normal (B), $\dot{V}E$-$\dot{V}CO_2$ slope >34 (C), $\dot{V}O_2$ at the anaerobic threshold (*AT*) <11 mL/kg/min (D), the combination of peak $\dot{V}O_2$ ≤14 and $\dot{V}E$-$\dot{V}CO_2$ slope >34 (E), as well as $\dot{V}O_2$ at *AT* <11 and $\dot{V}E$-$\dot{V}CO_2$ slope >34 (F) as stratification points. Significant differences in survival were found at 6 months after the initial evaluation in A, C, D, E, and F. *(Reprinted with permission from Gitt AK, Wasserman K, Kilkowski C, et al. Exercise anaerobic threshold and ventilatory efficiency identify heart failure patients for high risk of early death.* Circulation. *2002;106[24]:3079-3084.)*

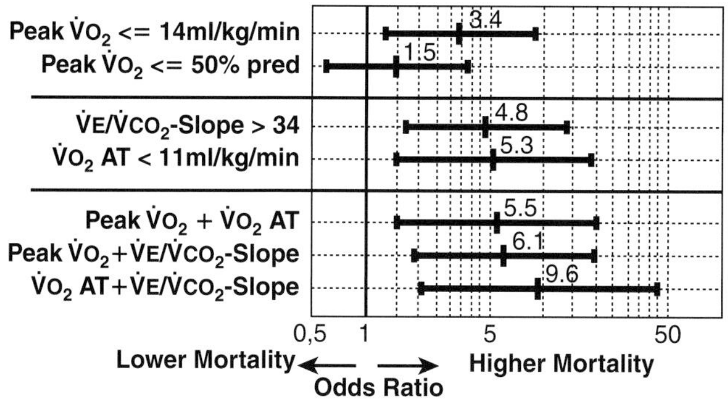

FIGURE 8.4. Cardiopulmonary predictors of early death within 6 months: univariate analysis. Numbers are odd ratios. Bars are 95% confidence interval. *(Reprinted with permission from Gitt AK, Wasserman K, Kilkowski C, et al. Exercise anaerobic threshold and ventilatory efficiency identify heart failure patients for high risk of early death.* Circulation. *2002;106[24]:3079-3084.)*

showing increased early death or hospitalization rates if values where beyond the threshold values for severity described in the preceding study. When adding oscillatory V̇E in assessing survival in stable patients with heart failure, death and early hospitalization rates within 6 months were even more marked (**Fig. 8.5**).

An interesting finding was reported by Agostoni et al,[71] who postulated that the gas exchange features that normally occur at or near the *AT* might be less clearly defined in patients with severe heart failure. If so, identification of the *AT* by gas exchange measurements would be less common in more severe patients. In 2137 heart failure patients who performed CPET, 562 total deaths and 87 heart transplants were performed during a mean follow-up of 3.4 years. In those in whom the *AT* could not identified, the V̇E-V̇CO2 slope was higher, peak V̇O2 was lower, and

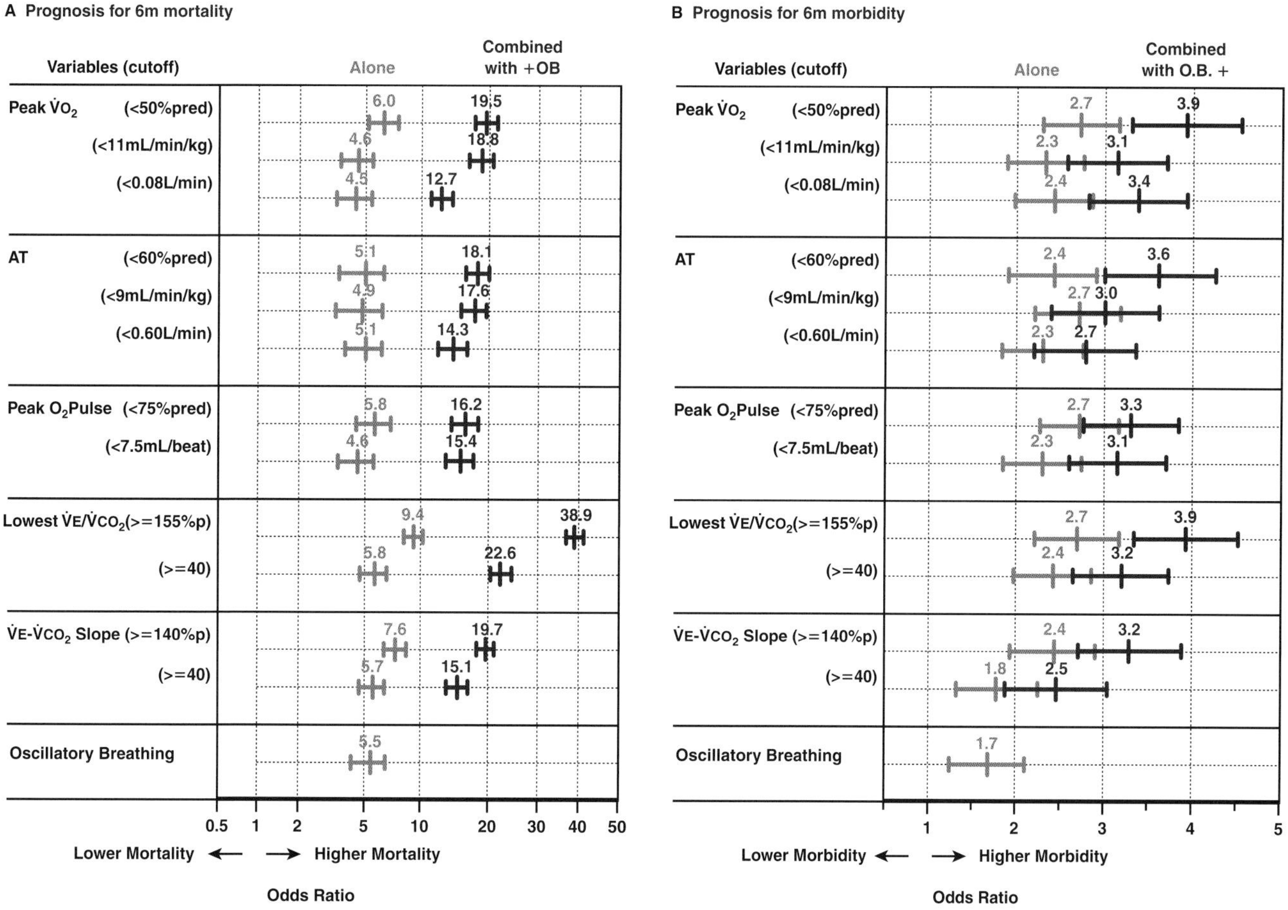

FIGURE 8.5. Odds ratio (OR) of cardiopulmonary exercise testing (CPET) variables, alone and combined with positive oscillatory breathing pattern (+OB), for 6-month mortality (A) and morbidity (B) in patients with New York Heart Association (NYHA) class III systolic left ventricular heart failure. A: The OR on the left show the mean and 95% confidence intervals of the individual CPET measurements, and the bars at the right are OR for the CPET measurements combined with oscillatory breathing pattern (+OB). The ORs for all CPET measurements and +OB alone and combined are significant. When each CPET index was combined with +OB, the OR values were significantly increased ($P < .05$ to $P < .001$). The best single predictor of 6-month mortality is the lowest V̇E/V̇CO2 (≥155% predicted) (OR = 9.4) and the best combination is lowest V̇E/V̇CO2 (≥155% predicted) with +OB (OR = 38.9). B: Although the OR values are lower, the trend agrees with the mortality data. *(Reprinted from Sun XG, Hansen JE, Beshai JF, Wasserman K. Oscillatory breathing and exercise gas exchange abnormalities prognosticate early mortality and morbidity in heart failure.* J Am Coll Cardiol. *2010;55[17]:1814-1823. Copyright © 2010 American College of Cardiology Foundation. With permission.)*

oscillatory breathing was more prevalent. With multivariable analysis, peak $\dot{V}O_2$, $\dot{V}E$-$\dot{V}CO_2$ slope, low hemoglobin, and low LVEF among other variables were significant, but nonidentification of the *AT* was found to have the highest hazard ratio for all-cause mortality and cardiovascular death or transplant. However, at least one caution has been raised about using *AT* for prognostic assessment in patients with chronic atrial fibrillation.[72] In this study, 2578 patients with heart failure in sinus rhythm were contrasted with 398 with atrial fibrillation during CPET. The best cutoff value of $\dot{V}O_2$ at the *AT* for prediction of cardiovascular death or urgent transplantation by receiver operating curve was 11.7 mL/kg/min for those with sinus rhythm but 12.8 mL/kg/min for those with atrial fibrillation.

Decreased "Ventilatory Efficiency" and Prognosis in Chronic Heart Failure

In view of the strong physiological rationale for peak $\dot{V}O_2$ and its success as a prognostic variable in chronic heart failure, it is very interesting that another and often independent predictor of outcome was identified. This concept has been termed either decreased "ventilatory efficiency" or "excess ventilation" during exercise. These terms reflect abnormally high $\dot{V}E$ relative to $\dot{V}CO_2$, most often expressed as an increased $\dot{V}E/\dot{V}CO_2$ at or close to the *AT* and/or an increase in $\dot{V}E$-$\dot{V}CO_2$ slope below the *AT* or VCP during a rapid incremental exercise test. As discussed in Chapter 2 ("Ventilatory Determinants" section), the relationship between $\dot{V}E$ and $\dot{V}CO_2$ at any particular work rate is given by

$$\dot{V}E = \dot{V}CO_2 \times 863 / [PaCO_2 \times (1 - VD/VT)] \quad (1)$$

Rearranging gives

$$\dot{V}E/\dot{V}CO_2 = 863 / [PaCO_2 \times (1 - VD/VT)] \quad (2)$$

The relationship between $\dot{V}E$ and $\dot{V}CO_2$ over its linear range (ie, typically up to the VCP) is given by

$$\dot{V}E = m \times \dot{V}CO_2 + c \quad (3)$$

where m and c are the $\dot{V}E$-$\dot{V}CO_2$ slope and $\dot{V}E$-intercept parameters, respectively. Similar to $\dot{V}E/\dot{V}CO_2$, m depends on the response trajectories of $PaCO_2$ and VD/VT.

An elevated $\dot{V}E$-$\dot{V}CO_2$ slope thus means that either $PaCO_2$ is decreased (hyperventilation due to augmented ventilatory drive) or VD/VT is increased, or both. This is also the case for an elevated $\dot{V}E/\dot{V}CO_2$ at the *AT* or at its nadir. In general, elevated VD/VT comes close to indicating "ventilatory inefficiency," whereas a low $PaCO_2$, in and of itself, does not (in some ways rather, a low $PaCO_2$ suggests quite efficient $\dot{V}E$). Nevertheless, the concept of ventilatory inefficiency has become adopted for either an increased $\dot{V}E$-$\dot{V}CO_2$ slope or an increased $\dot{V}E/\dot{V}CO_2$ near the *AT* or at its nadir.[73] It is not clear which of high VD/VT or low $PaCO_2$ contributes most to increased $\dot{V}E$ during exercise in chronic heart failure, and there are data supporting both mechanisms.[17,74-77]

Chua et al[78] were among the first to point out the prognostic value of excess ventilation. Eighty-three out of 173 patients had an elevated $\dot{V}E$-$\dot{V}CO_2$ slope (>34, mean 43.1) with an 18-month survival of 69% compared to 95% for heart failure patients with a lower slope. An elevated $\dot{V}E$-$\dot{V}CO_2$ slope was an independent predictor of survival in addition to peak $\dot{V}O_2$. Corrà et al[79] pointed out that peak $\dot{V}O_2$ has less value in those with intermediate peak $\dot{V}O_2$ and found that mortality during the study period was 30% in those with a $\dot{V}E$-$\dot{V}CO_2$ slope ≥35 compared with only 10% with a slope <35. Patients with a $\dot{V}E$-$\dot{V}CO_2$ slope >35 had similar mortality those with a peak $\dot{V}O_2$ <10 mL/kg/min. Nadruz et al[19] found that both peak $\dot{V}O_2$ and $\dot{V}E$-$\dot{V}CO_2$ slope were associated with composite poor outcome (death, LV assist device use, or heart transplantation) but were better predictors in HFpEF than HFrEF. A meta-analysis of 12 studies with 2628 patients and a mean follow-up of 31 months showed that slope of $\dot{V}E$-$\dot{V}CO_2$ was as effective for estimating prognosis as peak $\dot{V}O_2$.[80]

Recently, Kee et al[75] found a correlation between increased dead space ventilation during exercise and peak $\dot{V}O_2$, although for the dead space calculation, $PaCO_2$ was estimated using a published prediction equation rather than measured directly. On the other hand, Guazzi et al[81] also shed some light on the mechanism of "ventilatory inefficiency" in a study of 128 stable heart failure patients, of whom 24 died during the observation period for cardiac causes. Several predictors of death were found during univariate analysis including, as expected, low peak $\dot{V}O_2$ and high $\dot{V}E$-$\dot{V}CO_2$ slope. However, multivariate analysis determined that a low peak $PaCO_2$ (less than 35 mm Hg) was the strongest independent prognostic indicator. These data suggest increased ventilatory drive and hyperventilation as the prime cause of "ventilatory inefficiency" in heart failure rather than high VD/VT.

Prognosis in Heart Failure Based on Oscillatory Breathing During Exercise

A cyclical or periodic breathing pattern has long been observed in patients with heart failure at rest and during sleep. More recently, cyclic variation in breathing during exercise, termed exercise oscillatory breathing (EOV), has been reported during CPET, and the presence, amplitude, and periodicity of EOV has been associated with prognosis in heart failure patients. An American Heart Association consensus statement proposed an operational definition for EOV as a periodic breathing pattern that persists for at least 60% of the exercise test at an amplitude 15% or more the average resting value[5] while others have used other definitions. This phenomenon is usually readily recognized by the interpreter of the CPET. Whereas EOV may actually interfere with the measurements of peak $\dot{V}O_2$ and, to a lesser extent, $\dot{V}E$-$\dot{V}CO_2$ slope, the finding of EOV may serve as a submaximal predictor of poor outcome. For example, Dhakal and Lewis[82] reviewed 15 studies showing associations of EOV with other CPET markers of poor prognosis.

Corrà et al[83] found that 35% of stable heart failure patients had EOV, and 54% of these had elevated $\dot{V}E$-$\dot{V}CO_2$ slope, and presence of EOV was the strongest predictor of cardiac-related death, with higher predictive value than $\dot{V}E$-$\dot{V}CO_2$ slope. Leite et al[84] found that about 30% of heart failure patients had periodic breathing during exercise, and this was the only independent marker of mortality (30.9% died during observation). Guazzi et al[85] found that 35% of heart failure patients had EOV. Sixty-two out of 288 patients died during observation. Fifty-four percent of those with EOV had an elevated $\dot{V}E$-$\dot{V}CO_2$ slope, and a $\dot{V}E$-$\dot{V}CO_2$ slope >36.2 had 77% sensitivity and 64% specificity for mortality prediction. The combination of elevated $\dot{V}E$-$\dot{V}CO_2$ slope and presence of EOV resulted in a hazard ratio of 11.4.

Cardiopulmonary Exercise Testing and Evolving Management of Chronic Heart Failure

The use of CPET for prognostication has evolved as noted in the previous section, with at first the use of peak $\dot{V}O_2$ then the addition of ventilatory inefficiency, oscillatory $\dot{V}E$, and other variables. Similarly, management of heart failure has evolved with associated improvement in prognosis. The widespread addition of β-blockers was notable for having a major benefit on survival but less clear effects on CPET variables. This has been addressed by several investigators. O'Neill et al[86] found that a decrease in peak $\dot{V}O_2$ of 1 mL/kg/min was associated with an adjusted hazard ratio for transplant of 1.13 in those not on β-blockers but 1.27 in those on β-blockers. Adjusted 5-year survival was better for those on β-blockers at all levels of peak $\dot{V}O_2$ and did not become equal for the two groups until peak $\dot{V}O_2$ was 10 mL/min/kg. A cut point value of peak $\dot{V}O_2$ 14 mL/kg/min was thus considered too high for referral for possible transplant for patients receiving β-blockers. Agostoni et al[87] in a study of 572 stable heart failure patients with LVEF <50% of whom 81 were not treated with a β-blocker, 304 were given carvedilol, and 187 were treated with bisoprolol. Those given carvedilol were found to have a reduction in $\dot{V}E$-$\dot{V}CO_2$ slope compared to nontreated and bisoprolol-treated patients, as well as a higher P_{ETCO_2} during isocapnic buffering, suggesting that carvedilol was associated with reduction of ventilatory insufficiency and possible degree of hyperventilation compared with bisoprolol.

The study by Paolillo et al[57] and a large group of European investigators (MECKI Score Research Group) provides valuable insight. They noted that prognosis in heart failure has improved markedly during the last two-and-half decades and retrospectively analyzed cohorts taken from 6083 heart failure patients enrolled over successive blocks of time between 1993 and 2015. Members of later enrolled groups had progressively better outcomes compared to earlier groups, which were assumed to be due to improvements in management. These differences remained after correction for peak $\dot{V}O_2$ and $\dot{V}E$-$\dot{V}CO_2$ slope. Importantly, the authors found that the cutoff values for peak $\dot{V}O_2$ and $\dot{V}E$-$\dot{V}CO_2$ slope that would identify a 10% or 20% risk of a composite endpoint of cardiac death, urgent heart transplantation, of LV assist device differed between groups. For example, a 20% risk cutoff for peak $\dot{V}O_2$ was 15 mL/min/kg in 1993-2000, but was 9 mL/min/kg for those from 2001-2005, and as low as 5 mL/min/kg for the most recently enrolled subjects (2011-2015). Similarly, a $\dot{V}E$-$\dot{V}CO_2$ slope greater than 32 predicted a 20% risk of the composite endpoint for those from the 1993-2000 group, but much higher values were needed for the same risk in 2006-2010 (>59) and 2011-2015 (>57). Thus, the significance of CPET variables measured in patients with heart failure and their use in clinical decision making are dependent on the context of background therapies and prognosis.

Prognosis in Structural Heart Diseases

In the special case of valvular heart disease, there is consensus that patients with *symptomatic* aortic stenosis should not undergo exercise testing because of risks of complications. The role of CPET in assessment of prognosis and management of patients with asymptomatic or mildly symptomatic valvular aortic stenosis, while not fully defined, has been the focus of a number of studies. Dhoble and colleagues[88] found that in 155 patients with aortic valve area ≤1.5 cm^2 referred for testing, peak $\dot{V}O_2$ was <80% predicted in 54% of patients. During follow-up, 41 patients died and 72 underwent valve replacement. Survival was better in those with higher peak $\dot{V}O_2$ and O_2 pulse. The study by Le et al[89] looked at asymptomatic or questionably symptomatic mostly elderly patients with aortic valve area index ≤0.6 cm^2/m^2 and LV ejection fraction ≥0.50. If patients had normal peak $\dot{V}O_2$ (>83% predicted) and normal peak O_2 pulse (>95% predicted) or these variables were abnormal but had data suggesting nonhemodynamic limitations, the patients were managed conservatively. During a mean of 24 months follow-up, all-cause mortality was 4% compared with 8% in an age- and gender-matched population. For the patients with normal peak $\dot{V}O_2$ and O_2 pulse, 37% had cardiac death, heart failure hospitalization, or valve replacement; for those with abnormal variables but were otherwise managed conservatively, the composite poor outcome was 38.7%. Domanski et al[90] showed that in 51 asymptomatic patients with moderate to severe aortic stenosis by echocardiogram, there was 97% negative predictive value for cardiac events in patients with peak $\dot{V}O_2$ ≥85% predicted. In a small study of 43 patients without symptoms but aortic valve area <1 cm^2, a $\dot{V}E$-$\dot{V}CO_2$ slope >34 and peak $\dot{V}O_2$ <14 mL/kg/min were independently associated with symptoms during exercise that met criteria for valve replacement.[91] Thus, there are accumulating data to suggest a role for CPET in evaluation of patients with minimally symptomatic aortic stenosis. There are a few similar studies for chronic mitral regurgitation,[92,93] but these are mostly in conjunction with exercise echocardiography.

Congenital heart diseases, of course, are highly diverse in terms of the nature of the anatomic abnormality, evolution over time, and medical treatments or surgical repair or palliation. Nevertheless, there are data supporting the value of CPET in assessment of prognosis in these patients. Inuzuka et al[94] evaluated intermediate-term (5-year) mortality in a series of 1375 adult (mean age 33 years) congenital heart disease patients who had CPET at a single center. Low peak $\dot{V}O_2$, high $\dot{V}E$-$\dot{V}CO_2$ slope, and lower heart rate responsiveness were associated with increased risk for death over a median follow-up of 5.8 years. In another series, Dimopoulos et al[95] evaluated the $\dot{V}_E$-$\dot{V}CO_2$ slope and found it to be particularly high in patients with Eisenmenger physiology, but the strongest CPET variable in terms of prediction of survival only among non-cyanotic patients. Cyanosis was the strongest predictor of abnormal $\dot{V}_E$-$\dot{V}CO_2$ slope, and the quartile of patients with $\dot{V}_E$-$\dot{V}CO_2$ slope $\geq$38 had the worst prognosis.

Recommendations for Prognostic Evaluation for Potential Cardiac Transplantation

Since the late 1980s, heart transplant cardiologists have appreciated that peak $\dot{V}O_2$ more sensitively predicts prognosis than more classic heart failure risk factors such as LVEF, NYHA class IV symptoms, and neurohormonal markers (**Table 8.3**). Increasing experience has confirmed the prognostic value of peak $\dot{V}O_2$ in the evaluation of patients with heart failure.[44,46-48,66,96,97]

The 1993 Bethesda Conference for Cardiac Transplantation[44] provided indications for heart transplantation shown in **Table 8.3**. A low peak $\dot{V}O_2$ was the primary criterion, provided that at peak $\dot{V}O_2$, anaerobic metabolism had been reached (ie, exercise above the *AT*). In 2016, the International Society for Heart & Lung Transplantation issued updated international guidelines for heart transplantation listing,[98] and CPET for assessment of prognosis was strongly recommended for guidance. Defining a "maximal" CPET as one with a respiratory exchange ratio >1.05 and achievement of *AT* while on optimal pharmacologic therapy, they recommended a cutoff of peak $\dot{V}O_2$ $\leq$14 mL/kg/min but $\leq$12 mL/kg/min for those on β-blockers. In patients younger than 50 years and women, an alternate standard might be considered, such as <50% of predicted peak $\dot{V}O_2$. They did not give equal weight to ventilatory efficiency (eg, $\dot{V}_E$-$\dot{V}CO_2$ slope), but, as an alternative, they noted that listing for transplantation should be considered for a $\dot{V}_E$-$\dot{V}CO_2$ slope >35, in the presence of a submaximal CPET (ie, peak respiratory exchange ratio <1.05). The guidelines also offered recommendations for subsets of patients, including cardiac amyloidosis, restrictive cardiomyopathy, hypertrophic cardiomyopathy, and patients with Chagas disease.

TABLE 8.3 1993 Bethesda Conference: Indications for Heart Transplantation[a]

I. Accepted indications for transplantation

A. Maximal $\dot{V}O_2$ less than 10 mL/kg/min with achievement of anaerobic metabolism

B. Severe ischemia consistently limiting routine activity not amenable to bypass surgery or angioplasty

C. Recurrent symptomatic ventricular arrhythmias refractory to all accepted therapeutic modalities

II. Probable indications for cardiac transplantation

A. Maximal $\dot{V}O_2$ less than 14 mL/kg/min and major limitation of the patient's daily activities

B. Recurrent unstable ischemia not amenable to bypass surgery or angioplasty

C. Instability of fluid balance and/or renal function not due to patient noncompliance with regimen of weight monitoring, flexible use of diuretic drugs, and salt restriction

III. Inadequate indications for transplantation

A. Ejection fraction less than 20%

B. History of functional class III or IV symptoms of heart failure

C. Previous ventricular arrhythmias

D. Maximal $\dot{V}O_2$ greater than 15 mL/kg/min without other indications

Abbreviation: $\dot{V}O_2$, oxygen uptake.

[a]Reprinted from Mudge GH, Goldstein S, Addonizio LJ, et al. 24th Bethesda conference: Cardiac transplantation. Task force 3: recipient guidelines/prioritization. *J Am Coll Cardiol*. 1993;22(1): 1-64. Copyright © 1993 Elsevier. With permission

Evaluation of chronic heart failure, including severity, risk assessment, and treatment guidance, has become likely the best studied clinical application of CPET. Based on sound physiological principles, especially those relating overall function of the heart and circulation to peak $\dot{V}O_2$, the finding of differences in the $\dot{V}_E$-$\dot{V}CO_2$ relationship, as well the strong prognostic value of oscillatory breathing, CPET has become indispensable for clinical assessment and a valuable tool for understanding pathophysiology. Moreover, because heart failure is a common condition causing significant impairment, experience in the study of exercise function in this population has contributed importantly to integration of CPET into clinical practice by raising awareness of the value of the measurements, demonstrating that CPET can be performed by patients over wide ranges of age and disease severity, and proving that the data derived from this testing are sufficiently robust to be used in clinical decision making.

Prognosis in Pulmonary Arterial Hypertension and Prioritizing Patients for Lung Transplantation

The revolution in pharmacologic treatment of PAH has led to improvement in survival and quality of life. However, there remain patients who are unresponsive to pulmonary hypertension therapy or who progress on treatment for whom lung transplantation is the only remaining treatment option. Therefore, much more of the decision process for lung transplantation focuses on assessment of severity in the face of optimal medical management.[99] The critical nature of this decision requires objective documentation that the medical therapy is not working and that the disease is so severe that the patient is at imminent risk of dying without this major intervention. Thus, reliable quantitative evaluation of the ability to increase pulmonary blood flow under exercise stress is essential.

Wensel et al[22] reported that reduced peak $\dot{V}O_2$ was a prognosticator of early death from PAH. Sun et al[21] studied the exercise pathophysiology in a cohort of 64 patients with PAH and showed that peak $\dot{V}O_2$ decreases in proportion to worsening NYHA symptom class. However, symptoms were viewed as too variable with respect to function to be relied on for making the decision to resort to lung transplantation. In their multivariable analysis, peak $\dot{V}O_2$, peak work rate, *AT*, peak O_2 pulse, $\dot{V}E$-$\dot{V}CO_2$ slope, and $\dot{V}E/\dot{V}CO_2$ at the *AT* were significantly correlated with NYHA symptom class. They provided a classification scheme for severity based on these variables. Woods et al[100] looked at submaximal measurements of gas exchange during exercise and found that $P_{ET}CO_2$ was lower in 40 patients with PAH than 25 matched controls, while $\dot{V}E/\dot{V}CO_2$ ratio at the *AT* was higher (mean 42 ± 10 versus 33 + 5). Additionally, there was a relationship between severity of PAH by clinical determination and severity of pulmonary gas exchange impairment. The same group developed a gas exchange score that was related to severity of PAH,[101] and Badagliacca et al[102] showed added benefit of adding peak $\dot{V}O_2$ during exercise to change in cardiac index in a variety of PAH patients.

Despite the existence of these excellent noninvasive descriptors of the abnormalities found in pulmonary hypertension, they have not been systematically used to prognosticate survival for the purpose of directing lung transplantation decisions. However, we have found that those patients with PAH with the shortest survival tend to have the lowest peak $\dot{V}O_2$, *AT*, and $P_{ET}CO_2$ at the *AT* and the highest $\dot{V}E/\dot{V}CO_2$ at the *AT*. From this experience and that of Wensel et al,[22] we believe that objective physiological measurements should be useful in the assessment of if and when the lung should be transplanted in patients with primary pulmonary hypertension.

Oudiz et al[103] hypothesized that several variables collected during CPET over time would predict outcomes better than single measurements alone. One hundred three patients with PAH who underwent serial CPET were followed for a mean of 4.7 years, during which 20 patients died and 3 underwent lung transplantation. Overall, higher $\dot{V}E/\dot{V}CO_2$ at the *AT*, lower *AT*, lower $P_{ET}CO_2$ at the *AT*, higher NYHA symptom class, and lower peak $\dot{V}O_2$ were associated with decreased survival. After a median of 0.7 years, a repeat CPET showed similar association. If the patient did not have gas exchange evidence of a right-to-left shunt during the baseline CPET, there was a 20% likelihood of death or transplantation but this decreased to 7% on the second CPET. Thus, development of shunting was a poor prognostic finding; only 25% of those who developed a shunt (2 of 8) survived, but 16 of 17 who had a disappearance of the shunt on the second CPET survived. In multivariate analysis, persistence or development of an exercise-induced right-to-left shunt strongly predicted death or transplantation, independent of peak $\dot{V}O_2$ and ventilatory inefficiency. In the absence of a shunt, ventilatory inefficiency was associated with poorer outcomes. The data of Schwaiblmair[104] and colleagues also showed major differences between survivors and nonsurvivors with pulmonary hypertension, finding higher $\dot{V}E/\dot{V}CO_2$ and $\dot{V}E/\dot{V}O_2$ at *AT*. Peak $\dot{V}O_2$ <10.4 mL/min/kg had a 1.5-fold increase in mortality over 24 months as well as those with $\dot{V}E$-$\dot{V}CO_2$ slope >60 having a 5.8-fold risk of death. Ferreira et al[105] studied 84 patients, both with PAH and those with other conditions associated with PAH, of whom 13 died and 3 had atrial septostomy. Multiple variable regression analysis demonstrated that the $\dot{V}E$-$\dot{V}CO_2$ slope estimated over the entire work rate range (ie, up to peak exercise) >55 or $\dot{V}E/\dot{V}CO_2$ at peak exercise >57 were best related to poor prognosis compared with the $\dot{V}E$-$\dot{V}CO_2$ estimated up to the VCP or $\dot{V}E/\dot{V}CO_2$ at the *AT*. The 96.9% of those with $\dot{V}E$-$\dot{V}CO_2$ slope up to peak exercise <55 were free of a PAH-related event, whereas those with $\dot{V}E$-$\dot{V}CO_2$ slope up to peak exercise >55 and $\Delta\dot{V}O_2/\Delta WR$ <5.5 mL/min/watt had a poorer outcome. Several noninvasive and invasive CPET variables that were independent predictors of outcome were identified by Wensel and colleagues,[106] who reported on 226 consecutive patients with PAH who underwent right heart catheterization and CPET. During a follow-up period of 1508 days, 72 patients died and 30 underwent lung transplantation. Variables that were independent predictors of outcome included low peak $\dot{V}O_2$ percentage predicted, high pulmonary vascular resistance, and low increase in heart rate with exercise. Peak $\dot{V}O_2$, percentage predicted, alone could be used for risk assessment. The highest quartile of patients (peak $\dot{V}O_2$ >65% predicted) had 1-year survival of 100%, whereas the lowest quartile with peak $\dot{V}O_2$ <34.1% predicted had only a 69.6% 1 year and 23% 5-year survival. Intermediate quartiles had corresponding 1- and 5-year outcomes. Similar to heart failure patients, Tang and colleagues[107] found that the oxygen uptake efficiency slope (OUES; slope of the $\dot{V}O_2$ versus log $\dot{V}E$ relationship) predicted a poor outcome in patients with PAH along with the usual predictive variables in univariate analysis and had potential for usefulness in patients who performed submaximal CPET studies.

Because response to therapy is key in PAH, the study by Groepenhoff et al[108] of a relatively small number of patients may be relevant. They studied 65 idiopathic PAH patients during CPET and again a mean 13 months later. Predictors of survival from the initial CPET included 6-minute walk distance, maximal heart rate, and $\dot{V}E$-$\dot{V}CO_2$ slope, but not peak $\dot{V}O_2$. After treatment was started, 6-minute walk distance, peak $\dot{V}O_2$, peak heart rate, and $\dot{V}E$-$\dot{V}CO_2$ slope remained as significant predictors, although only the change in 6-minute walk distance, peak $\dot{V}O_2$, maximal heart rate was significant, and not the change in $\dot{V}E$-$\dot{V}CO_2$ slope.

Prognosis in Lung Diseases

Chronic Obstructive Pulmonary Disease and Prioritizing Patients for Lung Volume Reduction Surgery

Oga et al[109] analyzed the relations among exercise capacity, health status, and mortality rate in 150 male patients with stable COPD with a mean postbronchodilator FEV_1 of 47.4% of predicted. Each patient was studied with pulmonary function testing, CPET, and health status questionnaires[110] at entry into the study. In a 5-year follow-up, 31 had died. Multivariate Cox proportional hazards analysis revealed that the peak $\dot{V}O_2$ was predictive of mortality independent of FEV_1 and age. Stepwise Cox proportional hazards analysis revealed that the peak $\dot{V}O_2$ was the most significant predictor of early mortality, Hiraga et al[111] also studied the relationship between physiological parameters (derived from CPET) and survival time, over a 3- to 5-year period in 120 patients with COPD; they had similar findings to Oga et al.[109]

Neder et al[30] recently reviewed the clinical relationship of ventilatory inefficiency in COPD to outcome and pointed out that ventilatory inefficiency as a predictor of outcome has become very useful but most often in disorders not usually associated with limited ventilatory capacity (heart failure and PAH). In a study looking at both dynamic hyperinflation and ventilatory inefficiency in COPD during exercise, Neder et al[112] reported on 288 patients followed for a median of 57 months. Of the 77 who died (26.7%), age, body mass index, and resting ratio of inspiratory capacity to total lung capacity (IC/TLC) predicted all-cause and respiratory mortality and only the nadir $\dot{V}E/\dot{V}CO_2$ >34 had further predictive value. Dynamic hyperinflation during exercise as determined by change in the IC/TLC ratio and exercise capacity by 6-minute walk distance were significantly related to all-cause and respiratory mortality.[113]

The National Emphysema Treatment Trial in the United States, the focus of which was treatment with pulmonary rehabilitation alone compared to with rehabilitation and lung reduction surgery, revealed that the only patient group that benefited from the surgery was the group with upper lung field emphysema and reduced exercise tolerance (40 W/min or less at peak).[114] If the patient did not have reduced exercise tolerance, regardless of the distribution of the emphysema, surgical resection did not improve the prognosis or exercise tolerance of the patient.

Use of CPET for Prognosis in Other Lung Diseases Including Idiopathic Pulmonary Fibrosis

Idiopathic pulmonary fibrosis is a chronic progressive disease and much has been written about diagnosis and differentiation from other interstitial lung diseases, including other idiopathic disorders and diseases secondary to other systemic diseases.[115-117] Because of the relentless progression of untreated interstitial pulmonary fibrosis (IPF) and newly approved pharmacologic therapies that appear to slow progression, risk stratification is important in selecting candidates for treatment, which also may include consideration of lung transplantation. Severity and risk assessment are mostly based on resting pulmonary function, but 6-minute walk distance and oxygen desaturation during exercise are most commonly used. Because early treatment is likely associated with improved survival, accurate risk stratification may be valuable. Because IPF is characteristically seen in an older population with comorbidities, CPET may also be of some help in assessing these patients.

Manali et al[118] found correlations between dyspnea scores and 6-minute walk distance and, during CPET, oxygen desaturation, elevated $\dot{V}E$-$\dot{V}CO_2$ slope, and $\dot{V}E/\dot{V}CO_2$ at the *AT*. In a small number of patients with IPF (22 men and 12 women), Vainshelboim et al[119] found that peak work rate <62 W, peak $\dot{V}O_2$ ≤13.8 mL/kg/min, $\dot{V}E/\dot{V}CO_2$ at the AT >34, and the lowest value of $\dot{V}E/\dot{V}O_2$ >34 were cutoff values that separated the 11 who died from the survivors. Nonsurvivors more often had pulmonary hypertension and more severe desaturation during exercise. van der Plas et al[120] found elevated systolic pulmonary artery pressure in 11 patients with IPF (>40 mm Hg) and compared these to 27 without elevated pressures. Only $\dot{V}E/\dot{V}CO_2$ at the *AT* was different between the two groups, and $\dot{V}E/\dot{V}CO_2$ at the *AT* >45 had significantly worse survival. In a small prospective study of 25 IPF patients of whom 17 patients survived during the observation period, Triantafillidou et al[121] found that $\dot{V}E$-$\dot{V}CO_2$ slope, peak $\dot{V}O_2$, and $\dot{V}E/\dot{V}CO_2$ at the *AT* along with other variables were predictive, but the $\dot{V}E$-$\dot{V}CO_2$ slope and peak $\dot{V}O_2$ had the strongest relationships. The combination of peak $\dot{V}O_2$ and diffusing capacity for carbon monoxide (DLCO) at rest was the strongest combined index. Among the largest studies relating pulmonary hypertension in IPF to CPET and prognosis is the study by Gläser et al.[122] Seventy-three out of 135 patients with IPF had pulmonary hypertension identified by right heart catheterization. Patients with pulmonary hypertension could be best identified by $\dot{V}E$-$\dot{V}CO_2$ slope (cutoff value ≥152.4% of predicted), peak $\dot{V}O_2$ (percentage predicted) ≤56%, and DLCO at rest. Sensitivity ranged from 59.7% to 88.9% and specificity from 56.4% to 88.4%. Survival over about a 48-month period was closely tied to presence of pulmonary hypertension diagnosed invasively.

In a multicenter study of 433 patients with cystic fibrosis who fulfilled criteria for a maximal test, time to death or lung transplantation was related to peak $\dot{V}O_2$ percentage predicted, peak work rate, $\dot{V}E/\dot{V}O_2$, and $\dot{V}E/\dot{V}CO_2$ at the *AT*, after adjustment for covariates that had been associated with poor outcomes previously, suggesting that CPET was a valuable addition to other prognostic indicators.[123]

Similar to patients with COPD, dynamic hyperinflation during exercise is a common finding in cystic fibrosis. Stevens et al[124] tested 109 adult patients and found that 58% demonstrated dynamic hyperinflation significantly related to severity of FEV_1 and forced vital capacity (FVC), but the presence of dynamic hyperinflation in this study was not associated with the likelihood of a pulmonary exacerbation over the next 2 years.

PREOPERATIVE EVALUATION OF SURGICAL RISK

Evaluating the risk of major surgery complications, particularly in the frail and elderly, is an important application of CPET. Older et al,[125] Ridgway et al,[8] and Wilson et al[126] have shown that the ability of the heart, lungs, pulmonary, and the peripheral circulations to support an increased metabolic rate in the postoperative period can be evaluated by preoperative CPET. In other words, a patient's capacity to increase oxygen delivery during exercise correlates with ability for maintaining organ system function after surgery. The CPET, especially determination of the peak $\dot{V}O_2$ and *AT*, and $\dot{V}E/\dot{V}CO_2$

at the *AT* has been shown to be useful in identifying high-risk surgical patients, including those judged to have normal cardiopulmonary function by clinical assessments and measurements made during rest. A CPET is useful, particularly in evaluating the elderly prior to surgery, for identifying patients with unsuspected heart, lung disease, and for quantifying cardiorespiratory reserve prior to lung resection surgery.

Thoracic Surgery

Patients being considered for noncardiac thoracic surgery, usually for resection for lung cancer, may be at particular risk of postoperative complications including cardiorespiratory insufficiency. The CPET has been suggested as a valuable adjunct because spirometry, radionuclide scanning, and arterial blood gases have not been completely successful in identifying all high-risk patients and, most important, may miss patients with significant cardiovascular disease. Conversely, and importantly, because resectional surgery remains the most effective therapy for lung cancer, CPET may identify patients who may be able to tolerate resection even though results of resting lung function alone might suggest otherwise.

Smith et al[127] retrospectively reported 22 patients who underwent elective thoracotomy and found 11 who had postoperative respiratory failure, myocardial infarction, arrhythmias, lobar atelectasis, pulmonary embolism, or death. These 11 patients had a significantly lower mean peak $\dot{V}O_2$ than those without complications after surgery. A total of 91% of patients with complications had a peak $\dot{V}O_2$ during cycle ergometry of less than 20 mL/kg/min. In this study, 6 of 6 patients who had a peak $\dot{V}O_2$ of less than 15 mL/min/kg and 4 of 6 patients who had a peak $\dot{V}O_2$ between 15 and 20 mL/min/kg had complications. Similarly, a peak $\dot{V}O_2$ of less than 10 mL/kg/min identified the 2 patients who died and the majority of postoperative complications among 50 patients reported by Bechard and Wetstein.[128]

Bolliger et al[129] found that peak $\dot{V}O_2$ during cycle ergometry, expressed as percentage predicted, was predictive of postresection complications such as CO_2 retention, prolonged mechanical ventilation, myocardial infarction, pneumonia, pulmonary embolism, and death. In a group of 80 patients, 8 of 9 patients with peak $\dot{V}O_2$ of less than 60% predicted had complications, whereas only 8 of the remaining 71 patients had complications. When patients had a peak $\dot{V}O_2$ greater than 75% of predicted, 90% were complication free. The same group used radionuclide scans based on projected loss of FEV_1 to estimate "postoperative" peak $\dot{V}O_2$. Patients with complications had a lower mean predicted postoperative peak $\dot{V}O_2$ (10.6 ± 3.6 mL/kg/min versus 14.8 ± 3.5 mL/kg/min), and, if <10 mL/kg/min, 100% mortality.[130]

A prospective study by Morice et al[131] provided additional evidence for the value of CPET in "high-risk" patients undergoing thoracotomy. A total of 37 patients had been considered inoperable because of a low FEV_1 (<40% predicted), an anticipated postsurgical FEV_1 of less than 33% predicted, an abnormal radionuclide scan, or a Pa_{CO_2} more than 45 mm Hg. Thirteen patients who underwent CPET had a peak $\dot{V}O_2$ greater than 15 mL/kg/min. Eight of these patients subsequently had resectional surgery. Although mean FEV_1 was poor in this group (mean 40% of predicted), 6 of 8 patients had an uncomplicated course, and all patients were discharged within 22 days of surgery. This study suggests that even some high-risk patients, based on resting lung function, can be more objectively assessed with data from CPET.

Current American College of Chest Physicians guidelines for physiological evaluation of lung resection candidates[132] recommend CPET with measurement of peak $\dot{V}O_2$ to define operative risk for patients with impaired lung function or with suspected comorbid cardiac disease. Peak $\dot{V}O_2$ measurements ≥20 mL/kg/min are associated with the lowest operative risks, and levels between 15 and 20 mL/kg/min with moderately increased risk. Levels of 10 to 15 mL/kg/min are predictive of increased incidence of perioperative complications, and levels of less than 10 mL/kg/min are generally felt to limit operative intervention due to high risk of morbidity and mortality from the procedure, regardless of the intensity of surgery.

Abdominal Surgery

Older et al[125] found, in a retrospective study of elderly patients undergoing major abdominal surgeries, that the *AT* obtained during CPET was particularly valuable in identifying risk of perioperative mortality. In 187 patients aged over 60 years, *AT* averaged 12.4 ± 2.7 mL/min/kg. If the *AT* was less than 11 mL/min/kg (found in 30% of the study patients), mortality from cardiovascular complications was 18%. On the other hand, if the *AT* was greater than 11 mL/min/kg, the cardiovascular death rate in the postoperative period was only 0.8%. Of interest, those patients who manifested evidence of myocardial ischemia in addition to having an *AT* of less than 11 mL/min/kg had a 42% mortality rate, whereas those with evidence of ischemia but with *AT* above 11 mL/min/kg had a mortality rate a tenth of that.

In a later prospective study of 548 patients over 60 years of age (or with ischemic heart disease), Older et al[133] used the *AT* to separate high from low risk for mortality following major surgery. Based on their earlier retrospective study, they used an *AT* of 11 mL/min/kg as the threshold for separating high from low risk. Patients without other predefined indications for monitoring were triaged to the ward for routine care if their *AT* was greater than 11 mL/min/kg, they had no ECG evidence of myocardial ischemia, and $\dot{V}E/\dot{V}O_2$ at the *AT* was less than 35. This represented 51% of the total population studied and none of these patients died of cardiovascular causes. A total of 21% of the population studied had an *AT* greater than 11 mL/min/kg but also had either ECG evidence of myocardial ischemia or $\dot{V}E/\dot{V}O_2$ at the *AT* of more than 35—a change found with heart failure. They were admitted to the intermediate care unit. Of this population, 1.7% (2 patients) died of cardiovascular causes. The remaining 28% (153 patients) of the starting population were identified as high risk based on an *AT* of less than 11 mL/min/kg or on the nature of the planned surgery.

These were triaged to the intensive care unit and had a 4.6% cardiovascular system mortality. Thus, use of CPET to determine the high-risk patient for major surgery allowed the services to use their high-care units for those people who were most ill and identified patients at low risk, as assessed by CPET, to be admitted directly to the ward. These observations triggered a number of subsequent studies of high risk surgical populations, which have broadly confirmed the prognostic value of exercise capacity in the context of high risk surgical candidates. These data were used as a basis for recommendations for preoperative CPET by the Preoperative Exercise Testing and Training Society.[134]

Current Recommendations for the Use of Preoperative Exercise Training ("PreHab") Prior to Thoracic or Abdominal Surgery

More recent reviews[134-137] and guidelines[2,132] have continued to help define the role of CPET in preoperative evaluation, including the potential role of preoperative rehabilitation training to reduce surgical complications. As such, there is an increasing literature on the role of 3 to 6 weeks of aerobic and strength exercise rehabilitation ("PreHab") in patients with suboptimal preoperative physiological studies to improve surgical outcomes.[138] However, this literature area at present suffers from several small "n," single-site studies, with nonstandard collection and assessment of operative and postoperative outcomes, and a lack of standardization of exercise training regiments, so that optimal use of exercise testing and training in this setting is not yet defined.

Who Should Undergo Cardiopulmonary Exercise Testing Preoperatively?

Several questions remain about the use of CPET in preoperative evaluation. First, who are the most suitable candidates? It is unlikely that all patients need to be tested, but patients with suspected cardiopulmonary disease (especially cardiac disease) may be confirmed with CPET. Older patients and those with marginal lung or cardiac function or limited exercise tolerance who might otherwise be excluded from major thoracic or abdominal surgery (as being at too high a risk for surgical complications) may be good candidates for CPET testing. Current European, American, and British guidelines differ in their recommendations for the physiological thresholds to perform CPET prior to lung resection surgery. Specifically, the European guidelines recommend CPET in any patient with an FEV_1 or D_{LCO} <80% predicted.[139] British guidelines recommend CPET when the patient's predicted postoperative FEV_1 or D_{LCO} are <40%.[140] Finally, the current American College of Chest Physicians guidelines[132] recommend CPET when either the predicted postoperative FEV_1 or D_{LCO} are <30% or the shuttle walk is <22 m. Each of these guidelines identifies a role for CPET in risk stratification, but there is not one unifying recommendation on selection of patients for testing at this time.

Second, there is the question about which CPET measures are useful for preoperative evaluation. Measurements of peak $\dot{V}O_2$ and *AT* provide objective data that can be used to identify high- and low-risk populations. Other measurements including $\dot{V}E/\dot{V}CO_2$ at the *AT*, $\dot{V}E$-$\dot{V}CO_2$ slope, and peak O_2 pulse have also been evaluated with conflicting results.

Third, there is a need to focus on postoperative complications relating to specific types of surgery, to standardize how these are categorized and documented, and to define the role of CPET in identifying those risks. The results of CPET in patients have been largely used in those undergoing thoracic (lung) and abdominal surgery. The value of CPET for predicting complications of other forms of surgery, such as heart or vascular surgery or orthopedic procedures, has not been well established. Finally, there is a need for more evidence that improvement in preoperative exercise capacity by smoking cessation, medical therapy, exercise training ("PreHab"), or other interventions can reduce peri- and postoperative risks.

DETERMINING IMPAIRMENT FOR DISABILITY EVALUATION

Impairment and Disability

The term *impairment*, as used in the United States, is a measurable, objective decrease in functional capacity, regardless of causation or situation, but not infrequently related to potential occupational exposures. *Disability* is an assessment of the impact of impairment on the individual and requires socioeconomic and environmental input, including factors such as age, gender, education, economic and social environment, and energy requirements of the occupation.[141] A World Health Organization statement[142] defined impairment as "any loss or abnormality of psychological, physiological, or anatomical structure or function," whereas disability was defined as "any restriction or lack (resulting from impairment) of ability to perform an activity within the range considered normal for a human being." Physicians are frequently asked to identify and measure impairment. Although medical opinions are often also sought about a patient's disability, such decisions are usually made through an administrative or legal process. The CPET permits objective measurement of physiological function, thereby determining impairment, not disability. The determination of disability is often even more complicated when attribution of cause leads to possible occupationally related lung or heart or other disease.

A CPET is indicated when a precise measurement of work capacity (work rate, peak $\dot{V}O_2$, or the *AT*) is required, or when symptoms or subjective exercise capacity are inconsistent with resting measurements. One potential advantage may be in evaluating people with one disorder (eg, heart disease, peripheral arterial disease) coexisting with another (eg, lung disease, increased blood carboxyhemoglobin from cigarette smoking or $\dot{V}A/\dot{Q}$ abnormality from pulmonary vascular occlusive disease in whom ventilatory drive is exceptionally high). In the case of the latter, mild to moderate defects in ventilatory mechanics might be sufficient to create intolerable dyspnea during mild exercise. In some patients, exercise capacity may be limited by a mechanism other than impairment in ventilatory mechanics detected by resting pulmonary function testing. Exercise-related abnormalities of arterial blood gas tensions and/or increased V_D/V_T may identify subtle evidence of respiratory disease as a cause of exercise limitation.

Assessing Impairment in Lung or Heart Disease Only Using Resting Measurements

In 1986, the American Thoracic Society statement on evaluation of impairment and disability secondary to respiratory disorders recommended a systematic evaluation process.[141] The statement was "concerned primarily with impairments related to reduced lung function," and presented a rating system for impairment from lung disease based on FVC, FEV_1, FEV_1/FVC, and single-breath D_{LCO}. It suggested that there was a well-documented relation between measurements made at rest (eg, FEV_1 and D_{LCO}) and measurements made during exercise (peak $\dot{V}O_2$ and work capacity) and that the majority of individuals undergoing an evaluation for impairment would not require CPET.

This conclusion can be challenged, however, by considering whether maximum work capacity can be predicted from resting pulmonary function. As an example, begin by assuming that an adult individual's $FEV_1 = 1.5$ L (moderately reduced for an average size adult). If FEV_1 is used to predict maximum exercise $\dot{V}E$ by using two reported estimates ($FEV_1 \times 35$ and $FEV_1 \times 40$),[143] maximum $\dot{V}E$ values would range from 52.5 L/min to 60 L/min. Next, assume that V_D/V_T at maximum exercise ranges from a low of 0.15 in a normal individual to 0.40 in a patient with moderate $\dot{V}A/\dot{Q}$ mismatching from lung disease. Using this range, the estimated maximum alveolar ventilation ($\dot{V}A$; ie, $\dot{V}A = \dot{V}E \times [1 - V_D/V_T]$) would range from 31.5 to 51 L/min for the maximum $\dot{V}E$ values calculated from the FEV_1 value of 1.5 L. Then, assuming that Pa_{CO_2} is between 25 to 35 mm Hg (not unusual numbers), one could estimate the extremes of $\dot{V}CO_2$ that could be present by the following equation:

$$\dot{V}CO_2 \text{ L/min (STPD)} = Pa_{CO_2} \times \dot{V}A \text{ L/min (BTPS)} / 863 \quad (4)$$

The estimated $\dot{V}CO_2$, using these example figures, ranges from 0.91 to 2.10 L/min. Finally, $\dot{V}O_2$ is related to $\dot{V}CO_2$ (as $\dot{V}O_2 = \dot{V}CO_2/R$), and R at maximum exercise typically ranges from about 0.9 to 1.2. Therefore, our hypothetical individual's peak $\dot{V}O_2$ might be as low as 0.76 L/min or as high as 2.33 L/min for the same FEV_1 using the extremes for each of the values identified (see **Table 8.4** and **8.5**).

TABLE 8.4 Potential Range of Peak $\dot{V}O_2$ and Peak Work Rate for a Hypothetical Individual With FEV_1 = 1.5 L[a,b]

FEV_1, L	Multiply by to estimate MVV	MVV or peak $\dot{V}E$, L/min	V_D/V_T	$\dot{V}A$, L/min	Pa_{CO_2}, mm Hg	$\dot{V}CO_2$, L/min	R	$\dot{V}O_2$, L/min	Est WR, Watts
1.5	35	52.5	0.30	36.8	25	1.06	1.2	0.89	32
							0.9	1.18	61
					35	1.49	1.2	1.24	67
							0.9	1.66	109
			0.15	44.6	25	1.29	1.2	1.08	51
							0.9	1.44	87
					35	1.81	1.2	1.51	94
							0.9	2.01	144
	40	60.0	0.30	42.0	25	1.22	1.2	1.01	44
							0.9	1.35	78
					35	1.70	1.2	1.42	85
							0.9	1.89	132
			0.15	51.0	25	1.48	1.2	1.23	66
							0.9	1.64	107
					35	2.07	1.2	1.72	115
							0.9	2.30	173

Abbreviations: Est WR, estimated work rate; FEV_1, forced expiratory volume in the first second of expiration; MVV, maximum voluntary ventilation. $\dot{V}A$, alveolar ventilation; $\dot{V}CO_2$, CO_2 output; V_D/V_T, dead space/tidal volume ratio; $\dot{V}E$, minute ventilation; $\dot{V}O_2$, O_2 uptake.

[a]An individual with an FEV_1 of 1.5 L may have a calculated MVV ("indirect MVV") typically = 35 × FEV_1 or 40 × FEV_1. Assuming he or she achieves this value at peak exercise, this would be the peak $\dot{V}E$. For plausible V_D/V_T values of 0.15 or 0.30, estimated peak alveolar ventilation is given by $\dot{V}A = \dot{V}E \times (1 - V_D/V_T)$. For a plausible Pa_{CO_2} at peak exercise of 25 or 35 mm Hg, $\dot{V}CO_2 = (\dot{V}A \times 863) / Pa_{CO_2}$. For these values with respiratory exchange ratio (RER) assumed to be either 0.9 or 1.2, estimated peak $\dot{V}O_2 = \dot{V}CO_2 / R$. Finally, the estimated peak work rate can be calculated as: (Peak $\dot{V}O_2$ minus the unloaded cycling $\dot{V}O_2$, in mL/min) / 10.1 mL/min/W. Unloaded cycling $\dot{V}O_2$ is estimated from weight as 151 + (6 × weight in kg) (see figure 4.2).

[b]The peak $\dot{V}O_2$ and peak WR extremes illustrate the concept that estimates of maximum work capacity (peak $\dot{V}O_2$) and work rate (peak WR) may vary considerably for individuals with the same FEV_1.

TABLE 8.5 Percentage of Diagnostic Causes of Reduced Work Capacity in 138 Workers With Impairment[a,b]

69% cardiovascular
41% cardiac
28% peripheral arterial or other
14% airway obstruction
4% restrictive lung disease
11% neurologic or musculoskeletal
2% obesity

[a]Impairment is defined as peak $\dot{V}O_2$ below the 95% confidence limit of predicted.

[b]Data from Oren A, Sue DY, Hansen JE, Torrance DJ, Wasserman K. The role of exercise testing in impairment evaluation. *Am Rev Respir Dis.* 1987;135(1):230-235.

In conclusion, although the *ventilatory capacity* of the respiratory system may be successfully predicted from resting FEV_1 ("estimated maximum voluntary ventilation," and this, too, is open to question), the *ventilatory requirement* for a given work rate during exercise cannot be accurately predicted from resting pulmonary function measurements in the face of disease. This is consistent with the experience in chronic heart failure, for which it is widely accepted that resting measurements are poor for assessment of prognosis and functional capacity.

Exercise Testing and Impairment Evaluation

A number of investigators have provided a foundation for the role of integrative CPET for determination of impairment due to lung or cardiovascular disease.[144-154] Exercise testing complements clinical evaluation and adds to resting pulmonary function and imaging studies. It increases diagnostic accuracy both quantitatively (measurement of work capacity, peak $\dot{V}O_2$, and progressively increasing or sustainable work capacity) and qualitatively (identification of the cause of exercise limitation).

The Committee on Social Security Cardiovascular Disability Criteria was tasked to assist the Social Security Administration with revising criteria for cardiovascular disability in its "Listing of Impairments."[155] In this detailed monograph, they determined that exercise tests are generally safe for patients with heart diseases. They recommended that determining peak $\dot{V}O_2$ during a symptom-limited treadmill or cycle-ergometer exercise test is the most objective method to assess exercise capacity in heart failure patients and stated that it was useful to determine both the severity of disease and whether heart failure is the cause of exercise limitation. They proposed that peak $\dot{V}O_2$ less than 15 mL/kg/min should be a criterion for exercise impairment. For tests conducted without gas exchange measurement, they estimated 5 metabolic equivalents (METs) (where 1 MET equals the resting metabolic rate, assumed by convention to be 3.5 mL/min/kg) or less would be consistent with that peak $\dot{V}O_2$. They provided recommendations for disability listing that included combinations of symptoms and resting ejection fraction, along with frequency of hospitalizations or objective measurement of exercise limitation (or cardiologist assessment of excessive risk of exercise testing).

Pulmonary function testing is the cornerstone of evaluation of impairment from any respiratory disease,[156] with guidance primarily based on the American Medical Association (AMA) *Guides to the Evaluation of Permanent Impairment*, sixth edition.[157] The AMA guide classifies resting pulmonary function into five classes of severity based primarily on vital capacity (VC), FEV_1, and D_{LCO}. The use of CPET should generally be considered when dyspnea is disproportionate to pulmonary function, concern is raised about subject effort, or when objective data is sought regarding specific job requirements. Sood[156] suggested that peak $\dot{V}O_2$ may be the "gold standard" for assessing impairment; however, it is difficult to understand how this value can be linked closely with sustained work capacity or the requirements of specific work tasks. Nevertheless, the sixth edition of the AMA guide provides a table associating "arduous work" with a peak $\dot{V}O_2$ >30 mL/kg/min down to "light work" at 7 mL/kg/min. It has been proposed that the basis for the commonly used peak $\dot{V}O_2$ <15 mL/kg/min for work limitation is likely related to the need for adequate sustained work capacity to travel to and from work.[156]

The potential for CPET to contribute to determination of the presence and the basis of work impairment is illustrated by our experience evaluating 490 current or retired shipyard workers.[149] Of this population, 348 men who had complaints of exercise limitation or who were suspected of having exercise limitation were studied using CPET with a 1-minute incremental cycle ergometry test. A conclusion was made by the physician referring the patient for exercise studies as to the likelihood of exercise limitation, if any, and the specific organ system limiting exercise. This determination was based on chest roentgenograms, resting pulmonary function tests, resting ECG, medical history, physical examination, and smoking history (**Fig. 8.6**) but not CPET. Following CPET, another conclusion was made but this time, using all data acquired during the evaluation, including the exercise test.

On the initial assessment, 148 subjects were predicted to have normal work capacity, but 46 of these subjects (31%) turned out to have a peak $\dot{V}O_2$ below the 95% confidence limit. The accuracy of the clinical prediction of a low work capacity was similar: 66 subjects were expected to have low work capacity; of these, only 43 (67%) were correctly categorized. Furthermore, the referring physicians could not judge whether the work capacity was normal or reduced in 134 subjects (38.5% of the total were evaluated to be indeterminate) without CPET.

Following CPET, 60% of the indeterminate group were found to have a normal peak $\dot{V}O_2$, and 37% had an abnormally low peak $\dot{V}O_2$. Although the magnitude of reduction of peak $\dot{V}O_2$ had a significant correlation with resting pulmonary function (VC, FEV_1, D_{LCO} as percentage predicted),

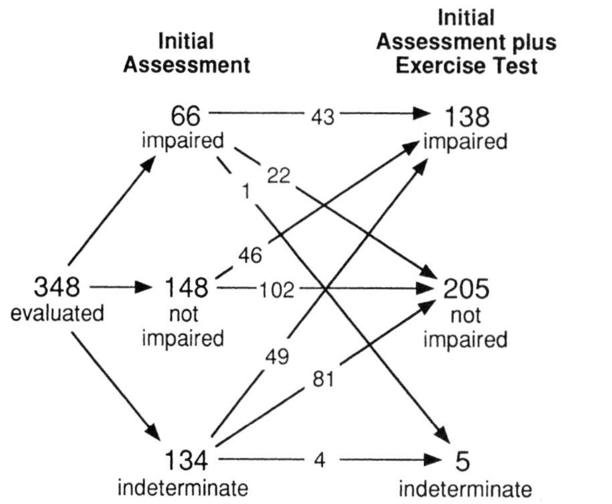

FIGURE 8.6. The influence of cardiopulmonary exercise testing on the evaluation of work impairment; 348 patients were initially referred for suspicion of functional impairment secondary to asbestos exposure. The initial assessment was done without exercise testing but with all other clinical modalities available to the evaluating physician. This assessment concluded that 66 were impaired, but no decision could be reached on 134 of the 348 patients being evaluated. In the final assessment, cardiopulmonary exercise data were added to the information available to the physician rendering the interpretation. This new information confirmed (cardiopulmonary exercise testing taken as the gold standard) impairment in 43 of the 66, with 22 going into the "not impaired" category and 1 into the indeterminate category. In contrast, 95 individuals were added to the impaired category: 46 from the "not impaired" category and 49 from the indeterminate category; 102 of the 148 individuals thought to be not impaired were confirmed as being not impaired. However, 81 were added to this category from the indeterminate category and 22 from the impaired category, making a total of 205 individuals for whom it was thought that there was no basis on which to conclude that the patient had a physiological impairment in the ability to perform physical work. Only 4 of the 134 individuals whose impairment was uncertain before cardiopulmonary exercise testing remained in this category after the cardiopulmonary exercise test.

prediction of reduced work capacity from resting pulmonary function was often unhelpful. Overall, 138 workers had abnormally low peak $\dot{V}O_2$. Of these, 43 were correctly predicted to be impaired without CPET, whereas a further 46 were incorrectly predicted to be normal without CPET, and 49 who had impairment by CPET were indeterminate without it (see **Fig. 8.6**). The sensitivity of resting pulmonary function tests, chest roentgenograms, and other studies for detecting low peak $\dot{V}O_2$ was only about 31%.

The cause of exercise limitation in this setting may not be reflected in resting studies, largely because the most often used resting data are the tests of pulmonary function. Among our 138 subjects with low peak $\dot{V}O_2$, only 25 were limited by obstructive or restrictive lung diseases, whereas in 95 (69%) of 138 cases, the exercise limitation was due to cardiovascular diseases (**Table 8.5**). The presence of a high proportion of cardiovascular disease in this patient population is not unique; Agostoni et al[144] similarly found that 37% of 120 asbestos workers had unexpected cardiac limitation rather than ventilatory limitation.

Oxygen Cost of Work

In approximate terms, the oxygen cost ($\dot{V}O_2$) for performing office work might be about 5 to 7 mL/kg/min, for moderate labor about 15 mL/kg/min, and for strenuous labor 20 to 30 mL/kg/min. Some guidelines suggest, in addition, that workers can perform manual labor at a comfortable work pace when this was approximately 40% of maximal $\dot{V}O_2$, a value approximating the $\dot{V}O_2$ average at the *AT* in sedentary normal adults.

Having obtained measurements of peak $\dot{V}O_2$ and *AT*, it might be tempting to relate these to the oxygen cost of specific work tasks. Estimates of the O_2 costs of various physical activities, occupations, and specific kinds of movements exist.[158] For given individuals who differ in age, weight, gender, rate of work, efficiency of movement, or degree of intermittency of the work task, however, the true metabolic cost of work ($\dot{V}O_2$) should vary greatly. For this reason, we recommend that the predicted metabolic cost of particular tasks be used as broad estimates rather than providing precise task-specific metabolic costs. For clinicians regularly performing assessments of occupational fitness or impairment, the use of exercise protocols designed to simulate occupational tasks or use of field testing with portable gas exchange measurement devices may have particular practical utility.

EXERCISE TRAINING OR REHABILITATION

Physiological Basis of Exercise Rehabilitation

Endurance exercise training is commonly used to improve exercise tolerance and quality of life. There are benefits to exercise training both in healthy individuals (including athletes) and in a number of patient groups. It is widely conceded that an aerobic exercise-training regimen is the most beneficial portion of rehabilitation programs, and CPET is uniquely suited to gauge the specific benefits of exercise training. In addition to helping one understand the specific physiological changes induced by the exercise training, CPET serves to rule out coexisting disease processes that could contraindicate a rigorous exercise program.

The beneficial effects of aerobic exercise training can include (see Chapter 2)[159-167]

1. Increasing muscle mass, capillary density, biochemical capacity, and mitochondrial number
2. Improving the distribution of blood and therefore O_2 flow to the contracting muscle, thereby reducing the cardiac (heart rate) stress
3. Reducing the lactic acidosis at a given supra-*AT* work rate, resulting in a decrease in CO_2 and H^+ production, ventilatory drive, and dyspnea at a given work rate
4. Improving the patient's sense of well-being

Understanding the physiological changes that occur in response to exercise training is important both for prescribing training and rehabilitation interventions and for interpreting CPET results for trained versus untrained individuals. These changes are discussed in the following sections.

Skeletal Muscle

An effective program of endurance training influences functions such as muscle hypertrophy, fiber type transformations, metabolic changes, and angiogenesis in the trained musculature via signaling pathways that regulate gene expression and protein turnover. A detailed discussion is beyond the scope of this chapter, but the interested reader is referred to these references.[161,168,169] As discussed in Chapter 2 ("Skeletal Muscle: Mechanical Properties and Fiber Types" section), skeletal muscles are composed of two major varieties of contractile cells. Type I, oxidative, or slow-twitch fibers are designed for prolonged repetitive contraction. The type IIb (or IIx), glycolytic, or fast-twitch fibers have rapid contractile properties but a limited capacity for prolonged repetitive contraction, while type IIa fibers represent an intermediate type II subpopulation having a degree of oxidative potential. The relative proportion of these two fiber types varies from muscle group to muscle group in a given individual and for the same muscle in different individuals. Type IIa fibers can be transformed into type I fibers, and type IIx fibers can remodel into type IIa fibers. These changes are reflected in an increased oxidative profile. For example, mitochondrial number and size increase in type I fibers. Enzyme activities in both the cytosol and the mitochondria are upregulated, facilitating Krebs (or tricarboxylic acid) cycle reactions and mitochondrial oxidative phosphorylation (see Chapter 2, "Bioenergetics" section). The capacity to oxidatively metabolize the end product of glycolysis (ie, pyruvate), fatty acids, and ketone bodies is therefore increased, resulting in less lactate production at a given submaximal work rate. In parallel with the increased ability to use oxygen, the ability to supply oxygen by improved blood flow to the muscle cells increases. Myoglobin levels in the trained type I muscle are higher; this may contribute to the ability to transport oxygen from the muscle capillary to the mitochondrial site of oxidative metabolism. If muscle capillaries proliferate out of proportion to the increase in muscle fiber size with training, the diffusion distance from the oxygen source (hemoglobin in the muscle capillary) to the oxygen sink (the mitochondrion in the muscle cell) is reduced, allowing a given level of mitochondrial oxygen consumption to be sustained at a lower capillary P_{O_2}. These structural and biochemical changes are seen only in the muscle groups involved in the training regimen; this is known as the "principle of specificity." For example, walking or running does not induce such changes in the arm muscles. Similarly, training on a stationary bicycle will not fully translate into improvements in running performance because different groups of muscles are involved. Also, body composition usually changes as a result of an effective program of endurance training. The size of the trained muscles increases with endurance training consequent to the hypertrophic response, which is reflected in an increased lean body mass.

Cardiac Output and Heart Rate

After an effective program of training in normal individuals (see Chapter 2, "Cardiac Output" section) and patients who had been physically inactive for prolonged periods, the cardiovascular system undergoes significant changes as a result of the training. The heart hypertrophies with increases in both ventricular wall thickness and chamber size, with stroke volume being higher at rest, at any given work rate, and at peak exercise. However, as cardiac output at rest and at a given work rate is unaffected after exercise training, the corresponding heart rate responses will be distinctly lower, although peak heart rate is unchanged. As a result, cardiac output at peak exercise is increased. Both systolic and diastolic blood pressures tend to be lower after training, especially in the hypertensive individual. Training may not increase cardiac output and stroke volume in patients with heart disease. However, heart rate is reduced at a given work rate after training, presumably due to better blood flow distribution to the working muscles and perhaps improved capillarization of muscle fibers, allowing an increase in O_2 extraction.[7,170]

Arterial Blood (Lactate)

The improved oxygen delivery to the more densely distributed mitochondria and the improved mitochondrial capability for aerobic metabolism that results from remodeling of the exercising muscles following an effective program of endurance training delays the onset of anaerobic metabolism. Thus, at any given work rate above the pretraining *AT*, arterial blood lactate levels are lower after exercise

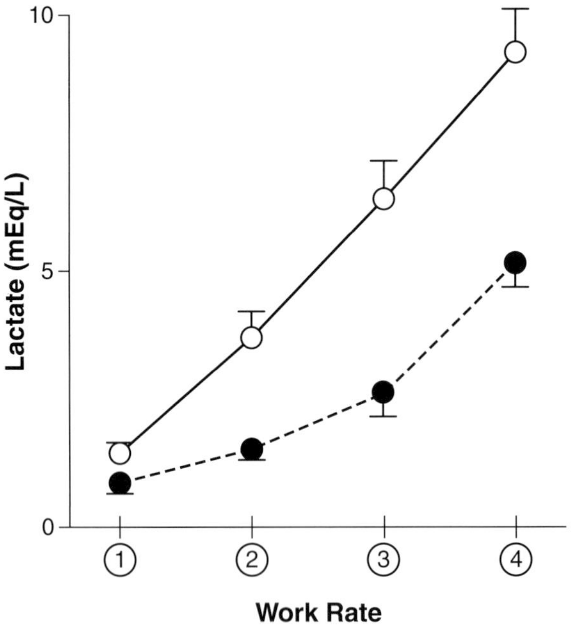

FIGURE 8.7. Effect of endurance training on end-exercise arterial blood lactate levels at four work rates. Values plotted are the average (± standard error) responses of 10 individuals before (solid line) and after (dashed line) endurance training. Individuals exercised for 15 minutes at work rates ranging from moderate (work rate 1) to very heavy intensity (work rate 4). After training, blood lactate levels are lower in response to identical exercise tasks. *(Reproduced with permission from Casaburi R, Storer TW, Ben-Dov I, Wasserman K. Effect of endurance training on possible determinants of $\dot{V}O_2$ during heavy exercise.* J Appl Physiol. *1987;62[1]:199-207. Copyright © 1987 American Physiological Society. All rights reserved.)*

training (**Fig. 8.7**).[171,172] Sullivan et al[173] demonstrated that knowledge of peak $\dot{V}O_2$ and *AT* allowed good prediction of an individual's blood lactate level in response to a given level of constant work rate exercise.

Oxygen Uptake

Endurance training increases maximal $\dot{V}O_2$, largely because maximal cardiac output increases with little or no widening of the maximal arteriovenous O_2 content difference. In healthy individuals, improvements on the order of 8% to 15% are commonly seen. For typical ramp-type incremental exercise tests, $\dot{V}O_2$ below the *AT* is not altered appreciably by training. Over the full work rate range for such tests, differences are difficult to discern (the overall $\Delta\dot{V}O_2/\Delta WR$ slope remains approximately 10 mL/min/W).

Effective exercise training typically results in more rapid phase II $\dot{V}O_2$ kinetics, thereby reducing the magnitude of the oxygen deficit at a given sub-*AT* work rate and reducing the size of the $\dot{V}O_2$ slow component at a given supra-*AT* work rate in close proportion to the associated decrease in arterial blood [lactate] (see Chapter 2, "Oxygen Uptake Kinetics" section).[171,172] Despite this close correlation, the mechanism of this decreased supra-*AT* oxygen requirement remains controversial (see Chapter 2, "Oxygen Uptake Kinetics" section).

Ventilation

In both the steady state and during exercise transients, $\dot{V}E$ responds in close proportion to CO_2 output (see Chapter 2, "Ventilatory Control" section). After training, at a given supra-*AT* work rate, $\dot{V}E$ is lower in proportion to the associated decrease in CO_2 output, the latter primarily due to the reduced bicarbonate (HCO_3^-) buffering of the lactic acidosis. Moreover, because of a less marked lactic acidosis, H^+ stimulation of the carotid bodies is reduced, resulting in less hyperventilation at a given supra-*AT* work rate (see Chapter 2 "Ventilatory Control" section). This means that $PaCO_2$ is higher at a given supra-*AT* work rate. **Figure 8.8** shows the responses to 15 minutes of exercise at four progressively higher work rates before and after a program of endurance training, there being an appreciably lower $\dot{V}E$ response at the supra-*AT* work rates posttraining.

Other Physiological Responses

Blood catecholamine and other hormonal responses to a given level of heavy exercise are often considerably lower after training.[172,174,175] The body temperature increase that occurs with exercise can also be attenuated.[171,176] The rating of perceived exertion is also generally reduced,[177] although whether this is predominantly linked to improved physiological function or to psychological factors is unclear.[178]

Exercise Rehabilitation in Heart Disease

The objective of exercise training is to improve both exercise tolerance and quality of life. Because patients with heart disease become physically inactive as a result of reduced ability to deliver blood to the muscles of locomotion, the skeletal muscles undergo change characteristic of detraining. The American Heart Association Committee on Exercise, Rehabilitation, and Prevention[179] wrote a comprehensive statement on the role of exercise in chronic heart failure. In contrast to the practice up until about 30 to 40 years ago, when patients with heart failure were put to bed to *rest* their hearts, patients with heart failure are now put on *exercise training* programs. The statement summarizes many studies showing the benefits of exercise training, in which exercise tolerance and peak $\dot{V}O_2$ are increased, the latter by 12% to 31%, depending on the study and the particular training schedule employed. The training effect was, however, consistently correlated with the duration of the program. No significant exercise-related complications were reported. Despite the

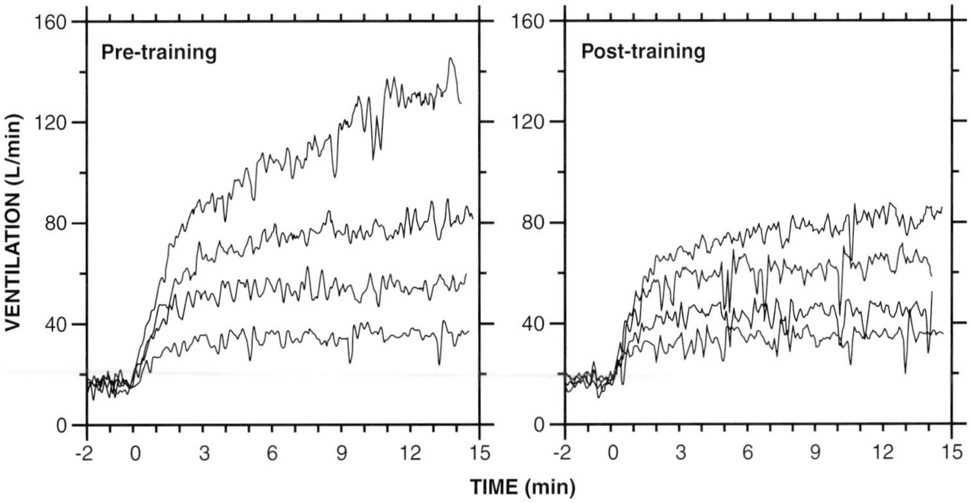

FIGURE 8.8. Effect of endurance training on the breath-by-breath time course of ventilation following the onset of constant work rate exercise in a healthy individual. Left: Pretraining responses to 95, 148, 191, and 233 W. Right: Posttraining responses to identical work rates after 8 weeks of endurance training. Note the marked decrease in ventilation at the higher work rates after training. *(Reproduced with permission from Casaburi R, Storer TW, Ben-Dov I, Wasserman K. Effect of endurance training on possible determinants of $\dot{V}O_2$ during heavy exercise.* J Appl Physiol. *1987;62[1]:199-207. Copyright © 1987 American Physiological Society. All rights reserved.)*

consistent increase in peak $\dot{V}O_2$ and exercise tolerance with training found in patients with heart failure, no consistent echocardiographic changes are demonstrable.

It has not been demonstrated that circulating catecholamine levels consistently decrease with exercise training in patients with heart failure, in contrast to normal individuals exercising above the pretraining *AT*.[171,172] However, as for normal individuals (see **Fig. 8.7**), exercise training in patients with heart failure reduces arterial [lactate] and its accompanying $[H^+]$ response at a given supra-*AT* work rate. Consequently, exercise ventilatory drive, as in normal individuals, is also decreased (see **Fig. 8.8**).[180,181] However, in contrast to the predominant mechanism for the decrease in $\dot{V}E$ with training in normal individuals, which is attributable to a delayed lactic acidosis, some of the decrease in $\dot{V}E$ in heart failure might be attributed to a decrease in the often markedly elevated VD/VT. Some investigators also attribute the decrease in $\dot{V}E$ to attenuation of an abnormally stimulated ergoreflex originating in skeletal muscle.[182]

Exercise training results in a decrease in heart rate at a given $\dot{V}O_2$. Some of this reduction in heart rate might be due to an increase in stroke volume, as reported in some studies, but most is thought to be due to peripheral changes and better perfusion of and O_2 extraction by the muscles involved in the exercise. When cardiac function and the ability to increase cardiac output improve, the changes in muscle that came about due to inactivity may be reversed. Thus, the contribution of muscle atrophy to the exercise limitation might be alleviated with exercise training.

With that logic in mind, Itoh and Kato[183] studied the effect of short-term training after cardiac surgery for valvular heart disease and coronary artery bypass graft surgery. As their training work rate, they used that at the *AT* rather than the level that was recommended by the American College of Sports Medicine,[184] which is 40% to 85% of the above-rest predicted maximum heart rate. They found the latter impractical both because of the range of recommended heart rate and also because most of the patients were receiving β-adrenergic receptor blockade therapy, thus limiting the heart rate response. Using peak $\dot{V}O_2$, *AT*, $\Delta\dot{V}O_2/\Delta WR$, and the time constant for the $\dot{V}O_2$ response to constant work rate exercise as outcome measures, they found significant improvement in aerobic function in the group of postsurgery patients who underwent exercise training but not in the control group of postsurgery patients who did not undergo exercise training. The authors reasoned that the work rate at the subject's *AT* would be a safe and effective work level for exercise training in these cardiac patients, specifically, because at the *AT* the O_2 requirements for the work would be met (ie, there was by definition no significant lactic acidosis), the heart would not be "overstressed." The sympathetic nervous system is not excessively stimulated at the *AT*, as evidenced by only minor changes in circulating norepinephrine and epinephrine levels, in contrast to the increases at higher work rates (see Chapter 2). Patients find this training program acceptable because they can maintain exercise at the *AT* over a prolonged period of time.

Using similar logic to Itoh and Kato,[183] Dubach et al[185] examined the effect of a 2-month endurance exercise training program using a combination of walking and cycling training at a work rate comparable to the subject's *AT*. Training was started approximately 36 days after myocardial infarction. Myocardial injury, as evaluated by magnetic resonance imaging of the heart, was not extended by the training program. The trained patients increased peak $\dot{V}O_2$ and *AT* by 26% and 39%, respectively, whereas there was no detectable improvement in the nontrained control group.

Belardinelli et al[186] studied the effect of exercise training on LV diastolic filling in patients with dilated cardiomyopathy using pulsed Doppler echocardiography. They found that exercise training increased the *AT* and peak $\dot{V}O_2$ by improving the impairment of LV relaxation via an improvement in peak early filling of the left ventricle.

The key physiological effect of training in the heart disease patient is the reduction in heart rate, thereby allowing increased blood flow through the coronary blood vessels and more time for cardiac filling during diastole. Also, because of more aerobic and less anaerobic regeneration of ATP after training, the lactic acidosis is less severe at a given level of supra-*AT* exercise. Thus, there is less ventilatory drive and therefore less ventilatory stress. Finally, of great importance is a greater sense of well-being in patients as they find that they are becoming physically stronger and, as a consequence, more active.

Exercise Rehabilitation in Chronic Obstructive Pulmonary Disease

The National Emphysema Treatment Trial and other randomized trials support the concept that exercise training improves exercise tolerance and reduces dyspnea on exertion in patients with COPD undergoing rehabilitation.[187,188] The CPET provides unequivocal evidence of the physiological benefits of training in these patients. Although most of the studies have been in patients with COPD, beneficial effects of exercise programs[188] have also been published in patients with cystic fibrosis,[189] interstitial lung disease,[190] and asthma.[191]

Patients with COPD are usually ventilatory limited, that is, their exercise tolerance is limited by the level of $\dot{V}E$ that they can attain and/or sustain. This occurs both because the $\dot{V}E$ that can be attained is low while the $\dot{V}E$ required for a given work rate is high (see **Fig. 4.6**). The low $\dot{V}E$ ceiling is related to the impaired lung mechanics and is manifest as a functionally zero breathing reserve (ie, when ventilatory capacity is measured by the maximum voluntary ventilation maneuver or $FEV_1 \times 40$; see **Fig. 4.9**). Although we can predict that respiratory muscle fatigue is induced by the high work of breathing resulting from high expiratory airway resistance and hyperinflation-induced mechanical disadvantage of the diaphragm and chest wall muscles,[192] the evidence for this is not straightforward. The tidal volume usually does not get smaller, and $\dot{V}E$ does not decrease as exercise is sustained. However, it is not unusual for $PaCO_2$ to increase as work rate increases, providing evidence that alveolar ventilation cannot keep pace with the CO_2 load.

The high $\dot{V}E$ requirement for a given level of exercise is dictated by inefficient gas exchange (high V_D/V_T), hypoxic and H^+ stimulation of $\dot{V}E$, resulting from the lactic acidosis and associated CO_2 production.[193,194] In some patients, lactic acidosis at a low work rate, as a result of detraining, is contributory to the increased ventilatory drive. But detraining does not reduce the ability of the muscles to extract and use O_2 from the blood. Maltais et al[195] showed that the leg muscles of COPD patients are capable of extracting O_2 normally, suggesting that a primary muscle-bioenergetic defect is not limiting exercise tolerance in these patients. Also, the studies of Richardson et al[196] demonstrate that if the ventilatory and cardiac requirements of exercise are reduced by exercising only one leg at a time, the exercising leg can increase its work capacity as compared with both legs performing the same exercise simultaneously. These studies suggest that defects in the leg muscles do not limit exercise capacity in COPD.

Because patients with moderate to severe COPD are typically ventilatory limited, it is logical to turn our attention to modalities that can reduce their abnormal increases in ventilatory drive during exercise. For example, the onset of lactic acidosis at a low work rate, coupled with arterial hypoxemia and decreased oxygen delivery to the tissues (due to increased pulmonary vascular resistance, decreased cardiac output as a result of the interference of lung mechanics on cardiac function,[197] or inefficient muscle perfusion) might all be expected to contribute to increase the exacerbated $\dot{V}E$ requirement. Although some of these abnormalities are likely related to severe deconditioning due to inactivity,[198] a myopathy related to corticosteroid use might also be a factor.

Although some doubt was at one time cast that COPD patients could or would gain physiological benefits from a program of exercise training, it is now generally viewed as one of the most effective interventions in this population.[187,199,200] Rational strategies—chief among them the use of work rates that are a high percentage of peak exercise tolerance[201]—have demonstrated that physiological benefits *are* achievable. Thus, it is possible to decrease the exercise lactic acidosis by exercise training (**Fig. 8.9**), thereby reducing H^+ and CO_2 production. The CPET shows that exercise tolerance is increased after a rigorous program of rehabilitative exercise training in COPD patients.[193,202] In a group of patients with predominantly moderate COPD, training-induced reductions in $\dot{V}E$ requirement were closely correlated with the reduction in arterial blood lactate levels (**Fig. 8.10**).[193] In a group of patients with more severe disease, the reduction in $\dot{V}E$ requirement was associated with the adoption of a more efficient (slower, deeper) breathing pattern.[203]

Besides determining the degree (and mechanism) of improvement in exercise tolerance that occurs as a result of an exercise program, CPET has other well-defined uses in the context of pulmonary rehabilitation[188]:

1. Identify contraindications to an exercise training program.

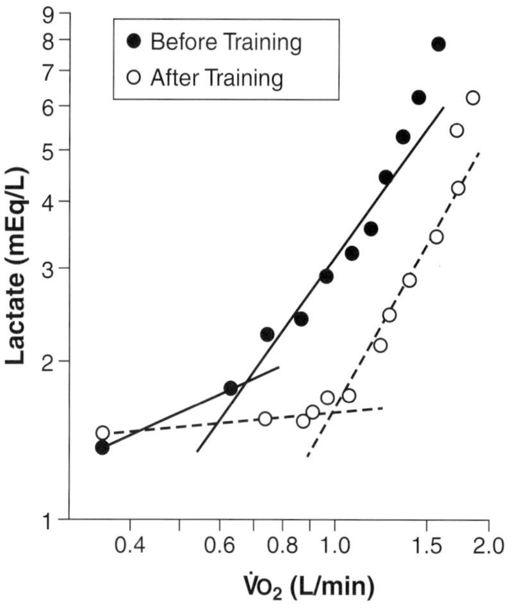

FIGURE 8.9. Arterial blood lactate levels, before and after training, during incremental exercise in a patient with chronic obstructive pulmonary disease undergoing rehabilitation. Arterial [lactate] is plotted versus oxygen uptake on a log-log scale. Closed circles are responses before training; open circles are responses after training. Before training, [lactate] rises very early in exercise. After training, the [lactate] rise is delayed, and the anaerobic threshold (point of intersection of two linear segments) occurs at a considerably higher $\dot{V}O_2$, indicating that a physiological training response has occurred. *(Reprinted with permission of the American Thoracic Society. Copyright © 2020 American Thoracic Society. All rights reserved. From Casaburi R, Patessio A, Ioli F, Zanaboni S, Donner CF, Wasserman K. Reductions in exercise lactic acidosis and ventilation as a result of exercise training in patients with obstructive lung disease.* Am Rev Respir Dis. *1991;143(1):9-18. The American Review of Respiratory Disease* is an official journal of the American Thoracic Society. [*Now titled The American Journal of Respiratory and Critical Care Medicine])*

2. Create precise exercise prescription guidelines for the patient based on his or her physiological capacity.
3. Determine what mechanism(s) of exercise intolerance are present and clarifying their contribution to exercise limitation.
4. Assess the effect of the rehabilitation program on aerobic and ventilatory responses.

A further modality to increase exercise tolerance might be O_2 breathing to provide additional O_2 during exercise to the COPD patient, even if there is a small degree of arterial hypoxemia.[204] This maneuver could potentially have up to four effects. First and most obvious, it inhibits the carotid bodies' responses to hypoxemia and H^+, thereby reducing $\dot{V}E$ and slowing breathing rate. Second, as a consequence of the slower breathing rate, expiratory duration is increased allowing the patient to exhale to a lower end-expiratory lung volume than during air breathing. Third, O_2 has some bronchodilator action. Fourth, it allows for washout of nitrogen (N_2) from low-$\dot{V}A/\dot{Q}$ areas of the lungs, thereby allowing end-expiratory lung volume to adjust downward because some of the O_2 replacing the N_2 will be absorbed.

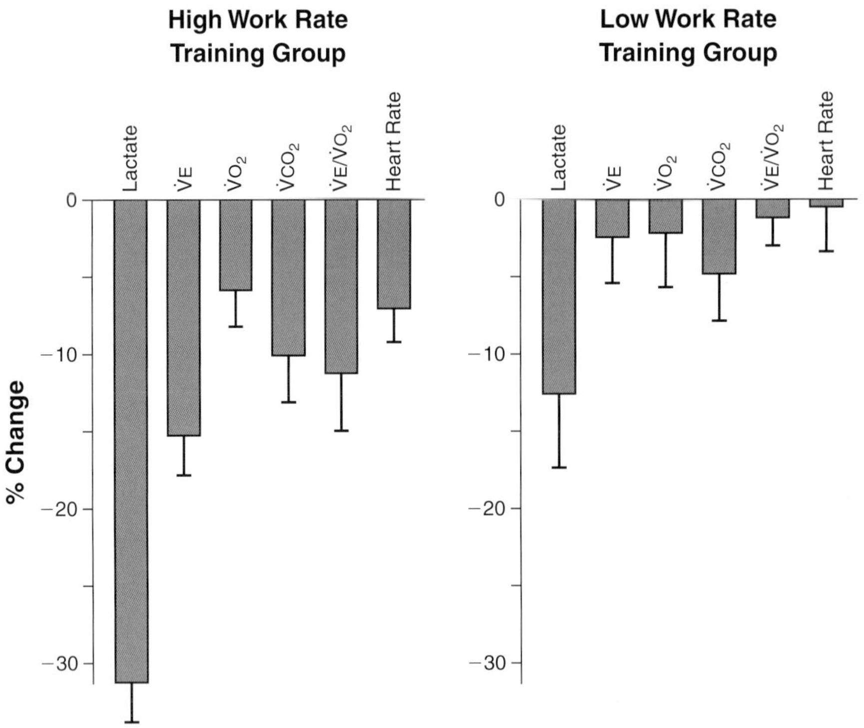

FIGURE 8.10. Changes in physiological responses to an identical exercise task produced by two exercise training strategies in patients with chronic obstructive pulmonary disease. Left: high work rate training group (n = 11). Right: low work rate training group (n = 8). Note that patients performed the same total work in their training program irrespective of group assignment. Percentage change is calculated from the average change in response at the time the pretraining study ended. Vertical lines represent 1 standard error of mean. Decreases in arterial [lactate], ventilation, O_2 uptake, CO_2 output, ventilatory equivalent for O_2, and heart rate are observed for both training regimens, but decreases are appreciably greater for the high work rate training group. *(Reprinted with permission of the American Thoracic Society. Copyright © 2020 American Thoracic Society. All rights reserved. From Casaburi R, Patessio A, Ioli F, Zanaboni S, Donner CF, Wasserman K. Reductions in exercise lactic acidosis and ventilation as a result of exercise training in patients with obstructive lung disease.* Am Rev Respir Dis. *1991;143[1]:9-18. The American Review of Respiratory Disease* is an official journal of the American Thoracic Society. [*Now titled The American Journal of Respiratory and Critical Care Medicine])*

ASSESSING THE EFFECTIVENESS OF TREATMENT

The major role of the heart, pulmonary circulation, cardiac, hematologic, and peripheral circulation systems is to cooperate in supporting cellular respiration at rest, and—specifically during exercise—the increased respiration of the involved skeletal muscles. That is, the skeletal muscle compartment undergoes the largest increase in respiration requirements of all the organs during exercise. Therefore, measurements of respiration and gas exchange in response to exercise should give the most direct global assessment of the function of these organ systems. Similarly, it can be expected that improvement in function related to effective treatment of the exercise-limiting disease, or conversely, worsening related to progression of disease, can be objectively documented with CPET.

To use CPET for the purpose of evaluating therapy, of course, it is necessary for the laboratory calibration to be accurate, to use sensitive end points, and to be consistent in methodology. The importance of quality control in CPET is well-illustrated by experience of clinical trialists. Cohn et al[205] emphasized the need for well-trained technicians and careful calibration of the cardiopulmonary exercise system in the context of the multicenter Vasodilator Heart Failure Trials of the Veterans Affairs Hospitals. Analysis of $\Delta\dot{V}O_2/\Delta WR$ values of control subjects in this trial led to discovery of problems related to measurement accuracy at some sites, which led to institution of appropriate quality control measures. Similar issues related to data quality were observed in a pulmonary hypertension trial[206] highlighting the importance of technical experience and quality control in the successful use of CPET in clinical research.

In contrast to clinical research trials, there is generally no external review of the accuracy of gas exchange data reported from a clinical laboratory, so it is particularly important that internal quality control processes are in place to identify the occurrence of measurement errors. **Figure 3.2** and the cases in Chapter 10 show the consistency of the value of $\Delta\dot{V}O_2/\Delta WR$ in normal individuals. This is best evaluated for quality control purposes by use of constant work rate tests with steady state measurement of $\dot{V}O_2$ at several different work rates of moderate intensity. Accuracy may be further validated when needed by using a metabolic simulator.[207]

Assuming measurements are made accurately, the physiological responses to exercise are highly reproducible in patients with stable pathophysiology. Hansen et al[208] studied patient performance reproducibility and reader reproducibility in 114 paired tests performed 1 to 3 days apart in 42 exercise-limited patients with PAH. Patient performance reproducibility rates were 5.8%, 6.5%, and 3.3%, and the reader reproducibility rates were 0.6%, 8.5%, and 2.1% for peak $\dot{V}O_2$, *AT*, and $\dot{V}E/\dot{V}CO_2$ at the *AT*, respectively.

Puente-Maestu et al[209] summarized the importance of exercise testing when used to assess outcomes of both pharmacologic and nonpharmacologic interventions in chronic lung diseases (eg, COPD, PAH, interstitial lung disease, cystic fibrosis). Their review summarized the use of incremental exercise tests, constant work rate (endurance) exercise tests performed to the limit of tolerance, incremental shuttle walk tests, endurance shuttle walk tests, and 6-minute walk tests as modalities used to assess the outcome of interventions. The authors concluded that high-intensity endurance constant work rate tests are more responsive to interventions than incremental exercise tests or 6-minute walk tests.

A number of cases are presented in Chapter 10 in which sequential studies documented that therapy-improved function and others in which therapy did not improve function significantly. Importantly, CPET provides the physician with reproducible and objective information needed to evaluate the clinical course of the patient and the effectiveness of therapeutic interventions.

SCREENING FOR DEVELOPMENT OF DISEASE IN AT-RISK PATIENTS

The intimate relationship between O_2 transport and exercise bioenergetics is clear. The normal gas exchange response to exercise is also well defined. Abnormal gas exchange responses to exercise are often characteristic for disease in a specific organ system. Thus, to detect disease of impaired coupling of external to cellular respiration at an early stage—and possibly prevent serious progression of the illness—a noninvasive CPET has potential to be a sensitive and comprehensive assessment tool.

Few investigative studies have been done that take advantage of noninvasive CPET to detect developing disease of the heart, lungs, pulmonary or systemic circulations, or the muscles. Because the normal range for peak $\dot{V}O_2$ is fairly wide, a single measure is not likely to be as useful in identifying early or mild disease as serial measures in which an individuals' capacity can be compared with their own prior performance. Other indices, such as $\dot{V}E/\dot{V}CO_2$ at the *AT*, $\dot{V}E$-$\dot{V}CO_2$ slope, the slope of heart rate relative to $\dot{V}O_2$, *AT*, and $\Delta\dot{V}O_2/\Delta WR$ would also be expected to be sensitively affected by a developing defect in the coupling of internal and external respiration. Thus, periodic CPETs may be valuable to perform, for example, in individuals with strong family histories of CAD, including silent myocardial ischemia.[210-213] Similarly, the measurement of the $\dot{V}E$-$\dot{V}CO_2$ slope and $\dot{V}E/\dot{V}CO_2$ at the *AT*, in view of the uniform predicted values of these measurements, would likely be sensitive noninvasive methods to detect and assess the severity of the development of heart failure[210,214] or pulmonary vascular disease due to connective tissue disease or familial forms of pulmonary hypertension among at-risk individuals.[215]

GRADED EXERCISE TESTING AND THE ATHLETE

Training for athletic competition, especially of the endurance kind, owes as much to the accumulated lore of the practices of previously successful athletes as to the application of training strategies based on the results of physiological experimentation. The underlying theme of the various approaches to endurance training, however, is that of stressing the system during training beyond the demands of the actual event. How far beyond the power demands of the event and with what patterns of work-rest repetition remain central issues.

Although many approaches will improve performance, the challenge is to determine the optimum pattern: the one that will achieve the greatest improvement in the available time. Laboratory exercise testing of the graded or incremental kind can provide a basis for establishing such a strategy,[216,217] ensuring that the chosen strategy is successfully accomplished during the training session, and establishing objective criteria to support the physiological benefits of the training scheme.

This is most clearly evident in considering the extremes of event duration: sprints and marathons (and beyond). That is, it is hard to see how knowledge of an individual's $\dot{V}O_2$max, critical power, and *AT* can possibly influence the choice of training speeds for a sprinter. Considerations of the recovery kinetics of, for example, muscle or blood [lactate] (which, for the purposes of this discussion, we use as proxy variables for the fatigue-inducing mechanisms) might be beneficial to the choice of interval strategy in the future. Indices of peak and mean power over a short maximum-effort sprint, such as provided by the Wingate test,[218] offer more in this regard. For example, if these indices show improvement as a result of the training program but performance at the event does not, this would suggest that the athlete's technique should be the focus of attention.

For events of marathon duration or longer, the glycogen-squandering aspects of anaerobic glycolysis and consequent increased rate of lactate and H^+ production are detrimental to performance. Consequently, a knowledge of the athlete's speed at the *AT*, by an appropriate measurement or estimation technique (including perceptual correlates[219]), can serve both as a means of optimizing the rate at which the event is actually performed[220] and as a frame of reference for a strategy for training at some higher speed that will induce a given degree of lactic acidemia—that is, one that is sustained at some target value aimed at inducing a training effect (in this case, to increase the *AT* and hence the potential optimum performance rate).

At the intervening middle distances, knowledge of the individual's profile of aerobic function is likely to be of considerably greater importance. Although it has been suggested that muscle glycogen depletion can contribute to fatigue at running events as short as 10 000 meters,[221] it is likely that in these events fatigue[162,222] is a result of metabolites increasing inexorably locally within muscle[223] and/or in sites within the brain[221,224] at a rate that causes them to attain a maximal, and limiting, value at the end of the race.

The upper limit of the work rate at which both $\dot{V}O_2$ and arterial blood [lactate] can be maintained at a high but constant level has been defined[225] to be, in general terms, the individual's critical power (see Chapter 2, "Power-Duration Curve and Critical Power" section).[226] In healthy young individuals, this occurs on average at a $\dot{V}O_2$ of approximately 50% of the difference between the *AT* and the peak $\dot{V}O_2$ and at a blood lactate level of approximately 4 to 5 mM. Presumably, this is the power output at which the rate of muscle lactate production is balanced by the rate of lactate consumed by other tissues and particularly by the liver (Cori cycle). However, these levels vary among individuals; hence, it is important to determine the specific level for a given athlete rather than relying on a group-mean value to guide training. These profiles will establish whether the training intensity is sufficiently high for the training target and also serve to monitor training-induced improvements. However, it is important to recognize that a particular level of blood lactate can be at resting levels or attained either by a relatively low constant work rate bout[227] or by work-recovery repetitions involving appreciably greater work rates.[228,229] This allows the recruitment pattern of muscle fibers and the metabolic and acid-base consequences of work to be proportionally manipulated for the training purpose.

The condition of "overtraining" is also important to the athlete because it can lead to increased risk of infections and depressed immunologic function, in addition to decrements of performance.[230,231] This appears to be a manifestation of prolonged high-intensity training, that is, lower levels can boost immune function. The use of graded exercise testing to establish the upper level of beneficial training intensities and duration should provide insight into the deleterious aspects of inappropriate training.

As more is learned about the physiological mechanisms that trigger "training effects" and how the variables of intensity, duration, and recovery interact to induce the effects,[232] laboratory testing will become even more useful in training prescriptions.

SUMMARY

Until the 1980s, CPET had not been applied in a general way in medicine because of the apparent complexity and time demands of the methods required to obtain the useful data. However, with the advent of automated gas analyzers, sensitive measuring devices, and computerized methods to calculate and display the massive amount of useful data that can be obtained from CPET, it is being recognized as an accurate, noninvasive technology with widespread applications at relatively low cost. We have used it most effectively for differential diagnosis, including unique diagnoses that cannot be made objectively without CPET. It takes the guesswork and bias out of differential diagnosis and effectiveness of therapy. It also makes impairment evaluation for disability more objective. It has been a very helpful guide in both cardiac and pulmonary rehabilitation for determining both the training work rate and whether improvement in exercise performance has occurred. In recent years, CPET has been shown to be a more accurate predictor of severity of disease and predictor of survival time in patients with heart failure than other techniques. Thus, it has been used in prioritizing patients for heart transplantation, with measured peak $\dot{V}O_2$ overriding measurements of resting function. It is likely that similar guidelines can be extended to other decisions regarding advanced therapies such as devise implantation, lung transplantation, and lung reduction surgery. The prognostic significance of cardiorespiratory function represented by measurements made during CPET extends to other contexts as well. It is now well established that exercise impairment predicts risk of complications among individuals who are candidates for major surgical interventions, so it is increasingly used to inform discussions of risk versus benefit for elective procedures. There are also increasing data that incorporate CPET data in prognostic assessments in congenital heart diseases, and this has potential to allow clinicians caring for these patients to better assess their tolerance for the cardiorespiratory stress of events such as elective surgeries or pregnancy.

The CPET has obvious applications in determining the therapeutic effectiveness of drugs and procedures in clinical cohorts and has similar potential for assessing individuals' responses to therapy or progression of disease. Less well documented, but obvious in application, is the use of this quantitative approach to detect disease early in its development—that is, before it is so advanced that abnormalities develop at rest and before they are reversible. The increasing number of applications for which CPET is currently employed attests to the growing recognition of its importance in medicine. It provides the potential to reduce health care costs by streamlining the diagnostic approach to disease and facilitating treatment decisions.

REFERENCES

1. Alison JA, McKeough ZJ, Johnston K, et al; for Lung Foundation Australia and the Thoracic Society of Australia and New Zealand. Australian and New Zealand pulmonary rehabilitation guidelines. *Respirology*. 2017;22:800-819.
2. American Thoracic Society, American College of Chest Physicians. ATS/ACCP statement on cardiopulmonary exercise testing. *Am J Respir Crit Care Med*. 2003;167:211-277.
3. Arena R, Myers J, Abella J, et al. Cardiopulmonary exercise testing is equally prognostic in young, middle-aged and older individuals diagnosed with heart failure. *Int J Cardiol*. 2011;151:278-283.
4. Arena R, Myers J, Guazzi M. The clinical and research applications of aerobic capacity and ventilatory efficiency in heart failure: an evidence-based review. *Heart Fail Rev*. 2008;13:245-269.

5. Balady GJ, Arena R, Sietsema K, et al. Clinician's guide to cardiopulmonary exercise testing in adults: a scientific statement from the American Heart Association. *Circulation*. 2010;122:191-225.
6. Forman DE, Myers J, Lavie CJ, Guazzi M, Celli B, Arena R. Cardiopulmonary exercise testing: relevant but underused. *Postgrad Med*. 2010;122:68-86.
7. Leon AS, Franklin BA, Costa F, et al. Cardiac rehabilitation and secondary prevention of coronary heart disease: an American Heart Association scientific statement from the Council on Clinical Cardiology (Subcommittee on Exercise, Cardiac Rehabilitation, and Prevention) and the Council on Nutrition, Physical Activity, and Metabolism (Subcommittee on Physical Activity), in collaboration with the American association of Cardiovascular and Pulmonary Rehabilitation. *Circulation*. 2005;111:369-376.
8. Ridgway ZA, Howell SJ. Cardiopulmonary exercise testing: a review of methods and applications in surgical patients. *Eur J Anaesthesiol*. 2010;27:858-865.
9. Stringer W. Cardiopulmonary exercise testing: current applications. *Expert Rev Respir Med*. 2010;4:179-188.
10. Chaudhry S, Arena R, Wasserman K, et al. Exercise-induced myocardial ischemia detected by cardiopulmonary exercise testing. *Am J Cardiol*. 2009;103:615-619.
11. Belardinelli R, Lacalaprice F, Tiano L, Muçai A, Perna GP. Cardiopulmonary exercise testing is more accurate than ECG-stress testing in diagnosing myocardial ischemia in subjects with chest pain. *Int J Cardiol*. 2014;174:337-342.
12. Chaudhry S, Arena R, Bhatt DL, Verma S, Kumar N. A practical clinical approach to utilize cardiopulmonary exercise testing in the evaluation and management of coronary artery disease: a primer for cardiologists. *Curr Opin Cardiol*. 2018;33:168-177.
13. Bishu K, Redfield MM. Acute heart failure with preserved ejection fraction: unique patient characteristics and targets for therapy. *Curr Heart Fail Rep*. 2013;10:190-197.
14. Reddy YNV, Carter RE, Obokata M, Redfield MM, Borlaug BA. A simple, evidence-based approach to help guide diagnosis of heart failure with preserved ejection fraction. *Circulation*. 2018;28;138:861-870.
15. Plitt GD, Spring JT, Moulton MJ, Agrawal DK. Mechanisms, diagnosis, and treatment of heart failure with preserved ejection fraction and diastolic dysfunction. *Expert Rev Cardiovasc Ther*. 2018;16:579-589.
16. Obokata M, Olson TP, Reddy YNV, Melenovsky V, Kane GC, Borlaug BA. Haemodynamics, dyspnoea, and pulmonary reserve in heart failure with preserved ejection fraction. *Eur Heart J*. 2018;39:2810-2821.
17. Van Iterson EH, Johnson BD, Borlaug BA, Olson TP. Physiological dead space and arterial carbon dioxide contributions to exercise ventilatory inefficiency in patients with reduced or preserved ejection fraction heart failure. *Eur J Heart Fail*. 2017;19:1675-1685.
18. Guazzi M, Myers J, Arena R. Cardiopulmonary exercise testing in the clinical and prognostic assessment of diastolic heart failure. *J Am Coll Cardiol*. 2005;46:1883-1890.
19. Nadruz W Jr, West E, Sengeløv M, et al. Prognostic value of cardiopulmonary exercise testing in heart failure with reduced, midrange, and preserved ejection fraction. *J Am Heart Assoc*. 2017;6(11):e006000.
20. Simonneau G, Montani D, Celermajer DS, et al. Haemodynamic definitions and updated clinical classification of pulmonary hypertension. *Eur Respir J*. 2019;53(1):1801913.
21. Sun XG, Hansen JE, Oudiz RJ, Wasserman K. Exercise pathophysiology in patients with primary pulmonary hypertension. *Circulation*. 2001;104:429-435.
22. Wensel R, Optiz CF, Anker SD, et al. Assessment of survival in patients with primary pulmonary hypertension: importance of cardiopulmonary exercise testing. *Circulation*. 2002;106:319-324.
23. Ting H, Sun XG, Chuang ML, Lewis DA, Hansen JE, Wasserman K. A noninvasive assessment of pulmonary perfusion abnormality in patients with primary pulmonary hypertension. *Chest*. 2001;119:824-832.
24. Waurick PE, Kleber FX. Cardiopulmonary exercise testing in pulmonary vascular disease: arterial and end-tidal CO_2 partial pressures in patients with acute and chronic pulmonary embolism and primary pulmonary hypertension. In: Wasserman K, ed. *Cardiopulmonary Exercise Testing and Cardiovascular Health*. Armonk, NY: Futura Publishing; 2002:178-173.
25. Davies H, Gazetopoulos N. Dyspnoea in cyanotic congenital heart disease. *Br Heart J*. 1965;27:28-41.
26. Sietsema KE, Cooper DM, Perloff SK, et al. Control of ventilation during exercise in patients with central venous-to-systemic arterial shunts. *J Appl Physiol (1985)*. 1988;64:234-242.
27. Schaeffer JP. *Morris' Human Anatomy*. New York, NY: The Blakiston Company; 1953.
28. Sun XG, Hansen JE, Oudiz R, Wasserman K. Gas exchange detection of exercise-induced right-to-left shunt in patients with primary pulmonary hypertension. *Circulation*. 2002;105:54-60.
29. Sietsema KE, Cooper DM, Perloff JK, et al. Dynamics of oxygen uptake during exercise in adults with cyanotic congenital heart disease. *Circulation*. 1986;73(6):1137-1144.
30. Neder JA, Berton DC, Arbex FF, et al. Physiological and clinical relevance of exercise ventilatory efficiency in COPD. *Eur Respir J*. 2017;49(3):1602036.
31. Boerrigter BG, Bogaard HJ, Trip P, et al. Ventilatory and cardiocirculatory exercise profiles in COPD: the role of pulmonary hypertension. *Chest*. 2012;142:1166-1174.
32. Holverda S, Bogaard HJ, Groepenhoff H, Postmus PE, Boonstra A, Vonk-Noordegraaf A. Cardiopulmonary exercise test characteristics in patients with chronic obstructive pulmonary disease and associated pulmonary hypertension. *Respiration*. 2008;76:160-167.
33. Vonbank K, Funk GC, Marzluf B, et al. Abnormal pulmonary arterial pressure limits exercise capacity in patients with COPD. *Wien Klin Wochenschr*. 2008;120(23-24):749-755.
34. Haller RG, Lewis SF, Estabrook RW, DiMauro S, Servidei S, Foster DW. Exercise intolerance, lactic acidosis, and abnormal cardiopulmonary regulation in exercise associated with adult skeletal muscle cytochrome c oxidase deficiency. *J Clin Invest*. 1989;84:155-161.
35. Riley M, Nugent A, Steele IC, et al. Gas exchange during exercise in McArdle's disease. *J Appl Physiol*. 1993;75:745-754.
36. Haller RG, Henriksson KG, Jorfeldt L, et al. Deficiency of skeletal muscle succinate dehydrogenase and aconitase. Pathophysiology of exercise in a novel human muscle oxidative defect. *J Clin Invest*. 1991;88:1197-1206.
37. Bogaard JM, Busch HFM, Scholte HR, Stam H, Versprille A. Exercise responses in patients with an enzyme deficiency in the mitochondrial respiratory chain. *Eur Respir J*. 1988;1:445-452.
38. Bogaard JM, Scholte HR, Busch FM, et al. Anaerobic threshold as detected from ventilatory and metabolic exercise responses in patients with mitochondrial respiratory chain defect. In: Tavassi L, DiPrampero PE, eds. *Advances in Cardiology. The Anaerobic Threshold: Physiological and Clinical Significance*. Basel, Switzerland: Karger; 1986:135-145.
39. Parsons JP, Hallstrand TS, Mastronarde JG, et al; for American Thoracic Society Subcommittee on Exercise-induced Bronchoconstriction. An official American Thoracic Society clinical practice guideline: exercise-induced bronchoconstriction. *Am J Respir Crit Care Med*. 2013;187:1016-1027.
40. Olin JT, Clary MS, Fan EM, et al. Continuous laryngoscopy quantitates laryngeal behaviour in exercise and recovery. *Eur Respir J*. 2016;48:1192-1200.
41. Criteria Committee of the New York Heart Association. In: New York Heart Association. *Diseases of the Heart and Blood Vessels: Nomenclature and Criteria for Diagnosis*. 6th ed. Boston, MA: Little, Brown and Co.; 1964.
42. Matsumura N, Nishijima H, Kojima S, Hashimoto F, Minami M, Yasuda H. Determination of anaerobic threshold for assessment of functional state in patients with chronic heart failure. *Circulation*. 1983;68:360-367.
43. Weber KT, Janicki JS. Cardiopulmonary exercise testing for evaluation of chronic cardiac failure. *Am J Cardiol*. 1985;55:22A-31A.

44. Mudge GH, Goldstein S, Addonizio LJ, et al. 24th Bethesda Conference: cardiac transplantation. Task force 3: recipient guidelines/prioritization. *J Am Coll Cardiol.* 1993;22:21-31.
45. Likoff MJ, Chandler SL, Kay HR. Clinical determinants of mortality in chronic congestive heart failure secondary to idiopathic dilated or to ischemic cardiomyopathy. *Am J Cardiol.* 1987;59:634-638.
46. Mancini DM, Eisen H, Kussmaul W, Mull R, Edmunds LH Jr, Wilson JR. Value of peak exercise oxygen consumption for optimal timing of cardiac transplantation in ambulatory patients with heart failure. *Circulation.* 1991;83:778-786.
47. Myers J, Gullestad L, Vagelos R, et al. Clinical, hemodynamic, and cardiopulmonary exercise test determinants of survival in patients referred for evaluation of heart failure. *Ann Intern Med.* 1998;129:286-293.
48. Stelken AM, Younis LT, Jennison SH, et al. Prognostic value of cardiopulmonary exercise testing using percent achieved of predicted peak oxygen uptake for patients with ischemic and dilated cardiomyopathy. *J Am Coll Cardiol.* 1996;27:345-352.
49. Cattadori G, Schmid JP, Brugger N, Gondoni E, Palermo P, Agostoni P. Hemodynamic effects of exercise training in heart failure. *J Card Fail.* 2011;17:916-922.
50. Metra M, Faggiano P, D'Aloia A, et al. Use of cardiopulmonary exercise testing with hemodynamic monitoring in the prognostic assessment of ambulatory patients with chronic heart failure. *J Am Coll Cardiol.* 1999;33:943-950.
51. Vignati C, Cattadori G. Measuring cardiac output during cardiopulmonary exercise testing. *Ann Am Thorac Soc.* 2017;14(suppl 1):S48-S52.
52. Wilson JR, Rayos G, Yeoh TK, Gothard P. Dissociation between peak exercise oxygen consumption and hemodynamic dysfunction in potential heart transplant candidates. *J Am Coll Cardiol.* 1995;26:429-435.
53. Bigi R, Desideri A, Rambaldi R, Cortigiani L, Sponzilli C, Fiorentini C. Angiographic and prognostic correlates of cardiac output by cardiopulmonary exercise testing in patients with anterior myocardial infarction. *Chest.* 2001;120:825-833.
54. Stringer W, Hansen J, Wasserman K. Cardiac output estimated noninvasively from oxygen uptake during exercise. *J Appl Physiol (1985).* 1997;82:908-912.
55. Paolillo S, Agostoni P. Prognostic role of cardiopulmonary exercise testing in clinical practice. *Ann Am Thorac Soc.* 2017;14(suppl 1):S53-S58.
56. Sullivan MJ, Hawthorne MH. Exercise intolerance in patients with chronic heart failure. *Prog Cardiovasc Dis.* 1995;38:1-22.
57. Paolillo S, Veglia F, Salvioni E, et al; for MECKI Score Research Group. Heart failure prognosis over time: how the prognostic role of oxygen consumption and ventilatory efficiency during exercise has changed in the last 20 years. *Eur J Heart Fail.* 2019;21:208-217.
58. Weber KT. Cardiopulmonary exercise testing and the evaluation of systolic dysfunction. In: Wasserman K, ed. *Exercise Gas Exchange in Heart Disease.* Armonk, NY: Futura Publishing; 1996:55-62.
59. Itoh H, Taniguichi K, Koike A, Doi M. Evaluation of severity of heart failure using ventilatory gas analysis. *Circulation.* 1990;81(suppl 1):II31-II37.
60. Koike A, Hiroe M, Adachi H, et al. Anaerobic metabolism as an indicator of aerobic function during exercise in cardiac patients. *J Am Coll Cardiol.* 1992;20:120-126.
61. Aaronson KD, Mancini DM. Is percentage of predicted maximal exercise oxygen consumption a better predictor of survival than peak exercise oxygen consumption for patients with severe heart failure? *J Heart Lung Transplant.* 1995;14:981-989.
62. Costanzo MR, Augustine S, Bourge R, et al. Selection and treatment of candidates for heart transplantation. A statement for health professionals from the Committee on Heart Failure and Cardiac Transplantation of the Council on Clinical Cardiology, American Heart Association. *Circulation.* 1995;92:3593-3612.
63. Rickenbacher PR, Trindade PT, Haywood GA, et al. Transplant candidates with severe left ventricular dysfunction managed with medical treatment: characteristics and survival. *J Am Coll Cardiol.* 1996;27:1192-1197.
64. Roul G, Moulichon ME, Bareiss P, et al. Exercise peak $\dot{V}O_2$ determination in chronic heart failure: is it still of value? *Eur Heart J.* 1994;15:495-502.
65. Szlachic J, Massie BM, Kramer BL, Topic N, Tubau J. Correlates and prognostic implication of exercise capacity in chronic congestive heart failure. *Am J Cardiol.* 1985;55:1037-1042.
66. Osada N, Chaitman BR, Miller LW, et al. Cardiopulmonary exercise testing identifies low risk patients with heart failure and severely impaired exercise capacity considered for heart transplantation. *J Am Coll Cardiol.* 1998;31:577-582.
67. Stevenson LW, Steimle AE, Fonarow G, et al. Improvement in exercise capacity of candidates awaiting heart transplantation. *J Am Coll Cardiol.* 1995;25:163-170.
68. Gitt AK, Wasserman K, Kilkowski C, et al. Exercise anaerobic threshold and ventilatory efficiency identify heart failure patients for high risk of early death. *Circulation.* 2002;106:3079-3084.
69. Elmariah S, Goldberg LR, Allen MT, Kao A. Effects of gender on peak oxygen consumption and the timing of cardiac transplantation. *J Am Coll Cardiol.* 2006;47(11):2237-2242.
70. Sun XG, Hansen JE, Beshai JF, Wasserman K. Oscillatory breathing and exercise gas exchange abnormalities prognosticate early mortality and morbidity in heart failure. *J Am Coll Cardiol.* 2010;55:1814-1823.
71. Agostoni P, Corrà U, Cattadori G, et al; for MECKI Score Research Group. Prognostic value of indeterminable anaerobic threshold in heart failure. *Circ Heart Fail.* 2013;6:977-987.
72. Magrì D, Agostoni P, Corrà U, et al; for Metabolic Exercise test data combined with Cardiac and Kidney Indexes (MECKI) Score Research Group. Deceptive meaning of oxygen uptake measured at the anaerobic threshold in patients with systolic heart failure and atrial fibrillation. *Eur J Prev Cardiol.* 2015;22:1046-1055.
73. Sun XG, Hansen JE, Garatachea N, Storer TW, Wasserman K. Ventilatory efficiency during exercise in healthy subjects. *Am J Respir Crit Care Med.* 2002;166:1443-1448.
74. Agostoni P, Guazzi M. Exercise ventilatory inefficiency in heart failure: some fresh news into the roadmap of heart failure with preserved ejection fraction phenotyping. *Eur J Heart Fail.* 2017;19:1686-1689.
75. Kee K, Stuart-Andrews C, Ellis MJ, et al. Increased dead space ventilation mediates reduced exercise capacity in systolic heart failure. *Am J Respir Crit Care Med.* 2016;193:1292-1300.
76. Sue DY. Excess ventilation during exercise and prognosis in chronic heart failure. *Am J Respir Crit Care Med.* 2011;183:1302-1310.
77. Van Iterson EH, Olson TP. Use of 'ideal' alveolar air equations and corrected end-tidal PCO_2 to estimate arterial PCO_2 and physiological dead space during exercise in patients with heart failure. *Int J Cardiol.* 2018;250:176-182.
78. Chua TP, Ponikowski P, Harrington D, et al. Clinical correlates and prognostic significance of the ventilatory response to exercise in chronic heart failure. *J Am Coll Cardiol.* 1997;29:1585-1590.
79. Corrà U, Mezzani A, Bosimini E, Scapellato F, Imparato A, Giannuzzi P. Ventilatory response to exercise improves risk stratification in patients with chronic heart failure and intermediate functional capacity. *Am Heart J.* 2002;143:418-426.
80. Poggio R, Arazi HC, Giorgi M, Miriuka SG. Prediction of severe cardiovascular events by $\dot{V}E/\dot{V}CO_2$ slope versus peak $\dot{V}O_2$ in systolic heart failure: a meta-analysis of the published literature. *Am Heart J.* 2010;160:1004-1014.
81. Guazzi M, Reina G, Tumminello G, Guazzi MD. Exercise ventilation inefficiency and cardiovascular mortality in heart failure: the critical independent prognostic value of the arterial CO_2 partial pressure. *Eur Heart J.* 2005;26:472-480.
82. Dhakal BP, Lewis GD. Exercise oscillatory ventilation: mechanisms and prognostic significance. *World J Cardiol.* 2016;8:258-266.
83. Corrà U, Giordano A, Bosimini E, et al. Oscillatory ventilation during exercise in patients with chronic heart failure: clinical correlates and prognostic implications. *Chest.* 2002;121:1572-1580.
84. Leite JJ, Mansur AJ, de Freitas HF, et al. Periodic breathing during incremental exercise predicts mortality in patients with chronic heart failure evaluated for cardiac transplantation. *J Am Coll Cardiol.* 2003;41:2175-2181.

85. Guazzi M, Arena R, Ascione A, Piepoli M, Guazzi MD; for Gruppo di Studio Fisiologia dell'Esercizio, Cardiologia dello Sport e Riabilitazione Cardiovascolare of the Italian Society of Cardiology. Exercise oscillatory breathing and increased ventilation to carbon dioxide production slope in heart failure: an unfavorable combination with high prognostic value. *Am Heart J*. 2007;153:859-867.
86. O'Neill JO, Young JB, Pothier CE, Lauer MS. Peak oxygen consumption as a predictor of death in patients with heart failure receiving beta-blockers. *Circulation*. 2005;111:2313-2318.
87. Agostoni P, Apostolo A, Cattadori G, et al. Effects of beta-blockers on ventilation efficiency in heart failure. *Am Heart J*. 2010;159:1067-1073.
88. Dhoble A, Enriquez-Sarano M, Kopecky SL, et al. Cardiopulmonary responses to exercise and its utility in patients with aortic stenosis. *Am J Cardiol*. 2014;113:1711-1716.
89. Le VD, Jensen GV, Kjøller-Hansen L. Prognostic usefulness of cardiopulmonary exercise testing for managing patients with severe aortic stenosis. *Am J Cardiol*. 2017;120:844-849.
90. Domanski O, Richardson M, Coisne A, et al. Cardiopulmonary exercise testing is a better outcome predictor than exercise echocardiography in asymptomatic aortic stenosis. *Int J Cardiol*. 2017;227:908-914.
91. Levy F, Fayad N, Jeu A, et al. The value of cardiopulmonary exercise testing in individuals with apparently asymptomatic severe aortic stenosis: a pilot study. *Arch Cardiovasc Dis*. 2014;107:519-528.
92. Bandera F, Generati G, Pellegrino M, et al. Mitral regurgitation in heart failure: insights from CPET combined with exercise echocardiography. *Eur Heart J Cardiovasc Imaging*. 2017;18:296-303.
93. Naji P, Griffin BP, Barr T, et al. Importance of exercise capacity in predicting outcomes and determining optimal timing of surgery in significant primary mitral regurgitation. *J Am Heart Assoc*. 2014;3(5):e001010.
94. Inuzuka R, Diller GP, Borgia F, et al. Comprehensive use of cardiopulmonary exercise testing identifies adults with congenital heart disease at increased mortality risk in the medium term. *Circulation*. 2012;125:250-259.
95. Dimopoulos K, Okonko DO, Diller GP, et al. Abnormal ventilatory response to exercise in adults with congenital heart disease relates to cyanosis and predicts survival. *Circulation*. 2006;113:2796-2802.
96. Cohn JN, Johnson GR, Shabetai R, et al. Ejection fraction, peak exercise oxygen consumption, cardiothoracic ratio, ventricular arrhythmias, and plasma norepinephrine as determinants of prognosis in heart failure. The V-HeFT VA Cooperative Studies Group. *Circulation*. 1993;87(6 suppl):V15-V16.
97. Stevenson LW. Role of exercise testing in the evaluation of candidates for cardiac transplantation. In: Wasserman K, ed. *Exercise Gas Exchange in Heart Disease*. Armonk, NY: Futura Publishing; 1996:271-186.
98. Mehra MR, Canter CE, Hannan MM, et al; for International Society for Heart Lung Transplantation Infectious Diseases Council; International Society for Heart Lung Transplantation Pediatric Transplantation Council; International Society for Heart Lung Transplantation Heart Failure and Transplantation Council. The 2016 International Society for Heart Lung Transplantation listing criteria for heart transplantation: a 10-year update. *J Heart Lung Transplant*. 2016;35:1-23.
99. Galiè N, Humbert M, Vachiery JL, et al; for ESC Scientific Document Group. 2015 ESC/ERS guidelines for the diagnosis and treatment of pulmonary hypertension: the Joint Task Force for the Diagnosis and Treatment of Pulmonary Hypertension of the European Society of Cardiology (ESC) and the European Respiratory Society (ERS): endorsed by: Association for European Paediatric and Congenital Cardiology (AEPC), International Society for Heart and Lung Transplantation (ISHLT). *Eur Heart J*. 2016;37:67-119.
100. Woods PR, Frantz RP, Taylor BJ, Olson TP, Johnson BD. The usefulness of submaximal exercise gas exchange to define pulmonary arterial hypertension. *J Heart Lung Transplant*. 2011;30:1133-1142.
101. Woods PR, Taylor BJ, Frantz RP, Johnson BD. A pulmonary hypertension gas exchange severity (PH-GXS) score to assist with the assessment and monitoring of pulmonary arterial hypertension. *Am J Cardiol*. 2012;109:1066-1072.
102. Badagliacca R, Papa S, Poscia R, et al. The added value of cardiopulmonary exercise testing in the follow-up of pulmonary arterial hypertension. *J Heart Lung Transplant*. 2019;38:306-314.
103. Oudiz RJ, Midde R, Hovenesyan A, et al. Usefulness of right-to-left shunting and poor exercise gas exchange for predicting prognosis in patients with pulmonary arterial hypertension. *Am J Cardiol*. 2010;105:1186-1191.
104. Schwaiblmair M, Faul C, von Scheidt W, Berghaus TM. Ventilatory efficiency testing as prognostic value in patients with pulmonary hypertension. *BMC Pulm Med*. 2012;12:23.
105. Ferreira EV, Ota-Arakaki JS, Ramos RP, et al. Optimizing the evaluation of excess exercise ventilation for prognosis assessment in pulmonary arterial hypertension. *Eur J Prev Cardiol*. 2014;21:1409-1419.
106. Wensel R, Francis DP, Meyer FJ, et al. Incremental prognostic value of cardiopulmonary exercise testing and resting haemodynamics in pulmonary arterial hypertension. *Int J Cardiol*. 2013;167:1193-1198.
107. Tang Y, Luo Q, Liu Z, et al. Oxygen uptake efficiency slope predicts poor outcome in patients with idiopathic pulmonary arterial hypertension. *J Am Heart Assoc*. 2017;6(7):e005037.
108. Groepenhoff H, Vonk-Noordegraaf A, van de Veerdonk MC, Boonstra A, Westerhof N, Bogaard HJ. Prognostic relevance of changes in exercise test variables in pulmonary arterial hypertension. *PLoS One*. 2013;8:e72013.
109. Oga T, Nishimura K, Tsukino M, Sato S, Hajiro T. Analysis of the factors related to mortality in chronic obstructive pulmonary disease: role of exercise capacity and health status. *Am J Respir Crit Care Med*. 2003;167:544-549.
110. Jones PW. Health status measurement in chronic obstructive pulmonary disease. *Thorax*. 2001;56:880-887.
111. Hiraga T, Maekura R, Okuda Y, et al. Prognostic predictors for survival in patients with COPD using cardiopulmonary exercise testing. *Clin Physiol Funct Imaging*. 2003;23:324-331.
112. Neder JA, Alharbi A, Berton DC, et al. Exercise ventilatory inefficiency adds to lung function in predicting mortality in COPD. *COPD*. 2016;13:416-424.
113. Ozgür ES, Nayci SA, Özge C, Taşdelen B. An integrated index combined by dynamic hyperinflation and exercise capacity in the prediction of morbidity and mortality in COPD. *Respir Care*. 2012;57:1452-1459.
114. Fishman A, Martinez F, Naunheim K, et al. A randomized trial comparing lung-volume-reduction surgery with medical therapy for severe emphysema. *N Engl J Med*. 2003;348:2059-2073.
115. Raghu G, Collard HR, Egan JJ, et al. An official ATS/ERS/JRS/ALAT statement: idiopathic pulmonary fibrosis: evidence-based guidelines for diagnosis and management. *Am J Respir Crit Care Med*. 2011;183:788-824.
116. Raghu G, Remy-Jardin M, Myers JL, et al; for American Thoracic Society, European Respiratory Society, Japanese Respiratory Society, and Latin American Thoracic Society. Diagnosis of idiopathic pulmonary fibrosis. An official ATS/ERS/JRS/ALAT clinical practice guideline. *Am J Respir Crit Care Med*. 2018;198:e44-e68.
117. Raghu G, Rochwerg B, Zhang Y, et al; for American Thoracic Society; European Respiratory Society; Japanese Respiratory Society; Latin American Thoracic Association. An official ATS/ERS/JRS/ALAT clinical practice guideline: treatment of idiopathic pulmonary fibrosis. An update of the 2011 clinical practice guideline. *Am J Respir Crit Care Med*. 2015;192(2):e3-e19.
118. Manali ED, Lyberopoulos P, Triantafillidou C, et al. MRC chronic Dyspnea Scale: relationships with cardiopulmonary exercise testing and 6-minute walk test in idiopathic pulmonary fibrosis patients: a prospective study. *BMC Pulm Med*. 2010;10:32.
119. Vainshelboim B, Oliveira J, Fox BD, Kramer MR. The prognostic role of ventilatory inefficiency and exercise capacity in idiopathic pulmonary fibrosis. *Respir Care*. 2016;61:1100-119.
120. van der Plas MN, van Kan C, Blumenthal J, Jansen HM, Wells AU, Bresser P. Pulmonary vascular limitation to exercise and survival in idiopathic pulmonary fibrosis. *Respirology*. 2014;19:269-275.
121. Triantafillidou C, Manali E, Lyberopoulos P, et al. The role of cardiopulmonary exercise test in IPF prognosis. *Pulm Med*. 2013;2013:514817.

122. Gläser S, Obst A, Koch B, et al. Pulmonary hypertension in patients with idiopathic pulmonary fibrosis—the predictive value of exercise capacity and gas exchange efficiency. *PLoS One*. 2013;8:e65643.
123. Hebestreit H, Hulzebos EH, Schneiderman JE, et al; for Prognostic Value of CPET in CF Study Group. Cardiopulmonary exercise testing provides additional prognostic information in cystic fibrosis. *Am J Respir Crit Care Med*. 2019;199:987-995.
124. Stevens D, Stephenson A, Faughnan ME, Leek E, Tullis E. Prognostic relevance of dynamic hyperinflation during cardiopulmonary exercise testing in adult patients with cystic fibrosis. *J Cyst Fibros*. 2013;12:655-661.
125. Older P, Smith R, Courtney P, Hone R. Preoperative evaluation of cardiac failure and ischemia in elderly patients by cardiopulmonary exercise testing. *Chest*. 1993;104:701-704.
126. Wilson RJT, Davies S, Yates D, Redman J, Stone M. Impaired functional capacity is associated with all-cause mortality after major elective intra-abdominal surgery. *Br J Anaesth*. 2010;105:297-303.
127. Smith TP, Kinasewitz GT, Tucker WY, Spillers WP, George RB. Exercise capacity as a predictor of post-thoracotomy morbidity. *Am Rev Respir Dis*. 1984;129:730-734.
128. Bechard D, Wetstein L. Assessment of exercise oxygen consumption as preoperative criterion for lung resection. *Ann Thor Surg*. 1987;44:344-349.
129. Bolliger CT, Jordan P, Solèr M, et al. Exercise capacity as a predictor of postoperative complications in lung resection candidates. *Am J Respir Crit Care Med*. 1995;151:1472-1480.
130. Bolliger CT, Wyser C, Roser H, Solèr M, Perruchoud AP. Lung scanning and exercise testing for the prediction of postoperative performance in lung resection candidates at increased risk for complications. *Chest*. 1995;108:341-348.
131. Morice RC, Peters EJ, Ryan MB, Putnam JB, Ali MK, Roth JA. Exercise testing in the evaluation of patients at high risk for complications from lung resection. *Chest*. 1992;101:356-361.
132. Brunelli A, Kim AW, Berger KI, Addrizzo-Harris DJ. Physiologic evaluation of the patient with lung cancer being considered for resectional surgery: diagnosis and management of lung cancer, 3rd ed: American College of Chest Physicians evidence-based clinical practice guidelines. *Chest*. 2013;143(5 suppl):e166S-e190S.
133. Older P, Hall A, Hader R. Cardiopulmonary exercise testing as a screening test for perioperative management of major surgery in the elderly. *Chest*. 1999;116:355-362.
134. Levett DZH, Jack S, Swart M, et al; for Perioperative Exercise Testing and Training Society. Perioperative cardiopulmonary exercise testing (CPET): consensus clinical guidelines on indications, organization, conduct, and physiological interpretation. *Br J Anaesth*. 2018;120:484-500.
135. Levett DZ, Edwards M, Grocott M, Mythen M. Preparing the patient for surgery to improve outcomes. *Best Pract Res Clin Anaesthesiol*. 2016;30:145-157.
136. Levett DZ, Grocott MP. Cardiopulmonary exercise testing, prehabilitation, and Enhanced Recovery After Surgery (ERAS). *Can J Anaesth*. 2015;62:131-142.
137. Stringer W, Casaburi R, Older P. Cardiopulmonary exercise testing: does it improve perioperative care and outcome? *Curr Opin Anaesthesiol*. 2012;25:178-184.
138. Barberan-Garcia A, Ubré M, Roca J, et al. Personalised prehabilitation in high-risk patients undergoing elective major abdominal surgery: a randomized blinded controlled trial. *Ann Surg*. 2018;267:50-56.
139. Brunelli A, Belardinelli R, Refai M, et al. Peak oxygen consumption during cardiopulmonary exercise test improves risk stratification in candidates to major lung resection. *Chest*. 2009;135:1260-1267.
140. British Thoracic Society, Society of Cardiothoracic Surgeons of Great Britain and Ireland Working Party. BTS guidelines: guidelines on the selection of patients with lung cancer for surgery. *Thorax*. 2001;56:89-108.
141. Renzetti AD, Bleecker ER, Epler GR, et al. Evaluation of impairment/disability secondary to respiratory disorders. *Am Rev Respir Dis*. 1986;133:1205-1209.
142. Wood PH. Appreciating the consequences of disease: the international classification of impairments, disabilities, and handicaps. *WHO Chron*. 1980;34:376-380.
143. Campbell SC. A comparison of the maximum voluntary ventilation with the forced expiratory volume in one second: an assessment of subject cooperation. *J Occup Med*. 1982;24:531-533.
144. Agostoni P, Smith DD, Schoene RGB, Robertson HT, Butler J. Evaluation of breathlessness in asbestos workers. Results of exercise testing. *Am Rev Respir Dis*. 1987;135:812-816.
145. Agusti AG, Roca J, Rodriguez-Roisin R, Xaubet A, Agusti-Vidal A. Different patterns of gas exchange response to exercise in asbestosis and idiopathic pulmonary fibrosis. *Eur Respir J*. 1988;1:510-516.
146. Cotes JE, Zejda J, King B. Lung function impairment as a guide to exercise limitation in work-related lung disorders. *Am Rev Respir Dis*. 1988;137:1089-1093.
147. Howard J, Mohsenifar Z, Brown HV, Koerner SK. Role of exercise testing in assessing functional respiratory impairment due to asbestos exposure. *J Occup Med*. 1982;24:685-689.
148. Markos J, Musk AW, Finucane KE. Functional similarities of asbestosis and cryptogenic fibrosing alveolitis. *Thorax*. 1988;43:708-714.
149. Oren A, Sue DY, Hansen JE, Torrance DJ, Wasserman K. The role of exercise testing in impairment evaluation. *Am Rev Respir Dis*. 1987;135:230-235.
150. Ortega F, Montemayor T, Sánchez A, Cabello F, Castillo J. Role of cardiopulmonary exercise testing and the criteria used to determine disability in patients with severe chronic obstructive pulmonary disease. *Am J Respir Crit Care Med*. 1994;150:747-751.
151. Pearle J. Exercise performance and functional impairment in asbestos-exposed workers. *Chest*. 1981;80:701-705.
152. Risk C, Epler GR, Gaensler EA. Exercise alveolar-arterial oxygen pressure difference in interstitial lung disease. *Chest*. 1984;85:69-74.
153. Sue DY, Oren A, Hansen JE, Wasserman K. Lung function and exercise performance in smoking and nonsmoking asbestos-exposed workers. *Am Rev Respir Dis*. 1985;132:612-618.
154. Wiedemann HP, Gee JBL, Balmes JR, Loke J. Exercise testing in occupational lung disease. *Clin Chest Med*. 1984;5:157-171.
155. Institute of Medicine. *Cardiovascular Disability: Updating the Social Security Listings*. Washington, DC: The National Academies Press; 2010.
156. Sood A. Performing a lung disability evaluation: how, when, and why? *J Occup Environ Med*. 2014;56(suppl 10):S23-S29.
157. American Medical Association. The pulmonary system. In: Rondinelli RD, ed. *Guides to the Evaluation of Permanent Impairment*. 6th ed. Chicago, IL: American Medical Association; 2008:77-99.
158. Ainsworth BE, Haskell WL, Herrmann SD, et al. 2011 Compendium of Physical Activities: a second update of codes and MET values. *Med Sci Sports Exerc*. 2011;43:1575-1581.
159. Egan B, Zierath JR. Exercise metabolism and the molecular regulation of skeletal muscle adaptation. *Cell Metab*. 2013;17:162-184.
160. Escobar KA, Cole NH, Mermier CM, VanDusseldorp TA. Autophagy and aging: maintaining the proteome through exercise and caloric restriction. *Aging Cell*. 2019;18:e12876.
161. Hawley JA, Hargreaves M, Joyner MJ, Zierath JR. Integrative biology of exercise. *Cell*. 2014;159:738-749.
162. Joyner MJ, Coyle EF. Endurance exercise performance: the physiology of champions. *J Physiol*. 2008;586:35-44.
163. Laughlin MH, Davis MJ, Secher NH, et al. Peripheral circulation. *Compr Physiol*. 2012;2:321-447.
164. Mueller PJ, Clifford PS, Crandall CG, Smith SA, Fadel PJ. Integration of central and peripheral regulation of the circulation during exercise: acute and chronic adaptations. *Compr Physiol*. 2017;8:103-151.
165. Rowell LB. *Human Cardiovascular Control*. New York, NY: Oxford University Press; 1993.
166. Sheel AW, Romer LM. Ventilation and respiratory mechanics. *Compr Physiol*. 2012;2:1093-1142.
167. Wilhelm EN, Mourot L, Rakobowchuk M. Exercise-derived microvesicles: a review of the literature. *Sports Med*. 2018;48:2025-2039.
168. Blaauw B, Schiaffino S, Reggiani C. Mechanisms modulating skeletal muscle phenotype. *Compr Physiol*. 2013;3:1645-1687.

169. Booth FW, Ruegsegger GN, Toedebusch RG, Yan Z. Endurance exercise and the regulation of skeletal muscle metabolism. *Prog Mol Biol Transl Sci*. 2015;135:129-151.
170. Belardinelli R. Exercise training in heart failure patients. In: Wasserman K, ed. *Cardiopulmonary Exercise Testing and Cardiovascular Health*. Armonk, NY: Futura Publishing; 2002:209-220.
171. Casaburi R, Storer TW, Ben-Dov I, Wasserman K. Effect of endurance training on possible determinants of $\dot{V}O2$ during heavy exercise. *J Appl Physiol (1985)*. 1987;62:199-207.
172. Poole DC, Ward SA, Whipp BJ. The effects of training on the metabolic and respiratory profile of high-intensity cycle ergometer exercise. *Eur J Appl Physiol Occup Physiol*. 1990;59:421-429.
173. Sullivan CS, Casaburi R, Storer TW, Wasserman K. Non-invasive prediction of blood lactate response to constant power outputs from incremental exercise tests. *Eur J Appl Physiol Occup Physiol*. 1995;71: 349-354.
174. Human adaptation to acute and chronic physical activity. In: Bouchard C, Shephard RJ, Stephens T, eds. *Physical Activity, Fitness and Health*. 2nd ed. Champaign, IL: Human Kinetics Books; 1993:41-60.
175. Winder WW, Hickson RC, Hagberg JA, Ehsani AA, McLane JA. Training-induced changes in hormonal and metabolic responses to submaximal exercise. *J Appl Physiol Respir Environ Exerc Physiol*. 1979;46:766-771.
176. Gisolfi C, Robinson S. Relations between physical training, acclimatization, and heat tolerance. *J Appl Physiol*. 1969;26:530-534.
177. Hill DW, Cureton KJ, Grisham SC, Collins MA. Effect of training on the rating of perceived exertion at the ventilatory threshold. *Eur J Appl Physiol Occup Physiol*. 1987;56:206-211.
178. Haas F, Schicchi JS, Axen K. Desensitization to dyspnea in chronic obstructive pulmonary disease. In: Casaburi R, Petty TL, eds. *Principles and Practice of Pulmonary Rehabilitation*. Philadelphia, PA: WB Saunders; 1993:242-251.
179. Piña IL, Apstein CS, Balady GJ, et al. Exercise and heart failure: a statement from the American Heart Association Committee on Exercise, Rehabilitation, and Prevention. *Circulation*. 2003;107:1210-1225.
180. Casaburi R, Storer TW, Wasserman K. Mediation of reduced ventilatory response to exercise after endurance training. *J Appl Physiol (1985)*. 1987;63:1533-1538.
181. Reindl I, Kleber FX. Exertional hyperpnea in patients with chronic heart failure is a reversible cause of exercise intolerance. *Basic Res Cardiol*. 1996;91(suppl 1):37-41.
182. Ponikowski PP, Chua TP, Francis DP, Capucci A, Coats AJ, Piepoli MF. Muscle ergoreceptor overactivity reflects deterioration in clinical status and cardiorespiratory reflex control in chronic heart failure. *Circulation*. 2001;104:2324-2330.
183. Itoh H, Kato K. Short-term exercise training after cardiac surgery. In: Wasserman K, ed. *Exercise Gas Exchange in Heart Disease*. Armonk, NY: Futura Publishing; 1996:229-244.
184. American College of Sports Medicine. *ACSM's Guidelines for Exercise Testing and Prescription*. Baltimore, MD: Williams & Wilkins; 1995.
185. Dubach P, Myers J, Dziekan G, et al. Effect of exercise training on myocardial remodeling in patients with reduced left ventricular function after myocardial infarction: application of magnetic resonance imaging. *Circulation*. 1997;95:2060-2067.
186. Belardinelli R, Georgiou D, Cianci G, Berman N, Ginzton L, Purcaro A. Exercise training improves left ventricular diastolic filling in patients with dilated cardiomyopathy. Clinical and prognostic implications. *Circulation*. 1995;91:2775-2784.
187. Garvey C, Bayles MP, Hamm LF, et al. Pulmonary rehabilitation exercise prescription in chronic obstructive pulmonary disease: review of selected guidelines: an official statement from the American Association of Cardiovascular and Pulmonary Rehabilitation. *J Cardiopulm Rehabil Prev*. 2016;36:75-83.
188. Ries AL, Bauldoff GS, Carlin BW, et al. Pulmonary rehabilitation: joint ACCP/AACVPR evidence-based clinical practice guidelines. *Chest*. 2007;131(5 suppl):4S-42S.
189. Orenstein DM, Noyes BE. Cystic fibrosis. In: Casaburi R, Petty TL, eds. *Principles and Practice of Pulmonary Rehabilitation*. Philadelphia, PA: Saunders; 1993:439-458.
190. Kenn K, Gloeckl R, Behr J. Pulmonary rehabilitation in patients with idiopathic pulmonary fibrosis—a review. *Respiration*. 2013;86: 89-99.
191. Clark CJ. The role of physical training in asthma. In: Casaburi R, Petty TL, eds. *Principles and Practice of Pulmonary Rehabilitation*. Philadelphia, PA: Saunders; 1993:424-438.
192. Whipp BJ, Pardy R. Breathing during exercise. In: Macklem P, Mead J, eds. *Handbook of Physiology, Respiration: Pulmonary Mechanics*. Washington, DC: American Physiological Society; 1986: 605-629.
193. Casaburi R, Patessio A, Ioli F, Zanaboni S, Donner CF, Wasserman K. Reductions in exercise lactic acidosis and ventilation as a result of exercise training in patients with obstructive lung disease. *Am Rev Respir Dis*. 1991;143:9-18.
194. Wasserman K, Sue DY, Casaburi R, Moricca RB. Selection criteria for exercise training in pulmonary rehabilitation. *Eur Respir J Suppl*. 1989;7:604S-610S.
195. Maltais F, Jobin J, Sullivan MJ, et al. Metabolic and hemodynamic responses of lower limb during exercise in patients with COPD. *J Appl Physiol (1985)*. 1998;84:1573-1580.
196. Richardson R, Leak B, Haseler L, et al. Normal skeletal muscle function in patients with COPD when exercise is not centrally limited. *Med Sci Sports Exerc*. 1999;31:S277.
197. Butler J, Schrijen F, Henriquez A, Polu JM, Albert RK. Cause of the raised wedge pressure on exercise in chronic obstructive pulmonary disease. *Am Rev Respir Dis*. 1988;138:350-354.
198. Casaburi R. Deconditioning. In: Fishman AP, ed. *Pulmonary Rehabilition. Lung Biology in Health and Disease Series*. New York, NY: Marcel Dekker; 1996:213-227.
199. Rochester CL, Vogiatzis I, Holland AE, et al; for ATS/ERS Task Force on Policy in Pulmonary Rehabilitation. An official American Thoracic Society/European Respiratory Society policy statement: enhancing implementation, use, and delivery of pulmonary rehabilitation. *Am J Respir Crit Care Med*. 2015;192:1373-1386.
200. Spruit MA, Singh SJ, Garvey C, et al; for ATS/ERS Task Force on Pulmonary Rehabilitation. An official American Thoracic Society/European Respiratory Society statement: key concepts and advances in pulmonary rehabilitation. *Am J Respir Crit Care Med*. 2013;188: e13-e64.
201. Punzal PA, Ries AL, Kaplan RM, Prewitt LM. Maximum intensity exercise training in patients with chronic obstructive pulmonary disease. *Chest*. 1991;100:618-623.
202. Stringer W, Marciniuk D. The role of cardiopulmonary exercise testing (CPET) in pulmonary rehabilitation (PR) of chronic obstructive pulmonary disease (COPD) patients. *COPD*. 2018;15(6): 621-631.
203. Casaburi R, Porszasz J, Burns MR, Carithers ER, Chang RS, Cooper CB. Physiologic benefits of exercise training in rehabilitation of patients with severe chronic obstructive pulmonary disease. *Am J Respir Crit Care Med*. 1997;155:1541-1551.
204. Somfay A, Pórszász J, Lee S-M, Casaburi R. Effect of hyperoxia on gas exchange and lactate kinetics following exercise onset in nonhypoxemic COPD patients. *Chest*. 2002;121:393-400.
205. Cohn JN, Ziesche S, Johnson G, et al. Use of exercise gas exchange measurements in multicenter drug studies. In: Wasserman K, ed. *Exercise Gas Exchange in Heart Disease*. Armonk, NY: Futura Publishing; 1996:245-256.
206. Oudiz RJ, Barst RJ, Hansen JE, et al. Cardiopulmonary exercise testing and six-minute walk correlations in pulmonary arterial hypertension. *Am J Cardiol*. 2006;97:123-126.
207. Huszczuk A, Whipp BJ, Wasserman K. A respiratory gas exchange simulator for routine calibration in metabolic studies. *Eur Respir J*. 1990;3:465-468.
208. Hansen JE, Sun X-G, Yasunobu Y, et al. Reproducibility of cardiopulmonary exercise measurements in patients with pulmonary arterial hypertension. *Chest*. 2004;126:816-824.
209. Puente-Maestu L, Palange P, Casaburi R, et al. Use of exercise testing in the evaluation of interventional efficacy: an official ERS statement. *Eur Respir J*. 2016;47:429-460.

210. Guazzi M, Arena R, Halle M, Piepoli MF, Myers J, Lavie CJ. 2016 Focused update: clinical recommendations for cardiopulmonary exercise testing data assessment in specific patient populations. *Eur Heart J*. 2018;39:1144-1161.
211. Guazzi M, Bandera F, Ozemek C, Systrom D, Arena R. Cardiopulmonary exercise testing: what is its value? *J Am Coll Cardiol*. 2017;70:1618-1636.
212. Marcadet DM, Pavy B, Bosser G, et al. French Society of Cardiology guidelines on exercise tests (part 1): methods and interpretation. *Arch Cardiovasc Dis*. 2018;111:782-790.
213. Marcadet DM, Pavy B, Bosser G, et al. French Society of Cardiology guidelines on exercise tests (part 2): indications for exercise tests in cardiac diseases. *Arch Cardiovasc Dis*. 2019;112:56-66.
214. Corrà U, Agostoni PG, Anker SD, et al. Role of cardiopulmonary exercise testing in clinical stratification in heart failure. A position paper from the Committee on Exercise Physiology and Training of the Heart Failure Association of the European Society of Cardiology. *Eur J Heart Fail*. 2018;20:3-15.
215. Dumitrescu D, Oudiz R, Karpouzas G, et al. Developing pulmonary vasculopathy in systemic sclerosis, detected with non-invasive cardiopulmonary exercise testing. *PLoS One*. 2010;5:e14293.
216. James DVB, Sandals LE, Wood DM, Jones AM. Pulmonary gas exchange. In: Winter EM, Jones AM, Davison RCR, Bromley PD, Mercer TH, eds. *Sport and Exercise Physiology Testing Guidelines. Vol 1: Sport Testing*. Abingdon, United Kingdom: Routledge; 2007:101-111.
217. Tanner RK, Gore CJ, eds. Determination of maximal oxygen consumption ($\dot{V}O_2$max) In: *Physiological Tests for Elite Athletes*. 2nd ed. Champaign, IL: Australian Institute of Sport; 2013:103-122.
218. Bar-Or O. The Wingate anaerobic test. An update on methodology, reliability and validity. *Sports Med*. 1987;4:381-394.
219. Noble BJ, Noble JM. Perception of effort during endurance training and performance. In: Shephard RJ, Astrand PO, eds. *Endurance in Sport*. Oxford, United Kingdom: Blackwell Scientific; 2nd Ed, 2000; 375-395.
220. Zoladz JA, Sargeant AJ, Emmerich J, Stoklosa J, Zychowski A. Changes in acid-base status of marathon runners during incremental field test. Relationship to mean competitive marathon velocity. *Eur J Appl Physiol Occup Physiol*. 1993;67:71-76.
221. Newsholme E, Castell LM. Can amino acids influence exercise performance in athletes? In: Steinacker J, Ward SA, eds. *The Physiology and Pathophysiology of Exercise Tolerance*. New York, NY: Plenum Press; 1996:269-274.
222. Noakes TD. Physiological models to understand exercise fatigue and the adaptations that predict or enhance athletic performance. *Scand J Med Sci Sports*. 2000;10:123-145.
223. Sargeant AJ, Beelen A. Human muscle fatigue in dynamic exercise. In: Sargeant AJ, Kernell D, eds. *Neuromuscular Fatigue*. Amsterdam, Netherlands: North Holland Publishers; 1992.
224. Khong TK, Selvanayagam VS, Sidhu SK, Yusof A. Role of carbohydrate in central fatigue: a systematic review. *Scand J Med Sci Sports*. 2017;27:376-384.
225. Poole DC, Ward SA, Gardner GW, Whipp BJ. Metabolic and respiratory profile of the upper limit for prolonged exercise in man. *Ergonomics*. 1988;31:1265-1279.
226. Hill DW. The critical power concept. A review. *Sports Med*. 1993;16:237-254.
227. Wasserman K, VanKessel A, Burton GB. Interaction of physiological mechanisms during exercise. *J Appl Physiol*. 1967;22:71-85.
228. Astrand I, Astrand PO, Christensen EH, Hedman R. Myohemoglobin as an oxygen-store in man. *Acta Physiol Scand*. 1960;48:454-460.
229. Turner AP, Cathcart AJ, Parker ME, Butterworth C, Wilson J, Ward SA. Oxygen uptake and muscle desaturation kinetics during intermittent cycling in humans. *Med Sci Sports Exerc*. 2006;38:492-503.
230. Cadegiani FA, Kater CE. Hormonal aspects of overtraining syndrome: a systematic review. *BMC Sports Sci Med Rehabil*. 2017;9:14.
231. Hoffman-Goetz L, Pedersen BK. Exercise and the immune system: a model of the stress response? *Immunol Today*. 1994;15:382-387.
232. Banister EW, Morton RH, Fitz-Clarke JR. Clinical dose-response effects of exercise. In: Steinacker J, Ward SA, eds. *The Physiology and Pathophysiology of Exercise Tolerance*. New York, NY: Plenum Press; 1996:297-309.

CHAPTER 9

Diagnostic Specificity of Exercise Intolerance: A Flowchart Approach

There are many indications for cardiopulmonary exercise testing (CPET), including quantifying exercise impairment in a patient with a known diagnosis, planning rehabilitation interventions, and assessing potential outcomes with medical management or in the postoperative period. In other patients, especially those who complain of exercise intolerance without a clear etiology, identifying the cause of intolerance is the major indication for exercise testing.

INTRODUCTION TO FLOWCHARTS

When patients complain of exercise intolerance, it is usually because they are unable to accomplish a task that they expect to complete with comparative ease and without unusual effort or undue feelings of fatigue or shortness of breath. This chapter introduces one strategy intended to show how physiological measurements made during exercise may be used to deduce, systematically, the potential pathophysiology that may be seen in a range of common disorders.

The approach outlined in this chapter uses flowcharts with sequential branch points based on physiological variables obtained during an incremental or ramp increase in work rate on a cycle ergometer to guide the interpreter to a potential conclusion that best fit the results. Major early branch points lead the interpreter to different flow charts. Each decision branch point is numbered, and the letter *R* refers to the right branch of the numbered branch point, and *L* to the left branch. Each final branch point leads to a box suggesting a common category of diagnosis that could account for the measurements found in the decision-making process, in addition to a list of additional measurements that further support the diagnosis. In contrast to earlier editions of this book, the current flowcharts deemphasize the need for arterial blood gas (ABG) measurements during testing, consistent with more frequently used noninvasive CPET studies.

The branch points were developed as dichotomous choices that facilitate decision making, but each branch-point decision should not be rigidly applied. For example, if the physiologic variable addressed at a particular branch point does not strongly favor one or the other branch, or if further measurements described do not adequately or consistently support that diagnosis, both branches of a branch point should be considered. Thus, the flowcharts should be used with some degree of flexibility and consideration of sound physiological principles. Finally, the CPET data should not be interpreted in isolation; other clinical information such as the history, pulmonary function tests, and lung and heart imaging should be included as well.

This flowchart method is certainly not the only approach for interpreting cardiopulmonary exercise tests and does not necessarily lead one to discrete clinical diagnoses. Indeed, there are conditions limiting exercise tolerance that are not specifically identified among the diagnostic end points of these flow charts, and there are many individuals who have more than one condition affecting exercise function which will result in a mixed set of responses. Rather, the flowcharts serve as the foundation for a structured approach to a physiologically based interpretation of exercise intolerance, and the resulting categorization highlights the pathophysiological defects or conditions limiting exercise function, which may sometimes span a number of specific clinical diagnoses.

The contribution to this chapter of Dr. Karlman Wasserman, its original author, could not be overstated and is gratefully acknowledged.

PEAK $\dot{V}O_2$ AND ANAEROBIC THRESHOLD (FLOWCHART 1)

Two physiological variables during CPET, the peak O_2 uptake ($\dot{V}O_2$) and the $\dot{V}O_2$ at the anaerobic threshold (*AT*), provide the first major decision break points for this flowchart approach (**Fig. 9.1**). The first question to address is whether the peak $\dot{V}O_2$ is normal or decreased (below 95% confidence limit for normal), thereby establishing if the patient's subjective exercise intolerance is associated with objective reduction in exercise capacity. At this step in particular, it is important to appreciate that the ranges of normal for peak $\dot{V}O_2$ and *AT* are fairly wide and can vary somewhat depending on the selection of reference values used by the laboratory. There are therefore circumstances in which it is difficult to classify these variables as being normal or reduced **for the particular individual** being tested. Consideration of their exercise habits and history as well as the source of the reference values is helpful in this. An individual with a normal peak $\dot{V}O_2$ may still have exercise intolerance, and it will be helpful to look at Flowchart 2 (**Fig. 9.2**) to explore possible reasons.

If the peak $\dot{V}O_2$ is low, the second question asked is whether the $\dot{V}O_2$ at the *AT* is normal, decreased, or indeterminate. A low peak $\dot{V}O_2$ with a normal *AT* leads the interpreter to Flowchart 3 (**Fig. 9.3**); these findings suggest that O_2 flow at a submaximal exercise level is within normal limits (at least up to and at the *AT*), but maximum exercise capacity is limited by one of a variety of other causes. A low peak $\dot{V}O_2$ with a low *AT* leads to Flowchart 4 (**Fig. 9.4**); this combination of both low peak $\dot{V}O_2$ and low *AT* suggest several disorders that limit the capacity to transport oxygen. Finally, low peak $\dot{V}O_2$ but with an indeterminate *AT* leads to Flowchart 5 (**Fig. 9.5**), where various combinations of variables lead to a variety of suggested diagnoses.

EXERCISE INTOLERANCE WITH NORMAL PEAK OXYGEN UPTAKE (FLOWCHART 2)

When peak $\dot{V}O_2$ is apparently normal but the patient complains of exercise intolerance, the main diagnostic possibilities are as follows:

1. The patient is normal but has anxiety about failing health or decreased fitness.
2. The patient is obese to the point of requiring an increased metabolic and cardiopulmonary response to perform a given activity.
3. The patient, previously healthy, has developed early cardiovascular or lung disease. Thus, despite a reduced ability to comfortably do the physical work to which he or she is accustomed, the peak $\dot{V}O_2$ still falls within the normal range of predicted values.

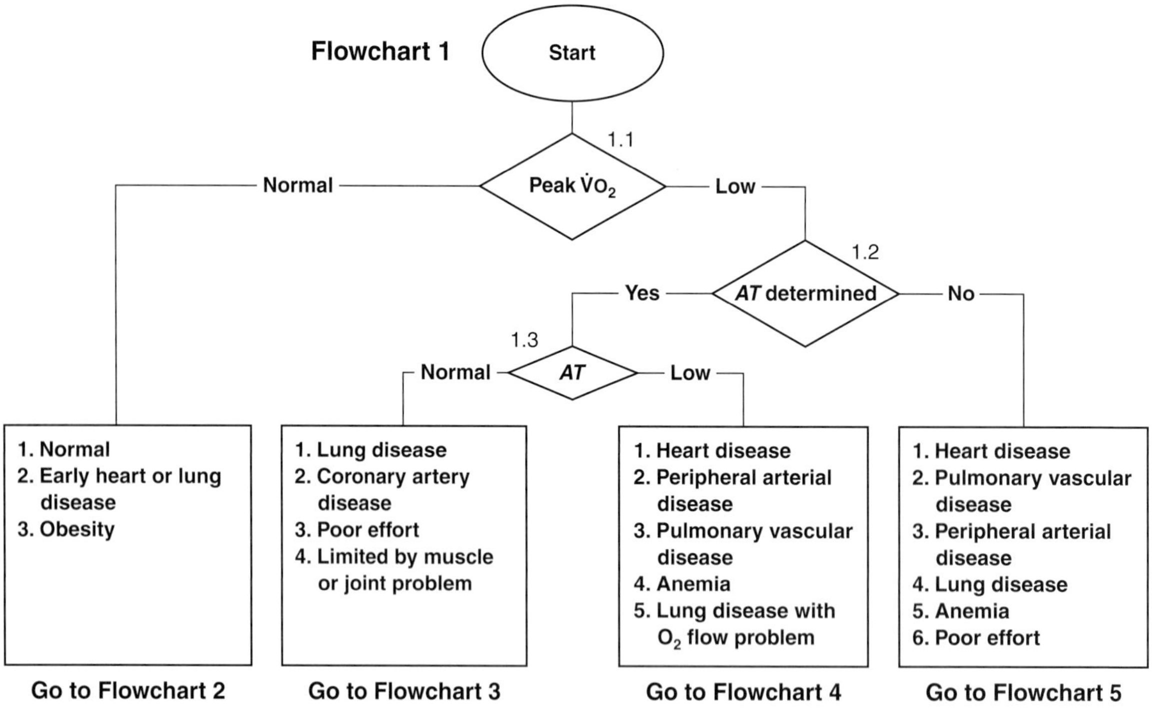

FIGURE 9.1. Flowchart for the differential diagnosis of the cause of exercise limitation. Analysis starts with the measurement of peak oxygen (O_2) uptake ($\dot{V}O_2$). Ellipsoids indicate starting points highlighting a question. The diamonds indicate branch points in the decision logic based on further questions. The boxes provide potential diagnoses (listed above the horizontal dashed line) and measurements that support the diagnosis (below the horizontal dashed line). If the supporting measurements do not fit well, try a closely related branch point leading to a different diagnosis in which the supporting measurements fit better. Branch points are numbered to correspond to the text. Abbreviations: N, Normal; unl, unloaded.

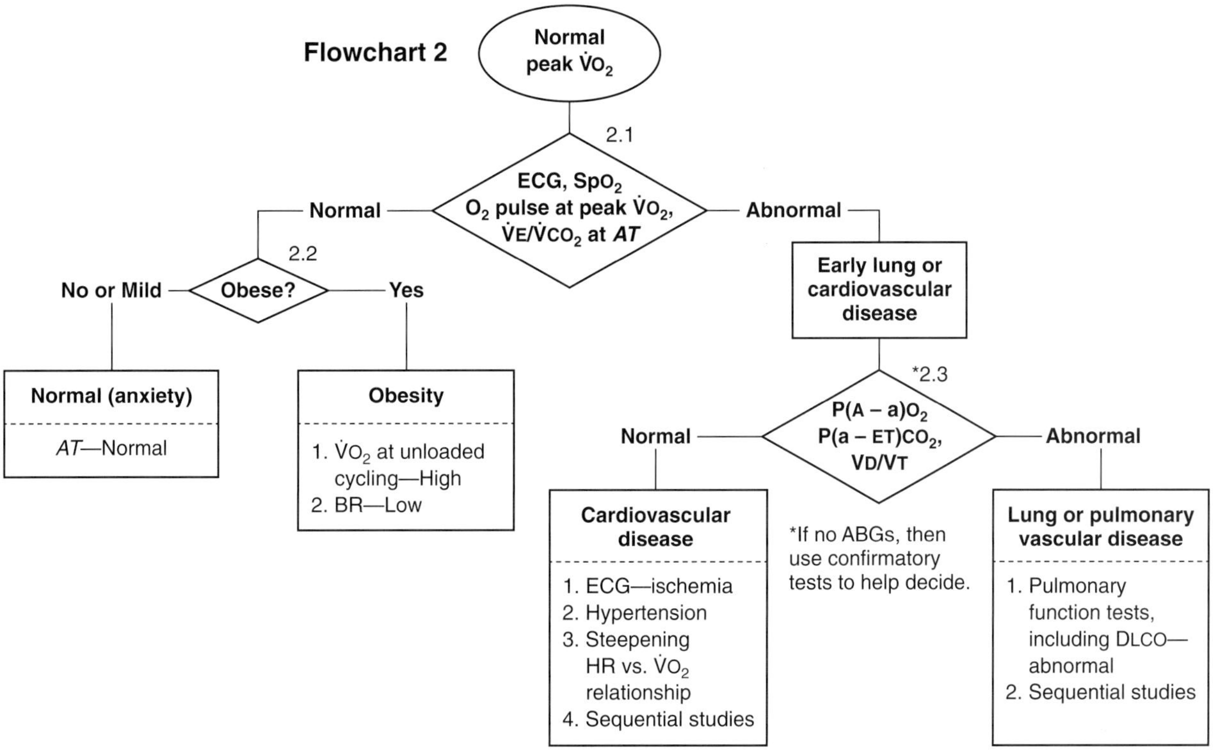

FIGURE 9.2. Flowchart for conditions in which peak oxygen (O_2) uptake ($\dot{V}O_2$) is normal, but the patient feels limited during exercise. If the supporting measurements do not fit well, try a closely related branch point leading to a different diagnosis in which the confirmatory measurements fit better. Symbols and use of flowchart are as described in "Introduction to Flowcharts" and legend for Figure 9.1.

The diagnostic flowchart leading to each of these diagnoses is shown in **Figure 9.2**.

A normal peak $\dot{V}O_2$ (greater than or equal to predicted peak $\dot{V}O_2$) with a low *AT* is unusual. However, it might be found in exceptionally sedentary subjects or patients with very mild disease that compromises O_2 transport to muscle cells.

LOW PEAK OXYGEN UPTAKE WITH NORMAL ANAEROBIC THRESHOLD (FLOWCHART 3)

A low peak $\dot{V}O_2$ but with a normal *AT* would indicate that O_2 transport is adequate during submaximal exercise, but some factor is causing the subject to stop exercise prior to reaching the normal predicted peak $\dot{V}O_2$ Because ventilatory limitation is an important cause of this pathophysiologic pattern, looking at breathing reserve is a good first branch point (Branch Point 3.1, see **Fig. 9.3**). A low breathing reserve would generally lead toward lung disease, obstructive or restrictive. A normal breathing reserve might suggest in this situation myocardial ischemia or a noncardiopulmonary reason (such as poor effort or musculoskeletal disorder) to stop exercise at a low peak $\dot{V}O_2$ after achieving a normal *AT*. Myocardial ischemia during exercise may be demonstrated on the electrocardiogram, but on occasions, evidence for ischemia may be reflected by evidence of the onset of left ventricular (LV) dysfunction due to ischemia.

LOW PEAK OXYGEN UPTAKE WITH LOW ANAEROBIC THRESHOLD (FLOWCHART 4)

In these patients, a low peak $\dot{V}O_2$ indicates decreased maximum exercise performance and a low *AT* indicates a problem with O_2 flow at submaximal exercise. The challenge is to identify which of many possible systems is responsible for this combination of abnormalities.

At the first branch point (see **Fig. 9.4**), low breathing reserve (Branch Point 4.1-L) leads toward lung disease or, unusually, to a low "set-point" for $Pa{CO_2}$, such as chronically low HCO_3^- or due to high altitude. If breathing reserve is normal or high (Branch Point 4.1-R), there are multiple reasons for this combination of findings, including lung and heart disease, peripheral arterial disease, and anemia. Branch points to help separate these disorders rely on ventilatory equivalent for CO_2 ($\dot{V}E/\dot{V}CO_2$) (or, with ABG, dead space/tidal volume ratio [VD/VT]) to distinguish pulmonary vascular disease or heart failure[1] (Branch Point 4.3-R) from those disorders that demonstrate an O_2 flow problem of nonpulmonary origin (Branch Point 4.3-L). The latter include anemia, peripheral arterial disease, and some forms of heart disease. Further branch points will lead to suggested disorders, and confirmatory data should prove helpful.

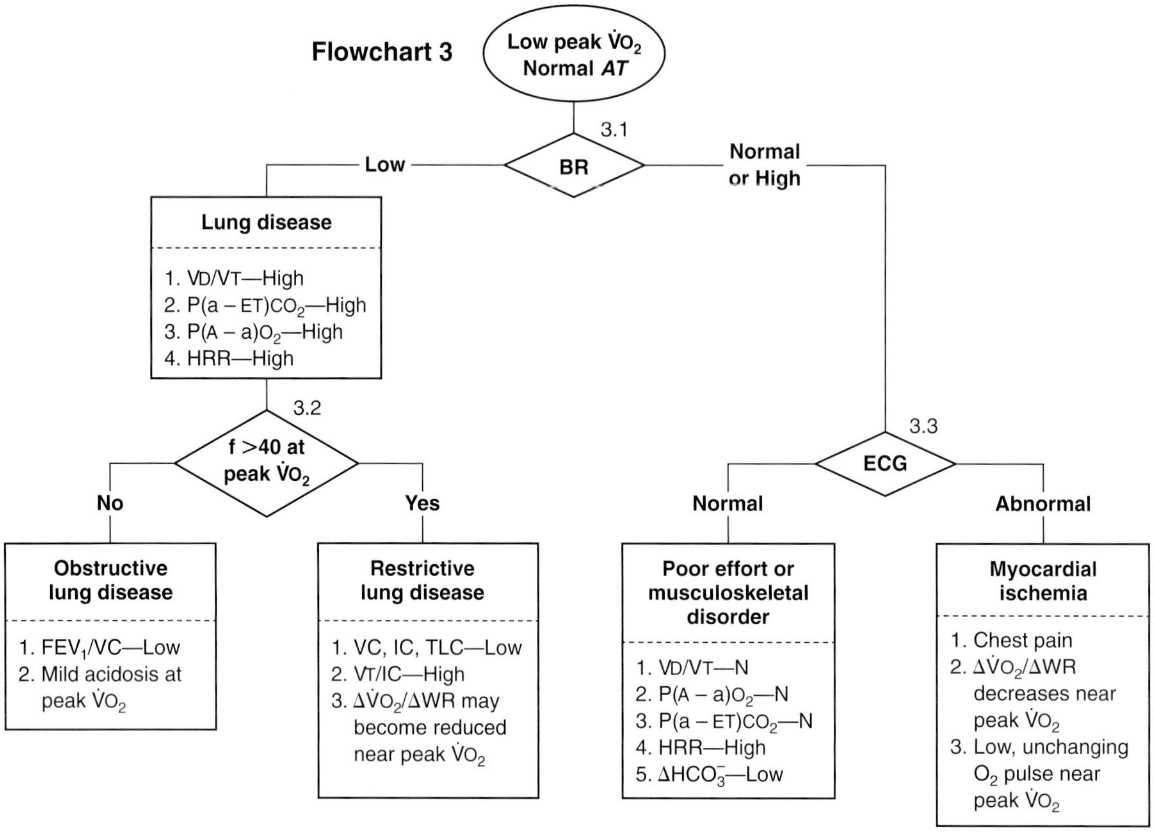

FIGURE 9.3. Flowchart for conditions in which peak oxygen (O_2) uptake ($\dot{V}O_2$) is low, but the anaerobic threshold (*AT*) is normal. If the supporting measurements do not fit well, try a closely related branch point leading to a different diagnosis in which the supporting measurements fit better. Symbols and use of flowchart are as described in "Introduction to Flowcharts" and legend for Figure 9.1.

LOW PEAK OXYGEN UPTAKE WITH ANAEROBIC THRESHOLD NOT DETERMINED (FLOWCHART 5)

The importance of the *AT* in deciding the cause of exercise limitation is demonstrated in the previous flowcharts. However, in some patients, the *AT* may not be clearly identified by gas exchange measurements because the rate of increase in work rate was too slow relative to the subject's work capacity. Also, the interpreter may feel that the *AT* is unreliable or indistinct because of breathing irregularities. Failure to identify an *AT* may also result from the patient stopping exercise before the *AT* is reached, either volitionally or due to breathing restriction secondary to abnormal lung mechanics.

An alternative strategy to using the *AT* as the second major branch point in the decision-making process (Flowchart 1, see **Fig. 9.1**) is described in Flowchart 5 (see **Fig. 9.5**). First, a reduced peak $\dot{V}O_2$ indicates that the patient's maximum exercise capacity is reduced. Second, in the absence of a determination of the *AT*, it is suggested that tests that suggest mismatching of ventilation to perfusion may make it possible to distinguish disorders associated with inefficiency of lung gas exchange from disorders associated with normal lung function and pulmonary circulation. Thus, Branch Point 5.1 (see **Fig 9.5**) uses ABG, if available, or pulmonary gas exchange measurements to identify the presence of mismatching of ventilation to perfusion (normal or high $\dot{V}E/\dot{V}CO_2$ measured at its nadir value or near the *AT*). These measurements have a narrow normal range, and, in addition, the higher the $\dot{V}E/\dot{V}CO_2$ measured at or near the *AT*, the higher the likelihood that VD/VT is abnormal. Thus, when $\dot{V}E/\dot{V}CO_2$ at this point was greater or equal than 39, VD/VT was abnormal 87% of the time.[2] Acute hyperventilation can also elevate the $\dot{V}E/\dot{V}CO_2$. However, if the respiratory exchange ratio is not abnormally elevated (below 1.0), then these surrogate markers of uneven ventilation relative to perfusion are most likely reliable reflections of abnormal lung gas exchange.

Diseases associated with abnormal ventilation–perfusion relationships (Branch Point 5.1-R) include lung diseases, pulmonary vascular diseases, and LV failure. Patients with myocardial ischemia without chronic heart failure, mild LV failure, anemia, peripheral arterial disease, and poor effort

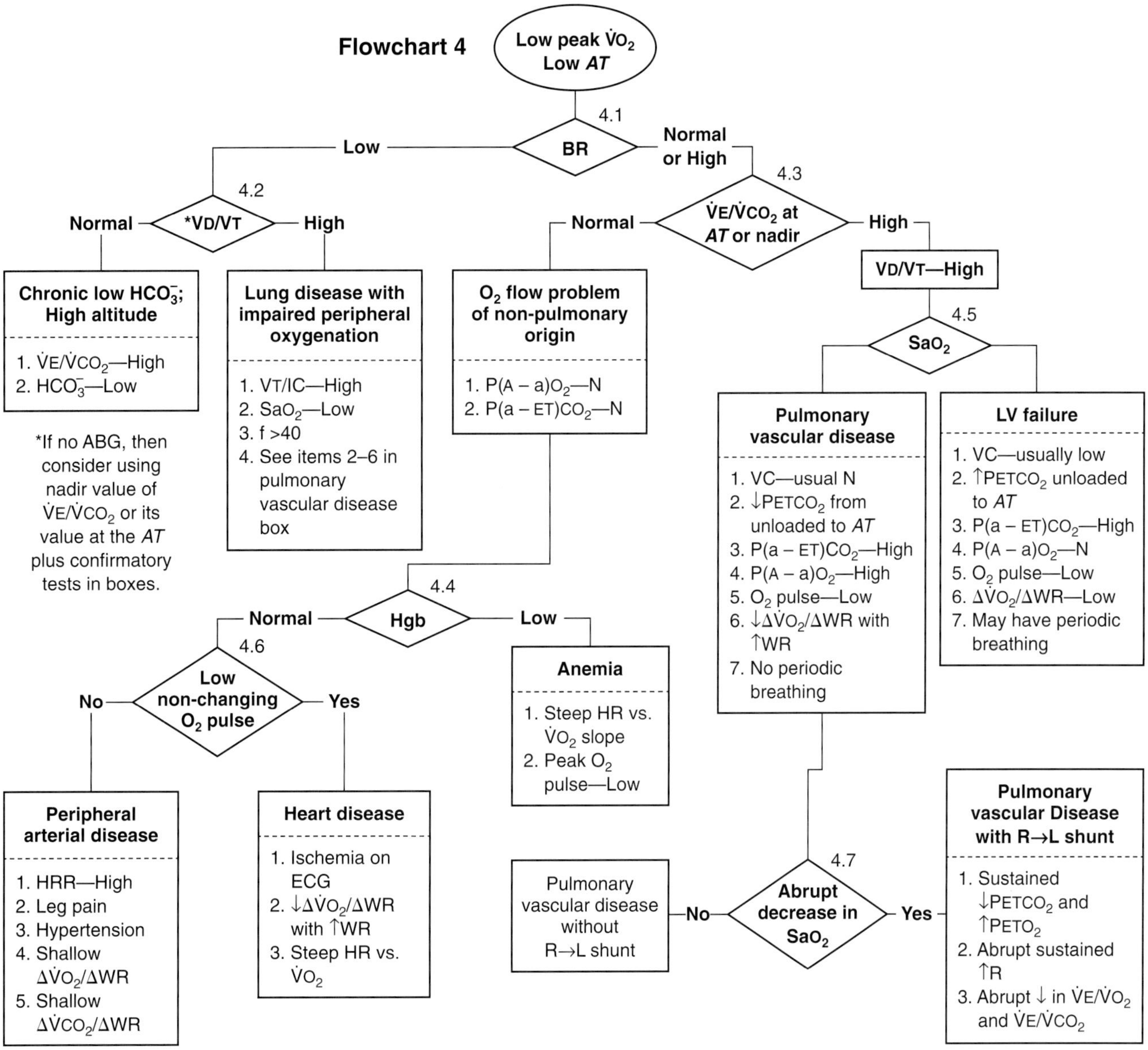

FIGURE 9.4. Flowchart for conditions in which both peak oxygen (O_2) uptake ($\dot{V}O_2$) and anaerobic threshold (*AT*) are reduced. If the supporting measurements do not fit well, try a closely related branch point leading to a different diagnosis in which the supporting measurements fit better. Symbols and use of flowchart are as described in "Introduction to Flowcharts" and legend for Figure 9.1.

alone would generally have normal ventilation–perfusion relationships (Branch Point 5.1-L).

Subsequent branch points separate those studies with abnormal gas exchange (Branch Point 5.1-R) from those with normal gas exchange (Branch Point 5.1-L). Low breathing reserve in the former group suggests obstructive or restrictive lung diseases, whereas a normal breathing reserve suggests LV failure or pulmonary vascular disease. Those with normal gas exchange (Branch Point 5.1-L) can have a variety of problems that range from myocardial ischemia, anemia, poor effort, peripheral arterial disease, and chronotropic incompetence. Variables that help distinguish these include heart rate reserve, hemoglobin concentration, and $\Delta\dot{V}O_2/\Delta WR$ at subsequent branch points.

SUMMARY

To determine the likely pathophysiological causes of exercise limitation, we found that a logical and useful approach can be developed and displayed in five flowcharts. Each flowchart starts with a question regarding whether the peak $\dot{V}O_2$ is normal or abnormal. Other

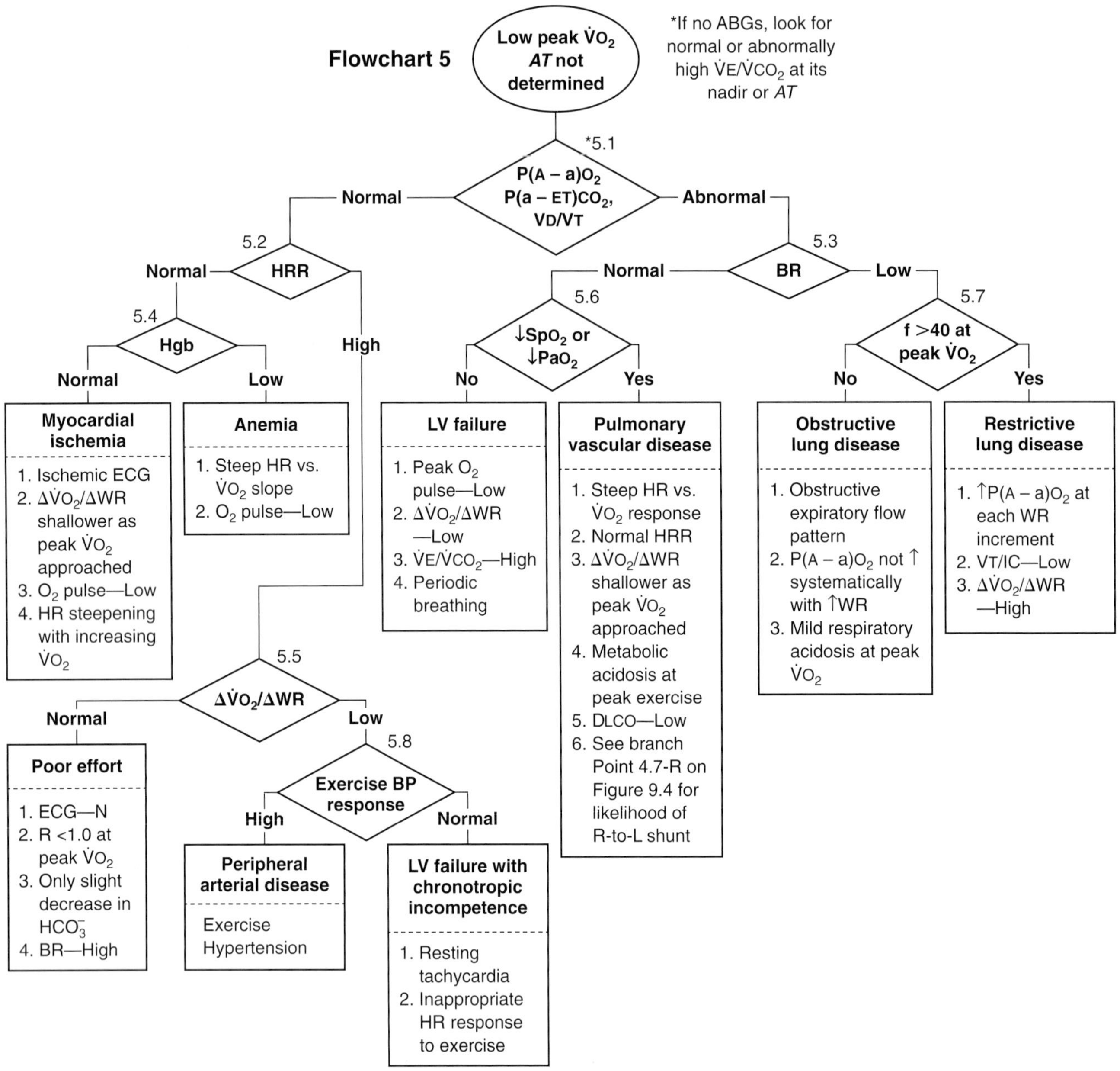

FIGURE 9.5. Flowchart for conditions in which peak oxygen (O_2) uptake ($\dot{V}O_2$) is low, but the anaerobic threshold (*AT*) has not been measured or cannot be reliably determined. If the supporting measurements do not fit well, try a closely related branch point leading to a different diagnosis in which the supporting measurements fit better. Symbols and use of flowchart are as described in "Introduction to Flowcharts" and the legend for Figure 9.1.

physiological measurements relating *AT*, breathing reserve, heart rate and $\dot{V}O_2$, ventilation–perfusion relationship, and $\Delta\dot{V}O_2/\Delta WR$ are then used to define the pathophysiological sites in the gas transport coupling of muscle metabolism to gas exchange at the airway. The identified pathophysiology can be used to establish the likely clinical diagnosis.

REFERENCES

1. Hansen JE, Ulubay G, Chow BF, Sun XG, Wasserman K. Mixed-expired and end-tidal CO_2 distinguish between ventilation and perfusion defects during exercise testing in patients with lung and heart diseases. *Chest*. 2007;132:977-983.
2. Roman MA, Casaburi JD, Porszasz J, Casaburi R. Noninvasive assessment of normality of VD/VT in clinical cardiopulmonary exercise testing utilizing incremental cycle ergometry. *Eur J Appl Physiol*. 2013;113:33-40.

CHAPTER 10

Case Presentations

PURPOSE AND MATERIAL

This chapter consists of a collection of examples of cardiopulmonary exercise tests (CPETs) along with discussion of the data and their interpretation. Cases were selected to illustrate both the range of normal cardiorespiratory responses during CPET, and how these are affected by chronic diseases that cause exercise intolerance. Because most of these examples are drawn from real clinical practice, there are some in which patient performance was less than optimal or the data, although we believe accurate, were not completely free of noise or artifacts. The cases also do not necessarily represent the "best" example of a particular condition. In fact, although underlying physiology dictates that impairment in a given organ system will have primary effects on a particular aspect of the exercise response, meaning that different diseases have typical findings on CPET, individuals are nevertheless unique. Characterizing the effect of a disease on the functional capacity of an individual, rather than on the disease category in general, is a major purpose of CPET. For the more common heart and lung diseases, therefore, several case examples are included to reflect that variation.

In successive editions of this text, cases have been added to and subtracted from this chapter to reflect evolving experience and applications of CPET. Some of the older cases that remain in the collection will be found not to reflect current medical practice, because they were conducted when the standard of care for a particular medical condition differed from the present. Those that have nevertheless been carried forward have been retained because the data are viewed as unique or instructive. In some cases, this is because they contain results of arterial blood gases measured during exercise, including some for individuals that would not have them measured currently. In other cases, the tests were performed by individuals who had previously undiagnosed disease, so the CPETs provide characterization of untreated conditions. Not surprisingly, interpretation of these early cases placed particular emphasis on diagnostic assessment, which prompted development of the flow chart analyses presented in Chapter 9. Tracing the results of exercise tests through the flowchart analyses reinforces the most common features of different categories of disease and can be especially useful as a learning exercise. Some of the case discussions in this chapter therefore reference the flow charts in the interpretation of the data. Others do not, either because of the personal approach of the interpreter or because the test was conducted, for example, for grading severity of impairment due to a known disease, planning rehabilitation, or some other indication other than diagnosis.

For reasons identified above, the vintage of cases included in this edition ranges from a few months to several decades prior to the publication date. There is therefore variability, not only in the subjects and purposes of the tests, but also in the technical specifications of equipment used and the complement of measurements obtained. The range of variables and data processing are therefore not entirely uniform from case to case, and this is reflected in the discussions.

FORMAT FOR CASE PRESENTATIONS

Cases are all presented in the same general format, beginning with an abbreviated clinical history limited to information necessary to appreciate the context of the test and the results. Pertinent demographic and respiratory function data are shown in the first table for each case, and a summary of key variables from the exercise data in a second table. A third table (and sometimes fourth if more than one test is presented) shows the exercise data in tabular form as 30-second averages of breath-by-breath measurements from rest through recovery. A graphical display of the data is presented in the form of a

The authors wish to acknowledge the enduring contributions of Drs. James E. Hansen and Karlman Wasserman, who authored some of these cases for earlier editions of this book and designed the format used throughout the chapter.

nine-panel array of graphs. Findings on exercise electrocardiograms are briefly described in the test results, but tracings are not reproduced in the interest of space.

Graphing Conventions

Case discussions are centered on review of the graphs, which are organized as detailed in Chapter 6. A number of formatting conventions are observed to facilitate data interpretation, also described in Chapter 6. The predicted value for peak oxygen uptake ($\dot{V}O_2$) is shown along with the test data on the panel 1 graph and for both peak $\dot{V}O_2$ and peak heart rate on the panel 3 graph. For cycle ergometry tests, work rate is plotted on panel 1 and scaled on the right y-axis such that each 100 W corresponds to 1 L of $\dot{V}O_2$ on the left y-axis. This results in the $\dot{V}O_2$ and work rate data increasing in parallel on the graph if their relationship ($\Delta\dot{V}O_2/\Delta WR$) is normal (10 mL/min $\dot{V}O_2$/Watt), which facilitates identification of deviations from normal. The relationship of carbon dioxide output ($\dot{V}CO_2$) as a function of $\dot{V}O_2$ (V-slope) is plotted in panel 3 with equal scaling on the x- and y-axes, and a diagonal line is superimposed on the plot that identifies the slope of 1 (45°) to facilitate identification of the anaerobic threshold. In panel 6, minute ventilation ($\dot{V}E$) on the y-axis is scaled with a 30:1 ratio to $\dot{V}CO_2$ on the x-axis so that data having a graphed slope of less than 45° represent a $\dot{V}E$-$\dot{V}CO_2$ slope of less than 30, which is approximately normal. When arterial blood gases are available, they are included in the third table and the gas tensions are plotted in panel 7 of the nine-panel figure.

For most cases, the graphs use the same 30-second averages of breath-by-breath data as shown in the third table of the case presentation; however, for the most recently added cases, the graphs use 10-second averages.

CHARACTERISTICS OF CASES

Scope

These cases reflect the range of patients encountered in the collective experience of the authors, which may differ from the profile of other practices or laboratories. For example, the patients represented are almost exclusively adults. Aside from children, there are undoubtedly many other populations and many conditions affecting exercise function that are not represented. It is hoped that the general approach to organizing and interpreting data will allow the reader to extrapolate to other populations and contexts in which the information provided by CPET is of value.

Conditions

One hundred cases are presented. The majority of these are presented in detail in the print version of this text; these are supplemented by additional cases identified by title in the print version and detailed in the on-line version. Cases are grouped for convenience into primary diagnostic categories, recognizing that many of the cases could easily be included under any of several different designations.

- Cases 1 to 14 were chosen to illustrate normal findings of persons of differing ages, levels of fitness, and testing conditions.
- Cases 15 to 25 are examples of common cardiovascular disorders, including chronic left ventricular heart failure (cases 15-19) and atherosclerotic cardiovascular disease (cases 20-25).
- Cases 26 to 38 are examples of structural heart diseases, including valvular disorders, congenital, and infiltrative processes.
- In cases 39 to 44, the primary findings are related to cardiac rate or rhythm.
- Cases 45 and 46 are examples of patients with impaired cardiovascular responses best characterized as inadequate preload.
- Cases 47 to 55 illustrate findings from patients with primary or secondary pulmonary vascular disorders.
- Common pulmonary diseases are represented in cases 56 to 71 including interstitial lung diseases (56-62) and chronic obstructive airways disease (cases 63-71).
- Cases 72 to 76 illustrate findings of extrapulmonary restriction of exercise ventilation.
- Cases 77 to 82 are of patients with neuromuscular disorders, including myopathic conditions.
- Cases 83 to 91 focus on discussion of how coexisting conditions, including heart and lung disease, cigarette smoking, and obesity, may affect exercise function and CPET variables. It should be noted that many cases in the preceding categories also have more than a single isolated disorder affecting the test results.
- Cases 92 to 100 were chosen as examples of a number of established or evolving applications of CPET in clinical practice. Each of these could have been included in one or more of the other diagnostic categories.

SYMBOLS, ABBREVIATIONS, AND CALCULATIONS

The symbols and abbreviations used in the case presentations and tables reflect standard usage in medical journals and prior sections of this book. *Symbols and Abbreviations* are identified in Appendix A, and their meanings defined in Appendix B, in the *Glossary*. Formulas used for deriving values for calculated variables are presented in Appendix C, *Calculations, Formulas, and Examples*. Predicted values used for reference in the cases are based on formulas detailed in Chapter 7. Within each case presentation, definitions of the abbreviations used for the core measurements can also be found in the legends for Figure 1 of that case.

CASE 1

Normal Man

CLINICAL FINDINGS

A 55-year-old executive was referred for exercise testing after complaining of decreased exercise tolerance. He noted weakness, fatigue, and some dyspnea after jogging one block, but he could walk 3 miles on a level surface without difficulty. He had become symptomatic after a period of inactivity due to an ankle injury 2 years earlier and felt he never returned to his former exercise tolerance. He did not report chest pain, syncope, palpitations, coughing, or wheezing. He had smoked half a pack of cigarettes per day for 10 years but had reduced his smoking to three to four cigarettes per week. He took no medications. Physical examination, chest roentgenograms, and resting electrocardiogram (ECG) were normal. For this and all following cases, the data are presented using standard abbreviations and symbols as defined in Appendices A, B, and C of this book.

EXERCISE FINDINGS

The patient performed exercise on a cycle ergometer. He pedaled at 60 rpm without added load for 3 minutes, and then the work rate was increased 20 W/min to his symptom-limited maximum. Arterial blood was sampled every second minute, and intra-arterial blood pressure was recorded from a percutaneously placed brachial artery catheter. The patient stopped exercise because of thigh fatigue. Twelve-lead ECG recordings remained normal during exercise. Selected pulmonary function data are shown in **Table 10.1.1** and selected exercise data in **Table 10.1.2** and **Figure 10.1.1**.

TABLE 10.1.1 Selected Respiratory Function Data

Measurement	Predicted	Measured
Age (y)		55
Sex		Male
Height (cm)		182
Weight (kg)	83	80
Hematocrit (%)		41
VC (L)	4.75	6.06
IC (L)	3.17	4.16
TLC (L)	7.08	8.24
FEV_1 (L)	3.76	4.52
FEV_1/VC (%)	79	75
MVV (L/min)	151	200
D_{LCO} (mL/mm Hg/min)	28.8	28.30

Abbreviations: D_{LCO}, diffusing capacity of lung for carbon monoxide; FEV_1, forced expiratory volume in 1 second; IC, inspiratory capacity; MVV, maximum voluntary ventilation; TLC, total lung capacity; VC, vital capacity.

INTERPRETATION

Comments

The results of the respiratory function studies are within normal limits.

Analysis

Peak oxygen (O_2) uptake ($\dot{V}O_2$) and anaerobic threshold are normal. The ECG and arterial blood gases are normal throughout exercise. The O_2 pulse at the maximum work rate is normal, as are the ventilatory equivalent for carbon dioxide ($\dot{V}E/\dot{V}CO_2$) at its lowest value and the slope of $\dot{V}E/\dot{V}CO_2$.

TABLE 10.1.2 Selected Exercise Data

Measurement	Predicted	Measured
Peak $\dot{V}O_2$ (L/min)	2.47	2.53
Maximum heart rate (beats/min)	165	176
Maximum O_2 pulse (mL/beat)	15.0	14.5
$\Delta\dot{V}O_2/\Delta WR$ (mL/min/W)	10.3	9.8
AT (L/min)	>1.07	1.2
Blood pressure (mm Hg [rest, max])		144/81, 225/87
Maximum $\dot{V}E$ (L/min)		107
Exercise breathing reserve (L/min)	>15	93
$\dot{V}E/\dot{V}CO_2$ @ *AT* or lowest	27.2	25.7
PaO_2 (mm Hg [rest, max ex])		98, 110
$P(A - a)O_2$ (mm Hg [rest, max ex])		5, 15
$PaCO_2$ (mm Hg [rest, max ex])		39, 32
$P(a - ET)CO_2$ (mm Hg [rest, max ex])		0, −5
V_D/V_T (rest, heavy ex)		0.26, 0.15
HCO_3^- (mEq/L [rest, 2-min recov])		25, 12

Abbreviations: *AT*, anaerobic threshold; $\Delta\dot{V}O_2/\Delta WR$, change in $\dot{V}O_2$/change in work rate; ex, exercise; HCO_3^-, bicarbonate; O_2, oxygen; $P(A - a)O_2$, alveolar-arterial PO_2 difference; $P(a - ET)CO_2$, arterial-end-tidal PCO_2 difference; recov, recovery; V_D/V_T, physiological dead space-tidal volume ratio; $\dot{V}E$, minute ventilation; $\dot{V}E/\dot{V}CO_2$, ventilatory equivalent for carbon dioxide; $\dot{V}O_2$, oxygen uptake.

TABLE 10.1.3 Air Breathing

Time (min)	Work rate (W)	BP (mm Hg)	HR (min^{-1})	f (min^{-1})	$\dot{V}E$ (L/min BTPS)	$\dot{V}CO_2$ (L/min STPD)	$\dot{V}O_2$ (L/min STPD)	$\frac{\dot{V}O_2}{HR}$ (mL/beat)	R	pH	HCO_3^- (mEq/L)	PO_2, mm Hg ET	PO_2, mm Hg a	PO_2, mm Hg (A − a)	PCO_2, mm Hg ET	PCO_2, mm Hg a	PCO_2, mm Hg (a − ET)	$\frac{\dot{V}E}{\dot{V}CO_2}$	$\frac{\dot{V}E}{\dot{V}O_2}$	$\frac{V_D}{V_T}$
0	Rest	153/87								7.42	25		97			39				
0.5	Rest		74	14	12.2	0.32	0.34	4.6	0.94			112			35			34	32	
1.0	Rest		78	13	9.8	0.25	0.31	4.0	0.81			105			38			35	28	
1.5	Rest		78	13	9.9	0.26	0.32	4.1	0.81			105			37			34	27	
2.0	Rest	144/81	80	11	9.2	0.26	0.34	4.3	0.76	7.42	24	103	98	5	38	38	0	32	24	0.26
2.5	Rest		79	12	11.4	0.32	0.42	5.3	0.76			102			38			32	25	
3.0	Rest		76	10	13.2	0.38	0.43	5.7	0.88			106			37			33	29	
3.5	Unloaded		93	16	18.2	0.56	0.66	7.1	0.85			105			38			30	26	
4.0	Unloaded		91	12	17.1	0.58	0.69	7.6	0.84			104			38			28	23	
4.5	Unloaded		87	19	16.2	0.48	0.57	6.6	0.84			104			40			30	26	
5.0	Unloaded		83	19	14.5	0.42	0.53	6.4	0.79			103			39			31	24	
5.5	Unloaded		85	22	16.9	0.48	0.59	6.9	0.81			102			40			31	25	
6.0	Unloaded	171/87	85	25	16.4	0.50	0.62	7.3	0.81	7.41	25	101	100	2	40	40	0	29	23	0.21
6.5	20		84	24	19.7	0.65	0.80	9.5	0.81			100			41			27	22	
7.0	20		86	28	18.1	0.58	0.67	7.8	0.87			104			40			27	23	
7.5	40		92	23	21.6	0.73	0.87	9.5	0.84			99			43			27	23	
8.0	40	183/84	93	18	19.9	0.69	0.82	8.8	0.84	7.40	24	101	99	5	42	40	−2	27	22	0.18
8.5	60		101	17	26.7	0.92	1.06	10.5	0.87			101			41			27	24	
9.0	60		104	17	26.0	0.91	1.03	9.9	0.88			102			42			27	24	
9.5	80		108	16	25.8	0.93	1.03	9.5	0.90			100			44			26	24	
10.0	80	195/81	110	16	28.4	1.07	1.16	10.5	0.92	7.38	23	103	98	9	43	40	−3	25	23	0.14
10.5	100		116	16	37.3	1.38	1.37	11.8	1.01			107			41			26	26	
11.0	100		123	17	38.1	1.44	1.41	11.5	1.02			107			43			25	26	
11.5	120		131	18	42.0	1.54	1.45	11.1	1.06			106			43			26	28	
12.0	120	207/87	135	19	44.5	1.67	1.62	12.0	1.03	7.37	23	107	103	7	43	41	−2	26	26	0.17
12.5	140		142	18	49.4	1.83	1.67	11.8	1.10			108			43			26	29	
13.0	140		146	20	49.4	1.87	1.74	11.9	1.07			109			42			26	27	
13.5	160		152	20	55.5	2.09	1.88	12.4	1.11			110			42			26	29	
14.0	160	213/90	155	19	58.3	2.23	1.99	12.8	1.12	7.35	21	110	101	13	42	39	−3	25	28	0.13
14.5	180		160	20	67.7	2.51	2.18	13.6	1.15			106			45			26	30	
15.0	180		163	22	69.5	2.55	2.16	13.3	1.18			112			42			27	31	
15.5	200		167	24	77.3	2.74	2.26	13.5	1.21			112			42			27	33	
16.0	200	225/87	170	27	90.7	3.10	2.42	14.2	1.28	7.31	18	115	105	15	40	36	−4	29	37	0.16
16.5	220		174	31	107.2	3.40	2.53	14.5	1.34			119			37			31	41	
17.0	220	216/90	176	30	102.9	3.20	2.36	13.4	1.36	7.30	15	118	110	15	37	32	−5	31	43	0.14
17.5	Recovery		162	24	84.3	2.64	1.93	11.9	1.37			114			41			31	43	
18.0	Recovery		158	21	71.5	2.10	1.26	8.0	1.67			124			35			33	55	
18.5	Recovery		151	18	57.6	1.67	1.02	6.8	1.64			126			34			34	55	
19.0	Recovery	165/75	149	19	52.7	1.44	0.91	6.1	1.58	7.22	12	126	124	5	32	30	−2	35	56	0.18

Abbreviations: BP, blood pressure; BTPS, body temperature pressure saturated; f, frequency; HCO_3^-, bicarbonate; HR, heart rate; $P(A - a)O_2$, alveolar-arterial PO_2 difference; $P(a - ET)CO_2$, arterial-end-tidal PCO_2 difference; $PETCO_2$, end-tidal PCO_2; $PETO_2$, end-tidal PO_2; R, respiratory exchange ratio; STPD, standard temperature pressure dry; $\dot{V}CO_2$, carbon dioxide output; V_D/V_T, physiological dead space–tidal volume ratio; $\dot{V}E$, minute ventilation; $\dot{V}E/\dot{V}CO_2$, ventilatory equivalent for carbon dioxide; $\dot{V}E/\dot{V}O_2$, ventilatory equivalent for oxygen; $\dot{V}O_2$, oxygen uptake.

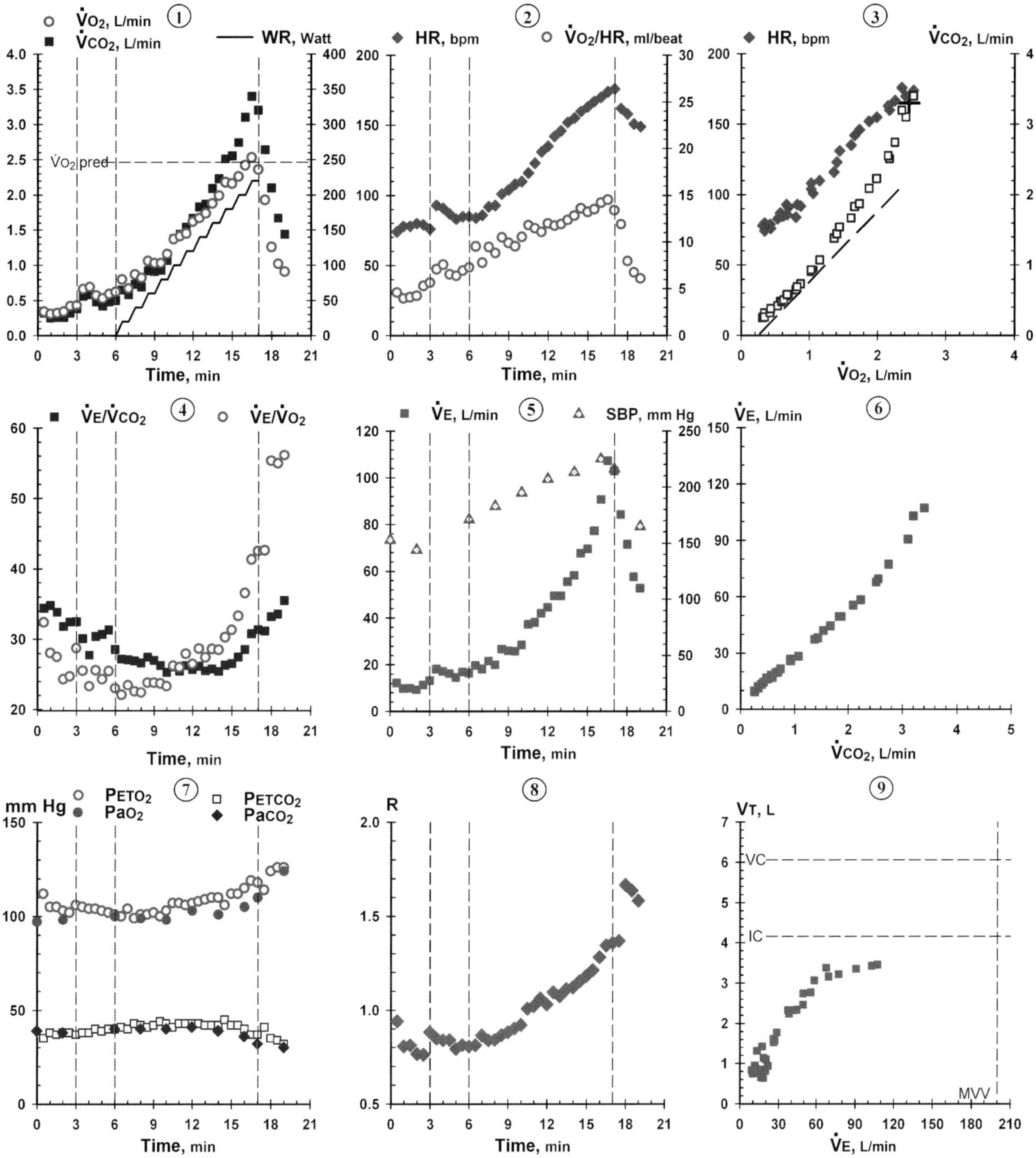

FIGURE 10.1.1. Vertical dashed lines in the panels in the left and middle columns indicate, from left to right, the beginning of unloaded cycling, start of increasing work rate (WR) at 20 W/min, and start of recovery. In **panel 1**, the increase in WR (right y-axis) is plotted with a scale of 100 W to 1 L of oxygen uptake ($\dot{V}O_2$) (left y-axis) such that WR is plotted parallel to a $\dot{V}O_2$ slope of 10 mL/min/W. In **panel 3**, carbon dioxide output ($\dot{V}CO_2$) (right y-axis) is plotted as a function of $\dot{V}O_2$ (x-axis) with identical scales so that the diagonal dashed line has a slope of 1 (45°). The $\dot{V}CO_2$ increasing more steeply than $\dot{V}O_2$ defines carbon dioxide (CO_2) derived from bicarbonate buffer, as long as ventilatory equivalent for CO_2 ($\dot{V}E/\dot{V}CO_2$) (**panel 4**) is not increasing and end-tidal PCO_2 ($PETCO_2$) (**panel 7**) is not decreasing, simultaneously. The black + symbol in **panel 3** indicates predicted values of heart rate (HR) (left y-axis) and $\dot{V}O_2$ for this individual. Abbreviations: IC, inspiratory capacity; MVV, maximum voluntary ventilation; $PETO_2$, end-tidal PO_2; R, respiratory exchange ratio; SBP, systolic blood pressure; VC, vital capacity; $\dot{V}E$, minute ventilation; $\dot{V}E/\dot{V}O_2$, ventilatory equivalent for oxygen; V_T, tidal volume.

Conclusion

This man has normal exercise function based on predicted values for his age and size. Given that he has been less active, his complaints could reflect anxiety regarding his physical status or residual deconditioning after a period of inactivity. Note that a test for a subject with these complaints would be most commonly performed noninvasively, and an arterial catheter with blood gases would be used only if necessary to resolve unexplained findings.

CASE 2

Normal Athletic Man

To view this case please access the eBook bundled with this text. Instructions are located on the inside front cover.

CASE 3

Normal Woman: Air and Oxygen Breathing Studies

CLINICAL FINDINGS

A 45-year-old woman was referred for evaluation of dyspnea. She had recently begun to increase her physical activities and felt that she had more shortness of breath than she should have. She had no significant medical problems, and physical and laboratory examinations revealed no abnormalities.

EXERCISE FINDINGS

The patient performed exercise on a cycle ergometer. She pedaled at 60 rpm without added load for 2 minutes. The work rate was then increased 10 W/min to her symptom-limited maximum. Arterial blood was sampled every second minute, and intra-arterial blood pressure was recorded

TABLE 10.3.1 Selected Respiratory Function Data

Measurement	Predicted	Measured
Age (y)		45
Sex		Female
Height (cm)		165
Weight (kg)	64	61
Hematocrit (%)		40
VC (L)	3.30	3.21
IC (L)	2.20	1.99
FEV_1 (L)	2.68	2.71
FEV_1/VC (%)	81	84
MVV (L/min)	112	117
D_{LCO} (mL/mm Hg/min)	24.1	21.1

Abbreviations: D_{LCO}, diffusing capacity of lung for carbon monoxide; FEV_1, forced expiratory volume in 1 second; FEV_1/VC, ; IC, inspiratory capacity; MVV, maximum voluntary ventilation; VC, vital capacity.

TABLE 10.3.2 Selected Exercise Data

Measurement	Predicted	Room air	O_2
Peak work rate (W)		130	160
Peak $\dot{V}O_2$ (L/min)	1.60	1.71	
Maximum heart rate (beats/min)	175	160	155
Maximum O_2 pulse (mL/beat)	9.1	10.7	
$\Delta\dot{V}O_2/\Delta WR$ (mL/min/W)	10.3	11.9	
AT (L/min)	>0.78	0.9	
Blood pressure (mm Hg [rest, max])		138/81, 194/81	106/75, 181/88
Maximum $\dot{V}E$ (L/min)		70	54
Exercise breathing reserve (L/min)	>15	47	63
$\dot{V}E/\dot{V}CO_2$ @ *AT* or lowest	27.8	23.3	21.3
PaO_2 (mm Hg [rest, max ex])		105, 108	643, 552
$P(A-a)O_2$ (mm Hg [rest, max ex])		5, 16	33, 117
$PaCO_2$ (mm Hg [rest, max ex])		38, 33	37, 44
$P(a-ET)CO_2$ (mm Hg [rest, max ex])		−1, −6	4, −3
VD/VT (rest, heavy ex)		0.21, 0.11	0.34, 0.18
HCO_3^- (mEq/L [rest, 2-min recov])		25, 13	25, NA

Abbreviations: *AT*, anaerobic threshold; $\Delta\dot{V}O_2/\Delta WR$, change in $\dot{V}O_2$/change in work rate; ex, exercise; HCO_3^-, bicarbonate; NA, not available; O_2, oxygen; $P(A-a)O_2$, alveolar-arterial PO_2 difference; $P(a-ET)CO_2$, arterial-end-tidal PCO_2 difference; VD/VT, physiological dead space-tidal volume ratio; $\dot{V}E$, minute ventilation; $\dot{V}E/\dot{V}CO_2$, ventilatory equivalent for carbon dioxide; $\dot{V}O_2$, oxygen uptake.

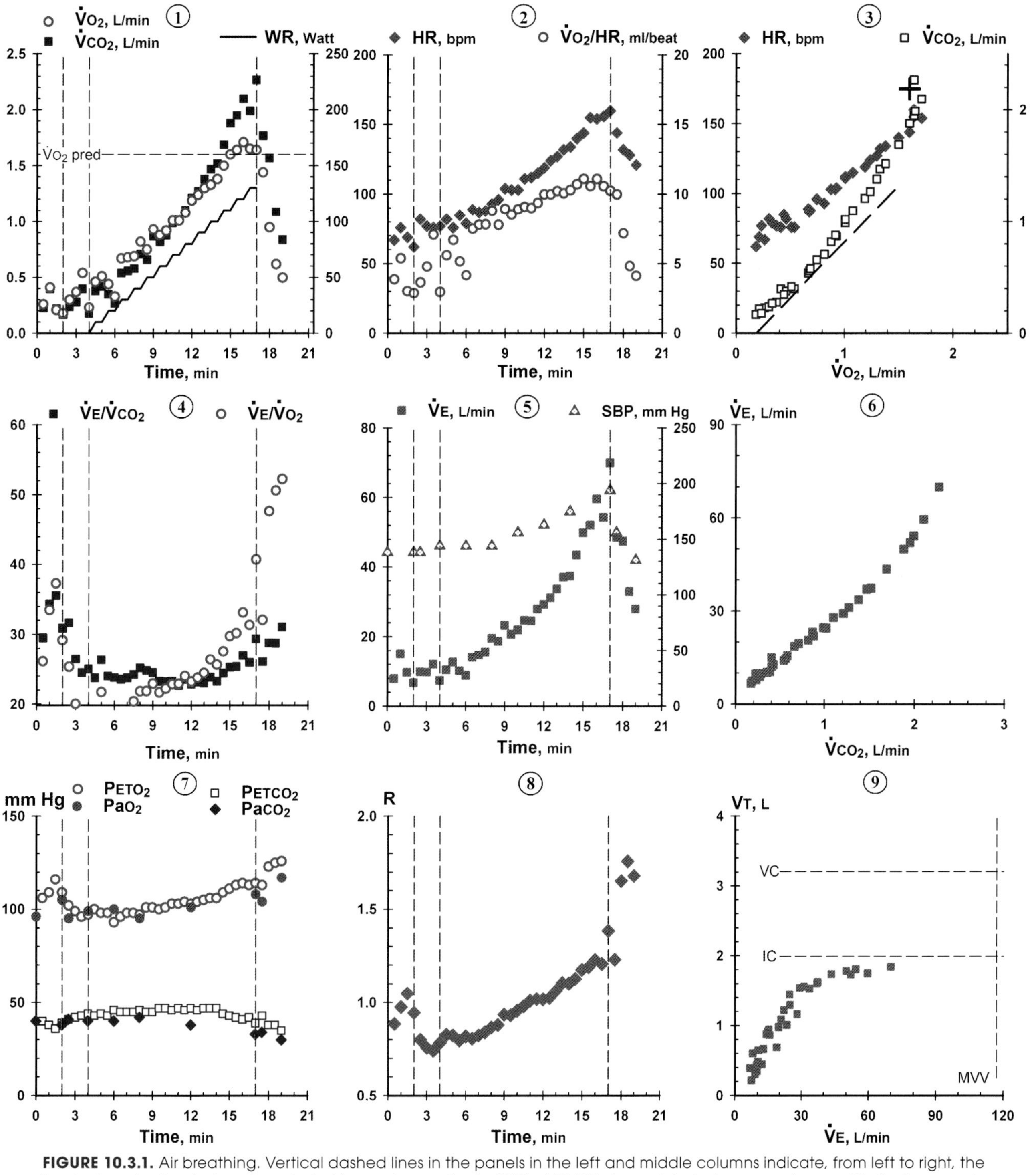

FIGURE 10.3.1. Air breathing. Vertical dashed lines in the panels in the left and middle columns indicate, from left to right, the beginning of unloaded cycling, start of increasing work rate (WR) at 10 W/min, and start of recovery. In **panel 1**, the increase in WR (right y-axis) is plotted with a scale of 100 W to 1 L of oxygen uptake ($\dot{V}O_2$) (left y-axis) such that WR is plotted parallel to a $\dot{V}O_2$ slope of 10 mL/min/W. In **panel 3**, carbon dioxide output ($\dot{V}CO_2$) (right y-axis) is plotted as a function of $\dot{V}O_2$ (x-axis) with identical scales so that the diagonal dashed line has a slope of 1 (45°). The $\dot{V}CO_2$ increasing more steeply than $\dot{V}O_2$ defines carbon dioxide CO_2) derived from bicarbonate buffer, as long as ventilatory equivalent for CO_2 ($\dot{V}E/\dot{V}CO_2$) (**panel 4**) is not increasing and end-tidal P_{CO_2} (P_{ETCO_2}) (**panel 7**) is not decreasing, simultaneously. The black + symbol in **panel 3** indicates predicted values of heart rate (HR) (left y-axis) and $\dot{V}O_2$ for this individual. Abbreviations: IC, inspiratory capacity; MVV, maximum voluntary ventilation; P_{ETO_2}, end-tidal partial P_{O_2}; R, respiratory exchange ratio; SBP, systolic blood pressure; VC, vital capacity; $\dot{V}E$, minute ventilation; $\dot{V}E/\dot{V}O_2$, ventilatory equivalent for oxygen; V_T, tidal volume.

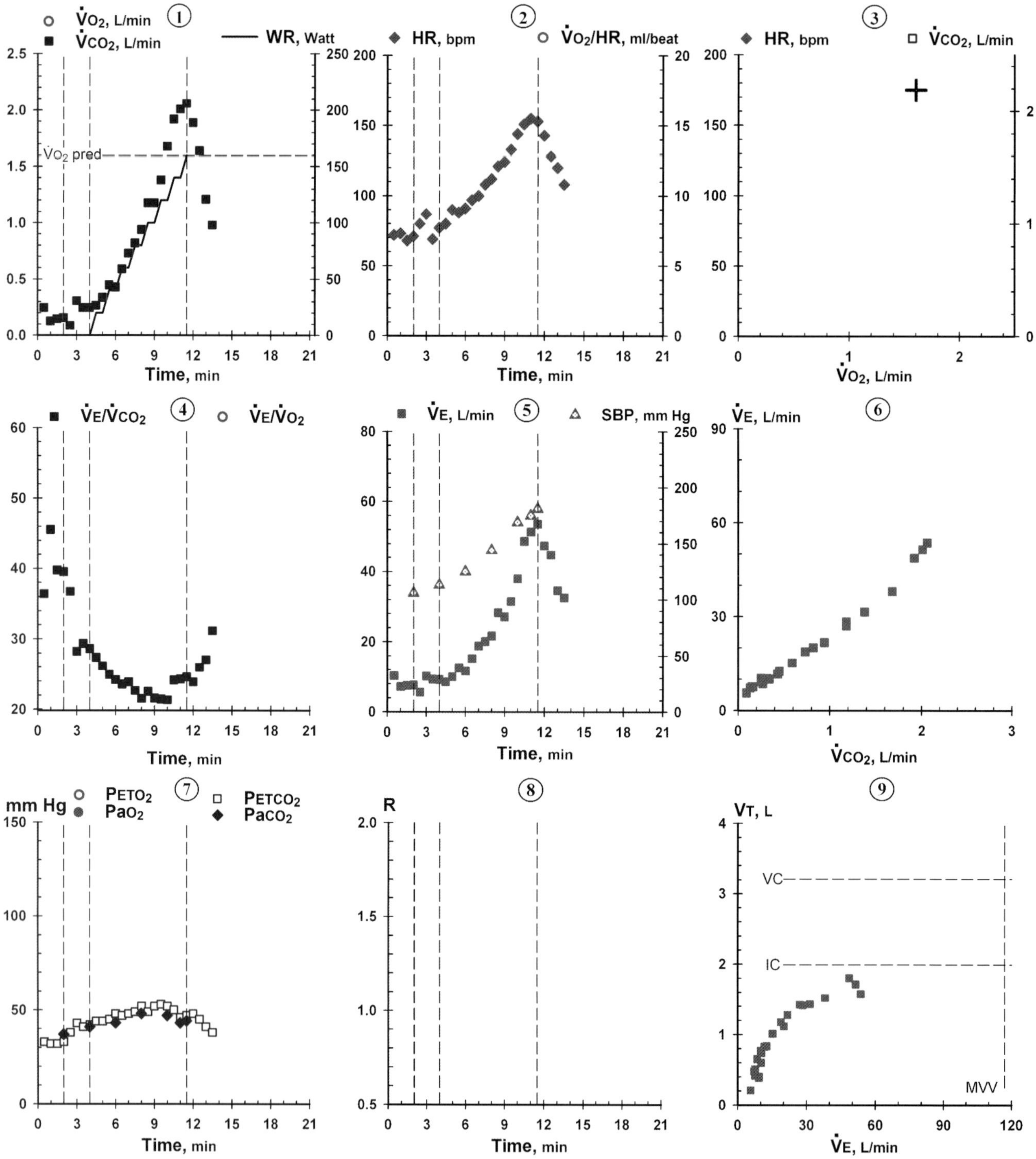

FIGURE 10.3.2. 100% Oxygen breathing. Vertical dashed lines in the panels in the left and middle columns indicate the beginning of unloaded cycling, start of increasing work rate (WR) at 20 W/min, and start of recovery. Oxygen uptake ($\dot{V}O_2$) data are not shown because of technical limitations of calculation with very high inspired oxygen levels. Abbreviations: HR, heart rate; IC, inspiratory capacity; MVV, maximum voluntary ventilation; P_{ETCO_2}, end-tidal P_{CO_2}; P_{ETO_2}, end-tidal P_{O_2}; R, respiratory exchange ratio; SBP, systolic blood pressure; VC, vital capacity; $\dot{V}CO_2$, carbon dioxide output; $\dot{V}E$, minute ventilation; $\dot{V}E/\dot{V}CO_2$, ventilatory equivalent for carbon dioxide; $\dot{V}E/\dot{V}O_2$, ventilatory equivalent for oxygen; V_T, tidal volume.

TABLE 10.3.3 Air Breathing

Time (min)	Work rate (W)	BP (mm Hg)	HR (min^{-1})	f (min^{-1})	$\dot{V}E$ (L/min BTPS)	$\dot{V}CO_2$ (L/min STPD)	$\dot{V}O_2$ (L/min STPD)	$\frac{\dot{V}O_2}{HR}$ (mL/beat)	R	pH	HCO_3^- (mEq/L)	PO_2, mm Hg ET	a	(A − a)	PCO_2, mm Hg ET	a	(a − ET)	$\frac{\dot{V}E}{\dot{V}CO_2}$	$\frac{\dot{V}E}{\dot{V}O_2}$	$\frac{V_D}{V_T}$
0.5	Rest	138/81								7.42	25		96			40				
1.0	Rest		67	13	7.9	0.23	0.26	3.9	0.88			106			40			30	26	
1.5	Rest		76	16	15.1	0.40	0.41	5.4	0.98			109			38			34	34	
2.0	Rest		69	22	9.7	0.22	0.21	3.0	1.05			116			36			36	37	
2.5	Rest	138/75	62	17	6.7	0.17	0.18	2.9	0.94	7.43	25	109	105	5	39	38	−1	31	29	0.21
3.0	Unloaded	138/81	82	27	9.9	0.24	0.30	3.7	0.80	7.41	26	102	95	6	41	41	0	32	25	0.26
3.5	Unloaded		77	28	9.8	0.28	0.37	4.8	0.76			99			42			27	20	
4.0	Unloaded		76	27	12.1	0.40	0.54	7.1	0.74			96			43			25	18	
4.5	Unloaded	144/75	77	34	7.4	0.18	0.23	3.0	0.78	7.41	25	97	99	2	44	40	−4	25	20	0.08
5.0	10		82	16	10.4	0.38	0.46	5.6	0.83			100			43			24	20	
5.5	10		76	19	12.7	0.42	0.51	6.7	0.82			98			44			26	22	
6.0	20		85	21	10.2	0.35	0.44	5.2	0.80			98			43			24	19	
6.5	20	144/75	79	29	8.9	0.27	0.33	4.2	0.82	7.41	25	93	100	3	46	40	−6	24	20	0.07
7.0	30		89	16	14.1	0.54	0.67	7.5	0.81			96			45			24	19	
7.5	30		87	16	14.7	0.56	0.68	7.8	0.82			98			45			24	20	
8.0	40		88	18	15.6	0.58	0.69	7.8	0.84			98			45			24	20	
8.5	40	144/75	93	20	19.6	0.71	0.82	8.8	0.87	7.39	25	97	95	8	46	42	−4	25	22	0.17
9.0	50		96	27	18.7	0.66	0.75	7.8	0.88			101			45			25	22	
9.5	50		104	23	23.3	0.87	0.93	8.9	0.94			101			45			25	23	
10.0	60		103	19	20.7	0.82	0.88	8.5	0.93			100			47			23	22	
10.5	60	156/75	103	18	22.0	0.88	0.92	8.9	0.96			101			47			23	22	
11.0	70		111	19	24.7	0.99	1.01	9.0	0.99			103			46			23	23	
11.5	70		112	17	24.6	1.02	1.01	9.0	1.01			103			47			23	23	
12.0	80		115	24	28.0	1.10	1.08	9.4	1.02			104			46			24	24	
12.5	80	163/75	119	19	29.3	1.21	1.19	10.0	1.02	7.37	22	103	101	11	47	38	−9	23	23	0.01
13.0	90		124	20	31.2	1.27	1.24	10.0	1.02			104			46			23	24	
13.5	90		127	22	33.7	1.38	1.30	10.2	1.06			105			47			23	24	
14.0	100		132	23	37.1	1.47	1.33	10.1	1.11			106			47			24	26	
14.5	100	175/81	134	23	37.4	1.52	1.38	10.3	1.10			106			47			23	26	
15.0	110		140	25	43.5	1.69	1.50	10.7	1.13			109			44			24	28	
15.5	110		144	28	50.0	1.88	1.60	11.1	1.18			111			43			25	30	
16.0	120		155	30	52.1	1.95	1.64	10.6	1.19			113			42			25	30	
16.5	120		154	34	59.6	2.10	1.71	11.1	1.23			114			41			27	33	
17.0	130		156	30	54.3	1.99	1.65	10.6	1.21			113			42			26	31	
17.5	130	194/81	160	38	70.0	2.27	1.64	10.3	1.38	7.31	16	114	108	16	39	33	−6	29	41	0.11
18.0	Recovery	156/69	144	28	48.6	1.77	1.44	10.0	1.23	7.28	16	113	104	17	43	34	−9	26	32	0.03
18.5	Recovery		132	26	47.5	1.57	0.95	7.2	1.65			123			38			29	48	
19.0	Recovery		128	19	33.0	1.09	0.62	4.8	1.76			125			38			29	51	
19.5	Recovery	131/63	121	22	28.0	0.84	0.50	4.1	1.68	7.26	13	126	117	13	35	30	−5	31	52	0.07

Abbreviations: BP, blood pressure; BTPS, body temperature pressure saturated; f, frequency; HCO_3^-, bicarbonate; HR, heart rate; $P(A - a)O_2$, alveolar-arterial PO_2 difference; $P(a - ET)CO_2$, arterial-end-tidal PCO_2 difference; $PETCO_2$, end-tidal PCO_2; $PETO_2$, end-tidal PO_2; R, respiratory exchange ratio; STPD, standard temperature pressure dry; $\dot{V}CO_2$, carbon dioxide output; V_D/V_T, physiological dead space-tidal volume ratio; $\dot{V}E$, minute ventilation; $\dot{V}E/\dot{V}CO_2$, ventilatory equivalent for carbon dioxide; $\dot{V}E/\dot{V}O_2$, ventilatory equivalent for oxygen; $\dot{V}O_2$, oxygen uptake.

from a percutaneously placed brachial artery catheter. A second incremental exercise test was performed with 100% oxygen (O_2) breathing 1.5 hours after recovery from the first test, with work rate increments of 20 W/min. She stopped exercise in each case complaining of general fatigue and shortness of breath. Resting and exercise electrocardiograms (ECGs) were normal. Selected demographic and pulmonary function data are shown in **Table 10.3.1**. Selected exercise data are shown in **Tables 10.3.2, 10.3.3,** and **10.3.4**, and in **Figures 10.3.1** and **10.3.2**.

TABLE 10.3.4 Oxygen Breathing

Time (min)	Work rate (W)	BP (mm Hg)	HR (min^{-1})	f (min^{-1})	$\dot{V}E$ (L/min BTPS)	$\dot{V}CO_2$ (L/min STPD)	$\dot{V}O_2$ (L/min STPD)	$\frac{\dot{V}O_2}{HR}$ (mL/beat)	R	pH	HCO_3^- (mEq/L)	PO_2, mm Hg ET	PO_2, mm Hg a	PO_2, mm Hg (A − a)	PCO_2, mm Hg ET	PCO_2, mm Hg a	PCO_2, mm Hg (a − ET)	$\frac{\dot{V}E}{\dot{V}CO_2}$	$\frac{\dot{V}E}{\dot{V}O_2}$	$\frac{V_D}{V_T}$
0.5	Rest		72	14	10.3	0.25									33			36		
1.0	Rest		73	15	7.2	0.13									32			46		
1.5	Rest		68	18	7.5	0.15									32			40		
2.0	Rest	106/75	71	15	7.6	0.16				7.44	25		643	33	33	37	4	40		0.34
2.5	Unloaded		80	27	5.6	0.09									38			37		
3.0	Unloaded		87	17	10.2	0.31									43			28		
3.5	Unloaded		69	23	9.3	0.25									41			29		
4.0	Unloaded	113/69	77	24	9.2	0.25				7.39	24		605	67	42	41	−1	29		0.21
4.5	20		80	13	8.5	0.27									44			27		
5.0	20		90	13	10.0	0.34									44			26		
5.5	40		88	15	12.5	0.45									45			25		
6.0	40	125/69	91	14	11.6	0.43				7.39	26		595	75	48	43	−5	24		0.15
6.5	60		97	15	15.2	0.59									47			24		
7.0	60		100	16	18.8	0.73									48			24		
7.5	80		108	18	20.1	0.82									49			23		
8.0	80	144/75	112	17	21.7	0.94				7.34	25		601	64	52	48	−4	22		0.15
8.5	100		121	20	28.3	1.18									49			23		
9.0	100		124	19	27.1	1.18									52			22		
9.5	120		133	22	31.5	1.38									53			21		
10.0	120	169/81	144	25	38.0	1.68				7.29	22		587	79	52	47	−5	21		0.13
10.5	140		151	27	48.7	1.92									50			24		
11.0	140	175/81	155	30	51.4	2.01				7.30	21		564	106	46	43	−3	24		0.17
11.5	160	181/88	153	34	53.6	2.06				7.28	20		552	117	47	44	−3	25		0.19
12.0	Recovery		143	26	47.4	1.89									48			24		
12.5	Recovery		128	26	44.8	1.64									45			26		
13.0	Recovery		120	22	34.6	1.21									41			27		
13.5	Recovery		108	23	32.5	0.98									38			31		

Abbreviations: BP, blood pressure; BTPS, body temperature pressure saturated; f, frequency; HCO_3^-, bicarbonate; HR, heart rate; P(A − a)O_2, alveolar-arterial PO_2 difference; P(a − ET)CO_2, arterial-end-tidal PCO_2 difference; $PETCO_2$, end-tidal PCO_2; $PETO_2$, end-tidal PO_2; R, respiratory exchange ratio; STPD, standard temperature pressure dry; $\dot{V}CO_2$, carbon dioxide output; VD/VT, physiological dead space–tidal volume ratio; $\dot{V}E$, minute ventilation; $\dot{V}E/\dot{V}CO_2$, ventilatory equivalent for carbon dioxide; $\dot{V}E/\dot{V}O_2$, ventilatory equivalent for oxygen; $\dot{V}O_2$, oxygen uptake.

INTERPRETATION

Comments

Resting respiratory function and ECG are normal. This set of tests illustrates rest and exercise blood gas values for an individual with essentially normal pulmonary gas exchange. For technical reasons, $\dot{V}O_2$ is not measured during the 100% O_2 breathing study, explaining the absence of some data in **Figure 10.3.2**.

Analysis

During the room air test, peak $\dot{V}O_2$ and anaerobic threshold are normal. There are no ECG abnormalities, and arterial blood gas values and VD/VT are normal throughout exercise. The patient is not obese. Thus, this patient has normal exercise capacity for her age and size, and there is no physiologic evidence of cardiovascular or pulmonary impairment.

The PaO_2 is normal during 100% O_2 breathing (**Table 10.3.4**), and PaO_2 values in excess of 550 mm Hg throughout exercise on O_2 breathing exclude a right-to-left shunt. Of note is that the patient was able to exercise to a higher work rate with a slightly lower heart rate during O_2 breathing compared to air breathing. Moreover, respiratory compensation for the metabolic acidosis (decrease in $PaCO_2$) was less evident during the O_2 breathing study, which may reflect decreased carotid body chemoreceptor stimulation due to hyperoxia.

Conclusion

Our final assessment is that this patient was normal and that her symptoms arose from her previously sedentary activity pattern.

CASE 4

Normal Man

CLINICAL FINDINGS

A 37-year-old shipyard machinist was evaluated because of complaints of dyspnea. He stated that he has been unable to play a full game of baseball for the last 6 years. He gets out of breath and has to stop after climbing three to four flights of stairs when working on shipboard. He never smoked. He denied cough, chest pain, edema, or other symptoms. Physical, roentgenographic, and laboratory examinations were normal.

EXERCISE FINDINGS

The patient performed exercise on a cycle ergometer. He pedaled at 60 rpm without added load for 3 minutes. The work rate was then increased 25 W/min to his symptom-limited maximum. Arterial blood was sampled every second minute, and intra-arterial blood pressure was recorded from a percutaneously placed brachial artery catheter. He stopped exercise because of general fatigue. Resting and exercise electrocardiograms (ECGs) were normal. Selected demographic and pulmonary function data are shown in **Table 10.4.1**. Selected exercise data are shown in **Tables 10.4.2** and **10.4.3** and in **Figure 10.4.1**.

INTERPRETATION

Comments

The results of this patient's resting respiratory function studies are normal. The resting ECG is normal.

TABLE 10.4.1 Selected Respiratory Function Data

Measurement	Predicted	Measured
Age (y)		37
Sex		Male
Height (cm)		157
Weight (kg)	63	67
Hematocrit (%)		45
VC (L)	3.30	4.38
IC (L)	2.20	2.80
TLC (L)	4.52	5.30
FEV_1 (L)	2.66	3.52
FEV_1/VC (%)	81	80
MVV (L/min)	127	124
D_{LCO} (mL/mm Hg/min)	22.4	29.8

Abbreviations: D_{LCO}, diffusing capacity of lung for carbon monoxide; FEV_1, forced expiratory volume in 1 second; IC, inspiratory capacity; MVV, maximum voluntary ventilation; TLC, total lung capacity; VC, vital capacity.

Analysis

Peak $\dot{V}O_2$ and the anaerobic threshold are below average, but within normal limits. Exercise ECG is normal. The O_2 pulse at peak $\dot{V}O_2$ and arterial blood gases are normal. The patient is not obese. Because of normal breathing reserve (MVV − $\dot{V}E$), he was not considered to be ventilatory limited.

Conclusion

This is a normal 37-year-old man. Symptoms probably relate to lack of fitness. Had the test been performed noninvasively (without arterial catheter), normal pulmonary gas exchange would be inferred by normal $\dot{V}E/\dot{V}CO_2$ at the anaerobic threshold or lowest value and normal $\dot{V}E$ versus $\dot{V}CO_2$ slope.

TABLE 10.4.2 Selected Exercise Data

Measurement	Predicted	Measured
Peak $\dot{V}O_2$ (L/min)	2.36	2.23
Maximum heart rate (beats/min)	183	188
Maximum O_2 pulse (mL/beat)	12.9	11.9
$\Delta\dot{V}O_2/\Delta WR$ (mL/min/W)	10.3	10.4
AT (L/min)	>0.99	1.1
Blood pressure (mm Hg [rest, max])		125/75, 188/94
Maximum $\dot{V}E$ (L/min)		90
Exercise breathing reserve (L/min)	>15	34
$\dot{V}E/\dot{V}CO_2$ @ *AT* or lowest	26.2	25.8
PaO_2 (mm Hg [rest, max ex])		84, 114
$P(A-a)O_2$ (mm Hg [rest, max ex])		7, 2
$PaCO_2$ (mm Hg [rest, max ex])		40, 38
$P(a-ET)CO_2$ (mm Hg [rest, max ex])		0, −4
V_D/V_T (rest, heavy ex)		0.31, 0.16
HCO_3^- (mEq/L [rest, 2-min recov])		24, 16

Abbreviations: *AT*, anaerobic threshold; $\Delta\dot{V}O_2/\Delta WR$, change in $\dot{V}O_2$/change in work rate; ex, exercise; HCO_3^-, bicarbonate; O_2, oxygen; $P(A-a)O_2$, alveolar-arterial PO_2 difference; $P(a-ET)CO_2$, arterial-end-tidal PCO_2 difference; V_D/V_T, physiological dead space-tidal volume ratio; $\dot{V}E$, minute ventilation; $\dot{V}E/\dot{V}CO_2$, ventilatory equivalent for carbon dioxide; $\dot{V}O_2$, oxygen uptake.

TABLE 10.4.3 Air Breathing

Time (min)	Work rate (W)	BP (mm Hg)	HR (min^{-1})	f (min^{-1})	$\dot{V}_E$ (L/min BTPS)	$\dot{V}CO_2$ (L/min STPD)	$\dot{V}O_2$ (L/min STPD)	$\frac{\dot{V}O_2}{HR}$ (mL/beat)	R	pH	HCO_3^- (mEq/L)	PO_2, mm Hg ET	a	(A − a)	PCO_2, mm Hg ET	a	(a − ET)	$\frac{\dot{V}_E}{\dot{V}CO_2}$	$\frac{\dot{V}_E}{\dot{V}O_2}$	$\frac{V_D}{V_T}$
0	Rest	125/75	7.41	24						7.41	24		103			39				
0.5	Rest		77	11	6.4	0.16	0.29	2.5	0.84			108			37			34	29	
1.0	Rest		78	14	7.5	0.18	0.23	2.9	0.78			107			36			35	27	
1.5	Rest		72	15	9.0	0.22	0.29	4.0	0.76			106			36			35	27	
2.0	Rest		78	13	7.1	0.16	0.20	2.6	0.80			108			35			37	30	
2.5	Rest		78	11	6.0	0.16	0.23	2.9	0.70			98			39			32	22	
3.0	Rest	125/81	82	13	6.9	0.17	0.27	3.3	0.63	7.39	24	94	84	7	40	40	0	34	21	0.31
3.5	Unloaded		83	21	9.0	0.26	0.40	4.8	0.65			80			47			28	18	
4.0	Unloaded		94	28	16.7	0.53	0.46	4.9	1.15			93			42			27	31	
4.5	Unloaded		93	38	12.1	0.32	0.44	4.7	0.73			92			44			28	20	
5.0	Unloaded		95	31	14.4	0.41	0.57	6.0	0.72			95			44			29	21	
5.5	Unloaded		93	23	11.5	0.34	0.45	4.8	0.76			96			44			28	21	
6.0	Unloaded	144/81	96	28	15.6	0.49	0.61	6.4	0.80	7.37	24	98	91	8	43	43	0	27	22	0.22
6.5	25		98	25	17.5	0.53	0.66	6.7	0.80			97			43			29	23	
7.0	25		102	26	16.6	0.50	0.67	6.6	0.75			96			43			29	21	
7.5	50		109	28	21.6	0.69	0.92	8.4	0.75			97			42			28	21	
8.0	50	150/81	117	25	23.5	0.82	1.08	9.2	0.76	7.38	25	95	95	1	44	43	−1	26	20	0.21
8.5	75		126	26	25.5	0.91	1.12	8.9	0.81			98			44			26	21	
9.0	75		127	27	27.7	1.01	1.19	9.4	0.85			99			45			25	21	
9.5	100		138	29	33.6	1.26	1.39	10.1	0.91			101			45			25	22	
10.0	100	181/94	141	32	38.6	1.47	1.54	10.9	0.95	7.37	24	102	104	2	45	42	−3	24	23	0.15
10.5	125		151	41	49.7	1.74	1.68	11.1	1.04			108			43			27	28	
11.0	125		162	40	53.5	1.92	1.78	11.0	1.08			110			42			26	28	
11.5	150		169	39	60.2	2.17	1.94	11.5	1.12			111			42			26	29	
12.0	150	188/94	176	46	68.8	2.36	2.04	11.6	1.16	7.37	22	112	114	2	42	38	−4	27	32	0.16
12.5	175		182	50	76.0	2.51	2.11	11.6	1.19			114			41			29	34	
13.0	175		188	51	89.7	2.84	2.23	11.9	1.27			118			38			30	38	
13.5	Recovery		178	31	59.6	2.17	1.83	10.3	1.19			111			43			26	31	
14.0	Recovery		161	29	47.5	1.66	1.19	7.4	1.39			116			41			27	38	
14.5	Recovery		144	27	42.0	1.37	0.84	5.8	1.63			123			37			29	47	
15.0	Recovery	181/100	136	28	37.5	1.08	0.62	4.6	1.74	7.30	16	127	126	2	35	33	−2	33	57	0.18
15.5	Recovery		135	24	23.9	0.68	0.44	3.3	1.55			124			36			32	50	

Abbreviations: BP, blood pressure; BTPS, body temperature pressure saturated; f, frequency; HCO_3^-, bicarbonate; HR, heart rate; $P(A - a)O_2$, alveolar-arterial PO_2 difference; $P(a - ET)CO_2$, arterial-end-tidal PCO_2 difference; $PETCO_2$, end-tidal PCO_2; $PETO_2$, end-tidal PO_2; R, respiratory exchange ratio; STPD, standard temperature pressure dry; $\dot{V}CO_2$, carbon dioxide output; V_D/V_T, physiological dead space–tidal volume ratio; $\dot{V}_E$, minute ventilation; $\dot{V}_E/\dot{V}CO_2$, ventilatory equivalent for carbon dioxide; $\dot{V}_E/\dot{V}O_2$, ventilatory equivalent for oxygen; $\dot{V}O_2$, oxygen uptake.

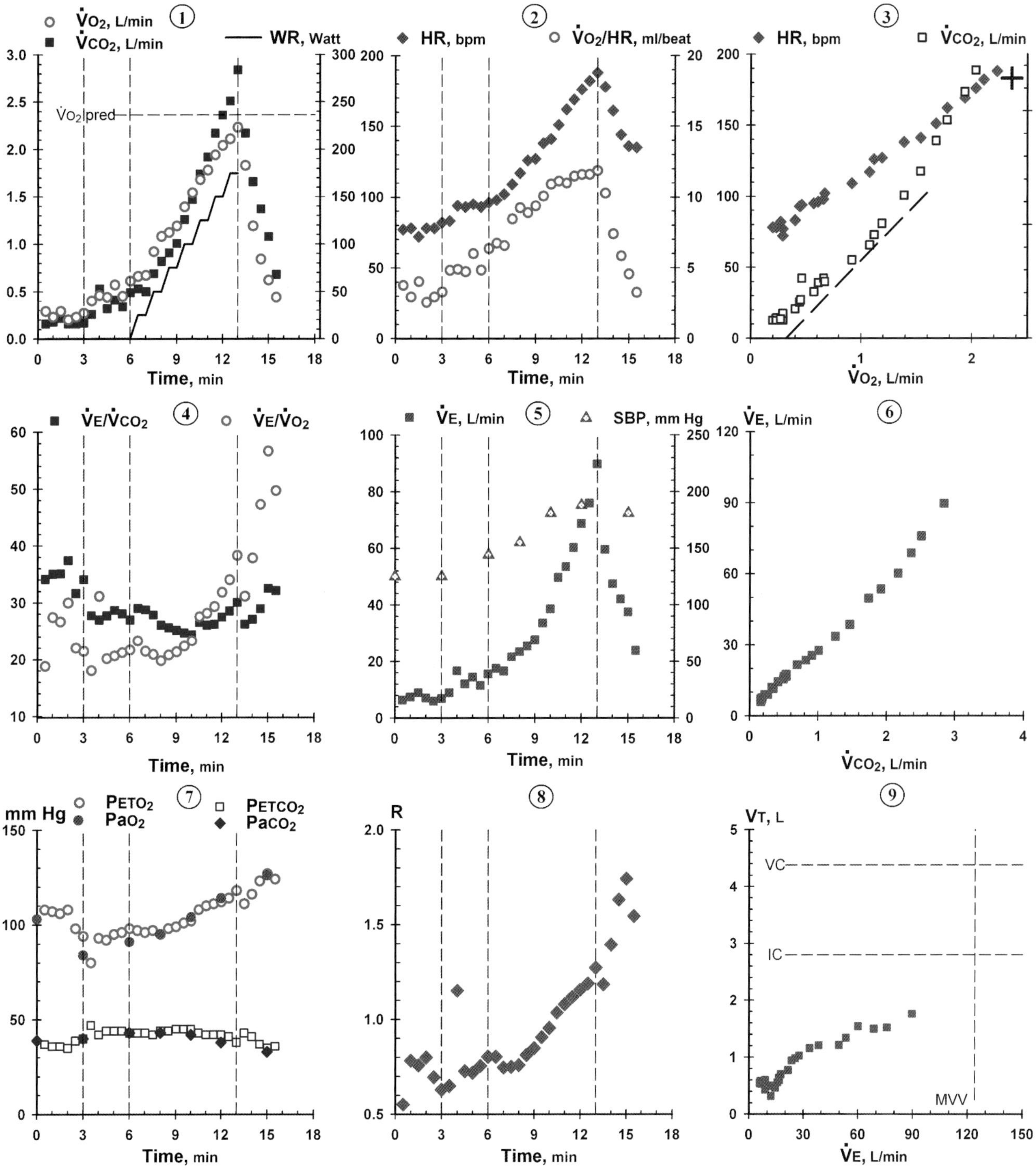

FIGURE 10.4.1. Vertical dashed lines in the panels in the left and middle columns indicate, from left to right, the beginning of unloaded cycling, start of increasing work rate (WR) at 25 W/min, and start of recovery. In **panel 1**, the increase in WR (right y-axis) is plotted with a scale of 100 W to 1 L of oxygen uptake ($\dot{V}O_2$) (left y-axis) such that WR is plotted parallel to a $\dot{V}O_2$ slope of 10 mL/min/W. In **panel 3**, carbon dioxide output ($\dot{V}CO_2$) (right y-axis) is plotted as a function of $\dot{V}O_2$ (x-axis) with identical scales so that the diagonal dashed line has a slope of 1 (45°). The $\dot{V}CO_2$ increasing more steeply than $\dot{V}O_2$ defines carbon dioxide (CO_2) derived from bicarbonate buffer, as long as ventilatory equivalent for CO_2 ($\dot{V}E/\dot{V}CO_2$) (**panel 4**) is not increasing and end-tidal PCO_2 ($PETCO_2$) (**panel 7**) is not decreasing, simultaneously. The black + symbol in **panel 3** indicates predicted values of heart rate (HR) (left y-axis) and $\dot{V}O_2$ for the individual. Abbreviations: IC, inspiratory capacity; MVV, maximum voluntary ventilation; $PETO_2$, end-tidal PCO_2; R, respiratory exchange ratio; SBP, systolic blood pressure; VC, vital capacity; $\dot{V}E$, minute ventilation; $\dot{V}E/\dot{V}O_2$, ventilatory equivalent for oxygen; V_T, tidal volume.

CASE 5

Fit Cyclist

CLINICAL FINDINGS

A 40-year-old man volunteered to perform an exercise test for demonstration purposes. He had been an avid cyclist in previous years but described himself as noncompetitive at the time of testing. He had no exercise-related symptoms and denied any chronic medical problems. His resting electrocardiogram was normal. He was taking no medications. Physical examination revealed a healthy-appearing man. Selected demographic and respiratory function data are shown in **Table 10.5.1**.

EXERCISE FINDINGS

Exercise was done on a cycle ergometer beginning with 3 minutes of unloaded pedaling at 60 rpm followed by continuous increase in work rate by 25 W/min. Exercise electrocardiogram showed no significant changes relative to rest. Key variables from the exercise test are summarized in **Table 10.5.2**. Thirty-second averages of exercise data are shown in **Table 10.5.3**, and data are displayed graphically as 10-second averages in **Figure 10.5.1**.

INTERPRETATION

Comment

This test is included as a demonstration of a fit individual reaching limitations of the pulmonary system under circumstances of high capacity for delivery and utilization of oxygen by the cardiovascular system and skeletal muscles, respectively.

TABLE 10.5.1 Selected Pulmonary Function Data

Measurement	Predicted	Measured
Age (y)		40
Sex		Male
Height (cm)		175
Weight (kg)		86.4
VC (L)	4.95	4.07
IC (L)	3.30	3.32
ERV (L)	1.65	0.48
FEV_1 (L)	3.95	3.22
FEV_1/VC (%)	80	80
MVV (L/min)	155	120

Abbreviations: ERV, expiratory reserve volume; FEV_1, forced expiratory volume in 1 second; IC, inspiratory capacity; MVV, maximum voluntary ventilation; VC, vital capacity.

Analysis

Cardiovascular and metabolic responses: Peak $\dot{V}O_2$ and *AT* were both above average predicted values. The $\Delta\dot{V}O_2/\Delta WR$ was normal. The heart rate was shallow relative to $\dot{V}O_2$ (panel 3), but the peak heart rate was close to predicted; peak oxygen pulse was therefore high. These findings are typical of cardiovascular conditioning with high cardiac stroke volume.

Ventilatory responses: The breathing reserve was small, indicating that he was at, or approaching, the limits of his breathing capacity at end exercise. He was therefore ventilatory limited in this test, albeit at a high level of exercise.

Gas exchange efficiency: The relationship of $\dot{V}E$ to $\dot{V}CO_2$ was normal, with normal $\dot{V}E/\dot{V}CO_2$ at the *AT*. The VD/VT, calculated using transcutaneous PCO_2 as an estimate of arterial values, was normal at rest and decreased appropriately during exercise. Consistent with this, in panel 7, it can be seen that the end-tidal PCO_2 values increased considerably from rest to midexercise, while transcutaneous PCO_2 remained close to resting level until late in the test when they began to decrease reflecting respiratory compensation for metabolic acidosis. It is normal for the arterial–end-tidal PCO_2 difference to become negative during exercise

TABLE 10.5.2 Selected Exercise Data

Measurement	Predicted	Measured
Peak $\dot{V}O_2$ (L/min)	2.83	3.85
Maximum heart rate (beats/min)	180	174
Maximum O_2 pulse (mL/beat)	15.7	22.1
$\Delta\dot{V}O_2/\Delta WR$ (mL/min/W)	10.3	10.1
AT (L/min)	>1.25	2.25
Blood pressure (mm Hg [rest, max])		154/72, 192/50
Maximum $\dot{V}E$ (L/min)		118
Breathing reserve (L/min)		2
$\dot{V}E/\dot{V}CO_2$ @ *AT*	<34	25
SpO_2 (% [rest, max ex])		98, 92
VD/VT (rest, max ex)		0.25, 0.10

Abbreviations: *AT*, anaerobic threshold; $\Delta\dot{V}O_2/\Delta WR$, change in $\dot{V}O_2$/change in work rate; ex, exercise; O_2, oxygen; SpO_2, oxygen saturation as measured by pulse oximetry; VD/VT, physiological dead space-tidal volume ratio; $\dot{V}E$, minute ventilation; $\dot{V}E/\dot{V}CO_2$, ventilatory equivalent for carbon dioxide; $\dot{V}O_2$, oxygen uptake.

TABLE 10.5.3 Air Breathing

Time (min)	Work rate (W)	BP (mm Hg)	HR (min^{-1})	f (min^{-1})	$\dot{V}E$ (L/min BTPS)	$\dot{V}CO_2$ (L/min STPD)	$\dot{V}O_2$ (L/min STPD)	$\frac{\dot{V}O_2}{HR}$ (mL/beat)	R	pH	HCO_3^- (mEq/L)	PO_2, mm Hg and SpO_2 % ET	SpO_2	(A − a)	PCO_2, mm Hg ET	tc	(a − ET)	$\frac{\dot{V}E}{\dot{V}CO_2}$	$\frac{\dot{V}E}{\dot{V}O_2}$	$\frac{VD^a}{VT}$
0.5	Rest		53	16.48	10.4	0.31	0.33	6.3	0.93			106	98		40	39.0		34	31	0.29
1.0	Rest		64	16.69	11.3	0.37	0.44	6.9	0.84			101	97		41	39.2		31	26	0.24
1.5	Rest		85	26.69	21.5	0.73	0.92	10.8	0.80			99	98		41	39.5		29	23	0.23
2.0	Rest		78	26.02	19.6	0.64	0.70	8.9	0.92			105	97		41	39.8		30	28	0.26
2.5	Rest		72	21.42	16.7	0.55	0.57	7.9	0.97			107	98		40	39.8		30	29	0.25
3.0	Rest	154/72	66	12.11	9.8	0.33	0.37	5.6	0.89			101	98		42	39.8		29	26	0.24
3.5	Rest		63	18.64	13.0	0.41	0.44	6.9	0.93			106	98		40	39.8		32	30	0.28
4.0	Unloaded		77	27.16	19.9	0.67	0.76	9.8	0.88			103	96		41	39.8		30	26	0.23
4.5	Unloaded		89	23.97	27.7	0.95	0.98	11.1	0.97			105	97		41	39.8		29	28	0.25
5.0	Unloaded		82	28.58	21.0	0.70	0.78	9.6	0.89			103	98		41	39.6		30	27	0.24
5.5	Unloaded		80	23.44	24.1	0.80	0.81	10.1	0.99			105	99		40	39.5		30	30	0.26
6.0	Unloaded		79	24.35	19.6	0.67	0.77	9.7	0.88			102	98		41	39.3		29	26	0.22
6.5	Unloaded		81	24.97	19.1	0.64	0.71	8.8	0.90			103	99		41	39.3		30	27	0.23
7.0	11		80	22.94	20.5	0.71	0.77	9.6	0.92			104	98		41	39.5		29	27	0.22
7.5	24		86	26.42	22.6	0.77	0.83	9.6	0.93			105	98		41	39.3		29	27	0.23
8.0	37	157/75	89	25.81	21.9	0.77	0.87	9.8	0.88			101	98		42	39.3		29	25	0.20
8.5	49		90	24.99	23.8	0.88	1.02	11.4	0.86			99	98		43	39.3		27	23	0.17
9.0	62		95	27.37	29.2	1.08	1.27	13.3	0.85			99	98		43	39.5		27	23	0.18
9.5	74		101	30.93	31.8	1.17	1.29	12.8	0.91			102	98		43	39.5		27	25	0.18
10.0	87		104	32.61	35.4	1.30	1.46	14.1	0.89			101	98		43	39.5		27	24	0.19
10.5	99		106	29.88	35.7	1.40	1.55	14.6	0.90			100	98		44	39.5		26	23	0.14
11.0	112		111	28.15	39.8	1.55	1.65	14.9	0.94			101	98		44	39.5		26	24	0.15
11.5	123		115	29.85	39.2	1.59	1.76	15.3	0.90			98	98		46	39.5		25	22	0.11
12.0	136		119	29.69	44.4	1.79	1.88	15.8	0.95			101	97		45	39.6		25	24	0.13
12.5	148		120	25.68	44.9	1.86	1.94	16.2	0.96			100	97		46	39.8		24	23	0.11
13.0	160		126	35.06	51.8	2.10	2.13	16.9	0.98			102	97		46	39.6		25	24	0.12
13.5	173		132	32.78	56.4	2.31	2.30	17.4	1.01			103	96		46	39.5		24	25	0.12
14.0	185		134	29.29	55.3	2.36	2.35	17.5	1.00			101	97		47	39.5		23	24	0.08
14.5	198		138	30.61	59.2	2.52	2.46	17.9	1.03			102	97		47	39.5		23	24	0.08
15.0	210	157/73	139	28.65	57.9	2.58	2.52	18.2	1.02			99	97		49	39.5		22	23	0.04
15.5	223		146	26.26	61.8	2.83	2.74	18.7	1.04			98	96		50	39.7		22	23	0.03
16.0	236		149	31.32	70.5	3.13	2.91	19.5	1.08			102	95		49	39.8		23	24	0.06
16.5	248		152	30.75	74.0	3.30	3.09	20.3	1.07			101	95		49	39.8		22	24	0.05
17.0	260		158	30.11	78.3	3.51	3.23	20.5	1.09			102	94		49	39.8		22	24	0.05
17.5	273		162	30.8	80.9	3.67	3.36	20.8	1.09			102	94		49	39.8		22	24	0.04
18.0	286		165	34.05	91.7	4.00	3.51	21.3	1.14			105	93		48	39.8		23	26	0.08
18.5	298		168	34.11	94.3	4.17	3.59	21.4	1.16			105	93		48	39.7		23	26	0.06
19.0	311		170	35.99	100.2	4.36	3.63	21.4	1.20			107	94		48	39.5		23	28	0.07
19.5	323		172	41.56	108.8	4.59	3.74	21.8	1.23			109	93		47	39.3		24	29	0.09
20.0	309		174	43.30	117.6	4.85	3.85	22.1	1.26			110	93		46	39.2		24	31	0.11
20.5	Recovery		172	37.69	102.0	4.37	3.33	19.3	1.31			109	92		48	38.8		23	31	0.07
21.0	Recovery	192/43	159	33.92	84.2	3.36	2.05	12.9	1.63			117	94		45	38.8		25	41	0.13
21.5	Recovery		147	28.57	67.5	2.55	1.61	10.9	1.59			118	98		42	38.5		26	42	0.17
22.0	Recovery		131	29.24	57.9	2.01	1.30	10.0	1.54			120	98		39	38.2		29	44	0.22
22.5	Recovery		124	30.44	47.2	1.56	1.13	9.1	1.39			118	98		38	37.7		30	42	0.24
23.0	Recovery		118	25.23	44.3	1.51	1.16	9.8	1.30			116	98		39	37.3		29	38	0.22

Abbreviations: BP, blood pressure; BTPS, body temperature pressure saturated; f, frequency; HCO_3^-, bicarbonate; HR, heart rate; $P(A - a)O_2$, alveolar-arterial PO_2 difference; $P(a - ET)CO_2$, arterial-end-tidal PCO_2 difference; $PETCO_2$, end-tidal PCO_2; $PETO_2$, end-tidal PO_2; R, respiratory exchange ratio; SpO_2, oxygen saturation as measured by pulse oximetry; STPD, standard temperature pressure dry; $\dot{V}CO_2$, carbon dioxide output; VD/VT, physiological dead space-tidal volume ratio; $\dot{V}E$, minute ventilation; $\dot{V}E/\dot{V}CO_2$, ventilatory equivalent for carbon dioxide; $\dot{V}E/\dot{V}O_2$, ventilatory equivalent for oxygen; $\dot{V}O_2$, oxygen uptake.

[a]VD/VT was calculated using transcutaneous PCO_2 ($PtcCO_2$) as an estimate of arterial carbon dioxide.

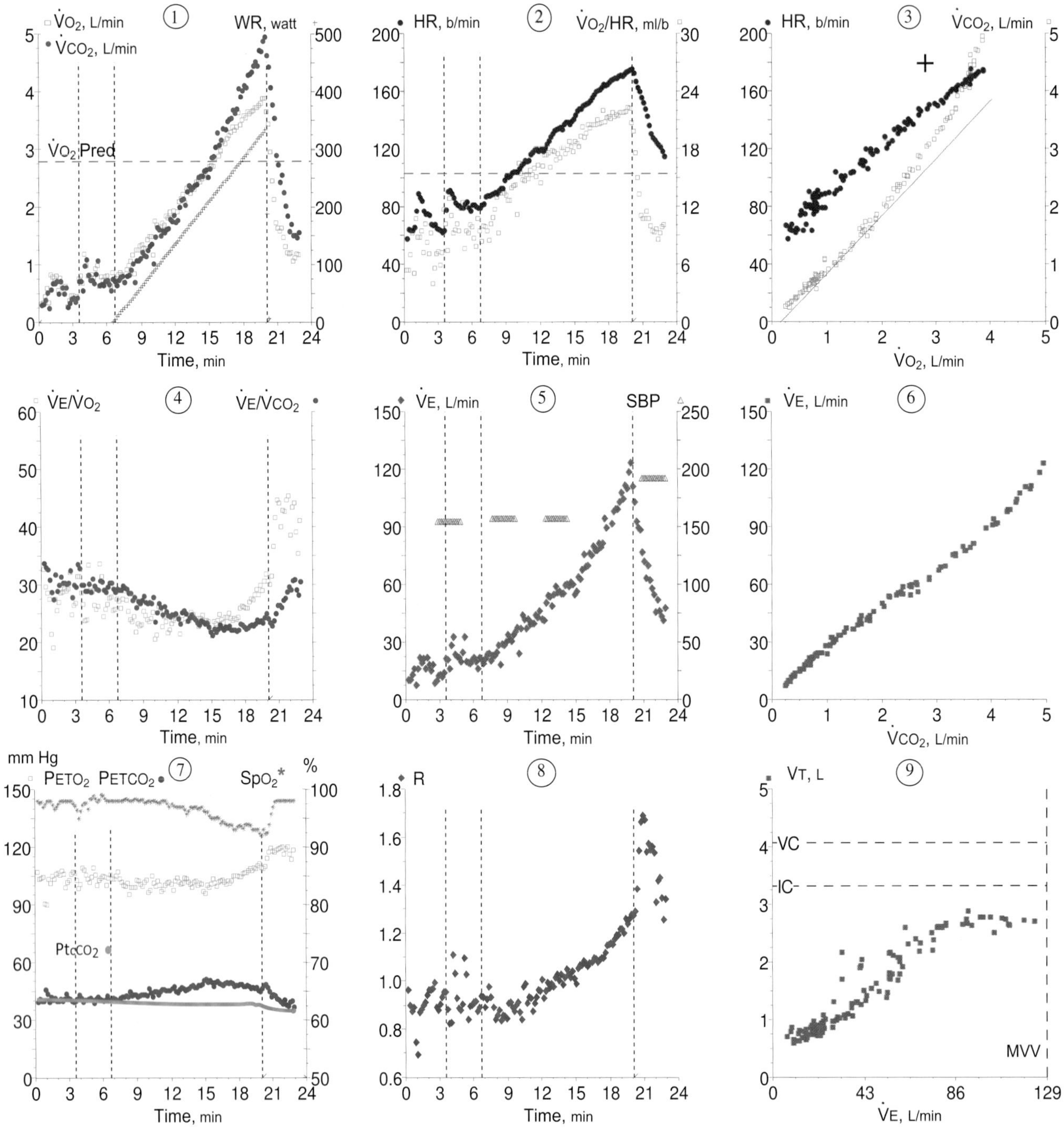

FIGURE 10.5.1. Vertical dashed lines in the panels in the left and middle columns indicate, from left to right, the beginning of unloaded cycling, start of increasing work rate (WR) at 25 W/min, and start of recovery. In **panel 1**, the increase in WR (right y-axis) is plotted with a scale of 100 W to 1 L of oxygen uptake ($\dot{V}O_2$) (left y-axis) such that WR is plotted parallel to a $\dot{V}O_2$ slope of 10 mL/min/W. Predicted peak $\dot{V}O_2$ is shown as a dashed horizontal line. In **panel 3**, carbon dioxide output ($\dot{V}CO_2$) (right y-axis) is plotted as a function of $\dot{V}O_2$ (x-axis) with identical scales so that the diagonal blue line has a slope of 1 (45°). The $\dot{V}CO_2$ increasing more steeply than $\dot{V}O_2$ defines carbon dioxide (CO_2) derived from bicarbonate buffer, as long as ventilatory equivalent for CO_2 ($\dot{V}E/\dot{V}CO_2$) (**panel 4**) is not increasing and end-tidal P_{CO_2} (P_{ETCO_2}) (**panel 7**) is not decreasing, simultaneously. The black + symbol in **panel 3** indicates predicted values of heart rate (HR) (left y-axis) and $\dot{V}O_2$ for this individual. Abbreviations: IC, inspiratory capacity; MVV, maximum voluntary ventilation; P_{ETO_2}, end-tidal P_{O_2}; P_{tcCO_2}, transcutaneous P_{CO_2}; R, respiratory exchange ratio; SBP, systolic blood pressure; Sp_{O_2}, oxygen saturation as measured by pulse oximetry; VC, vital capacity; $\dot{V}E$, minute ventilation; $\dot{V}E/\dot{V}O_2$, ventilatory equivalent for oxygen; V_T, tidal volume.

because P_{ETCO_2} increases, whereas arterial values remain stable up until the respiratory compensation point. In this case, the increase in P_{ETCO_2} was particularly marked. Also seen in panel 7 is a decrease in the pulse oximeter estimate of arterial oxygen saturation from 98% at rest to a nadir of 92% at end exercise. Although it is possible that this was artifact of the oximeter signal, arterial oxygen desaturation is a recognized phenomenon in well-conditioned athletes, the mechanism for which is not fully understood. Failure of pulmonary arterial blood to be fully oxygenated either due to microcirculatory shunts or to short pulmonary circulation transit time has been postulated.

Conclusion

This test demonstrates a high degree of cardiovascular fitness. For this individual, a high capacity for cardiovascular work, coupled with pulmonary function values that were in the lower range of normal, resulted in his using his maximal capacity for ventilation and pulmonary oxygen exchange during this incremental test.

CASE 6

Normal Individual: Cycle and Treadmill Studies

CLINICAL FINDINGS

A 37-year-old hospital employee was asymptomatic and volunteered for an exercise study. He did not exercise regularly or smoke. Physical examination, chest roentgenograms, and resting electrocardiogram (ECG) were normal. Demographic and respiratory function data are shown in **Table 10.6.1**.

EXERCISE FINDINGS

On 2 separate days, 1 month apart, the subject exercised to maximum tolerance using incremental exercise protocols, first on the cycle and second on the treadmill. He stopped on both occasions because of calf fatigue. There were no arrhythmias or abnormalities in the ECG. Exercise data are summarized in **Table 10.6.2** and shown in **Tables 10.6.3** and **10.6.4** and **Figures 10.6.1** and **10.6.2**.

INTERPRETATION

Comments

This study is presented to contrast the results when the same subject performed on the cycle and on the treadmill.

TABLE 10.6.1 Selected Respiratory Function Data

Measurement	Predicted	Measured
Age (y)		37
Sex		Male
Height (cm)		161
Weight (kg)	66	53
Hematocrit (%)		45
VC (L)	3.56	3.21
IC (L)	2.37	2.51
TLC (L)	4.90	5.01
FEV_1 (L)	2.87	2.64
FEV_1/VC (%)	81	82
MVV (L/min)	132	107
D_{LCO} (mL/mm Hg/min)	23.1	22.3

Abbreviations: D_{LCO}, diffusing capacity of lung for carbon monoxide; FEV_1, forced expiratory volume in 1 second; IC, inspiratory capacity; MVV, maximum voluntary ventilation; TLC, total lung capacity; VC, vital capacity.

The results of this subject's resting respiratory function studies were normal.

Analysis

Peak oxygen uptake ($\dot{V}O_2$) and the anaerobic threshold were normal for both cycle and treadmill exercise. The ECG and O_2 pulse were normal at maximum work rate. The peak $\dot{V}O_2$ was about 10% higher on the treadmill than on the cycle. Using the flowcharts in Chapter 9, the normal peak $\dot{V}O_2$ would lead to Flowchart 2, where normal ECG, SpO_2, O_2 pulse at peak $\dot{V}O_2$, and ventilatory equivalent for CO_2 ($\dot{V}E/\dot{V}CO_2$) at the anaerobic threshold would confirm a normal study.

Conclusion

This subject has exercise capacity in the lower range of normal. The finding of slightly higher peak $\dot{V}O_2$ on treadmill testing compared to cycle testing is typical for subjects who do not cycle regularly.

TABLE 10.6.2 Selected Exercise Data

	Predicted		Measured	
Measurement	Cycle	Treadmill	Cycle	Treadmill
Peak $\dot{V}O_2$ (L/min)	2.21	2.45	1.87	2.07
Maximum heart rate (beats/min)	183	183	173	183
Maximum O_2 pulse (mL/beat)	12.1	13.4	10.8	11.3
$\Delta\dot{V}O_2/\Delta WR$ (mL/min/W)	10.3		8.4	
AT (L/min)	>0.93	>1.03	1.1	1.15
Maximum $\dot{V}E$ (L/min)			76	85
Exercise breathing reserve (L/min)	>15	>15	31	22
$\dot{V}E/\dot{V}CO_2$ @ *AT* or lowest	26.1	26.1	21.7	23.8

Abbreviations: *AT*, anaerobic threshold; $\Delta\dot{V}O_2/\Delta WR$, change in $\dot{V}O_2$/change in work rate; O_2, oxygen; $\dot{V}E$, minute ventilation; $\dot{V}E/\dot{V}CO_2$, ventilatory equivalent for carbon dioxide; $\dot{V}O_2$, oxygen uptake.

TABLE 10.6.3 Cycle Ergometry

Time (min)	Work rate (W)	BP (mm Hg)	HR (min^{-1})	f (min^{-1})	$\dot{V}E$ (L/min BTPS)	$\dot{V}CO_2$ (L/min STPD)	$\dot{V}O_2$ (L/min STPD)	$\frac{\dot{V}O_2}{HR}$ (mL/beat)	R	pH	HCO_3^- (mEq/L)	PO_2, mm Hg ET	PO_2, mm Hg a	PO_2, mm Hg (A – a)	PCO_2, mm Hg ET	PCO_2, mm Hg a	PCO_2, mm Hg (a – ET)	$\frac{\dot{V}E}{\dot{V}CO_2}$	$\frac{\dot{V}E}{\dot{V}O_2}$	$\frac{VD}{VT}$
0.5	Rest		79	15	9.5	0.28	0.33	4.2	0.85			99			44			29	25	
1.0	Rest		95	14	11.1	0.36	0.42	4.4	0.86			97			45			28	24	
1.5	Rest		78	13	7.8	0.23	0.26	3.3	0.88			101			44			29	26	
2.0	Rest		74	14	7.3	0.19	0.21	2.8	0.90			102			43			32	29	
2.5	Unloaded		109	18	17.3	0.58	0.55	5.0	1.05			105			44			27	29	
3.0	Unloaded		97	8	11.1	0.44	0.52	5.4	0.85			96			46			24	20	
3.5	Unloaded		103	17	14.3	0.53	0.63	6.1	0.84			92			48			24	20	
4.0	Unloaded		104	16	15.1	0.56	0.65	6.3	0.86			94			47			25	21	
4.5	Unloaded		108	16	17.7	0.67	0.71	6.6	0.94			97			47			24	23	
5.0	Unloaded		97	16	14.8	0.55	0.55	5.7	1.00			103			46			24	24	
5.5	25		107	16	16.4	0.61	0.60	5.6	1.02			104			46			25	25	
6.0	25		108	18	16.2	0.57	0.57	5.3	1.00			103			45			26	26	
6.5	50		113	18	15.8	0.58	0.64	5.7	0.91			96			47			25	22	
7.0	50		110	17	17.1	0.67	0.74	6.7	0.91			94			50			23	21	
7.5	75		122	19	22.0	0.86	0.89	7.3	0.97			99			48			24	23	
8.0	75		129	17	19.8	0.85	0.90	7.0	0.94			93			52			22	20	
8.5	100		132	21	26.4	1.07	1.04	7.9	1.03			99			50			23	24	
9.0	100		133	17	22.9	1.07	1.12	8.4	0.96			89			57			20	19	
9.5	125		143	21	31.1	1.40	1.29	9.0	1.09			97			55			21	23	
10.0	125		147	22	35.1	1.64	1.50	10.2	1.09			95			56			20	22	
10.5	150		155	26	41.1	1.82	1.52	9.8	1.20			102			53			22	26	
11.0	150		159	27	44.4	1.94	1.58	9.9	1.23			103			53			22	27	
11.5	175		168	31	53.2	2.24	1.71	10.2	1.31			107			53			23	30	
12.0	175		173	44	75.8	2.79	1.87	10.8	1.49			114			46			26	29	
12.5	Recovery		167	34	60.1	2.31	1.67	10.0	1.38			109			50			25	34	
13.0	Recovery		158	30	49.5	1.88	1.29	8.2	1.46			112			49			25	36	
13.5	Recovery		146	31	48.8	1.68	0.98	6.7	1.71			118			44			27	47	
14.0	Recovery		140	27	40.1	1.30	0.73	5.2	1.78			121			42			29	52	

Abbreviations: BP, blood pressure; BTPS, body temperature pressure saturated; ET, f, frequency; HCO_3^-, bicarbonate; HR, heart rate; $P(A-a)O_2$, alveolar-arterial PO_2 difference; $P(a-ET)CO_2$, arterial-end-tidal PCO_2 difference; $PETCO_2$, end-tidal PCO_2; $PETO_2$, end-tidal PO_2; R, respiratory exchange ratio; STPD, standard temperature pressure dry; $\dot{V}CO_2$, carbon dioxide output; VD/VT, physiological dead space-tidal volume ratio; $\dot{V}E$, minute ventilation; $\dot{V}E/\dot{V}CO_2$, ventilatory equivalent for carbon dioxide; $\dot{V}E/\dot{V}O_2$, ventilatory equivalent for oxygen; $\dot{V}O_2$, oxygen uptake.

TABLE 10.6.4 Treadmill Ergometry

Time (min)	Treadmill grade (%)	BP (mm Hg)	HR (min^{-1})	f (min^{-1})	$\dot{V}E$ (L/min BTPS)	$\dot{V}CO_2$ (L/min STPD)	$\dot{V}O_2$ (L/min STPD)	$\frac{\dot{V}O_2}{HR}$ (mL/beat)	R	pH	HCO_3^- (mEq/L)	PO_2, mm Hg ET	PO_2, mm Hg a	PO_2, mm Hg (A − a)	PCO_2, mm Hg ET	PCO_2, mm Hg a	PCO_2, mm Hg (a − ET)	$\frac{\dot{V}E}{\dot{V}CO_2}$	$\frac{\dot{V}E}{\dot{V}O_2}$	$\frac{VD}{VT}$
0.5	Rest		87	16	8.0	0.20	0.21	2.4	0.95			105			40			33	32	
1.0	Rest		85	19	12.2	0.34	0.37	4.4	0.92			105			40			31	29	
1.5	Rest		81	19	8.6	0.20	0.23	2.8	0.87			106			40			35	30	
2.0	Rest		95	20	13.0	0.34	0.37	3.9	0.92			105			40			33	31	
2.5	0		107	22	14.6	0.47	0.45	4.2	1.04			103			44			27	28	
3.0	0		109	23	19.4	0.62	0.71	6.5	0.87			100			43			28	25	
3.5	3		109	22	19.1	0.63	0.76	7.0	0.83			97			44			27	23	
4.0	3		113	22	22.1	0.77	0.93	8.2	0.83			90			47			26	22	
4.5	6		116	23	21.9	0.77	0.88	7.6	0.88			97			47			26	23	
5.0	6		120	22	25.1	0.94	1.05	8.8	0.90			97			47			25	22	
5.5	9		124	22	27.5	1.06	1.11	9.0	0.95			98			48			24	23	
6.0	9		129	24	30.4	1.17	1.20	9.3	0.98			101			47			24	24	
6.5	12		138	28	35.0	1.31	1.30	9.4	1.01			102			47			25	25	
7.0	12		141	25	35.6	1.43	1.38	9.8	1.04			101			48			23	24	
7.5	15		144	27	38.6	1.53	1.45	10.1	1.06			100			50			24	25	
8.0	15		150	26	39.8	1.59	1.44	9.6	1.10			102			49			24	26	
8.5	18		155	29	45.6	1.82	1.58	10.2	1.15			104			49			24	27	
9.0	18		160	27	47.8	1.98	1.67	10.4	1.19			106			48			23	27	
9.5	21		166	30	53.3	2.14	1.73	10.4	1.24			108			48			24	29	
10.0	21		168	32	59.0	2.33	1.85	11.0	1.26			107			48			24	30	
10.5	24		175	37	67.3	2.54	1.89	10.8	1.34			113			45			25	34	
11.0	24		178	39	71.7	2.69	1.99	11.2	1.35			113			45			25	34	
11.5	27		183	43	84.9	2.97	2.07	11.3	1.43			116			43			27	39	
12.0	Recovery		178	28	47.8	1.75	1.26	7.1	1.39			109			49			26	36	
12.5	Recovery		175	37	68.8	2.60	1.85	10.6	1.41			114			46			25	35	
13.0	Recovery		171	37	68.3	2.40	1.57	9.2	1.53			116			45			27	42	
13.5	Recovery		163	35	58.1	1.84	1.20	7.4	1.53			119			40			30	46	
14.0	Recovery		151	37	49.2	1.41	0.86	5.7	1.64			122			38			33	54	

Abbreviations: BP, blood pressure; BTPS, body temperature pressure saturated; f, frequency; HCO_3^-, bicarbonate; HR, heart rate; $P(A - a)O_2$, alveolar-arterial PO_2 difference; $P(a - ET)CO_2$, arterial-end-tidal PCO_2 difference; $PETCO_2$, end-tidal PCO_2; $PETO_2$, end-tidal PO_2; R, respiratory exchange ratio; STPD, standard temperature pressure dry; $\dot{V}CO_2$, carbon dioxide output; VD/VT, physiological dead space-tidal volume ratio; $\dot{V}E$, minute ventilation; $\dot{V}E/\dot{V}CO_2$, ventilatory equivalent for carbon dioxide; $\dot{V}E/\dot{V}O_2$, ventilatory equivalent for oxygen; $\dot{V}O_2$, oxygen uptake.

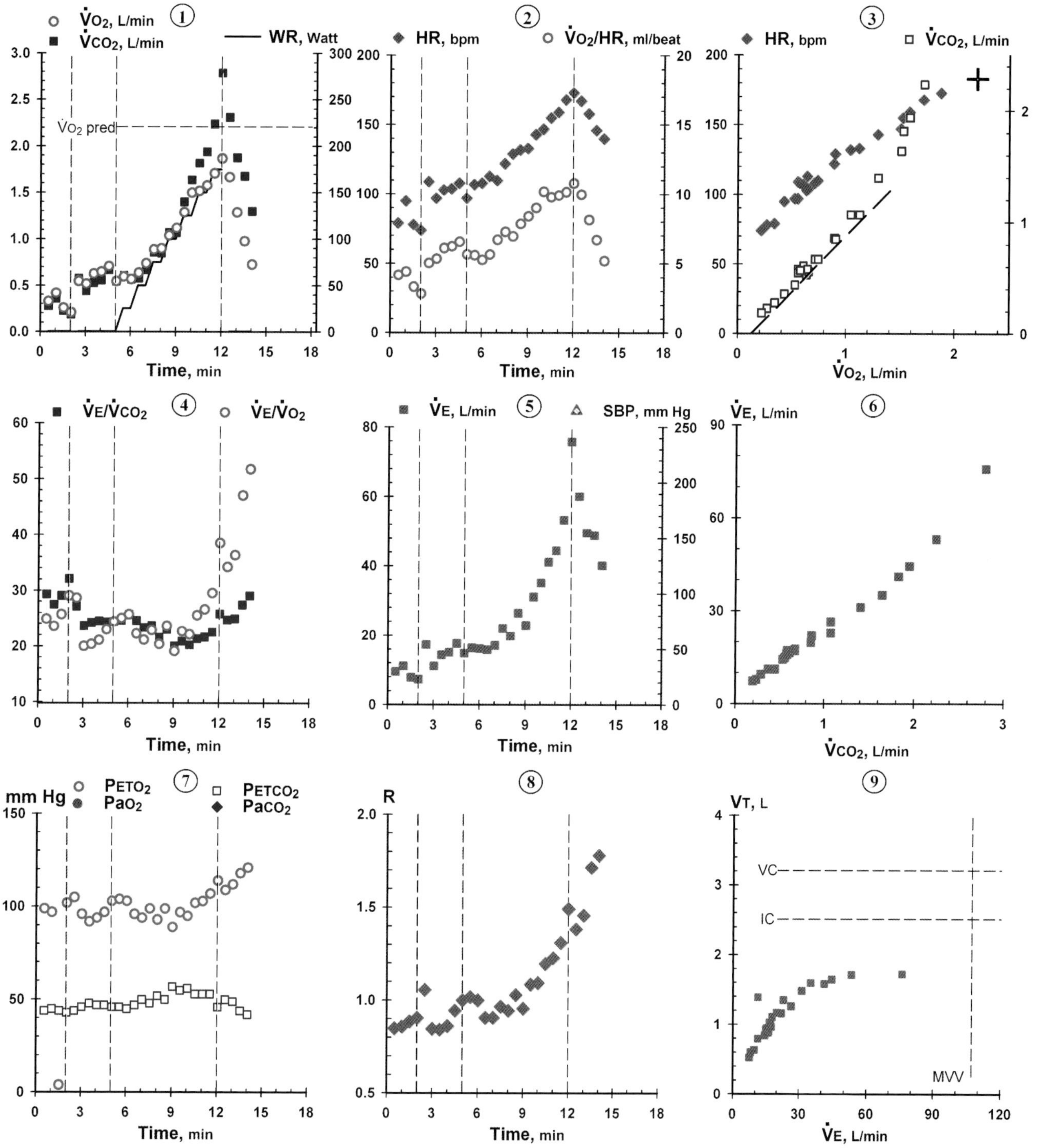

FIGURE 10.6.1. Cycle ergometry. Vertical dashed lines in the panels in the left and middle columns indicate, from left to right, the beginning of unloaded cycling, start of increasing work rate (WR) at 25 W/min, and start of recovery. In **panel 1**, the increase in WR (right y-axis) is plotted with a scale of 100 W to 1 L of oxygen uptake ($\dot{V}O_2$) (left y-axis) such that WR is plotted parallel to a $\dot{V}O_2$ slope of 10 mL/min/W. In **panel 3**, carbon dioxide output ($\dot{V}CO_2$) (right y-axis) is plotted as a function of $\dot{V}O_2$ (x-axis) with identical scales so that the diagonal dashed line has a slope of 1 (45°). The $\dot{V}CO_2$ increasing more steeply than $\dot{V}O_2$ defines carbon dioxide (CO_2) derived from bicarbonate buffer, as long as ventilatory equivalent for CO_2 ($\dot{V}E/\dot{V}CO_2$) (**panel 4**) is not increasing and end-tidal PCO_2 ($PETCO_2$) (**panel 7**) is not decreasing, simultaneously. The black + symbol in **panel 3** indicates predicted values of heart rate (HR) (left y-axis) and $\dot{V}O_2$ for the individual. Abbreviations: IC, inspiratory capacity; MVV, maximum voluntary ventilation; $PETO_2$, end-tidal PO_2; R, respiratory exchange ratio; SBP, systolic blood pressure; VC, vital capacity; $\dot{V}E$, minute ventilation; $\dot{V}E/\dot{V}O_2$, ventilatory equivalent for oxygen; VT, tidal volume.

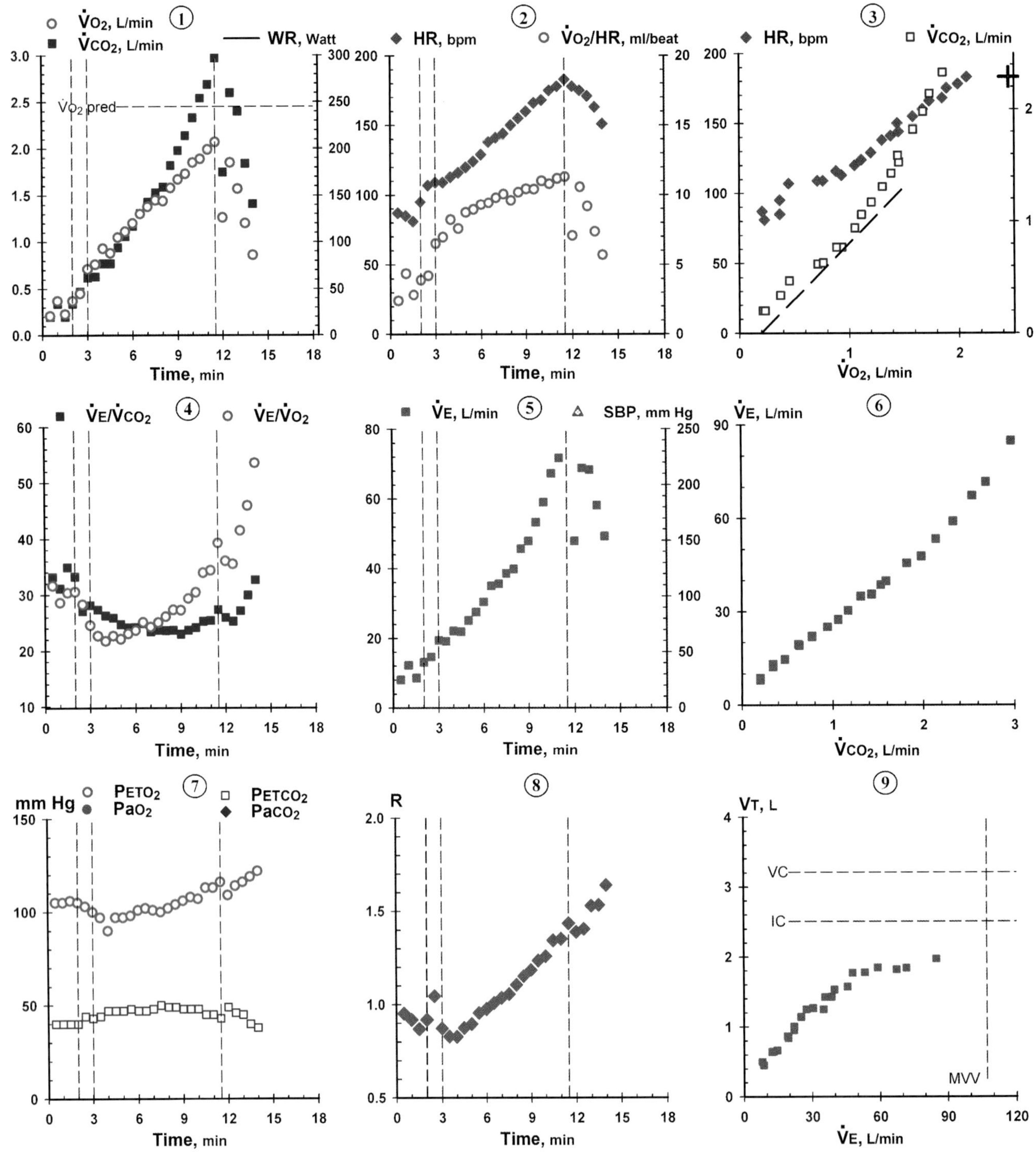

FIGURE 10.6.2. Treadmill ergometry. Vertical dashed lines in the panels in the left and middle columns indicate the beginning and end of the incremental exercise period. For 1 min prior to the first vertical line, the subject walked at zero grade at a speed of 3.0 mph. Thereafter, the speed remained constant and grade was increased by 3% each minute. In **panel 3**, carbon dioxide output ($\dot{V}CO_2$) (right y-axis) is plotted as a function of oxygen uptake ($\dot{V}O_2$) (x-axis) with identical scales so that the diagonal dashed line has a slope of 1 (45°). The $\dot{V}CO_2$ increasing more steeply than $\dot{V}O_2$ defines carbon dioxide (CO_2) derived from bicarbonate buffer, as long as ventilatory equivalent for CO_2 ($\dot{V}E/\dot{V}CO_2$) (**panel 4**) is not increasing and end-tidal PCO_2 ($PETCO_2$) (**panel 7**) is not decreasing, simultaneously. The black + symbol in **panel 3** indicates predicted values of heart rate (HR) (left y-axis) and $\dot{V}O_2$ for the individual. Abbreviations: IC, inspiratory capacity; MVV, maximum voluntary ventilation; $PETO_2$, end-tidal PO_2; R, respiratory exchange ratio; SBP, systolic blood pressure; VC, vital capacity; $\dot{V}E$, minute ventilation; $\dot{V}E/\dot{V}O_2$, ventilatory equivalent for oxygen; VT, tidal volume; WR, work rate.

CASE 7

Normal Individual: With and Without β-Adrenergic Blockade

CLINICAL FINDINGS

A 23-year-old student with stable asthma volunteered for a study evaluating the effect of a β-adrenergic blocker, pindolol, on exercise-induced asthma. He had had hay fever and asthma since childhood but was otherwise in excellent health. He was taking no medications. Physical examination, chest roentgenograms, electrocardiogram (ECG), and hemogram were normal. Demographic and respiratory function data are shown in **Table 10.7.1**.

EXERCISE FINDINGS

Two identical cycle exercise studies were performed a week apart. On each occasion, after baseline spirometry, 0.4 mg of pindolol or placebo was given intravenously over a 20-minute period. After repeat spirometry, the subject pedaled without added resistance at 60 rpm for 3 minutes and at 60 W for an additional 3 minutes. Thereafter, the work rate was increased 20 W every minute. On both occasions, the subject stopped because of fatigue. The ECG pattern remained normal. Repeat spirometry performed 2, 7, 12, 17, 22, and 27 minutes after exercise did not reveal exercise-induced bronchospasm after either study. Exercise data are summarized in **Table 10.7.2** and shown in **Tables 10.7.3** and **10.7.4** and **Figures 10.7.1** and **10.7.2**.

INTERPRETATION

Comments

This study is presented to demonstrate the effect of β-adrenergic blockade on exercise in a healthy person. Results of respiratory function testing are near normal at the time of study. The exercise testing protocol was modified to increase the likelihood of inducing postexercise bronchospasm. After unloaded cycling, the work rate was increased immediately to 60 W, followed by 1-minute increments of 20 W to achieve high-intensity exercise more quickly. This large initial increase in the work rate increment resulted in the unusually large increase in oxygen uptake ($\dot{V}O_2$) at the start of exercise, which is usually not desirable in most clinical testing circumstances.

Analysis

Peak $\dot{V}O_2$ and AT are within normal limits on both pre- and post-β-adrenergic blockade exercise tests. The ECG and oxygen (O_2) pulse at maximum work rate are normal. The large reduction in maximum heart rate, with slight reduction in peak $\dot{V}O_2$ and increase in maximum O_2 pulse, is typical of the effect of β-adrenergic blockade. The negative chronotropic effect of the β-blockade increases the time for ventricular filling, leading to a larger stroke volume as reflected in a larger O_2 pulse at the same work rate. Note the large increase in $\dot{V}O_2$ due to the increase from unloaded pedaling to 60 W, followed by the expected increase in $\dot{V}O_2$ with each subsequent 20 W increase in work rate (ie, normal; $\Delta\dot{V}O_2/\Delta WR$).

Conclusion

These studies are normal and demonstrate the decrease in heart rate, lesser decrease in peak $\dot{V}O_2$, and higher maximum O_2 pulse following β-adrenergic blockade.

TABLE 10.7.1 Selected Respiratory Function Data

Measurement	Predicted	Measured
Age (y)		23
Sex		Male
Height (cm)		170
Weight (kg)	68	64
Hematocrit (%)		45
VC (L)	47.9	4.86
IC (L)	3.21	3.40
TLC (L)	6.46	6.72
FEV_1 (L)	4.04	3.58
FEV_1/VC (%)	84	74
MVV (L/min)	175	142
DLCO (mL/mm Hg/min)	33.2	32.5

Abbreviations: DLCO, diffusing capacity of lung for carbon monoxide; FEV_1, forced expiratory volume in 1 second; IC, inspiratory capacity; MVV, maximum voluntary ventilation; TLC, total lung capacity; VC, vital capacity.

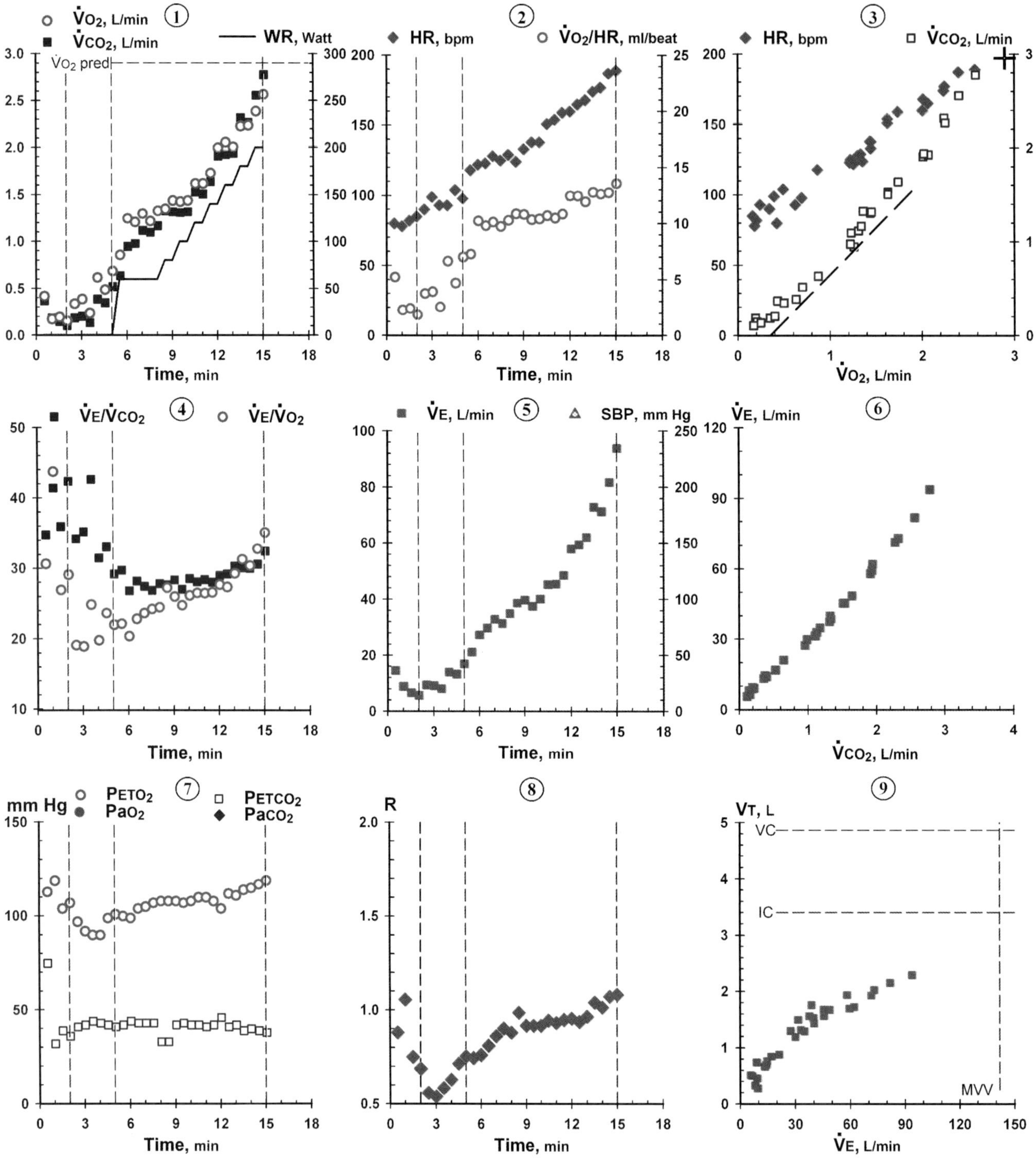

FIGURE 10.7.1. Before β-adrenergic blockade. Vertical dashed lines in the panels in the left and middle columns indicate, from left to right, the beginning of unloaded cycling, start of increasing work rate (WR), and start of recovery. Following unloaded cycling, the WR increased to 60 W for 3 minutes prior to progressively increasing by 20 W/min. In **panel 1**, the increase in WR (right y-axis) is plotted with a scale of 100 W to 1 L of oxygen uptake ($\dot{V}O_2$) (left y-axis) such that WR is plotted parallel to a $\dot{V}O_2$ slope of 10 mL/min/W. In **panel 3**, carbon dioxide output ($\dot{V}CO_2$) (right y-axis) is plotted as a function of $\dot{V}O_2$ (x-axis) with identical scales so that the diagonal dashed line has a slope of 1 (45°). The $\dot{V}CO_2$ increasing more steeply than $\dot{V}O_2$ defines carbon dioxide (CO_2) derived from bicarbonate buffer, as long as ventilatory equivalent for CO_2 ($\dot{V}E/\dot{V}CO_2$) (**panel 4**) is not increasing and end-tidal PCO_2 ($PETCO_2$) (**panel 7**) is not decreasing, simultaneously. The black + symbol in **panel 3** indicates predicted values of heart rate (HR) (left y-axis) and $\dot{V}O_2$ for this individual. Abbreviations: IC, inspiratory capacity; MVV, maximum voluntary ventilation; $PETO_2$, end-tidal PO_2; R, respiratory exchange ratio; SBP, systolic blood pressure; VC, vital capacity; $\dot{V}E$, minute ventilation; $\dot{V}E/\dot{V}O_2$, ventilatory equivalent for oxygen; V_T, tidal volume.

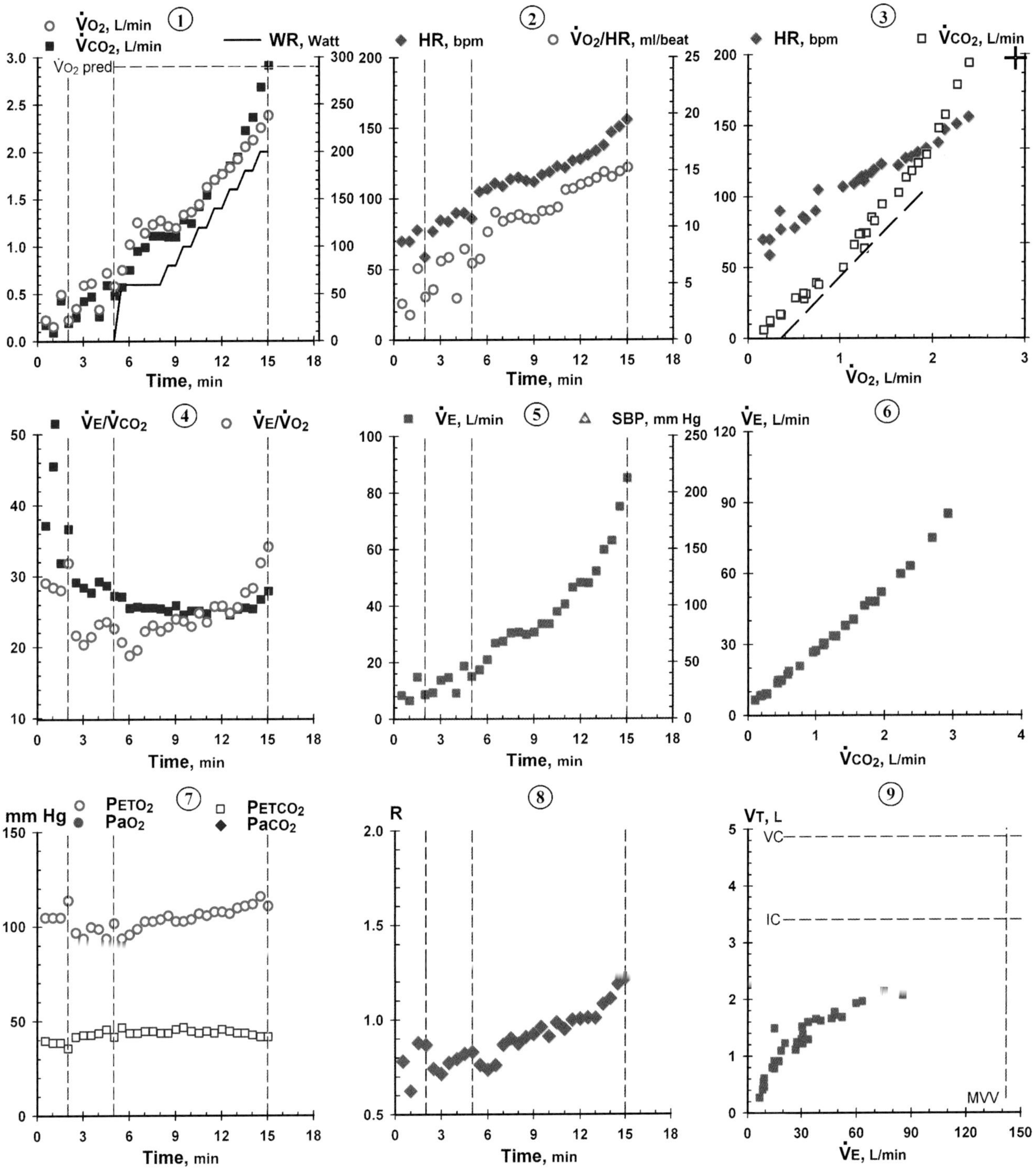

FIGURE 10.7.2. After β-adrenergic blockade. Vertical dashed lines in the panels in the left and middle columns indicate, from left to right, the beginning of unloaded cycling, start of increasing work rate (WR), and start of recovery. Following unloaded cycling, the WR was increased to 60 W for 3 minutes prior to progressively increasing by 20 W/min. In **panel 1**, the increase in WR (right y-axis) is plotted with a scale of 100 W to 1 L of oxygen uptake ($\dot{V}O_2$) (left y-axis) such that WR is plotted parallel to a $\dot{V}O_2$ slope of 10 mL/min/W. In **panel 3**, carbon dioxide output ($\dot{V}CO_2$) (right y-axis) is plotted as a function of $\dot{V}O_2$ (x-axis) with identical scales so that the diagonal dashed line has a slope of 1 (45°). The $\dot{V}CO_2$ increasing more steeply than $\dot{V}O_2$ defines carbon dioxide (CO_2) derived from bicarbonate buffer, as long as ventilatory equivalent for CO_2 ($\dot{V}E/\dot{V}CO_2$) (**panel 4**) is not increasing and end-tidal PCO_2 ($PETCO_2$) (**panel 7**) is not decreasing, simultaneously. The black + symbol in **panel 3** indicates predicted values of heart rate (HR) (left y-axis) and $\dot{V}O_2$ for this individual. Abbreviations: IC, inspiratory capacity; MVV, maximum voluntary ventilation; $PETO_2$, end-tidal PO_2; R, respiratory exchange ratio; SBP, systolic blood pressure; VC, vital capacity; $\dot{V}E$, minute ventilation; $\dot{V}E/\dot{V}O_2$, ventilatory equivalent for oxygen; V_T, tidal volume.

TABLE 10.7.2 Selected Exercise Data

Measurement	Predicted	Placebo	Pindolol
Peak $\dot{V}O_2$ (L/min)	2.90	2.57	2.39
Maximum heart rate (beats/min)	197	189	156
Maximum O_2 pulse (mL/beat)	14.7	13.6	15.3
$\Delta\dot{V}O_2/\Delta WR$ (mL/min/W)	10.3	10.5	9.7
AT (L/min)	>1.16	1.5	1.4
Maximum $\dot{V}E$ (L/min)		94	85
Exercise breathing reserve (L/min)	>15	48	57
$\dot{V}E/\dot{V}CO_2$ @ *AT* or lowest	24.3	27.7	25.2

Abbreviations: *AT*, anaerobic threshold; $\Delta\dot{V}O_2/\Delta WR$, change in $\dot{V}O_2$/change in work rate; O_2, oxygen; $\dot{V}E/\dot{V}CO_2$, ventilatory equivalent for carbon dioxide; $\dot{V}O_2$, oxygen uptake.

TABLE 10.7.3 Pre-β-Adrenergic Blockade

Time (min)	Work rate (W)	BP (mm Hg)	HR (min^{-1})	f (min^{-1})	$\dot{V}E$ (L/min BTPS)	$\dot{V}CO_2$ (L/min STPD)	$\dot{V}O_2$ (L/min STPD)	$\dot{V}O_2$/HR (mL/beat)	R	pH	HCO_3^- (mEq/L)	PO_2, mm Hg ET	PO_2, mm Hg a	PO_2, mm Hg (A − a)	PCO_2, mm Hg ET	PCO_2, mm Hg a	PCO_2, mm Hg (a − ET)	$\dot{V}E/\dot{V}CO_2$	$\dot{V}E/\dot{V}O_2$	V_D/V_T
0.5	Rest		80	19	14.5	0.37	0.42	5.3	0.88			113			75			35	31	
1.0	Rest		78	12	8.9	0.19	0.18	2.3	1.06			119			32			41	44	
1.5	Rest		82	13	6.5	0.15	0.20	2.4	0.75			104			39			36	27	
2.0	Rest		85	11	5.6	0.11	0.16	1.9	0.69			107			36			42	29	
2.5	Unloaded		90	34	9.4	0.19	0.34	3.8	0.56			97			41			34	19	
3.0	Unloaded		99	20	9.1	0.21	0.39	3.9	0.54			92			42			35	19	
3.5	Unloaded		93	25	8.1	0.14	0.24	2.6	0.58			90			44			43	25	
4.0	Unloaded		93	20	14.0	0.39	0.62	6.7	0.63			90			43			32	20	
4.5	Unloaded		104	20	13.3	0.35	0.49	4.7	0.71			99			42			33	24	
5.0	Unloaded		98	20	16.9	0.52	0.69	7.0	0.75			101			41			29	22	
5.5	60		118	24	21.1	0.64	0.86	7.3	0.74			100			42			30	22	
6.0	60		122	21	27.3	0.95	1.25	10.2	0.76			99			44			27	20	
6.5	60		123	25	29.8	0.98	1.21	9.8	0.81			104			43			28	23	
7.0	60		128	25	32.9	1.12	1.30	10.2	0.86			105			43			27	24	
7.5	60		125	21	31.4	1.10	1.22	9.8	0.90			107			43			27	24	
8.0	60		129	27	34.9	1.17	1.33	10.3	0.88			108			33			28	25	
8.5	80		124	22	38.7	1.33	1.35	10.9	0.99			108			33			28	27	
9.0	80		133	26	39.7	1.32	1.44	10.8	0.92			108			42			28	26	
9.5	100		138	24	37.5	1.31	1.43	10.4	0.92			107			43			27	25	
10.0	100		138	28	40.1	1.32	1.44	10.4	0.92			108			42			29	26	
10.5	120		151	27	45.3	1.53	1.62	10.7	0.94			110			42			28	27	
11.0	120		154	29	45.4	1.51	1.62	10.5	0.93			110			41			28	27	
11.5	140		159	29	48.5	1.64	1.73	10.9	0.95			108			42			28	27	
12.0	140		160	30	58.0	1.91	2.00	12.5	0.96			104			46			29	28	
12.5	160		165	35	59.4	1.93	2.06	12.5	0.94			112			41			29	27	
13.0	160		168	36	61.0	1.94	2.01	12.0	0.97			111			42			30	29	
13.5	180		174	36	72.9	2.32	2.23	12.8	1.04			114			39			30	31	
14.0	180		177	37	71.3	2.27	2.24	12.7	1.01			115			40			30	30	
14.5	200		187	38	81.7	2.56	2.39	12.8	1.07			117			39			31	33	
15.0	200		189	41	93.8	2.78	2.57	13.6	1.08			119			38			32	35	

Abbreviations: BP, blood pressure; BTPS, body temperature pressure saturated; f, frequency; HCO_3^-, bicarbonate; HR, heart rate; $P(A - a)O_2$, alveolar-arterial PO_2 difference; $P(a - ET)CO_2$, arterial-end-tidal PCO_2 difference; $PETCO_2$, end-tidal PCO_2; $PETO_2$, end-tidal PO_2; R, respiratory exchange ratio; STPD, standard temperature pressure dry; $\dot{V}CO_2$, carbon dioxide output; V_D/V_T, physiological dead space-tidal volume ratio; $\dot{V}E$, minute ventilation; $\dot{V}E/\dot{V}CO_2$, ventilatory equivalent for carbon dioxide; $\dot{V}E/\dot{V}O_2$, ventilatory equivalent for oxygen; $\dot{V}O_2$, oxygen uptake.

TABLE 10.7.4 Post-β-Adrenergic Blockade

Time (min)	Work rate (W)	BP (mm Hg)	HR (min^{-1})	f (min^{-1})	$\dot{V}_E$ (L/min BTPS)	$\dot{V}CO_2$ (L/min STPD)	$\dot{V}O_2$ (L/min STPD)	$\frac{\dot{V}O_2}{HR}$ (mL/beat)	R	pH	HCO_3^- (mEq/L)	PO_2, mm Hg ET	PO_2, mm Hg a	PO_2, mm Hg (A – a)	PCO_2, mm Hg ET	PCO_2, mm Hg a	PCO_2, mm Hg (a – ET)	$\frac{\dot{V}_E}{\dot{V}CO_2}$	$\frac{\dot{V}_E}{\dot{V}O_2}$	$\frac{V_D}{V_T}$
0.5	Rest		70	20	8.4	0.18	0.23	3.3	0.78			105			40			37	29	
1.0	Rest		70	24	6.6	0.10	0.16	2.3	0.63			105			39			46	29	
1.5	Rest		78	10	14.9	0.44	0.50	6.4	0.88			105			39			32	28	
2.0	Rest		59	16	8.7	0.20	0.23	3.9	0.87			114			36			37	32	
2.5	Unloaded		77	20	9.3	0.26	0.35	4.5	0.74			97			42			29	22	
3.0	Unloaded		85	17	13.7	0.43	0.60	7.1	0.72			94			43			29	20	
3.5	Unloaded		84	16	14.7	0.48	0.62	7.4	0.77			100			43			28	22	
4.0	Unloaded		90	15	9.2	0.27	0.34	3.8	0.79			99			44			29	23	
4.5	Unloaded		90	17	18.7	0.60	0.73	8.1	0.82			94			46			29	24	
5.0	Unloaded		86	19	15.0	0.49	0.59	6.9	0.83			102			42			27	23	
5.5	60		105	19	17.4	0.58	0.76	7.2	0.76			94			47			27	21	
6.0	60		107	17	20.9	0.76	1.03	9.6	0.74			96			44			26	19	
6.5	60		111	24	26.8	0.96	1.26	11.4	0.76			99			44			26	20	
7.0	60		109	22	27.5	1.00	1.15	10.6	0.87			103			45			26	22	
7.5	60		114	20	30.4	1.12	1.24	10.9	0.90			103			45			26	23	
8.0	60		115	25	30.7	1.12	1.28	11.1	0.88			104			44			26	22	
8.5	80		113	23	29.9	1.11	1.22	10.8	0.91			106			44			25	23	
9.0	80		112	22	30.7	1.11	1.20	10.7	0.93			103			46			26	24	
9.5	100		117	21	33.6	1.29	1.34	11.5	0.96			103			47			25	24	
10.0	100		119	26	33.7	1.25	1.37	11.5	0.91			104			45			25	23	
10.5	120		123	23	38.0	1.43	1.45	11.8	0.99			107			44			25	25	
11.0	120		122	25	40.6	1.55	1.63	13.4	0.95			106			45			25	24	
11.5	140		127	28	46.5	1.71	1.71	13.5	1.00			108			44			26	26	
12.0	140		128	28	48.2	1.78	1.77	13.8	1.01			108			46			26	26	
12.5	160		131	27	48.1	1.86	1.84	14.0	1.01			107			45			25	25	
13.0	160		134	31	52.2	1.95	1.93	14.4	1.01			110			44			25	26	
13.5	180		138	31	59.8	2.23	2.06	14.9	1.08			111			44			26	28	
14.0	180		147	32	63.1	2.37	2.13	14.5	1.11			112			43			25	28	
14.5	200		151	35	75.1	2.69	2.26	15.0	1.19			116			42			27	32	
15.0	200		156	41	85.2	2.92	2.39	15.3	1.22			111			42			28	34	

Abbreviations: BP, blood pressure; BTPS, body temperature pressure saturated; f, frequency; HCO_3^-, bicarbonate; HR, heart rate; $P(A - a)O_2$, alveolar-arterial PO_2 difference; $P(a - ET)CO_2$, arterial-end-tidal PCO_2 difference; $PETCO_2$, end-tidal PCO_2; $PETO_2$, end-tidal PO_2; R, respiratory exchange ratio; STPD, standard temperature pressure dry; $\dot{V}CO_2$, carbon dioxide output; V_D/V_T, physiological dead space–tidal volume ratio; $\dot{V}_E$, minute ventilation; $\dot{V}_E/\dot{V}CO_2$, ventilatory equivalent for carbon dioxide; $\dot{V}_E/\dot{V}O_2$, ventilatory equivalent for oxygen; $\dot{V}O_2$, oxygen uptake.

CASE 8

Normal Man With and Without Acute Cigarette Smoking

CLINICAL FINDINGS

A 27-year-old man volunteered for a research study to investigate the acute effect of cigarette smoking on cardiovascular and respiratory function during exercise. He was in excellent general health but had smoked cigarettes for 10 years. Physical examination, chest roentgenogram, and electrocardiogram (ECG) were normal. Demographic and respiratory function data are shown in **Table 10.8.1**.

EXERCISE FINDINGS

Two identical exercise studies were performed 6 days apart on a cycle ergometer. In the 5 hours before the first study, the subject smoked 15 medium-tar cigarettes. In the second study, he was under observation for 5 hours without smoking and breathed supplemental oxygen for the first 3 hours to hasten reduction of any carboxyhemoglobin in his blood. On both tests, he pedaled without added load at 60 rpm for 3 minutes. The work rate was then increased 25 W every minute to his symptom-limited maximum. On both occasions, the subject stopped exercise because of fatigue. The ECG remained normal. Carboxyhemoglobin levels were 6.1% at the start of the first study and 1.5% at the start of the second study. Exercise test data are summarized in **Table 10.8.2** and shown in **Tables 10.8.3** and **10.8.4** and **Figures 10.8.1** and **10.8.2**.

INTERPRETATION

Comments

This study is presented because it illustrates the small but significant effects of short-term cigarette smoking (or other cause of carboxyhemoglobinemia) on the peak oxygen uptake ($\dot{V}O_2$) and the anaerobic threshold. It also illustrates the reproducibility of the cardiac and gas exchange responses to exercise performed on different days and the effects of moderate obesity on the test results.

Resting respiratory function studies and the resting ECG were normal.

Analysis

Peak $\dot{V}O_2$ was clearly normal without prior smoking but was reduced to a marginally normal level in the setting of prior smoking. The anaerobic threshold was reduced after smoking but was normal without prior smoking. The subject

TABLE 10.8.1 Selected Respiratory Function Data

Measurement	Predicted	With prior smoking	Without smoking
Age (y)		27	27
Sex		Male	Male
Height (cm)		168	168
Weight (kg)	69	83	83
Hematocrit (%)		47	47
VC (L)	4.65	4.18	4.20
IC (L)	3.10	3.43	3.43
TLC (L)	6.19	6.26	6.68
FEV_1 (L)	3.79	3.57	3.55
FEV_1/VC (%)	81	85	85
MVV (L/min)	168	149	163
D_{LCO} (mL/mm Hg/min)	31.2	34.7	37.4

Abbreviations: D_{LCO}, diffusing capacity of lung for carbon monoxide; FEV_1, forced expiratory volume in 1 second; IC, inspiratory capacity; MVV, maximum voluntary ventilation; TLC, total lung capacity; VC, vital capacity.

TABLE 10.8.2 Selected Exercise Data

Measurement	Predicted	With prior smoking	Without smoking
Peak $\dot{V}O_2$ (L/min)	2.99	2.55	2.73
Maximum heart rate (beats/min)	193	178	182
Maximum O_2 pulse (mL/beat)	15.5	14.3	15.0
$\Delta\dot{V}O_2/\Delta WR$ (mL/min/W)	10.3	9.0	9.9
AT (L/min)	>1.23	1.1	1.25
Blood pressure (mm Hg [rest, max])		138/84, 183/110	132/84, 186/105
Maximum $\dot{V}E$ (L/min)		110	121
Exercise breathing reserve (L/min)	>15	39	42
$\dot{V}E/\dot{V}CO_2$ @ *AT* or lowest	24.8	24.6	24.3
PaO_2 (mm Hg [rest, max ex])		102, 103	109, 106
$P(A - a)O_2$ (mm Hg [rest, max ex])		5, 19	−1, 16
$PaCO_2$ (mm Hg [rest, max ex])		39, 34	39, 34
$P(a - ET)CO_2$ (mm Hg [rest, max ex])		−1, −3	−2, −3
VD/VT (rest, heavy ex)		0.37, 0.18	0.27, 0.20
HCO_3^- (mEq/L [rest, 2-min recov])		25, 14	26, 15
COHb (%)	<2	6.1	1.5

Abbreviations: AT, anaerobic threshold; COHb, carboxyhemoglobin; $\Delta\dot{V}O_2/\Delta WR$, change in $\dot{V}O_2$/change in work rate; HCO_3^-, bicarbonate; O_2, oxygen; $P(A - a)O_2$, alveolar-arterial PO_2 difference; $P(a - ET)CO_2$, arterial-end-tidal PCO_2 difference; VD/VT, physiological dead space–tidal volume ratio; $\dot{V}E$, minute ventilation; $\dot{V}E/\dot{V}CO_2$, ventilatory equivalent for carbon dioxide; $\dot{V}O_2$, oxygen uptake.

is about 20% overweight, and this likely contributed to the higher than normal $\dot{V}O_2$ measured during unloaded cycling, approximately 0.95 L/min. Notably, during the incremental phase of test, when the work rate was increased each minute by 25 W, the change in $\dot{V}O_2$/change in work rate ($\Delta\dot{V}O_2/\Delta WR$) slope increased normally.

Indices other than peak $\dot{V}O_2$ and anaerobic threshold that might reflect the effect of the increased carboxyhemoglobin during exercise are the O_2 pulse and $\Delta\dot{V}O_2/\Delta WR$. These are both reduced after cigarette smoking compared to without smoking in this subject, although still within normal limits. Although indices of ventilation–perfusion matching ($P[a - ET]CO_2$ and VD/VT) are normal at maximum exercise in this subject, abnormal exercise gas exchange may be seen after recent smoking.

Conclusion

Cigarette smoking affected exercise performance in this otherwise normal subject, likely due to increased carboxyhemoglobin. He also demonstrates the effect of obesity; higher $\dot{V}O_2$ than expected during unloaded cycling but a normal $\Delta\dot{V}O_2/\Delta WR$ thereafter.

TABLE 10.8.3 With Prior Smoking

Time (min)	Work rate (W)	BP (mm Hg)	HR (min^{-1})	f (min^{-1})	$\dot{V}E$ (L/min BTPS)	$\dot{V}CO_2$ (L/min STPD)	$\dot{V}O_2$ (L/min STPD)	$\dot{V}O_2/HR$ (mL/beat)	R	pH	HCO_3^- (mEq/L)	PO_2, mm Hg ET	a	(A − a)	PCO_2, mm Hg ET	a	(a − ET)	$\dot{V}E/\dot{V}CO_2$	$\dot{V}E/\dot{V}O_2$	V_D/V_T
	Rest	138/84								7.42	24		98			38				
0.5	Rest		76	26	12.1	0.24	0.31	4.1	0.77			100			41			41	32	
1.0	Rest		77	27	13.4	0.27	0.31	4.0	0.87			106			39			41	36	
1.5	Rest		76	27	11.1	0.21	0.27	3.6	0.78			97			42			42	33	
2.0	Rest	138/84	77	25	13.2	0.28	0.32	4.2	0.88	7.42	25	107	102	5	40	39	−1	40	35	0.37
2.5	Rest		76	25	12.4	0.26	0.30	3.9	0.87			105			40			40	34	
3.0	Rest		75	25	11.7	0.23	0.26	3.5	0.88			104			41			42	37	
3.5	Unloaded		99	19	15.8	0.50	0.51	5.2	0.98			104			43			28	2	8
4.0	Unloaded		101	20	17.1	0.56	0.65	6.4	0.86			97			43			28	24	
4.5	Unloaded		103	21	19.2	0.69	0.89	8.6	0.78			93			46			25	20	
5.0	Unloaded		103	21	23.6	0.87	0.96	9.3	0.91			97			45			25	23	
5.5	Unloaded		102	24	21.8	0.76	0.84	8.2	0.90			100			45			26	24	
6.0	Unloaded	156/96	105	23	23.8	0.85	0.92	8.8	0.92	7.39	24	102	98	8	45	41	−4	26	24	0.17
6.5	25		107	22	22.5	0.81	0.89	8.3	0.91			99			45			25	23	
7.0	25		109	21	24.0	0.90	0.99	9.1	0.91			100			44			25	22	
7.5	50		113	25	27.0	0.97	1.03	9.1	0.94			99			46			26	24	
8.0	50	165/93	115	23	32.1	1.16	1.17	10.2	0.99	7.38	24	101	95	13	45	41	−3	26	26	0.20
8.5	75		123	25	31.6	1.20	1.24	10.1	0.97			100			46			25	24	
9.0	75		124	25	35.4	1.36	1.33	10.7	1.02			103			46			24	25	
9.5	100		129	27	36.8	1.42	1.38	10.7	1.03			102			47			24	25	
10.0	100	177/96	135	26	43.4	1.68	1.53	11.3	1.10	7.36	24	102	94	16	47	43	−4	25	27	0.17
10.5	125		145	29	43.0	1.70	1.61	11.1	1.06			103			47			24	25	
11.0	125		150	30	50.8	2.01	1.88	12.5	1.07			103			48			24	26	
11.5	150		154	33	57.5	2.21	1.99	12.9	1.11			105			47			25	27	
12.0	150	177/99	162	36	66.6	2.47	2.09	12.9	1.18	7.33	22	107	95	18	46	42	−4	26	30	0.19
12.5	175		171	36	70.4	2.66	2.24	13.1	1.19			108			46			25	30	
13.0	175		172	43	84.8	2.95	2.34	13.6	1.26			112			43			28	35	
13.5	200		176	51	101.2	3.27	2.51	14.3	1.30			115			41			30	39	
14.0	200		178	62	110.6	3.36	2.55	14.3	1.32	7.32	17	119	103	19	37	34	−3	31	41	0.18
14.5	Recovery		176	45	95.2	2.99	2.18	12.4	1.37			119			39			31	42	
15.0	Recovery		164	43	81.4	2.46	1.49	9.1	1.65			123			37			32	52	
15.5	Recovery		160	43	70.6	1.93	1.15	7.2	1.68			125			36			35	58	
16.0	Recovery	165/84	153	35	53.3	1.46	0.98	6.4	1.49	7.27	14	123	112	14	35	32	−3	34	51	0.21

Abbreviations: BP, blood pressure; BTPS, body temperature pressure saturated; f, frequency; HCO_3^-, bicarbonate; HR, heart rate; $P(A - a)O_2$, alveolar-arterial PO_2 difference; $P(a - ET)CO_2$, arterial-end-tidal PCO_2 difference; $PETCO_2$, end-tidal PCO_2; $PETO_2$, end-tidal PO_2; R, respiratory exchange ratio; STPD, standard temperature pressure dry; $\dot{V}CO_2$, carbon dioxide output; V_D/V_T, physiological dead space-tidal volume ratio; $\dot{V}E$, minute ventilation; $\dot{V}E/\dot{V}CO_2$, ventilatory equivalent for carbon dioxide; $\dot{V}E/\dot{V}O_2$, ventilatory equivalent for oxygen; $\dot{V}O_2$, oxygen uptake.

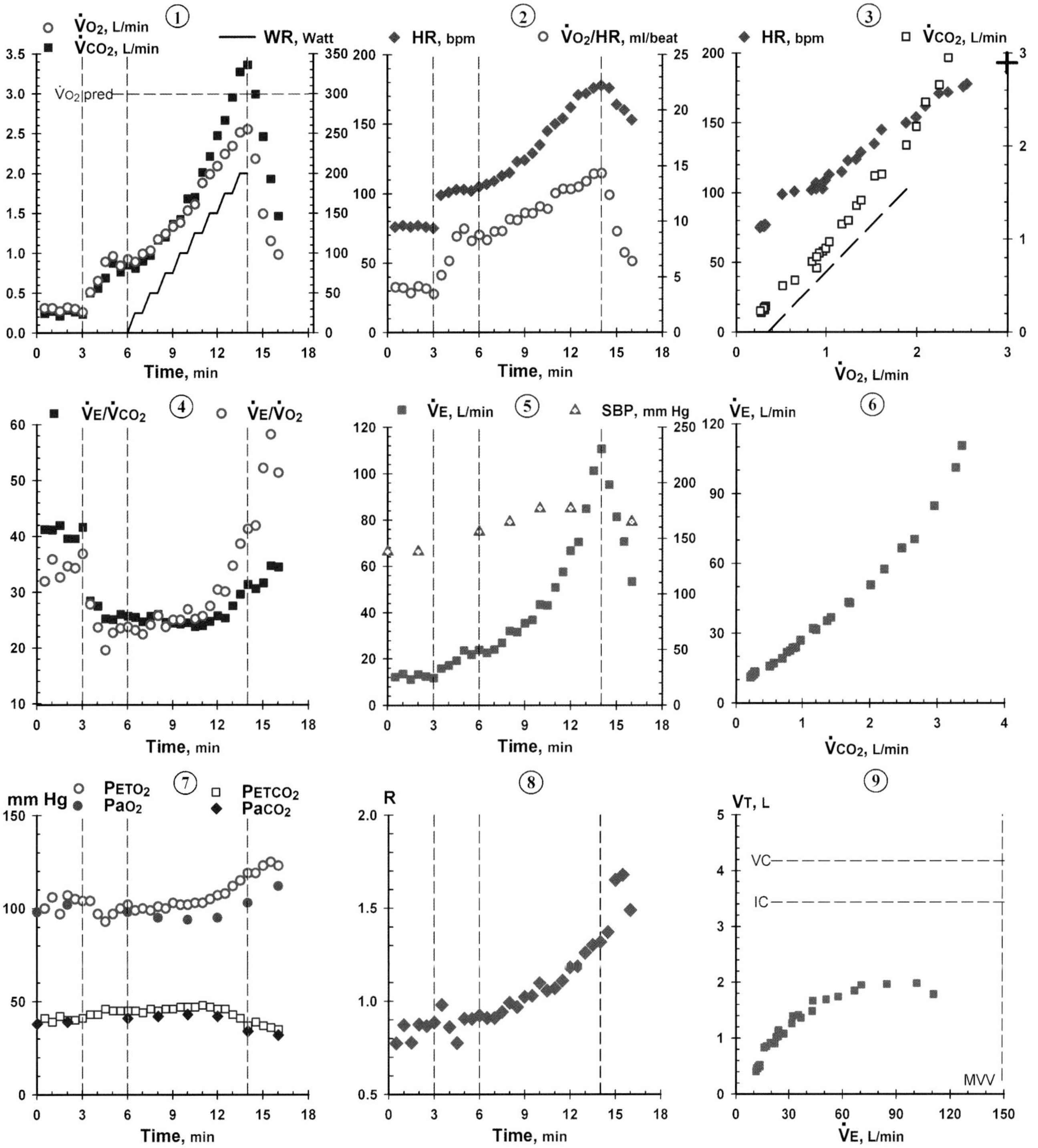

FIGURE 10.8.1. With prior cigarette smoking. Vertical dashed lines in the panels in the left and middle columns indicate, from left to right, the beginning of unloaded cycling, start of increasing work rate (WR) at 25 W/min, and start of recovery. In **panel 1**, the increase in WR (right y-axis) is plotted with a scale of 100 W to 1 L of oxygen uptake ($\dot{V}O_2$) (left y-axis) such that WR is plotted parallel to a $\dot{V}O_2$ slope of 10 mL/min/W. In **panel 3**, carbon dioxide output ($\dot{V}CO_2$) (right y-axis) is plotted as a function of $\dot{V}O_2$ (x-axis) with identical scales so that the diagonal dashed line has a slope of 1 (45°). The $\dot{V}CO_2$ increasing more steeply than $\dot{V}O_2$ defines carbon dioxide (CO_2) derived from bicarbonate buffer, as long as ventilatory equivalent for CO_2 ($\dot{V}E/\dot{V}CO_2$) (**panel 4**) is not increasing and end-tidal PCO_2 ($PETCO_2$) (**panel 7**) is not decreasing, simultaneously. The black + symbol in **panel 3** indicates predicted values of heart rate (HR) (left y-axis) and $\dot{V}O_2$ for this individual. Abbreviations: IC, inspiratory capacity; MVV, maximum voluntary ventilation; $PETO_2$, end-tidal PO_2; R, respiratory exchange ratio; SBP, systolic blood pressure; VC, vital capacity; $\dot{V}E$, minute ventilation; $\dot{V}E/\dot{V}O_2$, ventilatory equivalent for oxygen; V_T, tidal volume.

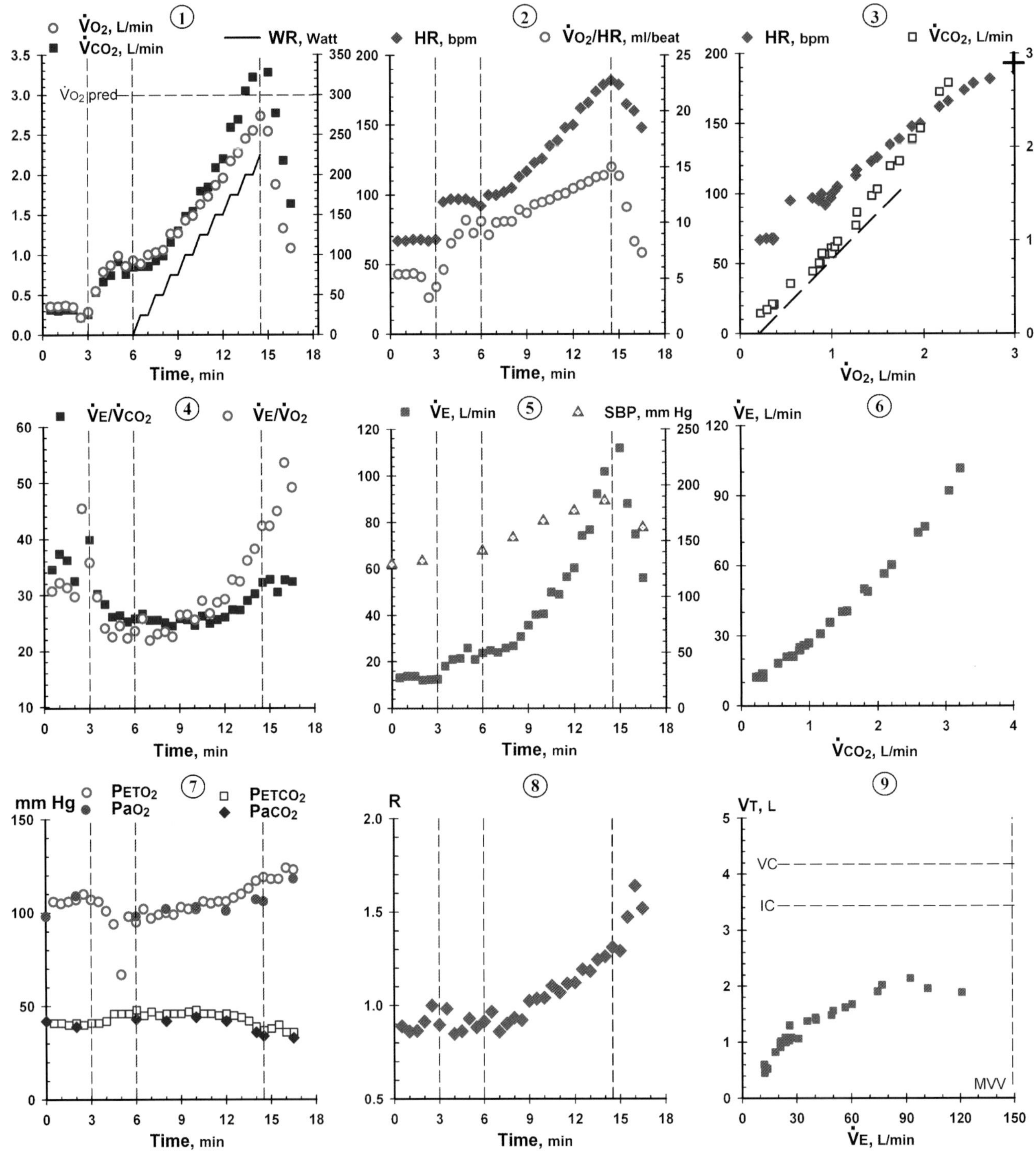

FIGURE 10.8.2. Without prior cigarette smoking. Vertical dashed lines in the panels in the left and middle columns indicate, from left to right, the beginning of unloaded cycling, start of increasing work rate (WR) at 25 W/min, and start of recovery. In **panel 1**, the increase in WR (right y-axis) is plotted with a scale of 100 W to 1 L of oxygen uptake ($\dot{V}O_2$) (left y-axis) such that WR is plotted parallel to a $\dot{V}O_2$ slope of 10 mL/min/W. In **panel 3**, carbon dioxide output ($\dot{V}CO_2$) (right y-axis) is plotted as a function of $\dot{V}O_2$ (x-axis) with identical scales so that the diagonal dashed line has a slope of 1 (45°). The $\dot{V}CO_2$ increasing more steeply than $\dot{V}O_2$ defines carbon dioxide (CO_2) derived from bicarbonate buffer, as long as ventilatory equivalent for CO_2 ($\dot{V}E/\dot{V}CO_2$) (**panel 4**) is not increasing and end-tidal PCO_2 ($PETCO_2$) (**panel 7**) is not decreasing, simultaneously. The black + symbol in **panel 3** indicates predicted values of heart rate (HR) (left y-axis) and $\dot{V}O_2$ for this individual. Abbreviations: IC, inspiratory capacity; MVV, maximum voluntary ventilation; $PETO_2$, end-tidal PO_2; R, respiratory exchange ratio; SBP, systolic blood pressure; VC, vital capacity; $\dot{V}E$, minute ventilation; $\dot{V}E/\dot{V}O_2$, ventilatory equivalent for oxygen; V_T, tidal volume.

TABLE 10.8.4 Without Prior Smoking

Time (min)	Work rate (W)	BP (mm Hg)	HR (min^{-1})	f (min^{-1})	$\dot{V}E$ (L/min BTPS)	$\dot{V}CO_2$ (L/min STPD)	$\dot{V}O_2$ (L/min STPD)	$\frac{\dot{V}O_2}{HR}$ (mL/beat)	R	pH	HCO_3^- (mEq/L)	PO_2, mm Hg ET	a	(A − a)	PCO_2, mm Hg ET	a	(a − ET)	$\frac{\dot{V}E}{\dot{V}CO_2}$	$\frac{\dot{V}E}{\dot{V}O_2}$	$\frac{V_D}{V_T}$
	Rest	129/84								7.40	26		99			42				
0.5	Rest		67	24	13.1	0.32	0.36	5.4	0.89			106			41			35	31	
1.0	Rest		67	26	13.8	0.31	0.36	5.4	0.86			105			41			37	32	
1.5	Rest		68	26	13.8	0.32	0.37	5.4	0.86			106			40			36	31	
2.0	Rest	132/84	68	20	12.1	0.32	0.35	5.1	0.91	7.43	25	107	109	−1	41	39	−2	33	30	0.27
2.5	Rest		67	27	12.3	0.22	0.22	3.3	1.00			110			40			45	45	
3.0	Rest		68	25	12.5	0.26	0.29	4.3	0.9			107			41			40	36	
3.5	Unloaded		95	22	18.2	0.54	0.55	5.8	0.98			106			41			30	30	
4.0	Unloaded		97	23	21.0	0.67	0.79	8.1	0.85			101			42			28	24	
4.5	Unloaded		97	21	21.4	0.75	0.87	9.0	0.86			94			46			26	23	
5.0	Unloaded		97	20	26.0	0.92	0.99	10.2	0.93			67			46			26	25	
5.5	Unloaded		95	21	21.0	0.76	0.86	9.1	0.88			98			46			25	22	
6.0	Unloaded	141/87	92	22	23.8	0.85	0.93	10.1	0.91	7.39	26	95	98	6	48	43	−5	26	24	0.20
6.5	25		100	24	25.0	0.86	0.89	8.9	0.97			102			45			27	26	
7.0	25		100	24	24.0	0.86	1.00	10.0	0.86			97			47			26	22	
7.5	50		102	25	25.9	0.93	1.03	10.1	0.90			99			45			26	23	
8.0	50	153/90	105	25	27.0	0.99	1.06	10.1	0.93	7.39	25	100	102	4	46	42	−4	25	23	0.17
8.5	75		113	29	30.9	1.16	1.26	11.2	0.92			99			46			25	23	
9.0	75		117	26	35.8	1.30	1.27	10.9	1.02			103			46			26	26	
9.5	100		123	28	40.3	1.48	1.43	11.6	1.03			102			47			26	27	
10.0	100	168/93	126	29	40.6	1.55	1.49	11.8	1.04	7.37	25	102	103	4	48	44	−4	25	26	0.19
10.5	125		135	32	50.0	1.80	1.63	12.1	1.10			106			46			26	29	
11.0	125		139	33	49.0	1.85	1.73	12.4	1.07			105			46			25	27	
11.5	150		148	35	56.6	2.09	1.87	12.6	1.12			106			45			26	29	
12.0	150	177/99	150	36	60.4	2.20	1.96	13.1	1.12	7.36	23	106	101	11	46	42	−4	26	29	0.20
12.5	175		162	39	74.3	2.59	2.17	13.4	1.19			108			45			27	33	
13.0	175		166	38	76.8	2.69	2.27	13.7	1.19			110			44			27	32	
13.5	200		174	43	92.2	3.05	2.45	14.1	1.24			113			42			29	36	
14.0	200	186/105	179	52	101.8	3.22	2.55	14.2	1.26	7.35	20	117	107	13	39	36	−3	30	38	0.20
14.5	225		182	64	121.0	3.58	2.73	15.0	1.31	7.32	17	119	106	16	37	34	−3	32	42	0.20
15.0	Recovery		179	52	111.9	3.28	2.54	14.2	1.29			118			38			33	42	
15.5	Recovery	165		41	88.0	2.77	1.88	11.4	1.47			118			40			31	45	
16.0	Recovery		160	43	74.9	2.18	1.33	8.3	1.64			124			36			33	54	
16.5	Recovery	162/90	148	35	56.1	1.64	1.08	7.3	1.52	7.26	15	123	118	8	36	33	−3	32	49	0.18

Abbreviations: BP, blood pressure; BTPS, body temperature pressure saturated; f, frequency; HCO_3^-, bicarbonate; HR, heart rate; $P(A - a)O_2$, alveolar-arterial PO_2 difference; $P(a - ET)CO_2$, arterial-end-tidal PCO_2 difference; $PETCO_2$, end-tidal PCO_2; $PETO_2$, end-tidal PO_2; R, respiratory exchange ratio; STPD, standard temperature pressure dry; $\dot{V}CO_2$, carbon dioxide output; V_D/V_T, physiological dead space-tidal volume ratio; $\dot{V}E$, minute ventilation; $\dot{V}E/\dot{V}CO_2$, ventilatory equivalent for carbon dioxide; $\dot{V}E/\dot{V}O_2$, ventilatory equivalent for oxygen; $\dot{V}O_2$, oxygen uptake.

CASE 9

Active Man With Dyspnea at High Altitude

CLINICAL FINDINGS

A 65-year-old self-employed man underwent cardiopulmonary exercise testing to evaluate exertional dyspnea that he had experienced when hiking at an altitude of 10 000 ft (3000 m). He had been an avid hiker for years but had noted a decreased ability to hike at high altitudes over the last 3 to 4 years. Of note, he was accustomed to taking the lead on hiking trips even as he aged and became progressively older compared to other hikers on the outings. He was referred to a cardiologist, who performed an extensive workup, including treadmill exercise tests (without gas exchange measurements), a nuclear medicine cardiac scan, echocardiogram, and coronary angiogram. The results of these tests were negative, but he was nevertheless told that he probably had an occult cardiomyopathy and was prescribed an angiotensin-converting enzyme inhibitor. The patient referred himself for a cardiopulmonary exercise test because he believed that the drug did not help him. Demographic and respiratory function data are shown in **Table 10.9.1**.

EXERCISE FINDINGS

Because his symptoms were limited to when he was hiking at altitude, the patient performed exercise on a cycle ergometer, first while breathing room air and then while breathing 15% oxygen (O_2) (equivalent to an 8000-ft altitude).

TABLE 10.9.1 Selected Respiratory Function Data

Measurement	Predicted	Measured
Age (y)		65
Sex		Male
Height (cm)		183
Weight (kg)	83	83
Hematocrit (%)		44
VC (L)	4.60	4.70
IC (L)	3.06	3.70
FEV_1 (L)	3.45	3.47
FEV_1/VC (%)	75	74
MVV (L/min)	142	129
D_{LCO} (mL/mm Hg/min)	28.0	28.6

Abbreviations: D_{LCO}, diffusing capacity of lung for carbon monoxide; FEV_1, forced expiratory volume in 1 second; IC, inspiratory capacity; MVV, maximum voluntary ventilation; VC, vital capacity.

On both occasions, he pedaled at 60 rpm without an added load for 3 minutes, followed by an increase in work rate by 20 W/min to tolerance. Arterial blood was sampled every second minute, and intra-arterial pressure was recorded from a percutaneously placed brachial artery catheter. The patient stopped exercise because of fatigue and shortness of breath. No electrocardiogram abnormalities were noted at rest or during exercise. Exercise data are summarized in **Table 10.9.2**, and shown in **Tables 10.9.3** and **10.9.4** and **Figures 10.9.1** and **10.9.2**.

TABLE 10.9.2 Selected Exercise Data

Measurement	Predicted (room air)	Measured	
		Air	15% O_2
Peak $\dot{V}O_2$ (L/min)	2.21	2.69	2.19
Maximum heart rate (beats/min)	155	175	172
Maximum O_2 pulse (mL/beat)	14.3	15.9	12.9
$\Delta\dot{V}O_2/\Delta WR$ (mL/min/W)	10.3	10.3	7.8
AT (L/min)	>0.99	1.9	1.2
Blood pressure (mm Hg [rest, max])		132/72, 210/90	114/66, 198/96
Maximum $\dot{V}E$ (L/min)		115	108
Exercise breathing reserve (L/min)	>15	14	21
$\dot{V}E/\dot{V}CO_2$ @ *AT* or lowest	28.2	30.2	29.9
PaO_2 (mm Hg [rest, max ex])		113, 106	77, 52
$P(A-a)O_2$ (mm Hg [rest, max ex])		−1, 16	0, 27
$PaCO_2$ (mm Hg [rest, max ex])		35, 33	32, 32
$P(a-ET)CO_2$ (mm Hg [rest, max ex])		1, −3	2, 0
V_D/V_T (rest, heavy ex)		0.25, 0.21	0.36, 0.19
HCO_3^- (mEq/L [rest, 2-min recov])		21, 15	21, 17

Abbreviations: *AT*, anaerobic threshold; $\Delta\dot{V}O_2/\Delta WR$, change in $\dot{V}O_2$/change in work rate; ex, exercise; HCO_3^-, bicarbonate; O_2, oxygen; $P(A-a)O_2$, alveolar-arterial PO_2 difference; $P(a-ET)CO_2$, arterial-end-tidal PCO_2 difference; recov, recovery; V_D/V_T, physiological dead space-tidal volume ratio; $\dot{V}E$, minute ventilation; $\dot{V}E/\dot{V}CO_2$, ventilatory equivalent for carbon dioxide; $\dot{V}O_2$, oxygen uptake.

TABLE 10.9.3 Room Air

Time (min)	Work rate (W)	BP (mm Hg)	HR (min^{-1})	f (min^{-1})	$\dot{V}_E$ (L/min BTPS)	$\dot{V}CO_2$ (L/min STPD)	$\dot{V}O_2$ (L/min STPD)	$\frac{\dot{V}O_2}{HR}$ (mL/beat)	R	pH	HCO_3^- (mEq/L)	PO_2, mm Hg ET	a	(A − a)	PCO_2, mm Hg ET	a	(a − ET)	$\frac{\dot{V}_E}{\dot{V}CO_2}$	$\frac{\dot{V}_E}{\dot{V}O_2}$	$\frac{V_D}{V_T}$
0.5	Rest		68	24	15.6	0.33	0.31	4.6	1.06			119			30			41	44	
1.0	Rest		68	16	17.5	0.40	0.33	4.9	1.21			119			30			40	49	
1.5	Rest		77	17	14.4	0.31	0.27	3.5	1.15			118			31			42	48	
2.0	Rest		83	22	17.8	0.39	0.33	4.0	1.18			114			32			41	48	
2.5	Unloaded		83	19	19.9	0.53	0.55	6.6	0.96			113			33			35	33	
3.0	Unloaded		80	21	21.3	0.53	0.49	6.1	1.08			115			32			37	40	
3.5	Unloaded		80	19	19.9	0.55	0.52	6.5	1.06			111			34			33	35	
4.0	Unloaded		76	19	21.2	0.58	0.63	8.3	0.92			112			33			34	31	
4.5	Unloaded		75	19	21.0	0.55	0.58	7.7	0.95			113			33			35	33	
5.0	Unloaded	135/72	81	23	19.8	0.52	0.58	7.2	0.90	7.40	21	110	113	−1	34	35	−1	34	31	0.25
5.5	20		81	18	24.5	0.67	0.65	8.0	1.03			109			34			34	35	
6.0	20		85	20	22.8	0.63	0.71	8.4	0.89			111			34			33	30	
6.5	40		87	21	27.1	0.81	0.85	9.8	0.95			105			33			31	30	
7.0	40	144/75	88	19	25.1	0.75	0.79	9.0	0.95	7.40	21	111	120	−6	36	35	−1	31	30	0.20
7.5	60		98	19	28.0	0.81	0.87	8.9	0.93			112			34			33	30	
8.0	60		100	20	29.4	0.91	1.10	11.0	0.83			107			35			30	25	
8.5	80		99	21	33.7	1.04	1.24	12.5	0.84			108			36			31	26	
9.0	80	144/75	112	21	34.5	1.07	1.23	11.0	0.87	7.40	21	108	106	5	36	35	−1	31	27	0.18
9.5	100		110	23	33.3	1.20	1.39	12.6	0.86			109			36			26	23	
10.0	100	162/84	113	23	42.6	1.33	1.50	13.3	0.89	7.40	22	110	109	1	35	36	−1	31	27	0.21
10.5	120		120	25	45.6	1.43	1.57	13.1	0.91			109			36			30	28	
11.0	120	168/84	124	24	49.6	1.57	1.69	13.6	0.93	7.40	23	110	107	4	36	37	1	30	28	0.22
11.5	140		130	24	51.2	1.67	1.84	14.2	0.91			108			37			29	27	
12.0	140		135	27	59.8	1.81	1.99	14.7	0.91			111			36			32	29	
12.5	160		140	29	61.2	1.87	2.03	14.5	0.92			109			38			31	29	
13.0	160	174/84	149	32	66.7	2.14	2.18	14.6	0.98	7.40	21	113	107	−7	36	35	−1	30	29	0.17
13.5	180		152	27	64.3	2.12	2.14	14.1	0.99			108			39			29	29	
14.0	180		154	31	73.7	2.45	2.45	15.9	1.00			112			37			29	29	
14.5	200		160	33	78.7	2.61	2.54	15.9	1.03			110			38			29	30	
15.0	200	207/84	172	36	91.8	2.91	2.60	15.1	1.12	7.40	21	117	100	18	35	35	0	30	34	0.19
15.5	220		175	42	102.1	3.09	2.69	15.4	1.15			118			34			32	37	
16.0	220	210/90	174	49	115.3	3.25	2.69	15.5	1.21	7.40	20	121	106	15	32	33	−1	34	41	0.23
16.5	Recovery		162	34	92.9	2.94	2.24	13.8	1.31	7.30	16	119	107	16	36	33	−3	31	40	0.14
17.0	Recovery		154	36	87.3	2.44	1.58	10.3	1.54			125			32			35	53	
17.5	Recovery		140	29	62.8	1.73	1.07	7.6	1.62			107			32			35	56	
18.0	Recovery		125	24	49.1	1.39	0.89	7.1	1.56	7.30	15	125	132	−4	33	31	−2	34	53	0.17

Abbreviations: BP, blood pressure; BTPS, body temperature pressure saturated; f, frequency; HCO_3^-, bicarbonate; HR, heart rate; $P(A-a)O_2$, alveolar-arterial PO_2 difference; $P(a-ET)CO_2$, arterial–end-tidal PCO_2 difference; $P_{ET}CO_2$, end-tidal PCO_2; $P_{ET}O_2$, end-tidal PO_2; R, respiratory exchange ratio; STPD, standard temperature pressure dry; $\dot{V}CO_2$, carbon dioxide output; V_D/V_T, physiological dead space–tidal volume ratio; $\dot{V}_E$, minute ventilation; $\dot{V}_E/\dot{V}CO_2$, ventilatory equivalent for carbon dioxide; $\dot{V}_E/\dot{V}O_2$, ventilatory equivalent for oxygen; $\dot{V}O_2$, oxygen uptake.

INTERPRETATION

Comments

Resting respiratory function studies were normal.

Analysis

On the room air exercise test, peak $\dot{V}O_2$ and anaerobic threshold are normal, in fact, well above predicted values for sedentary men. The low breathing reserve is compatible with high cardiovascular capacity and good motivation. While the patient was breathing 15% O_2, PaO_2 was reduced due to the lower FIO_2 and decreased further with exercise. Peak $\dot{V}O_2$, peak O_2 pulse, and anaerobic threshold all decreased relative to the room air study. These decreases were expected because all of these measurements are O_2 transport-dependent. The $\Delta\dot{V}O_2/\Delta WR$ was also somewhat reduced.

Conclusion

This man had excellent cardiovascular function with no evidence to support the diagnosis of cardiomyopathy. His symptoms were most likely due to the decrease in cardiovascular function associated with aging, which were highlighted when he tried to continue his physical feats of earlier years at the pace of younger colleagues, especially with the added physiological stress of high altitude.

TABLE 10.9.4 15% Oxygen

Time (min)	Work rate (W)	BP (mm Hg)	HR (min^{-1})	f (min^{-1})	$\dot{V}E$ (L/min BTPS)	$\dot{V}CO_2$ (L/min STPD)	$\dot{V}O_2$ (L/min STPD)	$\frac{\dot{V}O_2}{HR}$ (mL/beat)	R	pH	HCO_3^- (mEq/L)	PO_2, mm Hg ET	PO_2, mm Hg a	PO_2, mm Hg (A − a)	PCO_2, mm Hg ET	PCO_2, mm Hg a	PCO_2, mm Hg (a − ET)	$\frac{\dot{V}E}{\dot{V}CO_2}$	$\frac{\dot{V}E}{\dot{V}O_2}$	$\frac{VD}{VT}$
0.5	Rest		73	17	12.7	0.24	0.22	3.0	1.08			81			28			47	51	
1.0	Rest		67	14	12.1	0.30	0.28	4.2	1.07			78			31			36	39	
1.5	Rest		69	14	13.9	0.32	0.32	4.6	1.00			76			31			40	40	
2.0	Rest	114/56	67	15	9.1	0.17	0.16	2.4	1.07	7.44	21	79	77	0	30	32	−2	46	49	0.36
2.5	Rest		66	11	16.0	0.42	0.37	5.5	1.15			80			31			36	41	
3.0	Rest		75	16	10.3	0.17	0.15	2.0	1.16			82			29			53	61	
3.5	Unloaded		76	19	15.8	0.37	0.31	4.0	1.20			82			30			38	46	
4.0	Unloaded		81	14	17.5	0.48	0.45	5.6	1.07			76			33			34	36	
4.5	Unloaded		82	19	23.1	0.63	0.59	7.2	1.07			76			33			34	36	
5.0	Unloaded		84	15	18.4	0.53	0.54	6.5	0.97			72			34			32	31	
5.5	Unloaded		79	17	20.8	0.59	0.59	7.5	1.00			73			34			33	33	
6.0	Unloaded	132/36	73	15	19.8	0.55	0.51	7.1	1.07	7.39	20	77	76	0	32	33	1	34	36	0.21
6.5	20		84	22	15.7	0.45	0.46	5.5	0.97			70			36			31	30	
7.0	20		85	18	22.2	0.64	0.64	7.5	1.00			73			34			32	32	
7.5	40		85	18	23.6	0.73	0.73	8.6	1.00			72			35			30	30	
8.0	40	114/60	92	16	24.2	0.75	0.75	8.1	1.00	7.41	22	72	68	4	35	35	0	30	30	0.18
8.5	60		95	18	26.8	0.81	0.81	8.5	1.00			72			35			31	31	
9.0	60		102	22	29.4	0.89	0.86	8.5	1.03			72			36			31	32	
9.5	80		105	19	33.0	1.04	0.98	9.3	1.06			73			36			30	32	
10.0	80	144/66	105	22	36.0	1.11	1.01	9.7	1.10	7.42	22	75	66	9	35	35	0	31	34	0.19
10.5	100		108	23	38.9	1.20	1.10	10.1	1.10			75			35			31	34	
11.0	100		115	22	41.5	1.30	1.19	10.3	1.10			75			35			30	33	
11.5	120		114	24	45.7	1.43	1.23	10.8	1.16			76			36			31	36	
12.0	120	144/66	124	25	49.2	1.53	1.40	11.3	1.10	7.42	22	75	60	15	35	34	−1	31	34	0.17
12.5	140		124	28	54.5	1.65	1.45	11.7	1.14			77			34			32	36	
13.0	140		129	28	59.4	1.80	1.49	11.5	1.21			78			35			32	38	
13.5	160		140	28	65.7	2.00	1.71	12.2	1.17			77			35			32	37	
14.0	160	174/73	148	30	72.0	2.15	1.77	11.9	1.22	7.41	21	79	57	21	34	34	0	32	39	0.21
14.5	180		150	30	73.6	2.21	1.88	12.5	1.17			78			34			32	38	
15.0	180		152	28	74.6	2.29	1.83	12.0	1.25			79			35			32	39	
15.5	200		152	28	75.6	2.36	1.88	12.4	1.25			79			35			31	39	
16.0	200	195/84	160	33	84.8	2.57	1.98	12.4	1.30	7.38	19	80	52	28	35	33	−2	32	41	0.17
16.5	220		170	44	101.6	2.78	2.19	12.9	1.27			81			33			35	45	
17.0	220	198/96	172	45	107.9	3.03	2.15	12.5	1.41	7.33	17	85	56	27	31	32	1	34	49	0.21
17.5	Recovery		172	41	97.3	2.77	1.93	11.2	1.44			84			33			34	49	
18.0	Recovery		154									91			33					

Abbreviations: BP, blood pressure; BTPS, body temperature pressure saturated; f, frequency; HCO_3^-, bicarbonate; HR, heart rate; $P(A - a)O_2$, alveolar-arterial PO_2 difference; $P(a - ET)CO_2$, arterial-end-tidal PCO_2 difference; $PETCO_2$, end-tidal PCO_2; $PETO_2$, end-tidal PO_2; R, respiratory exchange ratio; STPD, standard temperature pressure dry; $\dot{V}CO_2$, carbon dioxide output; VD/VT, physiological dead space-tidal volume ratio; $\dot{V}E$, minute ventilation; $\dot{V}E/\dot{V}CO_2$, ventilatory equivalent for carbon dioxide; $\dot{V}E/\dot{V}O_2$, ventilatory equivalent for oxygen; $\dot{V}O_2$, oxygen uptake.

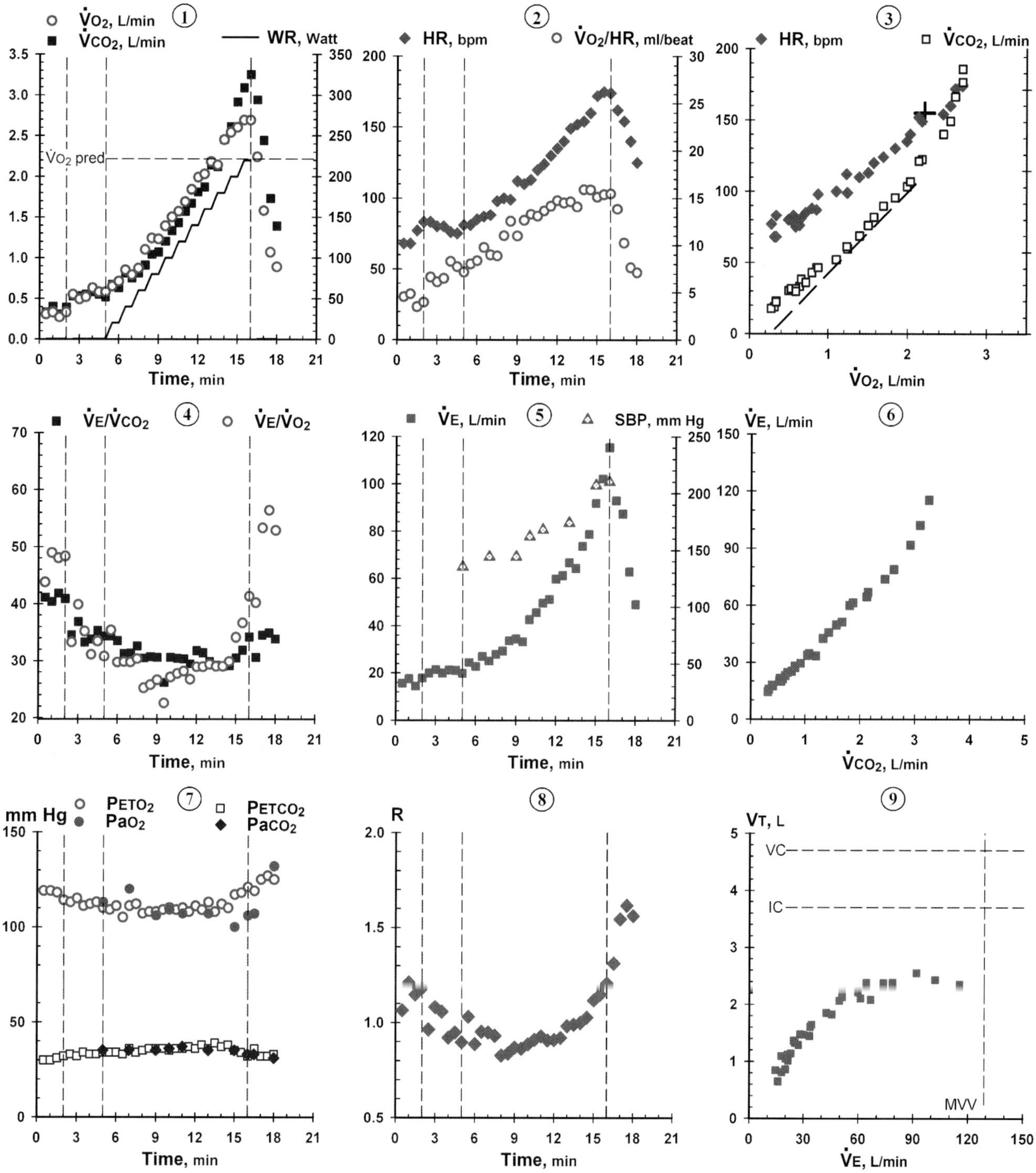

FIGURE 10.9.1. Air breathing. Vertical dashed lines in the panels in the left and middle columns indicate, from left to right, the beginning of unloaded cycling, start of increasing work rate (WR) at 20 W/min, and start of recovery. In **panel 1**, the increase in WR (right y-axis) is plotted with a scale of 100 W to 1 L of oxygen uptake ($\dot{V}O_2$) (left y-axis) such that WR is plotted parallel to a $\dot{V}O_2$ slope of 10 mL/min/W. In **panel 3**, carbon dioxide output ($\dot{V}CO_2$) (right y-axis) is plotted as a function of $\dot{V}O_2$ (x-axis) with identical scales so that the diagonal dashed line has a slope of 1 (45°). The $\dot{V}CO_2$ increasing more steeply than $\dot{V}O_2$ defines carbon dioxide (CO_2) derived from bicarbonate buffer, as long as ventilatory equivalent for CO_2 ($\dot{V}E/\dot{V}CO_2$) (**panel 4**) is not increasing and end-tidal PCO_2 ($PETCO_2$) (**panel 7**) is not decreasing, simultaneously. The black + symbol in **panel 3** indicates predicted values of heart rate (HR) (left y-axis) and $\dot{V}O_2$ for this individual. Abbreviations: IC, inspiratory capacity; MVV, maximum voluntary ventilation; $PETO_2$, end-tidal PO_2; R, respiratory exchange ratio; SBP, systolic blood pressure; VC, vital capacity; $\dot{V}E$, minute ventilation; $\dot{V}E/\dot{V}O_2$, ventilatory equivalent for oxygen; VT, tidal volume.

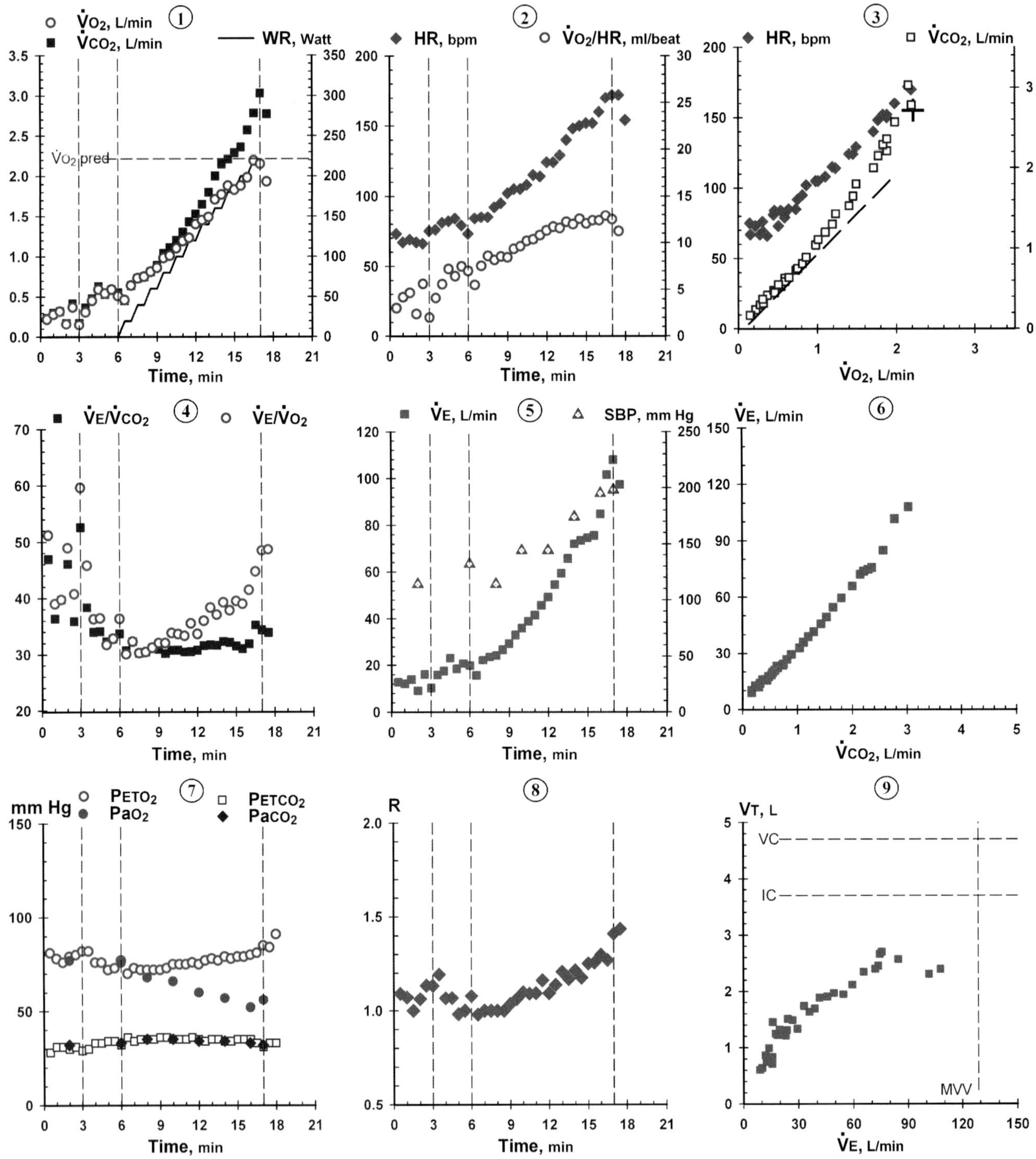

FIGURE 10.9.2. Fifteen percent oxygen breathing. Vertical dashed lines in the panels in the left and middle columns indicate, from left to right, the beginning of unloaded cycling, start of increasing work rate (WR) at 20 W/min, and start of recovery. In **panel 1**, the increase in WR (right y-axis) is plotted with a scale of 100 W to 1 L of oxygen uptake ($\dot{V}O_2$) (left y-axis) such that WR is plotted parallel to a $\dot{V}O_2$ slope of 10 mL/min/W. In **panel 3**, carbon dioxide output ($\dot{V}CO_2$) (right y-axis) is plotted as a function of $\dot{V}O_2$ (x-axis) with identical scales so that the diagonal dashed line has a slope of 1 (45°). The $\dot{V}CO_2$ increasing more steeply than $\dot{V}O_2$ defines carbon dioxide (CO_2) derived from bicarbonate buffer, as long as ventilatory equivalent for CO_2 ($\dot{V}E/\dot{V}CO_2$) (**panel 4**) is not increasing and end-tidal P_{CO_2} (P_{ETCO_2}) (**panel 7**) is not decreasing, simultaneously. The black + symbol in **panel 3** indicates predicted values of heart rate (HR) (left y-axis) and $\dot{V}O_2$ for this individual. Abbreviations: IC, inspiratory capacity; MVV, maximum voluntary ventilation; P_{ETO_2}, end-tidal P_{O_2}; R, respiratory exchange ratio; SBP, systolic blood pressure; VC, vital capacity; $\dot{V}E$, minute ventilation; $\dot{V}E/\dot{V}O_2$, ventilatory equivalent for oxygen; V_T, tidal volume.

CASE 10

Active Woman With Patent Foramen Ovale

CLINICAL FINDINGS

A 68-year-old woman was referred for exercise testing because she had been found to have a patent foramen ovale on an echocardiogram. The imaging had been performed following a peripheral retinal artery occlusion several months previously suspected to be of embolic origin. She described herself as nonathletic but had no exercise symptoms and regularly enjoyed activities such as biking, walking, and tap dancing. Her medical history was otherwise notable for systemic hypertension and migraine. Medications on the day of testing were aspirin and hydrochlorothiazide. Physical examination showed a healthy-appearing woman with normal findings on heart and lung examination. Resting electrocardiogram had findings of right atrial enlargement but was otherwise normal. Selected demographic and pulmonary function data are in **Table 10.10.1**.

EXERCISE FINDINGS

The patient exercised on a cycle ergometer beginning with 3 minutes of unloaded pedaling at 60 rpm followed by continuous increase in work rate by 10 W/min until the test ended with symptoms of leg fatigue. There were no arrhythmias or ST segment changes on exercise electrocardiogram. Key exercise findings are summarized in **Table 10.10.2**. Data are shown in **Table 10.10.3** and in **Figure 10.10.1**.

TABLE 10.10.1 Demographics and Selected Respiratory Function Data

Measurement	Predicted	Measured
Age (y)		68
Sex		Female
Height (cm)		157.5
Weight (kg)		53
VC (L)	3.0	2.79
IC (L)	2.05	1.66
ERV	0.74	1.35
FEV_1 (L)	2.11	2.47
FEV_1/VC (%)	76	82
MVV (L/min)	82	84

Abbreviations: ERV, expiratory reserve volume; FEV_1, forced expiratory volume in 1 second; IC, inspiratory capacity; MVV, maximum voluntary ventilation; VC, vital capacity.

TABLE 10.10.2 Selected Exercise Data

Measurement	Predicted	Measured
Peak $\dot{V}O_2$ (L/min)	1.11	1.30
Maximum heart rate (beats/min)	152	171
Maximum O_2 pulse (mL/beat)	7.3	8.0
$\Delta\dot{V}O_2/\Delta WR$ (mL/min/W)	10	10.3
AT (L/min)	>0.6	0.8
Blood pressure (mm Hg [rest, max ex])		100/70, 146/75
Maximum $\dot{V}E$ (L/min)		49
Breathing reserve (L/min)	>15	35
$\dot{V}E/\dot{V}CO_2$ @ *AT*	<34.4	27
SpO_2 (% [rest, max ex])		98, 98

Abbreviations: *AT*, anaerobic threshold; $\Delta\dot{V}O_2/\Delta WR$, change in $\dot{V}O_2$/change in work rate; ex, exercise; O_2, oxygen; SpO_2, oxygen saturation as measured by pulse oximetry; $\dot{V}E$, minute ventilation; $\dot{V}E/\dot{V}CO_2$, ventilatory equivalent for carbon dioxide; $\dot{V}O_2$, oxygen uptake.

INTERPRETATION

Comment

This test is presented as an example of normal exercise function in an older active woman.

Analysis

Cardiovascular and metabolic responses: $\dot{V}O_2$ increased appropriately relative to work rate and at peak exercise was above the average predicted value. Anaerobic threshold was also normal. The heart rate increased appropriately relative to $\dot{V}O_2$. Peak heart rate and peak O_2 pulse were also above average. Blood pressure (not graphed) was normal at rest and increased normally with exercise.

Ventilation: There was a normal breathing reserve. Of particular note in this patient was the absence of findings that are typical of exercise-induced right-to-left shunt in patients with pulmonary arterial hypertension who also have patent foramen ovale.

Gas exchange efficiency: Oxygenation appears normal and the relationship of $\dot{V}E$ to $\dot{V}CO_2$ was normal. This implies that $\dot{V}/\dot{Q}$ matching was within normal limits.

Conclusion

This was a normal exercise test demonstrating above-average exercise capacity for a woman of this age. Although it was still suspected that she had suffered paradoxical embolization to a retinal artery, there was no evidence to suggest exercise induced right-to-left shunting at the time of this exercise test.

TABLE 10.10.3 Air Breathing

Time (min)	Work rate (W)	BP (mm Hg)	HR (min^{-1})	f (min^{-1})	$\dot{V}E$ (L/min BTPS)	$\dot{V}CO_2$ (L/min STPD)	$\dot{V}O_2$ (L/min STPD)	$\frac{\dot{V}O_2}{HR}$ (mL/beat)	R	pH	HCO_3^- (mEq/L)	PO_2, mm Hg and SpO_2, % ET	SpO_2	(A − a)	PCO_2, mm Hg ET	a	(a − ET)	$\frac{\dot{V}E}{\dot{V}CO_2}$	$\frac{\dot{V}E}{\dot{V}O_2}$	$\frac{VD}{VT}$
0.5	Rest		64	17	6.7	0.15	0.15	2.3	0.98			109	98		37			46	45	
1.0	Rest		83	15	6.1	0.15	0.18	2.1	0.86			102	97		40			40	35	
1.5	Rest	100/70	86	17	7.8	0.19	0.22	2.5	0.87			103	96		40			41	36	
2.0	Rest		83	17	7.4	0.18	0.20	2.5	0.87			102	96		40			42	36	
2.5	Rest		87	16	8.1	0.20	0.21	2.4	0.94			107	96		38			40	38	
3.0	Rest		84	18	8.4	0.20	0.22	2.7	0.90			103	96		40			42	38	
3.5	Unloaded		91	21	11.4	0.32	0.38	4.2	0.85			99	97		42			36	30	
4.0	Unloaded		95	21	11.2	0.30	0.32	3.4	0.93			104	96		40			37	35	
4.5	Unloaded		94	19	10.4	0.30	0.35	3.7	0.86			98	97		44			35	30	
5.0	Unloaded		97	23	12.7	0.36	0.41	4.2	0.88			100	96		42			35	31	
5.5	Unloaded		98	20	12.2	0.36	0.41	4.2	0.88			99	97		44			34	30	
6.0	Unloaded		98	24	13.6	0.38	0.42	4.2	0.92			102	96		42			35	32	
6.5	3		99	24	13.5	0.38	0.42	4.3	0.90			100	97		43			35	32	
7.0	8		99	25	14.0	0.39	0.42	4.3	0.92			102	97		42			36	33	
7.5	13	112/72	99	26	13.3	0.37	0.39	3.9	0.95			102	97		43			36	35	
8.0	18		102	26	14.7	0.44	0.48	4.7	0.92			100	97		44			34	31	
8.5	23		108	20	16.1	0.53	0.55	5.1	0.96			101	97		44			31	29	
9.0	28		109	22	14.6	0.48	0.5	4.6	0.95			100	97		45			31	29	
9.5	33		113	25	17.2	0.58	0.62	5.4	0.93			99	97		46			30	28	
10.0	38		116	20	17.4	0.65	0.68	5.8	0.95			97	97		48			27	26	
10.5	43		123	25	20.4	0.73	0.72	5.9	1.00			101	97		46			28	28	
11.0	48		128	26	22.1	0.80	0.79	6.2	1.01			101	97		47			28	28	
11.5	53	122/80	132	26	23.1	0.87	0.83	6.3	1.04			101	97		47			27	28	
12.0	58		137	28	25.0	0.93	0.87	6.4	1.07			102	97		47			27	29	
12.5	63		136	29	28.3	1.06	0.97	7.2	1.09			103	97		47			27	29	
13.0	68		145	24	29.0	1.14	1.00	6.9	1.14			105	97		47			25	29	
13.5	73		148	30	32.8	1.23	1.07	7.2	1.15			106	97		46			27	31	
14.0	78		152	31	32.6	1.23	1.07	7.0	1.16			106	97		47			26	31	
14.5	83		156	29	36.6	1.39	1.16	7.5	1.20			107	97		46			26	31	
15.0	88		160	29	39.2	1.49	1.21	7.6	1.23			109	97		45			26	32	
15.5	93	146/75	163	33	41.5	1.51	1.24	7.6	1.22			109	97		45			27	34	
16.0	98		166	32	44.2	1.58	1.24	7.5	1.27			112	97		43			28	36	
16.5	103		168	33	49.0	1.74	1.35	8.1	1.29			113	97		42			28	36	
17.0	108		171	33	48.3	1.69	1.30	7.6	1.30			113	98		42			29	37	
17.5	Recovery		171	35	44.3	1.58	1.24	7.2	1.27			112	98		43			28	36	
18.0	Recovery		160	26	34.7	1.29	0.87	5.5	1.48			114	98		44			27	40	
18.5	Recovery		151	27	27.4	0.93	0.60	4.0	1.54			116	98		43			30	46	
19.0	Recovery		145	23	23.1	0.79	0.54	3.7	1.46			115	98		43			29	43	

Abbreviations: BP, blood pressure; BTPS, body temperature pressure saturated; f, frequency; HCO_3^-, bicarbonate; HR, heart rate; $P(A - a)O_2$, alveolar-arterial PO_2 difference; $P(a - ET)CO_2$, arterial-end-tidal PCO_2 difference; $PETCO_2$, end-tidal PCO_2; $PETO_2$, end-tidal PO_2; R, respiratory exchange ratio; SpO_2, oxygen saturation as measured by pulse oximetry; STPD, standard temperature pressure dry; $\dot{V}CO_2$, carbon dioxide output; VD/VT, physiological dead space-tidal volume ratio; $\dot{V}E$, minute ventilation; $\dot{V}E/\dot{V}CO_2$, ventilatory equivalent for carbon dioxide; $\dot{V}E/\dot{V}O_2$, ventilatory equivalent for oxygen; $\dot{V}O_2$, oxygen uptake.

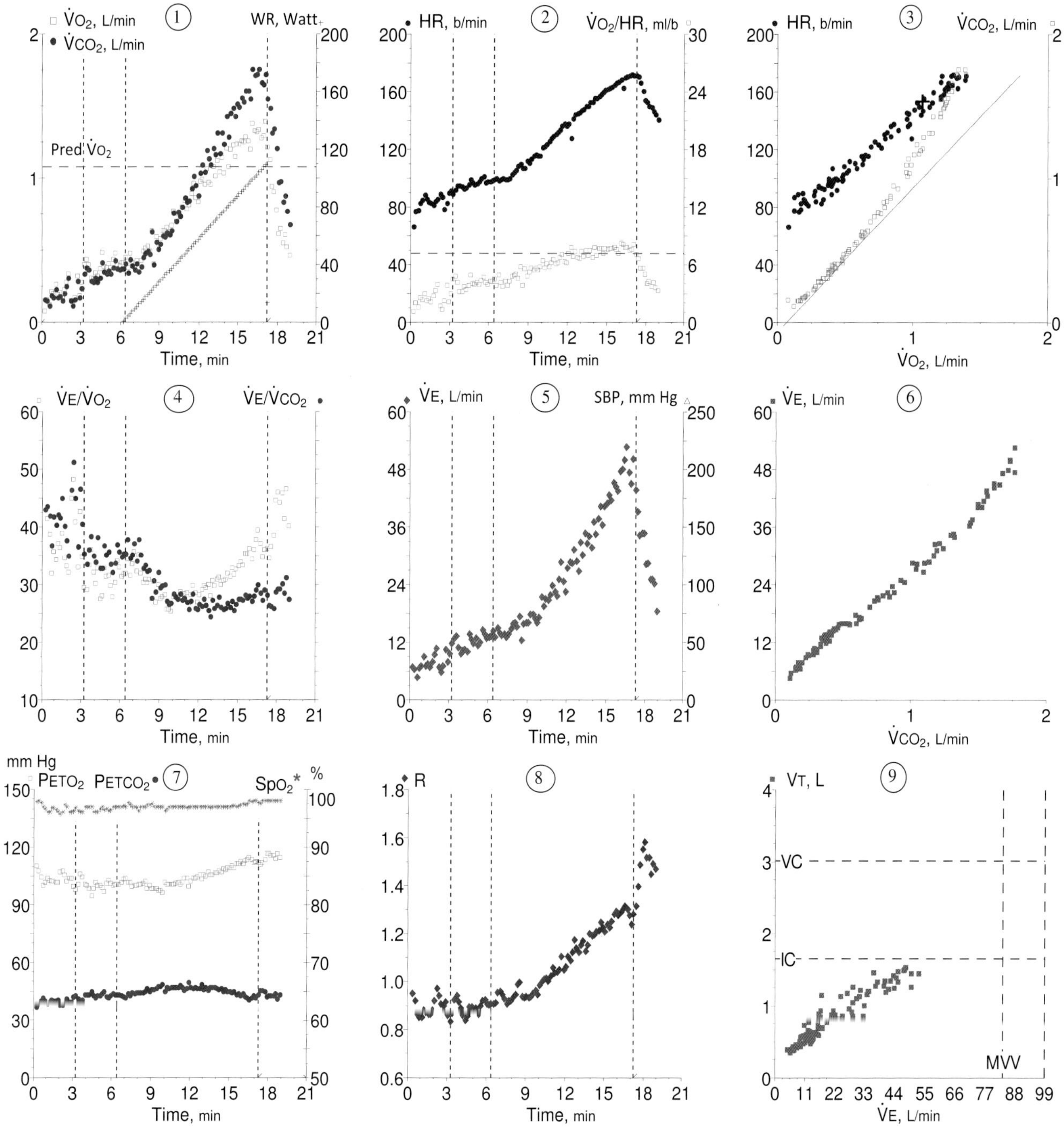

FIGURE 10.10.1. Vertical dashed lines in the panels in the left and middle columns indicate, from left to right, the beginning of unloaded cycling, start of increasing work rate (WR) at 10 W/min, and start of recovery. In **panel 1**, the increase in WR (right y-axis) is plotted with a scale of 100 W to 1 L of oxygen uptake ($\dot{V}O_2$) (left y-axis) such that WR is plotted parallel to a $\dot{V}O_2$ slope of 10 mL/min/W. Predicted peak $\dot{V}O_2$ is shown as a dashed horizontal line. In **panel 3**, carbon dioxide output ($\dot{V}CO_2$) (right y-axis) is plotted as a function of $\dot{V}O_2$ (x-axis) with identical scales so that the diagonal blue line has a slope of 1 (45°). The $\dot{V}CO_2$ increasing more steeply than $\dot{V}O_2$ defines carbon dioxide (CO_2) derived from bicarbonate buffer, as long as ventilatory equivalent for CO_2 ($\dot{V}E/\dot{V}CO_2$) (**panel 4**) is not increasing and end-tidal PCO_2 ($PETCO_2$) (**panel 7**) is not decreasing, simultaneously. The black + symbol in **panel 3** indicates predicted values of heart rate (HR) (left y-axis) and $\dot{V}O_2$ for this individual. Abbreviations: IC, inspiratory capacity; MVV, maximum voluntary ventilation; $PETO_2$, end-tidal PO_2; R, respiratory exchange ratio; SBP, systolic blood pressure; SpO_2, oxygen saturation as measured by pulse oximetry; VC, vital capacity; $\dot{V}E$, minute ventilation; $\dot{V}E/\dot{V}O_2$, ventilatory equivalent for oxygen; V_T, tidal volume.

CASE 11

Normal Aging Athletic Man: Serial Tests Between Age 66 and 76

To view this case please access the eBook bundled with this text. Instructions are located on the inside front cover.

CASE 12

Mild Airflow Obstruction and Hyperventilation

CLINICAL FINDINGS

A 47-year-old woman was referred for exercise testing to evaluate the cause of persistent dyspnea. She had a history of intermittent asthma as a child, which had resolved as a young adult. In recent years, she experienced dyspnea, which had progressed to being present almost constantly, along with an intermittent nonproductive cough. Pulmonary function tests had shown mild reversible airflow obstruction. Allergy testing had confirmed allergy to common pollens, dusts, and molds. She had taken extensive measures to remove potential allergens from her home and diet but had not been using prescribed asthma medications because she felt that they were ineffective and made her jittery. She had undergone computed tomography angiogram of the chest, nuclear stress test, upper endoscopy, and direct laryngoscopy, which were all reported as normal. She denied wheezing, stridor, hoarseness, or nighttime awakening. She also denied history of panic attacks or anxiety.

TABLE 10.12.1 Selected Respiratory Function Data

Measurement	Predicted	Measured
Age (y)		47
Sex		Female
Height (cm)		170
Weight (kg)		61.4
VC (L)	3.97	4.56
IC (L)	3.11	2.41
ERV (L)	1.48	1.56
FEV_1 (L)	3.10	3.16
FEV_1/VC (%)	81	68
MVV (L/min)	107	105

Abbreviations: ERV, expiratory reserve volume; FEV_1, forced expiratory volume in 1 second; IC, inspiratory capacity; MVV, maximum voluntary ventilation; VC, vital capacity.

On the day of testing, she was taking no medications and had not used any asthma medications for over 4 weeks. Examination revealed normal breath sounds and heart tones. Resting electrocardiogram was normal, and spirometry showed mild expiratory airflow obstruction (**Table 10.12.1**).

EXERCISE FINDINGS

The patient exercised on a cycle ergometer beginning with 2 minutes of rest and 3 minutes of unloaded pedaling at 60 rpm followed by continuous increase in work rate by 15 W/min until she ended exercise with symptoms of both leg fatigue and shortness of breath. There were no arrhythmias or ischemic changes on electrocardiogram. There was no wheezing or stridor on exam and postexercise spirometry showed a 10% increase in forced expiratory volume in 1 second compared to preexercise. The most notable findings on the test were evidence of pretest hyperventilation, which resolved over the course of the test. Data are shown in **Tables 10.12.2** and **10.12.3** and **Figure 10.12.1**.

INTERPRETATION

Comment

This test is presented to illustrate how hyperventilation can affect subsequent patterns of pulmonary gas exchange. The pattern of change of carbon dioxide output ($\dot{V}CO_2$) during reestablishment of the body's carbon dioxide (CO_2) stores after a period of hyperventilation may mimic occurrence of the anaerobic threshold (*AT*). This phenomenon has thus been termed a "pseudothreshold" pattern.[1]

Analysis

Cardiovascular and metabolic responses: Peak oxygen uptake ($\dot{V}O_2$) was normal, and the rate of increase of $\dot{V}O_2$ was appropriate for the increase in work rate (panel 1). Heart

TABLE 10.12.2 Selected Exercise Data

Measurement	Predicted	Measured
Peak $\dot{V}O_2$ (L/min)	1.59	1.76
Maximum heart rate (beats/min)	173	160
Maximum O_2 pulse (mL/beat)	9.2	11.0
$\Delta\dot{V}O_2/\Delta WR$ (mL/min/W)	10	10.9
AT (L/min)	>0.77	1.1
Blood pressure (mm Hg [rest, max])		114/79, 146/79
Maximum $\dot{V}E$ (L/min)		57
Breathing reserve (L/min)	>31.8	48
$\dot{V}E/\dot{V}CO_2$ @ *AT*	<31	25
SpO_2 (% [rest, max ex])		98, 98
$PtcCO_2$ (mm Hg [rest, *AT*, max ex])		26, 40, 34
V_D/V_T (rest, max ex)		0.25, 0.21

Abbreviations: *AT*, anaerobic threshold; $\Delta\dot{V}O_2/\Delta WR$, change in $\dot{V}O_2$/change in work rate; ex, exercise; O_2, oxygen; $PtcCO_2$, PCO_2 measured by transcutaneous electrode; SpO_2, oxygen saturation as measured by pulse oximetry; V_D/V_T, physiological dead space–tidal volume ratio; $\dot{V}E$, minute ventilation; $\dot{V}E/\dot{V}CO_2$, ventilatory equivalent for carbon dioxide; $\dot{V}O_2$, oxygen uptake.

rate similarly increased normally and with a normal relationship to $\dot{V}O_2$ (panel 3). The end-exercise oxygen (O_2) pulse was normal (panel 2). Blood pressure also increased appropriately with exercise. The *AT* also appears normal, although its identification is complicated by the changes associated with recovery from acute hyperventilation prior to the onset of lactic acidosis. In panel 3, the slope of $\dot{V}CO_2$ relative to $\dot{V}O_2$ early in the test is considerably less than the expected value of approximately 1.0. Although CO_2 production rate was increasing during this time, some of the CO_2 produced was retained to reestablish stores that had been washed out during a preceding period of hyperventilation so that the measured $\dot{V}CO_2$ was an underestimate of the rate of change of production. This was evidenced by the transcutaneous PCO_2 values monitored throughout the test, which were initially around 26 mm Hg at rest and rose progressively to 40 by the middle of the test. Once CO_2 stores were repleted, the slope of $\dot{V}CO_2$ relative to $\dot{V}O_2$ (panel 3) increased to approximately 1.0. The resulting upward inflection of $\dot{V}CO_2$, at a $\dot{V}O_2$ of about 750 mL/min, could be mistaken for the *AT*. However, in this case, there is a brief period of around 1 minute following that point during which $\dot{V}CO_2$ and $\dot{V}O_2$ both increase with the expected slope of about 1.0 and then another inflection point in $\dot{V}CO_2$ consistent with the actual onset of lactate accumulation at a $\dot{V}O_2$ of slightly more than 1.0 L/min.

Ventilatory responses: The breathing reserve was normal. However, as identified earlier, evidence of hypocapnia was present at rest prior to starting exercise with both end-tidal PCO_2 (P_{ETCO_2}) and transcutaneous PCO_2 values of 26 mm Hg. The R values (panel 8) were not abnormally elevated at rest, indicating that hyperventilation had been present for long enough for stabilization of CO_2 balance. Once the test began, transcutaneous PCO_2 and P_{ETCO_2} values progressively rose to around 40 mm Hg as CO_2 stores in tissue and blood reaccumulated. The relative hypoventilation was reflected in the unusually low R, which dipped to as low as 0.6 in early exercise, and in the shallow initial slope of $\dot{V}CO_2$ versus $\dot{V}O_2$ (panel 3) as described earlier. Once PCO_2 values returned to the normal range, $\dot{V}O_2$ and $\dot{V}CO_2$ resumed a more normal relationship. Inspiratory capacity was measured repeatedly throughout exercise and increased modestly from resting levels, excluding dynamic hyperinflation. Postexercise spirometry showed a 10% increase in forced expiratory volume in 1 second compared to preexercise (data not shown), consistent with exercise-induced bronchodilation. Thus, the only ventilatory abnormality demonstrated was hyperventilation.

Efficiency of pulmonary gas exchange: Although the ventilatory equivalents were high at the beginning of data collection, the values decreased to the normal range as hyperventilation fully resolved. There was no desaturation by pulse oximetry. Gas exchange efficiency therefore appears normal.

Conclusion

This patient may be particularly sensitive to symptoms of dyspnea related to untreated asthma. There is no finding on the exercise test to suggest a more serious underlying cardiorespiratory disorder. The possibility of idiopathic hyperventilation as a cause of her symptoms was suggested by the finding of hyperventilation prior to exercise, although her history lacked other typical characteristics of this, so it is difficult to be certain of the causation.

Hyperventilation in the early part of an exercise test is not uncommon and is usually transient. It is important to recognize that hyperventilation, and also recovery from hyperventilation, can affect the pattern of the gas exchange data. A "pseudothreshold" can result when relative hypoventilation results in pulmonary $\dot{V}CO_2$ lagging the rate of metabolic CO_2 production. The acceleration of $\dot{V}CO_2$ once CO_2 stores have been restored can be mistaken for the *AT*. This may be suspected when there is a very shallow slope of $\dot{V}CO_2$ versus $\dot{V}O_2$ in early exercise. In the case presented here, this was distinct from the later inflection in $\dot{V}CO_2$, which represented the *AT*. Transcutaneous measures of PCO_2 were particularly useful in this case in confirming the presence and extent of the initial hypocapnia. Although P_{ETCO_2} values were also consistent with this, the P_{ETCO_2} often differs from arterial and needs to be interpreted with caution.

REFERENCE

1. Ozcelik O, Ward SA, Whipp BJ. Effect of altered body CO_2 stores on pulmonary gas exchange dynamics during incremental exercise in humans. *Exp Physiol*. 1999;84(5):999-1011.

TABLE 10.12.3 Air Breathing

Time (min)	Work rate (W)	BP (mm Hg)	HR (min^{-1})	f (min^{-1})	$\dot{V}E$ (L/min BTPS)	$\dot{V}CO_2$ (L/min STPD)	$\dot{V}O_2$ (L/min STPD)	$\dot{V}O_2$/HR (mL/beat)	R	pH	HCO_3^- (mEq/L)	PO_2, mm Hg and SpO_2, % ET	SpO_2	(A − a)	PCO_2, mm Hg ET	tc	(a − ET)	$\dot{V}E/\dot{V}CO_2$	$\dot{V}E/\dot{V}O_2$	VD/VT
0.5	Rest		48	10	10.5	0.25	0.30	6.4	0.83			120	98		26	26.3		42	35	0.25
1.0	Rest	114/79	66	13	9.6	0.22	0.27	4.1	0.80			120	99		25	26.3		45	36	0.27
1.5	Rest		67	10	9.6	0.23	0.29	4.3	0.81			120	99		26	26.6		41	33	0.25
2.0	Rest		66	5	4.4	0.11	0.15	2.3	0.73			113	99		29	27.2		40	29	0.23
2.5	Unloaded		67	12	11.8	0.25	0.33	4.9	0.76			119	99		25	27.8		47	36	0.37
3.0	Unloaded		70	14	10.7	0.25	0.34	4.8	0.75			115	98		28	28.4		42	32	0.32
3.5	Unloaded		73	12	9.2	0.26	0.42	5.8	0.62			106	99		31	28.7		35	22	0.18
4.0	Unloaded		73	11	7.8	0.22	0.35	4.8	0.62			104	99		31	29.6		35	22	0.21
4.5	Unloaded		72	10	9.1	0.26	0.42	5.8	0.61			102	99		32	30.4		35	22	0.22
5.0	Unloaded	132/75	71	12	8.2	0.22	0.36	5.2	0.62			102	99		33	31.4		36	22	0.29
5.5	Unloaded		73	12	11.5	0.33	0.49	6.7	0.68			107	98		32	32.3		35	23	0.26
6.0	8		71	11	7.8	0.24	0.34	4.7	0.70			106	97		33	32.6		33	23	0.21
6.5	15		71	12	11.2	0.34	0.49	7.0	0.69			106	98		33	32.8		33	23	0.23
7.0	23		72	11	8.1	0.23	0.33	4.5	0.69			105	98		33	33.1		36	25	0.29
7.5	30		76	15	8.9	0.28	0.49	6.5	0.56			91	98		37	33.2		32	18	0.21
8.0	38		82	9	12.4	0.41	0.68	8.3	0.60			91	98		38	34.3		30	18	0.20
8.5	44		85	15	15.5	0.49	0.81	9.6	0.61			94	98		36	35		31	19	0.25
9.0	53		88	12	10.9	0.41	0.68	7.7	0.60			88	98		41	36.1		27	16	0.13
9.5	59	125/68	94	13	17.2	0.63	0.92	9.8	0.68			99	98		38	36.9		27	19	0.18
10.0	68		97	12	18.3	0.70	0.94	9.7	0.75			97	97		42	37.8		26	19	0.16
10.5	75		102	13	18.3	0.75	0.94	9.2	0.80			98	97		44	38.5		25	20	0.12
11.0	82		105	17	23.8	0.93	1.09	10.4	0.85			102	98		42	39		26	22	0.17
11.5	90		111	15	25.3	0.98	1.06	9.6	0.92			106	98		42	39.5		26	24	0.19
12.0	98	138/79	113	18	29.7	1.19	1.28	11.3	0.93			105	98		42	39.6		25	23	0.16
12.5	105		119	20	32.2	1.30	1.33	11.2	0.98			107	98		43	39.9		25	24	0.16
13.0	113		127	22	40.4	1.54	1.43	11.3	1.07			113	98		40	40		26	28	0.21
13.5	120	146/79	135	21	43.7	1.61	1.46	10.9	1.10			114	98		40	39.5		27	30	0.23
14.0	128		140	24	45.5	1.69	1.53	10.9	1.10			114	98		39	38.6		27	30	0.20
14.5	135		148	30	57.9	1.95	1.70	11.5	1.15			119	98		36	37.6		30	34	0.26
15.0	143		155	26	56.9	1.98	1.69	10.9	1.17			118	98		37	36.5		29	34	0.21
15.5	Recovery		160	32	62.9	2.07	1.76	11.0	1.18			120	99		35	35.1		30	36	0.22
16.0	Recovery		151	26	48.1	1.73	1.41	9.3	1.23			119	98		38	34.3		28	34	0.13
16.5	Recovery	152/74	136	25	43.0	1.39	0.90	6.6	1.54			126	98		35	34.1		31	48	0.21

Abbreviations: BP, blood pressure; BTPS, body temperature pressure saturated; f, frequency; HCO_3^-, bicarbonate; HR, heart rate; $P(A-a)O_2$, alveolar-arterial PO_2 difference; $P(a-ET)CO_2$, arterial-end-tidal PCO_2 difference; $PETCO_2$, end-tidal PCO_2; $PETO_2$, end-tidal PO_2; R, respiratory exchange ratio; SpO_2, oxygen saturation as measured by pulse oximetry; STPD, standard temperature pressure dry; tc, transcutaneous; $\dot{V}CO_2$, carbon dioxide output; VD/VT, physiological dead space-tidal volume ratio; $\dot{V}E$, minute ventilation; $\dot{V}E/\dot{V}CO_2$, ventilatory equivalent for carbon dioxide; $\dot{V}E/\dot{V}O_2$, ventilatory equivalent for oxygen; $\dot{V}O_2$, oxygen uptake.

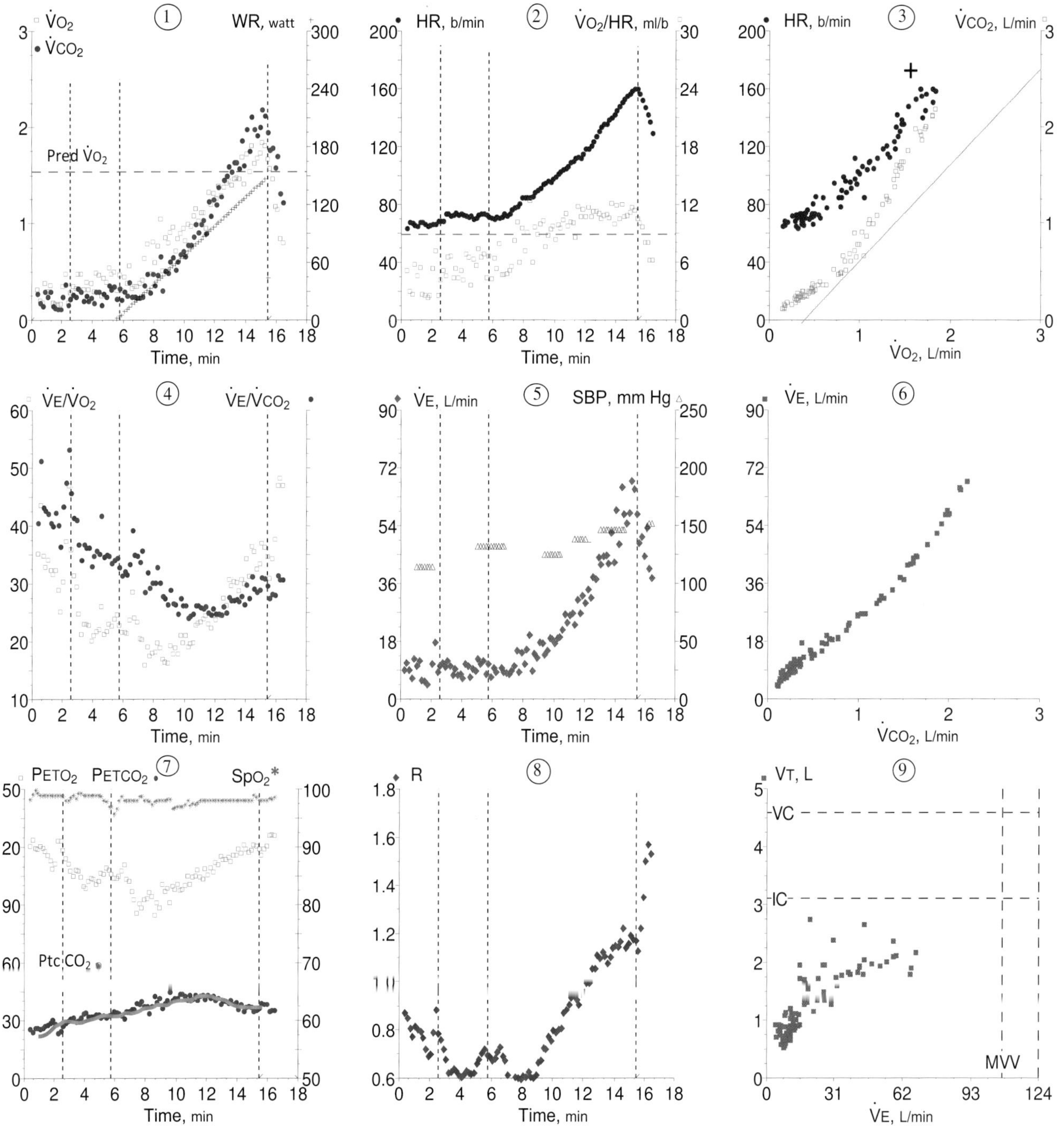

FIGURE 10.12.1. Vertical dashed lines in the panels in the left and middle columns indicate, from left to right, the beginning of unloaded cycling, start of increasing work rate (WR) at 10 W/min, and start of recovery. In **panel 1**, the increase in WR (right y-axis) is plotted with a scale of 100 W to 1 L of oxygen uptake ($\dot{V}O_2$) (left y-axis) such that WR is plotted parallel to a $\dot{V}O_2$ slope of 15 mL/min/W. Predicted peak $\dot{V}O_2$ is shown as a dashed horizontal line. In **panel 3**, carbon dioxide output ($\dot{V}CO_2$) (right y-axis) is plotted as a function of $\dot{V}O_2$ (x-axis) with identical scales so that the diagonal blue line has a slope of 1 (45°). The $\dot{V}CO_2$ increasing more steeply than $\dot{V}O_2$ defines carbon dioxide (CO_2) derived from bicarbonate buffer, as long as ventilatory equivalent for CO_2 ($\dot{V}E/\dot{V}CO_2$) (**panel 4**) is not increasing and end-tidal PCO_2 (P_{ETCO_2}) (**panel 7**) is not decreasing, simultaneously. The black + symbol in **panel 3** indicates predicted values of heart rate (HR) (left y-axis) and $\dot{V}O_2$ for this individual. Abbreviations: IC, inspiratory capacity; MVV, maximum voluntary ventilation; P_{ETO_2}, end-tidal PO_2; $PtcCO_2$, transcutaneous PCO_2; R, respiratory exchange ratio; SBP, systolic blood pressure; SpO_2, oxygen saturation as measured by pulse oximetry; $\dot{V}E$, minute ventilation; $\dot{V}E/\dot{V}O_2$, ventilatory equivalent for oxygen; V_T, tidal volume.

CASE 13

A Submaximal Test

CLINICAL FINDINGS

A 51-year-old man was referred for exercise testing to evaluate episodic shortness of breath. His symptoms could occur at rest and did not consistently occur with exercise. He had a history of polycythemia vera, which was evolving to myelofibrosis. This had previously been treated with phlebotomy, but recent hemoglobin values were stable at 12 g/dL without treatment. He had episodic pain in long bones attributed to his hematologic condition. There was a history of myocardial infarction several years previously but no recent chest pain and no orthopnea or heart failure. He worked as a truck driver and for exercise walked on a treadmill at a rate of 2.9 mph for 40 minutes without difficulty. At the time of testing, his medications include metoprolol, aspirin, and a statin. Physical examination was unremarkable. Resting electrocardiogram (ECG) showed Q waves in leads III and aVF. Demographic data are shown in **Table 10.13.1**.

EXERCISE FINDINGS

The patient exercised on a cycle ergometer beginning with 3 minutes of unloaded pedaling at 60 rpm followed by continuous increase in work rate by 10 W/min until the test ended due to symptoms of leg pain, which he described as bony and not muscular. The pain persisted into the recovery period and was consistent with his chronic bone pain. The exercise ECG showed occasional premature beats that resolved with exercise but no ischemic changes. Exercise data are shown in **Tables 10.13.2** and **10.13.3** and in **Figure 10.13.1**.

TABLE 10.13.1 Demographic Data

Measurement	Predicted	Measured
Age (y)		51
Sex		Male
Height (cm)		178
Weight (kg)		116
MVV (L/min)	165	NA
Hb (g/dL)		12

Abbreviations: Hb, hemoglobin; MVV, maximum voluntary ventilation; NA, not applicable.

INTERPRETATION

Comment

This case is presented as an example of a submaximal test in which cardiorespiratory findings were normal for the range of work performed and exercise was limited by symptoms attributable to other factors. Pulmonary function was not measured at the time of the test but was believed to be normal.

Analysis

Exercise performance was reduced relative to reference values but likely underestimates the patient's maximum cardiorespiratory capacity given that none of the measured variables were clearly maximal and the test ended with noncardiorespiratory symptoms.

Cardiovascular and metabolic responses: Peak oxygen uptake ($\dot{V}O_2$) was reduced compared to predicted, but this is likely due to exercise being ended due to leg pain prior to achieving cardiovascular or respiratory limits. The leg pain was not characteristic of claudication. The $\dot{V}O_2$ responses in the range of exercise that was accomplished were essentially normal, with normal $\Delta\dot{V}O_2/\Delta WR$ and a normal anaerobic threshold (*AT*). Exercise ended not long after attainment

TABLE 10.13.2 Selected Exercise Test Data

Measurement	Predicted	Measured
Peak $\dot{V}O_2$ (L/min)	2.86	1.71
Maximum heart rate (beats/min)	169	120
Heart rate reserve (beats/min)		49
Maximum O_2 pulse (mL/beat)	16.9	14.2
$\Delta\dot{V}O_2/\Delta WR$ (mL/min/W)	10	10
AT (L/min)	>1.29	1.45
Blood pressure (mm Hg [rest, max])		126/79, 171/92
Maximum $\dot{V}E$ (L/min)		40
Breathing reserve (L/min)		125 (estimated)
$\dot{V}E/\dot{V}CO_2$ @ *AT* (L/min)	<30.7	24
SpO_2 (% [rest, max ex])		100, 97

Abbreviations: *AT*, anaerobic threshold; $\Delta\dot{V}O_2/\Delta WR$, change in $\dot{V}O_2$/change in work rate; ex, exercise; O_2, oxygen; SpO_2, oxygen saturation as measured by pulse oximetry; $\dot{V}CO_2$, carbon dioxide output; $\dot{V}E$, minute ventilation; $\dot{V}O_2$, oxygen uptake.

TABLE 10.13.3 Air Breathing

Time (min)	Work rate (W)	BP (mm Hg)	HR (min^{-1})	f (min^{-1})	$\dot{V}E$ (L/min BTPS)	$\dot{V}CO_2$ (L/min STPD)	$\dot{V}O_2$ (L/min STPD)	$\frac{\dot{V}O_2}{HR}$ (mL/beat)	R	pH	HCO_3^- (mEq/L)	PO_2, mm Hg and SpO_2, % ET	a	(A − a)	PCO_2, mm Hg ET	a	(a − ET)	$\frac{\dot{V}E}{\dot{V}CO_2}$	$\frac{\dot{V}E}{\dot{V}O_2}$	$\frac{VD}{VT}$
0.5	Rest		92	11	14.1	0.49	0.51	5.5	0.96			107			40			29	28	
1.0	Rest	126/79	95	10	13.2	0.45	0.46	4.9	0.97			108	100		39			30	29	
1.5	Rest		97	10	14.6	0.45	0.44	4.6	1.02			111	100		38			32	33	
2.0	Rest		97	9	13.6	0.44	0.43	4.4	1.02			111	100		38			31	32	
2.5	Rest		97	9	10.6	0.37	0.42	4.3	0.88			105	100		40			29	25	
3.0	Unloaded		97	10	10.9	0.36	0.44	4.5	0.82			103	99		39			30	25	
3.5	Unloaded		104	9	17.4	0.67	0.75	7.2	0.89			101	98		42			26	23	
4.0	Unloaded		104	13	19.8	0.73	0.82	7.9	0.90			103	96		41			27	24	
4.5	Unloaded	130/76	102	12	19.1	0.73	0.82	8.0	0.89			101	96		42			26	23	
5.0	Unloaded		103	13	20.8	0.80	0.92	9.0	0.86			99	97		43			26	22	
5.5	Unloaded		102	13	19.2	0.75	0.88	8.7	0.85			98	97		44			26	22	
6.0	Unloaded		100	14	19.4	0.75	0.92	9.2	0.81			95	96		44			26	21	
6.5	8		100	14	20.6	0.80	0.98	9.8	0.82			96	97		44			26	21	
7.0	18		101	12	20.9	0.80	0.90	8.9	0.89			98	97		44			26	23	
7.5	24		100	13	18.6	0.74	0.91	9.1	0.81			93	98		46			25	20	
8.0	38		101	13	19.7	0.80	0.98	9.7	0.82			92	99		47			25	20	
8.5	44	154/80	103	14	20.7	0.84	1.02	9.9	0.83			93	98		46			25	20	
9.0	58		105	14	22.9	0.93	1.09	10.4	0.86			95	97		46			25	21	
9.5	68		105	15	23.9	0.99	1.18	11.2	0.84			92	96		47			24	20	
10.0	78		106	15	25.2	1.07	1.24	11.6	0.86			92	97		48			24	20	
10.5	88		107	17	27.4	1.14	1.30	12.1	0.88			94	97		48			24	21	
11.0	98		111	17	32.5	1.38	1.50	13.5	0.92			96	97		48			24	22	
11.5	108		115	18	37.9	1.58	1.60	13.9	0.99			99	97		47			24	24	
12.0	114	171/92	117	18	35.2	1.51	1.60	13.6	0.94			96	98		49			23	22	
12.5	128		120	18	39.5	1.71	1.71	14.2	1.00			99	97		48			23	23	
13.0	Recovery		117	19	38.6	1.60	1.53	13.1	1.05			102	98		47			24	25	
13.5	Recovery	152/75	109	16	31.8	1.31	1.20	11.0	1.09			104	98		47			24	27	
14.0	Recovery		106	16	26.5	1.05	0.95	9.0	1.10			105	98		45			25	28	
14.5	Recovery		104	14	19.8	0.78	0.74	7.2	1.04			105	98		45			26	27	

Abbreviations: BP, blood pressure; BTPS, body temperature pressure saturated; f, frequency; HCO_3^-, bicarbonate; HR, heart rate; $P(A - a)O_2$, alveolar-arterial PO_2 difference; $P(a - ET)CO_2$, arterial-end-tidal PCO_2 difference; $PETCO_2$, end-tidal PCO_2; $PETO_2$, end-tidal PO_2; R, respiratory exchange ratio; SpO_2, oxygen saturation as measured by pulse oximetry; STPD, standard temperature pressure dry; $\dot{V}CO_2$, carbon dioxide output; VD/VT, physiological dead space-tidal volume ratio; $\dot{V}E$, minute ventilation; $\dot{V}E/\dot{V}CO_2$, ventilatory equivalent for carbon dioxide; $\dot{V}E/\dot{V}O_2$, ventilatory equivalent for oxygen; $\dot{V}O_2$, oxygen uptake.

of the *AT*, so the *AT* was a relatively large percentage of the measured peak $\dot{V}O_2$, but when expressed as a percentage of the predicted maximal $\dot{V}O_2$ was near the lower limit of normal. The peak heart rate was low. Although this finding is sometimes attributable to β-blocker medication, the rate of increase in heart rate relative to $\dot{V}O_2$ toward their respective predicted maximal values (shown in panel 3 of **Fig. 10.13.1**) was not significantly shallower than average. The peak heart rate in this test thus seems to be due primarily to early termination of the test. Although the oxygen pulse at end exercise was also less than the predicted maximal value, it had not reached a clear asymptotic value, so was probably not a maximal measure. Peak oxygen pulse would also be expected to be below average due to the patient's anemia. As noted earlier, there was no evidence of ischemia on ECG up to a rate pressure product (heart rate times × blood pressure) of 20 570.

Ventilation and gas exchange efficiency: There was a large breathing reserve, so no indication that ventilation was limiting to exercise. Pulmonary gas exchange efficiency also appeared normal up to the level of exercise accomplished with normal $\dot{V}E/\dot{V}CO_2$ at the *AT* and normal pulse oximetry values.

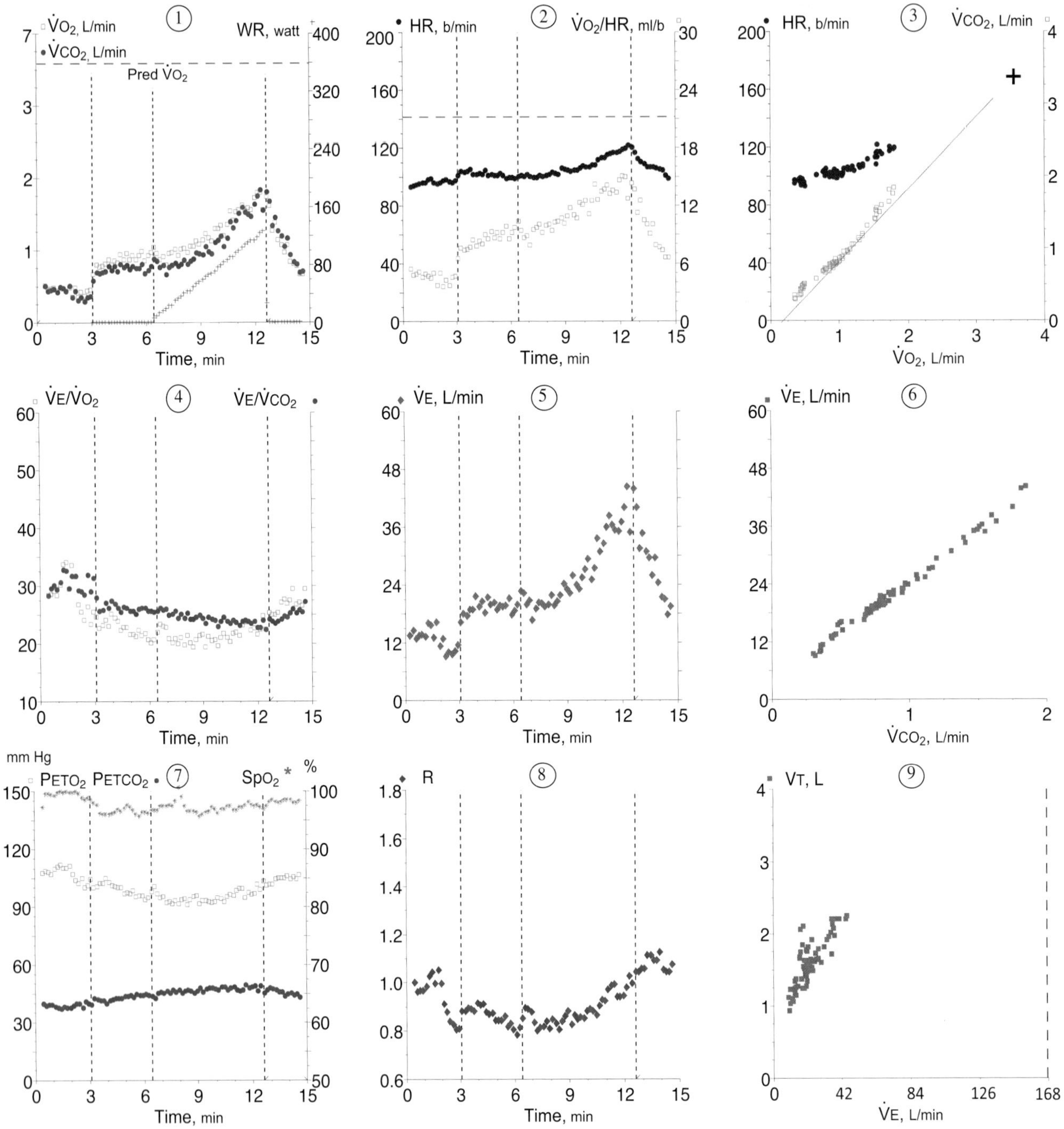

FIGURE 10.13.1. Vertical dashed lines in the panels in the left and middle columns indicate, from left to right, the beginning of unloaded cycling, start of increasing work rate (WR) at 10 W/min, and start of recovery. In **panel 1**, the increase in WR (right y-axis) is plotted with a scale of 100 W to 1 L of oxygen uptake ($\dot{V}O_2$) (left y-axis) such that WR is plotted parallel to a $\dot{V}O_2$ slope of 10 mL/min/W. Predicted peak $\dot{V}O_2$ is shown as a dashed horizontal line. In **panel 3**, carbon dioxide ($\dot{V}CO_2$) (right y-axis) is plotted as a function of $\dot{V}O_2$ (x-axis) with identical scales so that the diagonal blue line has a slope of 1 (45°). The $\dot{V}CO_2$ increasing more steeply than $\dot{V}O_2$ defines carbon dioxide (CO_2) derived from bicarbonate buffer, as long as ventilatory equivalent for CO_2 ($\dot{V}E/\dot{V}CO_2$) (**panel 4**) is not increasing and end-tidal P_{CO_2} (P_{ETCO_2}) (**panel 7**) is not decreasing, simultaneously. The black + symbol in **panel 3** indicates predicted values of heart rate (HR) (left y-axis) and $\dot{V}O_2$ for this individual. Abbreviations: IC, inspiratory capacity; MVV, maximum voluntary ventilation; P_{ETO_2}, end-tidal P_{O_2}; R, respiratory exchange ratio; SBP, systolic blood pressure; Sp_{O_2}, oxygen saturation as measured by pulse oximetry; VC, vital capacity; $\dot{V}E$, minute ventilation; $\dot{V}E/\dot{V}O_2$, ventilatory equivalent for oxygen; V_T, tidal volume.

Conclusion

Because the test ended with noncardiorespiratory symptoms prior to reaching objective cardiorespiratory limits, it was interpreted as a submaximal test. Submaximal tests can occur as a result of poor patient effort, although in this case, the patient exercised to the level of tolerable symptoms. The test could therefore represent a measure of his effective *functional* capacity, if these symptoms limit his usual activities, but should not be assumed to be a measure of his cardiorespiratory capacity. Significant limitation due to cardiovascular factors at higher levels of work could not be excluded.

CASE 14

A Long Test

CLINICAL FINDINGS

A 66-year-old woman was referred for testing because of exertional shortness of breath. She dates her symptoms back approximately 1 year, after an episode of influenza followed by bacterial pneumonia leading to a 9-day hospitalization. She had subsequently returned to work on a reduced schedule and was still short of breath with sustained activities that she had previously tolerated, such as walking at a fast pace. Ascending a flight of stairs caused shortness of breath, although she could do so without stopping. She did not do any recreational exercise. She was receiving physical therapy, but this constituted only stretching and mobility exercises. Her history was notable for chronic back pain related to disc disease, which limited her activities and for which she used a transcutaneous electrical nerve stimulation device. Medications were omeprazole, vitamins, and supplements. Physical examination was remarkable only for obesity. The electrocardiogram (ECG) showed a sinus rhythm with minor nonspecific ST segment changes. Demographic and respiratory function data are shown in **Table 10.14.1**.

EXERCISE FINDINGS

The patient exercised on a cycle ergometer beginning with 3 minutes of unloaded pedaling at 60 rpm followed by continuous increase in work rate by 5 W/min until the test ended with symptoms of shortness of breath. There were no significant ischemic changes or arrhythmia on exercise ECG.

TABLE 10.14.1 Selected Respiratory Function Data

Measurement	Predicted	Measured
Age (y)		66
Sex		Female
Height (cm)		161
Weight (kg)		91.1
VC (L)	3.06	2.70
IC (L)	2.15	2.61
ERV (L)	0.91	0.10
FEV_1 (L)	2.33	2.12
FEV_1/VC (%)	77	78
MVV (L/min)	87	94

Abbreviations: ERV, expiratory reserve volume; FEV_1, forced expiratory volume in 1 second; IC, inspiratory capacity; MVV, maximum voluntary ventilation; VC, vital capacity.

TABLE 10.14.2 Selected Exercise Data

Measurement	Predicted	Measured
Peak $\dot{V}O_2$ (L/min)	1.38	1.26
Maximum heart rate (beats/min)	154	153
Maximum O_2 pulse (mL/beat)	9.0	8.2
$\Delta\dot{V}O_2/\Delta WR$ (mL/min/W)	10	10
AT (L/min)	>0.74	0.65
Blood pressure (mm Hg [rest, max])		134/88, 180/100
Maximum $\dot{V}E$ (L/min)		48
Breathing reserve (L/min)		46
$\dot{V}E/\dot{V}CO_2$ @ *AT* (L/min)	<34	30
SpO_2 (% [rest, max ex])		95, 93

Abbreviations: *AT*, anaerobic threshold; $\Delta\dot{V}O_2/\Delta WR$, change in $\dot{V}O_2$/change in work rate; ex, exercise; O_2, oxygen; SpO_2, oxygen saturation as measured by pulse oximetry; $\dot{V}CO_2$, carbon dioxide output; $\dot{V}E$, minute ventilation; $\dot{V}O_2$, oxygen uptake.

Pulse oximeter showed decrement in estimated arterial oxygen saturation from 97% at rest to 93% at peak exercise. Additional data are shown in **Tables 10.14.2** and **10.14.3** and graphically in **Figure 10.14.1**.

INTERPRETATION

Comment

This case is presented as an example of a test that was longer than intended (25 min) due to selecting a relatively slow work rate increment. Test performance is generally best when the duration of incremental exercise is around 8 to 12 minutes. For this patient, predicted peak $\dot{V}O_2$ was 1.4 L/min, but because she reported exercise intolerance, it was expected that hers would be lower. In addition, because she was obese it was expected that $\dot{V}O_2$ would be higher than usual during the initial unloaded cycling period. Based on these two factors, it was expected that the increment in $\dot{V}O_2$ between unloaded cycling and peak effort would be around 500 to 700 mL/min. If this were the case, a work rate increment of 5 to 7 W/min would likely result in an incremental phase of around 10 minutes. Because the increase in $\dot{V}O_2$ during incremental exercise was actually around 1 L/min, the test took longer than planned. The patient nevertheless exercised to symptom-limited maximum and the resulting data are perfectly valid for interpretation.

TABLE 10.14.3 Air Breathing

Time (min)	Work rate (W)	BP (mm Hg)	HR (min^{-1})	f (min^{-1})	$\dot{V}_E$ (L/min BTPS)	$\dot{V}_{CO_2}$ (L/min STPD)	$\dot{V}_{O_2}$ (L/min STPD)	$\frac{\dot{V}_{O_2}}{HR}$ (mL/beat)	R	pH	HCO_3^- (mEq/L)	P_{O_2}, mm Hg and Sp_{O_2}, %: ET	Sp_{O_2}	(A − a)	P_{CO_2}, mm Hg: ET	a	(a − ET)	$\frac{\dot{V}_E}{\dot{V}_{CO_2}}$	$\frac{\dot{V}_E}{\dot{V}_{O_2}}$	$\frac{V_D}{V_T}$
0.5	Rest		83	9	12.5	0.35	0.37	4.4	0.96			110	95		36			36	34	
1.0	Rest		82	10	6.0	0.18	0.21	2.5	0.85			101	95		39			34	29	
1.5	Rest		83	9	7.5	0.22	0.25	3.0	0.88			106	95		37			34	30	
2.0	Rest		84	11	5.6	0.17	0.21	2.5	0.80			99	95		39			34	27	
2.5	Rest		85	11	7.7	0.23	0.28	3.3	0.82			101	94		39			33	27	
3.0	Rest		86	9	8.1	0.25	0.28	3.3	0.88			104	94		38			33	29	
3.5	Unloaded		84	12	8.0	0.25	0.31	3.7	0.83			99	95		40			31	26	
4.0	Unloaded	134/88	86	15	9.9	0.30	0.36	4.2	0.84			102	94		38			33	28	
4.5	Unloaded		88	11	11.1	0.35	0.41	4.6	0.86			101	93		39			32	27	
5.0	Unloaded		88	16	10.5	0.32	0.39	4.4	0.81			101	95		39			33	27	
5.5	Unloaded		87	16	11.4	0.36	0.44	5.0	0.82			99	93		40			32	26	
6.0	Unloaded		88	15	11.1	0.34	0.41	4.7	0.83			100	93		39			32	27	
6.5	1	130/80	87	16	12.1	0.37	0.45	5.1	0.84			101	93		39			32	27	
7.0	4		87	14	11.3	0.36	0.42	4.7	0.86			101	93		40			32	27	
7.5	6		88	15	12.5	0.39	0.45	5.1	0.87			103	94		38			32	28	
8.0	9		88	15	11.3	0.35	0.41	4.6	0.85			101	94		39			33	28	
8.5	11	130/100	89	14	11.9	0.38	0.46	5.1	0.84			99	94		40			31	26	
9.0	14		91	17	13.9	0.43	0.51	5.6	0.85			100	93		40			32	27	
9.5	16		94	15	13.4	0.43	0.49	5.2	0.88			101	92		40			31	27	
10.0	19		94	15	13.8	0.46	0.53	5.6	0.86			99	92		41			30	26	
10.5	21		98	14	14.4	0.48	0.56	5.7	0.87			99	92		41			30	26	
11.0	24	136/100	101	18	15.8	0.51	0.57	5.7	0.89			102	93		40			31	27	
11.5	26		104	17	17.8	0.58	0.64	6.2	0.91			102	93		40			30	28	
12.0	29		105	17	17.4	0.57	0.61	5.8	0.93			103	93		40			30	28	
12.5	32		106	18	17.7	0.60	0.65	6.1	0.92			102	93		41			30	27	
13.0	34	146/90	109	20	20.1	0.67	0.70	6.5	0.96			104	92		40			30	29	
13.5	36		111	21	21.2	0.70	0.70	6.3	0.99			105	92		40			30	30	
14.0	39		113	21	22.1	0.74	0.76	6.8	0.98			105	92		40			30	29	
14.5	42		114	22	23.0	0.78	0.77	6.7	1.01			106	93		40			30	30	
15.0	44		116	22	23.5	0.80	0.78	6.8	1.02			106	93		40			29	30	
15.5	47		118	22	25.8	0.86	0.82	7.0	1.04			107	93		40			30	31	
16.0	49		120	23	26.6	0.89	0.84	7.0	1.06			108	93		40			30	32	
16.5	51		122	23	27.5	0.93	0.88	7.2	1.06			108	93		40			30	31	
17.0	54		125	24	29.5	0.99	0.90	7.2	1.09			109	92		40			30	33	
17.5	57		98	25	30.1	1.01	0.94	9.6	1.08			109	93		40			30	32	
18.0	59	166/96	70	26	32.6	1.08	0.96	13.7	1.12			111	93		39			30	34	
18.5	61		105	26	34.2	1.12	1.00	9.6	1.12			111	93		39			30	34	
19.0	64		113	25	34.8	1.15	1.01	8.9	1.14			111	93		39			30	34	
19.5	66		125	27	35.8	1.18	1.03	8.2	1.14			111	93		39			30	35	
20.0	69		138	28	37.7	1.23	1.07	7.8	1.15			112	93		39			31	35	
20.5	71	160/90	141	28	40.4	1.30	1.11	7.8	1.18			113	93		38			31	37	
21.0	74		143	29	41.4	1.33	1.14	8.0	1.17			113	93		38			31	36	
21.5	76		147	31	44.1	1.40	1.19	8.1	1.18			114	92		38			31	37	
22.0	79		150	30	45.3	1.45	1.21	8.1	1.19			114	93		37			31	37	
22.5	81		153	32	47.3	1.50	1.26	8.2	1.19			115	93		37			32	38	
23.0	Recovery	180/100	155	38	55.6	1.60	1.24	8.0	1.30			120	92		34			35	45	
23.5	Recovery		145	30	42.4	1.27	0.96	6.6	1.32			118	94		36			33	44	
24.0	Recovery	158/94	135	27	34.5	1.02	0.74	5.5	1.38			119	95		35			34	47	
24.5	Recovery		130	25	31.2	0.90	0.63	4.9	1.43			120	95		35			35	49	

Abbreviations: BP, blood pressure; BTPS, body temperature pressure saturated; f, frequency; HCO_3^-, bicarbonate; HR, heart rate; $P(A - a)O_2$, alveolar-arterial P_{O_2} difference; $P(a - ET)CO_2$, arterial-end-tidal P_{CO_2} difference; P_{ETCO_2}, end-tidal P_{CO_2}; P_{ETO_2}, end-tidal P_{O_2}; R, respiratory exchange ratio; Sp_{O_2}, oxygen saturation as measured by pulse oximetry; STPD, standard temperature pressure dry; $\dot{V}_{CO_2}$, carbon dioxide output; V_D/V_T, physiological dead space–tidal volume ratio; $\dot{V}_E$, minute ventilation; $\dot{V}_E/\dot{V}_{CO_2}$, ventilatory equivalent for carbon dioxide; $\dot{V}_E/\dot{V}_{O_2}$, ventilatory equivalent for oxygen; $\dot{V}_{O_2}$, oxygen uptake.

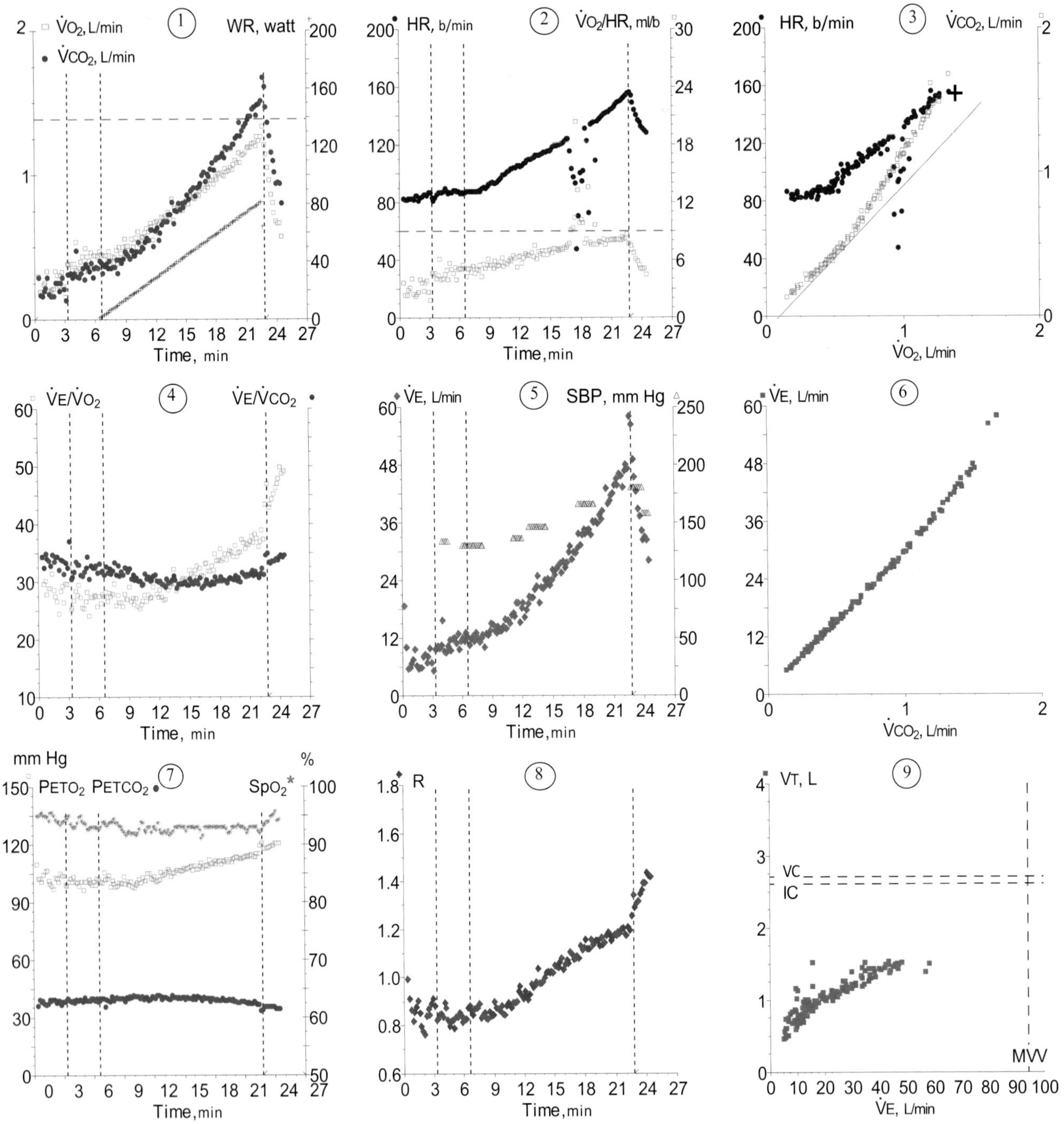

FIGURE 10.14.1. Vertical dashed lines in the panels in the left and middle columns indicate, from left to right, the beginning of unloaded cycling, start of increasing work rate (WR) at 5 W/min, and start of recovery. In **panel 1**, the increase in WR (right y-axis) is plotted with a scale of 100 W to 1 L of oxygen uptake ($\dot{V}O_2$) (left y-axis) such that WR is plotted parallel to a $\dot{V}O_2$ slope of 10 mL/min/W. Predicted peak $\dot{V}O_2$ is shown as a dashed horizontal line. In **panel 3**, carbon dioxide output ($\dot{V}CO_2$) (right y-axis) is plotted as a function of $\dot{V}O_2$ (x-axis) with identical scales so that the diagonal blue line has a slope of 1 (45°). The $\dot{V}CO_2$ increasing more steeply than $\dot{V}O_2$ defines carbon dioxide (CO_2) derived from bicarbonate buffer, as long as ventilatory equivalent for CO_2 ($\dot{V}E/\dot{V}CO_2$) (**panel 4**) is not increasing and end-tidal PCO_2 ($PETCO_2$) (**panel 7**) is not decreasing, simultaneously. The black + symbol in **panel 3** indicates predicted values of heart rate (HR) (left y-axis) and $\dot{V}O_2$ for this individual. Abbreviations: IC, inspiratory capacity; MVV, maximum voluntary ventilation; $PETO_2$, end-tidal PO_2; R, respiratory exchange ratio; SBP, systolic blood pressure; SpO_2, oxygen saturation as measured by pulse oximetry; VC, vital capacity; $\dot{V}E$, minute ventilation; $\dot{V}E/\dot{V}O_2$, ventilatory equivalent for oxygen; V_T, tidal volume.

Analysis

Cardiovascular and metabolic responses: The peak $\dot{V}O_2$ was within normal limits, but anaerobic threshold (*AT*) was lower than predicted. The $\dot{V}O_2$ during unloaded cycling was approximately double the resting $\dot{V}O_2$, which is typical for a normally proportioned individual, despite the fact that the patient was obese (body mass index 35). The $\dot{V}O_2$ subsequently increased appropriately relative to work rate (normal $\Delta\dot{V}O_2/\Delta WR$ in panel 1) and heart rate increased appropriately relative to $\dot{V}O_2$ (panel 3). Peak values for $\dot{V}O_2$, heart rate, and O_2 pulse were all normal. Noise in the heart rate and O_2 pulse data between minutes 16 and 19 in panels 2 and 3 resulted from transient motion artifact in the ECG signal.

The ventilatory response to exercise was normal with respect to breathing pattern and there was an ample breathing reserve.

Pulmonary gas exchange efficiency appeared grossly normal with a normal $\dot{V}E/\dot{V}CO_2$ at the *AT*. The estimated oxygen saturation was normal at rest but trended downward to 93% at peak exercise. As pulse oximeters do not provide precise measures of oxygen saturation, a mild abnormality in oxygenation cannot be known or excluded with certainty.

Conclusion

This was a good quality test, despite being somewhat long. Although exercise capacity was within the normal predicted range for a woman of this age and height, it could be that this was reduced relative to her capacity prior to her illness a year previously. Indexed to her body weight, peak $\dot{V}O_2$ and *AT* were consistent with her report of symptoms during modest activities. The low *AT* might be related to deconditioning related to her prior illness and subsequent reduced activity. Mildly abnormal oxygenation was also suggested, however, and could represent residua from her prior lung infection.

CASE 15

Chronic Heart Failure With Reduced Ejection Fraction

CLINICAL FINDINGS

A 71-year-old man was enrolled in a clinical trial investigating treatment of chronic left ventricular systolic heart failure. At the time of testing, his medical therapies had been optimized with treatment that included diuretics, an angiotensin-converting enzyme inhibitor, and β-adrenergic blocker. He was tested while in a well-compensated state without findings of overt volume overload. Resting electrocardiogram showed a sinus rhythm and intraventricular conduction delay. Demographic and respiratory function data are shown in **Table 10.15.1**.

EXERCISE FINDINGS

The patient exercised on a cycle ergometer beginning with 2 minutes of unloaded pedaling at 60 rpm followed by continuous increase in the work rate by 10 W/min until he stopped with symptoms of leg fatigue and shortness of breath. Blood pressure was measured intermittently by sphygmomanometer. There was no significant change in the electrocardiogram with exercise. Exercise data are summarized in **Table 10.15.2** and shown in **Table 10.15.3** and **Figure 10.15.1**.

INTERPRETATION

Comment

Resting spirometry showed mildly reduced volumes without evidence of airflow obstruction. This case is presented to illustrate common findings in the presence of chronic heart failure.

TABLE 10.15.1 Selected Respiratory Function Data

Measurement	Predicted	Measured
Age (y)		71
Sex		Male
Height (cm)		175
Weight (kg)		94
VC (L)	3.67	3.09
IC (L)	2.43	2.38
FEV_1 (L)	2.83	2.42
FEV_1/VC (%)	77	78
MVV (L/min)	110	98

Abbreviations: FEV_1, forced expiratory volume in 1 second; IC, inspiratory capacity; MVV, maximum voluntary ventilation; VC, vital capacity.

Analysis

Peak oxygen uptake ($\dot{V}O_2$) and anaerobic threshold were both low. Breathing reserve was normal despite the finding of high $\dot{V}E/\dot{V}CO_2$ and slope of $\dot{V}E$ versus $\dot{V}CO_2$, both consistent with chronic heart failure and linked to poorer prognosis. Characteristic of heart failure are the low $\Delta\dot{V}O_2/\Delta WR$, especially as $\dot{V}O_2$ appears to level off without further increase over the final 90 seconds of exercise despite increasing work rate, and low oxygen (O_2) pulse that also levels out near the end of exercise that probably indicates low stroke volume. In many patients, low stroke volume is compensated by higher heart rate, including peak heart rate, but his peak heart rate may be limited because of β-adrenergic blockade. Finally, in the early recovery period, there was a transient increase in O_2 pulse reflecting a delay in decrease in $\dot{V}O_2$ as heart rate rapidly began to decline. This suggests augmented stroke volume associated with the cessation of exercise.

Using the flowcharts, peak $\dot{V}O_2$ and anaerobic threshold were both low, which leads to Flowchart 4 (Chapter 9). At Branch Point 4.1, the normal breathing reserve branch is taken and then the branch point for high $\dot{V}E/\dot{V}CO_2$ at the anaerobic threshold (Branch Point 4.3). Because there is no evidence of O_2 desaturation, the tentative diagnosis is left ventricular failure with confirmatory data in the box below.

Conclusion

This test demonstrates findings typical of left ventricular systolic dysfunction. Impaired heart rate responsiveness—either due to heart failure, medication, or both—probably contributes to exercise limitation.

TABLE 10.15.2 Selected Exercise Data

Measurement	Predicted	Measured
Peak $\dot{V}O_2$ (L/min)	1.97	1.03
Maximum heart rate (beats/min)	149	83
Maximum O_2 pulse (mL/beat)	13.2	13.5
$\Delta\dot{V}O_2/\Delta WR$ (mL/min/W)	10.3	5.7
AT (L/min)	>0.93	0.75
Blood pressure (mm Hg [rest, max])		100/60, 160/70
Maximum $\dot{V}E$ (L/min)		59
Exercise breathing reserve (L/min)	>15	39
$\dot{V}E/\dot{V}CO_2$ @ *AT* or lowest	29.2	44.5

Abbreviations: *AT*, anaerobic threshold; $\Delta\dot{V}O_2/\Delta WR$, change in $\dot{V}O_2$/change in work rate; ex, exercise; O_2, oxygen; $\dot{V}E/\dot{V}CO_2$, ventilatory equivalent for carbon dioxide; $\dot{V}O_2$, oxygen uptake.

TABLE 10.15.3 Air Breathing

Time (min)	Work rate (W)	BP (mm Hg)	HR (min^{-1})	f (min^{-1})	$\dot{V}E$ (L/min BTPS)	$\dot{V}CO_2$ (L/min STPD)	$\dot{V}O_2$ (L/min STPD)	$\frac{\dot{V}O_2}{HR}$ (mL/beat)	R	pH	HCO_3^- (mEq/L)	PO_2, mm Hg ET	PO_2, mm Hg a	PO_2, mm Hg (A − a)	PCO_2, mm Hg ET	PCO_2, mm Hg a	PCO_2, mm Hg (a − ET)	$\frac{\dot{V}E}{\dot{V}CO_2}$	$\frac{\dot{V}E}{\dot{V}O_2}$	$\frac{VD}{VT}$
0.5	Rest	100/60	63	19	15.2	0.28	0.30	4.7	0.94			118			26			54	51	
1.0	Rest		64	18	14.3	0.26	0.26	4.1	0.98			119			26			56	54	
1.5	Rest		64	18	12.9	0.23	0.25	3.8	0.95			119			27			55	52	
2.0	Rest		64	19	14.8	0.26	0.26	4.1	0.97			120			25			58	56	
2.5	Rest		64	18	14.5	0.25	0.25	3.9	1.00			121			25			58	59	
3.0	Rest		63	19	13.7	0.24	0.25	4.0	0.96			120			26			57	55	
3.5	Unloaded	120/60	69	26	15.1	0.27	0.35	5.0	0.77			111			29			56	43	
4.0	Unloaded		73	29	26.1	0.48	0.52	7.1	0.92			118			26			54	50	
4.5	Unloaded		73	27	21.3	0.46	0.58	8.0	0.79			109			31			46	37	
5.0	Unloaded		76	29	28.2	0.60	0.68	8.9	0.88			114			28			47	42	
5.5	5		78	31	31.5	0.68	0.75	9.6	0.90			114			29			47	42	
6.0	10		77	32	33.9	0.76	0.79	10.3	0.95			114			29			45	43	
6.5	15		75	31	36.9	0.82	0.81	10.8	1.01			116			29			45	46	
7.0	20	122/68	73	31	39.1	0.88	0.85	11.6	1.04			116			29			45	46	
7.5	25		71	31	41.6	0.95	0.89	12.6	1.06			117			29			44	47	
8.0	30	130/64	75	31	45.8	1.03	0.93	12.3	1.11			118			29			45	49	
8.5	35		75	35	51.3	1.10	0.93	12.3	1.18			121			27			47	55	
9.0	40		78	33	50.3	1.12	0.97	12.4	1.16			120			28			45	52	
9.5	45	140/72	83	38	58.5	1.24	1.02	12.3	1.22			122			26			47	58	
10.0	50		83	38	57.2	1.22	1.02	12.3	1.19			122			27			47	56	
10.5	55	160/70	81	40	58.8	1.23	1.03	12.7	1.19			122			26			48	57	
11.0	Recovery	160/70	76	37	56.8	1.20	1.03	13.5	1.17			122			26			47	55	
11.5	Recovery		77	35	52.4	1.13	0.98	12.7	1.15			122			27			46	54	
12.0	Recovery		74	33	44.0	0.93	0.73	9.9	1.27			123			27			47	60	
12.5	Recovery		69	32	39.3	0.79	0.57	8.2	1.39			125			26			50	69	
13.0	Recovery	138/66	72	25	28.5	0.58	0.42	5.8	1.38			125			27			50	68	
13.5	Recovery		70	26	23.2	0.46	0.36	5.2	1.28			125			26			50	64	

Abbreviations: BP, blood pressure; BTPS, body temperature pressure saturated; f, frequency; HCO_3^-, bicarbonate; HR, heart rate; $P(A - a)O_2$, alveolar-arterial PO_2 difference; $P(a - ET)CO_2$, arterial-end-tidal PCO_2 difference; $PETCO_2$, end-tidal PCO_2; $PETO_2$, end-tidal PO_2; R, respiratory exchange ratio; STPD, standard temperature pressure dry; $\dot{V}CO_2$, carbon dioxide output; VD/VT, physiological dead space-tidal volume ratio; $\dot{V}E$, minute ventilation; $\dot{V}E/\dot{V}CO_2$, ventilatory equivalent for carbon dioxide; $\dot{V}E/\dot{V}O_2$, ventilatory equivalent for oxygen; $\dot{V}O_2$, oxygen uptake.

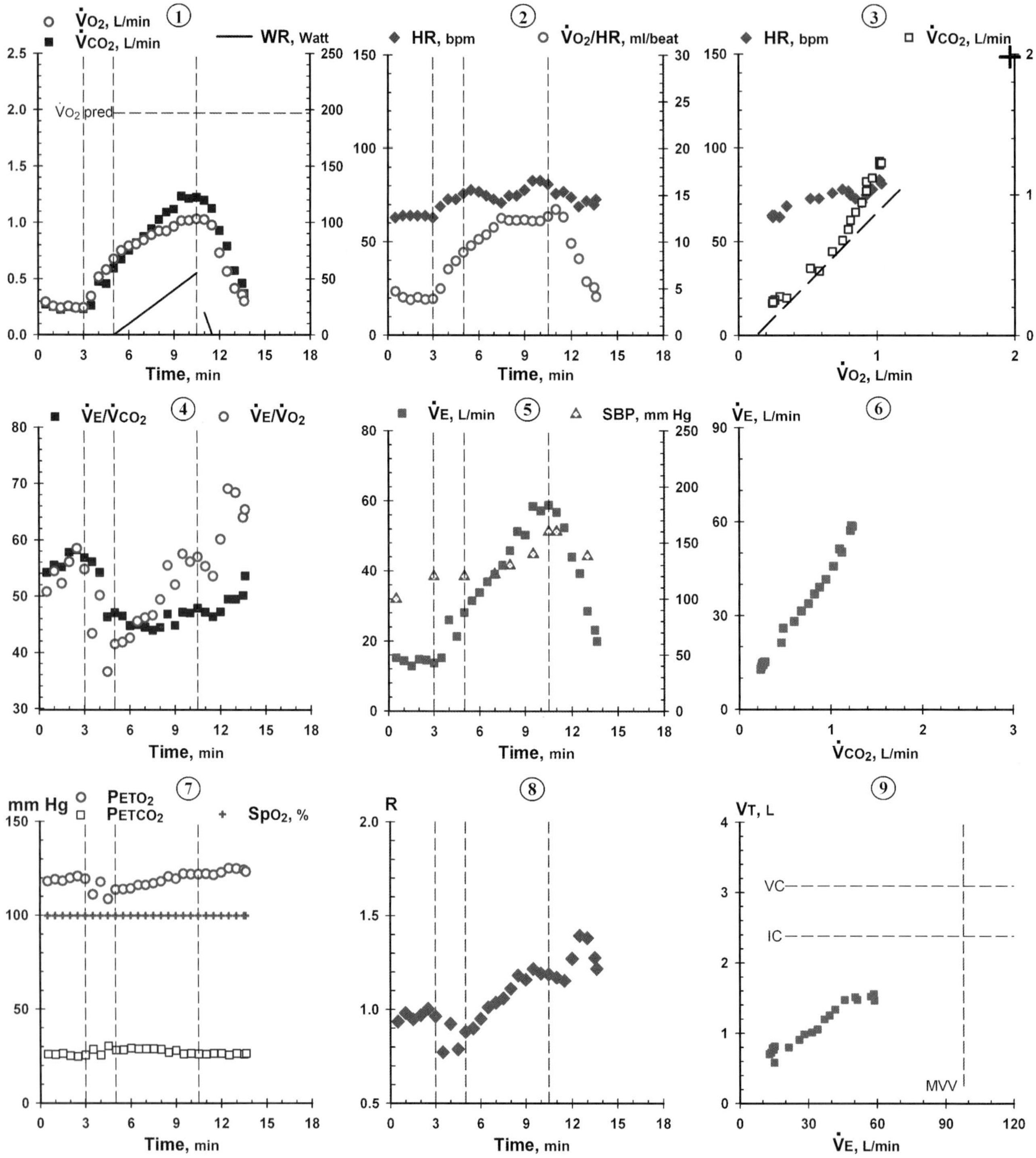

FIGURE 10.15.1. Vertical dashed lines in the panels in the left and middle columns indicate, from left to right, the beginning of unloaded cycling, start of increasing work rate (WR) at 10 W/min, and start of recovery. In **panel 1**, the increase in WR (right y-axis) is plotted with a scale of 100 W to 1 L of oxygen uptake ($\dot{V}O_2$) (left y-axis) such that WR is plotted parallel to a $\dot{V}O_2$ slope of 10 mL/min/W. In **panel 3**, carbon dioxide output ($\dot{V}CO_2$) (right y-axis) is plotted as a function of $\dot{V}O_2$ (x-axis) with identical scales so that the diagonal dashed line has a slope of 1 (45°). The $\dot{V}CO_2$ increasing more steeply than $\dot{V}O_2$ defines carbon dioxide CO_2 derived from bicarbonate buffer, as long as ventilatory equivalent for CO_2 ($\dot{V}E/\dot{V}CO_2$) (**panel 4**) is not increasing and end-tidal PCO_2 ($PETCO_2$) (**panel 7**) is not decreasing, simultaneously. The black + symbol in **panel 3** indicates predicted values of heart rate (HR) (left y-axis) and $\dot{V}O_2$ for this individual. Abbreviations: IC, inspiratory capacity; MVV, maximum voluntary ventilation; $PETO_2$, end-tidal PO_2; R, respiratory exchange ratio; SBP, systolic blood pressure; VC, vital capacity; $\dot{V}E$, minute ventilation; $\dot{V}E/\dot{V}O_2$, ventilatory equivalent for oxygen; V_T, tidal volume.

CASE 16

Chronic Heart Failure With Reduced Ejection Fraction

CLINICAL FINDINGS

A 41-year-old man had been disabled from prior work as a brickworker, woodworker, sandblaster, and security guard due to a back injury 9 years prior to this study. Exercise testing was requested as part of an evaluation for asbestos-related disease. He reported a 3-year history of dyspnea and productive cough and had been given diagnoses of asthmatic bronchitis and "probable" pulmonary asbestosis. He was diagnosed with hypertension 6 years earlier. He denied smoking but had repeated hospitalizations for alcoholism. Current medications included a β-blocker, hydrochlorothiazide, and a bronchodilator. Auscultation of the heart and lungs was normal, as were chest radiographs and the resting electrocardiogram (ECG).

EXERCISE FINDINGS

The patient performed exercise on a cycle ergometer. He pedaled at 60 rpm without added load for 3 minutes, after which the work rate was increased 20 W/min to his symptom-limited maximum. Arterial blood was sampled every second minute, and intra-arterial blood pressure was recorded from a percutaneously placed brachial artery catheter. He stopped exercise with complaints of shortness of breath, light-headedness, and leg fatigue. One premature ventricular contraction occurred during exercise, but ECGs were otherwise unchanged from rest.

INTERPRETATION

Comments

Resting pulmonary function (**Table 10.16.1**) was normal.

Analysis

Peak $\dot{V}O_2$ and anaerobic threshold (*AT*) were reduced, indicating abnormal exercise capacity. Because breathing reserve was normal, ventilatory limitation was unlikely. His peak heart rate (HR) did not reach predicted peak HR, indicating that he stopped before reaching his maximum or could be attributed to β-blockade. In the latter situation, oxygen (O_2) pulse is usually increased in normal subjects, so his low O_2 pulse may indicate a low stroke volume. This and the low $\Delta\dot{V}O_2/\Delta WR$ suggest a cardiovascular limitation, which is supported by normal $\dot{V}E/\dot{V}CO_2$ at the *AT* (decreased likelihood of pulmonary vascular disease) and absence of anemia.

Using the flowcharts, the low peak $\dot{V}O_2$ and *AT* leads to Flowchart 4 (Chapter 9). Normal breathing reserve (Branch Point 4.1) and ventilatory equivalent for carbon dioxide at the *AT* (Branch Point 4.3) suggest that the patient does not have an abnormal pulmonary circulation but rather a nonpulmonary O_2 flow problem. The hematocrit was normal (Branch Point 4.4), so this was most likely attributable to cardiovascular disease. There were no ECG changes to suggest acute ischemia. His $\Delta\dot{V}O_2/\Delta WR$ was low, and he had a low but rising O_2 pulse at maximum work rate (panel 2, **Fig. 10.16.1**). The patient's blood pressure response to exercise and HR reserve were normal (**Tables 10.16.2** and **10.16.3**), and he did not have leg pain with exercise, making

TABLE 10.16.1 Selected Respiratory Function Data

Measurement	Predicted	Measured
Age (y)		41
Sex		Male
Height (cm)		170
Weight (kg)	74	78
Hematocrit (%)		44
VC (L)	3.95	4.00
IC (L)	2.63	3.30
TLC (L)	5.58	5.28
FEV_1 (L)	3.16	3.43
FEV_1/VC (%)	80	86
MVV (L/min)	137	118
DLCO (mL/mm Hg/min)	25.8	24.7

Abbreviations: DLCO, diffusing capacity of the lung for carbon monoxide; FEV_1, forced expiratory volume in 1 second; IC, inspiratory capacity; MVV, maximum voluntary ventilation; VC, vital capacity.

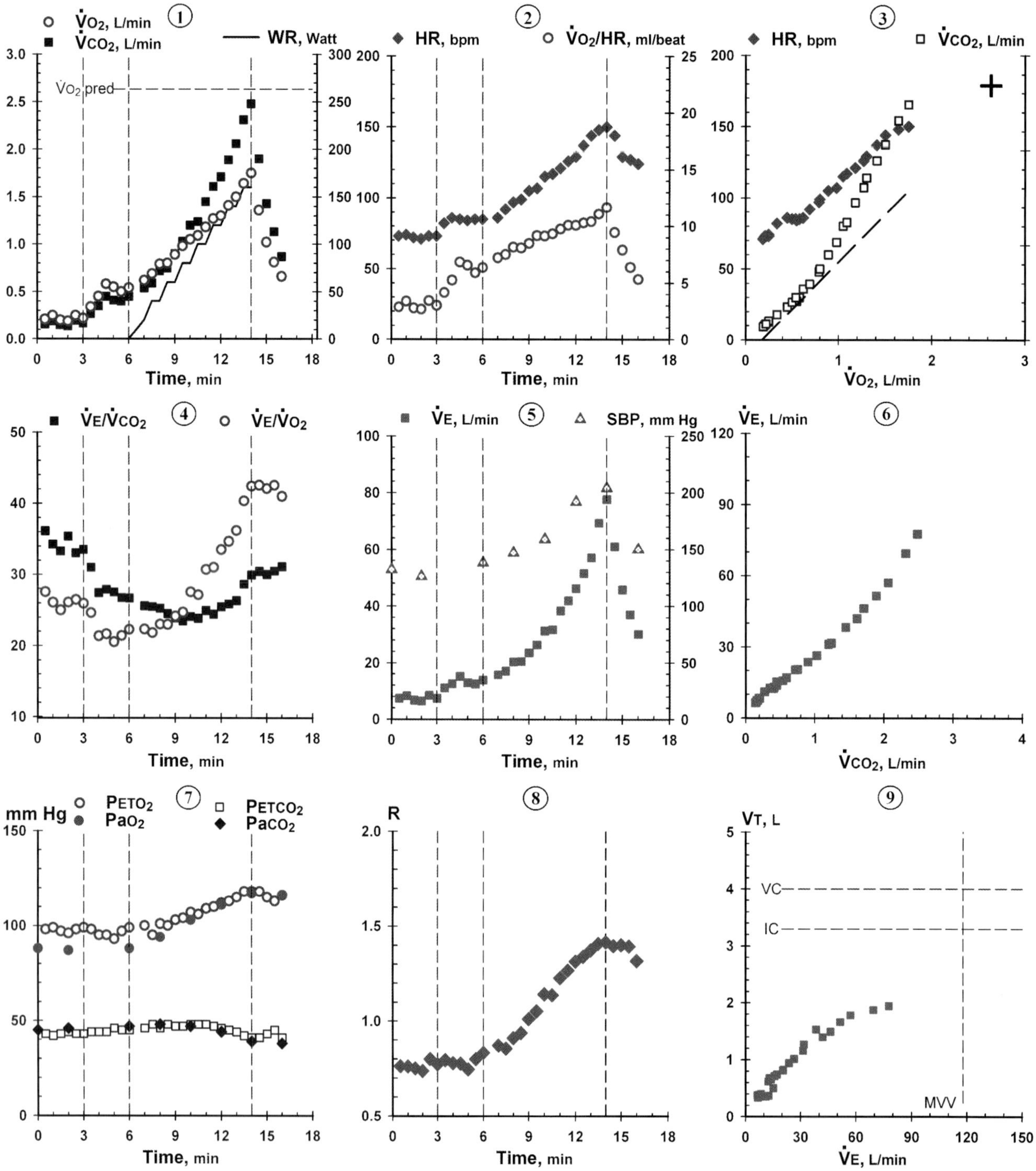

FIGURE 10.16.1. Vertical dashed lines in the panels in the left and middle columns indicate, from left to right, the beginning of unloaded cycling, start of increasing work rate (WR) at 20 W/min, and start of recovery. In **panel 1**, the increase in WR (right y-axis) is plotted with a scale of 100 W to 1 L of oxygen uptake ($\dot{V}O_2$) (left y-axis) such that WR is plotted parallel to a $\dot{V}O_2$ slope of 10 mL/min/W. In **panel 3**, carbon dioxide output ($\dot{V}CO_2$) (right y-axis) is plotted as a function of $\dot{V}O_2$ (x-axis) with identical scales so that the diagonal dashed line has a slope of 1 (45°). The $\dot{V}CO_2$ increasing more steeply than $\dot{V}O_2$ defines carbon dioxide (CO_2) derived from bicarbonate buffer, as long as ventilatory equivalent for CO_2 ($\dot{V}E/\dot{V}CO_2$) (**panel 4**) is not increasing and end-tidal PCO_2 ($PETCO_2$) (**panel 7**) is not decreasing, simultaneously. The black + symbol in **panel 3** indicates predicted values of heart rate (HR) (left y-axis) and $\dot{V}O_2$ for this individual. Abbreviations: IC, inspiratory capacity; MVV, maximum voluntary ventilation; $PETO_2$, end-tidal PO_2; R, respiratory exchange ratio; SBP, systolic blood pressure; VC, vital capacity; $\dot{V}E$, minute ventilation; $\dot{V}E/\dot{V}O_2$, ventilatory equivalent for oxygen; V_T, tidal volume.

TABLE 10.16.2 Selected Exercise Data

Measurement	Predicted	Measured
Peak $\dot{V}O_2$ (L/min)	2.64	1.75
Maximum heart rate (beats/min)	179	150
Maximum O_2 pulse (mL/beat)	14.7	11.7
$\Delta\dot{V}O_2/\Delta WR$ (mL/min/W)	10.3	8.3
AT (L/min)	>1.11	0.85
Blood pressure (mm Hg [rest, max ex])		132/87, 204/108
Maximum $\dot{V}E$ (L/min)		78
Exercise breathing reserve (L/min)	>15	40
$\dot{V}E/\dot{V}CO_2$ @ *AT* or lowest	26.2	24.1
PaO_2 (mm Hg [rest, max ex])		87, 117
$P(A - a)O_2$ (mm Hg [rest, max ex])		4, 3
$PaCO_2$ (mm Hg [rest, max ex])		46, 39
$P(a - ET)CO_2$ (mm Hg [rest, max ex])		2, −2
V_D/V_T (rest, heavy ex)		0.36, 0.23
HCO_3^- (mEq/L [rest, 2-min recov])		27, 18

Abbreviations: *AT*, anaerobic threshold; $\Delta\dot{V}O_2/\Delta WR$, change in $\dot{V}O_2$/change in work rate; ex, exercise; HCO_3^-, bicarbonate; O_2, oxygen; $P(A - a)O_2$, alveolar-arterial PO_2 difference; $P(a - ET)CO_2$, arterial-end-tidal PCO_2 difference; recov, recovery; V_D/V_T, physiological dead space–tidal volume ratio; $\dot{V}E$, minute ventilation; $\dot{V}E/\dot{V}CO_2$, ventilatory equivalent for carbon dioxide; $\dot{V}O_2$, oxygen uptake.

peripheral arterial disease unlikely. Because β-blocker therapy ordinarily results in a high O_2 pulse at peak exercise, the finding of a low O_2 pulse suggests a low stroke volume due to primary heart disease.

Conclusion

This patient had limitation to exercise at an abnormally low level due to cardiovascular dysfunction. A primary cardiac disorder was suspected because there were no specific findings to implicate pulmonary vascular, peripheral arterial, or coronary artery disease as the basis for the findings of impaired O_2 transport. Subsequent echocardiography confirmed the diagnosis of cardiomyopathy with left ventricular systolic dysfunction, perhaps due to alcoholism. There were no findings on this evaluation to support the prior suspicion of asbestosis.

TABLE 10.16.3 Air Breathing

Time (min)	Work rate (W)	BP (mm Hg)	HR (min^{-1})	f (min^{-1})	$\dot{V}E$ (L/min BTPS)	$\dot{V}CO_2$ (L/min STPD)	$\dot{V}O_2$ (L/min STPD)	$\frac{\dot{V}O_2}{HR}$ (mL/beat)	R	pH	HCO_3^- (mEq/L)	PO_2, mm Hg ET	a	(A − a)	PCO_2, mm Hg ET	a	(a − ET)	$\frac{\dot{V}E}{\dot{V}CO_2}$	$\frac{\dot{V}E}{\dot{V}O_2}$	$\frac{V_D}{V_T}$
0	Rest	132/87								7.39	27		88			45				
0.5	Rest		73	19	7.4	0.16	0.21	2.9	0.76			98			43			36	28	
1.0	Rest		74	21	8.3	0.19	0.25	3.4	0.76			99			42			34	26	
1.5	Rest		72	20	6.7	0.15	0.20	2.8	0.75			97			43			33	25	
2.0	Rest	126/84	71	17	6.4	0.14	0.19	2.7	0.74	7.39	27	96	87	4	44	46	2	35	26	0.36
2.5	Rest		73	21	8.4	0.20	0.25	3.4	0.80			98			43			33	26	
3.0	Rest		73	20	7.4	0.17	0.22	3.0	0.77			99			43			34	26	
3.5	Unloaded		82	31	11.0	0.27	0.34	4.1	0.79			98			44			31	25	
4.0	Unloaded		86	34	12.5	0.35	0.45	5.2	0.78			95			44			27	21	
4.5	Unloaded		85	30	15.1	0.45	0.58	6.8	0.78			95			44			28	22	
5.0	Unloaded		84	19	12.9	0.41	0.55	6.5	0.75			93			46			28	21	
5.5	Unloaded		85	20	12.4	0.40	0.50	5.9	0.80			97			45			27	21	
6.0	Unloaded	138/84	85	21	13.8	0.45	0.54	6.4	0.83	7.37	27	99	88	8	45	47	2	27	22	0.27
6.5	20		87	21	14.6	0.49	0.58	6.7	0.84			99			45			26	22	
7.0	20		86	22	15.7	0.54	0.62	7.2	0.87			100			46			26	22	
7.5	40	147/90	92	23	17.0	0.59	0.69	7.5	0.86	7.38	28	95	94	4	48	48	2	26	22	0.26
8.0	40		97	25	20.3	0.72	0.79	8.1	0.91			101			46			25	23	
8.5	60		99	25	20.5	0.75	0.80	8.1	0.94			100			48			25	23	
9.0	60		105	25	23.6	0.90	0.89	8.5	1.01			103			47			24	24	
9.5	80		107	26	26.4	1.03	0.98	9.2	1.05			104			47			23	25	
10.0	80	159/90	115	27	31.2	1.20	1.05	9.1	1.14	7.36	26	107	103	5	48	47	−1	24	28	0.22
10.5	100		117	25	31.7	1.24	1.09	9.3	1.14			106			48			24	27	
11.0	100		121	25	38.3	1.45	1.18	9.8	1.23			109			48			25	31	
11.5	120		126	30	41.9	1.61	1.27	10.1	1.27			110			47			24	31	
12.0	120	192/105	129	31	46.2	1.71	1.30	10.1	1.32	7.35	24	112	111	3	46	44	−2	25	34	0.22
12.5	140		137	31	51.5	1.89	1.41	10.3	1.34			113			45			26	35	
13.0	140		144	32	57.0	2.06	1.50	10.4	1.37			115			44			26	36	
13.5	160		148	37	69.3	2.31	1.64	11.1	1.41			118			42			29	40	
14.0	160	204/108	150	40	77.6	2.48	1.75	11.7	1.42	7.34	21	118	117	3	41	39	−2	30	42	0.25
14.5	Recovery		144	37	61.0	1.90	1.36	9.4	1.40			118			41			30	43	
15.0	Recovery		129	34	45.8	1.43	1.02	7.9	1.40			115			43			30	42	
15.5	Recovery		127	30	37.0	1.13	0.81	6.4	1.40			113			45			30	43	
16.0	Recovery	150/78	124	36	30.1	0.87	0.66	5.3	1.32	7.28	18	116	116	3	41	38	−3	31	41	0.24

Abbreviations: BP, blood pressure; BTPS, body temperature pressure saturated; f, frequency; HCO_3^-, bicarbonate; HR, heart rate; $P(A - a)O_2$, alveolar-arterial PO_2 difference; $P(a - ET)CO_2$, arterial-end-tidal PCO_2 difference; $PETCO_2$, end-tidal PCO_2; $PETO_2$, end-tidal PO_2; R, respiratory exchange ratio; STPD, standard temperature pressure dry; $\dot{V}CO_2$, carbon dioxide output; V_D/V_T, physiological dead space-tidal volume ratio; $\dot{V}E$, minute ventilation; $\dot{V}E/\dot{V}CO_2$, ventilatory equivalent for carbon dioxide; $\dot{V}E/\dot{V}O_2$, ventilatory equivalent for oxygen; $\dot{V}O_2$, oxygen uptake.

CASE 17

Chronic Heart Failure With Reduced Ejection Fraction and Pacemaker Dependence

CLINICAL FINDINGS

A 47-year-old man had exercise testing as part of the assessment of his chronic heart failure. He had a history of nonischemic cardiomyopathy with reduced ejection fraction, complete heart block, and ventricular arrhythmias. He had recently performed an exercise test on a cycle ergometer during which his heart rate was paced at a fixed rate of 60 beats/min, and peak oxygen uptake ($\dot{V}O_2$) was measured as 12.3 mL/min/kg. Retesting was conducted at this time using treadmill exercise, with the expectation that this might be more effective in stimulating an increase in pacemaker dependent heart rate.

He had a biventricular pacemaker and implantable cardioverter-defibrillator for the last 6 years and had undergone multiple ablative procedures for refractory arrhythmias. He lived independently and worked in an office, walking for 20 to 30 minutes most days for exercise. He had dyspnea when walking on any grade but was primarily limited in his daily activities by general fatigue. He denied orthopnea and had not had discharges of his implantable cardioverter-defibrillator over the previous 8 months. Medications at the time of testing were carvedilol, spironolactone, lisinopril, amiodarone, furosemide, and aspirin. Physical examination revealed a lean man with a surgical pacemaker site on the anterior chest. Lungs were clear to auscultation, heart tones were regular, and there was no peripheral edema. The resting electrocardiogram showed a ventricular paced rhythm at a rate of 60 beats/min. Demographic and respiratory function data are summarized in **Table 10.17.1**.

TABLE 10.17.1 Selected Respiratory Function Data

Measurement	Predicted	Measured
Age (y)		47
Sex		Male
Height (cm)		175
Weight (kg)		69
VC (L)	4.97	3.62
IC (L)	3.34	2.61
ERV (L)	1.63	0.96
FEV_1 (L)	3.89	2.91
FEV_1/VC (%)	78	80
MVV (L/min)	153	130

Abbreviations: ERV, expiratory reserve volume; FEV_1, forced expiratory volume in 1 second; IC, inspiratory capacity; MVV, maximum voluntary ventilation; VC, vital capacity.

EXERCISE FINDINGS

A modified Balke protocol was used for testing. The patient initially stood on the treadmill belt at rest for 2 minutes. Exercise began with walking at a speed of 2.4 mph with no grade. After 3 minutes of walking on level, the grade was increased by 1% per minute with no change in speed. The patient exercised for 9 minutes to peak settings of 2.4 mph and 7% grade and stopped with symptoms of leg fatigue. During the initial phase of zero-grade walking, there was an increase in the paced heart rate from 60 to 76 bpm and thereafter progressive increase to a peak of 90 bpm. No ectopy was seen. Exercise data are shown in **Tables 10.17.2** and **10.17.3** and shown graphically in **Figure 10.17.1**. For comparison, data from the prior cycle test are included in **Table 10.17.2** and the data from the cycle test are displayed graphically in **Figure 10.17.2**.

INTERPRETATION

Comments

This case is presented as an example of findings on exercise testing in heart failure. In addition, it highlights considerations for testing in individuals who are dependent on pacemakers for rate control during exercise. Rate adaptive pacemakers use a variety of strategies to identify need for increasing rate. Most include an accelerometer to sense motion, and these may be insensitive to exercise in a laboratory setting, particularly on a stationary cycle. Treadmill testing may also be preferred for testing patients with heart failure because much of the published data used for prognostic assessment in this clinical population were derived from treadmill exercise.

Analysis: Treadmill Test

Exercise capacity was severely reduced with a peak $\dot{V}O_2$ less than half of the reference value.

Variables reflecting cardiovascular capacity were abnormal with low values for peak $\dot{V}O_2$, anaerobic threshold, and peak heart rate, with electrocardiogram findings of pacemaker dependence as noted above. The peak $\dot{V}O_2$/HR (O_2 pulse) was normal, suggesting that he achieved an exercise stroke volume within the normal range. In the setting of isolated heart rate impairment, however, if cardiac function were otherwise normal, it would be expected that peak O_2 pulse would be higher than predicted, reflecting compensatory increase in stroke volume, so the peak O_2 pulse may

TABLE 10.17.2 Selected Exercise Data for Treadmill Test and Prior Cycle Test

Measurement	Predicted (cycle)	Measured (cycle)	Predicted (treadmill)	Measured (treadmill)
Peak $\dot{V}O_2$ (L/min)	2.44	0.83	2.68	1.32
Maximum heart rate (beats/min)	173	60	173	91
Maximum O_2 pulse (mL/beat)	14.1	13.9	15.5	14.4
$\Delta\dot{V}O_2/\Delta WR$ (mL/min/W)	10.3	8.0		NA
AT (L/min)	>1.09	0.75	>1.19	1.1
Blood pressure (mm Hg)		125/70, 115/67		89/48, 168/47
Maximum $\dot{V}E$ (L/min)		28		57
Breathing reserve (L/min)	>15	125		96
$\dot{V}E/\dot{V}CO_2$ @ *AT*	<31	33	<31	36
$\dot{V}E$ to $\dot{V}CO_2$ slope	<31	40	<31	39
SpO_2 (% [rest, max ex])		97, 97		98, 96

Abbreviations: *AT*, anaerobic threshold; $\Delta\dot{V}O_2/\Delta WR$, change in $\dot{V}O_2$/change in work rate; ex, exercise; O_2, oxygen; SpO_2, oxygen saturation as measured by pulse oximetry; $\dot{V}CO_2$, carbon dioxide output; $\dot{V}E$, minute ventilation; $\dot{V}E/\dot{V}CO_2$, ventilatory equivalent for carbon dioxide; $\dot{V}O_2$, oxygen uptake.

be considered abnormally constrained. Blood pressure was low at rest but did increase with exercise.

The ventilatory response to exercise was notable for an oscillatory pattern in ventilation and gas exchange variables. This is most evident in the graphs of R and the ventilatory equivalents. There was an ample breathing reserve.

Findings related to the efficiency of pulmonary gas exchange were notable for a steeper than normal relationship of $\dot{V}E$ to $\dot{V}CO_2$ but normal oxygenation as estimated by pulse oximetry.

Analysis: Cycle Test

From **Figure 10.17.2**, it is apparent that during the prior cycle test, the heart rate was fixed at a paced rate of 60 beats/min. The $\dot{V}O_2$ did not increase appropriately relative to work rate, and the peak $\dot{V}O_2$ was only a little more than triple the resting level (ie, 3 metabolic equivalents [METs]). Systolic blood pressure did not increase appreciably. The O_2 pulse increased to a peak value that was similar to what was measured on the treadmill test. The normal peak O_2 pulse values indicate that the *product* of stroke volume and $C(a - \bar{v})O_2$ reached normal maxima on both tests, although it cannot be known with certainly how much each of the two factors contributed to this. Normally, the increase in O_2 pulse is mediated by approximate tripling of the $C(a - \bar{v})O_2$ (which itself could account for 3 METs) and a smaller augmentation of stroke volume. Without an increase in heart rate, these are the only two variables that can support the increase of $\dot{V}O_2$. Oscillatory breathing was not evident on the cycle test, although the $\dot{V}E$ to $\dot{V}CO_2$ slope was steep and similar to that measured on the treadmill.

Conclusions

Although peak $\dot{V}O_2$ on treadmill testing was severely reduced relative to predicted values, it was higher than had been demonstrated on cycle testing and in the range of Weber class B for functional impairment in heart failure. The difference relative to the cycle test was attributable in part to the expected difference in peak $\dot{V}O_2$ between cycle and treadmill exercise, but, also undoubtedly reflects the better O_2 delivery associated with a higher heart rate response. Variables relevant to prognosis in heart failure were mixed in this case: the peak $\dot{V}O_2$ of 19.4 mL/min/kg is favorable; on the other hand, the elevated $\dot{V}E/\dot{V}CO_2$ and an oscillatory breathing pattern have both been identified as markers of poor prognosis. For this patient, complex arrhythmias not evident at the time of testing were also important in his clinical course and prognostic assessment.

TABLE 10.17.3 Treadmill Test[a]

Time (min)	Treadmill grade (%)	BP (mm Hg)	HR (min^{-1})	f (min^{-1})	$\dot{V}E$ (L/min BTPS)	$\dot{V}CO_2$ (L/min STPD)	$\dot{V}O_2$ (L/min STPD)	$\frac{\dot{V}O_2}{HR}$ (mL/beat)	R	pH	HCO_3^- (mEq/L)	Po_2, mm Hg or Spo_2, %			Pco_2, mm Hg			$\frac{\dot{V}E}{\dot{V}CO_2}$	$\frac{\dot{V}E}{\dot{V}O_2}$	$\frac{V_D}{V_T}$
												ET	Spo_2	(A − a)	ET	a	(a − ET)			
0.5	Rest		60	9	7.8	0.21	0.23	3.9	0.92			111	98		35			36	33	
1.0	Rest		60	8	8.3	0.24	0.27	4.6	0.87			109	98		35			35	30	
1.5	Rest		60	9	9.1	0.25	0.28	4.7	0.90			111	98		34			36	32	
2.0	Rest		60	9	7.5	0.21	0.23	3.9	0.90			110	98		35			36	32	
2.5	0		60	16	15.4	0.41	0.46	7.7	0.89			112	98		33			37	33	
3.0	0		68	17	18.9	0.48	0.48	7.1	1.00			117	98		31			39	39	
3.5	0		77	13	19.9	0.56	0.61	8.0	0.91			113	97		32			36	32	
4.0	0		77	17	26.2	0.72	0.82	10.6	0.88			114	97		31			37	32	
4.5	0	89/48	77	18	29.2	0.78	0.82	10.7	0.95			116	97		30			37	36	
5.0	0		77	20	31.7	0.83	0.83	10.7	1.00			118	96		30			38	38	
5.5	1		79	28	29.9	0.76	0.82	10.4	0.93			115	96		32			39	36	
6.0	1		86	21	34.2	0.93	1.01	11.7	0.93			114	96		32			37	34	
6.5	2		85	26	39.2	1.02	0.99	11.6	1.03			119	97		30			39	40	
7.0	2		84	25	39.7	1.05	1.02	12.1	1.03			119	97		31			38	39	
7.5	3	168/47	83	23	37.4	1.04	1.04	12.5	1.00			116	96		32			36	36	
8.0	3		81	26	43.6	1.15	1.10	13.5	1.05			119	96		31			38	40	
8.5	4		82	26	43.6	1.17	1.11	13.5	1.06			119	97		31			37	39	
9.0	4		84	25	41.4	1.14	1.12	13.3	1.02			116	97		33			36	37	
9.5	5		86	28	50.0	1.31	1.20	13.9	1.09			120	97		31			38	42	
10.0	5		88	30	50.6	1.33	1.21	13.7	1.11			120	97		31			38	42	
10.5	6		89	30	52.9	1.42	1.29	14.4	1.10			120	96		31			37	41	
11.0	6		90	30	52.7	1.41	1.29	14.3	1.10			120	95		31			37	41	
11.5	7		91	33	56.7	1.48	1.32	14.4	1.13			121	95		31			38	43	
12.0	Recovery		91	32	56.1	1.48	1.33	14.6	1.12			120	97		31			38	42	
12.5	Recovery		89	25	41.0	1.29	1.26	14.1	1.02			113	98		37			32	32	
13.0	Recovery		86	25	45.6	1.35	1.17	13.6	1.16			118	100		35			34	39	
13.5	Recovery	113/60	79	24	42.7	1.22	0.96	12.1	1.27			121	100		34			35	45	
14.0	Recovery		75	24	39.1	1.07	0.83	11.1	1.28			122	98		32			37	47	
14.5	Recovery		73	24	38.7	1.06	0.83	11.4	1.28			122	97		32			36	47	

Abbreviations: BP, blood pressure; BTPS, body temperature pressure saturated; f, frequency; HCO_3^-, bicarbonate; HR, heart rate; $P(A - a)O_2$, alveolar-arterial Po_2 difference; $P(a - ET)CO_2$, arterial-end-tidal Pco_2 difference; P_{ETCO_2}, end-tidal Pco_2; P_{ETO_2}, end-tidal Po_2; R, respiratory exchange ratio; Spo_2, oxygen saturation as measured by pulse oximetry; STPD, standard temperature pressure dry; $\dot{V}CO_2$, carbon dioxide output; V_D/V_T, physiological dead space-tidal volume ratio; $\dot{V}E$, minute ventilation; $\dot{V}E/\dot{V}CO_2$, ventilatory equivalent for carbon dioxide; $\dot{V}E/\dot{V}O_2$, ventilatory equivalent for oxygen; $\dot{V}O_2$, oxygen uptake.

[a]From the start of exercise to the start of recovery, treadmill speed was kept constant at 2.4 mph.

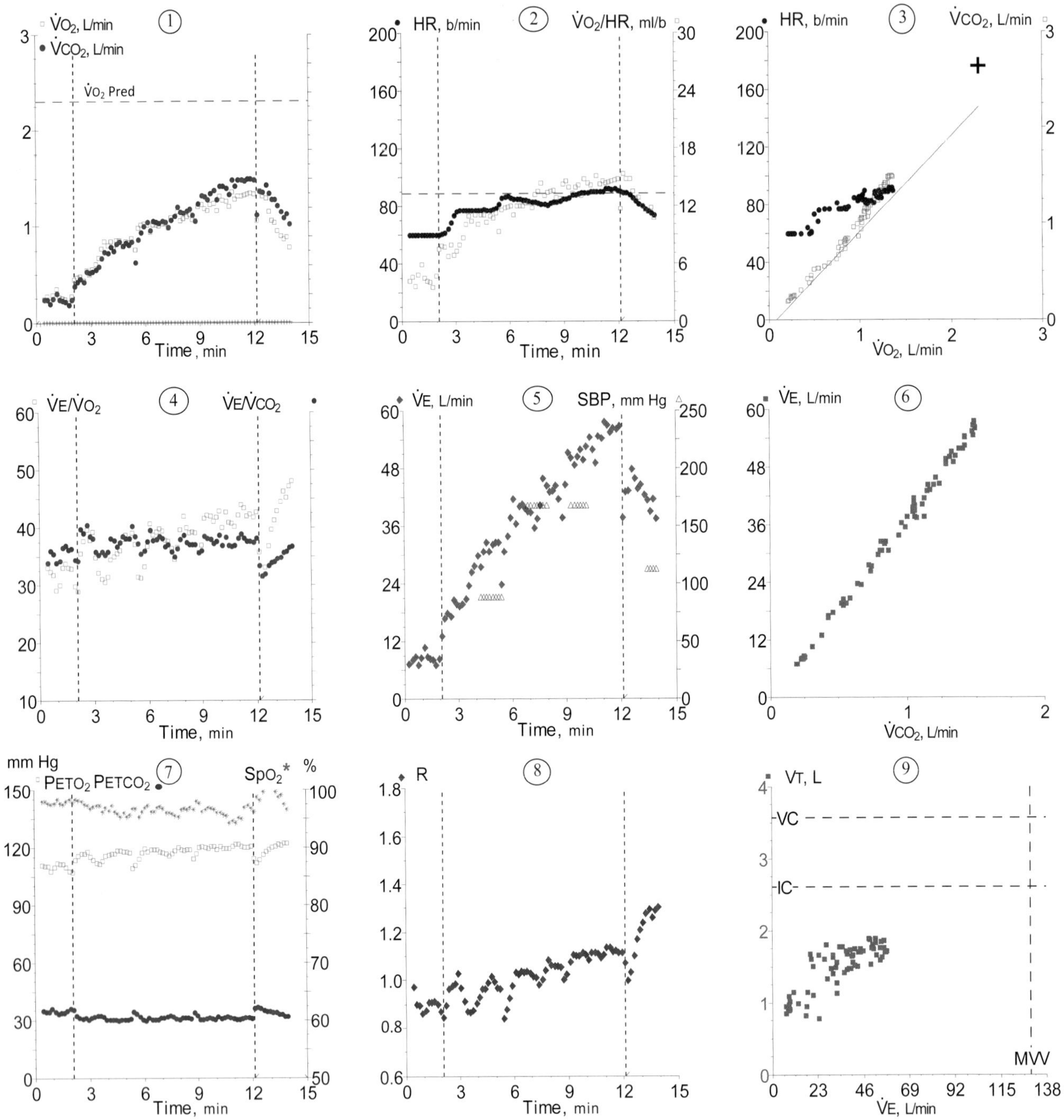

FIGURE 10.17.1. Treadmill test. Vertical dashed lines in the panels in the left and middle columns indicate, from left to right, the beginning of walking at 2.4 mph with no grade and the start of recovery. In **panel 1**, predicted peak oxygen uptake ($\dot{V}O_2$) is shown as a dashed horizontal line. Work rate is not displayed because of the difficulty in accurately determining work rate for treadmill exercise. In **panel 3**, carbon dioxide output ($\dot{V}CO_2$) (right y-axis) is plotted as a function of $\dot{V}O_2$ (x-axis) with identical scales so that the diagonal blue line has a slope of 1 (45°). The $\dot{V}CO_2$ increasing more steeply than $\dot{V}O_2$ defines carbon dioxide (CO_2) derived from bicarbonate buffer, as long as ventilatory equivalent for CO_2 ($\dot{V}E/\dot{V}CO_2$) (**panel 4**) is not increasing and end-tidal PCO_2 ($PETCO_2$) (**panel 7**) is not decreasing, simultaneously. The black + symbol in **panel 3** indicates predicted values of heart rate (HR) (left y-axis) and $\dot{V}O_2$ for this individual. Abbreviations: IC, inspiratory capacity; MVV, maximum voluntary ventilation; $PETO_2$, end-tidal PO_2; R, respiratory exchange ratio; SBP, systolic blood pressure; SpO_2, oxygen saturation as measured by pulse oximetry; VC, vital capacity; $\dot{V}E$, minute ventilation; $\dot{V}E/\dot{V}O_2$, ventilatory equivalent for oxygen; VT, tidal volume.

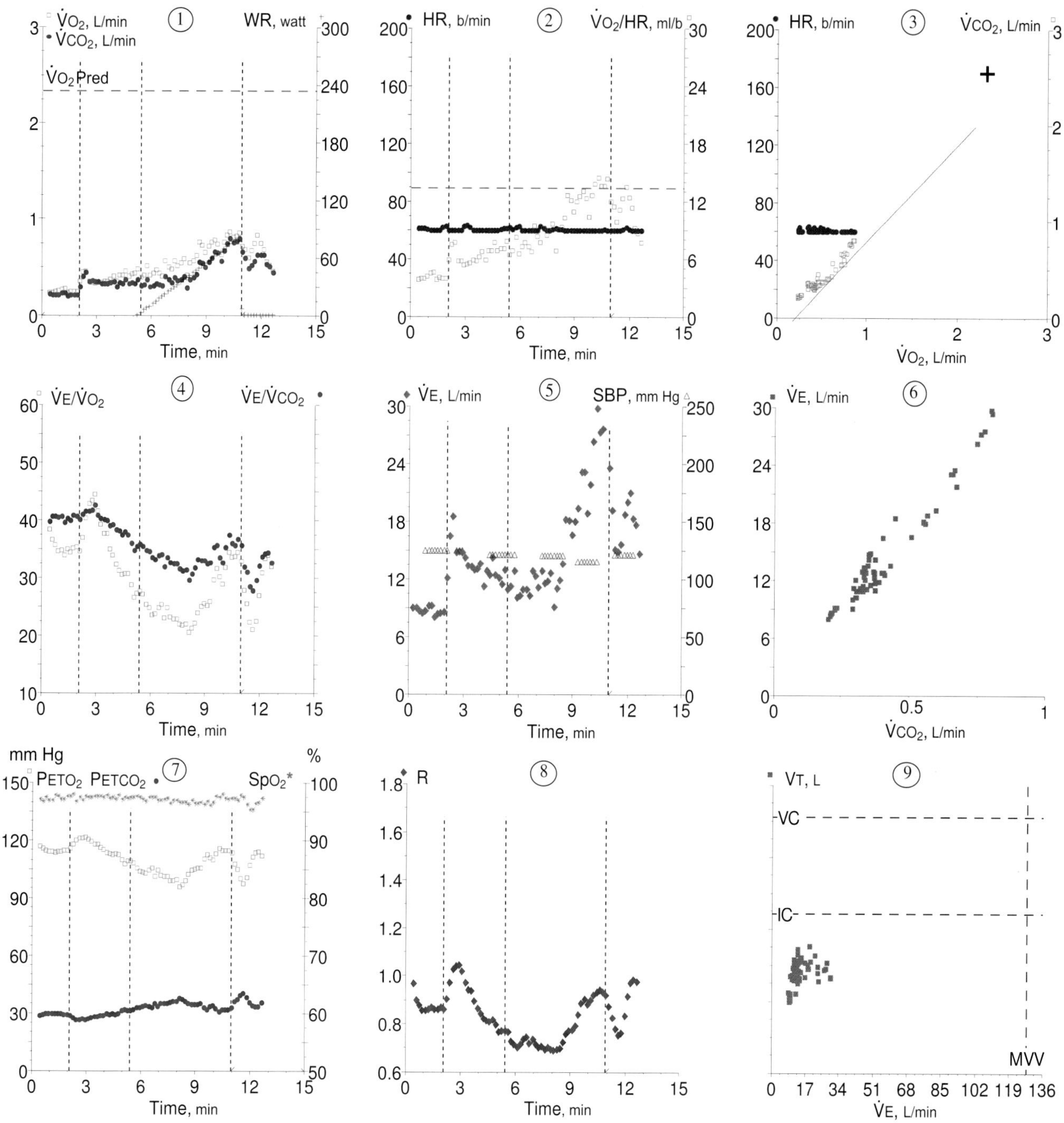

FIGURE 10.17.2. Cycle test. Vertical dashed lines in the panels in the left and middle columns indicate, from left to right, the beginning of unloaded cycling, start of increasing work rate (WR) at 10 W/min, and start of recovery. In **panel 1**, the increase in WR (right y-axis) is plotted with a scale of 100 W to 1 L of oxygen uptake ($\dot{V}O_2$) (left y-axis) such that WR is plotted parallel to a $\dot{V}O_2$ slope of 10 mL/min/W. Predicted peak $\dot{V}O_2$ is shown as a dashed horizontal line. In **panel 3**, carbon dioxide output ($\dot{V}CO_2$) (right y-axis) is plotted as a function of $\dot{V}O_2$ (x-axis) with identical scales so that the diagonal line has a slope of 1 (45°). The $\dot{V}CO_2$ increasing more steeply than $\dot{V}O_2$ defines carbon dioxide (CO_2) derived from bicarbonate buffer, as long as ventilatory equivalent for CO_2 ($\dot{V}E/\dot{V}CO_2$) (**panel 4**) is not increasing and end-tidal PCO_2 ($PETCO_2$) (**panel 7**) is not decreasing, simultaneously. The black + symbol in **panel 3** indicates predicted values of heart rate (HR) (left y-axis) and $\dot{V}O_2$ for this individual. Abbreviations: IC, inspiratory capacity; MVV, maximum voluntary ventilation; $PETO_2$, end-tidal PO_2; R, respiratory exchange ratio; SBP, systolic blood pressure; SpO_2, oxygen saturation as measured by pulse oximetry; VC, vital capacity; $\dot{V}E$, minute ventilation; $\dot{V}E/\dot{V}O_2$, ventilatory equivalent for oxygen; V_T, tidal volume.

CASE 18

Chronic Heart Failure: Oscillatory Ventilation and Gas Exchange

CLINICAL FINDINGS

A 57-year-old woman without prior medical history presented with complaints of 6 months of shortness of breath, exercise limitation, and easy fatigability. She had two-pillow orthopnea and paroxysmal nocturnal dyspnea. She did not experience exertional chest pain. An echocardiogram reported a dilated cardiomyopathy with a 15% left ventricular ejection fraction. She was treated with lisinopril, digoxin, warfarin, atorvastatin, and furosemide, and referred for exercise testing to quantify the severity of her heart failure. At the time of referral, she was symptomatically improved on therapy and had clear breath sounds and only trace pretibial edema. Chest radiographs were normal except for mild left ventricular enlargement. Resting electrocardiogram revealed sinus rhythm and left bundle branch block with rare premature ventricular contractions.

EXERCISE FINDINGS

The patient was studied during exercise on a cycle ergometer (**Fig. 10.18.1**). After 3 minutes of rest, she pedaled at 60 rpm without added load for 3 minutes. The work rate was then increased in a ramp pattern by 10 W/min to her symptom-limited maximum. Blood pressure was measured with a sphygmomanometer. Arterial oxyhemoglobin saturation was estimated by pulse oximeter. The patient stopped exercise on her own volition because of leg fatigue. During unloaded cycling, premature ventricular contractions occurred at about one per minute, but these resolved at higher work rates. The ST segments did not change with exercise. At rest and during early exercise, an oscillatory breathing pattern with a period of about 1 minute was observed (**Fig. 10.18.2**).

INTERPRETATION

Comments

This patient has an idiopathic cardiomyopathy and symptoms compatible with New York Heart Association class II to III. Respiratory function showed mild airway obstruction and mild reduction in diffusing capacity (**Table 10.18.1**). A distinctly oscillatory pattern of $\dot{V}O_2$, $\dot{V}CO_2$, and $\dot{V}E$ is seen at rest and at exercise intensities below the anaerobic threshold (*AT*) (see **Fig. 10.18.2**).

This patient's clinical diagnosis was not in question, as the exercise test was primarily done to assess prognosis and effectiveness of treatment. The test also demonstrates several of the features seen in chronic heart failure.

Analysis

Peak $\dot{V}O_2$ and *AT* are reduced, indicating abnormally low exercise capacity, but breathing reserve is normal (likely excluding ventilatory limitation). As the diagnosis of chronic heart failure is known, expected features might include low oxygen pulse at peak exercise, especially with flatter than normal rise with exercise, low $\Delta\dot{V}O_2/\Delta WR$, high $\dot{V}E/\dot{V}CO_2$ (at *AT* or its nadir value), high slope of $\dot{V}E$ versus $\dot{V}CO_2$, and low P_{ETCO_2}; this patient's exercise test demonstrated all of these features.

If using the flowcharts in Chapter 9 to establish a potential etiology of exercise limitation, the peak $\dot{V}O_2$ and *AT* are reduced (**Tables 10.18.2** and **10.18.3**), leading to Flowchart 4 (**Fig. 9.4**). Next the breathing reserve is normal (Branch Point 4.1), but the ventilatory equivalent for CO_2 at the *AT* is high (Branch Point 4.3), implying an increased V_D/V_T.[1] This leads to a presumed diagnostic category of *abnormal pulmonary circulation* (Branch Point 4.5). To help distinguish between $\dot{V}A/\dot{Q}$ mismatch due to primary pulmonary vascular disease (left branch) and high $\dot{V}A/\dot{Q}$ mismatch due to relative stasis of pulmonary blood flow caused by left ventricular failure (right branch), consider the arterial saturation (Branch Point 4.5). The normal arterial oxyhemoglobin saturation throughout exercise is more characteristic of the slow pulmonary blood flow (long transit time) of left ventricular dysfunction (right branch) as opposed to the shortened transit time associated with exercise arterial hypoxemia of primary pulmonary vascular disease (left branch).

The data in the nine-panel plots are graphed as 30-second averages, which is insufficient time resolution to fully appreciate the temporal pattern of change in $\dot{V}O_2$, $\dot{V}CO_2$, and $\dot{V}E$. When these variables are plotted using a moving average, a systematic oscillatory pattern is evident at rest and at low levels of exercise. This finding is seen in some patients with left ventricular failure and has features similar to Cheyne-Stokes respiration. The periodic (oscillatory) gas exchange pattern is analyzed in greater detail in **Figure 10.18.2**. The oscillations have a period of 1 minute from peak to peak and are greatest at rest and during mild-to-moderate exercise. The rise in $\dot{V}O_2$ begins first, followed by $\dot{V}CO_2$, $\dot{V}E$, and finally respiratory exchange ratio.

We postulate that the oscillation in gas exchange is caused by oscillating pulmonary blood flow due to cyclic

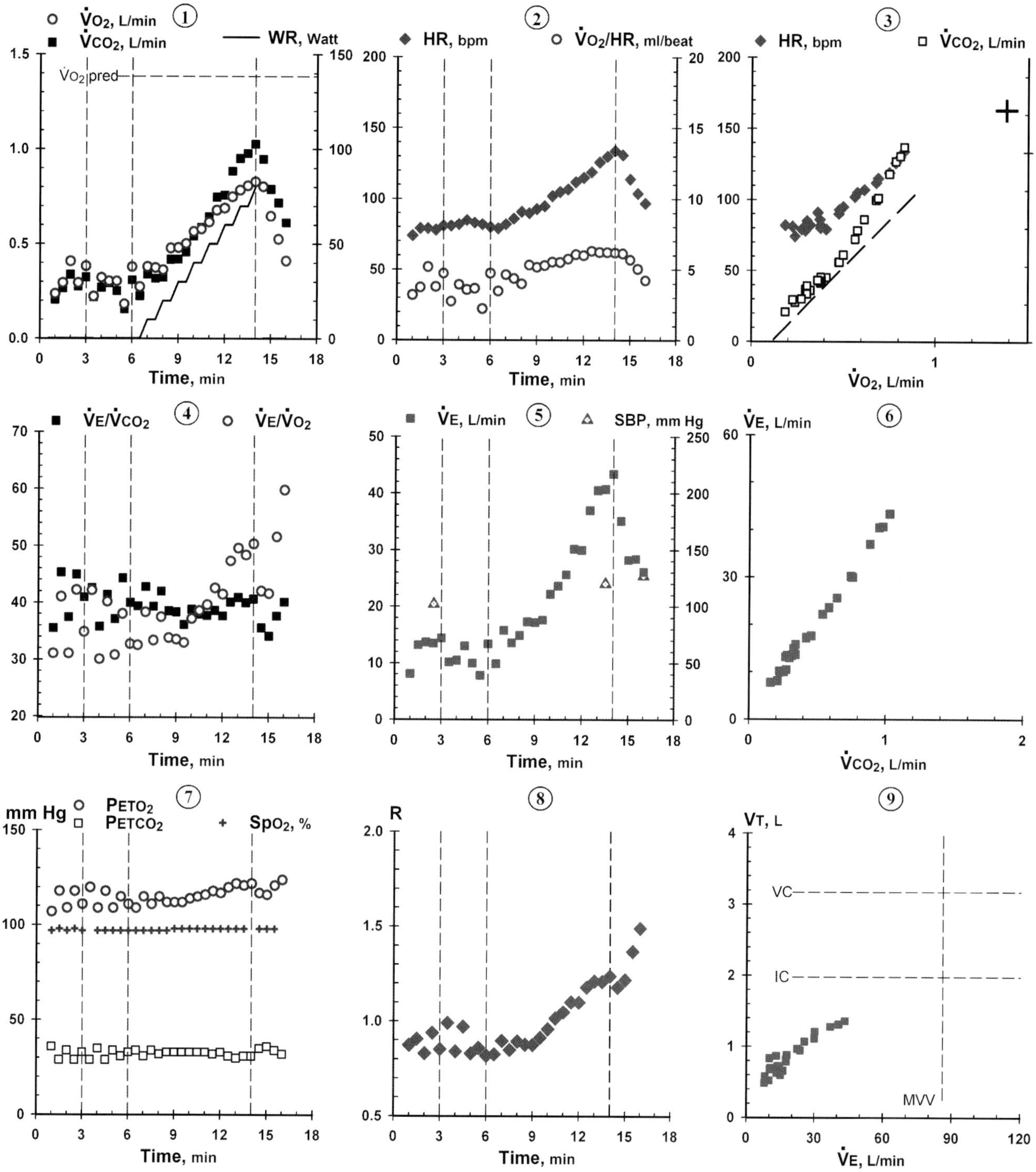

FIGURE 10.18.1. Vertical dashed lines in the panels in the left and middle columns indicate, from left to right, the beginning of unloaded cycling, start of increasing work rate (WR) at 10 W/min, and start of recovery. In **panel 1**, the increase in WR (right y-axis) is plotted with a scale of 100 W to 1 L of oxygen saturation ($\dot{V}O_2$) (left y-axis) such that WR is plotted parallel to a $\dot{V}O_2$ slope of 10 mL/min/W. In **panel 3**, carbon dioxide output ($\dot{V}CO_2$) (right y-axis) is plotted as a function of $\dot{V}O_2$ (x-axis) with identical scales so that the diagonal dashed line has a slope of 1 (45°). The $\dot{V}CO_2$ increasing more steeply than $\dot{V}O_2$ defines carbon dioxide (CO_2) derived from bicarbonate buffer, as long as ventilatory equivalent for CO_2 $\dot{V}E/\dot{V}CO_2$ (**panel 4**) is not increasing and end-tidal PCO_2 (P_{ETCO_2}) (**panel 7**) is not decreasing, simultaneously. The black + symbol in **panel 3** indicates predicted values of heart rate (HR) (left y-axis) and $\dot{V}O_2$ for this individual. Abbreviations: IC, inspiratory capacity; MVV, maximum voluntary ventilation; P_{ETO_2}, end-tidal PO_2; R, respiratory exchange ratio; SBP, systolic blood pressure; SpO_2, oxygen saturation as measured by pulse oximetry; VC, vital capacity; $\dot{V}E$, minute ventilation; $\dot{V}E/\dot{V}O_2$, ventilatory equivalent for oxygen; V_T, tidal volume.

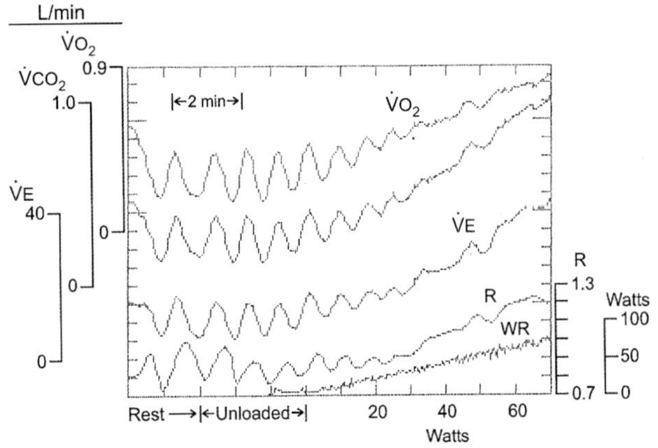

FIGURE 10.18.2. Oxygen uptake ($\dot{V}O_2$), carbon dioxide output ($\dot{V}CO_2$), minute ventilation ($\dot{V}E$), respiratory exchange ratio (R), and work rate (WR), from top to bottom, during rest and incremental exercise. Oscillations in the data have a period of 1 min from peak to peak and are most prominent at rest and during moderate exercise. The interbreath noise is reduced in this display by use of a moving interval (MI) average type of filtering. The breath-by-breath data were first converted into time-based data of 0.1-s time intervals by interpolation. For each data point, the data in the MI window were fitted by a fifth-order polynomial, and the center point of the MI is given by the center point of the polynomial. This provides superior fitting of data with rapid changes in slope. Analysis of the sinusoid-like patterns showed that the peak-to-peak interval for oscillations of $\dot{V}O_2$ was 1 min. The time delay following a $\dot{V}O_2$ peak to the peak of the other measured variables was 0.05 min for $\dot{V}CO_2$, 0.1 min for $\dot{V}E$, and 0.34 min for R. These times are compatible with a primary oscillation of pulmonary blood flow followed by secondary changes in ventilation. See the Interpretation section for further discussion.

changes in systemic blood pressure in the presence of a heart that is functioning on the flat or descending limb of the Frank–Starling curve. The cyclic changes in arterial pressure are known as *Traube–Hering waves* and have a period of 0.75 to 1.5 minutes. These changes in arterial tone do not affect cardiac output (and therefore pulmonary blood flow)

TABLE 10.18.1 Selected Respiratory Function Data

Measurement	Predicted	Measured
Age (y)		57
Sex		Female
Height (cm)		168
Weight (kg)		59.1
Hematocrit (%)		38.5
VC (L)	3.27	3.17
IC (L)	2.18	1.98
ERV (L)	1.09	1.19
FEV_1 (L)	2.64	2.17
FEV_1/VC (%)	81	69
MVV (L/min)	97	86
D_{LCO} (mL/mm Hg/min)	22.7	17.8

Abbreviations: D_{LCO}, diffusing capacity of the lung for carbon monoxide; ERV, expiratory reserve volume; FEV_1, forced expiratory volume in 1 second; IC, inspiratory capacity; MVV, maximum voluntary ventilation; VC, vital capacity.

TABLE 10.18.2 Selected Exercise Data

Measurement	Predicted	Measured
Peak $\dot{V}O_2$ (L/min)	1.35	0.83
Maximum heart rate (beats/min)	163	134
Maximum O_2 pulse (mL/beat)	8.3	6.2
$\Delta\dot{V}O_2/\Delta WR$ (mL/min/W)	10.3	6.9
AT (L/min)	>0.70	0.53
Blood pressure (mm Hg [rest, max])		102/66, 120/85
Maximum $\dot{V}E$ (L/min)		43
Exercise breathing reserve (L/min)	>15	43
$\dot{V}E/\dot{V}CO_2$ @ *AT* or lowest	28.9	38.2
P_{ETCO_2} @ *AT*	>40	33
$\dot{V}E$ versus $\dot{V}CO_2$	<32	38
Sa_{O_2} (pulse oximeter, % [rest, ex])	>95	98, 98

Abbreviations: *AT*, anaerobic threshold; $\Delta\dot{V}O_2/\Delta WR$, change in $\dot{V}O_2$/change in work rate; ex, exercise; O_2, oxygen; P_{ETCO_2}, end-tidal P_{CO_2}; Sa_{O_2}, arterial oxygen saturation; $\dot{V}CO_2$, carbon dioxide output; $\dot{V}E$, minute ventilation; $\dot{V}E/\dot{V}CO_2$, ventilatory equivalent for carbon dioxide; $\dot{V}O_2$, oxygen uptake.

in normal individuals because cardiac output normally depends most on venous return (ascending limb of the Frank–Starling curve). With left ventricular failure, however, the cardiac output is less dependent on cardiac preload (Starling's law of the heart) and more critically dependent on afterload. Thus, cardiac output and $\dot{V}O_2$ in patients with heart failure may vary with oscillations in vasomotor tone in the systemic arterial bed. The $\dot{V}E$ may oscillate secondary to the pulmonary blood flow oscillation if arterial Pa_{CO_2}, Pa_{O_2}, and H^+ oscillate as a result of cyclic changes in pulmonary blood flow–alveolar ventilation mismatch. It is thought that the increased production of catecholamines during heavy exercise obliterates the changing vasomotor tone stimulus from the central nervous system.

An oscillatory gas exchange pattern is characteristic of some patients with more severe forms of left ventricular failure[2] and is an independent predictor of mortality in this population.

Conclusion

This patient is presented to illustrate the oscillatory pattern in $\dot{V}O_2$ and other abnormalities that are common findings during exercise among patients with left ventricular failure.

REFERENCES

1. Wasserman K, Zhang Y-Y, Gitt A, et al. Lung function and exercise gas exchange in chronic heart failure. *Circulation*. 1997;96:2221-2227.
2. Ben-Dov I, Sietsema KE, Casaburi R, Wasserman K. Evidence that circulatory oscillations accompany ventilatory oscillations during exercise in patients with heart failure. *Am Rev Respir Dis*. 1992;145:776-781.

TABLE 10.18.3 Air Breathing

Time (min)	Work rate (W)	BP (mm Hg)	HR (min^{-1})	f (min^{-1})	$\dot{V}E$ (L/min BTPS)	$\dot{V}CO_2$ (L/min STPD)	$\dot{V}O_2$ (L/min STPD)	$\frac{\dot{V}O_2}{HR}$ (mL/beat)	R	pH	HCO_3^- (mEq/L)	PO_2, mm Hg ET	PO_2, mm Hg a	PO_2, mm Hg (A − a)	PCO_2, mm Hg ET	PCO_2, mm Hg a	PCO_2, mm Hg (a − ET)	$\frac{\dot{V}E}{\dot{V}CO_2}$	$\frac{\dot{V}E}{\dot{V}O_2}$	$\frac{V_D}{V_T}$
0.5	Rest		74	14	8.1	0.21	0.24	3.2	0.87			107			36			36	31	
1.0	Rest		79	21	13.2	0.27	0.30	3.7	0.91			118			29			45	41	
1.5	Rest		79	19	13.7	0.34	0.41	5.2	0.83			109			34			38	31	
2.0	Rest	102/66	78	20	13.5	0.28	0.30	3.8	0.94			118			29			45	42	
2.5	Rest		81	20	14.4	0.33	0.38	4.7	0.85			111			33			41	35	
3.0	Rest		81	15	10.2	0.22	0.22	2.8	0.99			120			29			43	42	
3.5	Unloaded		82	15	10.5	0.27	0.32	4.0	0.84			109			35			36	30	
4.0	Unloaded		85	15	13.0	0.30	0.31	3.6	0.97			118			29			41	40	
4.5	Unloaded		83	12	10.0	0.25	0.31	3.7	0.83			109			34			37	31	
5.0	Unloaded		82	16	7.8	0.16	0.18	2.2	0.86			115			31			44	38	
5.5	Unloaded		80	19	13.4	0.31	0.38	4.8	0.82			111			33			40	33	
6.0	Unloaded		79	19	9.9	0.23	0.28	3.5	0.83			109			34			39	33	
6.5	5		82	24	15.8	0.34	0.38	4.6	0.90			115			31			43	38	
7.0	10		86	21	13.6	0.32	0.38	4.4	0.85			111			34			39	33	
7.5	15		91	25	14.9	0.33	0.36	4.0	0.89			115			32			42	38	
8.0	20		90	22	17.3	0.42	0.48	5.3	0.88			112			33			39	34	
8.5	25		93	21	17.2	0.42	0.48	5.2	0.88			112			33			38	34	
9.0	30		95	20	17.6	0.46	0.50	5.3	0.91			112			33			36	33	
9.5	35		102	23	22.2	0.54	0.57	5.5	0.96			114			33			39	37	
10.0	40		105	25	23.6	0.59	0.58	5.5	1.02			115			33			38	39	
10.5	45		107	24	25.6	0.65	0.62	5.8	1.05			116			33			38	40	
11.0	50		112	25	30.2	0.75	0.68	6.1	1.10			118			32			39	43	
11.5	55		115	27	30.0	0.76	0.69	6.0	1.10			117			33			38	41	
12.0	60		119	29	37.0	0.89	0.75	6.3	1.18			120			31			40	47	
12.5	65		126	31	40.5	0.95	0.79	6.2	1.21			122			30			41	50	
13.0	70	120/85	130	31	40.7	0.98	0.81	6.2	1.21			121			31			40	48	
13.5	75		134	32	43.4	1.03	0.83	6.2	1.24			122			31			41	50	
14.0	Recovery		131	26	35.1	0.95	0.80	6.1	1.18			117			35			36	42	
14.5	Recovery		114	24	28.2	0.79	0.65	5.7	1.22			116			36			34	42	
15.0	Recovery		104	25	28.4	0.72	0.53	5.1	1.37			121			34			38	52	
15.5	Recovery	127/75	97	29	26.1	0.61	0.41	4.2	1.49			124			32			40	60	

Abbreviations: BP, blood pressure; BTPS, body temperature pressure saturated; f, frequency; HCO_3^-, bicarbonate; HR, heart rate; $P(A - a)O_2$, alveolar-arterial PO_2 difference; $P(a - ET)CO_2$, arterial-end-tidal PCO_2 difference; $PETCO_2$, end-tidal PCO_2; $PETO_2$, end-tidal PO_2; R, respiratory exchange ratio; STPD, standard temperature pressure dry; $\dot{V}CO_2$, carbon dioxide output; V_D/V_T, physiological dead space-tidal volume ratio; $\dot{V}E$, minute ventilation; $\dot{V}E/\dot{V}CO_2$, ventilatory equivalent for carbon dioxide; $\dot{V}E/\dot{V}O_2$, ventilatory equivalent for oxygen; $\dot{V}O_2$, oxygen uptake.

CASE 19

Chronic Heart Failure With Preserved Ejection Fraction (Exercise-Induced Pulmonary Venous Hypertension)

CLINICAL FINDINGS

This 67-year-old woman presented with 2 years of exertional dyspnea. She was previously quite physically active and first noted symptoms during her regular dance classes. She eventually discontinued dancing due to progressive dyspnea but continued to be as active as her symptoms would allow. By the time of this evaluation, she was short of breath walking on a level grade. She monitored her heart rate while active and reported that she was severely short of breath when her heart rate rose above 120 to 130 beats/min, requiring that she stop to rest and recover before resuming activities. She had no symptoms at rest. She was a lifelong nonsmoker and had a stable weight. Her medical history was significant for hypothyroidism well managed on levothyroxine, and osteoporosis treated with alendronate sodium. Physical examination and chest radiographs were normal. An electrocardiogram showed a right bundle branch block. An echocardiogram obtained 1 year prior to evaluation had shown normal left ventricular function (ejection fraction 65% to 70%), mild mitral regurgitation, and aortic sclerosis without stenosis. There was no evidence of pulmonary hypertension, but mild-to-moderate left ventricular diastolic dysfunction by transmitral flow indices was noted.

EXERCISE FINDINGS

The patient performed exercise on a cycle ergometer beginning with 3 minutes of pedaling at 60 rpm without added load, followed by continuous increase in work rate of 10 W/min until she stopped due to leg fatigue, marked dyspnea, and an inability to maintain a cadence above 40 rpm. There were no arrhythmias or ischemic changes on electrocardiogram. Exercise data are summarized in **Table 10.19.1** and shown in **Table 10.19.2** and **Figure 10.19.1**.

INTERPRETATION

Comments

The pulmonary function tests were normal. Demographic and respiratory function data are shown in **Table 10.19.1**.

Analysis

Despite her complaints of exercise intolerance and technical problems performing the test, this patient reached her predicted peak oxygen uptake ($\dot{V}O_2$) and peak heart rate, although she had a somewhat low anaerobic threshold (*AT*). The oxygen pulse at peak exercise was borderline low. These findings could be consistent with either below-average fitness or early cardiovascular dysfunction. There were no arrhythmias or repolarization abnormalities to suggest myocardial ischemia as the basis for these findings. With respect to ventilation, there was a large breathing reserve, indicating that she was not limited by lung mechanics. The ventilatory equivalents decreased normally during exercise; however, ventilatory equivalent for CO_2 ($\dot{V}E/\dot{V}CO_2$) at the *AT* remained above expected. This finding, along with the low *AT* and probably abnormal $\Delta\dot{V}O_2/\Delta WR$, raised the question of a pulmonary vascular abnormality. Diastolic dysfunction, which had been identified on her prior echocardiogram, could account for exertional symptoms, the abnormalities in the $\dot{V}O_2$ response to exercise, and the above-average $\dot{V}E/\dot{V}CO_2$. Based on this suspicion, a right heart catheterization was performed for measurement of central vascular pressures at rest and during exercise. At rest, pulmonary capillary wedge pressure was normal at 8 mm Hg. Immediately after a brief period of arm exercise (raising and lowering both arms holding a 1-L saline bag in each hand), however, the pulmonary capillary wedge pressure increased markedly to 24 mm Hg. The exercise-induced pulmonary venous hypertension was attributed to impaired diastolic relaxation of the left ventricle and was the probable basis of her exertional symptoms.

TABLE 10.19.1 Selected Respiratory Function Data

Measurement	Predicted	Measured
Age (y)		67
Sex		Female
Height (cm)		157
Weight (kg)		60
Hematocrit (%)		39.4
VC (L)	2.67	3.02
IC (L)	1.78	2.33
FEV_1 (L)	2.13	2.26
FEV_1/VC (%)	83	75
MVV (L/min)	98	90

Abbreviations: FEV_1, forced expiratory volume in 1 second; IC, inspiratory capacity; MVV, maximum voluntary ventilation; VC, vital capacity.

TABLE 10.19.2 Selected Exercise Data

Measurement	Predicted	Measured
Peak $\dot{V}O_2$ (L/min)	1.16	1.08
Maximum heart rate (beats/min)	153	157
Maximum O_2 pulse (mL/beat)	7.6	6.9
$\Delta\dot{V}O_2/\Delta WR$ (mL/min/W)	10.3	
AT (L/min)	>0.64	0.60
Blood pressure (mm Hg [rest, max])		107/90, 182/115
Maximum $\dot{V}E$ (L/min)		56
Exercise breathing reserve (L/min)	>15	34
$\dot{V}E/\dot{V}CO_2$ @ *AT* or lowest	30.4	33.2

Abbreviations: *AT*, anaerobic threshold; $\Delta\dot{V}O_2/\Delta WR$, change in $\dot{V}O_2$/change in work rate; O_2, oxygen; $\dot{V}E$, minute ventilation; $\dot{V}E/\dot{V}CO_2$, ventilatory equivalent for carbon dioxide; $\dot{V}O_2$, oxygen uptake.

Conclusion

Although this patient's peak $\dot{V}O_2$ was in the normal range, the *AT* was low. These findings, in the context of the clinical history, raised suspicion for early cardiovascular disease, arguably more likely than a low level of fitness. This was further supported by the finding of a borderline high $\dot{V}E/\dot{V}CO_2$ at the *AT*. Exercise-induced pulmonary venous hypertension due to heart failure with preserved ejection fraction was confirmed on follow-up cardiac catheterization.

TABLE 10.19.3 Air Breathing

Time (min)	Work rate (W)	BP (mm Hg)	HR (min^{-1})	f (min^{-1})	$\dot{V}E$ (L/min BTPS)	$\dot{V}CO_2$ (L/min STPD)	$\dot{V}O_2$ (L/min STPD)	$\frac{\dot{V}O_2}{HR}$ (mL/beat)	R	pH	HCO_3^- (mEq/L)	PO_2, mm Hg			PCO_2, mm Hg			$\frac{\dot{V}E}{\dot{V}CO_2}$	$\frac{\dot{V}E}{\dot{V}O_2}$	$\frac{VD}{VT}$
												ET	a	(A − a)	ET	a	(a − ET)			
0.5	Rest	107/90	103	19	12.0	0.30	0.29	2.8	1.04			117			32			40	41	
1.0	Rest		104	23	10.8	0.24	0.27	2.6	0.88			110			35			46	41	
1.5	Rest		95	20	13.2	0.36	0.38	4.0	0.95			113			34			37	35	
2.0	Rest		99	21	10.7	0.26	0.28	2.8	0.95			112			35			41	39	
2.5	Rest	130/89	102	21	11.8	0.30	0.32	3.1	0.95			113			34			39	37	
3.0	Rest		102	22	11.5	0.30	0.32	3.1	0.96			113			35			38	36	
3.5	Unloaded	130/89	104	24	14.8	0.38	0.41	4.0	0.92			110			36			39	36	
4.0	Unloaded		121	31	21.5	0.58	0.64	5.3	0.91			112			34			37	34	
4.5	Unloaded		126	32	20.4	0.57	0.60	4.8	0.95			112			35			36	34	
5.0	Unloaded		122	34	25.8	0.72	0.71	5.8	1.02			116			33			36	36	
5.5	Unloaded	154/96	127	29	22.2	0.66	0.68	5.4	0.97			112			36			33	32	
6.0	Unloaded		130	25	24.3	0.75	0.73	5.6	1.02			113			36			33	33	
6.5	3		122	32	23.6	0.68	0.64	5.3	1.05			115			35			35	37	
7.0	8		120	25	21.4	0.66	0.66	5.5	1.01			113			36			32	33	
7.5	13		121	26	21.0	0.62	0.63	5.2	0.98			111			36			34	33	
8.0	18		120	26	22.8	0.68	0.66	5.5	1.03			115			35			34	35	
8.5	23	156/107	126	23	17.7	0.55	0.60	4.8	0.91			107			38			32	29	
9.0	27		131	28	27.3	0.81	0.81	6.2	1.00			114			35			34	34	
9.5	33		133	29	29.4	0.87	0.79	6.0	1.10			118			33			34	37	
10.0	37		133	24	27.2	0.80	0.71	5.4	1.13			119			32			34	38	
10.5	42		135	30	30.3	0.86	0.78	5.7	1.11			119			31			35	39	
11.0	48	161/115	140	29	28.5	0.85	0.80	5.7	1.07			117			33			34	36	
11.5	52		142	26	32.4	0.96	0.85	6.0	1.12			119			32			34	38	
12.0	57		145	25	32.6	1.00	0.89	6.2	1.12			118			33			33	37	
12.5	62		147	39	37.4	1.03	0.88	6.0	1.17			122			30			36	43	
13.0	67		150	39	42.3	1.16	1.01	6.7	1.15			121			30			36	42	
13.5	72	182/85	153	30	40.4	1.15	0.95	6.2	1.22			122			31			35	43	
14.0	77		155	38	48.3	1.26	1.06	6.8	1.19			123			29			38	46	
14.5	82		157	48	55.8	1.34	1.08	6.9	1.24			126			27			42	52	
15.0	Recovery	182/85	156	58	56.0	1.21	0.97	6.2	1.25			128			25			46	58	
15.5	Recovery		154	43	44.2	1.04	0.81	5.3	1.29			127			26			42	55	
16.0	Recovery		147	47	47.0	0.93	0.60	4.1	1.55			133			22			51	78	
16.5	Recovery		131	51	39.1	0.69	0.45	3.4	1.53			134			21			57	87	

Abbreviations: BP, blood pressure; BTPS, body temperature pressure saturated; f, frequency; HCO_3^-, bicarbonate; HR, heart rate; $P(A - a)O_2$, alveolar-arterial PO_2 difference; $P(a - ET)CO_2$, arterial-end-tidal PCO_2 difference; $PETCO_2$, end-tidal PCO_2; $PETO_2$, end-tidal PO_2; R, respiratory exchange ratio; STPD, standard temperature pressure dry; $\dot{V}CO_2$, carbon dioxide output; VD/VT, physiological dead space-tidal volume ratio; $\dot{V}E$, minute ventilation; $\dot{V}E/\dot{V}CO_2$, ventilatory equivalent for carbon dioxide; $\dot{V}E/\dot{V}O_2$, ventilatory equivalent for oxygen; $\dot{V}O_2$, oxygen uptake.

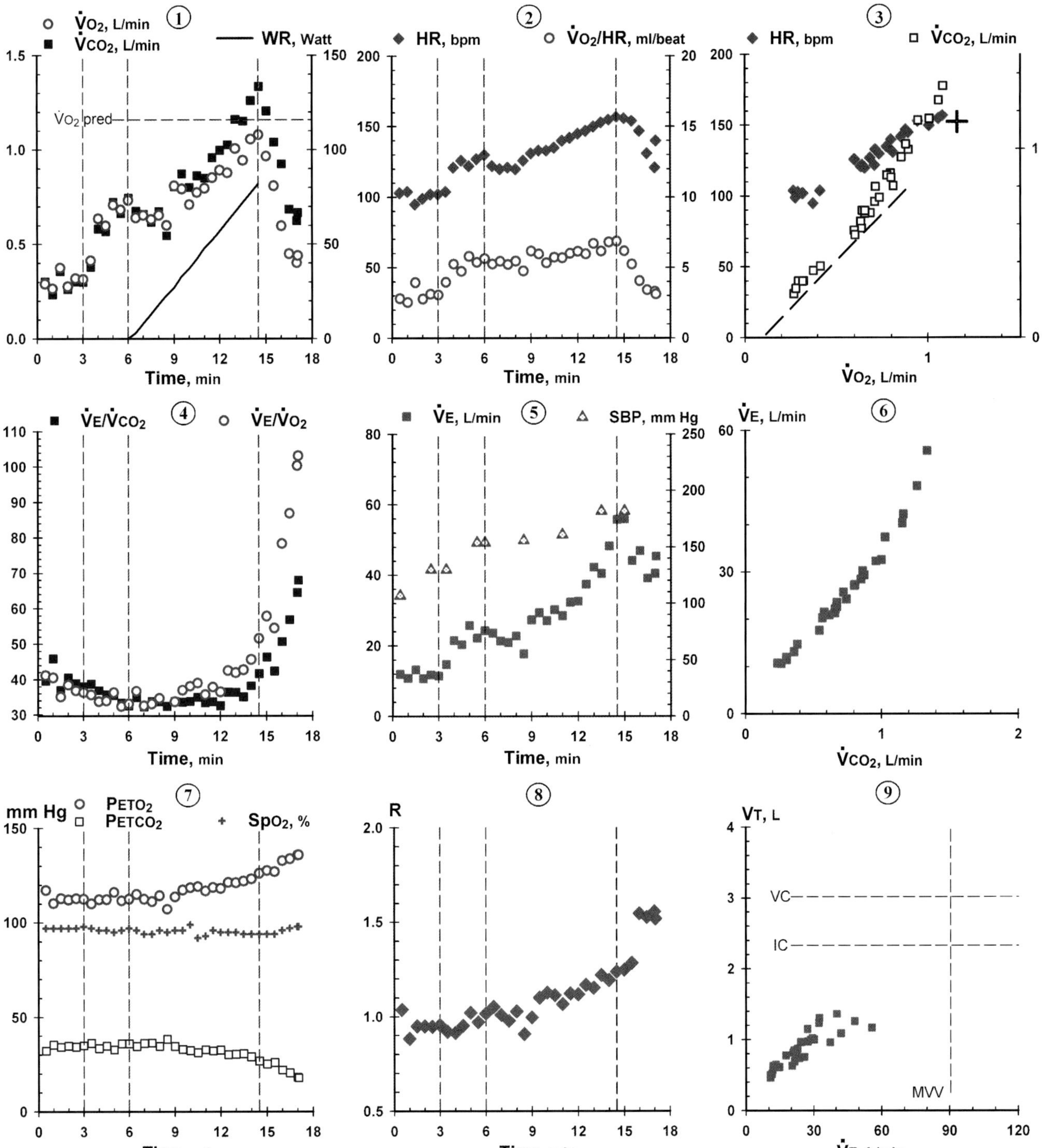

FIGURE 10.19.1. Vertical dashed lines in the panels in the left and middle columns indicate, from left to right, the beginning of unloaded cycling, start of increasing work rate (WR) at 10 W/min, and start of recovery. In **panel 1**, the increase in WR (right y-axis) is plotted with a scale of 100 W to 1 L of oxygen uptake ($\dot{V}O_2$) (left y-axis) such that WR is plotted parallel to a $\dot{V}O_2$ slope of 10 mL/min/W. In **panel 3**, carbon dioxide output ($\dot{V}CO_2$) (right y-axis) is plotted as a function of $\dot{V}O_2$ (x-axis) with identical scales so that the diagonal dashed line has a slope of 1 (45°). The $\dot{V}CO_2$ increasing more steeply than $\dot{V}O_2$ defines carbon dioxide (CO_2) derived from bicarbonate buffer, as long as ventilatory equivalent for CO_2 ($\dot{V}E/\dot{V}CO_2$) (**panel 4**) is not increasing and end-tidal PCO_2 ($PETCO_2$) (**panel 7**) is not decreasing, simultaneously. The black + symbol in **panel 3** indicates predicted peak values of heart rate (HR) (left y-axis) and $\dot{V}O_2$ for this individual. Abbreviations: IC, inspiratory capacity; MVV, maximum voluntary ventilation; $PETO_2$, end-tidal PO_2; R, respiratory exchange ratio; SBP, systolic blood pressure; VC, vital capacity; $\dot{V}E$, minute ventilation; $\dot{V}E/\dot{V}O_2$, ventilatory equivalent for oxygen; V_T, tidal volume.

CASE 20

Gas Exchange Evidence of Myocardial Ischemia

A healthy 65-year-old man (previously described as Case 9 of this chapter) enjoyed hiking in the mountains and had normal exercise findings with above-average exercise capacity. Seven years later, at age 72, he still enjoyed hiking, although he no longer did so at high altitude. He had returned to his cardiologist complaining that he had fatigue with exertion and could no longer keep pace when walking on level grade with his female companion. An exercise echocardiogram study was done without gas exchange measurements and reportedly showed ST-segment depression in the left precordial leads and a run of three premature ventricular contractions near the end of the test. The estimated pulmonary artery pressure during exercise by echocardiography was 70 mm Hg. Because the patient's overall exercise tolerance was good and the echocardiogram was otherwise normal, the electrocardiogram (ECG) changes were discounted as a "false-positive ECG response." However, because of the suggestion of possible pulmonary hypertension, further studies were done. Pulmonary function tests and a ventilation-perfusion ($\dot{V}/\dot{Q}$) scan revealed no abnormalities to account for the echocardiogram findings, and the patient was referred for cardiopulmonary exercise testing for further evaluation.

TABLE 10.20.1 Selected Respiratory Function Data

Measurement	Predicted	Measured
Age (y)		72
Sex		Male
Height (cm)		184
Weight (kg)	83	84
Hematocrit (%)		47
VC (L)	4.61	4.39
IC (L)	3.08	3.82
FEV_1 (L)	3.29	2.94
FEV_1/VC (%)	75	68
MVV (L/min)	134	130
D_{LCO} (mL/mm Hg/min)	27.0	19.2

Abbreviations: D_{LCO}, diffusing capacity of the lung for carbon monoxide; FEV_1, forced expiratory volume in 1 second; IC, inspiratory capacity; MVV, maximum voluntary ventilation; VC, vital capacity.

EXERCISE FINDINGS

The patient was tested using the same protocol as that used in his initial evaluation at age 65, including arterial blood sampling and blood pressure measurements. After 3 minutes of rest and 3 minutes of unloaded cycling, work rate increased by 20 W/min until symptomatic maximum. On ECG monitoring, there was ST-segment depression in leads aVF, III, and V_5, first noted at a heart rate of around 125 beats/min and progressing to a maximum of 2 mm at a heart rate of 137 beats/min. He had no ectopic beats or chest pain and the repolarization abnormalities resolved in the recovery period.

INTERPRETATION

Comments

Resting respiratory function studies were normal (**Table 10.20.1**).

Analysis

Compared to the study performed at age 65, the predicted peak $\dot{V}O_2$ for this patient had decreased by 0.2 L/min, but his measured peak $\dot{V}O_2$ had decreased by 0.7 L/min, still within normal limits (**Tables 10.20.2** and **10.20.3** and **Figs. 10.20.1** and **10.20.2**). However, the abnormal ECG findings were suggestive of exercise-induced myocardial ischemia, which was consistent with a decrease in the slope of $\Delta\dot{V}O_2/\Delta WR$ and steepening of the heart rate–$\dot{V}O_2$ relationship. Corresponding to this, the rise in oxygen (O_2) pulse flattens and even decreases with the onset of myocardial ischemia. This patient probably developed significant myocardial ischemia starting at a $\dot{V}O_2$ about 1.4 L/min and a heart rate of about 110 beats/min (the point at which the heart rate–$\dot{V}O_2$ relationship began to steepen and O_2 pulse no longer increased). Because $C(a - \bar{v})O_2$ increases with increasing $\dot{V}O_2$, the constant O_2 pulse could indicate that the stroke volume was decreasing above the work rate at which the O_2 pulse became constant.

As to consideration of pulmonary vascular disease, his V_D/V_T, $P(A - a)O_2$, and $P(a - ET)CO_2$ were normal, indicating that he did not have functionally significant impairment in either breathing mechanics or pulmonary gas exchange, making pulmonary vascular disease unlikely, despite the echocardiogram findings.

Conclusion

This man's aerobic function decreased more rapidly than predicted with age despite his maintenance of an active lifestyle. He had physiologic and ECG evidence of myocardial ischemia during exercise above a $\dot{V}O_2$ of 1.4 L/min and heart rate of 110 beats/min. He did not have evidence of significant pulmonary vascular disease, based on the blood gas and V_D/V_T data during exercise and the normal $\dot{V}E/\dot{V}CO_2$ at the anaerobic threshold.

TABLE 10.20.2 Selected Exercise Data

Measurement	Predicted	Measured
Peak $\dot{V}O_2$ (L/min)	2.02	1.99
Maximum heart rate (beats/min)	148	152
Maximum O_2 pulse (mL/beat)	13.6	13.1
$\Delta\dot{V}O_2/\Delta WR$ (mL/min/W)	10.3	8.6
AT (L/min)	>0.95	1.4
Blood pressure (mm Hg [rest, max])		110/60, 200/75
Maximum $\dot{V}E$ (L/min)		85
Exercise breathing reserve (L/min)	>15	46
$\dot{V}E/\dot{V}CO_2$ @ *AT* or lowest	28.2	30.9
PaO_2 (mm Hg [rest, max ex])		102, 105
$P(A - a)O_2$ (mm Hg [rest, max ex])		15, 21
$PaCO_2$ (mm Hg [rest, max ex])		37, 34
$P(a - ET)CO_2$ (mm Hg [rest, max ex])		5, −2
VD/VT (rest, heavy ex)		0.53, 0.18
HCO_3^- (mEq/L [rest, 2-min recov])		24, 20

Abbreviations: *AT*, anaerobic threshold; $\Delta\dot{V}O_2/\Delta WR$, change in $\dot{V}O_2$/change in work rate; ex, exercise; HCO_3^-, bicarbonate; O_2, oxygen; $P(A - a)O_2$, alveolar-arterial PO_2 difference; $P(a - ET)CO_2$, arterial-end-tidal PCO_2 difference; recov, recovery; VD/VT, physiological dead space-tidal volume ratio; $\dot{V}E$, minute ventilation; $\dot{V}E/\dot{V}CO_2$, ventilatory equivalent for carbon dioxide; $\dot{V}O_2$, oxygen uptake.

TABLE 10.20.3 Air Breathing

Time (min)	Work rate (W)	BP (mm Hg)	HR (min^{-1})	f (min^{-1})	$\dot{V}E$ (L/min BTPS)	$\dot{V}CO_2$ (L/min STPD)	$\dot{V}O_2$ (L/min STPD)	$\frac{\dot{V}O_2}{HR}$ (mL/beat)	R	pH	HCO_3^- (mEq/L)	PO_2, mm Hg ET	PO_2, mm Hg a	PO_2, mm Hg (A − a)	PCO_2, mm Hg ET	PCO_2, mm Hg a	PCO_2, mm Hg (a − ET)	$\frac{\dot{V}E}{\dot{V}CO_2}$	$\frac{\dot{V}E}{\dot{V}O_2}$	$\frac{V_D}{V_T}$
0.5	Rest		65	24	15.9	0.26	0.21	3.3	1.20			139			29			55	67	
1.0	Rest		65	24	12.9	0.23	0.22	3.4	1.03			134			32			48	50	
1.5	Rest	110/60	65	18	10.6	0.20	0.21	3.3	0.93	7.42	24	130	102	9	33	37	4	46	43	0.43
2.0	Rest		63	21	17.1	0.37	0.39	6.2	0.96			131			33			42	40	
2.5	Rest		72	26	19.3	0.39	0.37	5.2	1.04			136			31			45	46	
3.0	Rest		67	23	18.4	0.35	0.32	4.8	1.08			136			30			48	52	
3.5	Unloaded		75	24	22.0	0.49	0.49	6.5	1.00			132			31			41	41	
4.0	Unloaded		77	17	21.1	0.53	0.51	6.6	1.04			133			33			38	39	
4.5	Unloaded		70	17	24.2	0.58	0.55	7.8	1.06			132			32			39	42	
5.0	Unloaded		69	18	17.3	0.41	0.41	5.9	1.01			133			33			39	39	
5.5	Unloaded		68	21	21.8	0.50	0.46	6.8	1.08			132			31			41	44	
6.0	Unloaded	130/65	66	19	16.2	0.34	0.34	5.2	0.99	7.40	22	135	103	11	33	36	3	44	43	0.41
6.5	7		65	25	19.4	0.40	0.40	6.2	1.00			133			32			43	44	
7.0	18		70	31	19.6	0.39	0.42	6.0	0.93			130			33			44	41	
7.5	29		75	22	21.7	0.54	0.60	8.0	0.90			127			34			37	33	
8.0	39	105/40	76	20	20.5	0.50	0.52	6.8	0.97	7.47	23	129	110	7	34	32	−2	38	37	0.27
8.5	50		77	19	22.5	0.59	0.68	8.8	0.87			125			35			36	31	
9.0	62	105/40	84	20	27.4	0.75	0.85	10.2	0.88	7.41	24	123	97	10	36	39	3	35	30	0.34
9.5	71		86	22	32.4	0.88	0.92	10.7	0.95			127			35			35	33	
10.0	80	120/50	89	23	33.7	0.97	1.07	12.0	0.90	7.42	24	123	103	7	37	37	0	33	30	0.28
10.5	90		99	26	43.9	1.18	1.18	11.9	1.01			129			34			36	36	
11.0	100	115/40	94	23	45.7	1.29	1.31	13.9	0.98	7.41	24	127	99	12	36	39	3	34	34	0.34
11.5	109		101	23	45.5	1.35	1.41	13.9	0.96			125			37			33	31	
12.0	120	135/50	108	25	50.0	1.46	1.47	13.6	0.99	7.43	24	126	107	6	36	37	1	33	33	0.28
12.5	129		111	27	53.9	1.60	1.57	14.1	1.02			127			36			32	33	
13.0	141	145/55	114	25	55.8	1.70	1.65	14.4	1.03	7.42	23	126	106	9	37	36	−1	32	33	0.23
13.5	149		118	24	54.7	1.71	1.63	13.8	1.04			126			38			31	32	
14.0	162	150/55	123	27	61.7	1.91	1.81	14.7	1.05	7.40	22	126	106	9	38	36	−2	31	33	0.23
14.5	169		130	30	71.3	2.10	1.84	14.2	1.14			130			36			33	38	
15.0	177	175/65	136	32	71.2	2.14	1.89	13.9	1.14	7.40	21	129	103	15	37	35	−2	32	36	0.22
15.5	192		143	32	79.1	2.34	1.95	13.7	1.20			132			36			33	39	
16.0	201	180/65	150	32	81.1	2.34	1.94	12.9	1.21	7.40	21	132	100	21	35	34	−1	34	41	0.24
16.5	Recovery		154	29	74.5	2.31	1.95	12.7	1.18	7.39	20	129	105	15	39	34	−5	31	37	0.18
17.0	Recovery		138	29	74.7	2.13	1.47	10.7	1.44			136			36			34	49	
17.5	Recovery		121	30	61.2	1.62	0.97	8.0	1.67			141			34			36	61	
18.0	Recovery		108	32	47.3	1.17	0.70	6.5	1.66			142			32			38	64	
18.5	Recovery		101	27	44.1	1.07	0.67	6.6	1.60			142			31			40	63	

Abbreviations: BP, blood pressure; BTPS, body temperature pressure saturated; f, frequency; HCO_3^-, bicarbonate; HR, heart rate; $P(A - a)O_2$, alveolar-arterial PO_2 difference; $P(a - ET)CO_2$, arterial-end-tidal PCO_2 difference; $PETCO_2$, end-tidal PCO_2; $PETO_2$, end-tidal PO_2; R, respiratory exchange ratio; STPD, standard temperature pressure dry; $\dot{V}CO_2$, carbon dioxide output; V_D/V_T, physiological dead space-tidal volume ratio; $\dot{V}e$, minute ventilation; $\dot{V}E/\dot{V}CO_2$, ventilatory equivalent for carbon dioxide; $\dot{V}E/\dot{V}O_2$, ventilatory equivalent for oxygen; $\dot{V}O_2$, oxygen uptake.

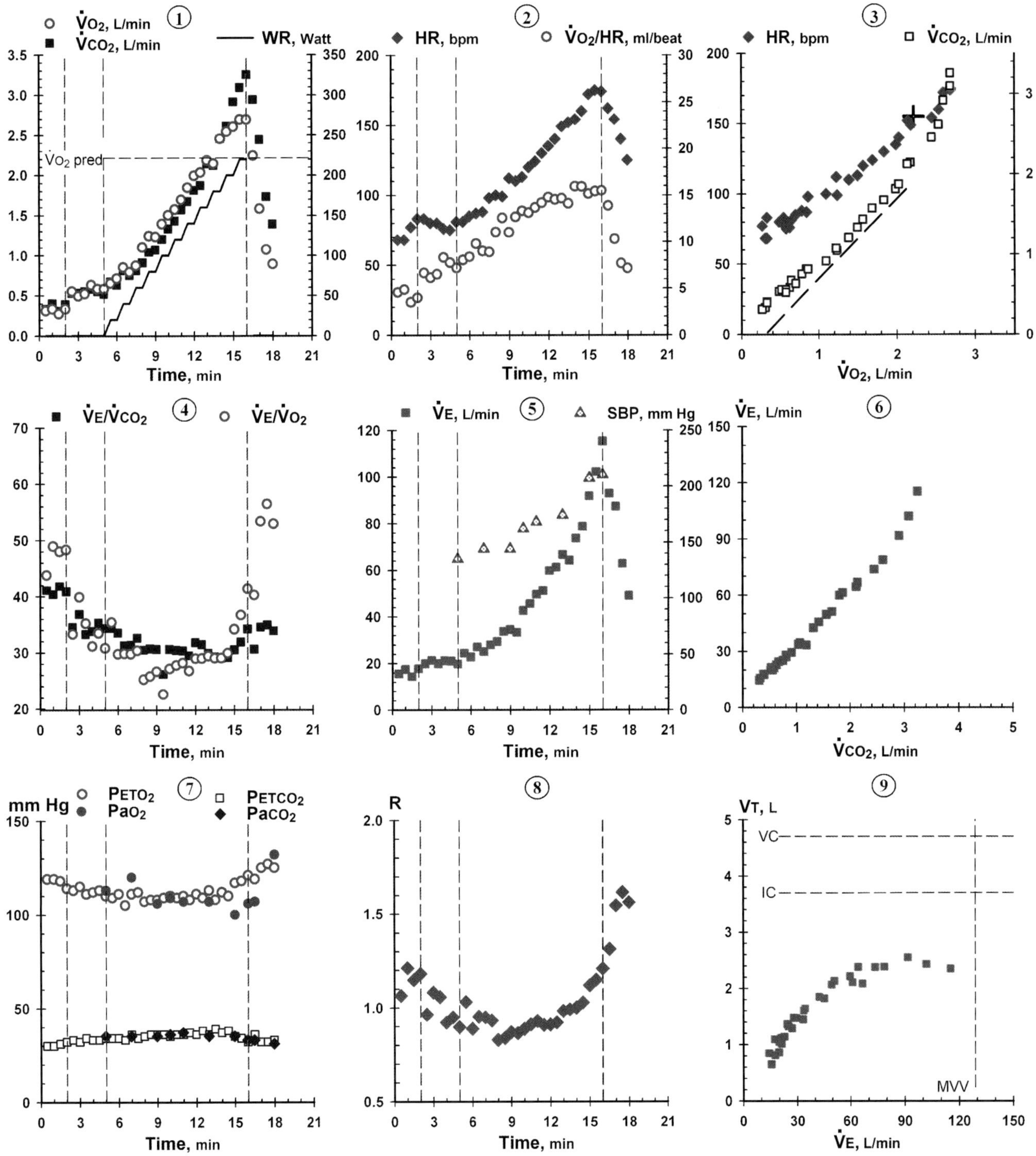

FIGURE 10.20.1. Test performed at age 65. Vertical dashed lines in the panels in the left and middle columns indicate, from left to right, the beginning of unloaded cycling, start of increasing work rate (WR) at 20 W/min, and start of recovery. In **panel 1**, the increase in WR (right y-axis) is plotted with a scale of 100 W to 1 L of oxygen uptake ($\dot{V}O_2$) (left y-axis) such that WR is plotted parallel to a $\dot{V}O_2$ slope of 10 mL/min/W. In **panel 3**, carbon dioxide output $\dot{V}CO_2$ (right y-axis) is plotted as a function of $\dot{V}O_2$ (x-axis) with identical scales so that the diagonal dashed line has a slope of 1 (45°). The $\dot{V}CO_2$ increasing more steeply than $\dot{V}O_2$ defines carbon dioxide (CO_2) derived from bicarbonate buffer, as long as ventilatory equivalent for CO_2 ($\dot{V}E/\dot{V}CO_2$) (**panel 4**) is not increasing and end-tidal PCO_2 ($PETCO_2$) (**panel 7**) is not decreasing, simultaneously. The black + symbol in **panel 3** indicates predicted values of heart rate (HR) (left y-axis) and $\dot{V}O_2$ for this individual. Abbreviations: IC, inspiratory capacity; MVV, maximum voluntary ventilation; $PETO_2$, end-tidal PO_2; R, respiratory exchange ratio; SBP, systolic blood pressure; VC, vital capacity; $\dot{V}E$, minute ventilation; $\dot{V}E/\dot{V}O_2$, ventilatory equivalent for oxygen; VT, tidal volume.

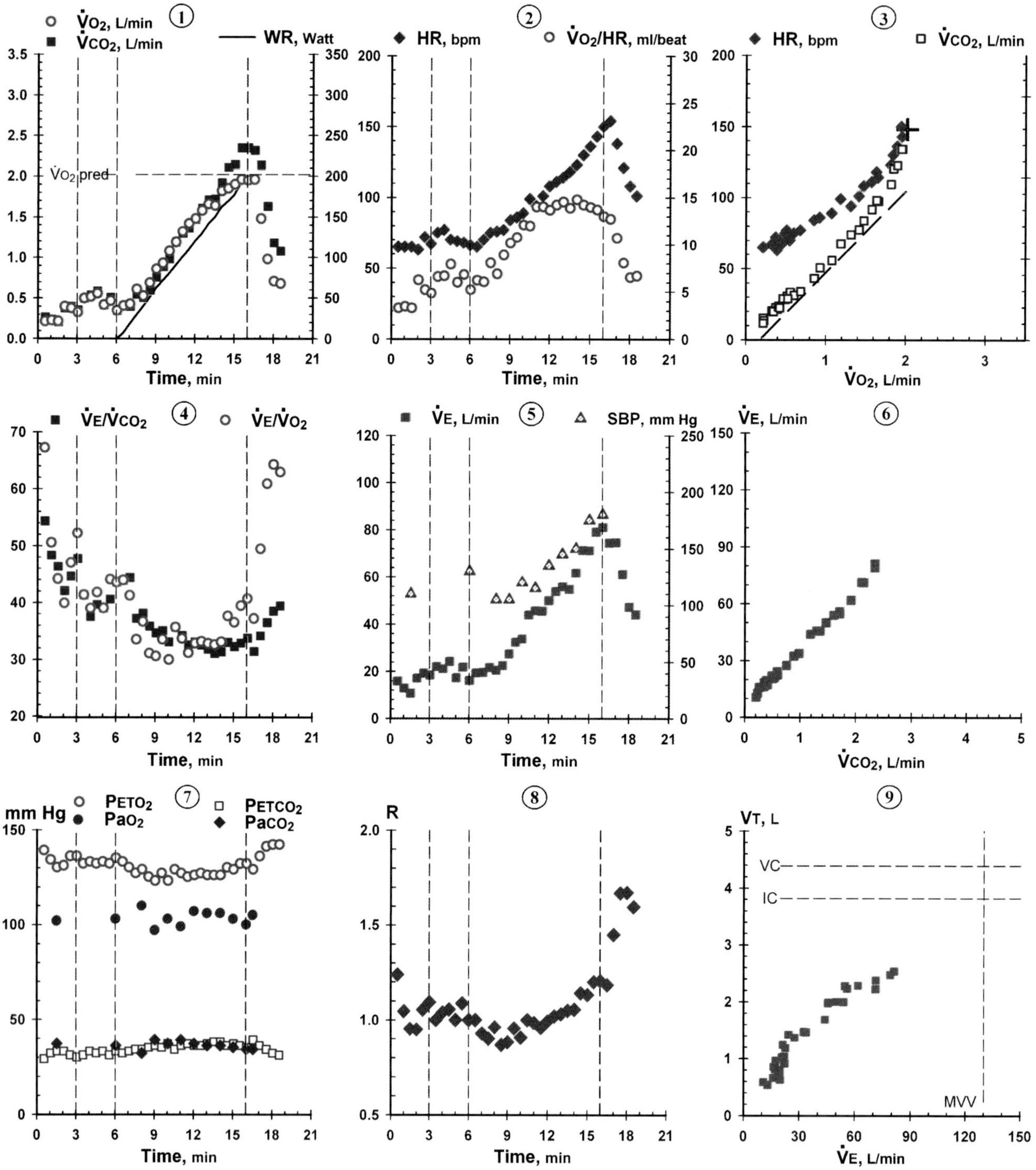

FIGURE 10.20.2. Test performed at age 72. Vertical dashed lines in the panels in the left and middle columns indicate, from left to right, the beginning of unloaded cycling, start of increasing work rate (WR) at 20 W/min, and start of recovery. In **panel 1**, the increase in WR (right y-axis) is plotted with a scale of 100 W to 1 L of oxygen uptake ($\dot{V}O_2$) (left y-axis) such that WR is plotted parallel to a $\dot{V}O_2$ slope of 10 mL/min/W. In **panel 3**, carbon dioxide output ($\dot{V}CO_2$) (right y-axis) is plotted as a function of $\dot{V}O_2$ (x-axis) with identical scales so that the diagonal dashed line has a slope of 1 (45°). The $\dot{V}CO_2$ increasing more steeply than $\dot{V}O_2$ defines carbon dioxide (CO_2) derived from bicarbonate buffer, as long as ventilatory equivalent for CO_2 ($\dot{V}E/\dot{V}CO_2$) (**panel 4**) is not increasing and end-tidal PCO_2 ($PETCO_2$) (**panel 7**) is not decreasing, simultaneously. The black + symbol in **panel 3** indicates predicted values of heart rate (HR) (left y-axis) and $\dot{V}O_2$ for this individual. Abbreviations: IC, inspiratory capacity; MVV, maximum voluntary ventilation; $PETO_2$, end-tidal PO_2; R, respiratory exchange ratio; SBP, systolic blood pressure; VC, vital capacity; $\dot{V}E$, minute ventilation; $\dot{V}E/\dot{V}O_2$, ventilatory equivalent for oxygen; VT, tidal volume.

CASE 21

Claudication: Gas Exchange Findings in Peripheral Arterial Disease

CLINICAL FINDINGS

A 65-year-old, cigarette-smoking man was evaluated as part of a research study related to coronary artery calcification. He had been overweight and diabetic for approximately 6 years. He walked regularly for exercise but had been limited in his speed of walking for approximately 5 years due to pain in his thighs and calves, especially on the right side. He had some cough and sputum production for a decade. He denied chest pain, shortness of breath, wheezing, edema, or skin problems. Pulses could not be palpated in the legs except for a faint right femoral artery pulse. The patient had no edema; skin warmth and color were good. Demographic and respiratory function data are shown in **Table 10.21.1**.

EXERCISE FINDINGS

The patient performed exercise on a cycle ergometer. He pedaled at 60 rpm without an added load for 3 minutes. The work rate was then increased 15 W/min to tolerance. Heart rate and rhythm were continuously monitored; 12-lead electrocardiograms (ECGs) were obtained during rest, exercise, and recovery. Blood pressure was measured with a sphygmomanometer. The patient appeared to give an excellent effort and stopped exercise because of bilateral thigh and calf pain, similar to his usual symptoms. He denied chest pain or discomfort during or after the study. The ECGs showed occasional premature ventricular contractions both at rest and during exercise but were otherwise normal. No abnormal ST segments or T waves were noted before, during, or after exercise. Exercise data are summarized in **Table 10.21.2** and shown in **Table 10.21.3** and graphically in **Figure 10.21.1**.

INTERPRETATION

Comments

The patient has mild, asymptomatic airway obstruction; diabetes mellitus; obesity; and clinical evidence of peripheral arterial disease. Of note, his cardiac scan had shown no coronary artery calcification.

Analysis

Peak oxygen uptake ($\dot{V}O_2$) and the anaerobic threshold were reduced, indicating a problem with oxygen (O_2) flow of some kind. Normal breathing reserve and normal $\dot{V}E/\dot{V}CO_2$ at the anaerobic threshold makes a pulmonary problem unlikely and would be consistent with stopping exercise because of leg pain/claudication. The patient's limiting symptoms were typical of claudication due to peripheral arterial disease. Confirmatory findings include exercise-induced systemic hypertension, low $\Delta\dot{V}O_2/\Delta WR$, low $\Delta\dot{V}CO_2/\Delta WR$, and high heart rate reserve. The absence of ECG changes indicative of myocardial ischemia, despite the exaggerated

TABLE 10.21.1 Selected Respiratory Function Data

Measurement	Predicted	Measured
Age (y)		65
Sex		Male
Height (cm)		170
Weight (kg)	74	88
Hematocrit (%)		42
VC (L)	3.43	3.65
IC (L)	2.44	3.20
FEV_1 (L)	2.74	2.48
FEV_1/VC (%)	79	68
MVV (L/min)	110	92

Abbreviations: FEV_1, forced expiratory volume in 1 second; IC, inspiratory capacity; MVV, maximum voluntary ventilation; VC, vital capacity.

TABLE 10.21.2 Selected Exercise Data

Measurement	Predicted	Measured
Peak $\dot{V}O_2$ (L/min)	2.04	1.06
Maximum heart rate (beats/min)	155	135
Maximum O_2 pulse (mL/beat)	13.2	7.9
$\Delta\dot{V}O_2/\Delta WR$ (mL/min/W)	10.3	6.9
AT (L/min)	>0.95	0.8
Blood pressure (mm Hg [rest, max])		164/88, 278/110
Maximum $\dot{V}E$ (L/min)		33
Exercise breathing reserve (L/min)	>15	59
$\dot{V}E/\dot{V}CO_2$ @ *AT* or lowest	28.7	25.2

Abbreviations: *AT*, anaerobic threshold; $\Delta\dot{V}O_2/\Delta WR$, change in $\dot{V}O_2$/change in work rate; O_2, oxygen; $\dot{V}E$, minute ventilation; $\dot{V}E/\dot{V}CO_2$, ventilatory equivalent for CO_2; $\dot{V}O_2$, oxygen uptake.

TABLE 10.21.3 Air Breathing

Time (min)	Work rate (W)	BP (mm Hg)	HR (min^{-1})	f (min^{-1})	$\dot{V}E$ (L/min BTPS)	$\dot{V}CO_2$ (L/min STPD)	$\dot{V}O_2$ (L/min STPD)	$\frac{\dot{V}O_2}{HR}$ (mL/beat)	R	pH	HCO_3^- (mEq/L)	PO_2, mm Hg ET	PO_2, mm Hg a	PO_2, mm Hg (A − a)	PCO_2, mm Hg ET	PCO_2, mm Hg a	PCO_2, mm Hg (a − ET)	$\frac{\dot{V}E}{\dot{V}CO_2}$	$\frac{\dot{V}E}{\dot{V}O_2}$	$\frac{VD}{VT}$
0	Rest	164/88																		
0.5	Rest		95	22	12.8	0.36	0.36	3.8	1.00			106			38			30	30	
1.0	Rest	188/80	93	21	11.1	0.32	0.36	3.9	0.89			110			41			29	26	
1.5	Rest		95	19	11.2	0.32	0.35	3.7	0.91			108			38			30	27	
2.0	Rest	218/80	94	20	10.6	0.30	0.33	3.5	0.91			105			39			30	27	
2.5	Rest		97	22	8.0	0.20	0.23	2.4	0.87			105			40			31	27	
3.0	Rest	198/82	98	20	10.3	0.29	0.35	3.6	0.83			105			40			30	25	
3.5	Unloaded		110	20	14.1	0.46	0.52	4.7	0.88			104			41			27	24	
4.0	Unloaded	214/100	110	20	13.5	0.44	0.54	4.9	0.81			100			42			27	22	
4.5	Unloaded		113	20	13.4	0.39	0.49	4.3	0.80			108			37			30	24	
5.0	Unloaded	239/96	112	20	17.3	0.62	0.72	6.4	0.86			100			43			25	22	
5.5	Unloaded		113	19	17.8	0.63	0.72	6.4	0.88			101			44			26	22	
6.0	Unloaded	254/90	111	22	17.1	0.59	0.68	6.1	0.87			101			44			26	22	
6.5	7.5		115	20	19.2	0.69	0.75	6.5	0.92			102			44			25	23	
7.0	15	255/100	117	20	19.2	0.70	0.76	6.5	0.92			103			43			25	23	
7.5	22.5		119	22	20.6	0.74	0.79	6.6	0.94			103			43			25	24	
8.0	30	245/114	121	19	23.7	0.88	0.94	7.8	0.94			103			43			25	23	
8.5	37.5		122	21	23.7	0.88	0.91	7.5	0.97			103			44			25	24	
9.0	45	252/110	125	21	24.7	0.91	0.94	7.5	0.97			103			44			25	24	
9.5	52.5		127	19	24.8	0.92	0.92	7.2	1.00			105			44			25	25	
10.0	60	256/114	130	21	29.7	1.08	1.04	8.0	1.04			107			43			26	27	
10.5	67.5		131	21	32.7	1.15	1.07	8.2	1.07			109			42			27	29	
11.0	75	278/110	135	24	32.6	1.13	1.06	7.9	1.07			111			42			27	29	
11.5	Recovery		126	21	28.4	1.02	0.95	7.5	1.07			108			44			26	26	
12.0	Recovery	269/90	124	20	26.5	0.95	0.86	6.9	1.10			109			44			26	29	
12.5	Recovery		119	26	22.6	0.71	0.63	5.3	1.13			115			40			29	32	
13.0	Recovery	241/86	113	23	21.2	0.72	0.64	5.7	1.13			111			42			27	30	

Abbreviations: BP, blood pressure; BTPS, body temperature pressure saturated; f, frequency; HCO_3^-, bicarbonate; HR, heart rate; $P(A - a)O_2$, alveolar-arterial PO_2 difference; $P(a - ET)CO_2$, arterial-end-tidal PCO_2 difference; $PETCO_2$, end-tidal PCO_2; $PETO_2$, end-tidal PO_2; R, respiratory exchange ratio; STPD, standard temperature pressure dry; $\dot{V}CO_2$, carbon dioxide output; VD/VT, physiological dead space-tidal volume ratio; $\dot{V}E$, minute ventilation; $\dot{V}E/\dot{V}CO_2$, ventilatory equivalent for carbon dioxide; $\dot{V}E/\dot{V}O_2$, ventilatory equivalent for oxygen; $\dot{V}O_2$, oxygen uptake.

exercise blood pressure response, suggests that the coronary vessels are relatively uninvolved.

Using the flowcharts (Chapter 9) to reach a tentative diagnosis, low peak $\dot{V}O_2$ and low anaerobic threshold would lead to Flowchart 4. Here, the high breathing reserve (Branch Point 4.1) and normal $\dot{V}E/\dot{V}CO_2$ at the anaerobic threshold (Branch Point 4.3) lead to the category of "O_2 flow problem of nonpulmonary origin." Given a normal hematocrit (Branch Point 4.4), this indicates a cardiovascular disorder with a low nonchanging O_2 pulse (Branch Point 4.6) most consistent with peripheral arterial disease, as likely expected.

Conclusion

This patient has typical symptoms of peripheral arterial disease reflecting impaired O_2 supply to exercising muscle. Not surprisingly, this impairment is reflected in abnormalities of $\dot{V}O_2$. In addition, in contrast to other cardiovascular diseases, the increase in $\dot{V}CO_2$ relative to work rate was reduced as well ($\Delta\dot{V}CO_2/\Delta WR$), similar to the lower $\Delta\dot{V}O_2/\Delta WR$. This may be a reflection of diffuse lower extremity vascular disease constraining leg blood flow so severely that it constituted an abnormally low proportion of the total circulation perfusing the exercising muscles. Consequently, in the venous return, less CO_2 appeared as well as less O_2 extracted. This would be consistent with the patient's bilateral symptoms affecting both proximal and distal muscle groups. Although many patients with peripheral arterial disease are limited by associated coronary artery disease, this does not seem to be true for this man.

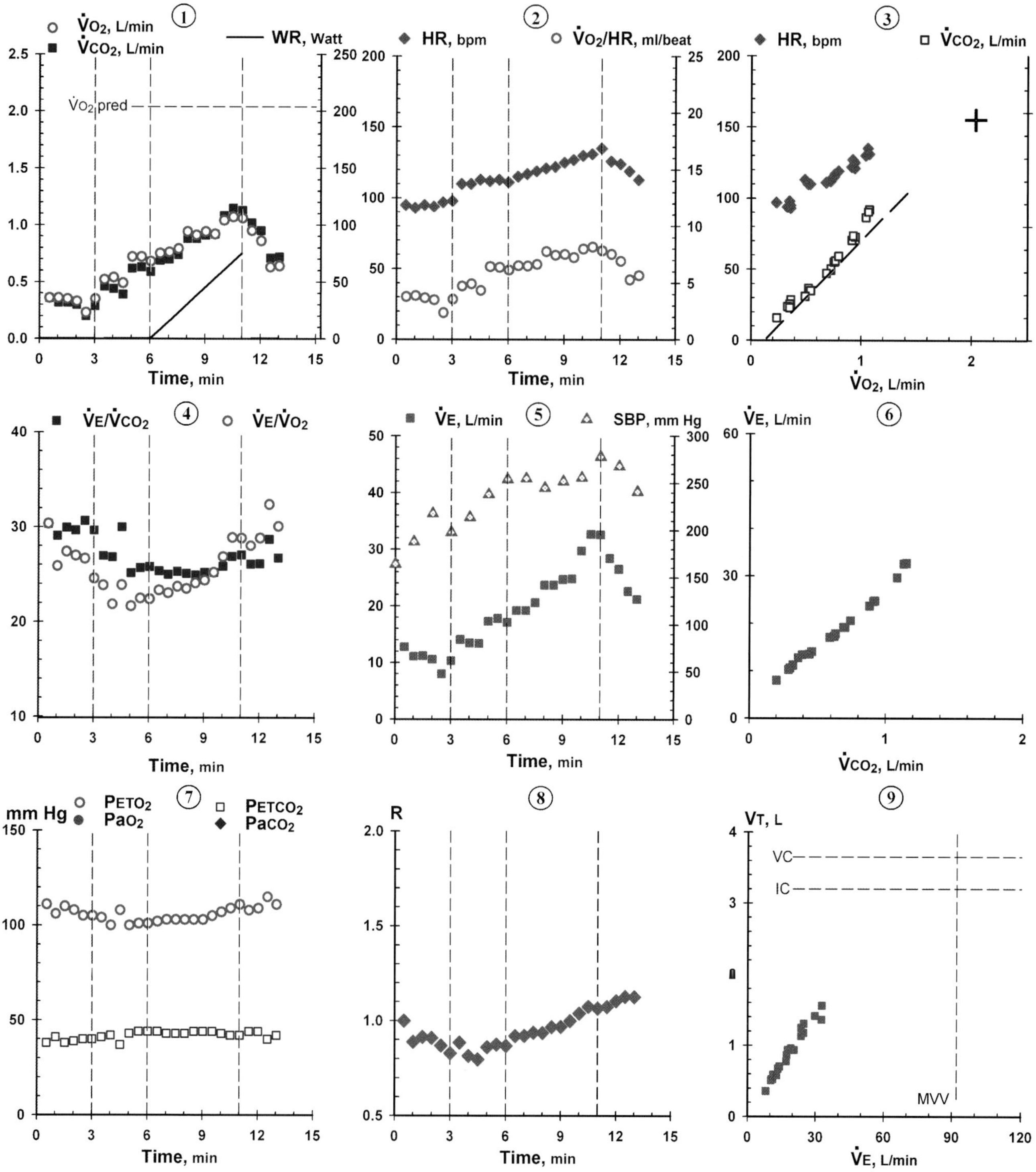

FIGURE 10.21.1. Vertical dashed lines in the panels in the left and middle columns indicate, from left to right, the beginning of unloaded cycling, start of increasing work rate (WR) at 15 W/min, and start of recovery. In **panel 1**, the increase in WR (right y-axis) is plotted with a scale of 100 W to 1 L of oxygen uptake ($\dot{V}O_2$) (left y-axis) such that WR is plotted parallel to a $\dot{V}O_2$ slope of 10 mL/min/W. In **panel 3**, carbon dioxide output ($\dot{V}CO_2$) (right y-axis) is plotted as a function of $\dot{V}O_2$ (x-axis) with identical scales so that the diagonal dashed line has a slope of 1 (45°). The $\dot{V}CO_2$ increasing more steeply than $\dot{V}O_2$ defines carbon dioxide (CO_2) derived from bicarbonate buffer, as long as ventilatory equivalent for CO_2 ($\dot{V}E/\dot{V}CO_2$) (**panel 4**) is not increasing and P_{CO_2} (P_{ETCO_2}) (**panel 7**) is not decreasing, simultaneously. The black + symbol in **panel 3** indicates predicted values of heart rate (HR) (left y-axis) and $\dot{V}O_2$ for this individual. Abbreviations: IC, inspiratory capacity; MVV, maximum voluntary ventilation; P_{ETO_2}, end-tidal P_{O_2}; R, respiratory exchange ratio; SBP, systolic blood pressure; VC, vital capacity; $\dot{V}E$, minute ventilation; $\dot{V}E/\dot{V}O_2$, ventilatory equivalent for oxygen; V_T, tidal volume.

CASE 22

Exertional Chest Pain With Gas Exchange Evidence of Myocardial Ischemia

To view this case please access the eBook bundled with this text. Instructions are located on the inside front cover.

CASE 23

Exercise-Induced Myocardial Ischemia

CLINICAL FINDINGS

A 61-year-old, retired man complained of breathing difficulties that he could not quantify or describe well. He denied shortness of breath but stated that he stopped using stairs because of a "peculiar feeling in his chest." He also complained of a stabbing substernal and right flank pain not associated with exertion or stress and of neck pain associated with movement of the head attributed to degenerative cervical spine arthritis. He had never smoked cigarettes. Examination revealed psoriasis and normal blood pressure, heart sounds, and peripheral pulses. He had electrocardiogram (ECG) findings suggestive of left ventricular hypertrophy.

TABLE 10.23.1 Selected Respiratory Function Data

Measurement	Predicted	Measured
Age (y)		61
Sex		Male
Height (cm)		176
Weight (kg)	78	70
Hematocrit (%)		39
VC (L)	4.23	3.95
IC (L)	2.82	2.60
TLC (L)	6.47	6.01
FEV_1 (L)	3.32	3.25
FEV_1/VC (%)	78	82
MVV (L/min)	137	121
D_{LCO} (mL/mm Hg/min)	25.5	33.3

Abbreviations: D_{LCO}, diffusing capacity of lung for carbon monoxide; FEV_1, forced expiratory volume in 1 second; IC, inspiratory capacity; MVV, maximum voluntary ventilation; TLC, total lung capacity; VC, vital capacity.

TABLE 10.23.2 Selected Exercise Data

Measurement	Predicted	Measured
Peak $\dot{V}O_2$ (L/min)	2.08	1.90
Maximum heart rate (beats/min)	159	180
Maximum O_2 pulse (mL/beat)	13.1	10.6
$\Delta\dot{V}O_2/\Delta WR$ (mL/min/W)	10.3	7.5
AT (L/min)	>0.91	1.1
Blood pressure (mm Hg [rest, max])		144/75, 246/108
Maximum $\dot{V}E$ (L/min)		86
Exercise breathing reserve (L/min)	>15	35
$\dot{V}E/\dot{V}CO_2$ @ *AT* or lowest	28.1	27.1
PaO_2 (mm Hg [rest, max ex])		87, 103
$P(A - a)O_2$ (mm Hg [rest, max ex])		5, 15
$PaCO_2$ (mm Hg [rest, max ex])		41, 40
$P(a - ET)CO_2$ (mm Hg [rest, max ex])		2, −1
V_D/V_T (rest, heavy ex)		0.48, 0.24
HCO_3^- (mEq/L [rest, 2-min recov])		26, 20

Abbreviations: *AT*, anaerobic threshold; $\Delta\dot{V}O_2/\Delta WR$, change in $\dot{V}O_2$/change in work rate; ex, exercise; HCO_3^-, bicarbonate; O_2, oxygen; $P(A - a)O_2$, alveolar-arterial PO_2 difference; $P(a - ET)CO_2$, arterial-end-tidal PCO_2 difference; recov, recovery; V_D/V_T, physiological dead space-tidal volume ratio; $\dot{V}E$, minute ventilation; $\dot{V}E/\dot{V}CO_2$, ventilatory equivalent for carbon dioxide; $\dot{V}O_2$, oxygen uptake.

TABLE 10.23.3 Air Breathing

Time (min)	Work rate (W)	BP (mm Hg)	HR (min^{-1})	f (min^{-1})	$\dot{V}E$ (L/min BTPS)	$\dot{V}CO_2$ (L/min STPD)	$\dot{V}O_2$ (L/min STPD)	$\frac{\dot{V}O_2}{HR}$ (mL/beat)	R	pH	HCO_3^- (mEq/L)	PO_2, mm Hg			PCO_2, mm Hg			$\frac{\dot{V}E}{\dot{V}CO_2}$	$\frac{\dot{V}E}{\dot{V}O_2}$	$\frac{VD}{VT}$
												ET	a	(A − a)	ET	a	(a − ET)			
	Rest	144/75								7.48	26		106			36				
0.5	Rest		66	20	7.4	0.12	0.17	2.6	0.71			104			37			48	34	
1.0	Rest		67	16	9.1	0.19	0.27	4.0	0.70			101			37			41	29	
1.5	Rest		68	19	11.9	0.28	0.42	6.2	0.67			93			41			37	24	
2.0	Rest		70	14	7.6	0.13	0.20	2.9	0.65	7.44	27	37	87	5	39	41	2	49	32	0.48
2.5	Rest		70	15	7.9	0.13	0.17	2.4	0.76			101			37			51	39	
3.0	Rest	150/75	70	15	13.2	0.28	0.40	5.7	0.70			91			42			43	30	
3.5	Unloaded		84	14	8.5	0.23	0.35	4.2	0.66			90			43			32	21	
4.0	Unloaded		88	17	13.2	0.34	0.52	5.9	0.65			90			42			35	23	
4.5	Unloaded		85	21	15.4	0.37	0.58	6.8	0.64			91			42			37	23	
5.0	Unloaded		86	17	14.2	0.39	0.59	6.9	0.66			89			43			33	22	
5.5	Unloaded		89	15	17.7	0.55	0.80	9.0	0.69			86			44			30	21	
6.0	Unloaded	171/78	88	17	15.0	0.43	0.63	7.2	0.68	7.41	29	90	83	4	45	46	1	32	22	0.37
6.5	20		95	20	17.2	0.54	0.76	8.0	0.71			91			45			29	20	
7.0	20		93	19	17.9	0.52	0.68	7.3	0.76			95			44			31	24	
7.5	40		95	15	17.6	0.60	0.78	8.2	0.77			93			46			27	21	
8.0	40	192/78	102	17	24.3	0.85	1.03	10.1	0.83	7.40	29	94	83	11	45	48	3	27	22	0.31
8.5	60		104	17	26.0	0.90	1.02	9.8	0.88			97			46			27	24	
9.0	60		105	22	26.9	0.92	1.05	10.0	0.88			97			46			27	24	
9.5	80		122	32	34.2	1.14	1.18	9.7	0.97			102			46			28	27	
10.0	80	216/87	127	25	36.1	1.26	1.29	10.2	0.98	7.40	28	101	94	9	47	46	−1	27	26	0.29
10.5	100		132	27	40.8	1.39	1.31	9.9	1.06			107			44			28	29	
11.0	100		136	28	37.4	1.35	1.30	9.6	1.04			102			48			26	27	
11.5	120		144	29	51.4	1.78	1.58	11.0	1.13			107			45			27	31	
12.0	120	231/96	150	33	50.8	1.77	1.50	10.0	1.18	7.39	27	108	98	12	46	45	−1	27	32	0.28
12.5	140		156	30	58.1	2.04	1.69	10.8	1.21			110			44			27	33	
13.0	140		168	34	63.3	2.13	1.74	10.4	1.22			111			44			28	35	
13.5	160		172	35	72.8	2.38	1.84	10.7	1.29			113			43			29	38	
14.0	160	234/99	178	34	76.0	2.53	1.90	10.7	1.33	7.39	24	117	103	15	41	40	−1	29	38	0.24
14.5	180	246/108	180	47	85.6	2.62	1.85	10.3	1.42			118			41			31	44	
15.0	Recovery		171	35	71.3	2.46	1.90	11.1	1.29			114			43			28	36	
15.5	Recovery		160	36	66.6	2.15	1.45	9.1	1.48			118			41			30	44	
16.0	Recovery		143	20	47.5	1.53	1.03	7.2	1.49			116			43			30	44	
16.5	Recovery	192/78	135	29	49.6	1.51	1.00	7.4	1.51	7.30	20	117	107	13	42	41	−1	31	47	0.31

Abbreviations: BP, blood pressure; BTPS, body temperature pressure saturated; f, frequency; HCO_3^-, bicarbonate; HR, heart rate; $P(A - a)O_2$, alveolar-arterial PO_2 difference; $P(a - ET)CO_2$, arterial-end-tidal PCO_2 difference; $PETCO_2$, end-tidal PCO_2; $PETO_2$, end-tidal PO_2; R, respiratory exchange ratio; STPD, standard temperature pressure dry; $\dot{V}CO_2$, carbon dioxide output; VD/VT, physiological dead space-tidal volume ratio; $\dot{V}E$, minute ventilation; $\dot{V}E/\dot{V}CO_2$, ventilatory equivalent for carbon dioxide; $\dot{V}E/\dot{V}O_2$, ventilatory equivalent for oxygen; $\dot{V}O_2$, oxygen uptake.

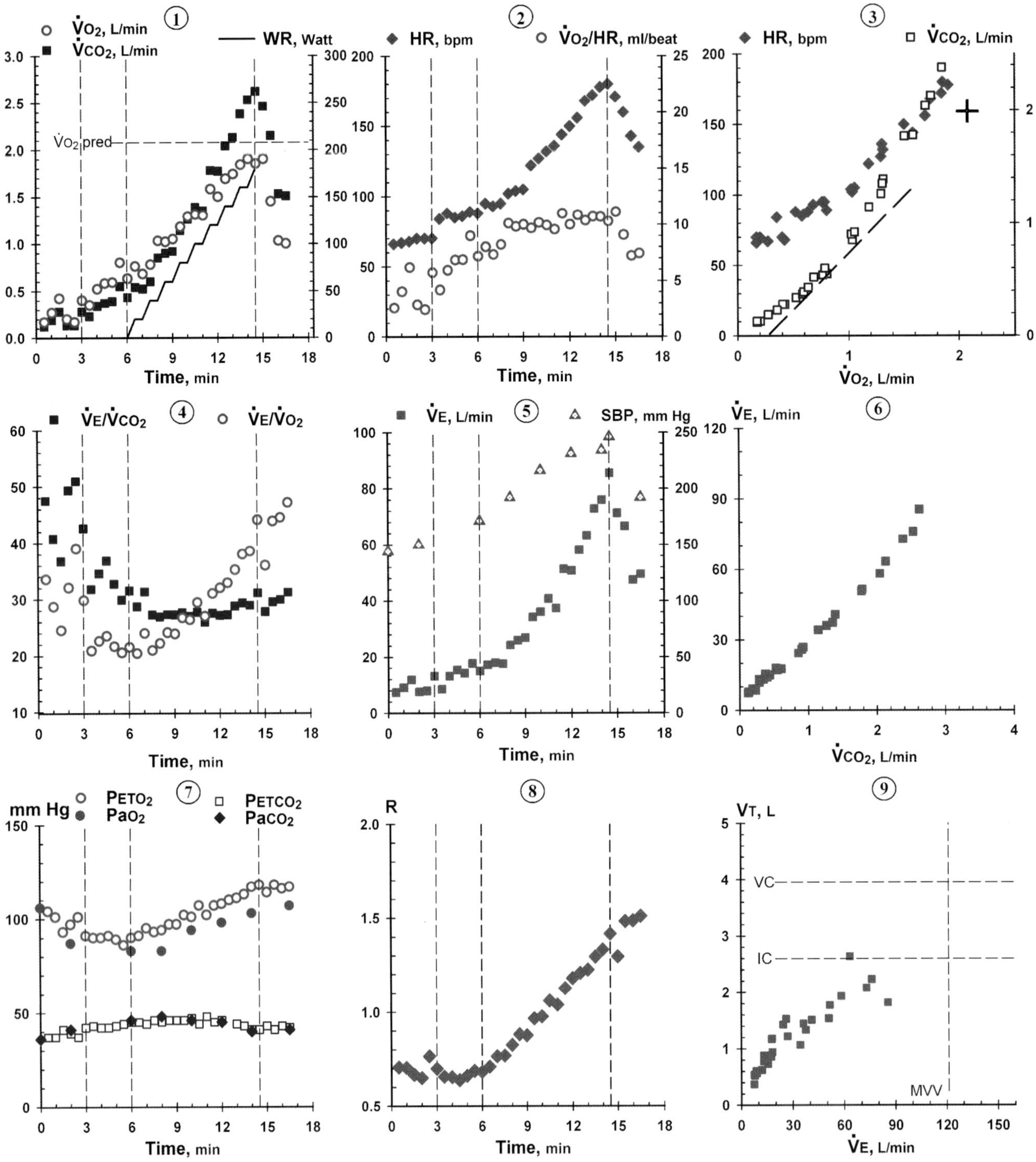

FIGURE 10.23.1. Vertical dashed lines in the panels in the left and middle columns indicate, from left to right, the beginning of unloaded cycling, start of increasing work rate (WR) at 20 W/min, and start of recovery. In **panel 1**, the increase in WR (right y-axis) is plotted with a scale of 100 W to 1 L of oxygen uptake ($\dot{V}O_2$) (left y-axis) such that WR is plotted parallel to a $\dot{V}O_2$ slope of 10 mL/min/W. In **panel 3**, carbon dioxide output ($\dot{V}CO_2$) (right y-axis) is plotted as a function of $\dot{V}O_2$ (x-axis) with identical scales so that the diagonal dashed line has a slope of 1 (45°). The $\dot{V}CO_2$ increasing more steeply than $\dot{V}O_2$ defines carbon dioxide (CO_2) derived from bicarbonate buffer, as long as ventilatory equivalent for CO_2 ($\dot{V}E/\dot{V}CO_2$) (**panel 4**) is not increasing and end-tidal PCO_2 ($PETCO_2$) (**panel 7**) is not decreasing, simultaneously. The black + symbol in **panel 3** indicates predicted values of heart rate (HR) (left y-axis) and $\dot{V}O_2$ for the subject. Abbreviations: IC, inspiratory capacity; MVV, maximum voluntary ventilation; $PETO_2$, end-tidal PO_2; R, respiratory exchange ratio; SBP, systolic blood pressure; VC, vital capacity; $\dot{V}E$, minute ventilation; $\dot{V}E/\dot{V}O_2$, ventilatory equivalent for oxygen; V_T, tidal volume.

EXERCISE FINDINGS

The patient performed exercise on a cycle ergometer. He pedaled at 60 rpm without added load for 3 minutes. The work rate was then increased 20 W/min to his symptom-limited maximum. Arterial blood was sampled every second minute, and intra-arterial blood pressure was recorded from a percutaneously placed brachial artery catheter. The patient stopped exercise because of shortness of breath and tired thighs. He denied chest pain. The ECG developed slight ST-segment depression in leads II, III, aVF, V_5, and V_6 at 120 W of exercise (heart rate 150), which progressed to maximum ST depression of 5 mm at the cessation of exercise (180 W). Rare, unifocal, premature ventricular contractions were noted. The ECG returned to baseline after 14 minutes of recovery.

INTERPRETATION

Comments

Resting respiratory function and ECG were normal (**Table 10.23.1**). Exercise data are summarized in **Table 10.23.2** and shown in **Table 10.23.3** and graphically in **Figure 10.23.1**.

Analysis

This patient complained of chest discomfort that might be considered atypical of myocardial ischemia but demonstrated significant ECG changes (ST-segment depression) during exercise. Despite normal peak oxygen uptake ($\dot{V}O_2$) and anaerobic threshold (*AT*), he showed features suggestive of acute onset of left ventricular dysfunction coincident with ST-segment depressions, including flattening of $\Delta\dot{V}O_2/\Delta WR$ and O_2 pulse that plateaued during the last stages of exercise. Findings that support relatively normal cardiovascular response to exercise prior to onset of presumed ischemia include the normal *AT*, normal $\dot{V}E/\dot{V}CO_2$ at the *AT*, and normal slope of $\dot{V}E$ versus $\dot{V}CO_2$. He was not ventilatory limited.

The flowcharts (Chapter 9) lead initially to Flowchart 2 (normal peak $\dot{V}O_2$ and *AT*), where the next branch point includes the ECG. Because the ECG is abnormal and consistent with ischemia, the likely diagnosis is myocardial ischemia.

Conclusion

This patient with atypical chest pain experienced exercise-induced myocardial ischemia. The low O_2 pulse, steep heart rate–$\dot{V}O_2$ relationship, and reduced $\Delta\dot{V}O_2/\Delta WR$ indicate that the ST-segment changes were significant—that is, they were consistent with the development of myocardial dysfunction due to exercise-induced ischemia.

CASE 24

Myocardial Ischemia With Diffuse Distal Coronary Artery Disease

CLINICAL FINDINGS

A 47-year-old asymptomatic man was referred for cardiopulmonary exercise testing because of a strong family history of coronary artery disease and the finding of coronary artery calcification on an ultrafast computed tomographic cardiac scan. Physical examination, chest radiographs, and resting electrocardiograms (ECGs) were normal.

EXERCISE FINDINGS

The patient performed exercise on a cycle ergometer. He pedaled at 60 rpm without an added load for 3 minutes. The work rate was then increased 25 W/min to tolerance. Heart rate and rhythm were continuously monitored; 12-lead ECGs were obtained during rest, exercise, and recovery. Blood pressure was measured with a sphygmomanometer and oxygen (O_2) saturation with pulse oximeter. The patient appeared to give an excellent effort and stopped exercise because of leg fatigue. He denied chest pain during or after the study. The ECGs showed progressive down sloping ST-segment depression in leads II, III, aVF, and V_3 to V_6 after 150 W of exercise, which reached approximately 3 mm in leads II and V_4 at the cessation of exercise. These changes resolved by 5 minutes of recovery; there was no ectopy.

TABLE 10.24.1 Selected Respiratory Function Data

Measurement	Predicted	Measured
Age (y)		47
Sex		Male
Height (cm)		175
Weight (kg)	78	64
Hematocrit (%)		42
VC (L)	4.78	5.04
IC (L)	3.19	3.70
FEV_1 (L)	3.91	4.03
FEV_1/VC (%)	81	80
MVV (L/min)	153	180

Abbreviations: FEV_1, forced expiratory volume in 1 second; IC, inspiratory capacity; MVV, maximum voluntary ventilation; VC, vital capacity.

INTERPRETATION

Comments

Spirometry was normal (**Table 10.24.1**). Exercise data are summarized in **Table 10.24.2** and shown in **Table 10.24.3** and graphically in **Figure 10.24.1**.

Analysis

Flowchart analysis (Chapter 9): Referring to Flowchart 1, peak oxygen uptake ($\dot{V}O_2$) was reduced, but the anaerobic threshold was within normal limits. Proceeding next to Flowchart 3, the high breathing reserve (Branch Point 3.1) and abnormal ECG that developed during exercise (Branch Point 3.3) lead to the diagnosis of myocardial ischemia. The low O_2 pulse and failure of $\dot{V}O_2$ and O_2 pulse to rise appropriately for the last 2.5 minutes of exercise indicate that an O_2 delivery problem developed at that time. The constant O_2 pulse indicates that the product of the arterial–mixed venous O_2 content difference and stroke volume reached its maximum value prematurely. This constant value might reflect a decreasing stroke volume while arteriovenous difference is increasing.

TABLE 10.24.2 Selected Exercise Data

Measurement	Predicted	Measured
Peak $\dot{V}O_2$ (L/min)	2.35	1.88
Maximum heart rate (beats/min)	173	181
Maximum O_2 pulse (mL/beat)	13.6	10.4
$\Delta\dot{V}O_2/\Delta WR$ (mL/min/W)	10.3	6.4
AT (L/min)	>1.01	1.3
Blood pressure (mm Hg [rest, max])		125/82, 160/90
Maximum $\dot{V}E$ (L/min)		78
Exercise breathing reserve (L/min)	>15	102
$\dot{V}E/\dot{V}CO_2$ @ *AT* or lowest	26.6	19.6
O_2 saturation, oximeter (rest, max ex)		99, 95

Abbreviations: *AT*, anaerobic threshold; $\Delta\dot{V}O_2/\Delta WR$, change in $\dot{V}O_2$/change in work rate; ex, exercise; O_2, oxygen; $\dot{V}E$, minute ventilation; $\dot{V}E/\dot{V}CO_2$, ventilatory equivalent for carbon dioxide; $\dot{V}O_2$, oxygen uptake.

TABLE 10.24.3 Air Breathing

Time (min)	Work rate (W)	BP (mm Hg)	HR (min^{-1})	f (min^{-1})	$\dot{V}E$ (L/min BTPS)	$\dot{V}CO_2$ (L/min STPD)	$\dot{V}O_2$ (L/min STPD)	$\frac{\dot{V}O_2}{HR}$ (mL/beat)	R	pH	HCO_3^- (mEq/L)	PO_2, mm Hg ET	a	(A − a)	PCO_2, mm Hg ET	a	(a − ET)	$\frac{\dot{V}E}{\dot{V}CO_2}$	$\frac{\dot{V}E}{\dot{V}O_2}$	$\frac{VD}{VT}$
	Rest	125/82																		
0.5	Rest		86	11	5.4	0.15	0.21	2.4	0.71			89			44			30	21	
1.0	Rest		89	14	3.4	0.06	0.09	1.0	0.67			86			46			37	25	
1.5	Rest		80	10	6.0	0.20	0.29	3.6	0.69			83			47			26	18	
2.0	Rest	110/60	80	8	3.6	0.09	0.13	1.6	0.69			90			46			32	22	
2.5	Rest		81	12	4.6	0.14	0.19	2.3	0.74			91			46			26	19	
3.0	Rest		98	8	4.6	0.14	0.16	1.6	0.88			89			47			28	25	
3.5	Unloaded		105	12	9.2	0.36	0.43	4.1	0.84			87			49			23	19	
4.0	Unloaded		103	12	9.5	0.35	0.46	4.5	0.76			89			48			24	18	
4.5	Unloaded		103	14	11.0	0.41	0.51	5.0	0.80			90			48			24	19	
5.0	Unloaded		105	12	11.9	0.47	0.56	5.3	0.84			90			48			23	19	
5.5	Unloaded		105	17	9.7	0.37	0.45	4.3	0.82			87			51			22	18	
6.0	Unloaded	120/82	106	13	12.2	0.48	0.56	5.3	0.86			93			49			23	20	
6.5	25		106	13	8.0	0.32	0.37	3.5	0.86			89			52			22	19	
7.0	20		109	12	13.6	0.55	0.59	5.4	0.93			95			50			23	21	
7.5	50		114	12	14.1	0.61	0.63	5.5	0.97			92			51			21	21	
8.0	50	130/90	119	13	16.3	0.70	0.75	6.3	0.93			93			51			22	20	
8.5	75		122	14	17.3	0.77	0.84	6.9	0.92			92			52			21	19	
9.0	75		131	14	18.7	0.88	0.88	6.7	1.00			92			53			20	20	
9.5	100		137	16	22.2	1.05	1.09	8.0	0.96			92			54			20	19	
10.0	100	130/90	140	15	23.3	1.13	1.19	8.5	0.95			91			55			19	19	
10.5	125		145	17	26.3	1.20	1.24	8.6	0.97			94			55			21	20	
11.0	125		152	17	29.5	1.47	1.35	8.9	1.09			95			56			19	21	
11.5	150		158	18	32.8	1.66	1.50	9.5	1.11			95			56			19	21	
12.0	150	145/90	163	19	37.7	1.88	1.56	9.6	1.21			100			55			19	23	
12.5	175		167	22	44.8	2.13	1.73	10.4	1.23			101			55			20	25	
13.0	175		169	22	45.1	2.23	1.76	10.4	1.27			102			56			19	25	
13.5	200		173	22	53.4	2.52	1.85	10.7	1.36			103			54			20	28	
14.0	200	160/90	176	26	62.5	2.76	1.87	10.6	1.48			111			49			22	32	
14.5	225		181	32	77.5	3.00	1.87	10.3	1.60			113			48			25	40	
15.0	225		181	31	77.8	2.95	1.88	10.4	1.57			113			47			25	40	
15.5	Recovery		167	22	53.4	2.37	1.62	9.7	1.46			110			50			22	32	
16.0	Recovery		152	21	40.2	1.71	1.06	7.0	1.61			114			48			22	36	
16.5	Recovery		140	20	39.1	1.57	0.92	6.6	1.71			116			47			24	41	
17.0	Recovery	160/75	131	17	28.9	1.10	0.59	4.5	1.86			120			44			25	47	

Abbreviations: BP, blood pressure; BTPS, body temperature pressure saturated; f, frequency; HCO_3^-, bicarbonate; HR, heart rate; $P(A - a)O_2$, alveolar-arterial PO_2 difference; $P(a - ET)CO_2$, arterial-end-tidal PCO_2 difference; $PETCO_2$, end-tidal PCO_2; $PETO_2$, end-tidal PO_2; R, respiratory exchange ratio; STPD, standard temperature pressure dry; $\dot{V}CO_2$, carbon dioxide output; VD/VT, physiological dead space–tidal volume ratio; $\dot{V}E$, minute ventilation; $\dot{V}E/\dot{V}CO_2$, ventilatory equivalent for carbon dioxide; $\dot{V}E/\dot{V}O_2$, ventilatory equivalent for oxygen; $\dot{V}O_2$, oxygen uptake.

Conclusion

The abrupt change in a previously normal pattern of utilization of O_2 (normal $\Delta\dot{V}O_2/\Delta WR$) after which $\dot{V}O_2$ fails to keep pace with increasing work rate suggests exercise-induced myocardial ischemia. The combination of O_2 delivery abnormalities (which imply a failure of cardiac output to increase appropriately for the work rate) and ECG findings consistent with myocardial ischemia suggests that the patient had functionally important coronary artery disease. Follow-up coronary angiograms showed diffuse distal coronary artery disease not amenable to bypass. The patient was treated medically.

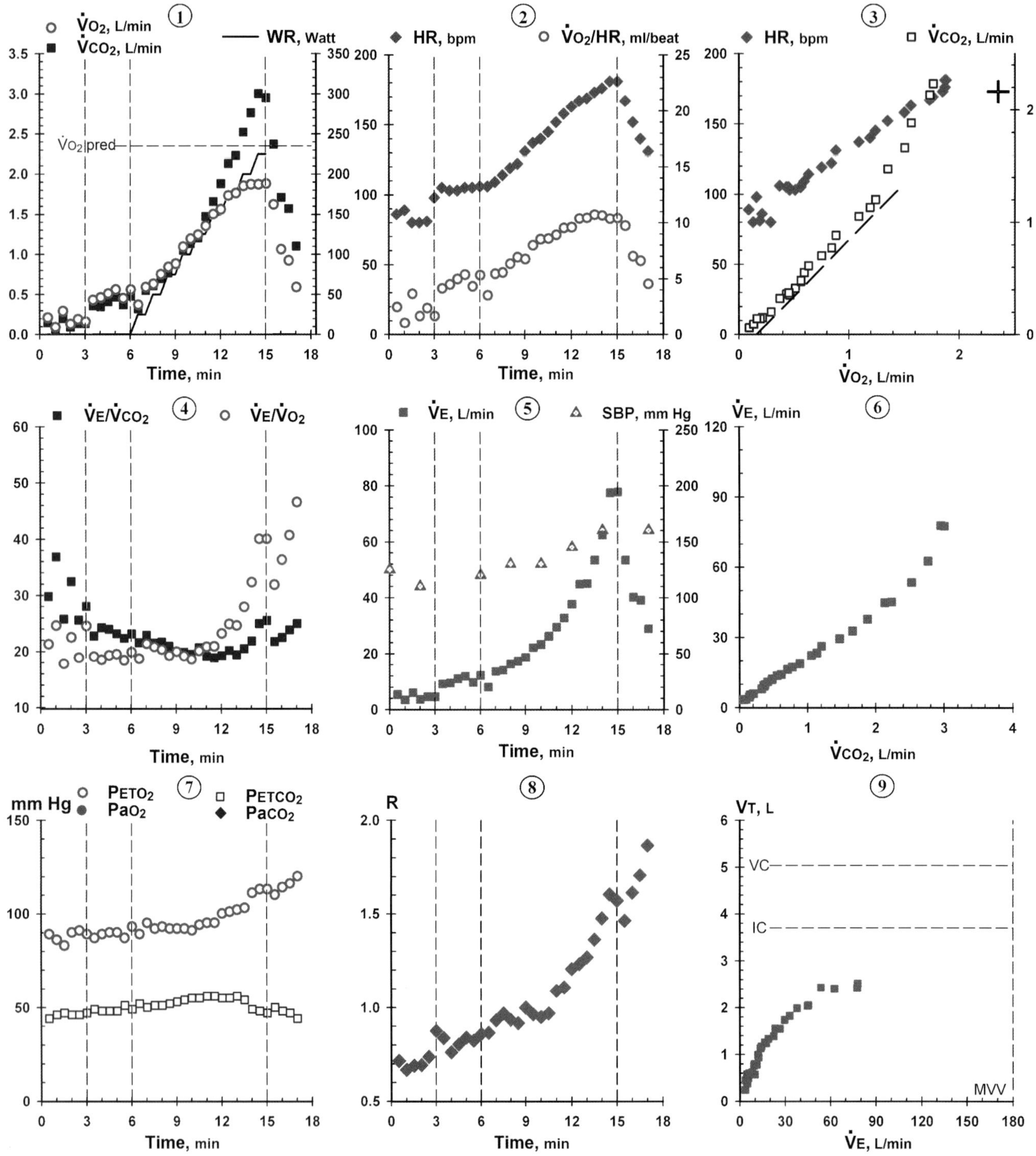

FIGURE 10.24.1. Vertical dashed lines in the panels in the left and middle columns indicate, from left to right, the beginning of unloaded cycling, start of increasing work rate (WR) at 25 W/min, and start of recovery. In **panel 1**, the increase in WR (right y-axis) is plotted with a scale of 100 W to 1 L of oxygen uptake ($\dot{V}O_2$) (left y-axis) such that WR is plotted parallel to a $\dot{V}O_2$ slope of 10 mL/min/W. In **panel 3**, carbon dioxide output ($\dot{V}CO_2$) (right y-axis) is plotted as a function of $\dot{V}O_2$ (x-axis) with identical scales so that the diagonal dashed line has a slope of 1 (45°). The $\dot{V}CO_2$ increasing more steeply than $\dot{V}O_2$ defines carbon dioxide (CO_2) derived from bicarbonate buffer, as long as ventilatory equivalent for CO_2 ($\dot{V}E/\dot{V}CO_2$) (**panel 4**) is not increasing and end-tidal PCO_2 ($PETCO_2$) (**panel 7**) is not decreasing, simultaneously. The black + symbol in **panel 3** indicates predicted values of heart rate (HR) (left y-axis) and $\dot{V}O_2$ for this individual. Abbreviations: IC, inspiratory capacity; MVV, maximum voluntary ventilation; $PETO_2$, end-tidal PO_2; R, respiratory exchange ratio; SBP, systolic blood pressure; VC, vital capacity; $\dot{V}E$, minute ventilation; $\dot{V}E/\dot{V}O_2$, ventilatory equivalent for oxygen; V_T, tidal volume.

CASE 25

Myocardial Ischemia: Development of Inducible Myocardial Ischemia Over 3 Years

CLINICAL FINDINGS

A 57-year-old man with suspected asbestos-associated disease had exercise tests performed at a 3-year interval to monitor his respiratory function. When first evaluated, he had a several year history of diabetes mellitus treated with insulin, hypertension treated with hydrochlorothiazide, obesity, arthritis of the hip, and moderate exertional dyspnea. He had never smoked tobacco. Examination at that time revealed moderate obesity and minimal pleural thickening on his chest radiographs. The respiratory function and exercise study data of that evaluation are shown in **Tables 10.25.1** to **10.25.3** and **Figure 10.25.1**. When evaluated 3 years later (**Tables 10.25.4** to **10.25.6** and **Fig. 10.25.2**), he was being treated with cimetidine for symptoms of "gas" pain in his left anterior chest associated with exercise.

EXERCISE FINDINGS

On both occasions, the patient performed exercise on a cycle ergometer. He pedaled at 60 rpm without an added load for 2 or 3 minutes. The work rate was then increased 20 W/min to tolerance. On the first occasion, arterial blood was sampled every second minute and intra-arterial pressure was recorded from a percutaneously placed brachial artery catheter.

TABLE 10.25.1 Selected Respiratory Function Data: First Study

Measurement	Predicted	Measured
Age (y)		57
Sex		Male
Height (cm)		171
Weight (kg)	74	96
Hematocrit (%)		46
VC (L)	3.99	4.25
IC (L)	2.66	3.37
TLC (L)	6.03	6.00
FEV_1 (L)	3.14	3.52
FEV_1/VC (%)	79	83
MVV (L/min)	134	135
D_{LCO} (mL/mm Hg/min)	26.4	36.4

Abbreviations: D_{LCO}, diffusing capacity of the lung for carbon monoxide; FEV_1, forced expiratory volume in 1 second; IC, inspiratory capacity; MVV, maximum voluntary ventilation; VC, vital capacity.

The patient stopped exercise because of thigh pain, without chest or abdominal pain. No electrocardiogram (ECG) abnormalities were noted at rest, but during high work levels, 1- to 2-mm J-point depression with upsloping ST segments was seen in noncontiguous leads.

On the second exercise test, the patient stopped exercise because of calf fatigue and an inability to maintain his cycling frequency. During the last 1 to 2 minutes of exercise, he noted left parasternal nonradiating "gas" pain, typical of his recent symptoms, which subsided within 3 minutes of recovery. He denied shortness of breath. The resting ECG was normal. However, at 120 W, 1.5 mm of ST-segment depression was evident in leads II, III, aVF, V_3, and V_4; by 140 W, the ST depression had progressed to 2.5 to 3 mm and had extended to include V_5 and V_6. The ECG returned to normal by 3 minutes after exercise.

TABLE 10.25.2 Selected Exercise Data: First Study

Measurement	Predicted	Measured
Peak $\dot{V}O_2$ (L/min)	2.32	2.20
Maximum heart rate (beats/min)	163	148
Maximum O_2 pulse (mL/beat)	14.2	14.9
$\Delta\dot{V}O_2/\Delta WR$ (mL/min/W)	10.3	10.3
AT (L/min)	>1.02	1.2
Blood pressure (mm Hg [rest, max])		156/94, 250/113
Maximum $\dot{V}E$ (L/min)		143
Exercise breathing reserve (L/min)	>15	−8
$\dot{V}E/\dot{V}CO_2$ @ *AT* or lowest	27.8	28.8
PaO_2 (mm Hg [rest, max ex])		100, 129
$P(A-a)O_2$ (mm Hg [rest, max ex])		10, 3
$PaCO_2$ (mm Hg [rest, max ex])		35, 23
$P(a-ET)CO_2$ (mm Hg [rest, max ex])		−4, −2
VD/VT (rest, heavy ex)		0.16, 0.19
HCO_3^- (mEq/L [rest, 2-min recov])		24, 15

Abbreviations: *AT*, anaerobic threshold; $\Delta\dot{V}O_2/\Delta WR$, change in $\dot{V}O_2$/change in work rate; ex, exercise, HCO_3^-, bicarbonate; O_2, oxygen; $P(A-a)O_2$, alveolar-arterial PO_2 difference; $P(a-ET)CO_2$, arterial-end-tidal PCO_2 difference; recov, recovery; VD/VT, physiological dead space-tidal volume ratio; $\dot{V}E$, minute ventilation; $\dot{V}E/\dot{V}CO_2$, ventilatory equivalent for carbon dioxide; $\dot{V}O_2$, oxygen uptake.

TABLE 10.25.3 First Study

Time (min)	Work rate (W)	BP (mm Hg)	HR (min^{-1})	f (min^{-1})	$\dot{V}_E$ (L/min BTPS)	$\dot{V}CO_2$ (L/min STPD)	$\dot{V}O_2$ (L/min STPD)	$\frac{\dot{V}O_2}{HR}$ (mL/beat)	R	pH	HCO_3^- (mEq/L)	PO_2, mm Hg ET	PO_2, mm Hg a	PO_2, mm Hg (A − a)	PCO_2, mm Hg ET	PCO_2, mm Hg a	PCO_2, mm Hg (a − ET)	$\frac{\dot{V}_E}{\dot{V}CO_2}$	$\frac{\dot{V}_E}{\dot{V}O_2}$	$\frac{V_D}{V_T}$
0.5	Rest	156/94								7.37	24		84			43				
1.0	Rest		80	10	11.9	0.36	0.40	5.0	0.90			109			36			31	28	
1.5	Rest		85	11	10.0	0.32	0.39	4.6	0.82			103			39			28	23	
2.0	Rest		87	7	9.4	0.30	0.36	4.1	0.83			104			39			29	24	
2.5	Rest	175/100	84	7	10.1	0.32	0.38	4.5	0.84	7.40	21	105	100	10	39	35	−4	30	25	0.16
3.0	Unloaded		97	21	21.8	0.65	0.85	8.8	0.76			94			43			31	24	
3.5	Unloaded		96	18	17.4	0.55	0.74	7.7	0.74			99			40			29	21	
4.0	Unloaded		100	22	23.7	0.77	1.01	10.1	0.76			99			40			28	22	
4.5	Unloaded	206/113	98	21	20.8	0.63	0.71	7.2	0.89	7.41	19	105	103	13	40	31	−9	30	27	0.07
5.0	20		101	21	28.3	0.91	1.01	10.0	0.90			104			39			29	26	
5.5	20		101	20	29.2	0.92	1.02	10.1	0.90			106			39			30	27	
6.0	40		102	16	29.4	0.96	1.07	10.5	0.90			104			40			29	26	
6.5	40	219/106	108	20	26.3	0.89	1.04	9.6	0.86	7.39	21	103	100	9	40	36	−4	28	24	0.12
7.0	60		111	21	30.3	1.01	1.14	10.3	0.89			104			41			28	25	
7.5	60		115	22	35.2	1.17	1.22	10.6	0.96			107			40			28	27	
8.0	80		117	25	40.7	1.36	1.36	11.6	1.00			110			39			28	28	
8.5	80	238/106	129	26	45.7	1.50	1.41	10.9	1.06	7.39	21	112	103	13	39	36	−3	29	31	0.16
9.0	100		123	28	50.9	1.65	1.53	12.4	1.08			114			38			29	32	
9.5	100		125	29	51.9	1.70	1.56	12.5	1.09			114			38			29	32	
10.0	120		127	32	67.8	2.02	1.68	13.2	1.20			119			35			32	39	
10.5	120	250/113	131	39	80.3	2.24	1.84	14.0	1.22	7.41	19	122	114	9	32	31	−1	34	42	0.18
11.0	140		131	41	91.5	2.42	1.99	15.2	1.22			120			34			36	44	
11.5	140		141	55	121.3	2.79	2.15	15.2	1.30			128			27			42	54	
12.0	160	235/110	148	59	142.8	2.95	2.20	14.9	1.34	7.42	15	130	129	3	25	23	−2	47	63	0.19
12.5	Recovery		131	39	80.8	2.04	1.73	13.2	1.18			124			30			38	45	
13.0	Recovery		119	33	50.4	1.18	0.98	8.2	1.20			127			27			40	49	

Abbreviations: BP, blood pressure; BTPS, body temperature pressure saturated; f, frequency; HCO_3^-, bicarbonate; HR, heart rate; $P(A - a)O_2$, alveolar-arterial PO_2 difference; $P(a - ET)CO_2$, arterial-end-tidal PCO_2 difference; $PETCO_2$, end-tidal PCO_2; $PETO_2$, end-tidal PO_2; R, respiratory exchange ratio; STPD, standard temperature pressure dry; $\dot{V}CO_2$, carbon dioxide output; V_D/V_T, physiological dead space-tidal volume ratio; $\dot{V}_E$, minute ventilation; $\dot{V}_E/\dot{V}CO_2$, ventilatory equivalent for carbon dioxide; $\dot{V}_E/\dot{V}O_2$, ventilatory equivalent for oxygen; $\dot{V}O_2$, oxygen uptake.

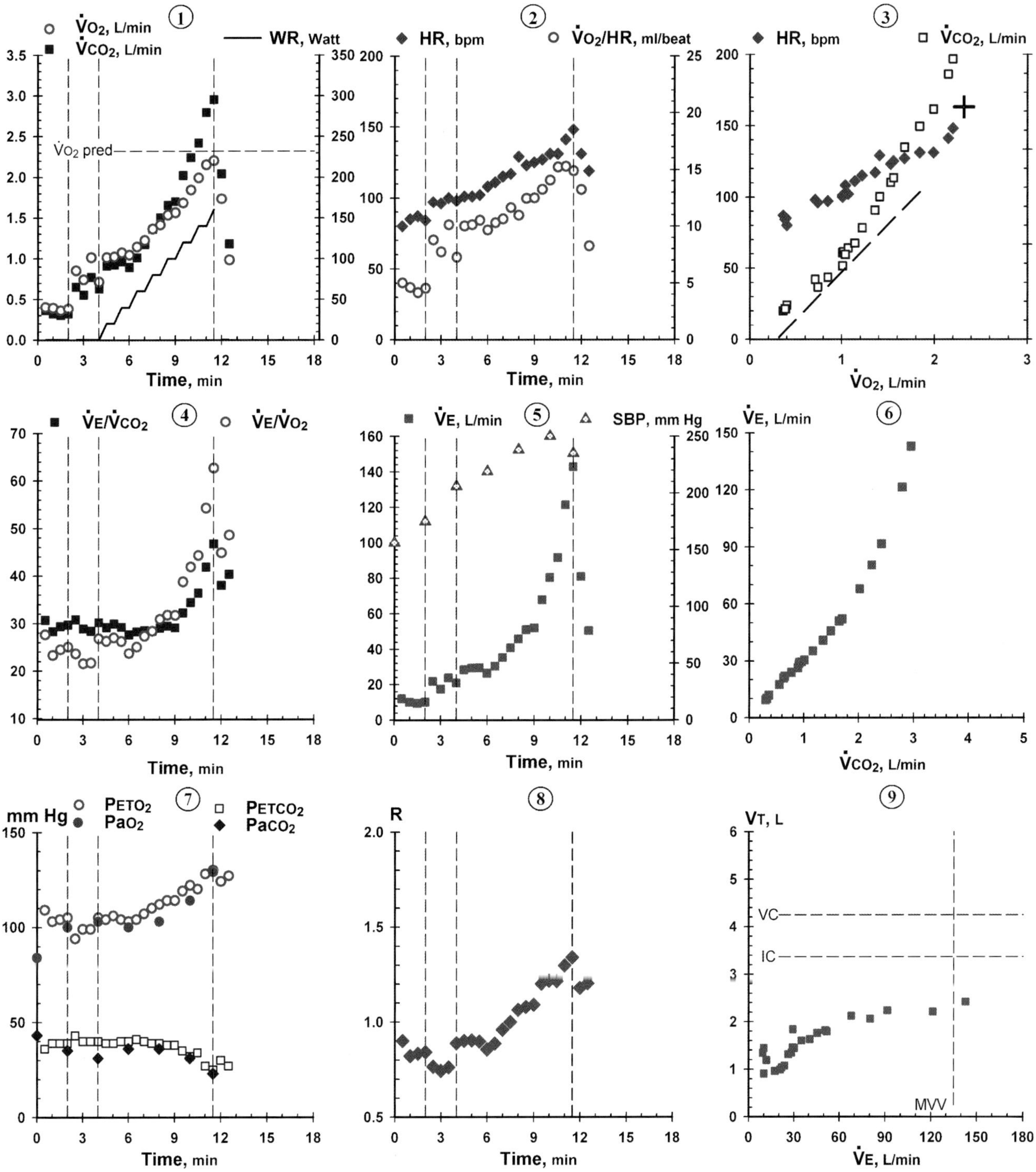

FIGURE 10.25.1. First study, age 57. Vertical dashed lines in the panels in the left and middle columns indicate, from left to right, the beginning of unloaded cycling, start of increasing work rate (WR) at 20 W/min, and start of recovery. In **panel 1**, the increase in WR (right y-axis) is plotted with a scale of 100 W to 1 L of oxygen uptake ($\dot{V}O_2$) (left y-axis) such that WR is plotted parallel to a $\dot{V}O_2$ slope of 10 mL/min/W. In **panel 3**, carbon dioxide output ($\dot{V}CO_2$) (right y-axis) is plotted as a function of $\dot{V}O_2$ (x-axis) with identical scales so that the diagonal dashed line has a slope of 1 (45°). The $\dot{V}CO_2$ increasing more steeply than $\dot{V}O_2$ defines carbon dioxide (CO_2) derived from bicarbonate buffer, as long as ventilatory equivalent for CO_2 ($\dot{V}E/\dot{V}CO_2$) (**panel 4**) is not increasing and end-tidal PCO_2 ($PETCO_2$) (**panel 7**) is not decreasing, simultaneously. The black + symbol in **panel 3** indicates predicted values of heart rate (HR) (left y-axis) and $\dot{V}O_2$ for this individual. Abbreviations: IC, inspiratory capacity; MVV, maximum voluntary ventilation; $PETO_2$, end-tidal PO_2; R, respiratory exchange ratio; SBP, systolic blood pressure; VC, vital capacity; $\dot{V}E$, minute ventilation; $\dot{V}E/\dot{V}O_2$, ventilatory equivalent for oxygen; VT, tidal volume.

TABLE 10.25.4 Selected Respiratory Function Data: Second Study

Measurement	Predicted	Measured
Age (y)		60
Sex		Male
Height (cm)		171
Weight (kg)	74	87
VC (L)	3.92	4.38
IC (L)	2.61	2.53
TLC (L)	6.11	5.87
FEV_1 (L)	3.06	3.59
FEV_1/VC (%)	78	81
MVV (L/min)	132	158
D_{LCO} (mL/mm Hg/min)	26.4	31.8

Abbreviations: D_{LCO}, diffusing capacity of the lung for carbon monoxide; FEV_1, forced expiratory volume in 1 second; IC, inspiratory capacity; MVV, maximum voluntary ventilation; TLC, total lung capacity; VC, vital capacity.

TABLE 10.25.5 Selected Exercise Data: Second Study

Measurement	Predicted	Measured
Peak $\dot{V}O_2$ (L/min)	2.19	1.63
Maximum heart rate (beats/min)	160	118
Maximum O_2 pulse (mL/beat)	13.7	14.2
$\Delta\dot{V}O_2/\Delta WR$ (mL/min/W)	10.3	6.8
AT (L/min)	>0.96	1.05
Blood pressure (mm Hg [rest, max])		140/80, 210/100
Maximum $\dot{V}_E$ (L/min)		79
Exercise breathing reserve (L/min)	>15	79
$\dot{V}_E/\dot{V}CO_2$ @ *AT* or lowest	28.1	28.3

Abbreviations: *AT*, anaerobic threshold; $\Delta\dot{V}O_2/\Delta WR$, change in $\dot{V}O_2$/change in work rate; O_2, oxygen; $\dot{V}_E$, minute ventilation; $\dot{V}_E/\dot{V}CO_2$, ventilatory equivalent for carbon dioxide; $\dot{V}O_2$, oxygen uptake.

INTERPRETATION

Comments

Resting respiratory function studies and arterial blood gases and pH were normal at both evaluations.

Analysis

In the first study, all findings were normal with the exception of inadequately controlled hypertension and a negative breathing reserve, the latter interpreted as indicating the patient's sensitive ventilatory response to the exercise-induced metabolic acidosis with precise pH regulation. To maintain normal pH, he lowered his Pa_{CO_2} from 35 to 23 mm Hg over a 3.5-minute period. He had no evidence of pulmonary or cardiovascular dysfunction, including findings at the time of the nonspecific ECG changes noted near the end of exercise.

In the second study, 3 years later, peak $\dot{V}O_2$ was reduced while the anaerobic threshold, although lower than that of the earlier study, remained within the normal range. The ECG during the second exercise study was clearly abnormal, leading to the diagnosis of myocardial ischemia, and the flattening of $\Delta\dot{V}O_2/\Delta WR$ and flat O_2 pulse during increasing work rate are consistent with this diagnosis.

Conclusion

This patient, with risk factors for coronary artery disease, initially had a normal gas exchange response to incremental exercise. Three years later, his oxygen flow became abnormal during incremental exercise coincident with ECG abnormalities and chest pain. These findings strongly supported the diagnosis of myocardial ischemia.

TABLE 10.25.6 Second Study

Time (min)	Work rate (W)	BP (mm Hg)	HR (min^{-1})	f (min^{-1})	$\dot{V}_E$ (L/min BTPS)	$\dot{V}CO_2$ (L/min STPD)	$\dot{V}O_2$ (L/min STPD)	$\frac{\dot{V}O_2}{HR}$ (mL/beat)	R	pH	HCO_3^- (mEq/L)	PO_2, mm Hg ET	PO_2, mm Hg a	PO_2, mm Hg (A − a)	PCO_2, mm Hg ET	PCO_2, mm Hg a	PCO_2, mm Hg (a − ET)	$\frac{\dot{V}_E}{\dot{V}CO_2}$	$\frac{\dot{V}_E}{\dot{V}O_2}$	$\frac{V_D}{V_T}$
	Rest	140/80																		
0.5	Rest		59	12	9.1	0.25	0.31	5.3	0.81			102			39			32	26	
1.0	Rest	140/900	57	12	9.6	0.25	0.29	5.1	0.86			106			37			34	30	
1.5	Rest		54	13	6.2	0.13	0.15	2.8	0.87			104			38			39	34	
2.0	Rest	140/90	55	15	7.7	0.16	0.22	4.0	0.73			99			39			40	39	
2.5	Rest		57	13	10.5	0.28	0.37	6.5	0.76			99			39			34	25	
3.0	Rest		57	19	10.8	0.27	0.34	6.0	0.79			101			39			34	27	
3.5	Unloaded		70	18	16.8	0.56	0.70	10.0	0.80			100			41			27	22	
4.0	Unloaded		70	13	16.7	0.52	0.58	8.3	0.90			108			38			30	27	
4.5	Unloaded		70	14	17.0	0.56	0.66	9.4	0.85			104			39			28	24	
5.0	Unloaded		72	19	21.3	0.65	0.69	9.6	0.94			109			38			30	29	
5.5	Unloaded		72	19	19.8	0.63	0.73	10.1	0.86			103			40			29	25	
6.0	Unloaded	145/90	76	16	21.2	0.68	0.80	10.5	0.85			100			41			29	25	
6.5	20		76	13	18.0	0.59	0.66	8.7	0.89			106			39			29	26	
7.0	20		76	15	19.9	0.66	0.76	10.0	0.87			103			40			28	25	
7.5	40		76	16	21.8	0.74	0.87	11.4	0.85			102			41			28	23	
8.0	40	180/90	83	19	28.2	0.92	0.98	11.8	0.94			104			41			29	27	
8.5	60		85	17	27.1	0.95	1.06	12.5	0.90			102			42			27	24	
9.0	60		88	20	36.8	1.23	1.23	14.0	1.00			102			42			29	29	
9.5	80		93	24	37.4	1.25	1.18	12.7	1.06			109			41			28	30	
10.0	80	195/85	100	23	42.1	1.38	1.26	12.6	1.10			113			38			29	32	
10.5	100		102	25	48.4	1.53	1.36	13.3	1.13			114			38			30	34	
11.0	100		105	29	57.6	1.72	1.42	13.5	1.21			118			35			32	39	
11.5	120		103	34	68.8	1.92	1.50	14.6	1.28			121			33			34	44	
12.0	120	210/100	113	49	79.3	2.02	1.54	13.6	1.31			121			33			37	49	
12.5	140		118	40	78.0	2.06	1.58	13.4	1.30			119			34			36	47	
13.0	140		115	42	76.5	2.16	1.63	14.2	1.33			119			33			34	45	
13.5	Recovery		98	27	66.8	1.89	1.35	13.8	1.40			120			34			34	48	
14.0	Recovery	210/90	97	27	61.9	1.71	1.23	12.7	1.39			123			32			35	48	
14.5	Recovery		91	20	45.6	1.27	0.94	10.3	1.35			122			33			34	46	
15.0	Recovery	180/90	91	23	41.9	1.16	0.88	9.7	1.32			122			33			34	45	

Abbreviations: BP, blood pressure; BTPS, body temperature pressure saturated; f, frequency; HCO_3^-, bicarbonate; HR, heart rate; $P(A - a)O_2$, alveolar-arterial PO_2 difference; $P(a - ET)CO_2$, arterial-end-tidal PCO_2 difference; $PETCO_2$, end-tidal PCO_2; $PETO_2$, end-tidal PO_2; R, respiratory exchange ratio; STPD, standard temperature pressure dry; $\dot{V}CO_2$, carbon dioxide output; V_D/V_T, physiological dead space-tidal volume ratio; $\dot{V}_E$, minute ventilation; $\dot{V}_E/\dot{V}CO_2$, ventilatory equivalent for carbon dioxide; $\dot{V}_E/\dot{V}O_2$, ventilatory equivalent for oxygen; $\dot{V}O_2$, oxygen uptake.

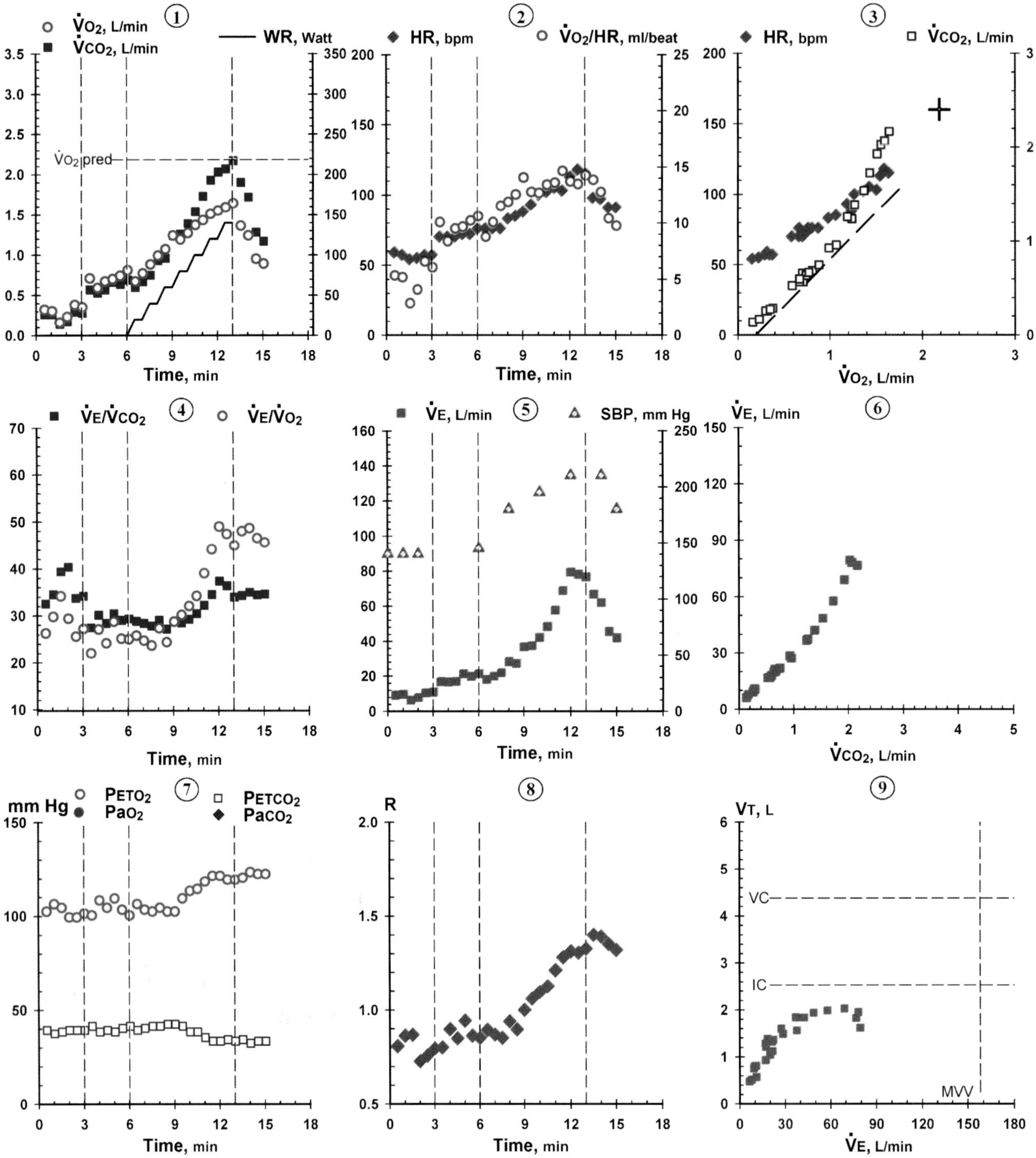

FIGURE 10.25.2. Second study, age 60. Vertical dashed lines in the panels in the left and middle columns indicate, from left to right, the beginning of unloaded cycling, start of increasing work rate (WR) at 20 W/min, and start of recovery. In **panel 1**, the increase in WR (right y-axis) is plotted with a scale of 100 W to 1 L of oxygen uptake ($\dot{V}O_2$) (left y-axis) such that WR is plotted parallel to a $\dot{V}O_2$ slope of 10 mL/min/W. In **panel 3**, carbon dioxide output ($\dot{V}CO_2$) (right y-axis) is plotted as a function of $\dot{V}O_2$ (x-axis) with identical scales so that the diagonal dashed line has a slope of 1 (45°). The $\dot{V}CO_2$ increasing more steeply than $\dot{V}O_2$ defines carbon dioxide (CO_2) derived from bicarbonate buffer, as long as ventilatory equivalent for CO_2 ($\dot{V}E/\dot{V}CO_2$) (**panel 4**) is not increasing and end-tidal PCO_2 ($PETCO_2$) (**panel 7**) is not decreasing, simultaneously. The black + symbol in **panel 3** indicates predicted values of heart rate (HR) (left y-axis) and $\dot{V}O_2$ for this individual. Abbreviations: IC, inspiratory capacity; MVV, maximum voluntary ventilation; $PETO_2$, end-tidal PO_2; R, respiratory exchange ratio; SBP, systolic blood pressure; VC, vital capacity; $\dot{V}E$, minute ventilation; $\dot{V}E/\dot{V}O_2$, ventilatory equivalent for oxygen; V_T, tidal volume.

CASE 26

Atrial Septal Defect and Hemochromatosis

CLINICAL FINDINGS

A 54-year-old man was found to have a small atrial septal defect (ASD) on echocardiogram after complaining of episodic dizziness and exertional shortness of breath. The ASD was believed to be hemodynamically insignificant. Magnetic resonance imaging of the brain showed small vessel disease. The medical history was notable for a diagnosis of hemochromatosis several years previously treated with serial phlebotomy. His last phlebotomy was several months prior to this test and recent hemoglobin had been stable at 14 g/dL. He worked on board a ship which involved being on his feet and climbing up and down ladders throughout the day. His only medication was aspirin, 81 mg/d. Physical examination revealed clear breath sounds and a regular cardiac rhythm without murmur. There was no edema. Resting electrocardiogram (ECG) showed a sinus rhythm with occasional premature ventricular contractions. Demographic and respiratory function data are shown in **Table 10.26.1**.

EXERCISE FINDINGS

The patient exercised on a cycle ergometer beginning with 3 minutes of unloaded pedaling at 60 rpm followed by continuous increase in work rate by 20 W/min. The test was terminated by examiners at a work rate of 182 W when there was a run of three ventricular premature beats. At the time the test ended, the patient endorsed some shortness of breath but no light-headedness, chest pain or palpitations, and stated he could have exercised further. On ECG, there were continued premature beats, which increased in frequency near peak exercise but no ischemic changes. Exercise data are shown in **Tables 10.26.2** and **10.26.3** and in **Figure 10.26.1**.

INTERPRETATION

Comment

This patient had two conditions that could affect cardiac function.

Analysis

Exercise capacity was within the normal range as the peak $\dot{V}O_2$ attained was low normal. Despite the fact that the test was stopped prior to symptom limitation, there appeared to be a plateau in $\dot{V}O_2$ during the last 1.5 minutes as work rate continued to increase by an additional 30 W (panel 1), suggesting that this was a true maximal value. Up until that point, the $\Delta\dot{V}O_2/\Delta WR$ was normal and anaerobic threshold was above the lower limit of normal. Blood pressure (not graphed) increased appropriately with exercise. The ECG findings of an increase in ventricular ectopy during exercise was abnormal, however.

Ventilatory responses to exercise did not appear to be limiting as there was an ample breathing reserve.

TABLE 10.26.1 Selected Respiratory Function Data

Measurement	Predicted	Measured
Age (y)		54
Sex		Male
Height (cm)		173
Weight (kg)		101
VC (L)	4.52	4.03
IC (L)	3.21	4.14
ERV (L)	1.31	0.18
FEV_1 (L)	3.53	3.08
FEV_1/VC (%)	78	76
MVV (L/min)	140	136

Abbreviations: ERV, expiratory reserve volume; FEV_1, forced expiratory volume in 1 second; IC, inspiratory capacity; MVV, maximum voluntary ventilation; VC, vital capacity.

TABLE 10.26.2 Selected Exercise Test Data

Measurement	Predicted	Measured
Peak $\dot{V}O_2$ (L/min)	2.49	2.14
Maximum heart rate (beats/min)	166	155
Maximum O_2 pulse (mL/beat)	15	14
$\Delta\dot{V}O_2/\Delta WR$ (mL/min/W)	10.3	10.4
AT (L/min)	>1.13	1.20
Blood pressure (mm Hg [rest, max ex])		118/72, 196/83
Maximum $\dot{V}E$ (L/min)		90
Breathing reserve (L/min)	>15	50
$\dot{V}E/\dot{V}CO_2$ @ *AT*	<31	32
$\dot{V}E$-$\dot{V}CO_2$ slope	<31	31
SpO_2 (% [rest, max ex])		99, 97
V_D/V_T (rest, max ex)		0.35, 0.29

Abbreviations: *AT*, anaerobic threshold; $\Delta\dot{V}O_2/\Delta WR$, change in $\dot{V}O_2$/change in work rate; ex, exercise; O_2, oxygen; SpO_2, oxygen saturation as measured by pulse oximetry; $\dot{V}CO_2$, carbon dioxide output; V_D/V_T, physiological dead space–tidal volume ratio; $\dot{V}E$, minute ventilation; $\dot{V}E/\dot{V}CO_2$, ventilatory equivalent for carbon dioxide; $\dot{V}O_2$, oxygen uptake.

TABLE 10.26.3 Air Breathing

Time (min)	Work rate (W)	BP (mm Hg)	HR (min^{-1})	f (min^{-1})	$\dot{V}E$ (L/min BTPS)	$\dot{V}CO_2$ (L/min STPD)	$\dot{V}O_2$ (L/min STPD)	$\frac{\dot{V}O_2}{HR}$ (mL/beat)	R	pH	HCO_3^- (mEq/L)	PO_2, mm Hg and SpO_2: ET	SpO_2	(A − a)	PCO_2, mm Hg: ET	tc	(a − ET)	$\frac{\dot{V}E}{\dot{V}CO_2}$	$\frac{\dot{V}E}{\dot{V}O_2}$	$\frac{VD}{VT}$
0.5	Rest		87	17	16.6	0.42	0.41	4.7	1.01			119	99		29	31.7		40	40	0.30
1.0	Rest		100	14	14.1	0.36	0.37	3.7	0.98			118	99		29	32.3		39	38	0.31
1.5	Rest		101	16	15.5	0.38	0.38	3.7	1.01			119	99		29	32.7		41	41	0.34
2.0	Rest	116/73	99	14	13.2	0.33	0.33	3.4	0.99			118	99		29	32.8		40	40	0.33
2.5	Rest		95	20	9.9	0.21	0.24	2.5	0.87			114	98		30	33.0		47	41	0.38
3.0	Rest		94	17	9.8	0.23	0.30	3.2	0.76			108	98		31	32.8		43	32	0.34
3.5	Rest		97	16	14.9	0.34	0.37	3.8	0.92			116	98		29	32.8		44	41	0.38
4.0	Unloaded		101	17	20.4	0.54	0.62	6.1	0.88			112	98		31	31.7		38	33	0.27
4.5	Unloaded		109	14	20.2	0.56	0.63	5.7	0.89			113	98		31	30.8		36	32	0.23
5.0	Unloaded		107	15	20.5	0.56	0.63	5.8	0.89			114	98		30	30.5		37	33	0.23
5.5	Unloaded		104	15	18.5	0.50	0.59	5.7	0.85			112	98		31	30.5		37	31	0.23
6.0	Unloaded		106	18	17.9	0.49	0.61	5.7	0.80			110	98		31	26.6		37	29	0.11
6.5	Unloaded		104	13	21.1	0.59	0.71	6.8	0.83			109	98		32	24.1		36	30	0.02
7.0	6		107	14	20.1	0.57	0.69	6.4	0.83			110	98		32	26.5		35	29	0.09
7.5	17		108	12	20.5	0.59	0.69	6.4	0.86			109	99		32	29.0		35	30	0.16
8.0	27		111	16	20.8	0.60	0.74	6.6	0.82			108	98		32	30.5		35	28	0.19
8.5	36		112	19	25.7	0.71	0.83	7.4	0.85			111	98		31	31.5		36	31	0.25
9.0	46	118/72	112	17	24.1	0.70	0.88	7.9	0.80			107	98		33	31.8		34	27	0.22
9.5	56		114	15	29.2	0.89	1.05	9.2	0.85			108	98		34	32.2		33	28	0.20
10.0	66		116	16	30.0	0.93	1.09	9.4	0.86			107	98		34	32.7		32	28	0.19
10.5	77		118	17	32.7	1.02	1.16	9.8	0.88			106	98		35	33.0		32	28	0.20
11.0	87		122	22	40.7	1.23	1.28	10.5	0.96			111	98		34	33.3		33	32	0.23
11.5	97	139/73	124	21	41.7	1.31	1.37	11.1	0.96			110	98		35	33.5		32	31	0.20
12.0	107		127	23	48.8	1.50	1.50	11.8	1.00			112	98		34	33.8		33	32	0.23
12.5	116		131	22	52.3	1.60	1.57	12.1	1.01			112	98		34	33.8		33	33	0.23
13.0	127	157/78	134	23	58.1	1.75	1.67	12.5	1.05			113	98		34	33.8		33	35	0.25
13.5	136		137	23	59.3	1.83	1.76	12.9	1.04			112	98		35	33.8		32	34	0.23
14.0	147		140	26	66.1	2.00	1.87	13.4	1.07			114	97		34	33.8		33	35	0.24
14.5	156		143	28	73.0	2.16	1.95	13.6	1.10			116	97		34	33.8		34	37	0.26
15.0	167	196/83	148	31	82.8	2.36	2.07	14.0	1.14			118	97		32	33.8		35	40	0.29
15.5	177		152	33	87.2	2.47	2.14	14.1	1.15			118	97		32	33.7		35	41	0.29
16.0	184		155	35	90.1	2.47	2.10	13.6	1.18			120	97		31	33.5		36	43	0.31
16.5	Recovery		151	34	86.0	2.30	1.87	12.4	1.23			121	97		30	33.2		37	46	0.32
17.0	Recovery	172/68	143	34	79.6	1.97	1.39	9.7	1.42			126	98		28	33.0		40	57	0.36
17.5	Recovery		137	28	55.7	1.42	1.09	8.0	1.30			123	98		29	32.8		39	51	0.34
18.0	Recovery		130	26	49.0	1.24	1.02	7.9	1.22			122	98		29	32.5		39	48	0.30
18.5	Recovery		128	29	50.6	1.22	0.98	7.7	1.24			123	98		28	32.5		41	52	0.31

Abbreviations: BP, blood pressure; BTPS, body temperature pressure saturated; f, frequency; HCO_3^-, bicarbonate; HR, heart rate; $P(A - a)O_2$, alveolar-arterial PO_2 difference; $P(a - ET)CO_2$, arterial-end-tidal PCO_2 difference; $PETCO_2$, end-tidal PCO_2; $PETO_2$, end-tidal PO_2; $PtcCO_2$, transcutaneous PCO_2; R, respiratory exchange ratio; SpO_2, oxygen saturation as measured by pulse oximetry; STPD, standard temperature pressure dry; $\dot{V}CO_2$, carbon dioxide output; VD/VT, physiological dead space-tidal volume ratio; $\dot{V}E$, minute ventilation; $\dot{V}E/\dot{V}CO_2$, ventilatory equivalent for carbon dioxide; $\dot{V}E/\dot{V}O_2$, ventilatory equivalent for oxygen; $\dot{V}O_2$, oxygen uptake.

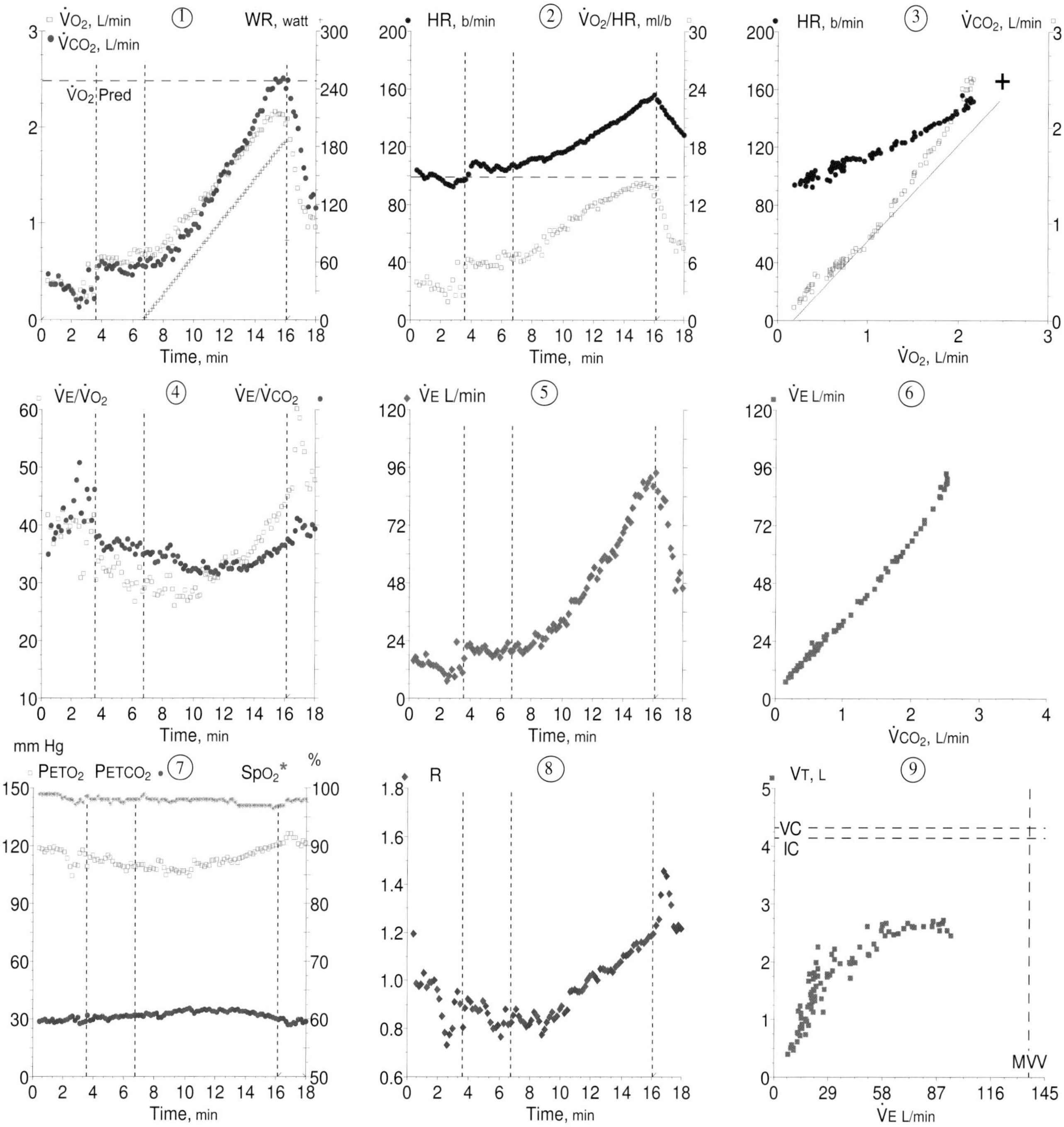

FIGURE 10.26.1. Vertical dashed lines in the panels in the left and middle columns indicate, from left to right, the beginning of unloaded cycling, start of increasing work rate (WR) at 20 W/min, and start of recovery. In **panel 1**, the increase in WR (right y-axis) is plotted with a scale of 100 W to 1 L of oxygen uptake ($\dot{V}O_2$) (left y-axis) such that WR is plotted parallel to a $\dot{V}O_2$ slope of 10 mL/min/W. Predicted peak $\dot{V}O_2$ is shown as a dashed horizontal line. In **panel 3**, carbon dioxide output ($\dot{V}CO_2$) (right y-axis) is plotted as a function of $\dot{V}O_2$ (x-axis) with identical scales so that the diagonal blue line has a slope of 1 (45°). The $\dot{V}CO_2$ increasing more steeply than $\dot{V}O_2$ defines carbon dioxide (CO_2) derived from bicarbonate buffer, as long as ventilatory equivalent for CO_2 ($\dot{V}E/\dot{V}CO_2$) (**panel 4**) is not increasing and end-tidal P_{CO_2} (P_{ETCO_2}) (**panel 7**) is not decreasing, simultaneously. The black + symbol in **panel 3** indicates predicted values of heart rate (HR) (left y-axis) and $\dot{V}O_2$ for this individual. Abbreviations: IC, inspiratory capacity; MVV, maximum ventilation; P_{ETO_2}, end-tidal P_{O_2}; R, respiratory exchange ratio; Sp_{O_2}, oxygen saturation as measured by pulse oximetry; VC, vital capacity; $\dot{V}E$, minute ventilation; $\dot{V}E/\dot{V}O_2$, ventilatory equivalent for oxygen; V_T, tidal volume.

The borderline elevation in $\dot{V}E/\dot{V}CO_2$ at the anaerobic threshold suggests some degree of high $\dot{V}/\dot{Q}$ relationships in the lung, but calculated V_D/V_T (**Table 10.26.3**) using transcutaneous PCO_2 values as a surrogate for $PaCO_2$ was not elevated and oxygenation by pulse oximetry was normal, so pulmonary gas exchange efficiency was normal.

Conclusion

This test demonstrated exercise capacity within the normal range but with abnormal development of increased ectopy with exercise. Although he had a finding of a small ASD by echocardiography, there was no suggestion of right to left shunting. If he had significant left to right shunting, exercise capacity could be reduced by reduction in systemic blood flow; however, this seemed unlikely based on the imaging assessment performed previously. Cardiac involvement by hemochromatosis can be associated with ectopy and this was postulated to be the most likely basis of the findings. This test did not reproduce the symptoms that had brought him to medical attention, but the findings on exercise ECG warrant follow-up.

CASE 27

Symptomatic Chronic Mitral Insufficiency

CLINICAL FINDINGS

This 43-year-old female electronics assembler had rheumatic fever at age 10. Over the 6 months prior to testing, she had developed increasing dyspnea and orthopnea, with intermittent atrial fibrillation and pleural effusion, requiring repeated hospitalizations. There was no evidence of mitral stenosis or coronary artery disease on catheterization, angiography, or echocardiography. At the time of exercise study, she had a sinus rhythm and findings of mitral regurgitation with left atrial and left ventricular enlargement but no pleural effusion or dependent edema. Her medications were digoxin, furosemide, and potassium chloride.

EXERCISE FINDINGS

The patient performed exercise on a cycle ergometer. She pedaled at 60 rpm without added load for 3 minutes, after which the work rate was increased 5 W/min to her symptom-limited maximum. She stopped cycling because of general fatigue. There were no ST-segment changes or arrhythmia on electrocardiogram.

INTERPRETATION

Comments

Respiratory function at rest was compatible with a mild restrictive defect, and the diffusing capacity of the lung for carbon monoxide was normal (**Table 10.27.1**). Exercise data are summarized in **Table 10.27.2** and shown in **Table 10.27.3** and graphically in **Figure 10.27.1**.

Analysis

This patient's peak $\dot{V}O_2$ and anaerobic threshold were quite low and the most striking feature was the very steep heart rate (HR) response during exercise. She exceeded predicted HR despite having a very low peak $\dot{V}O_2$; therefore, her oxygen (O_2) pulse was very low at maximum exercise and the O_2 pulse response was low and unchanging. This suggests very low forward stroke volume. In addition, she had a low $\Delta\dot{V}O_2/\Delta WR$, supporting poor O_2 delivery during exercise. The lack of evidence of ventilatory limitation and the relatively normal $\dot{V}E/\dot{V}CO_2$ and $\dot{V}E$ versus $\dot{V}CO_2$ slope make pulmonary vascular disease (a potential cause of low stroke volume) unlikely, and she is not anemic. It is unclear in this patient whether the high HR response contributed to the low stroke volume (inadequate time for diastolic filling) or was a compensatory mechanism because of the low stroke volume.

Similarly, using the flowcharts (Chapter 9) to establish a tentative diagnosis, the low peak $\dot{V}O_2$ and anaerobic threshold (Flowchart 1) lead to Flowchart 4. The breathing reserve was

TABLE 10.27.1 Selected Respiratory Function Data

Measurement	Predicted	Measured
Age (y)		43
Sex		Female
Height (cm)		160
Weight (kg)	61	56
VC (L)	2.88	2.03
IC (L)	1.92	1.49
TLC (L)	4.33	3.32
FEV_1 (L)	2.36	1.81
FEV_1/VC (%)	82	89
MVV (L/min)	90	90
D_{LCO} (mL/mm Hg/min)	21.7	23.5

Abbreviations: D_{LCO}, diffusing capacity of the lung for carbon monoxide; FEV_1, forced expiratory volume in 1 second; IC, inspiratory capacity; MVV, maximum voluntary ventilation; TLC, total lung capacity; VC, vital capacity.

TABLE 10.27.2 Selected Exercise Data

Measurement	Predicted	Measured
Peak $\dot{V}O_2$ (L/min)	1.57	0.79
Maximum heart rate (beats/min)	177	186
Maximum O_2 pulse (mL/beat)	8.9	4.2
$\Delta\dot{V}O_2/\Delta WR$ (mL/min/W)	10.3	5.6
AT (L/min)	>0.74	0.65
Maximum $\dot{V}E$ (L/min)		31
Exercise breathing reserve (L/min)	>15	59
$\dot{V}E/\dot{V}CO_2$ @ *AT* or lowest	26.8	31.6

Abbreviations: *AT*, anaerobic threshold; $\Delta\dot{V}O_2/\Delta WR$, change in $\dot{V}O_2$/change in work rate; O_2, oxygen; $\dot{V}E$, minute ventilation; $\dot{V}E/\dot{V}CO_2$, ventilatory equivalent for carbon dioxide; $\dot{V}O_2$, oxygen uptake.

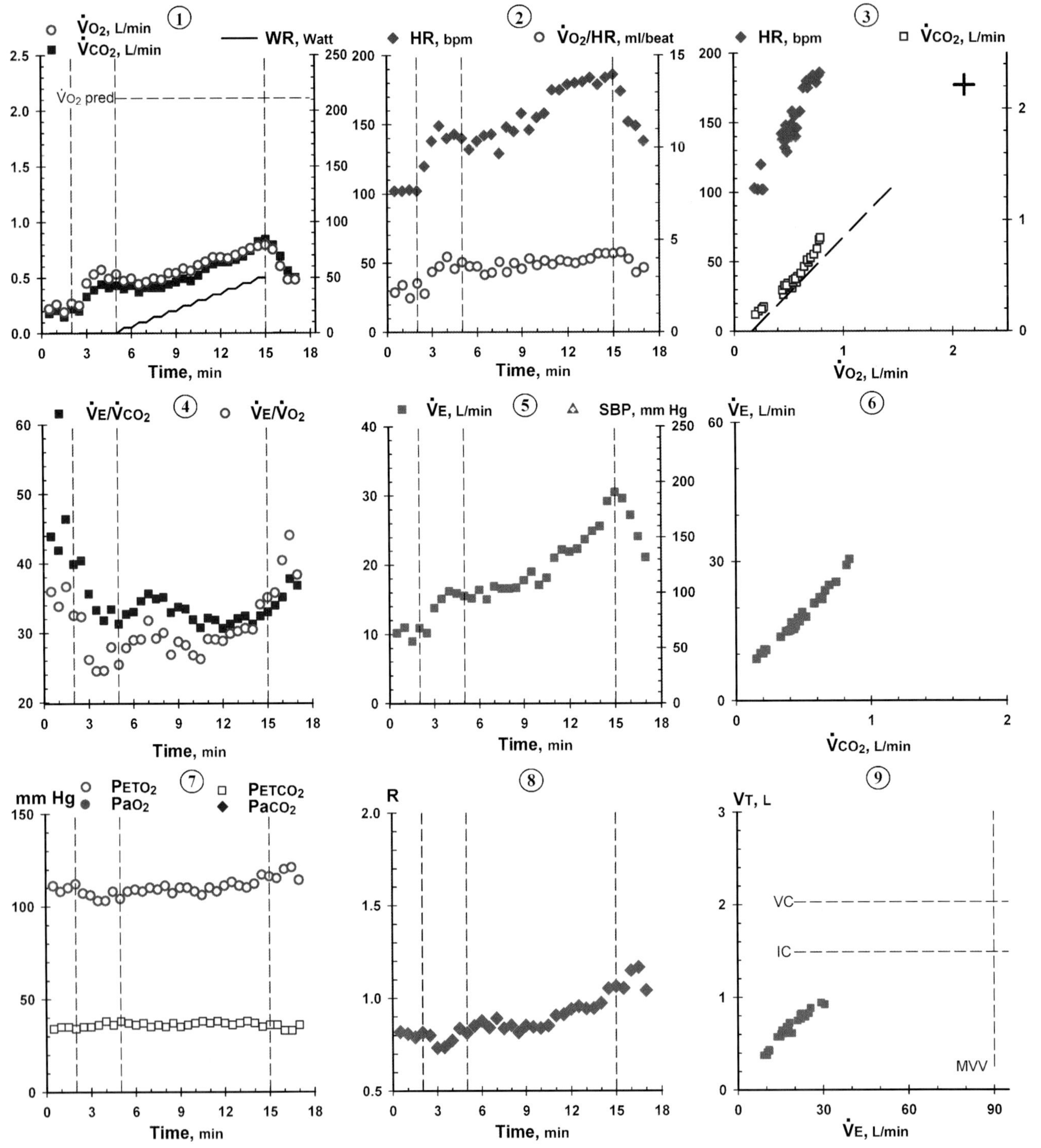

FIGURE 10.27.1. Vertical dashed lines in the panels in the left and middle columns indicate, from left to right, the beginning of unloaded cycling, start of increasing work rate (WR) at 5 W/min, and start of recovery. In **panel 1**, the increase in WR (right y-axis) is plotted with a scale of 100 W to 1 L of oxygen uptake ($\dot{V}O_2$) (left y-axis) such that WR is plotted parallel to a $\dot{V}O_2$ slope of 10 mL/min/W. In **panel 3**, carbon dioxide output ($\dot{V}CO_2$) (right y-axis) is plotted as a function of $\dot{V}O_2$ (x-axis) with identical scales so that the diagonal dashed line has a slope of 1 (45°). The $\dot{V}CO_2$ increasing more steeply than $\dot{V}O_2$ defines carbon dioxide (CO_2) derived from bicarbonate buffer, as long as ventilatory equivalent for CO_2 ($\dot{V}E/\dot{V}CO_2$) (**panel 4**) is not increasing and end-tidal P_{CO_2} (P_{ETCO_2}) (**panel 7**) is not decreasing, simultaneously. The black + symbol in **panel 3** indicates predicted values of heart rate (HR) (left y-axis) and $\dot{V}O_2$ for this individual. Abbreviations: IC, inspiratory capacity; MVV, maximum voluntary ventilation; P_{ETO_2}, end-tidal P_{O_2}; R, respiratory exchange ratio; SBP, systolic blood pressure; VC, vital capacity; $\dot{V}E$, minute ventilation; $\dot{V}E/\dot{V}O_2$, ventilatory equivalent for oxygen; VT, tidal volume.

TABLE 10.27.3 Air Breathing

Time (min)	Work rate (W)	BP (mm Hg)	HR (min^{-1})	f (min^{-1})	$\dot{V}E$ (L/min BTPS)	$\dot{V}CO_2$ (L/min STPD)	$\dot{V}O_2$ (L/min STPD)	$\frac{\dot{V}O_2}{HR}$ (mL/beat)	R	pH	HCO_3^- (mEq/L)	PO_2, mm Hg ET	PO_2, mm Hg a	PO_2, mm Hg (A − a)	PCO_2, mm Hg ET	PCO_2, mm Hg a	PCO_2, mm Hg (a − ET)	$\frac{\dot{V}E}{\dot{V}CO_2}$	$\frac{\dot{V}E}{\dot{V}O_2}$	$\frac{VD}{VT}$
0	Rest		102	27	10.2	0.18	0.22	2.2	0.82			111			34			44	36	
0.5	Rest		102	26	11.0	0.21	0.26	2.5	0.81			108			35			42	34	
1.0	Rest		103	24	9.0	0.15	0.19	1.8	0.79			110			35			46	37	
1.5	Rest		102	25	10.9	0.22	0.27	2.6	0.81			112			34			40	33	
2.0	Unloaded		120	25	10.2	0.20	0.25	2.1	0.80			107			35			40	32	
2.5	Unloaded		138	24	13.8	0.33	0.45	3.3	0.73			106			35			36	26	
3.0	Unloaded		149	25	15.1	0.39	0.53	3.6	0.74			103			36			33	24	
3.5	Unloaded		140	26	16.2	0.44	0.57	4.1	0.77			103			38			32	25	
4.0	Unloaded		143	26	15.9	0.41	0.49	3.4	0.84			108			36			33	28	
4.5	Unloaded		140	24	15.5	0.43	0.53	3.8	0.81			104			38			31	25	
5.0	5		132	25	15.2	0.40	0.47	3.6	0.85			108			37			33	28	
5.5	5		138	26	16.4	0.43	0.49	3.6	0.88			109			36			33	29	
6.0	10		142	26	15.0	0.37	0.44	3.1	0.84			108			37			35	29	
6.5	10		143	27	16.9	0.41	0.46	3.2	0.89			110			35			36	32	
7.0	15		129	27	16.6	0.41	0.49	3.8	0.84			109			36			35	29	
7.5	15		148	26	16.6	0.41	0.48	3.2	0.85			111			35			35	30	
8.0	20		145	26	16.7	0.44	0.54	3.7	0.81			107			37			33	27	
8.5	20		158	27	17.8	0.46	0.54	3.4	0.85			110			35			34	29	
9.0	25		146	31	19.0	0.49	0.58	4.0	0.84			110			36			33	28	
9.5	25		155	25	17.1	0.47	0.56	3.6	0.84			108			37			32	27	
10.0	30		158	25	18.1	0.52	0.61	3.9	0.85			106			38			31	26	
10.5	30		175	28	21.0	0.58	0.64	3.7	0.91			110			37			32	29	
11.0	35		175	29	22.2	0.62	0.68	3.9	0.91			108			38			32	29	
11.5	35		179	27	21.9	0.64	0.68	3.8	0.94			111			37			31	29	
12.0	40		180	28	22.3	0.64	0.67	3.7	0.96			113			36			31	30	
12.5	40		181	30	23.7	0.66	0.70	3.9	0.94			111			37			32	30	
13.0	45		184	30	24.9	0.69	0.73	4.0	0.95			110			38			32	31	
13.5	45		179	29	25.6	0.74	0.76	4.2	0.97			112			37			31	30	
14.0	50		184	31	29.2	0.82	0.78	4.2	1.05			117			35			32	34	
14.5	50		186	33	30.5	0.84	0.79	4.2	1.06			116			36			33	35	
15.0	Recovery		174	33	29.6	0.79	0.75	4.3	1.05			115			36			34	36	
15.5	Recovery		152	35	27.2	0.69	0.60	3.9	1.15			120			33			35	40	
16.0	Recovery		149	35	24.1	0.56	0.48	3.2	1.17			121			33			38	44	
16.5	Recovery		138	32	21.1	0.50	0.48	3.5	1.04			114			36			37	38	

Abbreviations: BP, blood pressure; BTPS, body temperature pressure saturated; f, frequency; HCO_3^-, bicarbonate; HR, heart rate; $P(A - a)O_2$, alveolar-arterial PO_2 difference; $P(a - ET)CO_2$, arterial-end-tidal PCO_2 difference; $PETCO_2$, end-tidal PCO_2; $PETO_2$, end-tidal PO_2; R, respiratory exchange ratio; STPD, standard temperature pressure dry; $\dot{V}CO_2$, carbon dioxide output; VD/VT, physiological dead space-tidal volume ratio; $\dot{V}E$, minute ventilation; $\dot{V}E/\dot{V}CO_2$, ventilatory equivalent for carbon dioxide; $\dot{V}E/\dot{V}O_2$, ventilatory equivalent for oxygen; $\dot{V}O_2$, oxygen uptake.

high/normal (Branch Point 4.1). The ventilatory equivalent for carbon dioxide was close to the upper limit of normal or perhaps slightly elevated at the anaerobic threshold, so both branches might be considered. If $\dot{V}E/\dot{V}CO_2$ were elevated, the flowchart leads to consideration of an abnormal pulmonary circulation, either due to primary pulmonary vascular disease or left heart failure. If not considered elevated, then an O_2 flow problem of nonpulmonary origin is considered, which does include heart disease as well. In this patient, low and flat O_2 pulse throughout exercise, steep HR-$\dot{V}O_2$ relationship, low HR reserve, and low $\Delta\dot{V}O_2/\Delta WR$ are all indicative of heart disease.

Conclusion

This patient has marked exercise intolerance due to mitral valve insufficiency leading to inadequate forward cardiac output response to exercise (heart failure).

CASE 28

Congenital Heart Disease: Coarctation and Ventricular Septal Defect Surgically Repaired

CLINICAL FINDINGS

This 21-year-old man had coarctation of the aorta and ventricular septal defect (VSD) identified at birth. In infancy, he underwent surgical repair of the coarctation and protective banding of the pulmonary artery, followed by a second procedure at 2 years of age to close the VSD and to release the pulmonary artery band. This procedure was complicated by complete heart block for which he received a permanent pacemaker. He had no specific restrictions as a child but was not athletic and was short of breath when running. He had minimal medical follow-up during his late teens. He was referred for exercise testing at the time of establishing care with an adult cardiologist who wished to quantify his functional capacity and evaluate him for possible biventricular pacing. He was working as a butcher and reported no difficulty in his daily activities, but he did not climb stairs or engage in sports. His only medication was carvedilol. He had a dual-chamber pacemaker operating in a VAT (ventricular paced, atrial sensed) mode. An echocardiogram performed just prior to referral had revealed the unexpected finding of global hypokinesis of the left ventricle with an ejection fraction of 35%. The right ventricle was enlarged with severe pulmonic valve regurgitation but normal estimated right ventricular pressures. On physical examination, the cardiac impulse was displaced laterally and there were murmurs in both midsystole and middiastole; breath sounds were clear. There was no peripheral edema or clubbing. The electrocardiogram showed P waves preceding each paced QRS with a PR interval of 260 ms and a QRS of 140 ms consistent with right ventricular pacing.

TABLE 10.28.1 Selected Demographic Data

Measurement	Predicted	Measured
Age (y)		21
Sex		Male
Height (cm)		183
Weight (kg)		84

EXERCISE FINDINGS

The patient performed exercise on a cycle ergometer beginning with 3 minutes of pedaling at 60 rpm without resistance, followed by continuous increase in work rate at a rate of 15 W/min. He ended the test at a work rate of 162 W with symptoms of leg fatigue. Heart rate increased progressively during exercise, without change in rhythm, and pulse oximetry remained normal.

Comments

Pulmonary function tests were not available. Demographic data are shown in **Table 10.28.1** and exercise data are summarized in **Table 10.28.2** and shown in **Table 10.28.3** and graphically in **Figure 10.28.1**.

Analysis

The exercise data show significant exercise impairment for a man of this age, with a peak oxygen uptake ($\dot{V}O_2$) that was only around 60% of the reference value and a reduced anaerobic threshold (*AT*). Although peak heart rate was also lower than predicted, it is apparent that he exercised well beyond his *AT*, which was abnormally low, and attained an end-exercise R of 1.1, so effort appears to have been good. The low peak heart rate may have been due to his β-blocker therapy. The slope of heart rate relative to $\dot{V}O_2$ was normal up to the level of exercise performed, reflecting intact sinus node function. With β-blockade in a healthy subject, this slope is usually shallow and the peak oxygen (O_2) pulse is above predicted, reflecting a partially compensatory increase in stroke volume. In this case, peak O_2 pulse was low, implying that while the offsetting effects of systolic dysfunction and β-blockade preserved stroke volume early in exercise, peak stroke volume was less than normal. The resting blood pressure was normal, and although only one repeat measure was recorded during exercise, it did not appear excessive. The ventilatory response to exercise was mildly abnormal with $\dot{V}E/\dot{V}CO_2$ values that are slightly higher than the upper limit of normal. The low peak $\dot{V}O_2$, peak O_2 pulse, and low *AT* are consistent with cardiac dysfunction limiting maximal cardiac output, and the modestly elevated ventilatory equivalents suggest

TABLE 10.28.2 Selected Exercise Data

Measurement	Predicted	Measured
Peak $\dot{V}O_2$ (L/min)	3.59	2.18
Maximum heart rate (beats/min)	199	148
Maximum O_2 pulse (mL/beat)	18.1	16.0
$\Delta\dot{V}O_2/\Delta WR$ (mL/min/W)	10.3	9.7
AT (L/min)	>1.51	1.39
Blood pressure (mm Hg [rest, max ex])		120/-,170/-
Maximum $\dot{V}E$ (L/min)		69
$\dot{V}E/\dot{V}CO_2$ @ *AT* or lowest	23.6	29.4

Abbreviations: *AT*, anaerobic threshold; $\Delta\dot{V}O_2/\Delta WR$, change in $\dot{V}O_2$/change in work rate; O_2, oxygen; $\dot{V}E$, minute ventilation; $\dot{V}E/\dot{V}CO_2$, ventilatory equivalent for carbon dioxide; $\dot{V}O_2$, oxygen uptake.

TABLE 10.28.3 Air Breathing

Time (min)	Work rate (W)	BP (mm Hg)	HR (min^{-1})	f (min^{-1})	$\dot{V}E$ (L/min BTPS)	$\dot{V}CO_2$ (L/min STPD)	$\dot{V}O_2$ (L/min STPD)	$\frac{\dot{V}O_2}{HR}$ (mL/beat)	R	pH	HCO_3^- (mEq/L)	PO_2, mm Hg ET	PO_2, mm Hg a	PO_2, mm Hg (A − a)	PCO_2, mm Hg ET	PCO_2, mm Hg a	PCO_2, mm Hg (a − ET)	$\frac{\dot{V}E}{\dot{V}CO_2}$	$\frac{\dot{V}E}{\dot{V}O_2}$	$\frac{VD}{VT}$
0.5	Rest	120/-	83	21	12.8	0.38	0.44	5.3	0.86			104			38			34	29	
1.0	Rest		85	22	16.0	0.46	0.52	6.1	0.89			108			36			35	31	
1.5	Rest		89	17	14.2	0.40	0.44	5.0	0.90			105			38			35	32	
2.0	Rest		84	21	13.8	0.39	0.46	5.4	0.87			107			37			35	30	
2.5	Rest		83	18	12.8	0.37	0.42	5.1	0.88			105			38			34	30	
3.0	Rest		86	18	14.3	0.41	0.45	5.2	0.91			108			36			35	32	
3.5	Unloaded		86	19	11.5	0.33	0.39	4.5	0.84			104			38			35	29	
4.0	Unloaded		93	29	15.4	0.42	0.48	5.1	0.88			107			37			37	32	
4.5	Unloaded		98	30	20.2	0.58	0.65	5.7	0.89			108			36			35	31	
5.0	Unloaded		100	32	20.7	0.61	0.73	7.3	0.84			105			37			34	29	
5.5	Unloaded		95	29	24.2	0.70	0.76	8.0	0.93			109			36			34	32	
6.0	Unloaded		93	29	21.8	0.67	0.80	8.6	0.84			104			37			32	27	
6.5	5		92	29	20.2	0.61	0.69	7.5	0.89			106			38			33	29	
7.0	13		92	29	22.2	0.69	0.79	8.5	0.88			106			37			32	28	
7.5	20		96	30	21.2	0.65	0.76	7.9	0.86			105			38			33	28	
8.0	27		96	31	22.6	0.97	0.76	7.9	0.89			107			37			34	30	
8.5	35		101	32	24.1	0.73	0.85	8.5	0.86			105			37			33	28	
9.0	43		100	28	23.4	0.75	0.89	8.9	0.84			103			39			31	26	
9.5	50		100	30	26.5	0.82	0.93	9.3	0.89			104			38			32	29	
10.0	57		106	34	29.7	0.94	1.06	10.0	0.89			106			37			32	28	
10.5	56		111	32	29.1	0.95	1.08	9.7	0.88			105			38			31	27	
11.0	72		108	32	34.5	1.10	1.17	10.8	0.95			109			37			31	30	
11.5	80		114	38	31.0	1.05	1.20	10.5	0.88			103			39			29	26	
12.0	87		120	35	36.8	1.22	1.29	10.8	0.94			108			38			30	28	
12.5	95		117	33	37.3	1.28	1.39	11.9	0.92			105			39			29	27	
13.0	103		122	37	44.9	1.49	1.51	12.4	0.99			110			37			30	30	
13.5	110		123	35	43.6	1.49	1.53	12.5	0.97			107			39			29	28	
14.0	118		131	38	46.2	1.57	1.58	12.0	1.00			109			38			29	29	
14.5	125		132	37	49.8	1.72	1.71	12.9	1.01			109			39			29	29	
15.0	132		130	[illegible]	[illegible]	1.70	1.74	12.8	1.02			109			39			29	29	
15.5	140		140	42	60.8	2.01	1.90	13.6	1.06			113			37			30	32	
16.0	148	170/-	142	40	61.9	2.06	1.92	13.5	1.07			113			37			30	32	
16.5	155		145	43	69.0	2.21	2.01	13.9	1.10			115			36			31	34	
17.0	162		148	45	68.8	2.19	1.98	13.4	1.11			115			35			31	35	
17.5	165		136	40	67.5	2.35	2.18	16.0	1.08			111			38			29	31	
18.0	Recovery		125	38	60.6	2.07	1.71	13.7	1.21			115			38			29	35	
18.5	Recovery		114	32	49.9	1.64	1.28	11.2	1.28			117			37			30	39	
19.0	Recovery		105	34	41.1	1.31	1.10	10.5	1.19			116			36			31	37	
19.5	Recovery		102	36	46.1	1.45	1.29	12.6	1.13			115			36			32	36	

Abbreviations: BP, blood pressure; BTPS, body temperature pressure saturated; f, frequency; HCO_3^-, bicarbonate; HR, heart rate; $P(A-a)O_2$, alveolar-arterial PO_2 difference; $P(a-ET)CO_2$, arterial-end-tidal PCO_2 difference; $PETCO_2$, end-tidal PCO_2; $PETO_2$, end-tidal PO_2; R, respiratory exchange ratio; STPD, standard temperature pressure dry; $\dot{V}CO_2$, carbon dioxide output; VD/VT, physiological dead space-tidal volume ratio; $\dot{V}E$, minute ventilation; $\dot{V}E/\dot{V}CO_2$, ventilatory equivalent for carbon dioxide; $\dot{V}E/\dot{V}O_2$, ventilatory equivalent for oxygen; $\dot{V}O_2$, oxygen uptake.

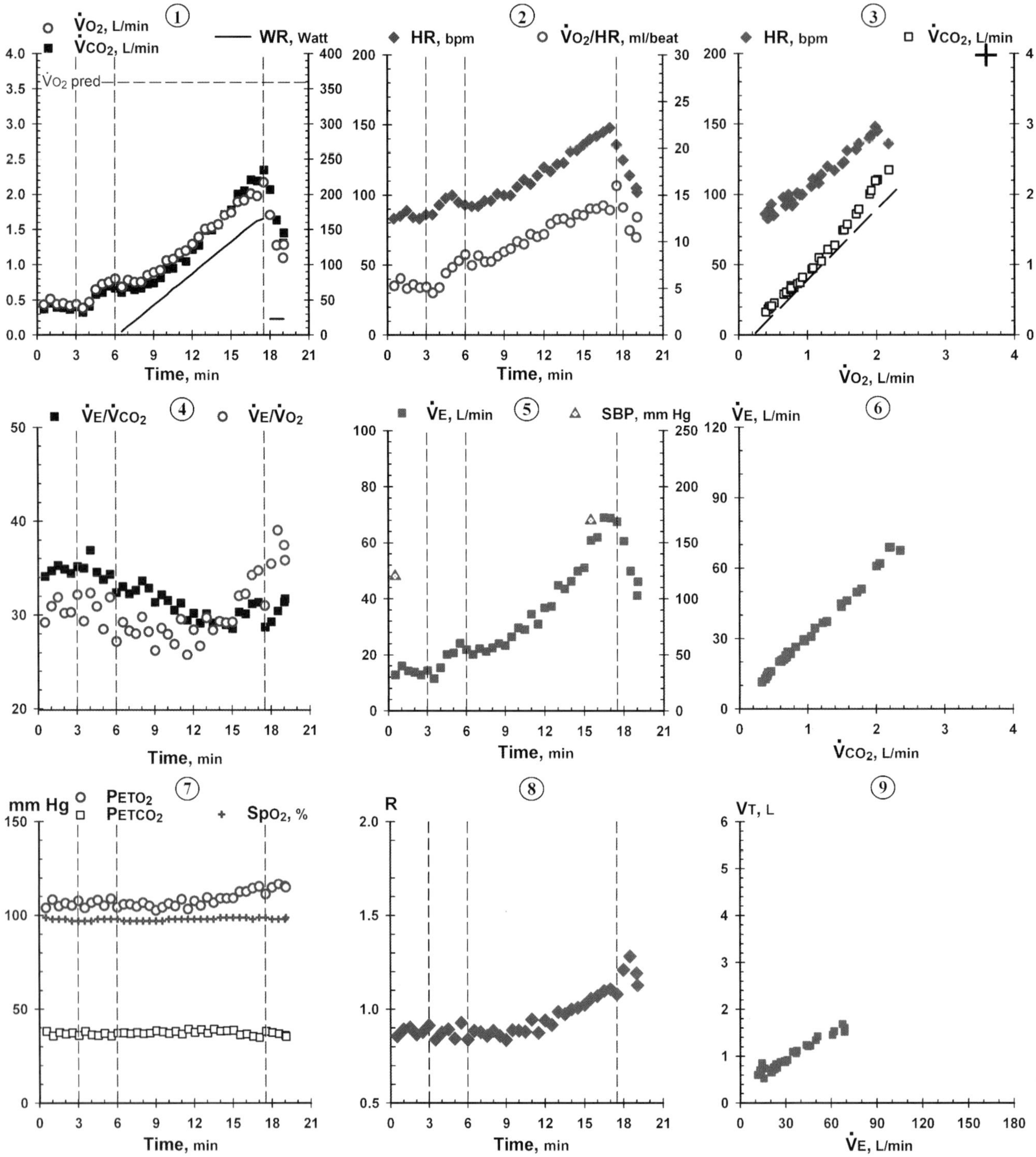

FIGURE 10.28.1. Vertical dashed lines in the panels in the left and middle columns indicate, from left to right, the beginning of unloaded cycling, start of increasing work rate (WR) at 15 W/min, and start of recovery. In **panel 1**, the increase in WR (right y-axis) is plotted with a scale of 100 W to 1 L of oxygen uptake ($\dot{V}O_2$) (left y-axis) such that WR is plotted parallel to a $\dot{V}O_2$ slope of 10 mL/min/W. In **panel 3**, carbon dioxide output ($\dot{V}CO_2$) (right y-axis) is plotted as a function of $\dot{V}O_2$ (x-axis) with identical scales so that the diagonal dashed line has a slope of 1 (45°). The $\dot{V}CO_2$ increasing more steeply than $\dot{V}O_2$ defines carbon dioxide (CO_2) derived from bicarbonate buffer, as long as ventilatory equivalent for CO_2 ($\dot{V}E/\dot{V}CO_2$) (**panel 4**) is not increasing and end-tidal P_{CO_2} (P_{ETCO_2}) (**panel 7**) is not decreasing, simultaneously. The black + symbol in **panel 3** indicates predicted values of heart rate (HR) (left y-axis) and $\dot{V}O_2$ for this individual. Abbreviations: P_{ETO_2}, end-tidal P_{O_2}; R, respiratory exchange ratio; SBP, systolic blood pressure; Sp_{O_2}, oxygen saturation as measured by pulse oximetry; $\dot{V}E$, minute ventilation; $\dot{V}E/\dot{V}O_2$, ventilatory equivalent for oxygen; VT, tidal volume.

early impairment in pulmonary $\dot{V}/\dot{Q}$ matching, even in the absence of overt findings of clinical heart failure.

Conclusion

Despite having early surgical therapy of congenital heart disease, this patient has significantly impaired exercise capacity, resulting from a number of residual or secondary processes. These include heart block with pacemaker dependence, the development of left ventricular systolic dysfunction, and pulmonic valve dysfunction. Typical of patients with congenital disorders, the extent of impairment was difficult to determine from history alone.

CASE 29

Congenital Heart Disease: Transposition of the Great Arteries With Surgical Repair

CLINICAL FINDINGS

This 22-year-old woman was referred for exercise testing as part of an evaluation for pulmonary hypertension reported on an echocardiogram. She was born with transposition of the great arteries and was treated with a palliative atrial septostomy shortly after birth, followed by an arterial switch procedure at 2 years of age. She was not restricted in her activities as a child and took part in gym classes along with her peers. She did not participate in sports, however, and maintained a sedentary lifestyle. Evidence of pulmonary hypertension was first noted 3 years prior to this referral on a routine echocardiogram performed during pregnancy. The findings were more pronounced on a follow-up echocardiogram, with a dilated right ventricle and an estimated pulmonary artery systolic pressure of 60 mm Hg. She was therefore referred to a pulmonary hypertension specialist who requested exercise testing. She admitted to shortness of breath when ascending stairs but did not think this was excessive. She denied syncope or chest pain. She was taking no medications. Examination was notable for a healed sternotomy scar, normal heart sounds, and clear lung fields. There was no cyanosis, clubbing, or edema of the extremities. An electrocardiogram showed a sinus rhythm with right ventricular hypertrophy and diffuse ST-T wave changes.

TABLE 10.29.1 Selected Respiratory Function Data

Measurement	Predicted	Measured
Age (y)		22
Sex		Female
Height (cm)		150
Weight (kg)		55
Hemoglobin (mg/dL)		14.3
VC (L)	3.09	3.10
IC (L)	2.06	2.26
TLC (L)	4.17	4.29
FEV_1 (L)	2.74	2.46
FEV_1/VC (%)	89	79
MVV (L/min)	103	80
D_{LCO} (mL/mm Hg/min)	23.8	21.5

Abbreviations: D_{LCO}, diffusing capacity of the lung for carbon monoxide; FEV_1, forced expiratory volume in 1 second; IC, inspiratory capacity; MVV, maximum voluntary ventilation; TLC, total lung capacity; VC, vital capacity.

EXERCISE FINDINGS

The patient performed exercise on a cycle ergometer beginning with 3 minutes of pedaling at 60 rpm without resistance, followed by a continuous increase in work rate by 10 W/min. She ended the test with the limiting symptom of leg fatigue. She also had shortness of breath but denied chest pain or light-headedness.

Comments

Resting pulmonary function, including lung mechanics and diffusing capacity, was essentially normal (**Table 10.29.1**). This case is presented because it reinforces the concept that the pulmonary gas exchange efficiency is to a great extent a reflection of regional ventilation–perfusion ($\dot{V}/\dot{Q}$) matching in the lung.

Analysis

Exercise capacity was low with the peak $\dot{V}O_2$ just over half of the predicted value and a similarly reduced anaerobic threshold (**Tables 10.29.2** and **10.29.3**). Peak heart rate was less than the predicted maximum, but heart rate accelerated steeply during the last minute of exercise, associated with a flat or declining oxygen pulse (**Fig. 10.29.1**). Because hemoglobin concentration and oxygen saturation were normal, the remarkably flat oxygen pulse pattern throughout exercise implies that maximal stroke volume and $C(a - \bar{v})O_2$ were attained early, and thereafter, $\dot{V}O_2$ increased by heart rate alone. This is indicative of cardiovascular impairment.

TABLE 10.29.2 Selected Exercise Data

Measurement	Predicted	Measured
Peak $\dot{V}O_2$ (L/min)	1.85	0.96
Maximum heart rate (beats/min)	198	141
Maximum O_2 pulse (mL/beat)	9.4	7.9
$\Delta\dot{V}O_2/\Delta WR$ (mL/min/W)	10.3	6.2
AT (L/min)	>0.77	0.57
Blood pressure (mm Hg [rest, max ex])		124/81, 195/151
Maximum $\dot{V}E$ (L/min)		31
Exercise breathing reserve (L/min)	>15	49
$\dot{V}E/\dot{V}CO_2$ @ *AT* or lowest	26.0	28.5

Abbreviations: *AT*, anaerobic threshold; $\Delta\dot{V}O_2/\Delta WR$, change in $\dot{V}O_2$/change in work rate; ex, exercise; O_2, oxygen; $\dot{V}E$, minute ventilation; $\dot{V}E/\dot{V}CO_2$, ventilatory equivalent for carbon dioxide; $\dot{V}O_2$, oxygen uptake.

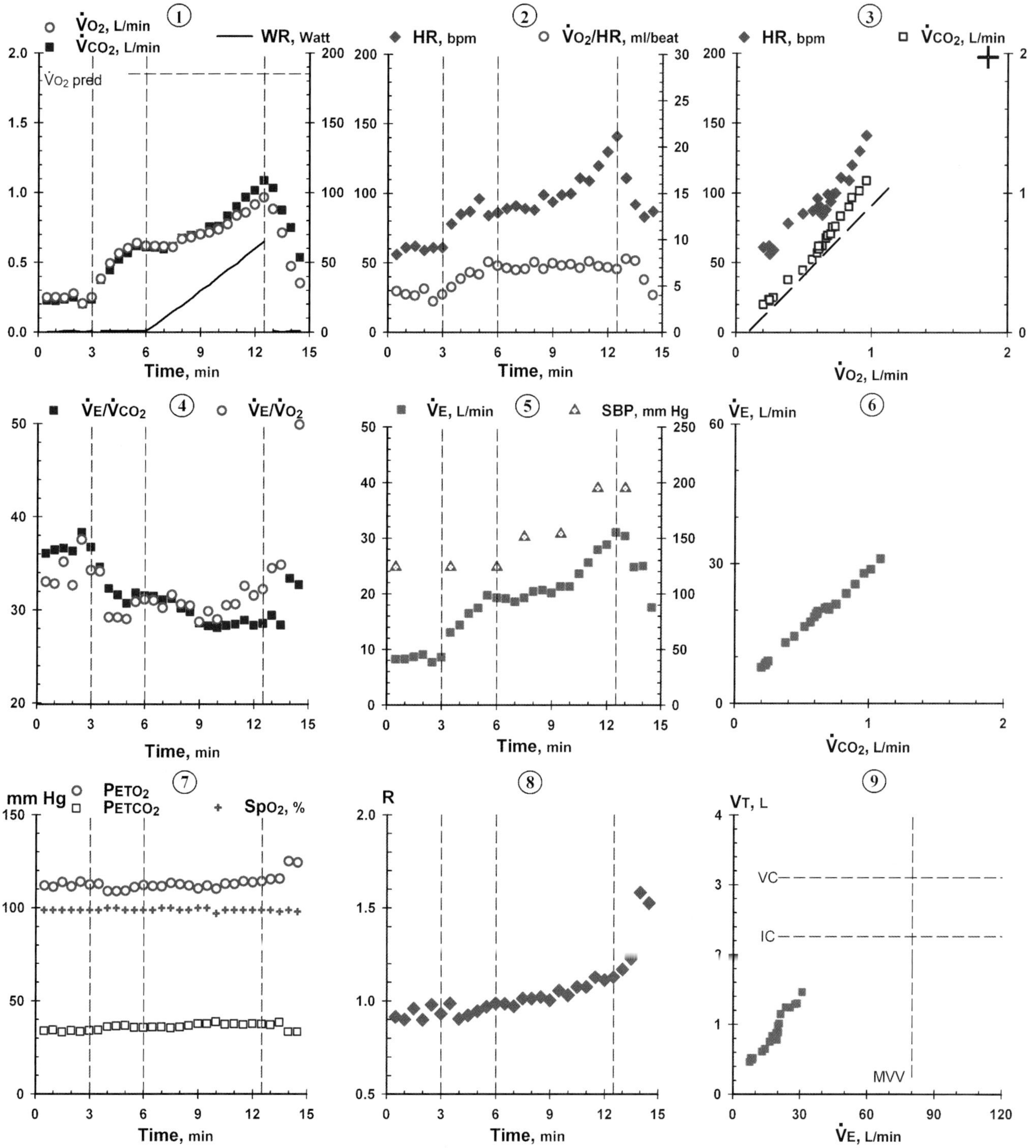

FIGURE 10.29.1. Vertical dashed lines in the panels in the left and middle columns indicate, from left to right, the beginning of unloaded cycling, start of increasing work rate (WR) at 10 W/min, and start of recovery. In **panel 1**, the increase in WR (right y-axis) is plotted with a scale of 100 W to 1 L of oxygen uptake ($\dot{V}O_2$) (left y-axis) such that WR is plotted parallel to a $\dot{V}O_2$ slope of 10 mL/min/W. In **panel 3**, carbon dioxide output ($\dot{V}CO_2$) (right y-axis) is plotted as a function of $\dot{V}O_2$ (x-axis) with identical scales so that the diagonal dashed line has a slope of 1 (45°). The $\dot{V}CO_2$ increasing more steeply than $\dot{V}O_2$ defines carbon dioxide (CO_2) derived from bicarbonate buffer, as long as ventilatory equivalent for CO_2 ($\dot{V}E/\dot{V}CO_2$) (**panel 4**) is not increasing and end-tidal PCO_2 ($PETCO_2$) (**panel 7**) is not decreasing, simultaneously. The black + symbol in **panel 3** indicates predicted values of heart rate (HR) (left y-axis) and $\dot{V}O_2$ for this individual. Abbreviations: IC, inspiratory capacity; MVV, maximum voluntary ventilation; $PETO_2$, end-tidal PO_2; R, respiratory exchange ratio; SBP, systolic blood pressure; SpO_2, oxygen saturation as measured by pulse oximetry; VC, vital capacity; $\dot{V}E$, minute ventilation; $\dot{V}E/\dot{V}O_2$, ventilatory equivalent for oxygen; VT, tidal volume.

TABLE 10.29.3 Air Breathing

Time (min)	Work rate (W)	BP (mm Hg)	HR (min^{-1})	f (min^{-1})	$\dot{V}E$ (L/min BTPS)	$\dot{V}CO_2$ (L/min STPD)	$\dot{V}O_2$ (L/min STPD)	$\frac{\dot{V}O_2}{HR}$ (mL/beat)	R	pH	HCO_3^- (mEq/L)	PO_2, mm Hg ET	PO_2, mm Hg a	PO_2, mm Hg (A − a)	PCO_2, mm Hg ET	PCO_2, mm Hg a	PCO_2, mm Hg (a − ET)	$\frac{\dot{V}E}{\dot{V}CO_2}$	$\frac{\dot{V}E}{\dot{V}O_2}$	$\frac{V_D}{V_T}$
0.5	Rest	124/81	56	16	8.2	0.23	0.25	4.4	0.92			112			34			36	33	
1.0	Rest		61	16	8.2	0.23	0.25	4.1	0.90			111			35			36	33	
1.5	Rest		62	17	8.7	0.24	0.25	4.0	0.96			114			33			37	35	
2.0	Rest		59	17	9.1	0.25	0.28	4.7	0.90			112			34			36	33	
2.5	Rest		61	17	7.7	0.20	0.21	3.4	0.98			114			34			38	38	
3.0	Rest		61	17	8.6	0.23	0.25	4.1	0.93			113			34			37	34	
3.5	Unloaded	124/81	78	21	13.1	0.38	0.38	4.9	0.99			113			34			35	34	
4.0	Unloaded		85	22	14.4	0.45	0.49	5.8	0.90			109			36			32	29	
4.5	Unloaded		87	22	16.5	0.52	0.57	6.5	0.92			109			37			32	29	
5.0	Unloaded		96	21	17.5	0.57	0.60	6.3	0.95			109			37			31	29	
5.5	Unloaded		84	25	19.7	0.62	0.64	7.6	0.97			111			36			32	31	
6.0	Unloaded		86	24	19.3	0.61	0.62	7.2	0.99			112			36			32	31	
6.5	5	124/81	89	24	19.2	0.61	0.62	6.9	0.99			112			36			31	31	
7.0	10		91	23	18.6	0.60	0.61	6.7	0.97			112			36			31	30	
7.5	15		89	22	19.3	0.62	0.61	6.9	1.01			113			36			31	32	
8.0	19	151/103	88	23	20.4	0.68	0.67	7.6	1.01			113			36			30	31	
8.5	24		99	21	20.7	0.69	0.68	6.9	1.02			112			37			30	30	
9.0	30		94	21	20.2	0.70	0.70	7.5	1.00			110			38			29	29	
9.5	34		99	19	21.3	0.71	0.71	7.2	1.06			112			38			28	30	
10.0	40	154/104	100	19	21.3	0.74	0.74	7.4	1.03			110			39			28	29	
10.5	45		111	19	23.6	0.83	0.77	7.0	1.08			113			38			28	31	
11.0	49		109	21	25.6	0.90	0.84	7.7	1.08			113			38			28	31	
11.5	55	195/151	120	22	27.9	0.97	0.86	7.1	1.13			114			37			29	33	
12.0	60		130	22	28.8	1.02	0.91	7.0	1.11			114			38			28	32	
12.5	65		141	21	31.1	1.09	0.96	6.8	1.13			114			38			29	32	
13.0	Recovery		111	24	30.4	1.03	0.88	7.9	1.17			115			37			29	34	
13.5	Recovery		92	20	24.8	0.87	0.71	7.7	1.23			116			39			28	35	
14.0	Recovery		83	22	25.0	0.75	0.47	5.7	1.58			125			35			33	53	
14.5	Recovery		87	15	17.6	0.54	0.35	4.0	1.53			124			34			33	50	

Abbreviations: BP, blood pressure; BTPS, body temperature pressure saturated; f, frequency; HCO_3^-, bicarbonate; HR, heart rate; $P(A - a)O_2$, alveolar-arterial PO_2 difference; $P(a - ET)CO_2$, arterial-end-tidal PCO_2 difference; $PETCO_2$, end-tidal PCO_2; $PETO_2$, end-tidal PO_2; R, respiratory exchange ratio; STPD, standard temperature pressure dry; $\dot{V}CO_2$, carbon dioxide output; V_D/V_T, physiological dead space-tidal volume ratio; $\dot{V}E$, minute ventilation; $\dot{V}E/\dot{V}CO_2$, ventilatory equivalent for carbon dioxide; $\dot{V}E/\dot{V}O_2$, ventilatory equivalent for oxygen; $\dot{V}O_2$, oxygen uptake.

In contrast, variables related to ventilation and pulmonary gas exchange were normal, including normal breathing reserve. In particular, the $\dot{V}E/\dot{V}CO_2$ ratio decreased into the high 20s during exercise, and oxygen saturation appeared normal (**Table 10.29.3**; **Fig. 10.29.1**), implying preserved $\dot{V}/\dot{Q}$ matching. This is in contrast to the typical findings of patients with obliterative pulmonary vascular disease in whom $\dot{V}E/\dot{V}CO_2$ is usually elevated. Although such pulmonary arterial disease can develop in a subset of patients after arterial switch procedures, the normal $\dot{V}E/\dot{V}CO_2$ ratio reflecting preserved pulmonary $\dot{V}/\dot{Q}$ matching suggests that, in this case, the elevated pressures reported on echocardiogram actually reflected *right ventricular* hypertension due to a proximal pulmonary arterial process without involvement of the more peripheral microcirculation. This can result from stenosis of the pulmonary outflow track or branch pulmonary arteries, which is a recognized late complication of the arterial switch procedure. This condition would normally be identified by a sonographer with expertise in congenital lesions but was missed in this case resulting in an initial misdiagnosis.

Conclusions

Exercise tolerance was reduced by cardiovascular factors, but pulmonary gas exchange was well preserved in this patient with congenital heart disease. The suspected cause of limitation and of her echocardiographic findings was pulmonary artery stenosis complicating the arterial switch procedure for transposition of the great arteries.

CASE 30

Patent Ductus Arteriosus With Left-to-Right Shunt, Presurgical Closure

CLINICAL FINDINGS

This 25-year-old man had recently developed exertional dyspnea and was found to have a patent ductus arteriosus (PDA). Cardiac catheterization demonstrated normal coronary arteries, a left ventricular ejection fraction of 56%, a large left-to-right shunt from the aorta through the patent ductus to the pulmonary artery, and normal pulmonary artery pressures at rest. The surgeon requested a preoperative cycle ergometer study with a pulmonary artery catheter in place to assess pulmonary artery pressures during exercise. The patient was sent to the exercise laboratory with a right radial artery and pulmonary artery catheters in place. Resting 12-lead electrocardiograms (ECGs) showed left atrial enlargement and left ventricular hypertrophy.

EXERCISE FINDINGS

The patient performed exercise on a cycle ergometer. He pedaled at 60 rpm without an added load for 3 minutes. The work rate was then increased 15 W/min to tolerance. Intra-arterial pressures were recorded continuously, and blood was intermittently sampled from both the systemic arterial and pulmonary arterial catheters. The patient stopped exercise because of calf and thigh fatigue. He had no chest pain and no further ECG abnormalities.

TABLE 10.30.1 Selected Respiratory Function Data

Measurement	Predicted	Measured
Age (y)		25
Sex		Male
Height (cm)		170
Weight (kg)	74	56
Hemoglobin (mg/dL)		14.6
VC (L)	4.39	4.27
IC (L)	2.93	2.42
TLC (L)	5.81	6.62
FEV_1 (L)	3.57	3.62
FEV_1/VC (%)	81	85
MVV (L/min)	156	158
D_{LCO} (mL/mm Hg/min)	29.6	35.6

Abbreviations: D_{LCO}, diffusing capacity of lung for carbon monoxide; FEV_1, forced expiratory volume in 1 second; IC, inspiratory capacity; MVV, maximum voluntary ventilation; TLC, total lung capacity; VC, vital capacity.

INTERPRETATION

Comments

Resting respiratory function studies were normal, with a high-normal D_{LCO} suggestive of an increase in pulmonary capillary blood volume (**Table 10.30.1**). The systemic blood pressure was high during exercise, but the pulmonary artery pressure remained normal. Exercise data are summarized in **Table 10.30.2** and shown in **Table 10.30.3** and graphically in **Figure 10.30.1**.

Analysis

Peak oxygen uptake ($\dot{V}O_2$) and anaerobic threshold were low, and there was a steeper than normal heart rate versus $\dot{V}O_2$ response. This was verified by a low and flat (unchanging) O_2 pulse; this could be explained by anemia (absent in this patient) or abnormally low $C(a - \bar{v})O_2$ or low stroke volume. The finding of low O_2 pulse throughout exercise indicates that the patient reached a maximum product of stroke volume × $C(a - \bar{v})O_2$ early in the exercise study. These findings would be characteristic of heart disease with low cardiac output. In the presence of a central circulatory shunt, however, there can be more than one cardiac output.

Cardiac output can be measured using the Fick equation. Usually, this formula is cardiac output = $\dot{V}O_2/[CaO_2 - C\bar{v}O_2]$, where the quantity in brackets is the difference between arterial O_2 content (CaO_2) and mixed venous O_2 content ($C\bar{v}O_2$). However, the formula can be used to estimate blood flow through any vascular bed from which O_2 is extracted ($\dot{V}O_2$) by using the difference in O_2 content from the beginning and at the end of that bed. In this patient, dividing $\dot{V}O_2$ by the difference between CaO_2 and $C\bar{v}O_2$, the blood flow determined would be the systemic blood flow. However, the left ventricle output in this patient with a left-to-right shunt from the aorta to the pulmonary artery must be greater than systemic blood flow, that is, equal to systemic blood flow plus flow through the left-to-right shunt. The total left ventricular output can be estimated by dividing $\dot{V}O_2$ by the difference between CaO_2 and the O_2 content of pulmonary artery blood (sampled after shunted blood from the aorta mixes with blood from the right ventricle). Because of the

TABLE 10.30.2 Selected Exercise Data

Measurement	Predicted	Measured
Peak $\dot{V}O_2$ (L/min)	2.68	1.68
Maximum heart rate (beats/min)	195	166
Maximum O_2 pulse (mL/beat)	13.7	10.1
$\Delta\dot{V}O_2/\Delta WR$ (mL/min/W)	10.3	8.2
AT (L/min)	>1.09	1.00
Systemic blood pressure (mm Hg [rest, max])		154/70, 228/105
Pulmonary artery pressure (mm Hg [rest, max])		20/10, 30/15
Maximum $\dot{V}E$ (L/min)		54
Exercise breathing reserve (L/min)	>15	104
$\dot{V}E/\dot{V}CO_2$ @ *AT* or lowest	24.5	24.3
PaO_2 (mm Hg [rest, max ex])		103, 95
$P(A - a)O_2$ (mm Hg [rest, max ex])		6, 17
$PaCO_2$ (mm Hg [rest, max ex])		39, 43
$P(a - ET)CO_2$ (mm Hg [rest, max ex])		0, −3
VD/VT (rest, max ex)		0.39, 0.20
HCO_3^- (mEq/L [rest, 2-min recov])		25, 18

Abbreviations: *AT*, anaerobic threshold; $\Delta\dot{V}O_2/\Delta WR$, change in $\dot{V}O_2$/change in work rate; ex, exercise; HCO_3^-, bicarbonate; O_2, oxygen; $P(A - a)O_2$, alveolar-arterial PO_2 difference; $P(a - ET)CO_2$, arterial-end-tidal PCO_2 difference; recov, recovery; VD/VT, physiological dead space–tidal volume ratio; $\dot{V}E$, minute ventilation; $\dot{V}E/\dot{V}CO_2$, ventilatory equivalent for carbon dioxide; $\dot{V}O_2$, oxygen uptake.

"step-up" in O_2 content due to mixing of well-oxygenated blood from the aorta, the difference between O_2 content in the pulmonary artery and CaO_2 would be small, thereby resulting in a high left ventricular total output even if systemic blood flow is normal or reduced. (In this patient, total left ventricular output was measured to be considerably elevated relative to $\dot{V}O_2$ [data not shown], consistent with the shunt.)

If using the flowcharts (Chapter 9), peak $\dot{V}O_2$ and the anaerobic threshold were low, leading to Flowchart 4. The high breathing reserve (Branch Point 4.1); normal $\dot{V}E/\dot{V}CO_2$ (Branch Point 4.3); normal hematocrit (Branch Point 4.4); and low, unchanging O_2 pulse (Branch Point 4.6) lead to the category of heart disease. The ECG did not show evidence of myocardial ischemia, but the low $\Delta\dot{V}O_2/\Delta WR$ and steep heart rate versus $\dot{V}O_2$ indicate impairment in effective cardiovascular function. The normal values for ventilatory equivalents, $P(A - a)O_2$, and VD/VT indicate that pulmonary $\dot{V}A/\dot{Q}$ matching was well maintained, arguing against significant pulmonary vascular disease.

Conclusion

The large left-to-right shunt through the PDA obligates an increased left ventricular output to support both the shunt and the systemic blood flow needed to meet peripheral O_2 requirements at rest. With exercise, increased cardiac output is normally directed to the exercising muscle by restriction of blood flow to other vascular beds. In this case, however, blood flow to the exercising muscle was compromised by unregulated recirculation of part of the left ventricular output though the ductus left-to-right shunt. Thus, O_2 delivery to the peripheral tissues was inadequate for the demands of exercise. These abnormalities should be correctable by closing the ductus left-to-right shunt. Following surgical closure of the PDA, this patient's dyspnea and exercise tolerance improved considerably.

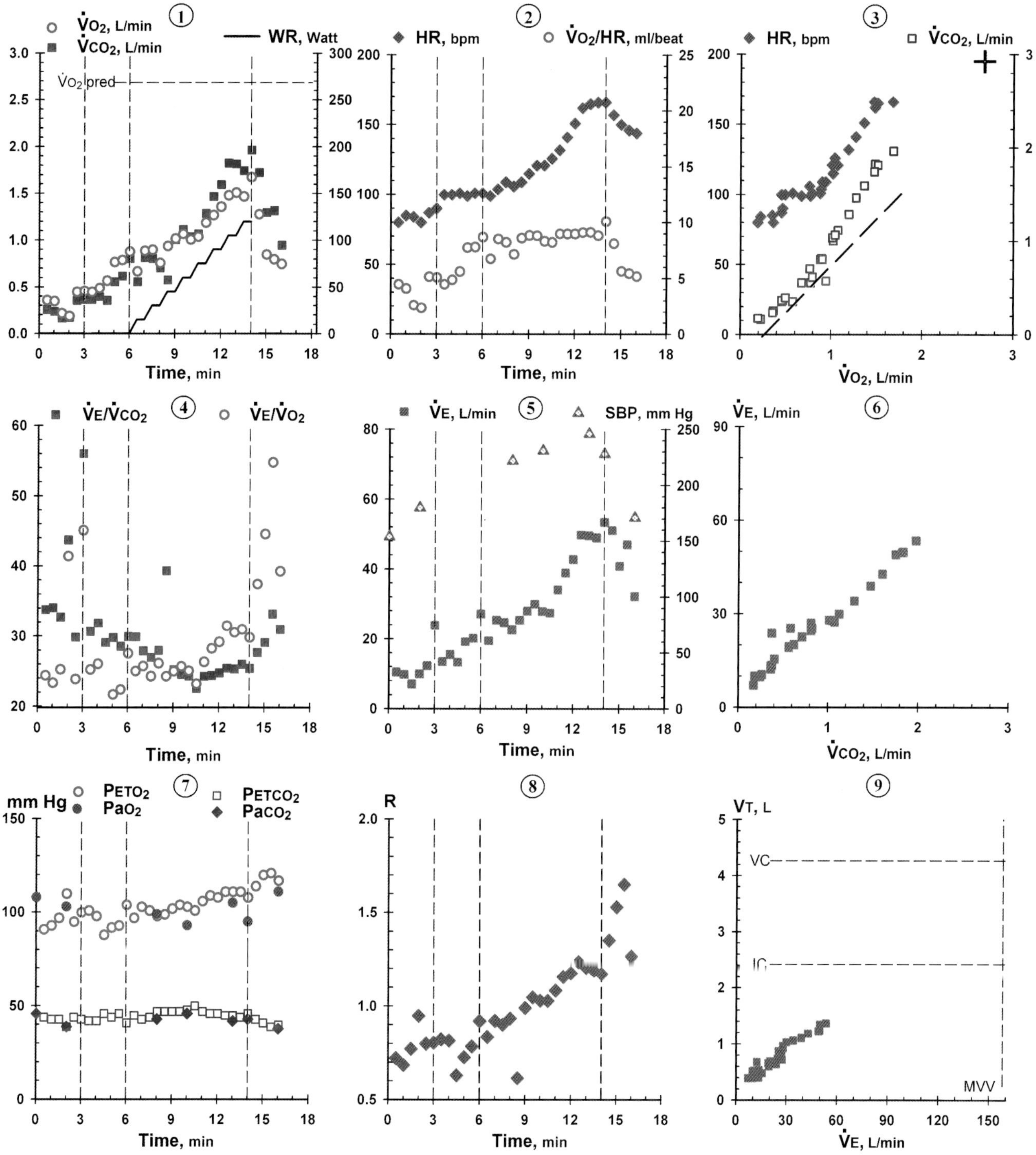

FIGURE 10.30.1. Vertical dashed lines in the panels in the left and middle columns indicate, from left to right, the beginning of unloaded cycling, start of increasing work rate (WR) at 15 W/min, and start of recovery. In **panel 1**, the increase in WR (right y-axis) is plotted with a scale of 100 W to 1 L of oxygen uptake ($\dot{V}O_2$) (left y-axis) such that WR is plotted parallel to a $\dot{V}O_2$ slope of 10 mL/min/W. In **panel 3**, carbon dioxide output ($\dot{V}CO_2$) (right y-axis) is plotted as a function of $\dot{V}O_2$ (x-axis) with identical scales so that the diagonal dashed line has a slope of 1 (45°). The $\dot{V}CO_2$ increasing more steeply than $\dot{V}O_2$ defines carbon dioxide (CO_2) derived from bicarbonate buffer, as long as ventilatory equivalent for CO_2 ($\dot{V}E/\dot{V}CO_2$) (**panel 4**) is not increasing and end-tidal PCO_2 ($PETCO_2$) (**panel 7**) is not decreasing, simultaneously. The black + symbol in **panel 3** indicates predicted values of heart rate (HR) (left y-axis) and $\dot{V}O_2$ for this individual. Abbreviations: IC, inspiratory capacity; MVV, maximum voluntary ventilation; $PETO_2$, end-tidal PO_2; R, respiratory exchange ratio; SBP, systolic blood pressure; VC, vital capacity; $\dot{V}E$, minute ventilation; $\dot{V}E/\dot{V}O_2$, ventilatory equivalent for oxygen; V_T, tidal volume.

TABLE 10.30.3 Air Breathing

Time (min)	Work rate (W)	BP (mm Hg)	HR (min^{-1})	f (min^{-1})	$\dot{V}E$ (L/min BTPS)	$\dot{V}CO_2$ (L/min STPD)	$\dot{V}O_2$ (L/min STPD)	$\frac{\dot{V}O_2}{HR}$ (mL/beat)	R	pH	HCO_3^- (mEq/L)	PO_2, mm Hg ET	a	(A − a)	PCO_2, mm Hg ET	a	(a − ET)	$\frac{\dot{V}E}{\dot{V}CO_2}$	$\frac{\dot{V}E}{\dot{V}O_2}$	$\frac{V_D}{V_T}$
0	Rest	154/69								7.32	23		108			46				
0.5	Rest		80	20	10.5	0.26	0.36	4.5	0.72			91			44			34	24	
1.0	Rest		85	19	9.8	0.24	0.35	4.1	0.69			93			43			34	23	
1.5	Rest		84	18	7.1	0.17	0.22	2.6	0.77			97			43			33	25	
2.0	Rest	180/87	80	25	10.0	0.18	0.19	2.4	0.95	7.42	25	110	103	6	39	39	0	44	41	0.39
2.5	Rest		87	18	12.3	0.36	0.45	5.2	0.80			95			44			30	24	
3.0	Rest		90	37	23.9	0.37	0.46	5.1	0.80			100			43			56	45	
3.5	Unloaded		100	25	13.5	0.37	0.45	4.5	0.82			101			42			31	25	
4.0	Unloaded		100	32	15.5	0.40	0.49	4.9	0.82			98			42			32	26	
4.5	Unloaded		101	33	13.5	0.36	0.57	5.6	0.63			88			46			29	18	
5.0	Unloaded		99	29	19.2	0.56	0.77	7.8	0.73			92			44			30	22	
5.5	Unloaded		101	29	20.2	0.62	0.79	7.8	0.78			93			46			29	22	
6.0	Unloaded		101	33	27.1	0.81	0.88	8.7	0.92			104			41			30	28	
6.5	15		99	32	19.5	0.56	0.67	6.8	0.84			97			45			30	25	
7.0	15		104	29	25.4	0.82	0.89	8.6	0.92			103			43			28	26	
7.5	30		109	33	24.7	0.81	0.90	8.3	0.90			101			44			27	24	
8.0	30	222/102	106	33	22.7	0.71	0.76	7.2	0.93	7.39	26	98	99	6	47	43	−4	28	26	0.28
8.5	45		109	30	25.4	0.58	0.94	8.6	0.62			99			47			39	24	
9.0	45		115	29	28.0	1.01	1.02	8.9	0.99			102			47			25	25	
9.5	60		121	29	30.0	1.12	1.07	8.8	1.05			104			47			25	26	
10.0	60	231/96	121	30	27.9	1.04	1.01	8.3	1.03	7.35	25	103	93	12	48	46	−2	24	25	0.24
10.5	75		126	38	27.4	1.07	1.04	8.3	1.03			101			50			23	23	
11.0	75		132	32	34.1	1.29	1.19	9.0	1.08			106			47			24	26	
11.5	90		141	35	38.9	1.47	1.27	9.0	1.16			109			46			24	28	
12.0	90		151	36	42.8	1.69	1.36	9.0	1.18			108			46			25	29	
12.5	105		162	37	49.8	1.83	1.48	9.1	1.24			111			45			25	32	
13.0	105	246/108	165	40	49.6	1.82	1.51	9.2	1.21	7.34	22	111	105	9	45	42	−3	25	31	0.21
13.5	120		166	40	49.0	1.75	1.47	8.9	1.19			111			44			26	31	
14.0	120	228/105	166	39	53.5	1.97	1.68	10.1	1.17	7.30	21	108	95	17	46	43	−3	25	30	0.24
14.5	Recovery		157	37	51.1	1.73	1.28	8.2	1.35			114			43			28	37	
15.0	Recovery		150	34	40.8	1.30	0.85	5.7	1.53			120			41			29	45	
15.5	Recovery		146	37	47.0	1.32	0.80	5.5	1.65			121			39			33	55	
16.0	Recovery	171/90	144	32	32.2	0.95	0.75	5.2	1.27	7.29	18	117	111	7	40	38	−2	31	39	0.31

Abbreviations: BP, blood pressure; BTPS, body temperature pressure saturated; f, frequency; HCO_3^-, bicarbonate; HR, heart rate; $P(A-a)O_2$, alveolar-arterial PO_2 difference; $P(a-ET)CO_2$, arterial-end-tidal PCO_2 difference; $PETCO_2$, end-tidal PCO_2; $PETO_2$, end-tidal PO_2; R, respiratory exchange ratio; STPD, standard temperature pressure dry; $\dot{V}CO_2$, carbon dioxide output; V_D/V_T, physiological dead space–tidal volume ratio; $\dot{V}E$, minute ventilation; $\dot{V}E/\dot{V}CO_2$, ventilatory equivalent for carbon dioxide; $\dot{V}E/\dot{V}O_2$, ventilatory equivalent for oxygen; $\dot{V}O_2$, oxygen uptake.

CASE 31

Patent Ductus Arteriosus With Right-to-Left Shunt (Eisenmenger Ductus Syndrome)

CLINICAL FINDINGS

This 37-year-old woman was identified as having a patent ductus arterious (PDA) as a child but had not undergone surgical repair. In early adulthood, she was told she had pulmonary hypertension. She reports being normally active while growing up and being able to ride a bicycle. Her sister describes her as less active than her peers, however, and having been protected from vigorous activities by her parents. She had worked for several years as an accountant but quit work at her parents' urging out of concern for her health. She stated that she could walk on level ground for extended periods at her own pace and ascend the stairs to her third floor apartment. She identified fatigue as her primary limiting symptom in her daily activities. She denied cough, wheezing, or syncope but sometimes noted cyanosis of her fingers. She was a nonsmoker but had exposure to secondhand smoke as a child. On examination, she was thin, with reduced muscle mass. Breath sounds were clear and cardiac examination was notable for a prominent S_2 and a III/VI holosystolic murmur. There was cyanosis and clubbing of the toes but not of the fingers. While seated at rest, pulse oximeter readings from the fingers of either hand were 93% to 94% and the toes were 60% to 65% bilaterally.

EXERCISE FINDINGS

Exercise testing was performed on a cycle ergometer. After pedaling at 60 rpm for 3 minutes, the work rate was increased continuously by 10 W/min until the patient stopped with symptoms of leg fatigue. Pulse oximetry was monitored on a right-hand finger and read 94% to 95% at rest and during the first several minutes of exercise. Thereafter, there was progressive decline in estimated saturation to 85% at end exercise with further decrease in the first 1 to 2 minutes of recovery.

TABLE 10.31.1 Selected Respiratory Function Data

Measurement	Predicted	Measured
Age (y)		37
Sex		Female
Height (cm)		166
Weight (kg)		49
VC (L)	3.91	1.96
IC (L)	2.36	1.53
FEV_1 (L)	3.22	0.95
FEV_1/VC (%)	83	48
MVV (L/min)	108	39

Abbreviations: FEV_1, forced expiratory volume in 1 second; IC, inspiratory capacity; MVV, maximum voluntary ventilation; VC, vital capacity.

INTERPRETATION

Comments

The differential cyanosis noted on physical examination is characteristic of PDA with a reversal of shunt due to pulmonary hypertension. A recent echocardiogram had demonstrated right ventricular hypertrophy, large PDA, and estimated pulmonary artery pressures at systemic levels. Spirometry showed a moderate ventilatory defect, which was partially due to airflow obstruction (**Table 10.31.1**).

Analysis

Peak $\dot{V}O_2$ and anaerobic threshold (*AT*) were both reduced (**Tables 10.31.2** and **10.31.3**). The abnormalities in the $\dot{V}O_2$ response to exercise are strikingly evident in the graphical displays (**Figure 10.31.1**), which demonstrate an abnormally slow increase in $\dot{V}O_2$ relative to work rate (panel 1) and subsequent delayed decrease in $\dot{V}O_2$ toward baseline in the recovery period. These indicate severely impaired oxygen delivery to the exercising muscle. Oxygen (O_2) pulse (panel 2) increased only marginally with exercise and actually decreased during the latter half of incremental work. This corresponds to the very steep increase in heart rate relative to $\dot{V}O_2$ (panel 3).

TABLE 10.31.2 Selected Exercise Data

Measurement	Predicted	Measured
Peak $\dot{V}O_2$ (L/min)	1.48	0.60
Maximum heart rate (beats/min)	183	157
Maximum O_2 pulse (mL/beat)	8.1	4.4
$\Delta\dot{V}O_2/\Delta WR$ (mL/min/W)	10.3	3.5
AT (L/min)	>0.68	0.50
Blood pressure (mm Hg [rest, max])		104/77, 175/105
Maximum $\dot{V}E$ (L/min)		24
Exercise breathing reserve (L/min)	>15	15
$\dot{V}E/\dot{V}CO_2$ @ *AT* or lowest	26.9	38.6
O_2 saturation, finger pulse oximetry (% [rest, max])		95, 85

Abbreviations: *AT*, anaerobic threshold; $\Delta\dot{V}O_2/\Delta WR$, change in $\dot{V}O_2$/change in work rate; O_2, oxygen; $\dot{V}E$, minute ventilation; $\dot{V}E/\dot{V}CO_2$, ventilatory equivalent for carbon dioxide; $\dot{V}O_2$, oxygen uptake.

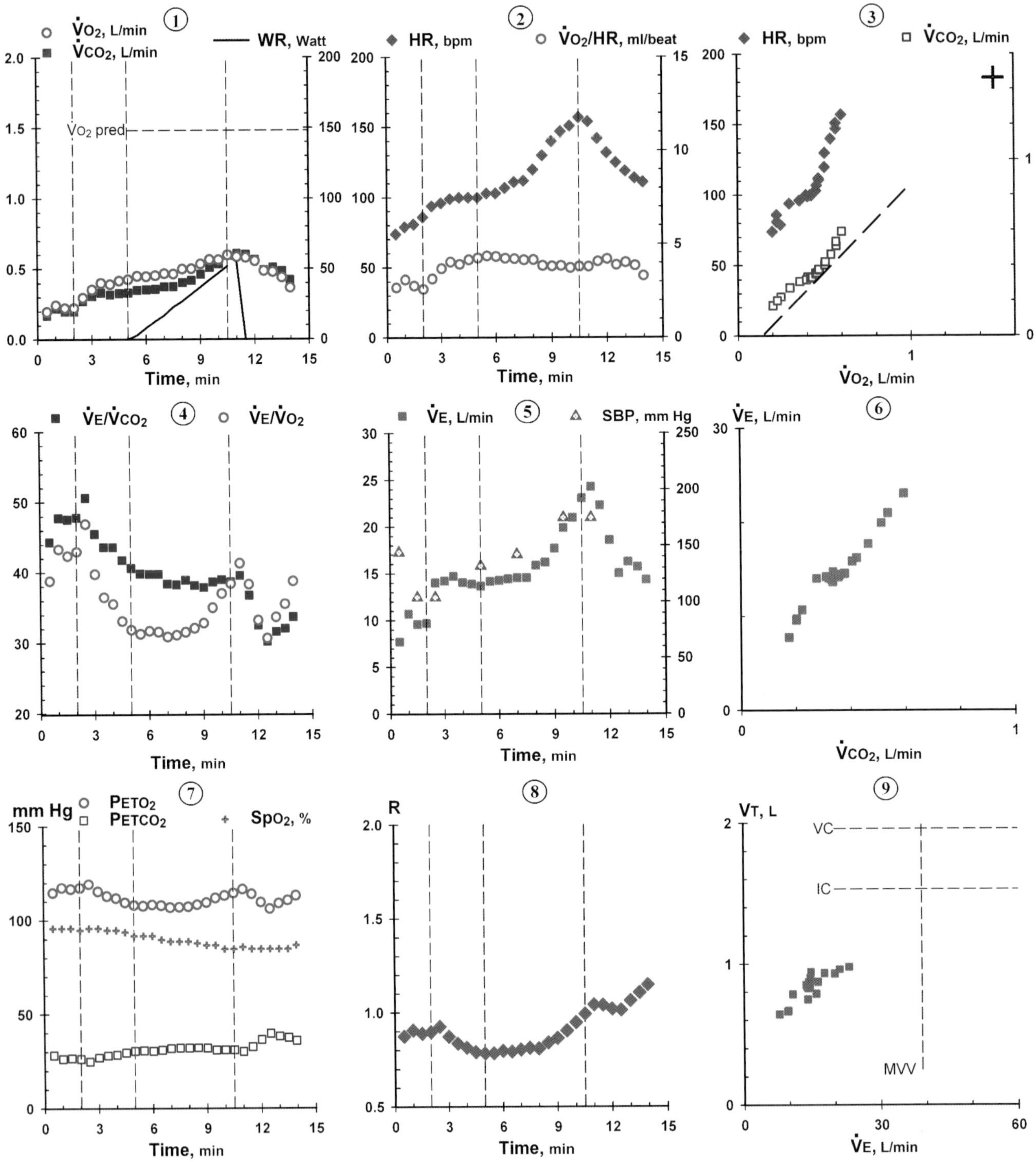

FIGURE 10.31.1. Vertical dashed lines in the panels in the left and middle columns indicate, from left to right, the beginning of unloaded cycling, start of increasing work rate (WR) at 10 W/min, and start of recovery. In **panel 1**, the increase in WR (right y-axis) is plotted with a scale of 100 W to 1 L of oxygen uptake ($\dot{V}O_2$) (left y-axis) such that WR is plotted parallel to a $\dot{V}O_2$ slope of 10 mL/min/W. In **panel 3**, carbon dioxide (CO_2) (right y-axis) is plotted as a function of $\dot{V}O_2$ (x-axis) with identical scales so that the diagonal dashed line has a slope of 1 (45°). The $\dot{V}CO_2$ increasing more steeply than $\dot{V}O_2$ defines carbon dioxide (CO_2) derived from bicarbonate buffer, as long as ventilatory equivalent for CO_2 ($\dot{V}E/\dot{V}CO_2$) (**panel 4**) is not increasing and end-tidal PCO_2 ($PETCO_2$) (**panel 7**) is not decreasing, simultaneously. The black + symbol in **panel 3** indicates predicted values of heart rate (HR) (left y-axis) and $\dot{V}O_2$ for this individual. Abbreviations: IC, inspiratory capacity; MVV, maximum voluntary ventilation; $PETO_2$, end-tidal PO_2; R, respiratory exchange ratio; SBP, systolic blood pressure; SpO_2, oxygen saturation as measured by pulse oximetry; VC, vital capacity; $\dot{V}E$, minute ventilation; $\dot{V}E/\dot{V}O_2$, ventilatory equivalent for oxygen; V_T, tidal volume.

TABLE 10.31.3 Air Breathing

Time (min)	Work rate (W)	BP (mm Hg)	HR (min^{-1})	f (min^{-1})	$\dot{V}_E$ (L/min BTPS)	$\dot{V}CO_2$ (L/min STPD)	$\dot{V}O_2$ (L/min STPD)	$\frac{\dot{V}O_2}{HR}$ (mL/beat)	R	pH	HCO_3^- (mEq/L)	PO_2, mm Hg ET	PO_2, mm Hg a	PO_2, mm Hg (A − a)	PCO_2, mm Hg ET	PCO_2, mm Hg a	PCO_2, mm Hg (a − ET)	$\frac{\dot{V}_E}{\dot{V}CO_2}$	$\frac{\dot{V}_E}{\dot{V}O_2}$	$\frac{V_D}{V_T}$
	Rest	144/105																		
0.5	Rest		74	12	7.8	0.18	0.20	2.7	0.88			115			29			44	39	
1.0	Rest		79	14	10.7	0.22	0.25	3.1	0.91			118			27			48	43	
1.5	Rest	104/77	81	15	9.6	0.20	0.23	2.8	0.89			117			27			48	42	
2.0	Rest		86	15	9.7	0.20	0.23	2.6	0.90			118			27			48	43	
2.5	Rest		94	19	14.1	0.28	0.30	3.2	0.93			120			25			51	47	
3.0	Unloaded		96	17	14.2	0.31	0.36	3.7	0.87			116			27			46	40	
3.5	Unloaded		99	16	14.7	0.34	0.40	4.1	0.84			113			28			44	37	
4.0	Unloaded		100	17	14.1	0.32	0.40	4.0	0.82			112			29			44	36	
4.5	Unloaded		100	17	13.9	0.33	0.42	4.2	0.79			110			30			42	33	
5.0	Unloaded		100	16	13.7	0.34	0.43	4.3	0.79			108			31			41	32	
5.0	Unloaded	132/87	100	16	13.7	0.34	0.43	4.3	0.79			108			31			41	32	
5.5	3		103	16	14.2	0.36	0.45	4.4	0.79			108			31			40	31	
6.0	8		103	17	14.3	0.36	0.45	4.4	0.80			109			31			40	32	
6.5	13		107	17	14.4	0.36	0.46	4.3	0.79			108			31			40	32	
7.0	17	142/88	111	16	14.6	0.38	0.47	4.2	0.80			107			32			38	31	
7.5	23		112	16	14.6	0.38	0.47	4.2	0.81			107			32			38	31	
8.0	27		120	20	15.9	0.41	0.50	4.2	0.81			108			32			39	32	
8.5	32		130	19	16.2	0.42	0.50	3.9	0.84			109			33			38	32	
9.0	37		140	19	17.7	0.47	0.54	3.8	0.87			110			32			38	33	
9.5	42	175/82	147	21	19.9	0.51	0.57	3.9	0.90			112			31			39	35	
10.0	47		151	22	21.0	0.54	0.57	3.8	0.95			113			31			39	37	
10.5	52		157	24	23.1	0.60	0.60	3.8	0.99			115			31			39	38	
11.0	56	175/82	154	25	24.3	0.61	0.59	3.8	1.04			117			31			40	41	
11.5	Recovery		142	20	22.3	0.61	0.58	4.1	1.04			114			33			37	38	
12.0	Recovery		132	16	18.6	0.57	0.56	4.2	1.02			110			37			33	33	
12.5	Recovery		125	15	15.0	0.50	0.49	3.9	1.01			106			40			30	31	
13.0	Recovery		119	15	16.3	0.51	0.48	4.1	1.06			109			39			32	34	
13.5	Recovery		114	15	15.7	0.49	0.44	3.9	1.11			111			38			32	36	
14.0	Recovery		111	16	14.4	0.43	0.37	3.3	1.15			113			36			34	39	

Abbreviations: BP, blood pressure; BTPS, body temperature pressure saturated; f, frequency; HCO_3^-, bicarbonate; HR, heart rate; $P(A - a)O_2$, alveolar-arterial PO_2 difference; $P(a - ET)CO_2$, arterial-end-tidal PCO_2 difference; P_{ETCO_2}, end-tidal PCO_2; P_{ETO_2}, end-tidal PO_2; R, respiratory exchange ratio; STPD, standard temperature pressure dry; $\dot{V}CO_2$, oxygen uptake; V_D/V_T, physiological dead space-tidal volume ratio; $\dot{V}_E$, minute ventilation; $\dot{V}_E/\dot{V}CO_2$, ventilatory equivalent for carbon dioxide; $\dot{V}_E/\dot{V}O_2$, ventilatory equivalent for oxygen; $\dot{V}O_2$, oxygen uptake.

Ventilation in response to exercise was higher than normal, as reflected in high $\dot{V}_E/\dot{V}CO_2$ at the *AT* and steep slope of $\dot{V}_E$ relative to $\dot{V}CO_2$. This is consistent with high $\dot{V}_A/\dot{Q}$ due to pulmonary vascular disease, which is intrinsic to Eisenmenger syndrome. The pattern of ventilation at the start of exercise differed from findings commonly observed with central circulatory right-to-left shunting, however, in that there was no acute increase in the ventilatory equivalents or decrease in end-tidal PCO_2. This is consistent with the ductus arteriosus being distal to the takeoff of the innominate and left common carotid arteries so that desaturation associated with right-to-left shunting affected blood flowing to the lower extremities but not blood flow to the carotid and central chemoreceptors. Nevertheless, this patient had gradual desaturation on finger pulse oximetry. Because brachial artery blood flow should leave the aorta proximal to the ductus, the exercise desaturation likely resulted from nonshunt mechanisms related to pulmonary vascular disease and very low central venous oxygenation. The finger pulse oximeter readings do not reflect the more severe desaturation of the lower extremity blood flow.

Abnormalities in $\dot{V}O_2$ resulted from impaired oxygen delivery to the exercising muscle due to a PDA. In the present case, the impairment was attributable to both the low O_2 content of the blood and the effect of pulmonary vascular disease on cardiac output, with inability to regulate distribution of blood with normal O_2 content to the legs. Despite abnormal lung function and moderately increased ventilatory equivalents observed in the test performed, she had a normal breathing reserve at end exercise and ended the test with leg fatigue, so she did not appear to be ventilatory limited.

Conclusion

This patient has severe exercise impairment due to the effects of reduced cardiac output due to pulmonary vascular disease and reduced arterial oxygen content due to right-to-left shunt. The latter is underestimated by her upper extremity pulse oximetry and does not result in the typical ventilatory responses of a central shunt due to the location of the PDA, which does not direct shunted blood to the ventilatory control centers.

CASE 32

Bicuspid Aortic Valve With Aortic Regurgitation

CLINICAL FINDINGS

A 25-year-old man with bicuspid aortic valve was referred for exercise testing to assess his exercise capacity as part of the monitoring of his valve disease. He had undergone a prior test 2 years earlier. He reported no limitations to his activities while growing up and denied any exercise-associated dyspnea, chest pain, or light-headedness. He played team sports in high school. Since graduating, he had continued to do some exercise, primarily resistance training with weights, and occasional running or cycling. At the time of testing, he worked in a sales position, which he described as sedentary but said he was interested in pursuing training as a firefighter. His medical history was otherwise unremarkable. Medications at the time of testing consisted of lisinopril. Physical examination was notable only for a grade II/VI diastolic murmur. Pulse pressure was normal. The resting electrocardiogram showed a regular sinus rhythm and was normal. Demographic and respiratory function data are shown in **Table 10.32.1**.

EXERCISE FINDINGS

The patient exercised on a cycle ergometer beginning with 3 minutes of unloaded pedaling at 60 rpm followed by continuous increase in work rate by 25 W/min until the test ended with symptoms of leg fatigue. Other than an increase in heart rate, there were no significant changes on the electrocardiogram. Results of the current and prior test are summarized in **Table 10.32.2** and data from the most recent test shown in **Table 10.32.3** and **Figure 10.32.1**.

TABLE 10.32.1 Selected Respiratory Function Data

Measurement	Predicted	Measured
Age (y)		25
Sex		Male
Height (cm)		178
Weight (kg)		87.2
VC (L)	5.54	5.12
IC (L)	3.55	3.79
ERV (L)	1.99	1.77
FEV_1 (L)	3.85	4.57
FEV_1/VC (%)	75	83
MVV (L/min)	192	184

Abbreviations: ERV, expiratory reserve volume; FEV_1, forced expiratory volume in 1 second; IC, inspiratory capacity; MVV, maximum voluntary ventilation; VC, vital capacity.

INTERPRETATION

Comment

This case is an illustration of the use of exercise testing for objective measure of functional capacity in patients with congenital heart disease. It also provides a basis for discussion of some practical issues related to calculating and using normal values, and the advantages of serial data, particularly in assessment of the clinical course of a patient with a progressive disorder.

Analysis

Exercise capacity was mildly reduced based on peak oxygen uptake ($\dot{V}O_2$) of 76% of the reference value. The anaerobic threshold was also below the lower limit of normal. The $\Delta\dot{V}O_2/\Delta WR$ was normal. The rate of increase of heart rate relative to $\dot{V}O_2$ was steeper than average and the end exercise O_2 pulse was lower than predicted. Blood pressure increased appropriately with exercise.

Ventilation increased normally and there was ample breathing reserve.

The efficiency of pulmonary gas exchange appeared normal with normal $\dot{V}E/\dot{V}CO_2$ values and normal pulse oximetry.

All these findings were quite similar to values measured 2 years previously (see **Table 10.32.2**).

The peak $\dot{V}O_2$ of 27.9 mL/min/kg body weight would likely be interpreted as below the normal predicted range regardless of which of several approaches were selected for calculating the normal value, but the exact percent of predicted would vary depending on these selections. As discussed in Chapter 7, for individuals who are overweight, we advocate using height rather than weight in calculating predicted normal values, assuming that excess weight is likely to be adipose tissue rather than muscle. In addition, we have found that predicted peak $\dot{V}O_2$ values calculated for sedentary young adults are often high, so to avoid overestimating the lower limits of normal, we recommend using an age of 30 years when calculating predicted peak $\dot{V}O_2$ for individuals in their 20s. These conventions were used in calculating the predicted values shown

TABLE 10.32.2 Selected Exercise Data Ages 25 and 23

Measurement	Predicted age 25	Measured age 25	Measured age 23
Peak $\dot{V}O_2$ (L/min)	3.2	2.43	2.51
Peak $\dot{V}O_2$ (mL/min/kg)		27.9	28.2
Maximum heart rate (beats/min)	195	174	177
Maximum O_2 pulse (mL/beat)	16.4	14.0	14.2
$\Delta\dot{V}O_2/\Delta WR$ (mL/min/W)	10.3	10.1	10.2
AT (L/min)	>1.38	1.2	1.25
Blood pressure (mm Hg [rest, max])		141/80, 207/80	122/75, 187/133
Maximum $\dot{V}E$ (L/min)		79	94
Breathing reserve (L/min)	>15	105	90
$\dot{V}E/\dot{V}CO_2$ @ *AT*	<29	25	26
SpO_2 (% [rest, max ex])		97, 97	97, 97

Abbreviations: *AT*, anaerobic threshold; $\Delta\dot{V}O_2/\Delta WR$, change in $\dot{V}O_2$/change in work rate; ex, exercise; O_2, oxygen; SpO_2, oxygen saturation as measured by pulse oximetry; $\dot{V}E$, minute ventilation; $\dot{V}E/\dot{V}CO_2$, ventilatory equivalent for carbon dioxide; $\dot{V}O_2$, oxygen uptake.

in **Table 10.32.2**. Of course, the predicted values would vary depending on which reference equations were used and how weight and age were treated in the calculations. Serial testing in patients with chronic and/or progressive conditions provides the interpreter with the advantage of comparing measured values with the patient's own historical values.

Conclusion

Exercise capacity of this young man was mildly reduced. The reductions of peak $\dot{V}O_2$ and O_2 pulse and steeper than average increase in heart rate relative to $\dot{V}O_2$ were all consistent with reduction in forward stroke volume and cardiac output, consistent with his known aortic insufficiency. These findings appeared relatively stable over a 2-year interval of time.

TABLE 10.32.3 Age 25

Time (min)	Work rate (W)	BP (mm Hg)	HR (min^{-1})	f (min^{-1})	$\dot{V}E$ (L/min BTPS)	$\dot{V}CO_2$ (L/min STPD)	$\dot{V}O_2$ (L/min STPD)	$\frac{\dot{V}O_2}{HR}$ (mL/beat)	R	pH	HCO_3^- (mEq/L)	PO_2, mm Hg and SpO_2, %			PCO_2, mm Hg			$\frac{\dot{V}E}{\dot{V}CO_2}$	$\frac{\dot{V}E}{\dot{V}O_2}$	$\frac{V_D}{V_T}$
												ET	SpO_2	(A − a)	ET	a	(a − ET)			
0.5	Rest		79	20	14.1	0.36	0.43	5.4	0.84			110	98		33			39	33	
1.0	Rest		88	21	10.5	0.24	0.31	3.6	0.76			104	97		35			45	34	
1.5	Rest		90	16	11.0	0.28	0.37	4.1	0.76			104	97		35			39	30	
2.0	Rest		88	17	9.6	0.23	0.31	3.5	0.75			102	97		36			42	31	
2.5	Rest		93	18	10.2	0.24	0.33	3.5	0.74			102	97		36			42	31	
3.0	Rest		91	18	11.8	0.30	0.39	4.3	0.76			102	97		36			40	30	
3.5	Rest	141/80	89	19	12.1	0.30	0.37	4.1	0.82			106	97		36			40	33	
4.0	Rest		87	18	10.7	0.26	0.34	4.0	0.76			102	97		37			41	31	
4.5	Unloaded		92	20	15.4	0.44	0.53	5.7	0.83			105	97		37			35	29	
5.0	Unloaded		107	19	15.2	0.45	0.55	5.1	0.83			103	98		38			33	28	
5.5	Unloaded		113	20	15.3	0.45	0.52	4.6	0.86			105	97		38			34	29	
6.0	Unloaded		97	19	14.3	0.43	0.51	5.3	0.83			102	97		39			33	28	
6.5	Unloaded	139/82	94	19	14.4	0.43	0.51	5.5	0.83			103	97		39			34	28	
7.0	Unloaded		93	19	13.9	0.41	0.50	5.4	0.83			103	97		39			34	28	
7.5	6		93	20	15.2	0.46	0.55	6.0	0.83			103	97		39			33	28	
8.0	17		94	18	14.2	0.42	0.51	5.4	0.83			102	97		39			33	28	
8.5	32		103	15	16.5	0.50	0.61	6.0	0.81			99	97		40			33	27	
9.0	43	149/82	106	19	17.5	0.57	0.75	7.0	0.77			96	97		41			31	23	
9.5	56		105	20	20.0	0.67	0.85	8.1	0.79			97	97		42			30	23	
10.0	69		113	21	22.8	0.79	0.96	8.4	0.83			97	97		43			29	24	
10.5	82		121	20	26.4	0.96	1.10	9.1	0.87			98	97		44			28	24	
11.0	94		130	21	29.4	1.08	1.15	8.8	0.94			101	98		44			27	25	
11.5	107		137	19	34.4	1.33	1.37	10.0	0.97			101	97		45			26	25	
12.0	120	183/77	133	22	36.6	1.41	1.39	10.4	1.01			102	97		46			26	26	
12.5	132		135	25	40.0	1.53	1.51	11.2	1.02			102	97		46			26	26	
13.0	144		141	20	43.3	1.73	1.63	11.6	1.07			103	97		46			25	27	
13.5	156		149	23	48.3	1.95	1.79	12.0	1.09			104	97		47			25	27	
14.0	168		149	24	54.1	2.13	1.86	12.5	1.15			106	97		46			25	29	
14.5	181	207/80	157	25	58.8	2.36	2.06	13.1	1.15			106	97		47			25	29	
15.0	195		165	26	59.3	2.43	2.16	13.1	1.13			104	97		48			24	27	
15.5	207		170	29	67.5	2.70	2.34	13.8	1.15			106	96		47			25	29	
16.0	219		174	35	78.8	2.98	2.43	14.0	1.23			110	97		45			26	32	
16.5	Recovery		176	36	84.2	3.01	2.32	13.2	1.29			113	96		43			28	36	
17.0	Recovery	172/52	170	33	75.6	2.62	1.55	9.1	1.69			119	97		42			29	49	
17.5	Recovery		160	22	54.9	1.86	1.06	6.6	1.76			120	97		40			29	52	
18.0	Recovery		150	28	55.0	1.62	0.95	6.4	1.70			123	97		36			34	58	
18.5	Recovery		146	30	44.8	1.26	0.84	5.7	1.50			121	97		36			35	53	

Abbreviations: BP, blood pressure; BTPS, body temperature pressure saturated; f, frequency; HCO_3^-, bicarbonate; HR, heart rate; $P(A - a)O_2$, alveolar-arterial PO_2 difference; $P(a - ET)CO_2$, arterial-end-tidal PCO_2 difference; $PETCO_2$, end-tidal PCO_2; $PETO_2$, end-tidal PO_2; R, respiratory exchange ratio; SpO_2, oxygen saturation as measured by pulse oximetry; STPD, standard temperature pressure dry; $\dot{V}CO_2$, carbon dioxide output; V_D/V_T, physiological dead space–tidal volume ratio; $\dot{V}E$, minute ventilation; $\dot{V}E/\dot{V}CO_2$, ventilatory equivalent for carbon dioxide; $\dot{V}E/\dot{V}O_2$, ventilatory equivalent for oxygen; $\dot{V}O_2$, oxygen uptake.

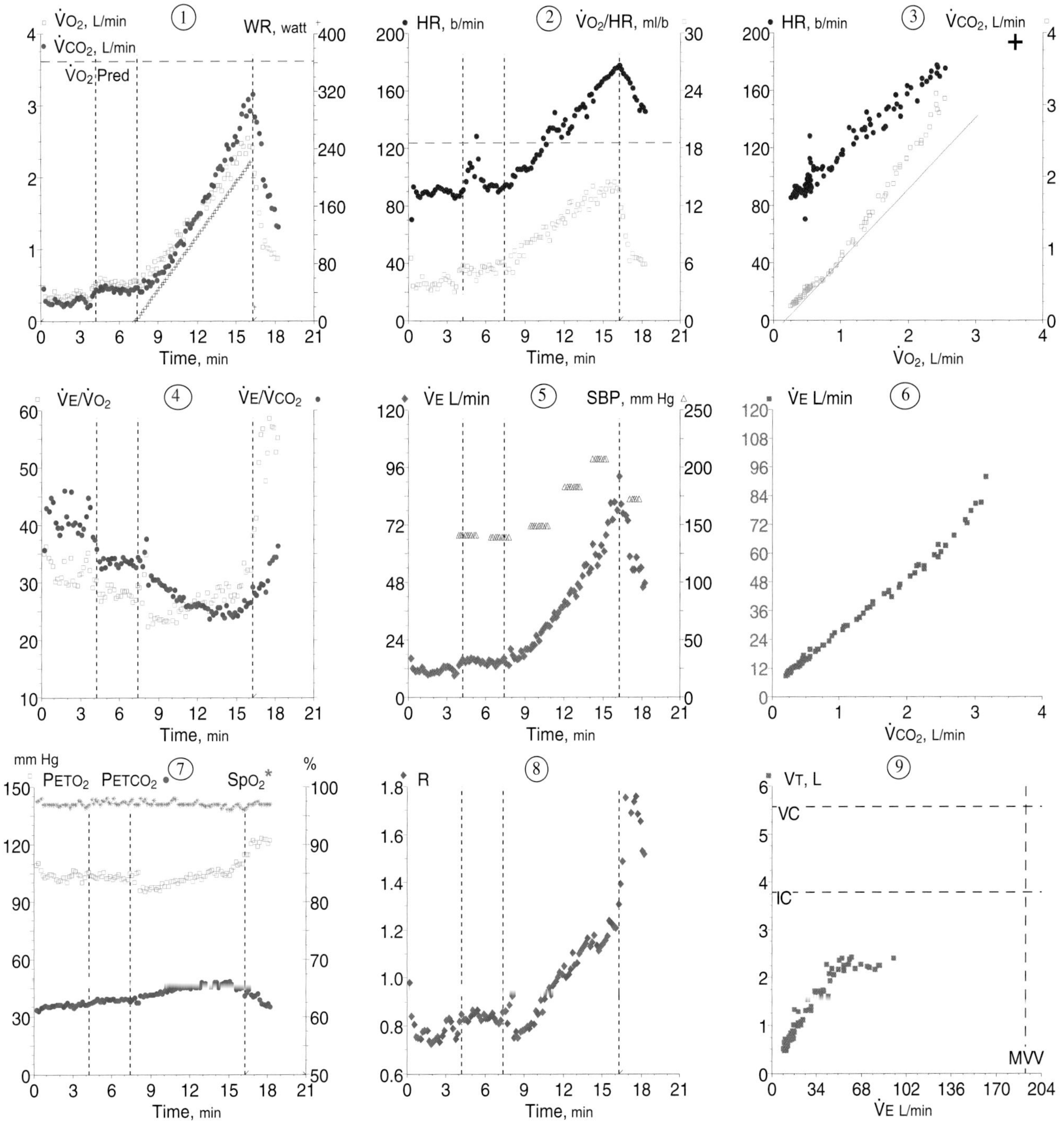

FIGURE 10.32.1. Vertical dashed lines in the panels in the left and middle columns indicate, from left to right, the beginning of unloaded cycling, start of increasing work rate (WR) at 25 W/min, and start of recovery. In **panel 1**, the increase in WR (right y-axis) is plotted with a scale of 100 W to 1 L of oxygen uptake ($\dot{V}O_2$) (left y-axis) such that WR is plotted parallel to a $\dot{V}O_2$ slope of 10 mL/min/W. Predicted peak $\dot{V}O_2$ is shown as a dashed horizontal line. In **panel 3**, carbon dioxide output ($\dot{V}CO_2$) (right y-axis) is plotted as a function of $\dot{V}O_2$ (x-axis) with identical scales so that the diagonal blue line has a slope of 1 (45°). The $\dot{V}CO_2$ increasing more steeply than $\dot{V}O_2$ defines carbon dioxide (CO_2) derived from bicarbonate buffer, as long as ventilatory equivalent for CO_2 ($\dot{V}E/\dot{V}CO_2$) (**panel 4**) is not increasing and end-tidal PCO_2 (P_{ETCO_2}) (**panel 7**) is not decreasing, simultaneously. The black + symbol in **panel 3** indicates predicted values of heart rate (HR) (left y-axis) and $\dot{V}O_2$ for this individual. Abbreviations: IC, inspiratory capacity; MVV, maximum voluntary ventilation; P_{ETO_2}, end-tidal PO_2; R, respiratory exchange ratio; SBP, systolic blood pressure; SpO_2, oxygen saturation as measured by pulse oximetry; VC, vital capacity; $\dot{V}E$, minute ventilation; $\dot{V}E/\dot{V}O_2$, ventilatory equivalent for oxygen; V_T, tidal volume.

CASE 33

Surgically Repaired Coarctation of the Aorta With Bicuspid Aortic Valve

To view this case please access the eBook bundled with this text. Instructions are located on the inside front cover.

CASE 34

Fontan Circulation

CLINICAL FINDINGS

An 18-year-old woman was referred for exercise testing at the time of her transition of care from pediatric to adult congenital heart disease providers. She was born with hypoplastic right ventricle and pulmonic atresia and underwent a number of palliative cardiac surgeries in infancy and early childhood including a Blalock-Taussig procedure, atrial septostomy, and bidirectional cavopulmonary shunts. At 3 years, she had an extracardiac Fontan procedure. She reports being normally active throughout childhood and having no restrictions on her activities or difficulty keeping up with her peers. She felt that she was more limited by back pain related to scoliosis and corrective back surgery performed at age 14 years than she was by her cardiac condition. She worked in a grocery store, standing for extended periods of time, lifting items, and pushing carts. Her history was otherwise notable for a diagnosis of attention deficit disorder. Her medications were lisinopril, aspirin, and methylphenidate. Physical examination was notable for multiple healed surgical scars on the thorax. Lungs were clear to auscultation and the cardiac examination notable for single S1 and S2. There was no cyanosis, clubbing, or edema. Pulse oximeter was 94% on the upper extremity digits bilaterally. Resting electrocardiogram showed a regular supraventricular rhythm at a rate of 107 and diffuse ST and T wave abnormalities. Demographic and respiratory function data are shown in **Table 10.34.1**.

TABLE 10.34.1 Selected Respiratory Function Data

Measurement	Predicted	Measured
Age (y)		18
Sex		Female
Height (cm)		162.5
Weight (kg)		59
VC (L)	3.81	2.65
IC (L)	2.35	1.7
ERV (L)	1.46	0.68
FEV_1 (L)	3.37	2.15
FEV_1/VC (%)	87	81
MVV (L)	116	54 (direct), 86 (indirect)

Abbreviations: ERV, expiratory reserve volume; FEV_1, forced expiratory volume in 1 second; IC, inspiratory capacity; MVV, maximum voluntary ventilation; VC, vital capacity.

EXERCISE FINDINGS

Testing was performed on a treadmill. After 2 minutes of standing on the treadmill at rest, the patient walked at a pace of 2.4 mph and zero grade for 3 minutes. The speed was then increased to comfortable tolerance, first to 3.0 mph for 1 minute and then 3.5 mph for 1 minute with the grade remaining zero. Thereafter, the speed was maintained at 3.5 mph and the grade was increased by 2% every minute until the patient signaled she was unable to continue exercise, with peak settings of 3.5 mph and 12% grade. She reported her limiting symptom as shortness of breath and trouble keeping pace with the treadmill belt. Exercise electrocardiogram showed a progressive rise in heart rate to 159 beats/min. There was no change in rhythm and no further change in the QRS-T complexes. Exercise data are shown in **Tables 10.34.2** and **10.34.3** and in **Figure 10.34.1**.

TABLE 10.34.2 Selected Exercise Data

Measurement	Predicted[a]	Measured
Peak $\dot{V}O_2$ (mL/min)	2.17	1.73
Peak $\dot{V}O_2$ (mL/min/kg)	36.7	29.3
Maximum heart rate (beats/min)	202	170
Maximum O_2 pulse (mL/beat)	10.7	10.2
$\Delta\dot{V}O_2/\Delta WR$	10.3	N/A
AT (mL/min)	>0.95	1.25
Blood pressure (mm Hg)		N/A
Maximum $\dot{V}E$ (L/min)	54 (direct MVV), 86 (indirect MVV)	74
Breathing reserve (L/min)	>15	−20, 12
$\dot{V}E/\dot{V}CO_2$ @ *AT*	<29	35
$\dot{V}E$-$\dot{V}CO_2$ slope	<29	33
SpO_2 (% [rest, max ex])		94, 92

Abbreviations: *AT*, anaerobic threshold; $\Delta\dot{V}CO_2/\Delta WR$, change in $\dot{V}CO_2$/change in work rate; ex, exercise; MVV, maximum voluntary ventilation; N/A, not available; O_2, oxygen; SpO_2, oxygen saturation as measured by pulse oximetry; $\dot{V}CO_2$, carbon dioxide output; $\dot{V}E$, minute ventilation; $\dot{V}E/\dot{V}CO_2$, ventilatory equivalent for carbon dioxide; $\dot{V}O_2$, oxygen uptake.

[a]Predicted peak $\dot{V}O_2$ and subsequently derived predicted values were calculated using pediatric equations (Cooper et al[3]) for cycle exercise as described in Chapter 7 and adjusted upward by 10% for treadmill exercise.

INTERPRETATION

Comment

The Fontan circulation is characterized by a single functioning ventricle, which is connected to the aorta to perfuse the systemic circulation. There is no subpulmonary ventricle, so pulmonary circulation has been described as "passive" and is aided by the peripheral muscle contractions pushing blood centrally and respiratory muscles pulling blood into the thorax by negative pressure. As in many other clinical populations, exercise capacity is among factors that are predictive of survival.[1]

Analysis

Exercise capacity was mildly reduced with a peak oxygen uptake ($\dot{V}O_2$) of just under 80% of predicted value.

Cardiovascular and metabolic responses: Anaerobic threshold was normal and O_2 pulse reached a normal peak value. The heart rate response to exercise was nonlinear, increasing more steeply at higher levels of $\dot{V}O_2$. Blood pressure measurements could not be accurately determined.

Ventilatory responses: There was some discrepancy between the maximum voluntary ventilation(MVV) measured directly versus calculated from the FEV_1. The patient exceeded the former during exercise and reached a peak $\dot{V}E$ that was only 12 L/min less than the calculated (indirect) MVV. She thus appeared either at, or approaching, the limits of her breathing capacity. This was attributable to a combination of reduced breathing capacity (low MVV) and elevated breathing requirements (high $\dot{V}E/\dot{V}CO_2$). The high ventilatory equivalents and mild resting hypoxemia could represent regional $\dot{V}/\dot{Q}$ mismatching in the lung or, less likely, could result from residual right to left shunting. There were no findings in the ventilation and gas exchange responses to suggest acute exercise-induced right to left shunting. Pulse oximetry was mildly reduced at rest and remained stable during the initial minutes of the test, but the instrument signal became inadequate during the latter part of the test so further desaturation may have not been detected.

Conclusion

This test demonstrated unusually good exercise capacity for an individual with Fontan circulation. Peak $\dot{V}O_2$ among patients with this condition averages 60% of the healthy age, sex, and size-based predicted values, although it varies widely among individuals.[1] Exercise limitation with Fontan circulation is usually attributable to cardiovascular factors; however, ventilatory restriction is not uncommon and can be a contributing factor to exercise limitation.[2] Impaired breathing mechanics can result from developmental factors, the effect of prior thoracic surgeries on chest wall mechanics, and/or phrenic nerve injury resulting in diaphragm paralysis. For this patient, scoliosis and prior back surgery are likely to have contributed to her restricted lung mechanics.

REFERENCES

1. Ohuchi H, Negishi J, Noritake K, et al. Prognostic value of exercise variables in 335 patients after the Fontan operation: a 23-year single-center experience of cardiopulmonary exercise testing. *Congenit Heart Dis*. 2015;10:105–116.
2. Takken T, Tacken MH, Blank AC, Hulzebos EH, Strengers JL, Helders PJ. Exercise limitation in patients with Fontan circulation: a review. *J Cardiovasc Med (Hagerstown)*. 2007;8:775–781.
3. Cooper DM, Weiler-Ravell D. Gas exchange response to exercise in children. *Am Rev Resp Dis*. 1984;129(2 pt 2):S47–S48.

TABLE 10.34.3 Treadmill Test

Time (min)	Treadmill speed (min/h)	Grade (%)	BP (mm Hg)	HR (min^{-1})	f (min^{-1})	$\dot{V}E$ (L/min BTPS)	$\dot{V}CO_2$ (L/min STPD)	$\dot{V}O_2$ (L/min STPD)	$\frac{\dot{V}O_2}{HR}$ (mL/beat)	R	pH	HCO_3^- (mEq/L)	PO_2, mm Hg and SpO_2, %			PCO_2, mm Hg			$\frac{\dot{V}E}{\dot{V}CO_2}$	$\frac{\dot{V}E}{\dot{V}O_2}$	$\frac{V_D}{V_T}$
													ET	SpO_2	(A − a)	ET	a	(a − ET)			
0.5	Rest			107	21	14.3	0.30	0.32	3.0	0.95			120	94		27			48	45	
1.0	Rest			104	20	13.6	0.29	0.30	2.9	0.95			120	94		27			47	45	
1.5	Rest			104	23	13.2	0.26	0.26	2.5	1.01			122	93		26			51	51	
2.0	Rest			104	21	12.9	0.26	0.26	2.5	0.99			121	94		27			49	49	
2.5	2.4	0		106	24	19.7	0.47	0.52	4.9	0.90			115	94		30			42	38	
3.0	2.4	0		113	29	23.3	0.59	0.62	5.4	0.96			116	94		30			39	38	
3.5	2.4	0		110	26	23.6	0.62	0.67	6.1	0.93			115	94		31			38	35	
4.0	2.4	0		111	27	24.3	0.65	0.74	6.7	0.88			112	94		32			37	33	
4.5	2.4	0		107	26	24.8	0.66	0.73	6.8	0.90			113	92		32			37	34	
5.0	2.4	0		107	28	26.0	0.68	0.74	6.9	0.92			115			31			38	35	
5.5	3.0	0		107	31	28.7	0.73	0.77	7.2	0.95			116			30			39	37	
6.0	3.0	0		113	29	27.6	0.75	0.82	7.2	0.91			113			32			37	34	
6.5	3.5	0		118	30	29.2	0.79	0.85	7.2	0.93			114			32			37	34	
7.0	3.5	0		119	30	32.1	0.88	0.95	8.0	0.93			114			32			36	34	
7.5	3.5	2		120	34	34.2	0.93	0.98	8.1	0.95			115			32			37	35	
8.0	3.5	2		122	35	37.1	1.03	1.09	8.9	0.95			115			32			36	34	
8.5	3.5	4		131	32	38.4	1.10	1.15	8.8	0.96			113			33			35	33	
9.0	3.5	4		131	33	40.4	1.18	1.19	9.0	0.99			114			34			34	34	
9.5	3.5	6		137	36	45.2	1.30	1.29	9.4	1.01			115			33			35	35	
10.0	3.5	6		136	39	49.5	1.43	1.38	10.1	1.04			116			33			35	36	
10.5	3.5	8		147	40	53.8	1.54	1.44	9.9	1.06			117			33			35	37	
11.0	3.5	8		156	38	52.7	1.57	1.53	9.8	1.03			115			34			33	34	
11.5	3.5	10		163	41	59.6	1.71	1.56	9.6	1.10			117			33			35	38	
12.0	3.5	10		168	42	63.4	1.81	1.64	9.8	1.10			118			33			35	39	
12.5	3.5	12		162	49	74.0	1.98	1.73	10.7	1.15			121			31			37	43	
13.0	Recovery			169	45	69.7	1.88	1.62	9.6	1.16			120			32			37	43	
13.5	Recovery			174	41	61.6	1.69	1.38	7.9	1.23			121	92		32			36	45	
14.0	Recovery			159	40	57.3	1.47	1.06	6.7	1.39			125	91		30			39	54	
14.5	Recovery			153	41	53.9	1.26	0.90	5.9	1.40			127	91		27			43	60	
15.0	Recovery			126	37	40.2	0.98	0.81	6.5	1.20			123	92		29			41	49	

Abbreviations: BP, blood pressure; BTPS, body temperature pressure saturated; f, frequency; HCO_3^-, bicarbonate; HR, heart rate; $P(A - a)O_2$, alveolar-arterial PO_2 difference; $P(a - ET)CO_2$, arterial-end-tidal PCO_2 difference; $PETCO_2$, end-tidal PCO_2; $PETO_2$, end-tidal PO_2; R, respiratory exchange ratio; SpO_2, oxygen saturation as measured by pulse oximetry; STPD, standard temperature pressure dry; $\dot{V}CO_2$, carbon dioxide output; V_D/V_T, physiological dead space-tidal volume ratio; $\dot{V}E$, minute ventilation; $\dot{V}E/\dot{V}CO_2$, ventilatory equivalent for carbon dioxide; $\dot{V}E/\dot{V}O_2$, ventilatory equivalent for oxygen; $\dot{V}O_2$, oxygen uptake.

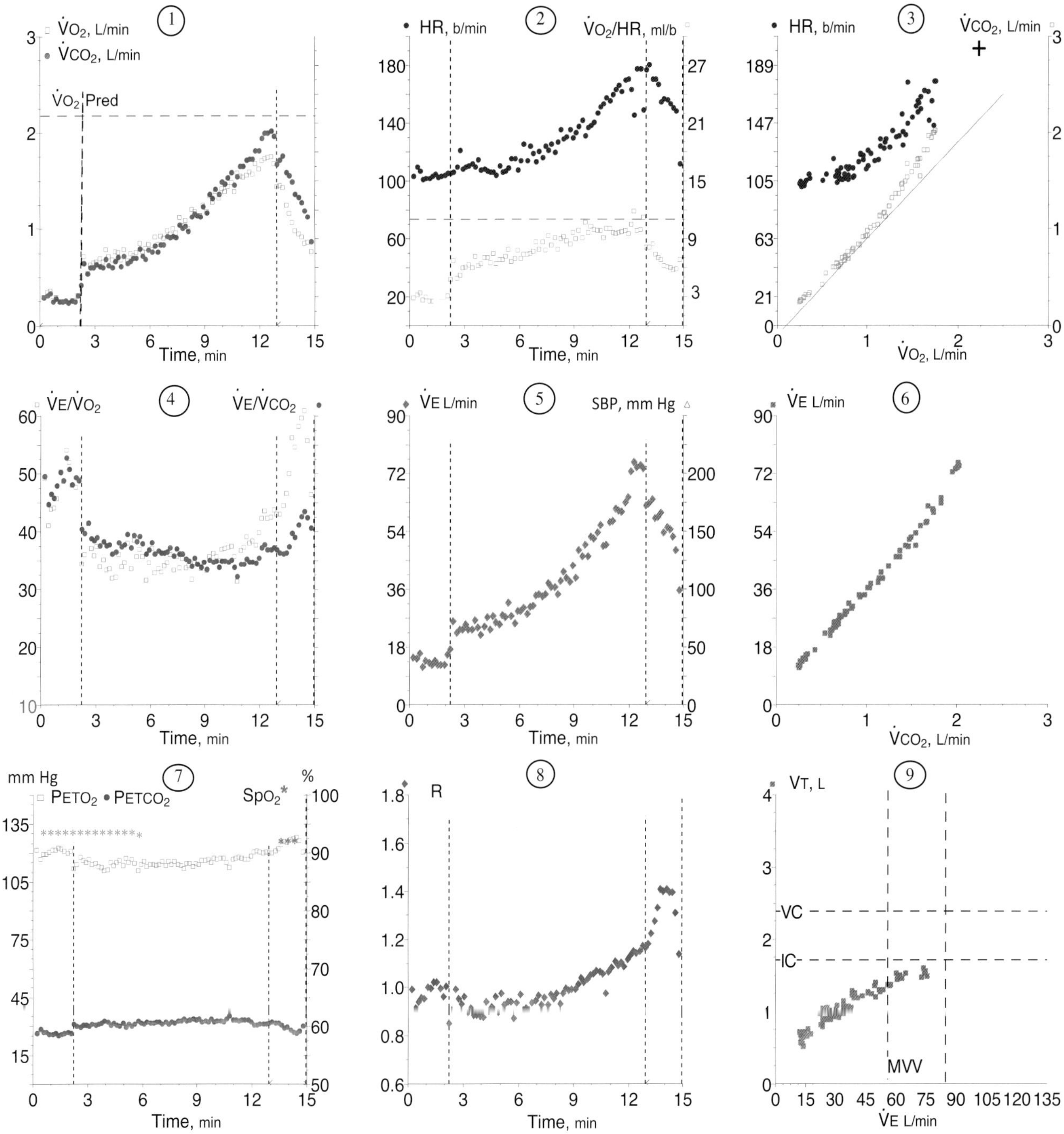

FIGURE 10.34.1. Vertical dashed lines in the panels in the left and middle columns indicate, from left to right, the beginning of treadmill walking at 2.4 mph, and the start of recovery. In **panel 1**, predicted peak oxygen uptake ($\dot{V}O_2$) is shown as a dashed horizontal line. Work rate is not plotted because of the difficulty of precisely estimating work rate from treadmill settings. In **panel 3**, carbon dioxide output ($\dot{V}CO_2$) (right y-axis) is plotted as a function of $\dot{V}O_2$ (x-axis) with identical scales so that the diagonal blue line has a slope of 1 (45°). The $\dot{V}CO_2$ increasing more steeply than $\dot{V}O_2$ defines carbon dioxide (CO_2) derived from bicarbonate buffer, as long as ventilatory equivalent for CO_2 ($\dot{V}E/\dot{V}CO_2$) (**panel 4**) is not increasing and end-tidal PCO_2 ($PETCO_2$) (**panel 7**) is not decreasing, simultaneously. The black + symbol in **panel 3** indicates predicted peak values of heart rate (HR) (left y-axis) and $\dot{V}O_2$ for this individual. Abbreviations: IC, inspiratory capacity; MVV, maximum voluntary ventilation; $PETO_2$, end-tidal PO_2; R, respiratory exchange ratio; SBP, systolic blood pressure; SpO_2, oxygen saturation as measured by pulse oximetry; VC, vital capacity; $\dot{V}E$, minute ventilation; $\dot{V}E/\dot{V}O_2$, ventilatory equivalent for oxygen; V_T, tidal volume.

CASE 35

Ventricular Septal Defect With Eisenmenger Syndrome

CLINICAL FINDINGS

A woman with Eisenmenger syndrome had serial exercise testing in her 60s. A ventricular septal defect had been identified at birth but not surgically repaired. She was not proscribed exercise as a child but recalled always having lower physical capacity than her peers. Cardiac catheterization in her teens identified pulmonary hypertension. Another catheterization had been performed at age 58 years at which time she was told that a heart-lung transplant would be her only surgical treatment option but that her age precluded consideration. Her daily activities were limited by fatigue, chest pressure, and breathlessness. She had variable cyanosis but denied edema or orthopnea. She lived independently and had worked in a clerical job prior to retiring on medical disability. She had noted gradually increasing shortness of breath and fatigue with household activities over several years. Treatment with an endothelin receptor antagonist was begun at age 62 years, and exercise testing was conducted periodically to track her functional capacity. The test presented herein was performed at age 66 years. Medications at the time of testing were bosentan, digoxin, thyroid replacement, and nocturnal supplemental oxygen. Physical examination was notable for a regular cardiac rhythm and holosystolic murmur. Breath sounds were clear. There was symmetric clubbing of the fingers but no peripheral edema. The resting electrocardiogram showed sinus rhythm, diffuse ST-T wave abnormalities, and occasional premature ventricular complexes. Demographic and respiratory function data are shown in **Table 10.35.1**.

TABLE 10.35.1 Selected Respiratory Function Data

Measurement	Predicted	Measured
Age (y)		66
Sex		Female
Height (cm)		164
Weight (kg)		51.8
VC (L)	3.19	2.13
IC (L)	2.21	1.38
ERV (L)	0.98	0.70
FEV_1 (L)	2.44	1.44
FEV_1/VC (%)	70	68
MVV (L/min)	89	56

Abbreviations: ERV, expiratory reserve volume; FEV_1, forced expiratory volume in 1 second; IC, inspiratory capacity; MVV, maximum voluntary ventilation; VC, vital capacity.

EXERCISE FINDINGS

The patient exercised on a cycle ergometer beginning with 3 minutes of unloaded pedaling at 60 rpm followed by continuous increase in work rate by 10 W/min until the test ended with the primary symptom of leg fatigue. During exercise, the electrocardiogram showed a decrease in ectopy and no other significant changes. Exercise data are shown in **Table 10.35.2** (key variables along with results from three prior tests), **Table 10.35.3**, and **Figure 10.35.1**.

INTERPRETATION

Comment

This patient had relatively mild hypoxemia by pulse oximetry at rest, although it worsened with exercise. Spirometry showed a restrictive defect, which is not uncommon among individuals with congenital heart disease. Results of the exercise test were characteristic of the effects of pulmonary hypertension secondary to congenital heart disease. Tests performed over a period of several years demonstrate the repeatability of the findings.

Analysis

Cardiovascular responses: There are marked abnormalities in the oxygen uptake oxygen uptake ($\dot{V}O_2$) response to exercise, consistent with severe cardiovascular impairment. Peak $\dot{V}O_2$ was less than half of the predicted value. In panel 1 of the figure, the change in $\dot{V}O_2$/change in WR ($\Delta\dot{V}O_2/\Delta WR$) appears to be shallow. Given the very small range of work rates and $\dot{V}O_2$ attained, however, it is difficult to calculate the $\Delta\dot{V}O_2/\Delta WR$ with confidence. In **Table 10.35.2**, $\Delta\dot{V}O_2/\Delta WR$ was therefore reported only as <5 mL/min/W. Evidence supporting the impression that it was abnormal is evident in the recovery period during which it appears that $\dot{V}O_2$ decreases back toward baseline more slowly than normal. Consistent with this, the R value (panel 8) declines in the early minutes of recovery rather than increasing, which would be the normal finding. This results from the time course of recovery of $\dot{V}O_2$ being slower than that of $\dot{V}CO_2$, rather than the reverse, consistent with accumulation of an abnormal "oxygen deficit" during the preceding exercise and need to replenish the energetic deficit with sustained elevation in $\dot{V}O_2$ in the early recovery period. The anaerobic threshold appears to be exceeded during the test, but this was likely during the initial phase of unloaded cycling and so was reported as lower than the $\dot{V}O_2$ measured during that period. In panel 3, it is apparent that heart rate increased

TABLE 10.35.2 Selected Exercise Data

Measurement	Predicted	Measured: Age 66 y	Age 65 y	Age 64 y	Age 63 y
Peak $\dot{V}O_2$ (L/min)	1.16	0.50	0.45	0.45	0.51
Maximum heart rate (beats/min)	154	118	103	94	107
Maximum O_2 pulse (mL/beat)	7.6	4.3	4.3	4.8	4.7
$\Delta\dot{V}O_2/\Delta WR$ (mL/min/W)	10.3	<5	<5	<5	<5
AT (L/min)	>0.62	<0.400	<0.400	<0.400	<0.400
Blood pressure (mm Hg [rest, max])		118/61, 162/82	112/63, 145/86	119/68, 136/78	128/85, 155/91
MVV (Maximum $\dot{V}E$ [L/min])		56, 24	61, 25	58, 20	60, 23
Breathing reserve (L/min)		32	36	38	36
$\dot{V}E/\dot{V}CO_2$ @ *AT*	<34	53	54	45	50
$\dot{V}E$-$\dot{V}CO_2$ slope	<33	52	50	45	48
SpO_2 (% [rest, max ex])		94, 88	91, 85	93, 85	92, 85

Abbreviations: *AT*, anaerobic threshold; $\Delta\dot{V}O_2/\Delta WR$, change in $\dot{V}O_2$/change in work rate; ex, exercise; MVV, maximum voluntary ventilation; O_2, oxygen; SpO_2, oxygen saturation as measured by pulse oximetry; $\dot{V}CO_2$, carbon dioxide output; $\dot{V}E$, minute ventilation; $\dot{V}E/\dot{V}CO_2$, ventilatory equivalent for carbon dioxide; $\dot{V}O_2$, oxygen uptake.

TABLE 10.35.3 Age 66 Years

Time (min)	Work rate (W)	BP (mm Hg)	HR (min⁻¹)	f (min⁻¹)	$\dot{V}E$ (L/min BTPS)	$\dot{V}CO_2$ (L/min STPD)	$\dot{V}O_2$ (L/min STPD)	$\frac{\dot{V}O_2}{HR}$ (mL/beat)	R	pH	HCO_3^- (mEq/L)	PO_2, mm Hg and SpO_2, %: ET	SpO_2	(A − a)	PCO_2, mm Hg: ET	a	(a − ET)	$\frac{\dot{V}E}{\dot{V}CO_2}$	$\frac{\dot{V}E}{\dot{V}O_2}$	$\frac{VD}{VT}$
0.5	Rest		83	15	8.1	0.16	0.20	2.4	0.80			116	77		27			51	41	
1.0	Rest		83	14	6.9	0.13	0.18	2.1	0.73			112	93		28			54	39	
1.5	Rest		86	13	7.8	0.16	0.22	2.6	0.71			110	93		29			49	35	
2.0	Rest		89	17	9.4	0.18	0.24	2.7	0.74			113	93		28			52	39	
2.5	Rest		87	13	6.6	0.13	0.17	2.0	0.75			111	94		29			51	38	
3.0	Rest	118/61	87	15	8.6	0.18	0.24	2.8	0.73			110	94		29			48	35	
3.5	Unloaded		88	18	9.7	0.20	0.25	2.9	0.77			112	93		28			50	38	
4.0	Unloaded		93	18	13.3	0.27	0.33	3.6	0.81			116	93		26			49	40	
4.5	Unloaded		97	20	15.2	0.31	0.36	3.7	0.85			117	91		26			49	42	
5.0	Unloaded		99	21	17.5	0.35	0.41	4.2	0.86			118	89		26			50	43	
5.5	Unloaded		100	22	18.7	0.38	0.41	4.1	0.91			119	88		26			50	45	
6.0	Unloaded	152/69	103	22	20.3	0.41	0.44	4.3	0.94			120	88		25			49	46	
6.5	3		105	24	21.7	0.44	0.47	4.4	0.94			120	89		25			49	47	
7.0	7		109	24	22.3	0.45	0.46	4.2	0.97			122	87		25			49	48	
7.5	12		116	24	23.1	0.48	0.49	4.2	0.97			121	87		25			48	47	
8.0	17		115	25	23.2	0.48	0.50	4.3	0.97			121	88		25			48	46	
8.5	22		118	25	23.0	0.48	0.49	4.1	0.98			121	88		25			48	47	
9.0	Recovery	162/82	116	26	24.2	0.50	0.52	4.4	0.97			121	88		25			48	47	
9.5	Recovery		99	26	23.1	0.46	0.46	4.7	1.00			123	88		24			50	50	
10.0	Recovery		94	24	18.3	0.37	0.39	4.2	0.96			121	84		26			49	47	
10.5	Recovery		90	24	16.0	0.33	0.35	3.9	0.93			119	88		26			49	46	
11.0	Recovery		85	20	11.5	0.23	0.25	2.9	0.92			118	91		27			50	46	
11.5	Recovery	133/78	86	21	13.2	0.27	0.30	3.4	0.92			118	92		27			49	45	
12.0	Recovery		80	18	8.7	0.17	0.18	2.3	0.92			117	93		28			52	48	

Abbreviations: BP, blood pressure; BTPS, body temperature pressure saturated; f, frequency; HCO_3^-, bicarbonate; HR, heart rate; $P(A - a)O_2$, alveolar-arterial PO_2 difference; $P(a - ET)CO_2$, arterial-end-tidal PCO_2 difference; $PETCO_2$, end-tidal PCO_2; $PETO_2$, end-tidal PO_2; R, respiratory exchange ratio; SpO_2, oxygen saturation as measured by pulse oximetry; STPD, standard temperature pressure dry; $\dot{V}CO_2$, carbon dioxide output; VD/VT, physiological dead space–tidal volume ratio; $\dot{V}E$, minute ventilation; $\dot{V}E/\dot{V}CO_2$, ventilatory equivalent for carbon dioxide; $\dot{V}E/\dot{V}O_2$, ventilatory equivalent for oxygen; $\dot{V}O_2$, oxygen uptake.

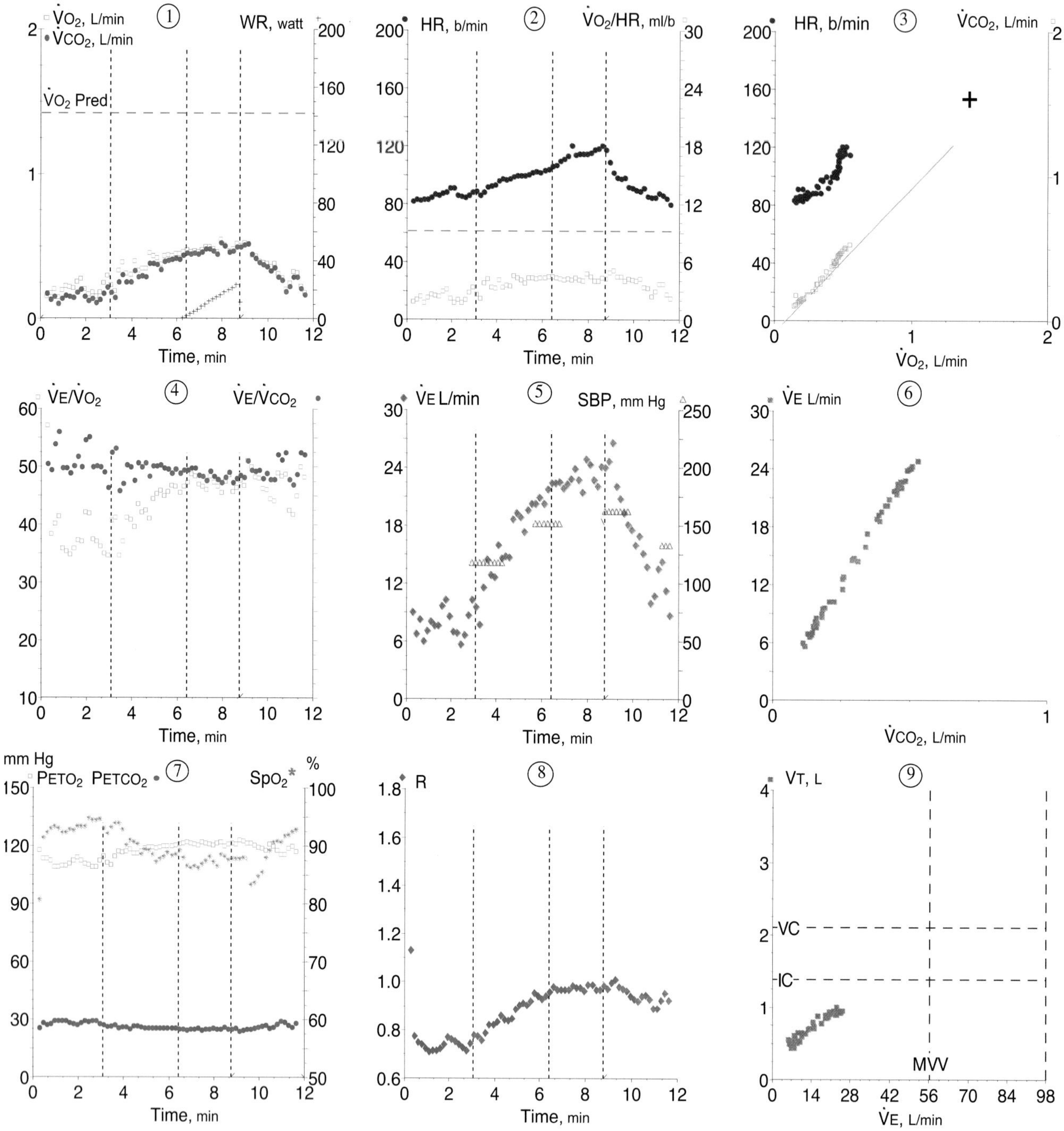

FIGURE 10.35.1. Vertical dashed lines in the panels in the left and middle columns indicate, from left to right, the beginning of unloaded cycling, start of increasing work rate (WR) at 10 W/min, and start of recovery. In **panel 1**, the increase in WR (right y-axis) is plotted with a scale of 100 W to 1 L of oxygen uptake ($\dot{V}O_2$) (left y-axis) such that WR is plotted parallel to a $\dot{V}O_2$ slope of 10 mL/min/W. Predicted peak $\dot{V}O_2$ is shown as a dashed horizontal line. In **panel 2**, predicted peak oxygen pulse is shown as a dashed horizontal line. In **panel 3**, carbon dioxide output ($\dot{V}CO_2$) (right y-axis) is plotted as a function of $\dot{V}O_2$ (x-axis) with identical scales so that the diagonal bue line has a slope of 1 (45°). The $\dot{V}CO_2$ increasing more steeply than $\dot{V}O_2$ defines carbon dioxide (CO_2) derived from bicarbonate buffer, as long as ventilatory equivalent for CO_2 ($\dot{V}E/\dot{V}CO_2$) (**panel 4**) is not increasing and end-tidal PCO_2 ($PETCO_2$) (**panel 7**) is not decreasing, simultaneously. The black + symbol in **panel 3** indicates predicted peak values of heart rate (HR) (left y-axis) and $\dot{V}O_2$ for this individual. Abbreviations: IC, inspiratory capacity; MVV, maximum voluntary ventilation; $PETO_2$, end-tidal PO_2; R, respiratory exchange ratio; SBP, systolic blood pressure; SpO_2, oxygen saturation as measured by pulse oximetry; $\dot{V}E$, minute ventilation; $\dot{V}E/\dot{V}O_2$, ventilatory equivalent for oxygen; V_T, tidal volume.

steeply relative to $\dot{V}O_2$, which is also reflected in the low and unchanging O_2 pulse in panel 2.

Ventilatory responses: There is an ample breathing reserve. The ventilatory pattern is characteristic of an increase in right-to-left intracardiac shunt with exercise. That is, ventilation increases more than gas exchange at exercise onset so that the ventilatory equivalents increase rather than decrease. The P_{ETCO_2} values also decrease, with reciprocal increase in P_{ETO_2}.

Efficiency of pulmonary gas exchange is clearly abnormal with progressive decrease in pulse oximeter values and high ratio of $\dot{V}E$ relative to $\dot{V}CO_2$. These findings could arise solely from $\dot{V}/\dot{Q}$ mismatching within the lung but also predictably result from the effects of right-to-left shunt on arterial oxygenation and the ventilatory demands needed to maintain arterial PCO_2 homeostasis.

Conclusion

Exercise capacity is severely limited in a pattern typical of limited cardiovascular function and right-to-left shunt. Despite the degree of the impairment, this patient has had fairly stable findings over a 3-year period of testing.

CASE 36

Tetralogy of Fallot, Surgically Repaired

CLINICAL FINDINGS

A 27-year-old man was referred for exercise testing at the time of transition to adult care of congenital heart disease. He was born with tetralogy of Fallot for which he underwent surgical repair at age 16 months. He had no restrictions on his physical activities while growing up and said he was able to keep up with his peers, playing team sports in high school and college. After college, he continued to exercise most days of the week, including running and working out in a gym, and his work in law enforcement was physically active. He denied any exercise related symptoms. He had an episode of atrial flutter at age 26 years, treated with cardioversion and a β-blocker. Recent echocardiography had demonstrated pulmonary valve stenosis and regurgitation, with enlargement of the right ventricle and dilatation of the outflow tract. Medications were low-dose aspirin and low-dose metoprolol. Physical examination revealed a normally developed young man with healed thoracotomy scar. There were systolic and diastolic murmurs; breath sounds were clear; and there was no cyanosis, clubbing, or edema. Resting electrocardiogram showed normal sinus rhythm and right bundle branch block with occasional premature ventricular contractions. Demographic and respiratory function data are shown in **Table 10.36.1**.

EXERCISE FINDINGS

The patient exercised on a cycle ergometer beginning with 3 minutes of unloaded pedaling at 60 rpm followed by continuous increase in work rate by 25 W/min until the test ended with symptoms of leg fatigue. Exercise electrocardiogram showed no evidence of ischemia or arrhythmia. Exercise data are summarized in **Tables 10.36.2** and **10.36.3** and in **Figure 10.36.1**.

INTERPRETATION

Comment

This patient had no subjective complaints of exercise intolerance and maintained a physically active lifestyle. Imaging studies demonstrated significant pulmonary valve and right ventricular outflow tract disorders, however, which occur commonly as late complications after surgical repair for tetralogy of Fallot. His providers requested exercise assessment to aid in decisions regarding timing of pulmonary valve replacement, although cardiopulmonary exercise testing criteria for this are not well defined.

Analysis

Cardiovascular and metabolic responses: Peak $\dot{V}O_2$ and peak heart rate were both mildly reduced relative to the reference values. The increase in heart rate relative to $\dot{V}O_2$ (panel 3)

TABLE 10.36.1 Selected Respiratory Function Data

Measurement	Predicted	Measured
Age (y)		27
Sex		Male
Height (cm)		183
Weight (kg)		90.5
VC (L)	5.52	4.5
IC (L)		3.06
ERV (L)		1.23
FEV_1 (L)	4.47	2.95
FEV_1/VC (%)	82	66
MVV (L/min)		118
TLC (L)	7.30	5.37
D_{LCO} (mL/mm Hg/min)	36.4	20.4

Abbreviations: D_{LCO}, diffusing capacity of the lung for carbon monoxide; ERV, expiratory reserve volume; FEV_1, forced expiratory volume in 1 second; IC, inspiratory capacity; MVV, maximum voluntary ventilation; TLC, total lung capacity; VC, vital capacity.

TABLE 10.36.2 Selected Exercise Data

Measurement	Predicted	Measured
Peak $\dot{V}O_2$ (L/min)	3.45	2.64
Maximum heart rate (beats/min)	195	164
Maximum O_2 pulse (mL/beat)	17.7	16.1
$\Delta\dot{V}O_2/\Delta WR$ (mL/min/W)	10.3	9.2
AT (L/min)	>1.47	1.75
Blood pressure (mm Hg [rest, max])		100/74, 151/81
Maximum $\dot{V}E$ (L/min)		77
Breathing reserve (L/min)	>15	41
$\dot{V}E/\dot{V}CO_2$ @ *AT* (L/min)	<28	28
$\dot{V}E$-$\dot{V}CO_2$ slope	<28	21
SpO_2 (% [rest, max ex])		98, 98

Abbreviations: *AT*, anaerobic threshold; $\Delta\dot{V}O_2/\Delta WR$, change in $\dot{V}O_2$/change in work rate; ex, exercise; O_2, oxygen; SpO_2, oxygen saturation as measured by pulse oximetry; $\dot{V}CO_2$, carbon dioxide output; $\dot{V}E$, minute ventilation; $\dot{V}E/\dot{V}CO_2$, ventilatory equivalent for carbon dioxide; $\dot{V}O_2$, oxygen uptake.

TABLE 10.36.3 Air Breathing

Time (min)	Work rate (W)	BP (mm Hg)	HR (min^{-1})	f (min^{-1})	$\dot{V}E$ (L/min BTPS)	$\dot{V}CO_2$ (L/min STPD)	$\dot{V}O_2$ (L/min STPD)	$\frac{\dot{V}O_2}{HR}$ (mL/beat)	R	pH	HCO_3^- (mEq/L)	PO_2, mm Hg and SpO_2, % ET	SpO_2	(A − a)	PCO_2, mm Hg ET	a	(a − ET)	$\frac{\dot{V}E}{\dot{V}CO_2}$	$\frac{\dot{V}E}{\dot{V}O_2}$	$\frac{VD}{VT}$
0.5	Rest		69	22	14.2	0.39	0.43	6.3	0.91			113	98		33			36	33	
1.0	Rest		77	18	16.3	0.43	0.44	5.7	0.99			118	99		30			38	37	
1.5	Rest	100/74	67	16	17.7	0.46	0.41	6.1	1.13			120	98		30			38	43	
2.0	Rest		72	19	14.2	0.36	0.37	5.2	0.97			116	99		31			39	38	
2.5	Rest		70	17	12.7	0.35	0.36	5.2	0.95			116	99		32			37	35	
3.0	Rest		75	20	13.7	0.35	0.37	4.9	0.96			117	99		30			39	37	
3.5	Unloaded		83	22	14.1	0.38	0.47	5.7	0.82			108	99		34			37	30	
4.0	Unloaded		79	17	17.9	0.54	0.75	9.5	0.72			101	99		36			33	24	
4.5	Unloaded		79	15	18.8	0.59	0.75	9.5	0.79			101	99		37			32	25	
5.0	Unloaded		79	17	17.2	0.53	0.63	8.0	0.84			104	98		37			33	27	
5.5	Unloaded		76	20	16.8	0.52	0.69	9.0	0.76			101	99		37			32	25	
6.0	Unloaded		78	17	22.6	0.70	0.80	10.2	0.87			107	99		36			32	28	
6.5	9	121/74	79	21	17.0	0.54	0.72	9.1	0.75			100	98		38			32	24	
7.0	20		79	17	16.9	0.55	0.73	9.2	0.76			99	99		39			31	23	
7.5	33		80	15	21.4	0.65	0.71	8.8	0.92			106	98		37			33	30	
8.0	45	110/73	86	18	20.4	0.69	0.91	10.6	0.75			99	99		38			30	22	
8.5	57		85	19	21.6	0.70	0.87	10.3	0.80			101	99		38			31	25	
9.0	70		89	20	23.9	0.83	1.12	12.6	0.74			97	99		40			29	21	
9.5	81		101	20	24.7	0.90	1.19	11.8	0.76			95	98		42			27	21	
10.0	95	109/74	101	24	30.2	1.07	1.34	13.3	0.80			98	98		41			28	22	
10.5	107		102	22	32.7	1.22	1.43	14.1	0.85			100	98		42			27	23	
11.0	118		110	24	33.0	1.31	1.59	14.4	0.83			98	98		43			25	21	
11.5	131		113	26	36.6	1.45	1.63	14.3	0.89			101	98		42			25	23	
12.0	144	121/73	116	18	39.7	1.65	1.77	15.2	0.93			98	98		47			24	22	
12.5	155		122	24	42.6	1.77	1.89	15.5	0.94			98	97		47			24	22	
13.0	168		114	20	44.5	1.92	1.97	17.2	0.98			97	97		49			23	23	
13.5	180		133	26	50.5	2.11	2.11	15.9	1.00			101	97		47			24	24	
14.0	191	151/81	139	31	54.6	2.26	2.20	15.8	1.03			103	97		46			24	25	
14.5	204		148	25	60.2	2.56	2.36	15.9	1.08			102	96		48			24	26	
15.0	217		157	31	68.7	[illegible]	[illegible]	16.1	1.12			105	96		47			24	27	
15.5	228		163	34	75.5	3.04	2.62	16.0	1.16			107	97		46			25	29	
16.0	Recovery		162	37	77.1	3.09	2.64	16.3	1.17			108	94		46			25	29	
16.5	Recovery	133/80	161	34	59.5	2.61	2.15	13.4	1.22			107	97		49			23	28	
17.0	Recovery		148	33	57.1	2.17	1.43	9.7	1.51			117	96		42			26	40	
17.5	Recovery		136	27	51.4	1.89	1.31	9.6	1.44			116	98		42			27	39	
18.0	Recovery		127	27	43.0	1.52	1.10	8.7	1.38			117	98		40			28	39	
18.5	Recovery		120	26	40.6	1.35	1.00	8.4	1.35			118	96		38			30	41	
19.0	Recovery		116	26	40.3	1.30	1.02	8.8	1.27			117	97		37			31	39	

Abbreviations: BP, blood pressure; BTPS, body temperature pressure saturated; f, frequency; HCO_3^-, bicarbonate; HR, heart rate; $P(A-a)O_2$, alveolar-arterial PO_2 difference; $P(a-ET)CO_2$, arterial-end-tidal PCO_2 difference; $PETCO_2$, end-tidal PCO_2; $PETO_2$, end-tidal PO_2; R, respiratory exchange ratio; SpO_2, oxygen saturation as measured by pulse oximetry; STPD, standard temperature pressure dry; $\dot{V}CO_2$, carbon dioxide output; VD/VT, physiological dead space–tidal volume ratio; $\dot{V}E$, minute ventilation; $\dot{V}E/\dot{V}CO_2$, ventilatory equivalent for carbon dioxide; $\dot{V}E/\dot{V}O_2$, ventilatory equivalent for oxygen; $\dot{V}O_2$, oxygen uptake.

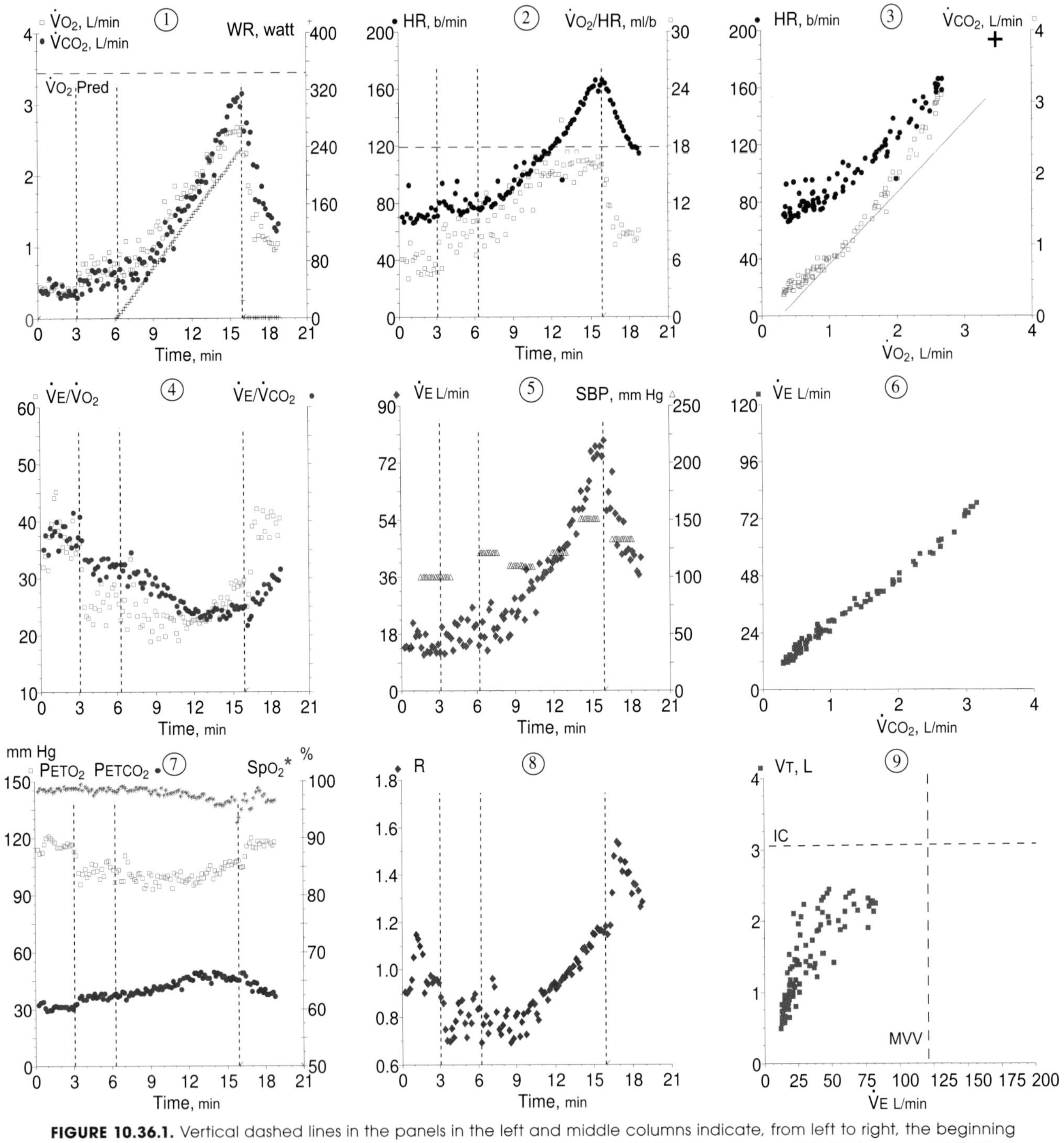

FIGURE 10.36.1. Vertical dashed lines in the panels in the left and middle columns indicate, from left to right, the beginning of unloaded cycling, start of increasing work rate (WR) at 25 W/min, and start of recovery. In **panel 1**, the increase in WR (right y-axis) is plotted with a scale of 100 W to 1 L of oxygen uptake ($\dot{V}O_2$) (left y-axis) such that WR is plotted parallel to a $\dot{V}O_2$ slope of 10 mL/min/W. Predicted peak $\dot{V}O_2$ is shown as a dashed horizontal line. In **panel 3**, carbon dioxide output ($\dot{V}CO_2$) (right y-axis) is plotted as a function of $\dot{V}O_2$ (x-axis) with identical scales so that the diagonal blue line has a slope of 1 (45°). The $\dot{V}CO_2$ increasing more steeply than $\dot{V}O_2$ defines carbon dioxide (CO_2) derived from bicarbonate buffer, as long as ventilatory equivalent for CO_2 ($\dot{V}E/\dot{V}CO_2$) (**panel 4**) is not increasing and end-tidal P_{CO_2} (P_{ETCO_2}) (**panel 7**) is not decreasing, simultaneously. The black + symbol in **panel 3** indicates predicted peak values of heart rate (HR) (left y-axis) and $\dot{V}O_2$ for this individual. Abbreviations: IC, inspiratory capacity; MVV, maximum voluntary ventilation; P_{ETO_2}, end-tidal P_{O_2}; R, respiratory exchange ratio; SBP, systolic blood pressure; Sp_{O_2}, oxygen saturation as measured by pulse oximetry; VC, vital capacity; $\dot{V}E$, minute ventilation; $\dot{V}E/\dot{V}O_2$, ventilatory equivalent for oxygen; V_T, tidal volume.

was initially normal but became somewhat steeper near peak exercise, despite the history of β-blocker therapy, and peak oxygen pulse was near normal but not elevated. The anaerobic threshold was within normal limits.

Ventilation and pulmonary gas exchange responses: There was a breathing reserve. Pulse oximetry was normal and the relationship of $\dot{V}E$ to $\dot{V}CO_2$ was normal, so there was no evidence for impairment in pulmonary gas exchange.

Conclusion

The findings indicate mild impairment in the cardiovascular response to exercise, presumably related to the right-sided cardiac abnormalities demonstrated on imaging, which were likely to be progressive. There was in addition impairment in pulmonary function testing with both mildly reduced lung volumes and mild airflow obstruction. These do not appear limiting to exercise, however.

CASE 37

Tetralogy of Fallot, Unrepaired

CLINICAL FINDINGS

A 23-year-old woman was referred for exercise testing at the time of transitioning care to an adult congenital heart disease provider. She was born with tetralogy of Fallot with pulmonary atresia and aortopulmonary collaterals. Between 6 and 10 years of age, she had staged surgeries, including a unifocalization procedure, which was intended to consolidate pulmonary vessels into conduits of large enough caliber for future surgical repair. Pulmonary vascular anatomy was never deemed sufficient for definitive surgical repair, however, so no additional interventions were performed. She was a college student and could walk on level ground at her own pace but could not keep pace with her peers. She was short of breath on ascending any stairs or inclines. She had episodes of light-headedness with exertion and one episode of syncope in the preceding year. She was most commonly limited in her activities by shortness of breath and general tiredness. She was prescribed atenolol and low-dose aspirin but was taking neither. On physical examination, breath sounds were clear and cardiac examination notable for continuous murmurs audible throughout the precordium and posterior thorax. There was clubbing of the digits and cyanosis of the nail beds. There was no peripheral edema. The electrocardiogram showed a sinus rhythm. Demographic and respiratory function information is shown in **Table 10.37.1**.

TABLE 10.37.1 Selected Respiratory Function Data

Measurement	Predicted	Measured
Age (y)		23
Sex		Female
Height (cm)		170
Weight (kg)		53.2
VC (L)	4.16	3.01
IC (L)	2.48	2.05
ERV (L)	1.68	1.11
FEV_1 (L)	3.58	2.3
FEV_1/VC (%)	86	76
MVV (L/min)		72

Abbreviations: ERV, expiratory reserve volume; FEV_1, forced expiratory volume in 1 second; IC, inspiratory capacity; MVV, maximum voluntary ventilation; VC, vital capacity.

EXERCISE FINDINGS

The patient exercised on a cycle ergometer beginning with 3 minutes of unloaded pedaling at 60 rpm followed by continuous increase in work rate by 10 W/min until exercise was ended with symptoms of general fatigue. Exercise data are summarized in **Tables 10.37.2** and **10.37.3** and in **Figure 10.37.1**.

INTERPRETATION

Comment

This patient's history of light-headedness and syncope are indications for caution in exercise testing. She was instructed to exert herself only to the level she normally tolerated in her daily activities and no attempt was made to encourage effort beyond that level.

Analysis

Cardiovascular and metabolic responses: Oxygen uptake ($\dot{V}O_2$) did not increase appropriately to the increase in work rate (shallow $\Delta\dot{V}O_2/\Delta WR$, panel 1) and the peak $\dot{V}O_2$ was very low relative to predicted maximal $\dot{V}O_2$. Heart rate in-

TABLE 10.37.2 Selected Exercise Data

Measurement	Predicted	Measured
Peak $\dot{V}O_2$ (L/min)	1.82	0.67
Maximum heart rate (beats/min)	190	115
Maximum O_2 pulse (mL/beat)	9.6	5.8
$\Delta\dot{V}O_2/\Delta WR$ (mL/min/W)	10.3	5.0
AT (L/min)	>0.8	<0.50
Blood pressure (mm Hg [rest, max])		110/60, 143/62
Maximum $\dot{V}E$ (L/min)		39
Breathing reserve (L/min)	>15	33
$\dot{V}E/\dot{V}CO_2$ @ *AT*	<30	~50
$\dot{V}E$-$\dot{V}CO_2$ slope	<30	60
SpO_2 (% [rest, max ex])		79, 59

Abbreviations: *AT*, anaerobic threshold; $\Delta\dot{V}O_2/\Delta WR$, change in $\dot{V}O_2$/change in work rate; ex, exercise; O_2, oxygen; SpO_2, oxygen saturation as measured by pulse oximetry; $\dot{V}CO_2$, carbon dioxide output; $\dot{V}E$, minute ventilation; $\dot{V}E/\dot{V}CO_2$, ventilatory equivalent for carbon dioxide; $\dot{V}O_2$, oxygen uptake.

TABLE 10.37.3 Air Breathing

Time (min)	Work rate (W)	BP (mm Hg)	HR (min⁻¹)	f (min⁻¹)	$\dot{V}E$ (L/min BTPS)	$\dot{V}CO_2$ (L/min STPD)	$\dot{V}O_2$ (L/min STPD)	$\frac{\dot{V}O_2}{HR}$ (mL/beat)	R	pH	HCO_3^- (mEq/L)	PO_2, mm Hg and SpO_2, % ET	SpO_2	(A − a)	PCO_2, mm Hg ET	a	(a − ET)	$\frac{\dot{V}E}{\dot{V}CO_2}$	$\frac{\dot{V}E}{\dot{V}O_2}$	$\frac{V_D}{V_T}$
0.5	Rest		75	14	10.5	0.22	0.25	3.3	0.87			118	79		26			48	42	
1.0	Rest	110/60	79	13	11.3	0.24	0.27	3.5	0.88			118	92		27			47	42	
1.5	Rest		78	14	11.4	0.25	0.28	3.6	0.88			117	90		27			46	41	
2.0	Rest		77	13	11.9	0.25	0.27	3.5	0.93			118	88		27			47	44	
2.5	Rest		79	8	10.7	0.24	0.26	3.3	0.91			117	78		27			44	40	
3.0	Rest		78	10	12.3	0.27	0.29	3.7	0.94			119	77		26			46	43	
3.5	Unloaded		79	18	14.7	0.30	0.31	3.9	0.98			121	79		26			49	48	
4.0	Unloaded		87	17	16.3	0.34	0.36	4.1	0.94			120	79		26			49	45	
4.5	Unloaded		87	22	19.9	0.39	0.40	4.7	0.96			122	78		24			51	49	
5.0	Unloaded		84	22	20.5	0.41	0.43	5.2	0.94			121	74		25			50	48	
5.5	Unloaded	125/62	85	20	19.6	0.39	0.42	4.9	0.94			121	69		25			50	47	
6.0	Unloaded		87	22	23.0	0.46	0.47	5.4	0.97			123	68		24			50	49	
6.5	3		88	18	19.6	0.40	0.41	4.7	0.97			123	68		24			49	48	
7.0	7		92	23	25.0	0.51	0.54	5.8	0.96			122	67		25			49	47	
7.5	12		92	25	26.9	0.52	0.50	5.5	1.03			125	65		23			52	53	
8.0	17	140/65	91	25	26.2	0.51	0.50	5.5	1.02			125	66		23			51	52	
8.5	22		94	24	28.0	0.54	0.52	5.5	1.05			125	65		23			52	54	
9.0	27		99	23	28.3	0.57	0.57	5.7	1.01			124	65		24			49	50	
9.5	32		102	24	30.9	0.61	0.57	5.6	1.05			125	63		23			51	54	
10.0	37	136/68	105	24	32.1	0.63	0.59	5.6	1.07			126	62		23			51	55	
10.5	42		109	25	33.9	0.66	0.62	5.7	1.07			125	61		23			51	55	
11.0	47		111	26	36.7	0.70	0.63	5.7	1.10			127	58		23			53	58	
11.5	52		115	26	39.1	0.75	0.67	5.8	1.12			127	59		23			52	59	
12.0	Recovery	143/62	105	26	36.3	0.70	0.64	6.0	1.10			126	57		23			52	57	
12.5	Recovery		95	21	29.9	0.62	0.57	6.0	1.08			124	53		25			48	52	
13.0	Recovery		94	20	26.1	0.55	0.52	5.5	1.07			123	50		26			47	50	
13.5	Recovery	129/67	95	18	22.9	0.50	0.48	5.1	1.04			122	53		27			46	47	
14.0	Recovery		89	21	22.3	0.47	0.44	4.9	1.06			122	57		26			48	51	
14.5	Recovery		85	21	22.5	0.46	0.44	5.1	1.07			123	60		26			48	52	

Abbreviations: BP, blood pressure; BTPS, body temperature pressure saturated; f, frequency; HCO_3^-, bicarbonate; HR, heart rate; $P(A - a)O_2$, alveolar-arterial PO_2 difference; $P(a - ET)CO_2$, arterial–end-tidal CO_2 difference; $PETCO_2$, end-tidal PCO_2; $PETO_2$, end-tidal PO_2; R, respiratory exchange ratio; SpO_2, oxygen saturation as measured by pulse oximetry; STPD, standard temperature pressure dry; $\dot{V}CO_2$, carbon dioxide output; V_D/V_T, physiological dead space–tidal volume ratio; $\dot{V}E$, minute ventilation; $\dot{V}E/\dot{V}CO_2$, ventilatory equivalent for carbon dioxide; $\dot{V}E/\dot{V}O_2$, ventilatory equivalent for oxygen; $\dot{V}O_2$, oxygen uptake.

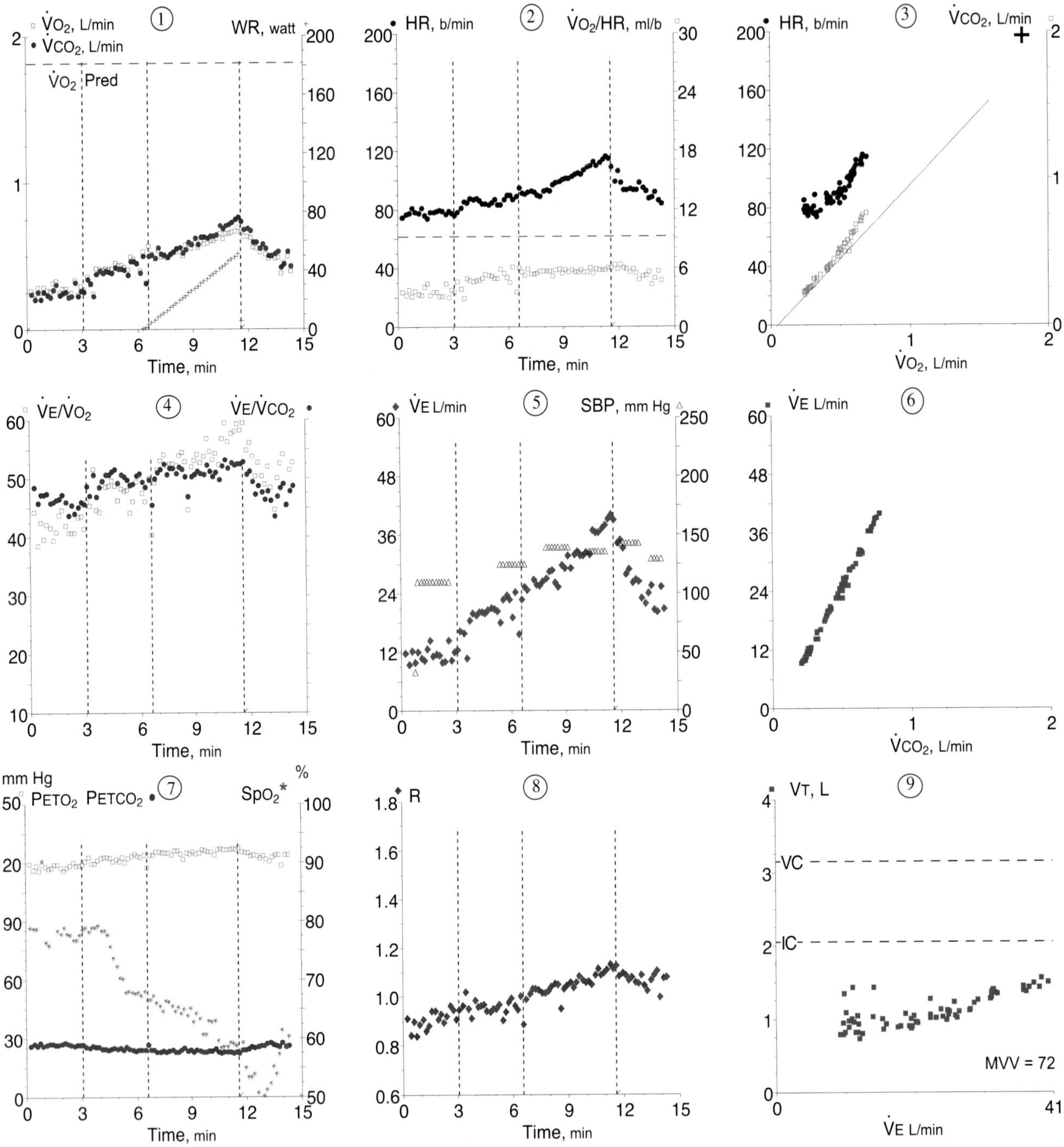

FIGURE 10.37.1. Vertical dashed lines in the panels in the left and middle columns indicate, from left to right, the beginning of unloaded cycling, start of increasing work rate (WR) at 10 W/min, and start of recovery. In **panel 1**, the increase in WR (right y-axis) is plotted with a scale of 100 W to 1 L of oxygen uptake ($\dot{V}O_2$) (left y-axis) such that WR is plotted parallel to a $\dot{V}O_2$ slope of 10 mL/min/W. Predicted peak $\dot{V}O_2$ is shown as a dashed horizontal line. In **panel 3**, carbon dioxide output ($\dot{V}CO_2$) (right y-axis) is plotted as a function of $\dot{V}O_2$ (x-axis) with identical scales so that the diagonal blue line has a slope of 1 (45°). The $\dot{V}CO_2$ increasing more steeply than $\dot{V}O_2$ defines carbon dioxide (CO_2) derived from bicarbonate buffer, as long as ventilatory equivalent for CO_2 ($\dot{V}E/\dot{V}CO_2$) (**panel 4**) is not increasing and end-tidal P_{CO_2} (P_{ETCO_2}) (**panel 7**) is not decreasing, simultaneously. The black + symbol in **panel 3** indicates predicted peak values of heart rate (HR) (left y-axis) and $\dot{V}O_2$ for this individual. Abbreviations: IC, inspiratory capacity; MVV, maximum voluntary ventilation; P_{ETO_2}, end-tidal P_{O_2}; R, respiratory exchange ratio; SBP, systolic blood pressure; Sp_{O_2}, oxygen saturation as measured by pulse oximetry; VC, vital capacity; $\dot{V}E$, minute ventilation; $\dot{V}E/\dot{V}O_2$, ventilatory equivalent for oxygen; V_T, tidal volume.

creased steeply relative to $\dot{V}O_2$ (panel 3), but the peak heart rate was low. The oxygen pulse (O_2 pulse) increased modestly at the start of exercise, reaching a plateau value, which was lower than the normal peak value. This implies that $C(a - \bar{v})O_2$ reached a maximal value early in exercise, and the falling arterial O_2 content offset any increase in venous extraction of O_2. In the early recovery period, $\dot{V}O_2$ recovered slowly, as evidenced by O_2 pulse remaining at the peak value for the first minute of recovery, as an abnormally large O_2 deficit was restored. A related finding was the decrease in R value in early recovery, resulting from $\dot{V}O_2$ returning back toward baseline values more slowly than carbon dioxide output ($\dot{V}CO_2$). Given the steady rise in R value (panel 8), and the inflection point in the V-slope (panel 3), it appears that lactic acidosis developed despite the low work rates attained. In fact, the patient was likely above anaerobic threshold during the initial phase of unloaded cycling, so it is not possible to identify an exact value and it was reported as less than the unloaded cycling value.

Ventilation did not appear limiting, as there was an ample breathing reserve. The increase in minute ventilation ($\dot{V}E$) at the start of exercise was disproportionate to $\dot{V}O_2$ and $\dot{V}CO_2$ (ventilatory equivalents increased at exercise onset, panel 4), and there was reciprocal increase in end tidal PO_2 and decrease in end tidal PCO_2 (panel 7) typical of the ventilatory effects of augmented right to left shunting.

Pulmonary gas exchange was abnormal, with low SpO_2 at rest, and marked decline in SpO_2 beginning shortly after the start of exercise. The SpO_2 decreased further in the early recovery period, which is not uncommon in cyanotic congenital heart diseases, and probably reflects further increase in shunting as systemic vascular resistance decreased at the end of exercise. Intracardiac shunt was undoubtedly the major cause of hypoxemia, but there may also be regional mismatching of pulmonary $\dot{V}/\dot{Q}$ given the abnormal pulmonary vascular anatomy. The increase of $\dot{V}E$ was steep relative to $\dot{V}CO_2$ and $\dot{V}E/\dot{V}CO_2$ remained high throughout the test. These too may be primarily due to the effect of central circulatory shunting on ventilation, with additional effect of regional $\dot{V}/\dot{Q}$ mismatching and high pulmonary V_D/V_T.

Conclusion

Even though no attempt was made to push the patient to maximal exertion, the shallow $\dot{V}O_2$ responses, flat O_2 pulse, and progressive hypoxemia suggest the peak $\dot{V}O_2$ measured was a realistic measure of her maximal exercise capacity. These $\dot{V}O_2$ findings could result from any severe impairment in exercise cardiac output and O_2 delivery. The pattern of ventilation and gas exchange in the setting of cyanosis, however, was characteristic of exercise-induced increase in systemic venous to arterial shunting. Both limitation of total systemic blood flow and marked O_2 desaturation contribute to limiting O_2 delivery.

CASE 38

Amyloid Cardiomyopathy

CLINICAL FINDINGS

The patient is an 88-year-old man with a recent diagnosis of amyloid cardiomyopathy. A pacemaker had been placed for bradycardia. His history was also notable for mild lower lobe interstitial fibrosis on imaging of his lungs and for spinal stenosis that had limited his tolerance for walking for a number of years. He also had shortness of breath that had been progressive over the previous 2 years to the point that he was dyspneic with any activity, even walking in his home. He endorsed orthopnea and occasional nocturnal wakening due to dyspnea. His examination was notable for focal fine crackles at the lung bases bilaterally, regular heart tones without murmur, and no peripheral edema. The electrocardiogram (ECG) showed a paced rhythm at a rate of 69 and low voltages in all leads. Medications on the day of testing were furosemide, carvedilol, quinapril, clopidogrel, potassium supplement, and aspirin. Demographic and respiratory function data are shown in **Table 10.38.1**.

EXERCISE FINDINGS

The patient exercised on a cycle ergometer beginning with 3 minutes of unloaded pedaling at 60 rpm followed by continuous increase in work rate by 10 W/min to a peak work rate of 32 W. He reported leg pain typical of his spinal stenosis but said the exercise was limited by both shortness of breath and leg fatigue. The ECG initially showed a paced rhythm, but as exercise progressed heart rate increased in an apparent native rhythm with a wide QRS complex. There was no ectopy noted. Exercise data are summarized in **Tables 10.38.2** and **10.38.3** and in **Figure 10.38.1**.

TABLE 10.38.1 Selected Respiratory Function Data

Measurement	Predicted	Measured
Age (y)		88
Sex		Male
Height (cm)		172
Weight (kg)		68.6
VC (L)	3.29	3.22
IC (L)	3.0	2.15
ERV (L)	0.29	1.1
FEV_1 (L)	2.24	2.52
FEV_1/VC (%)	70	78
MVV (L/min)	97	88

Abbreviations: ERV, expiratory reserve volume; FEV_1, forced expiratory volume in 1 second; IC, inspiratory capacity; MVV, maximum voluntary ventilation; VC, vital capacity.

INTERPRETATION

Comment

This case is presented as an example of heart failure due to a restrictive cardiomyopathy. Some of the gas exchange variables are difficult to quantify in this test because of a marked oscillatory breathing pattern.

Analysis

Exercise capacity was low with a peak $\dot{V}O_2$ of 12.4 mL/min/kg. This corresponds to around 3 metabolic equivalents (METs) or 3 times the resting metabolic rate. Even though the measured peak $\dot{V}O_2$ was 64% of the predicted value, because of his age, the predicted value itself was not high in absolute terms so that even modest reductions might be expected to

TABLE 10.38.2 Selected Exercise Data

Measurement	Predicted	Measured
Peak $\dot{V}O_2$ (L/min)	1.29	0.82
Maximum heart rate (beats/min)	132	109
Heart rate reserve (beats/min)	0	23
Maximum O_2 pulse (mL/beat)	9.8	7.5
$\Delta\dot{V}O_2/\Delta WR$ (mL/min/W)	10.3	NA
AT (L/min)	>0.63	NA
Blood pressure (mm Hg [rest, max])		110/64, 112/60
Maximum $\dot{V}E$ (L/min)		40
Breathing reserve (L/min)	>15	48
$\dot{V}E/\dot{V}CO_2$ @ *AT*	<35	Approximately 48
$\dot{V}E$-$\dot{V}CO_2$ slope	<34	Approximately 45
SpO_2 (% [rest, max ex])		100, 100

Abbreviations: *AT*, anaerobic threshold; $\Delta\dot{V}O_2/\Delta WR$, change in $\dot{V}O_2$/change in work rate; ex, exercise; NA, not applicable; O_2, oxygen; SpO_2, oxygen saturation as measured by pulse oximetry; $\dot{V}CO_2$, carbon dioxide output; $\dot{V}E$, minute ventilation; $\dot{V}E/\dot{V}CO_2$, ventilatory equivalent for carbon dioxide; $\dot{V}O_2$, oxygen uptake.

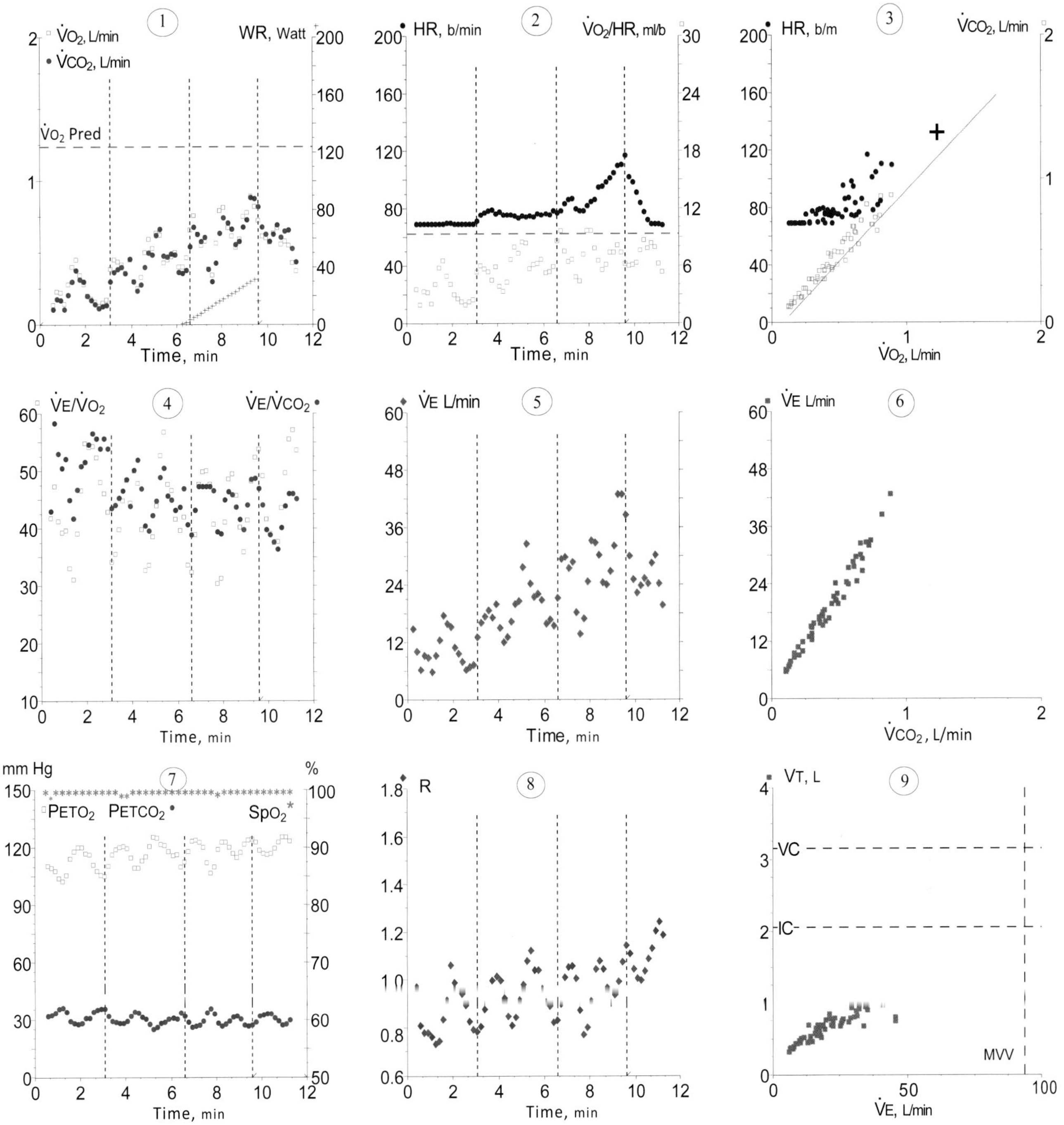

FIGURE 10.38.1. Vertical dashed lines in the panels in the left and middle columns indicate, from left to right, the beginning of unloaded cycling, start of increasing work rate (WR) at 10 W/min, and start of recovery. In **panel 1**, the increase in WR (right y-axis) is plotted with a scale of 100 W to 1 L of oxygen uptake ($\dot{V}O_2$) (left y-axis) such that WR is plotted parallel to a $\dot{V}O_2$ slope of 10 mL/min/W. Predicted peak $\dot{V}O_2$ is shown as a dashed horizontal line. In **panel 3**, carbon dioxide output ($\dot{V}CO_2$) (right y-axis) is plotted as a function of $\dot{V}O_2$ (x-axis) with identical scales so that the diagonal blue line has a slope of 1 (45°). The $\dot{V}CO_2$ increasing more steeply than $\dot{V}O_2$ defines carbon dioxide (CO_2) derived from bicarbonate buffer, as long as ventilatory equivalent for CO_2 ($\dot{V}E/\dot{V}CO_2$) (**panel 4**) is not increasing and end-tidal P_{CO_2} (P_{ETCO_2}) (**panel 7**) is not decreasing, simultaneously. The black + symbol in **panel 3** indicates predicted peak values of heart rate (left y-axis) and $\dot{V}O_2$ for this individual. Abbreviations: IC, inspiratory capacity; MVV, maximum voluntary ventilation; P_{ETO_2}, end-tidal P_{O_2}; R, respiratory exchange ratio; SBP, systolic blood pressure; Sp_{O_2}, oxygen saturation as measured by pulse oximetry; VC, vital capacity; $\dot{V}E$, minute ventilation; $\dot{V}E/\dot{V}O_2$, ventilatory equivalent for oxygen; V_T, tidal volume.

TABLE 10.38.3 Cycle Test

Time (min:sec)	Work rate (W)	BP (mm Hg)	HR (min⁻¹)	f (min⁻¹)	$\dot{V}E$ (L/min BTPS)	$\dot{V}CO_2$ (L/min STPD)	$\dot{V}O_2$ (L/min STPD)	$\frac{\dot{V}O_2}{HR}$ (mL/beat)	R	pH	HCO_3^- (mEq/L)	PO_2, mm Hg and SpO_2, % ET	SpO_2	(A − a)	PCO_2, mm Hg ET	a	(a − ET)	$\frac{\dot{V}E}{\dot{V}CO_2}$	$\frac{\dot{V}E}{\dot{V}O_2}$	$\frac{V_D}{V_T}$
0	Rest		69	21	11.5	0.26	0.32	4.7	0.80			110	100		33			45	36	
0.5	Rest		69	18	8.2	0.16	0.20	2.9	0.78			109	100		33			53	41	
1.0	Rest	110/64	69	19	9.6	0.22	0.30	4.3	0.74			104	100		35			43	32	
1.5	Rest		69	24	16.1	0.32	0.35	5.0	0.93			117	100		28			50	46	
2.0	Rest		69	20	9.5	0.17	0.18	2.5	0.97			118	100		30			55	54	
2.5	Rest		69	18	6.9	0.13	0.16	2.3	0.81			107	100		35			54	44	
3.0	Unloaded		75	26	15.8	0.35	0.43	5.7	0.83			111	100		32			45	37	
3.5	Unloaded		78	24	18.2	0.39	0.39	5.0	1.00			120	100		28			46	47	
4.0	Unloaded		76	27	13.2	0.27	0.29	3.8	0.92			114	100		32			50	45	
4.5	Unloaded	107/68	74	27	19.4	0.48	0.55	7.4	0.86			113	100		32			41	35	
5.0	Unloaded		75	33	28.0	0.58	0.54	7.2	1.07			124	100		26			49	52	
5.5	Unloaded		75	30	21.1	0.47	0.47	6.2	1.01			120	100		29			45	45	
6.0	2		77	28	16.8	0.39	0.46	6.0	0.86			114	100		32			43	37	
6.5	7		80	33	27.3	0.62	0.68	8.5	0.92			119	100		28			44	40	
7.0	12		85	33	24.9	0.52	0.50	5.9	1.05			122	100		27			48	50	
7.5	17		80	31	18.5	0.46	0.57	7.1	0.80			109	100		34			41	33	
8.0	22		88	34	32.0	0.70	0.69	7.8	1.01			121	100		27			46	46	
8.5	27	112/60	99	35	25.1	0.60	0.63	6.3	0.96			117	100		31			42	40	
9.0	32		109	53	39.5	0.83	0.82	7.5	1.00			121	100		28			48	48	
9.5	Recovery		106	34	30.8	0.71	0.64	6.1	1.10			122	100		29			44	48	
10.0	Recovery		84	28	23.5	0.63	0.62	7.4	1.01			117	100		33			37	38	
10.5	Recovery		70	30	27.8	0.63	0.55	8.0	1.14			123	100		29			44	50	
11.0	Recovery		69	28	21.0	0.46	0.38	5.5	1.21			124	100		29			46	56	

Abbreviations: BP, blood pressure; BTPS, body temperature pressure saturated; f, frequency; HCO_3^-, bicarbonate; HR, heart rate; $P(A - a)O_2$, alveolar-arterial PO_2 difference; $P(a - ET)CO_2$, arterial–end-tidal PCO_2 difference; $PETCO_2$, end-tidal PCO_2; $PETO_2$, end-tidal PO_2; R, respiratory exchange ratio; SpO_2, oxygen saturation as measured by pulse oximetry; STPD, standard temperature pressure dry; $\dot{V}CO_2$, carbon dioxide output; V_D/V_T, physiological dead space–tidal volume ratio; $\dot{V}E$, minute ventilation; $\dot{V}E/\dot{V}CO_2$, ventilatory equivalent for carbon dioxide; $\dot{V}E/\dot{V}O_2$, ventilatory equivalent for oxygen; $\dot{V}O_2$, oxygen uptake.

limit ability for routine activities. It is therefore not surprising that he was symptomatic with minimal activity.

Cardiovascular findings: The resting ECG was abnormal with findings consistent with his known infiltrative heart disease. Although heart rate was paced at rest, it appeared to increase intrinsically up to the level of work achieved; peak heart rate was low. Blood pressure did not increase appreciably during exercise (not graphed). At end exercise, the O_2 pulse was lower than the normal predicted peak value, which would be consistent with impaired stroke volume. It appears that he likely exceeded the lactate threshold during the test based on the trend in the R values, but it cannot be precisely quantified due to the irregular breathing pattern and limited range of gas exchange increase.

Ventilation: The ventilation pattern was dominated by regular oscillations having a periodicity of around 90 seconds, which may be seen in patients with heart failure of any cause. Oscillatory breathing is often best identified from display of a rolling average of breath-by-breath data. Depending on how time-averaged values correspond to the oscillatory cycle, the pattern may be difficult to identify in graphical displays, which may simply appear "noisy". In the 10-second average values shown in **Figure 10.38.1**, oscillations are most clearly demonstrated in panels 7 and 8. There was a substantial breathing reserve, so he does not appear to have been limited by the mechanics of breathing.

Pulmonary gas exchange efficiency: Gas exchange abnormalities were evident in the steep relationship of $\dot{V}E$ to $\dot{V}CO_2$, suggesting high dead space ventilation and/or some reduction in arterial PCO_2. There was very little decrease in the ventilatory equivalents between rest and exercise, which implies that the effective V_D/V_T did not decrease normally. Pulse oximetry was normal and remained close to 100% throughout the test.

Conclusion

The findings are consistent with severe cardiovascular limitation due to chronic heart failure. The peak $\dot{V}O_2$ of 12.4 mL/min/kg corresponds to Weber functional class C for chronic heart failure. The oscillatory ventilation and steep relationship of $\dot{V}E/\dot{V}CO_2$ have each been associated with poor prognosis in patients with other forms of heart failure.[1] Although he had an uncharacterized pulmonary process, with radiographic abnormalities and crackles on lung exam, this was not associated with oxygenation problems and did not appear to contribute to his limitation.

REFERENCE

1. Sun XG, Hansen JE, Beshai JF, Wasserman K. Oscillatory breathing and exercise gas exchange abnormalities prognosticate early mortality and morbidity in heart failure. *J Am Coll Cardiol.* 2010;55: 1814-1823.

CASE 39

Athletic Man With Tachyarrhythmia

CLINICAL FINDINGS

A 53-year-old man was referred for exercise testing because of symptoms of fatigue, dyspnea, and weakness. He competed regularly in ultramarathons and other endurance events. For several months while training or competing, he had occasionally felt that his "legs weren't getting enough oxygen." He denied chest pain, wheezing, syncope, or other associated symptoms. He was able to continue his activities by modifying his pace, but symptoms occurred sporadically even after scaling back his training routine. Evaluation by his primary care physician included normal findings on routine blood tests, spirometry, electrocardiogram (ECG), echocardiogram, and nuclear cardiac stress test. His medical history was unremarkable, and he was taking no medications. Resting spirometry was normal, and ECG was notable only for sinus bradycardia. Physical examination was without abnormalities. Demographic and respiratory function data are shown in **Table 10.39.1**.

EXERCISE FINDINGS

The patient exercised on a cycle ergometer beginning with 3 minutes of unloaded pedaling at 60 rpm followed by continuous increase in work rate by 25 W/min. Exercise ECG showed a progressive rise in heart rate up to 156 beats/min at which point the rhythm became irregular, immediately followed by an abrupt increase in rate to over 240 beats/min with wide QRS complexes. Coincident with this, the patient signaled the need to stop, later confirming that this was typical of the symptoms he had been experiencing. Work rate was reduced as soon as these events were recognized and because the patient was alert and responsive, he was allowed to continue pedaling without resistance for 2 minutes. Once the work rate was reduced, heart rate slowed progressively and QRS complexes narrowed, but the rhythm remained irregularly irregular, consistent with atrial fibrillation. There were no ischemic changes on the postexercise ECG and no symptoms of chest pain or lightheadedness. His symptoms resolved entirely within several minutes. Exercise data are summarized in **Tables 10.39.2** and **10.39.3** and in **Figure 10.39.1**.

TABLE 10.39.1 Selected Respiratory Function Data

Measurement	Predicted	Measured
Age (y)		53
Sex		Male
Height (cm)		183
Weight (kg)		87.1
VC (L)	5.32	4.9
IC (L)	3.56	3.21
ERV (L)	1.76	1.26
FEV_1 (L)	4.09	4.13
FEV_1/VC (%)	84	77
MVV, L/min	156	154

Abbreviations: ERV, expiratory reserve volume; FEV_1, forced expiratory volume in 1 second; IC, inspiratory capacity; MVV, maximum voluntary ventilation; VC, vital capacity.

TABLE 10.39.2 Selected Exercise Data

Measurement	Predicted	Measured
Peak $\dot{V}O_2$ (L/min)	2.62	2.93
Maximum heart rate (beats/min)	167	156 (in sinus rhythm)
Heart rate reserve (beats/min)	0	11
Maximum O_2 pulse (mL/beat)	15.7	18.8
$\Delta\dot{V}O_2/\Delta WR$ (mL/min/W)	10.3	9.8
AT (L/min)	>1.19	1.60
Blood pressure (mm Hg [rest, max])		133/94, 234/107
Maximum $\dot{V}E$ (L/min)		93
Breathing reserve (L/min)	>15	61
$\dot{V}E/\dot{V}CO_2$ @ *AT*	<31	24
$\dot{V}E$-$\dot{V}CO_2$ slope	<31	23
SpO_2 (% [rest, max ex])		97, 97

Abbreviations: *AT*, anaerobic threshold; $\Delta\dot{V}O_2/\Delta WR$, change in $\dot{V}O_2$/change in work rate; ex, exercise; O_2, oxygen; SpO_2, oxygen saturation as measured by pulse oximetry; $\dot{V}CO_2$, carbon dioxide output; $\dot{V}E$, minute ventilation; $\dot{V}E/\dot{V}CO_2$, ventilatory equivalent for carbon dioxide; $\dot{V}O_2$, oxygen uptake.

INTERPRETATION

Comment

Gas exchange measures were not essential to the diagnostic findings of this test, which came from the ECG. The case is presented nevertheless to demonstrate the marked effect that a sudden decrease in effective cardiac output has on pulmonary gas exchange. Indeed, the patient had indicated as much when he reported that his legs "weren't getting enough oxygen."

TABLE 10.39.3 Air Breathing

Time (min)	Work rate (W)	BP (mm Hg)	HR (min^{-1})	f (min^{-1})	$\dot{V}E$ (L/min BTPS)	$\dot{V}CO_2$ (L/min STPD)	$\dot{V}O_2$ (L/min STPD)	$\frac{\dot{V}O_2}{HR}$ (mL/beat)	R	pH	HCO_3^- (mEq/L)	PO_2, mm Hg and SpO_2, %: ET	SpO_2	(A − a)	PCO_2, mm Hg: ET	a	(a − ET)	$\frac{\dot{V}E}{\dot{V}CO_2}$	$\frac{\dot{V}E}{\dot{V}O_2}$	$\frac{VD}{VT}$
0.5	Rest		54	8	5.0	0.13	0.18	3.4	0.72			101	97		36			39	28	
1.0	Rest	133/94	54	10	7.1	0.18	0.26	4.8	0.70			99	97		36			39	27	
1.5	Rest		56	12	7.7	0.20	0.28	5.0	0.72			100	97		36			39	28	
2.0	Rest		50	10	6.9	0.18	0.25	5.0	0.71			100	98		36			39	28	
2.5	Unloaded		67	14	15.4	0.48	0.64	9.7	0.75			99	97		38			32	24	
3.0	Unloaded		64	13	14.9	0.47	0.63	9.8	0.75			98	95		38			32	24	
3.5	Unloaded		60	13	11.6	0.35	0.46	7.7	0.76			99			39			33	25	
4.0	Unloaded		57	13	12.2	0.37	0.48	8.4	0.78			100			38			33	26	
4.5	Unloaded	135/94	60	13	14.2	0.44	0.58	9.6	0.76			99			38			32	25	
5.0	Unloaded		59	14	11.7	0.35	0.45	7.7	0.78			99			39			33	26	
5.5	10		58	12	12.5	0.40	0.51	8.9	0.77			100			38			31	24	
6.0	23		60	13	12.7	0.39	0.51	8.5	0.78			100	97		39			32	25	
6.5	34		64	13	13.8	0.44	0.57	9.0	0.77			98	96		40			31	24	
7.0	47	146/98	65	13	14.3	0.48	0.62	9.6	0.76			96	97		41			30	23	
7.5	58		68	12	15.4	0.55	0.74	10.9	0.74			91	97		43			28	21	
8.0	71		74	14	18.7	0.67	0.89	12.1	0.75			95	97		41			28	21	
8.5	82		76	13	20.3	0.74	0.98	12.9	0.75			93	97		43			28	21	
9.0	94	162/90	78	15	23.1	0.86	1.10	14.0	0.78			93	98		43			27	21	
9.5	106		81	14	27.3	1.02	1.30	16.0	0.79			93	97		44			27	21	
10.0	120		85	15	27.7	1.09	1.36	16.0	0.80			91	97		45			25	20	
10.5	132		88	14	31.4	1.26	1.51	17.2	0.83			92	97		46			25	21	
11.0	144	178/90	95	15	36.2	1.47	1.65	17.4	0.89			94	98		47			25	22	
11.5	156		100	15	35.8	1.51	1.73	17.3	0.87			92	98		48			24	21	
12.0	168		106	16	42.4	1.76	1.87	17.7	0.94			95	98		48			24	23	
12.5	180		111	17	47.0	1.95	1.99	17.9	0.98			97	98		48			24	24	
13.0	193		116	17	48.9	2.04	2.05	17.7	0.99			97	98		48			24	24	
13.5	205	210/110	122	18	53.0	2.22	2.20	17.9	1.01			97	98		48			24	24	
14.0	217		129	20	57.2	2.40	2.34	18.2	1.02			99	98		48			24	24	
14.5	229		133	20	63.2	2.60	2.43	18.2	1.07			100	97		47			24	26	
15.0	242	213/111	139	22	69.2	2.84	2.62	18.9	1.08			101	97		47			24	26	
15.5	254		146	23	78.4	3.08	2.71	18.6	1.14			105	97		45			25	29	
16.0	266		151	25	82.5	3.20	2.79	18.5	1.14			106	97		44			26	30	
16.5	278	234/107	156	28	92.7	3.43	2.93	18.8	1.17			109	97		42			27	32	
17.0	Recovery		202	29	87.4	2.61	2.00	9.9	1.30			119	97		34			33	44	
17.5	Recovery		181	25	71.3	2.47	1.96	10.8	1.26			114	97		40			29	36	
18.0	Recovery		166	20	52.0	1.74	1.32	8.0	1.32			115	98		39			30	39	
18.5	Recovery	207/94	140	17	39.6	1.34	1.04	7.4	1.29			114	99		40			30	38	
19.0	Recovery		130	13	29.2	1.03	0.82	6.3	1.26			112	99		41			28	36	
19.5	Recovery		135	18	36.5	1.15	0.92	6.8	1.25			116	98		37			32	40	

Abbreviations: BP, blood pressure; BTPS, body temperature pressure saturated; f, frequency; HCO_3^-, bicarbonate; HR, heart rate; $P(A - a)O_2$, alveolar-arterial PO_2 difference; $P(a - ET)CO_2$, arterial-end-tidal PCO_2 difference; $PETCO_2$, end-tidal PCO_2; $PETO_2$, end-tidal PO_2; R, respiratory exchange ratio; SpO_2, oxygen saturation as measured by pulse oximetry; STPD, standard temperature pressure dry; $\dot{V}CO_2$, carbon dioxide output; VD/VT, physiological dead space-tidal volume ratio; $\dot{V}E$, minute ventilation; $\dot{V}E/\dot{V}CO_2$, ventilatory equivalent for carbon dioxide; $\dot{V}E/\dot{V}O_2$, ventilatory equivalent for oxygen; $\dot{V}O_2$, oxygen uptake.

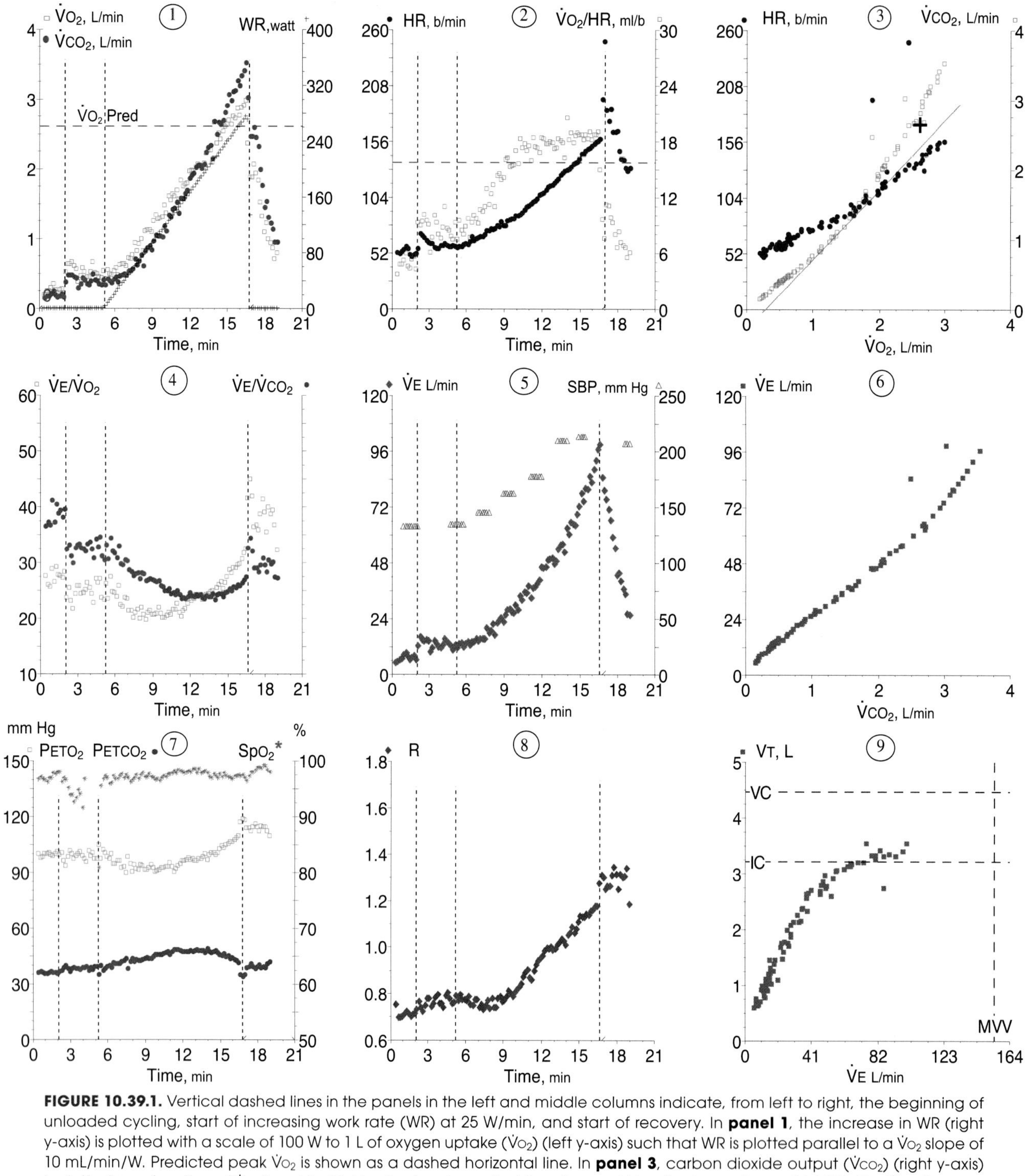

FIGURE 10.39.1. Vertical dashed lines in the panels in the left and middle columns indicate, from left to right, the beginning of unloaded cycling, start of increasing work rate (WR) at 25 W/min, and start of recovery. In **panel 1**, the increase in WR (right y-axis) is plotted with a scale of 100 W to 1 L of oxygen uptake ($\dot{V}O_2$) (left y-axis) such that WR is plotted parallel to a $\dot{V}O_2$ slope of 10 mL/min/W. Predicted peak $\dot{V}O_2$ is shown as a dashed horizontal line. In **panel 3**, carbon dioxide output ($\dot{V}CO_2$) (right y-axis) is plotted as a function of $\dot{V}O_2$ (x-axis) with identical scales so that the diagonal blue line has a slope of 1 (45°). The $\dot{V}CO_2$ increasing more steeply than $\dot{V}O_2$ defines carbon dioxide (CO_2) derived from bicarbonate buffer, as long as ventilatory equivalent for CO_2 ($\dot{V}E/\dot{V}CO_2$) (**panel 4**) is not increasing and end-tidal PCO_2 ($PETCO_2$) (**panel 7**) is not decreasing, simultaneously. The black + symbol in **panel 3** indicates predicted peak values of heart rate (HR) (left y-axis) and $\dot{V}O_2$ for this individual. Abbreviations: IC, inspiratory capacity; MVV, maximum voluntary ventilation; $PETO_2$, end-tidal PO_2; R, respiratory exchange ratio; SBP, systolic blood pressure; SpO_2, oxygen saturation as measured by pulse oximetry; VC, vital capacity; $\dot{V}E$, minute ventilation; $\dot{V}E/\dot{V}O_2$, ventilatory equivalent for oxygen; V_T, tidal volume.

Analysis

Cardiovascular and metabolic responses: The oxygen uptake ($\dot{V}O_2$) and oxygen (O_2) pulse just prior to stopping exercise were above the predicted maximal values. Blood pressure response to exercise was marked. Because exercise was interrupted by arrhythmia, it is possible that his true maximal values would be higher if he remained in sinus rhythm. The $\Delta\dot{V}O_2/\Delta WR$ and anaerobic threshold were both normal. Coincident with the onset of tachyarrhythmia, there was an immediate drop in $\dot{V}O_2$ and O_2 pulse (see panels 1 and 2) consistent with a reduction in the effective forward stroke volume and cardiac output. Although exercise also stopped immediately after this, it is apparent from the graphs that the gas exchange changes were more acute than what normally occurs at the end of a test. The event was so brief that the effect on gas exchange is only appreciated in the graphical data, which are displayed as 10-second averages whereas it is obscured in the 30-second averages shown in **Table 10.39.3**. Although cardiovascular capacity was at least above average, consistent with his athletic training, the nonlinear increase of heart rate relative to $\dot{V}O_2$ beginning around the anaerobic threshold (panel 3) and associated asymptote of O_2 pulse (panel 2) suggest the possibility that there was impairment of a previously higher cardiac stroke volume, perhaps related to hypertensive changes.

Ventilation, breathing reserve, and indices of pulmonary gas exchange efficiency were all normal across the range of exercise attained.

Conclusion

This patient's symptoms were reproduced by the occurrence of paroxysmal atrial fibrillation with rapid ventricular response during high-intensity exercise. It was fortuitous that this intermittent event was documented in the laboratory, but worth noting that had the test been stopped at 85% of predicted maximal heart rate, the arrhythmia would probably not have been seen. The wide complex tachycardia could not be immediately characterized when viewed on the monitor. However, because the postexercise rhythm was clearly atrial fibrillation, it was believed likely that the wide complexes represented rate-dependent conduction abnormalities rather than a primary ventricular arrhythmia. The patient was referred for further cardiac and electrophysiology evaluation.

CASE 40

Heart Rate Impairment Due to β-Adrenergic Blockade for Treatment of Hypertension

CLINICAL FINDINGS

A 60-year-old woman was evaluated because of chronic cough and moderate exertional dyspnea. She had systemic arterial hypertension, for which she was treated with a β-adrenergic blocker and diuretic. An angiotensin-converting enzyme inhibitor had not been prescribed because of the chronic cough. She had never smoked. Her resting electrocardiogram (ECG) was normal. At her initial exercise evaluation, she had a reduced exercise tolerance, with a reduced heart rate response and poor control of her hypertension. To determine whether the limited heart rate accounted for exercise intolerance, she had repeat testing performed after holding her β-blocker. Both tests are shown. The first was done while taking the β-blocker, and the second 2 days later after the β-adrenergic blocker had been withheld. Demographic and respiratory function data are shown in **Table 10.40.1**.

EXERCISE FINDINGS

On both tests, the patient performed exercise on a cycle ergometer. She cycled at 60 rpm without added load for 3 minutes, after which work rate was progressively increased by 10 W/min until she could not continue. Heart rate and rhythm were continuously monitored and arterial pressure was measured every 2 minutes by sphygmomanometer. The patient performed the tests with good effort and ended both with symptoms of leg fatigue. Exercise data for the two tests are summarized in **Table 10.40.2**. Data for the first and second tests are shown in **Table 10.40.3** and **Figure 10.40.1**, and in **Table 10.40.4** and **Figure 10.40.2**, respectively.

TABLE 10.40.1 Selected Respiratory Function Data

Measurement	Predicted	Measured
Age (y)		60
Sex		Female
Height (cm)		165
Weight (kg)		59
Hematocrit (%)		41
VC (L)	3.22	2.74
IC (L)	2.15	1.75
ERV (L)	1.07	1.00
FEV_1 (L)	2.53	1.76
FEV_1/VC (%)	78	64
MVV (L/min)	104	70
D_{LCO} (mL/mm Hg/min)	25.2	11.1

Abbreviations: D_{LCO}, diffusing capacity of the lung for carbon monoxide; ERV, expiratory reserve volume; FEV_1, forced expiratory volume in 1 second; IC, inspiratory capacity; MVV, maximum voluntary ventilation; VC, vital capacity.

INTERPRETATION

Comments

Resting pulmonary function showed moderate airway obstruction with significant reduction in her diffusing capacity. Her maximum heart rate on exercise testing was 113 beats/min with and 156 beats/min without β-adrenergic blockade (**Table 10.40.2**). Exercise ECGs were otherwise

TABLE 10.40.2 Selected Exercise Data

Measurement	Predicted	With β-blockade	Without β-blockade
Peak $\dot{V}O_2$ (L/min)	1.31	1.07	1.22
Maximum heart rate (beats/min)	160	113	156
Maximum O_2 pulse (mL/beat)	8.2	9.5	7.8
$\Delta\dot{V}O_2/\Delta WR$ (mL/min/W)	10.3	6.8	8.7
AT (L/min)	>0.68	0.50	0.80
Blood pressure (mm Hg [rest, max])		180/85, 200/100	170/90, 220/100
Maximum $\dot{V}E$ (L/min)		54	55
Exercise breathing reserve (L/min)	>15	16	15
$\dot{V}E/\dot{V}CO_2$ @ *AT* or lowest	29.4	31.5	29.2
P_{ETCO_2} at *AT*	>40	38	40
$\dot{V}E$ versus $\dot{V}CO_2$	<32	29	27
SaO_2 (pulse oximeter, % [rest, exercise])	>95	97, 97	95, 95

Abbreviations: *AT*, anaerobic threshold; $\Delta\dot{V}O_2/\Delta WR$, change in $\dot{V}O_2$/change in work rate; O_2, oxygen; P_{ETCO_2}, end-tidal PCO_2; SaO_2, arterial oxygen saturation; $\dot{V}CO_2$, carbon dioxide output; $\dot{V}E$, minute ventilation; $\dot{V}E/\dot{V}CO_2$, ventilatory equivalent for carbon dioxide; $\dot{V}O_2$, oxygen uptake.

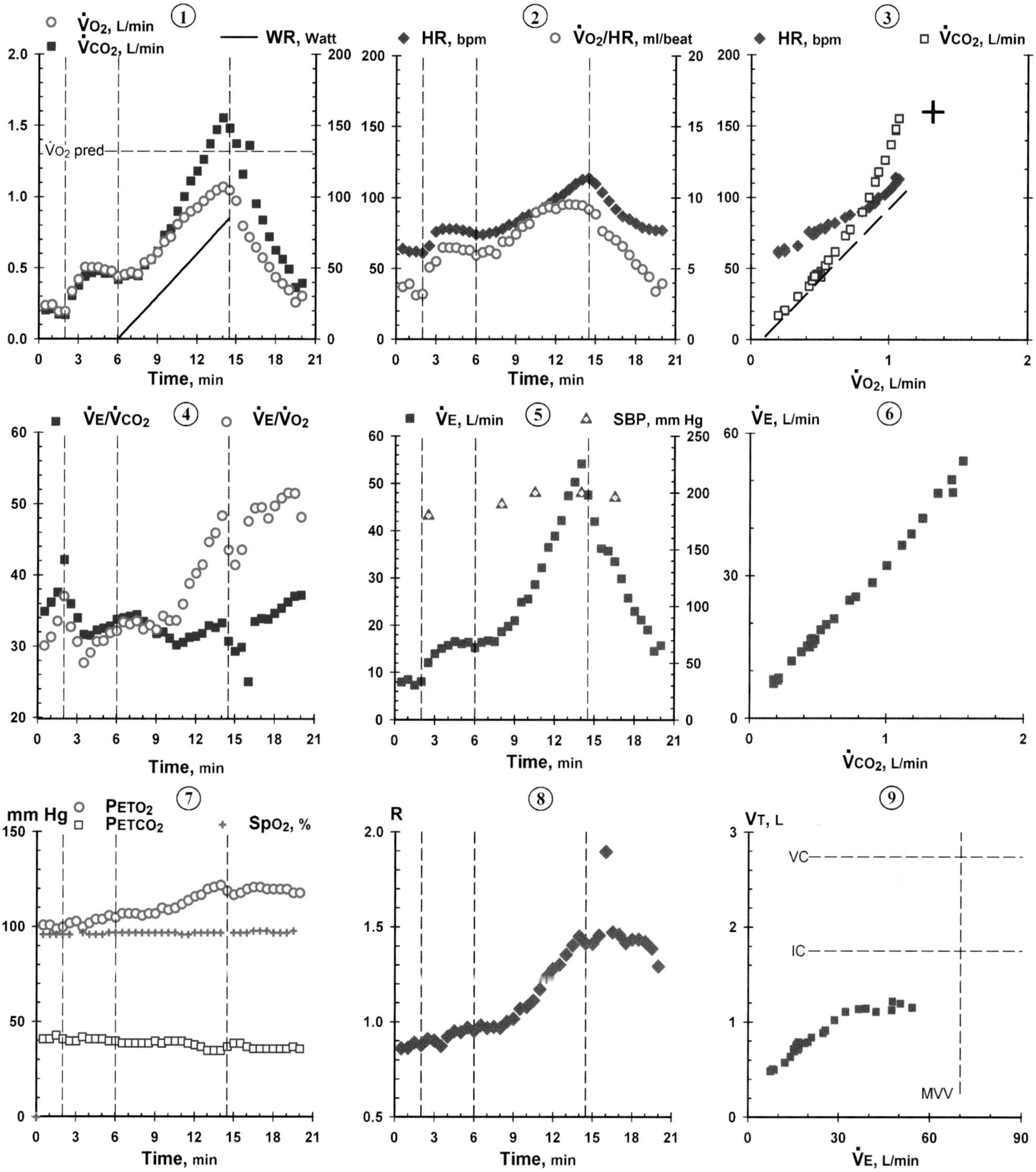

FIGURE 10.40.1. First study, while taking β-adrenergic blocker. Vertical dashed lines in the panels in the left and middle columns indicate, from left to right, the beginning of unloaded cycling, start of increasing work rate (WR) at 10 W/min, and start of recovery. In **panel 1**, the increase in WR (right y-axis) is plotted with a scale of 100 W to 1 L of oxygen uptake ($\dot{V}O_2$) (left y-axis) such that WR is plotted parallel to a $\dot{V}O_2$ slope of 10 mL/min/W. In **panel 3**, carbon dioxide output ($\dot{V}CO_2$ (right y-axis) is plotted as a function of $\dot{V}O_2$ (x-axis) with identical scales so that the diagonal dashed line has a slope of 1 (45°). The $\dot{V}CO_2$ increasing more steeply than $\dot{V}O_2$ defines carbon dioxide (CO_2) derived from bicarbonate buffer, as long as ventilatory equivalent for CO_2 ($\dot{V}E/\dot{V}CO_2$) (**panel 4**) is not increasing and end-tidal PCO_2 ($PETCO_2$) (**panel 7**) is not decreasing, simultaneously. The black + symbol in **panel 3** indicates predicted values of heart rate (HR) (left y-axis) and $\dot{V}O_2$ for this individual. Abbreviations: $PETO_2$, end-tidal PO_2; R, respiratory exchange ratio; SBP, systolic blood pressure; SpO_2, oxygen saturation as measured by pulse oximetry; VC, vital capacity; $\dot{V}E$; minute ventilation; $\dot{V}E/\dot{V}O_2$, ventilatory equivalent for oxygen; VT, tidal volume.

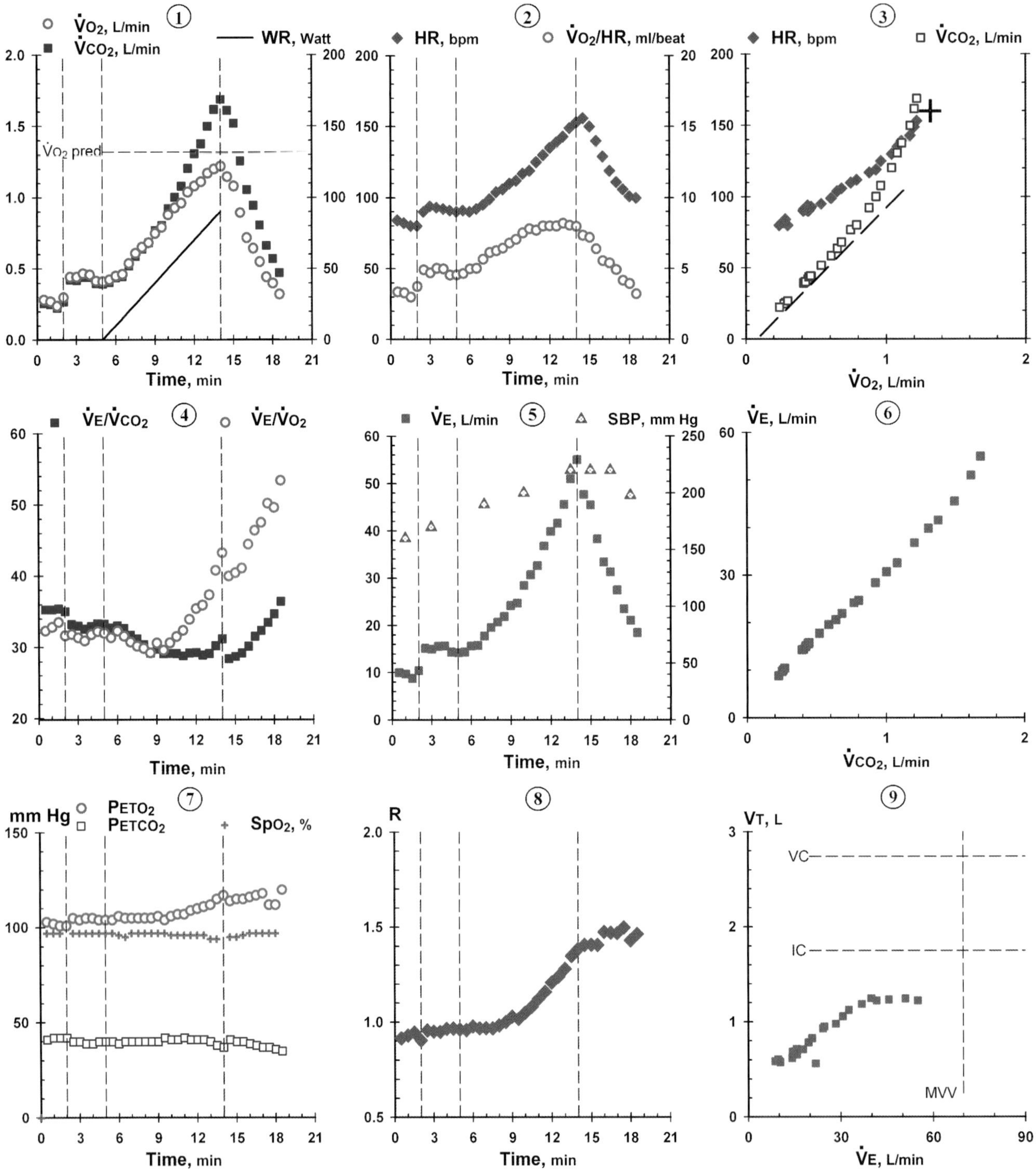

FIGURE 10.40.2. Second study, without β-adrenergic blocker. Vertical dashed lines in the panels in the left and middle columns indicate, from left to right, the beginning of unloaded cycling, start of increasing work rate (WR) at 10 W/min, and start of recovery. In **panel 1**, the increase in WR (right y-axis) is plotted with a scale of 100 W to 1 L of oxygen uptake ($\dot{V}O_2$) (left y-axis) such that WR is plotted parallel to a $\dot{V}O_2$ slope of 10 mL/min/W. In **panel 3**, carbon dioxide output ($\dot{V}CO_2$) (right y-axis) is plotted as a function of $\dot{V}O_2$ (x-axis) with identical scales so that the diagonal dashed line has a slope of 1 (45°). The $\dot{V}CO_2$ increasing more steeply than $\dot{V}O_2$ defines carbon dioxide (CO_2) derived from bicarbonate buffer, as long as ventilatory equivalent for CO_2 ($\dot{V}E/\dot{V}CO_2$) (**panel 4**) is not increasing and end-tidal PCO_2 ($PETCO_2$) (**panel 7**) is not decreasing, simultaneously. The black + symbol in **panel 3** indicates predicted values of heart rate (HR) (left y-axis) and $\dot{V}O_2$ for this individual. Abbreviations: IC, inspiratory capacity; MVV, maximum voluntary ventilation; $PETO_2$, end-tidal PO_2; R, respiratory exchange ratio; SBP, systolic blood pressure; SpO_2, oxygen saturation as measured by pulse oximetry; VC, vital capacity; $\dot{V}E$; minute ventilation; $\dot{V}E/\dot{V}O_2$, ventilatory equivalent for oxygen; V_T, tidal volume.

TABLE 10.40.3 On β-Adrenergic Blockade Medication

Time (min)	Work rate (W)	BP (mm Hg)	HR (min^{-1})	f (min^{-1})	$\dot{V}E$ (L/min BTPS)	$\dot{V}CO_2$ (L/min STPD)	$\dot{V}O_2$ (L/min STPD)	$\frac{\dot{V}O_2}{HR}$ (mL/beat)	R	pH	HCO_3^- (mEq/L)	PO_2, mm Hg			PCO_2, mm Hg			$\frac{\dot{V}E}{\dot{V}CO_2}$	$\frac{\dot{V}E}{\dot{V}O_2}$	$\frac{V_D}{V_T}$
												ET	a	(A − a)	ET	a	(a − ET)			
0.5	Rest		64	16	8.0	0.21	0.24	3.7	0.86			101			41			35	30	
1.0	Rest		62	17	8.5	0.21	0.24	3.9	0.86			101			41			36	31	
1.5	Rest		62	15	7.3	0.17	0.20	3.1	0.89			99			43			38	34	
2.0	Rest		61	16	8.1	0.17	0.20	3.2	0.88			100			41			42	37	
2.5	Rest	180/85	66	21	12.1	0.31	0.34	5.1	0.91			102			40			36	33	
3.0	Rest		76	22	14.0	0.38	0.42	5.5	0.90			103			40			34	31	
3.5	Unloaded		78	21	15.1	0.44	0.51	6.5	0.87			100			42			32	28	
4.0	Unloaded		78	21	15.8	0.47	0.51	6.5	0.92			102			41			32	29	
4.5	Unloaded		78	21	16.6	0.48	0.51	6.5	0.95			104			41			32	31	
5.0	Unloaded		77	21	16.1	0.46	0.49	6.3	0.95			104			41			33	31	
5.5	Unloaded		76	22	16.4	0.47	0.48	6.3	0.97			106			40			33	32	
6.0	Unloaded		74	22	15.3	0.42	0.44	6.0	0.95			105			40			34	32	
6.5	5		74	23	16.4	0.45	0.46	6.2	0.98			107			39			34	33	
7.0	10		75	23	16.8	0.46	0.47	6.3	0.97			107			39			34	33	
7.5	15		76	23	16.6	0.45	0.46	6.1	0.97			107			39			34	34	
8.0	20	190/90	78	24	18.7	0.52	0.54	6.9	0.97			106			39			34	32	
8.5	25		81	25	19.8	0.56	0.56	6.9	1.00			107			39			33	33	
9.0	30		82	25	21.0	0.62	0.61	7.4	1.02			107			40			32	32	
9.5	35		86	28	24.9	0.73	0.69	8.0	1.07			110			39			32	34	
10.0	40		88	28	25.6	0.78	0.72	8.2	1.08			109			40			31	34	
10.5	45	200/96	90	28	28.6	0.90	0.81	9.0	1.11			110			40			30	34	
11.0	50		93	29	32.2	1.00	0.86	9.2	1.17			112			40			31	36	
11.5	55		96	32	36.5	1.11	0.90	9.4	1.24			114			39			31	39	
12.0	60		100	34	38.9	1.18	0.92	9.2	1.28			116			38			31	40	
12.5	65		102	38	42.2	1.26	0.97	9.5	1.30			117			37			32	42	
13.0	70		106	42	47.4	1.37	1.01	9.6	1.36			120			35			33	45	
13.5	75		110	42	50.3	1.47	1.05	9.5	1.41			121			35			33	46	
14.0	80	200/100	113	47	54.2	1.56	1.07	9.5	1.45			122			35			33	48	
14.5	85		114	39	47.6	1.48	1.05	9.2	1.41			119			37			31	44	
15.0	90		110	33	42.0	1.38	0.97	8.0	1.41			117			30			29	41	
15.5	Recovery		104	29	36.2	1.16	0.80	7.7	1.46			118			39			30	44	
16.0	Recovery		98	30	35.7	1.36	0.72	7.3	1.90			120			37			25	48	
16.5	Recovery	196/90	92	30	33.5	0.95	0.65	7.0	1.47			121			36			34	49	
17.0	Recovery		87	29	29.9	0.84	0.57	6.6	1.46			121			36			34	50	
17.5	Recovery		85	27	25.8	0.72	0.51	6.0	1.42			120			36			34	48	
18.0	Recovery		82	25	23.0	0.63	0.44	5.3	1.43			120			36			35	50	
18.5	Recovery		79	24	21.2	0.56	0.39	5.0	1.44			120			36			35	51	
19.0	Recovery		78	23	19.1	0.50	0.35	4.5	1.42			120			36			36	52	
19.5	Recovery		77	21	14.6	0.37	0.26	3.4	1.39			118			37			37	52	
20.0	Recovery		77	21	15.8	0.40	0.31	4.0	1.29			118			36			37	48	

Abbreviations: BP, blood pressure; BTPS, body temperature pressure saturated; f, frequency; HCO_3^-, bicarbonate; HR, heart rate; $P(A-a)O_2$, alveolar-arterial PO_2 difference; $P(a-ET)CO_2$, arterial-end-tidal PCO_2 difference; $PETCO_2$, end-tidal PCO_2; $PETO_2$, end-tidal PO_2; R, respiratory exchange ratio; STPD, standard temperature pressure dry; $\dot{V}CO_2$, carbon dioxide output; V_D/V_T, physiological dead space–tidal volume ratio; $\dot{V}E$, minute ventilation; $\dot{V}E/\dot{V}CO_2$, ventilatory equivalent for carbon dioxide; $\dot{V}E/\dot{V}O_2$, ventilatory equivalent for oxygen; $\dot{V}O_2$, oxygen uptake.

TABLE 10.40.4 Off β-Adrenergic Blockade Medication

Time (min)	Work rate (W)	BP (mm Hg)	HR (min^{-1})	f (min^{-1})	$\dot{V}E$ (L/min BTPS)	$\dot{V}CO_2$ (L/min STPD)	$\dot{V}O_2$ (L/min STPD)	$\frac{\dot{V}O_2}{HR}$ (mL/beat)	R	pH	HCO_3^- (mEq/L)	PO_2, mm Hg ET	PO_2, mm Hg a	PO_2, mm Hg (A − a)	PCO_2, mm Hg ET	PCO_2, mm Hg a	PCO_2, mm Hg (a − ET)	$\frac{\dot{V}E}{\dot{V}CO_2}$	$\frac{\dot{V}E}{\dot{V}O_2}$	$\frac{V_D}{V_T}$
0.5	Rest		84	17	10.0	0.26	0.28	3.4	0.92			103			41			35	32	
1.0	Rest	160/80	82	16	9.7	0.25	0.27	3.3	0.93			102			42			35	33	
1.5	Rest		80	15	8.8	0.23	0.24	3.0	0.95			101			42			35	34	
2.0	Rest		80	18	10.4	0.27	0.30	3.8	0.90			101			42			35	32	
2.5	Unloaded		90	22	15.2	0.42	0.44	4.9	0.96			105			40			33	32	
3.0	Unloaded	170/90	94	22	15.0	0.42	0.44	4.7	0.95			104			40			33	31	
3.5	Unloaded		93	23	15.6	0.44	0.47	5.0	0.95			105			39			33	31	
4.0	Unloaded		92	22	15.7	0.44	0.46	5.0	0.97			105			39			33	32	
4.5	Unloaded		91	21	14.4	0.40	0.41	4.5	0.97			104			40			33	32	
5.0	Unloaded		90	23	14.3	0.40	0.41	4.6	0.96			104			40			33	32	
5.5	5		91	22	14.4	0.41	0.42	4.7	0.96			104			40			33	31	
6.0	10		90	24	15.7	0.44	0.45	5.0	0.98			106			39			33	32	
6.5	15		92	24	15.8	0.45	0.46	5.0	0.97			105			40			33	32	
7.0	20	190/90	95	25	17.8	0.52	0.54	5.7	0.97			105			40			32	31	
7.5	25		99	25	19.6	0.59	0.61	6.1	0.97			105			40			31	30	
8.0	30		104	25	20.7	0.64	0.65	6.3	0.98			105			40			30	30	
8.5	35		106	39	21.9	0.68	0.68	6.4	1.00			105			40			29	29	
9.0	40		110	26	24.2	0.77	0.75	6.8	1.03			106			40			30	31	
9.5	45		112	26	24.7	0.80	0.79	7.1	1.02			104			42			29	30	
10.0	50	200/100	117	29	28.4	0.92	0.88	7.5	1.05			106			41			29	31	
10.5	55		119	29	30.7	1.00	0.93	7.8	1.08			107			41			29	32	
11.0	60		125	29	32.6	1.08	0.96	7.7	1.12			107			42			29	32	
11.5	65		130	31	36.8	1.21	1.04	8.0	1.16			109			41			29	34	
12.0	70		135	32	39.9	1.31	1.08	8.0	1.21			110			41			29	35	
12.5	75		139	34	41.6	1.38	1.11	8.0	1.24			111			41			29	36	
13.0	80		143	37	45.6	1.50	1.17	8.2	1.28			112			40			29	37	
13.5	85	220/100	149	41	51.0	1.62	1.20	8.1	1.35			115			38			30	41	
14.0	90		153	45	55.0	1.69	1.22	8.0	1.39			117			37			31	43	
14.5	Recovery		156	37	47.7	1.61	1.15	7.3	1.41			114			41			28	40	
15.0	Recovery	220/100	150	36	45.5	1.52	1.08	7.2	1.41			115			40			29	40	
15.5	Recovery		140	31	38.3	1.26	0.89	6.4	1.41			115			40			29	41	
16.0	Recovery		129	30	33.4	1.06	0.72	5.6	1.47			116			39			30	44	
16.5	Recovery	220/100	119	29	31.3	0.95	0.64	5.4	1.47			117			38			32	46	
17.0	Recovery		111	28	27.5	0.81	0.55	4.9	1.47			118			37			32	48	
17.5	Recovery		106	25	23.5	0.66	0.44	4.2	1.50			112			37			34	50	
18.0	Recovery	198/90	101	25	21.1	0.57	0.40	4.0	1.43			112			36			35	50	
18.5	Recovery		100	25	18.5	0.47	0.32	3.2	1.46			120			35			36	53	

Abbreviations: BP, blood pressure; BTPS, body temperature pressure saturated; f, frequency; HCO_3^-, bicarbonate; HR, heart rate; $P(A - a)O_2$, alveolar-arterial PO_2 difference; $P(a - ET)CO_2$, arterial-end-tidal PCO_2 difference; $PETCO_2$, end-tidal PCO_2; $PETO_2$, end-tidal PO_2; R, respiratory exchange ratio; STPD, standard temperature pressure dry; $\dot{V}CO_2$, carbon dioxide output; V_D/V_T, physiological dead space-tidal volume ratio; $\dot{V}E$, minute ventilation; $\dot{V}E/\dot{V}CO_2$, ventilatory equivalent for carbon dioxide; $\dot{V}E/\dot{V}O_2$, ventilatory equivalent for oxygen; $\dot{V}O_2$, oxygen uptake.

unremarkable. Her blood pressure response was similar on the 2 days of testing.

Analysis

On the first test, while on β-blockade, peak $\dot{V}O_2$ and anaerobic threshold (*AT*) were low. A pulmonary cause of exercise intolerance was unlikely because breathing reserve was normal, and the normal ventilatory equivalent for $\dot{V}CO_2$ at the *AT* suggested no abnormalities in lung gas exchange. Of note, however, was the HR-$\dot{V}O_2$ response seen in panel 3, which was relatively flat. Also, the patient's *AT* was quite low. Finally, there may have been some flattening of the $\Delta\dot{V}O_2/\Delta WR$.

Using the flowcharts in Chapter 9, peak $\dot{V}O_2$ and *AT* were low, leading to Flowchart 4. The breathing reserve was borderline normal (Branch Point 4.1), and the ventilatory equivalent for $\dot{V}CO_2$ at the *AT* (Branch Point 4.3) was normal, leading to the category of oxygen (O_2) flow problem of nonpulmonary origin (anemia, heart disease, or peripheral arterial disease). She was not anemic, her ECG was normal during this test, and she had no symptoms of claudication. The increase in $\dot{V}O_2$, as related to work rate was normal at low work rates but became shallower, as peak $\dot{V}O_2$ was approached, making the calculated $\Delta\dot{V}O_2/\Delta WR$ slope low.

Two days later, after withholding her β-adrenergic blocker, the peak $\dot{V}O_2$ and *AT* were normal. The $\Delta\dot{V}O_2/\Delta WR$ also normalized. With these variables as well as the peak O_2 pulse, $\dot{V}E/\dot{V}CO_2$, $PETCO_2$ at the *AT*, and ECG all being normal, there are no findings to suggest cardiac or pulmonary vascular disease. She had inadequately controlled hypertension on both tests, but this did not appear to limit exercise tolerance as much as the drug that she was taking to treat it. Studies performed at rest suggested lung disease as the cause of her symptoms. Although the cause of her lung disease remained to be determined, it did not appear to be the proximal cause of her exercise limitation.

Conclusion

The patient was on a drug regimen that reduced her exercise tolerance without effectively controlling her hypertension. This case illustrates that cardiopulmonary exercise testing may help in the selection and dose titration of cardiovascular medications. Of note is the drop in O_2 pulse (still in the normal range) after cessation of β-blockade; a higher O_2 pulse is frequently seen with β-blockade.

CASE 41

Atrial Fibrillation With Rapid Ventricular Response During Exercise

CLINICAL FINDINGS

A 70-year-old woman was referred for exercise testing to follow up the suspicion of pulmonary hypertension reported on echocardiogram. The study had also demonstrated mitral and tricuspid regurgitation but normal right and left ventricular size and function. Both a sleep study and a computed tomography pulmonary angiogram were normal. She did not complain of exertional dyspnea during her normal activities, but she had a largely sedentary lifestyle and seldom did more than walk within her home and office. She did note that she was short of breath if walking up an incline. She had a history of systemic hypertension, hyperlipidemia, and chronic atrial fibrillation. Her medications included warfarin, atenolol, amlodipine, clonidine, simvastatin, and hydrochlorothiazide. Examination was notable for a holosystolic murmur at the cardiac apex. Lungs were clear to auscultation, and there was no peripheral edema. The resting electrocardiogram showed atrial fibrillation with a ventricular rate ranging from 80 to 90. There was no evidence of aberrant conduction.

EXERCISE FINDINGS

The patient exercised on a cycle ergometer. After 3 minutes of unloaded pedaling at 60 rpm, the work rate was increased progressively at a rate of 10 W/min until she stopped with the primary symptom of leg fatigue. During the initial phase of unloaded cycling, heart rate increased rapidly to about 150 beats/min. As work rate was increased, there was further increase of heart rate to 170 to 180 beats/min, which was well above the patient's predicted maximal heart rate. There were no ischemic changes noted. Exercise data are summarized in **Tables 10.41.2** and **10.41.3** and **Figure 10.41.1**.

INTERPRETATION

Comments

Spirometry was normal (**Table 10.41.1**).

Analysis

This patient demonstrated low peak $\dot{V}O_2$ and anaerobic threshold, along with a very high electrical heart rate response to exercise while remaining in atrial fibrillation. She had no evidence of ventilatory limitation but did have findings consistent with cardiovascular disease, including high $\dot{V}E/\dot{V}CO_2$, low O_2 pulse, and flat $\Delta\dot{V}O_2/\Delta WR$. Because she appeared to have normal left ventricular (LV) ejection fraction at rest when heart rate was lower, it is likely that her very high heart rate response was responsible for what appears to be low stroke volume due to inadequate ventricular filling during exercise. Mitral insufficiency could also

TABLE 10.41.1 Selected Respiratory Function Data

Measurement	Predicted	Measured
Age (y)		70
Sex		Female
Height (cm)		157
Weight (kg)		79
VC (L)	2.76	2.25
IC (L)	2.05	2.01
FEV_1 (L)	2.08	1.97
FEV_1/VC (%)	76	88
MVV (L/min)	82	87
D_{LCO} (mL/mm Hg/min)	18.7	17.22

Abbreviations: D_{LCO}, diffusing capacity of lung for carbon monoxide; FEV_1, forced expiratory volume in 1 second; IC, inspiratory capacity; MVV, maximum voluntary ventilation; VC, vital capacity.

TABLE 10.41.2 Selected Exercise Data

Measurement	Predicted	Measured
Peak $\dot{V}O_2$ (L/min)	1.22	0.82
Maximum heart rate (beats/min)	150	185
Maximum O_2 pulse (mL/beat)	8.1	4.9
$\Delta\dot{V}O_2/\Delta WR$ (mL/min/W)	10.3	5.3
AT (L/min)	>0.68	0.58
Blood pressure (mm Hg [rest, max])		157/92, 202/115
Maximum $\dot{V}E$ (L/min)		39
Exercise breathing reserve (L/min)	>15	48
$\dot{V}E/\dot{V}CO_2$ @ *AT* or lowest	30.8	39.2

Abbreviations: *AT*, anaerobic threshold; $\Delta\dot{V}O_2/\Delta WR$, change in $\dot{V}O_2$/change in work rate; ex, exercise; O_2, oxygen; $\dot{V}E$, minute ventilation; $\dot{V}E/\dot{V}CO_2$, ventilatory equivalent for carbon dioxide; $\dot{V}O_2$, oxygen uptake.

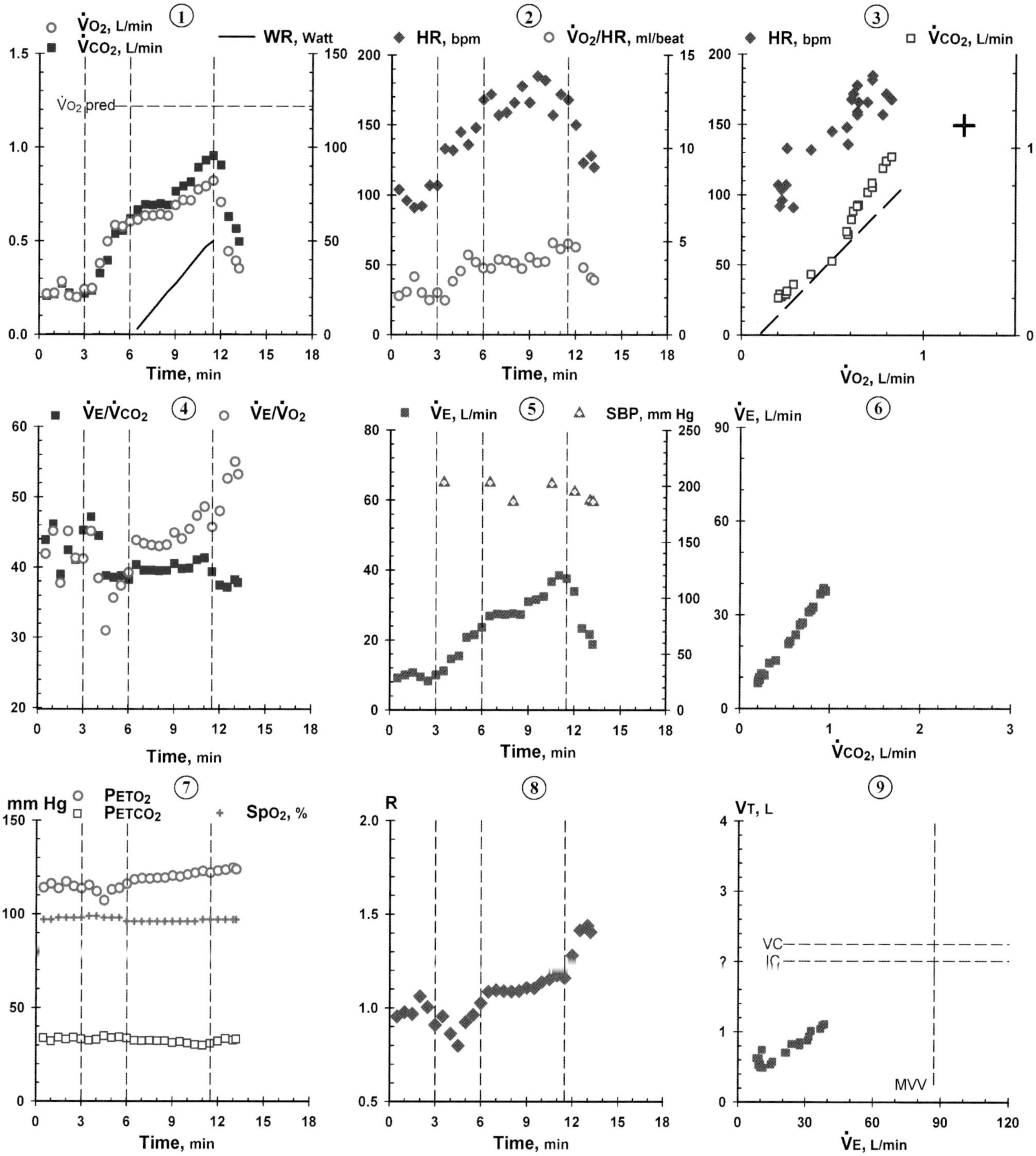

FIGURE 10.41.1. Vertical dashed lines in the panels in the left and middle columns indicate, from left to right, the beginning of unloaded cycling, start of increasing work rate (WR) at 10 W/min, and start of recovery. In **panel 1**, the increase in WR (right y-axis) is plotted with a scale of 100 W to 1 L of oxygen uptake ($\dot{V}O_2$) (left y-axis) such that WR is plotted parallel to a $\dot{V}O_2$ slope of 10 mL/min/W. In **panel 3**, carbon dioxide output ($\dot{V}CO_2$) (right y-axis) is plotted as a function of $\dot{V}O_2$ (x-axis) with identical scales so that the diagonal dashed line has a slope of 1 (45°). The $\dot{V}CO_2$ increasing more steeply than $\dot{V}O_2$ defines carbon dioxide (CO_2) derived from bicarbonate buffer, as long as ventilatory equivalent for CO_2 ($\dot{V}E/\dot{V}CO_2$) (**panel 4**) is not increasing and end-tidal PCO_2 ($PETCO_2$) (**panel 7**) is not decreasing, simultaneously. The black + symbol in **panel 3** indicates predicted values of heart rate (HR) (left y-axis) and $\dot{V}O_2$ for this individual. Abbreviations: IC, inspiratory capacity; MVV, maximum voluntary ventilation; $PETO_2$, end-tidal PO_2; R, respiratory exchange ratio; SBP, systolic blood pressure; SpO_2, oxygen saturation as measured by pulse oximetry; VC, vital capacity; $\dot{V}E$, minute ventilation; $\dot{V}E/\dot{V}O_2$, ventilatory equivalent for oxygen; VT, tidal volume.

TABLE 10.41.3 Air Breathing

Time (min)	Work rate (W)	BP (mm Hg)	HR (min^{-1})	f (min^{-1})	$\dot{V}E$ (L/min BTPS)	$\dot{V}CO_2$ (L/min STPD)	$\dot{V}O_2$ (L/min STPD)	$\frac{\dot{V}O_2}{HR}$ (mL/beat)	R	pH	HCO_3^- (mEq/L)	PO_2, mm Hg ET	PO_2, mm Hg a	PO_2, mm Hg (A − a)	PCO_2, mm Hg ET	PCO_2, mm Hg a	PCO_2, mm Hg (a − ET)	$\frac{\dot{V}E}{\dot{V}CO_2}$	$\frac{\dot{V}E}{\dot{V}O_2}$	$\frac{V_D}{V_T}$
0.5	Rest		104	17	9.1	0.21	0.22	2.1	0.95			114			34			44	42	
1.0	Rest		96	20	10.0	0.22	0.22	2.3	0.98			116			32			46	45	
1.5	Rest		91	14	10.7	0.28	0.28	3.1	0.97			114			34			39	38	
2.0	Rest		92	15	9.4	0.22	0.21	2.3	1.06			117			33			42	45	
2.5	Rest	157/92	107	13	8.3	0.20	0.20	1.9	1.01			115			34			41	41	
3.0	Rest		107	19	10.0	0.22	0.24	2.3	0.91			114			33			45	41	
3.5	Unloaded		133	23	11.2	0.24	0.25	1.9	0.96			115			33			47	45	
4.0	Unloaded		132	27	14.6	0.33	0.38	2.9	0.86			112			33			45	38	
4.5	Unloaded		145	27	15.4	0.40	0.50	3.4	0.80			107			35			39	31	
5.0	Unloaded		136	30	20.8	0.54	0.58	4.3	0.92			113			34			39	36	
5.5	Unloaded		148	31	21.6	0.56	0.58	3.9	0.96			114			34			39	37	
6.0	Unloaded		168	29	23.7	0.62	0.60	3.6	1.03			116			34			38	39	
6.5	3	203/113	172	32	26.9	0.67	0.61	3.6	1.09			118			33			40	44	
7.0	8		157	32	27.5	0.70	0.64	4.0	1.09			119			33			40	43	
7.5	13		159	33	27.4	0.69	0.64	4.0	1.09			119			33			40	43	
8.0	18	186/130	166	34	27.6	0.70	0.64	3.9	1.09			119			33			40	43	
8.5	23		178	33	27.4	0.69	0.63	3.6	1.09			119			32			40	43	
9.0	27		166	35	31.0	0.77	0.69	4.2	1.11			120			32			41	45	
9.5	32		185	34	31.6	0.79	0.72	3.9	1.11			120			32			40	44	
10.0	37		182	32	32.5	0.82	0.72	3.9	1.14			121			31			40	45	
10.5	42	202/115	157	35	36.7	0.89	0.78	4.9	1.15			122			31			41	47	
11.0	47		172	35	38.6	0.93	0.79	4.6	1.18			123			30			41	49	
11.5	50		168	34	37.6	0.96	0.82	4.9	1.16			122			31			39	46	
12.0	Recovery	195/157	150	31	34.0	0.91	0.71	4.7	1.28			123			32			37	48	
12.5	Recovery		123	23	23.4	0.63	0.45	3.6	1.42			124			34			37	53	
13.0	Recovery	187/140	128	24	21.7	0.57	0.39	3.1	1.44			125			33			38	55	
14.0	Recovery	186/138	120	21	18.8	0.50	0.35	3.0	1.41			124			33			38	53	

Abbreviations: BP, blood pressure; BTPS, body temperature pressure saturated; f, frequency; HCO_3^-, bicarbonate; HR, heart rate; $P(A-a)O_2$, alveolar-arterial PO_2 difference; $P(a-ET)CO_2$, arterial-end-tidal PCO_2 difference; $PETCO_2$, end-tidal PCO_2; $PETO_2$, end-tidal PO_2; R, respiratory exchange ratio; STPD, standard temperature pressure dry; $\dot{V}CO_2$, carbon dioxide output; V_D/V_T, physiological dead space–tidal volume ratio; $\dot{V}E$, minute ventilation; $\dot{V}E/\dot{V}CO_2$, ventilatory equivalent for carbon dioxide; $\dot{V}E/\dot{V}O_2$, ventilatory equivalent for oxygen; $\dot{V}O_2$, oxygen uptake.

contribute to lower effective LV stroke volume because of regurgitant flow.

Using the flowcharts in Chapter 9 for diagnostic purposes, peak $\dot{V}O_2$ and the anaerobic threshold were both low (Branch Points 1.1, 1.2, and 1.3), leading to Flowchart 4. Breathing reserve (Branch Point 4.1) was normal. The $\dot{V}E/\dot{V}CO_2$ was abnormally high. According to Branch Point 4.5, these findings, along with a normal pulse oximetry, suggest moderate-to-severe left ventricular heart failure, which is consistent with the other findings. However, the findings fit best with a diagnosis of poor forward LV stroke volume during exercise rather than "heart failure" because the low stroke volume is likely due to the marked tachycardia and absence of atrial contraction with this arrhythmia. To what extent she has pulmonary venous hypertension to account for the echocardiographic findings cannot be determined from these data, but the elevated ventilatory equivalents suggest this may be present, despite relatively little symptomatic complaints.

Conclusion

This test is presented to illustrate the finding of excessive atrio-ventricular (A-V) conduction and reduced stroke volume during exercise associated with rapid atrial fibrillation. Even though ventricular heart rate appeared reasonably well controlled at rest, it markedly accelerated during exercise, causing gas exchange abnormalities consistent with left ventricular failure. It would be interesting to repeat this study with better ventricular rate control.

CASE 42

Chronotropic Insufficiency With Escape Rhythm

To view this case please access the eBook bundled with this text. Instructions are located on the inside front cover.

CASE 43

Active Older Man With Second-Degree Heart Block

CLINICAL FINDINGS

A 90-year-old man was referred for exercise testing after an echocardiogram was reported to show elevated estimated pulmonary artery pressures. The echocardiogram had been done to evaluate a systolic murmur and did not demonstrate significant valve disease or other abnormalities. He was asymptomatic, without any exertional symptoms and was aware of having Wenckebach type heart block for many years. He worked full time, reported being a recreational runner since his 40s and routinely went for a weekly 2-mile jog. The medical history was also notable for hypothyroidism and anemia with hemoglobin values chronically in the range of 11 to 12 g/dL. His only regular medication was thyroid replacement. Physical examination revealed a regularly irregular cardiac rhythm and grade II/VI systolic ejection murmur at the left sternal border. Resting electrocardiogram showed a sinus rhythm with Mobitz type I (Wenckebach) second degree atrioventricular (A-V) block and average ventricular rate of 58. Demographic and respiratory function data are shown in **Table 10.43.1**.

TABLE 10.43.1 Selected Respiratory Function Data

Measurement	Predicted	Measured
Age (y)		90
Sex		Male
Height (cm)		173
Weight (kg)		72.7
VC (L)	3.22	3.27
IC (L)	3.22	3.46
ERV (L)	0.21	1.7
FEV_1 (L)	2.17	1.96
FEV_1/VC (%)	69	60
MVV (L/min)	95	94

Abbreviations: ERV, expiratory reserve volume; FEV_1, forced expiratory volume in 1 second; IC, inspiratory capacity; MVV, maximum voluntary ventilation; VC, vital capacity.

EXERCISE FINDINGS

The patient exercised on a cycle ergometer beginning with 3 minutes of unloaded pedaling at 60 rpm followed by continuous increase in work rate by 10 W/min until the test ended with symptoms of leg fatigue. With exercise, the cardiac rhythm became more regular, and there were no further nonconducted P waves above a heart rate of 75; however, peak heart rate was only 95 beats/min. There were no significant ST segment changes and the patient denied chest pain. Exercise data are summarized in **Tables 10.43.2** and **10.43.3** and in **Figure 10.43.1**.

TABLE 10.43.2 Selected Exercise Data

Measurement	Predicted	Measured
Peak $\dot{V}O_2$ (L/min)	1.28	1.33
Maximum heart rate (beats/min)	[illegible]	[illegible]
Heart rate reserve (beats/min)	0	35
Maximum O_2 pulse (mL/beat)	9.9	14.0
$\Delta\dot{V}O_2/\Delta WR$ (mL/min/W)	10.3	10.6
AT (L/min)	>0.63	0.875
Blood pressure (mm Hg [rest, max])		140/62, 171/54
Maximum $\dot{V}E$ (L/min)		44
Breathing reserve (L/min)	>15	50
$\dot{V}E/\dot{V}CO_2$ @ *AT*	<35	32
$\dot{V}E$-$\dot{V}CO_2$ slope	<34	30
SpO_2 (% [rest, max ex])		96, 98

Abbreviations: *AT*, anaerobic threshold; $\Delta\dot{V}O_2/\Delta WR$, change in $\dot{V}O_2$/change in work rate; ex, exercise; O_2, oxygen; SpO_2, oxygen saturation as measured by pulse oximetry; $\dot{V}CO_2$, carbon dioxide output; $\dot{V}E$, minute ventilation; $\dot{V}E/\dot{V}CO_2$, ventilatory equivalent for carbon dioxide; $\dot{V}O_2$, oxygen uptake.

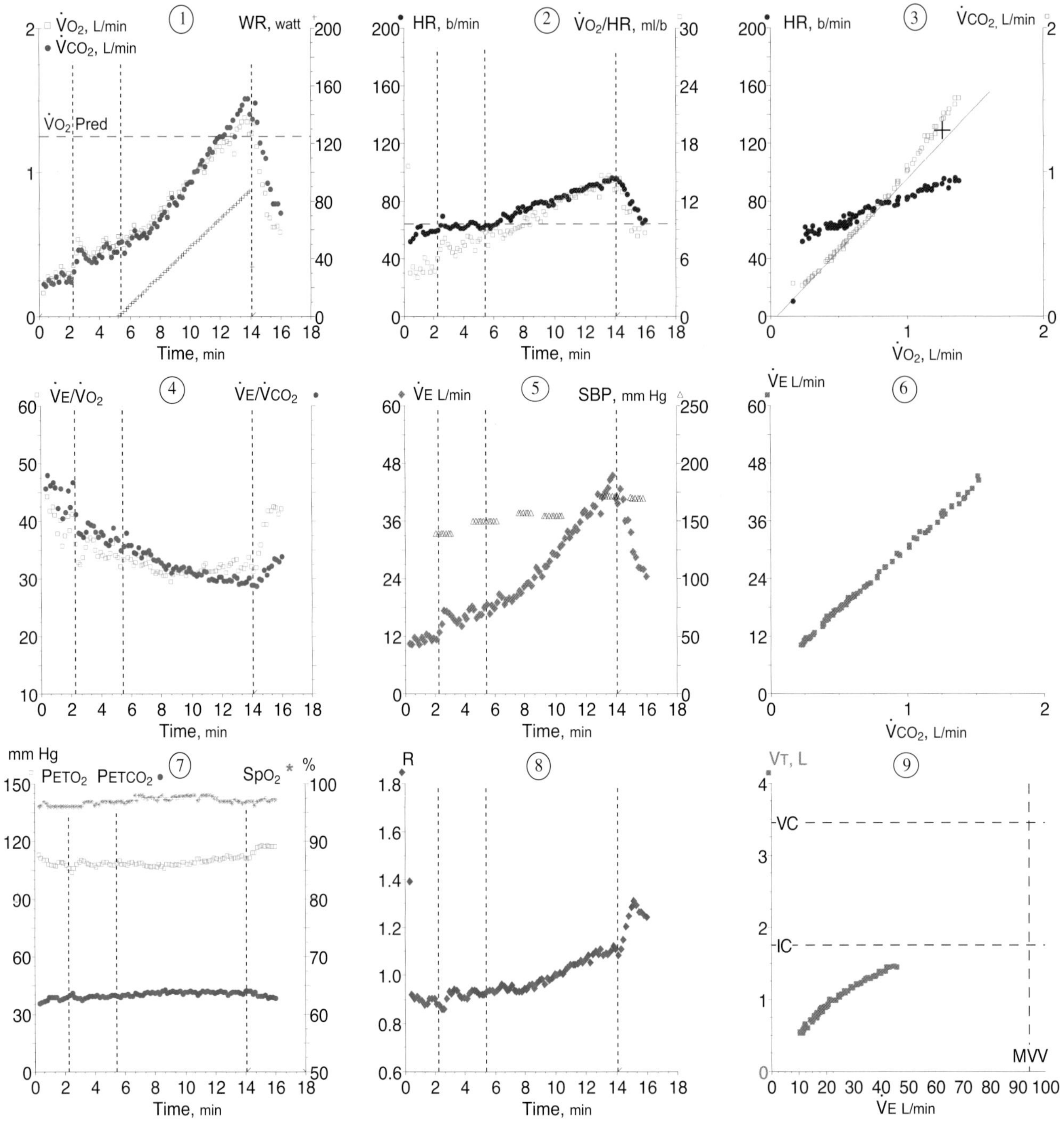

FIGURE 10.43.1. Vertical dashed lines in the panels in the left and middle columns indicate, from left to right, the beginning of unloaded cycling, start of increasing work rate (WR) at 10 W/min, and start of recovery. In **panel 1**, the increase in WR (right y-axis) is plotted with a scale of 100 W to 1 L of oxygen uptake ($\dot{V}O_2$) (left y-axis) such that WR is plotted parallel to a $\dot{V}O_2$ slope of 10 mL/min/W. Predicted peak $\dot{V}O_2$ is shown as a dashed horizontal line. In **panel 3**, carbon dioxide output ($\dot{V}CO_2$) (right y-axis) is plotted as a function of $\dot{V}O_2$ (x-axis) with identical scales so that the diagonal blue line has a slope of 1 (45°). The $\dot{V}CO_2$ increasing more steeply than $\dot{V}O_2$ defines carbon dioxide (CO_2) derived from bicarbonate buffer, as long as ventilatory equivalent for CO_2 ($\dot{V}E/\dot{V}CO_2$) (**panel 4**) is not increasing and end-tidal P_{CO_2} (P_{ETCO_2}) (**panel 7**) is not decreasing, simultaneously. The black + symbol in **panel 3** indicates predicted peak values of heart rate (HR) (left y-axis) and $\dot{V}O_2$ for this individual. Abbreviations: IC, inspiratory capacity; MVV, maximum voluntary ventilation; P_{ETO_2}, end-tidal P_{O_2}; R, respiratory exchange ratio; SBP, systolic blood pressure; Sp_{O_2}, oxygen saturation as measured by pulse oximetry; $\dot{V}E$, minute ventilation; $\dot{V}E/\dot{V}O_2$, ventilatory equivalent for oxygen; V_T, tidal volume.

TABLE 10.43.3 Air Breathing

Time (min)	Work rate (W)	BP (mm Hg)	HR (min^{-1})	f (min^{-1})	$\dot{V}E$ (L/min BTPS)	$\dot{V}CO_2$ (L/min STPD)	$\dot{V}O_2$ (L/min STPD)	$\frac{\dot{V}O_2}{HR}$ (mL/beat)	R	pH	HCO_3^- (mEq/L)	PO_2, mm Hg and SpO_2, % ET	SpO_2	(A − a)	PCO_2, mm Hg ET	a	(a − ET)	$\frac{\dot{V}E}{\dot{V}CO_2}$	$\frac{\dot{V}E}{\dot{V}O_2}$	$\frac{V_D}{V_T}$
0.5	Rest		30	19	10.3	0.21	0.23	7.7	0.92			112	96		36			49	45	
1.0	Rest		58	19	11.0	0.24	0.27	4.6	0.90			109	97		38			46	41	
1.5	Rest		59	20	11.6	0.27	0.31	5.2	0.88			107	96		39			43	38	
2.0	Rest	140/62	58	19	11.4	0.26	0.29	5.0	0.90			109	96		38			43	39	
2.5	Unloaded		61	21	13.0	0.32	0.36	6.0	0.87			106	96		40			41	36	
3.0	Unloaded		65	21	16.9	0.45	0.50	7.7	0.90			108	96		39			38	34	
3.5	Unloaded		63	21	15.3	0.39	0.41	6.6	0.94			110	97		38			40	37	
4.0	Unloaded		61	20	15.3	0.40	0.44	7.2	0.91			108	97		39			38	34	
4.5	Unloaded	150/60	64	20	17.1	0.47	0.51	8.0	0.92			108	97		39			36	34	
5.0	Unloaded		64	20	16.5	0.44	0.47	7.4	0.93			109	97		39			38	35	
5.5	3		62	20	17.7	0.50	0.54	8.6	0.93			108	97		40			36	33	
6.0	8		63	21	17.7	0.48	0.52	8.2	0.93			108	97		40			36	34	
6.5	13		66	21	19.9	0.57	0.60	9.2	0.95			109	97		40			35	33	
7.0	18		70	22	19.3	0.56	0.60	8.5	0.94			108	98		40			34	32	
7.5	23	157/64	70	21	19.8	0.58	0.61	8.8	0.94			108	98		41			34	32	
8.0	27		75	22	21.5	0.65	0.69	9.2	0.94			107	98		41			33	31	
8.5	33		75	23	22.9	0.71	0.75	10.0	0.95			107	98		42			32	31	
9.0	38	155/57	79	23	25.3	0.80	0.83	10.6	0.96			107	97		42			32	30	
9.5	43		79	24	25.8	0.81	0.83	10.4	0.98			108	98		42			32	31	
10.0	48		79	25	28.8	0.92	0.92	11.8	0.99			109	98		41			31	31	
10.5	53		83	25	30.3	0.99	0.98	11.9	1.01			109	98		42			31	31	
11.0	58		83	27	33.0	1.06	1.03	12.4	1.03			110	98		41			31	32	
11.5	63	154/56	88	26	34.2	1.15	1.10	12.5	1.05			110	98		42			30	31	
12.0	68		88	28	37.1	1.23	1.16	13.2	1.06			111	98		41			30	32	
12.5	73		91	28	37.8	1.28	1.19	13.1	1.07			111	97		42			30	32	
13.0	78	171/54	91	29	39.3	1.31	1.19	13.1	1.10			112	97		41			30	33	
13.5	83		93	29	42.1	1.45	1.33	14.4	1.09			111	97		42			29	32	
14.0	88		95	30	43.7	1.48	1.33	14.0	1.11			112	97		41			30	33	
14.5	Recovery		93	29	40.9	1.40	1.26	13.5	1.11			112	97		42			29	33	
15.0	Recovery	170/51	84	26	34.7	1.12	0.91	10.8	1.25			116	97		40			31	38	
15.5	Recovery		76	24	28.3	0.86	0.67	8.8	1.29			118	97		39			33	42	
16.0	Recovery		67	24	25.3	0.76	0.61	9.1	1.25			117	97		39			33	42	
16.5	Recovery		66	23	21.8	0.65	0.52	7.9	1.25			116	97		40			33	42	

Abbreviations: BP, blood pressure; BTPS, body temperature pressure saturated; f, frequency; HCO_3^-, bicarbonate; HR, heart rate; $P(A - a)O_2$, alveolar-arterial PO_2 difference; $P(a - ET)CO_2$, arterial-end-tidal PCO_2 difference; $PETCO_2$, end-tidal PCO_2; $PETO_2$, end-tidal PO_2; R, respiratory exchange ratio; SpO_2, oxygen saturation as measured by pulse oximetry; STPD, standard temperature pressure dry; $\dot{V}CO_2$, carbon dioxide output; V_D/V_T, physiological dead space-tidal volume ratio; $\dot{V}E$, minute ventilation; $\dot{V}E/\dot{V}CO_2$, ventilatory equivalent for carbon dioxide; $\dot{V}E/\dot{V}O_2$, ventilatory equivalent for oxygen; $\dot{V}O_2$, oxygen uptake.

INTERPRETATION

Comment

This case is presented as an example of maximal heart rate impairment in an older man with a long history of physical fitness. Although there was significant limitation of the chronotropic response to exercise, the finding of a high oxygen (O_2) pulse indicates that the patient had significant compensatory augmentation in stroke volume.

Analysis

Cardiovascular and metabolic: Oxygen uptake ($\dot{V}O_2$) increased appropriately relative to work rate and the peak value was above the average reference value. The rate of increase of heart rate relative to $\dot{V}O_2$ (panel 3) was shallow and the peak heart rate was below predicted. The end exercise O_2 pulse (panel 2) was well above predicted, consistent with high stroke volume. This is particularly notable because his mild anemia limited the peak $C(a - \bar{v})O_2$ value that could be attained.

Ventilation: The breathing reserve was normal. There was no evidence for respiratory compensation for metabolic acidosis (panel 6), but this is not a pathologic finding.

Gas exchange efficiency: Pulmonary gas exchange efficiency appeared normal with normal pulse oximetry and normal relationship between $\dot{V}E$ and $\dot{V}CO_2$.

Conclusion

Exercise capacity was normal and above the estimated average despite a limited peak heart rate response. The anaerobic threshold was a relatively high percentage of peak $\dot{V}O_2$, which is consistent with his age. The high O_2 pulse undoubtedly resulted from considerably increased exercise stroke volume, especially as this value would be constrained by the presence of anemia that limits the peak $C(a - \bar{v})O_2$. An augmented stroke volume is a normal response to impaired heart rate but requires that the ventricles be sufficiently compliant to accommodate increased diastolic filling and have intact inotropic function. This man's longstanding exercise history likely contributed to these characteristics. Despite the echocardiogram findings, none of the gas exchange abnormalities typical of pulmonary arterial hypertension or heart failure were evident on this test.

CASE 44

Active Man With Cardiac Conduction Defects

CLINICAL FINDINGS

A 76-year-old man had noted decreased exercise tolerance and dyspnea on exertion for 2 to 3 years. He had an active lifestyle that included swimming and fly fishing. Lately, on fishing trips at altitude, he became short of breath and could not keep pace with his companions. He swam each day for exercise, although had suspended his swimming for a time 2 years previously after rotator cuff surgery and since resuming had been unable to attain his prior work out distance of a mile due to shortness of breath. He was followed by his personal physicians with periodic cardiac imaging for a dilated aortic root without other structural abnormalities. He was aware that he had bradycardia and had been advised by his cardiologist that he might need a pacemaker, but there were no plans for the procedure. He had no history of light-headedness, syncope, orthopnea, or nocturnal dyspnea. His only medication was low-dose aspirin. Physical examination was notable for a slow cardiac rhythm with occasional irregularities, without murmur or gallop. Breath sounds were clear, and there was no peripheral edema. Resting electrocardiogram showed sinus bradycardia with a rate of 35 to 40 beats/min with first-degree atrioventricular block, occasional sinus pauses, and intraventricular conduction delay. Demographic and respiratory function data are shown in **Table 10.44.1**.

EXERCISE FINDINGS

The patient exercised on a cycle ergometer beginning with 3 minutes of unloaded pedaling at 60 rpm followed by continuous increase in work rate by 15 W/min until the test ended with symptoms of leg fatigue. On electrocardiogram, the heart rate remained relatively unchanged in the 40s up to a work rate of around 60 W at which point the rate began to accelerate and became more regular; the QRS complexes remained unchanged, but P waves were not discernible, suggesting a nonsinus rhythm. Heart rate at peak exercise was 94 beats/min. Exercise data are shown in **Tables 10.44.2** and **10.44.3** and in **Figures 10.44.1** and **10.44.2**.

TABLE 10.44.1 Selected Respiratory Function Data

Measurement	Predicted	Measured
Age (y)		76
Sex		Male
Height (cm)		175
Weight (kg)		92.7
VC (L)	4.0	4.88
IC (L)	3.18	4.46
ERV (L)	0.82	0.44
FEV_1 (L)	2.87	3.25
FEV_1/VC (%)	72	67
MVV (L/min)	142	165

Abbreviations: ERV, expiratory reserve volume; FEV_1, forced expiratory volume in 1 second; IC, inspiratory capacity; MVV, maximum voluntary ventilation; VC, vital capacity.

INTERPRETATION

Comment

This patient had an unusual combination of findings that included severe cardiac abnormalities and high exercise capacity. Because of the marked oscillations in the ventilation and gas exchange variables, quantifying many of the variables for this test was best accomplished from graphical displays rather than the tabular data.

Analysis

The scattered appearance of data from the first half of the exercise test resulted from an oscillatory breathing pattern, which was clearly evident when data were displayed as a rolling average during the test (see **Fig. 10.44.2**) but is less evident with the 10-second averaging used in **Figure 10.44.1**

TABLE 10.44.2 Selected Exercise Data

Measurement	Predicted	Measured
Peak $\dot{V}O_2$ (L/min)	1.83	2.35
Maximum heart rate (beats/min)	144	94
Heart rate reserve (beats/min)	0	50
Maximum O_2 pulse (mL/beat)	12.7	25
$\Delta\dot{V}O_2/\Delta WR$ (mL/min/W)	10.3	10.4
AT (L/min)	>0.87	~1.75
Blood pressure (mm Hg [rest, max])		132/70, 188/68
Maximum $\dot{V}E$ (L/min)		80
Breathing reserve (L/min)	>15	86
$\dot{V}E/\dot{V}CO_2$ @ *AT*	<34	35
$\dot{V}E$-$\dot{V}CO_2$ slope	<33	32.5
SpO_2 (% [rest, max ex])		96, 94

Abbreviations: *AT*, anaerobic threshold; $\Delta\dot{V}O_2/\Delta WR$, change in $\dot{V}O_2$/change in work rate; ex, exercise; O_2, oxygen; SpO_2, oxygen saturation as measured by pulse oximetry; $\dot{V}CO_2$, carbon dioxide output; $\dot{V}E$, minute ventilation; $\dot{V}E/\dot{V}CO_2$, ventilatory equivalent for carbon dioxide; $\dot{V}O_2$, oxygen uptake.

TABLE 10.44.3 Air Breathing

Time (min)	Work rate (W)	BP (mm Hg)	HR (min^{-1})	f (min^{-1})	$\dot{V}_E$ (L/min BTPS)	$\dot{V}_{CO_2}$ (L/min STPD)	$\dot{V}_{O_2}$ (L/min STPD)	$\frac{\dot{V}_{O_2}}{HR}$ (mL/beat)	R	pH	HCO_3^- (mEq/L)	P_{O_2}, mm Hg and Sp_{O_2}, %			P_{CO_2}, mm Hg			$\frac{\dot{V}_E}{\dot{V}_{CO_2}}$	$\frac{\dot{V}_E}{\dot{V}_{O_2}}$	$\frac{V_D}{V_T}$
												ET	Sp_{O_2}	(A − a)	ET	a	(a − ET)			
0.5	Rest		22	13	10.6	0.24	0.31	14.3	0.78			114	95		29			44	34	
1.0	Rest		38	16	16.3	0.38	0.52	13.7	0.73			112	97		29			43	31	
1.5	Rest		40	12	12.2	0.28	0.35	8.7	0.79			111	96		29			44	35	
2.0	Rest	132/70	40	15	18.4	0.43	0.61	15.3	0.71			113	96		28			43	30	
2.5	Unloaded		44	13	11.2	0.26	0.34	7.8	0.77			110	94		30			43	33	
3.0	Unloaded		46	16	26.6	0.58	0.74	16.2	0.78			117	96		26			46	36	
3.5	Unloaded		53	20	25.4	0.62	0.85	16.2	0.73			112	93		28			41	30	
4.0	Unloaded		49	16	18.8	0.46	0.65	13.3	0.70			109	96		30			41	29	
4.5	Unloaded		46	20	29.6	0.60	0.67	14.5	0.90			122	96		25			49	44	
5.0	Unloaded	157/67	44	14	21.6	0.52	0.69	15.7	0.75			111	96		29			42	31	
5.5	2		43	17	23.3	0.56	0.73	17.1	0.77			112	95		30			42	32	
6.0	9		50	15	17.9	0.40	0.44	8.9	0.91			114	96		30			45	40	
6.5	16		46	17	36.5	0.78	0.94	20.4	0.83			119	97		25			47	39	
7.0	25		46	13	22.3	0.58	0.76	16.7	0.76			109	95		30			39	29	
7.5	32	162/65	46	19	23.5	0.56	0.66	14.6	0.84			114	95		29			42	35	
8.0	39		46	19	32.5	0.80	1.05	22.8	0.76			112	96		30			40	31	
8.5	47		48	21	25.6	0.69	0.91	18.8	0.76			111	95		31			37	28	
9.0	54		57	18	32.8	0.87	1.09	19.2	0.80			114	96		30			38	30	
9.5	61	147/64	51	20	32.2	0.84	1.04	20.6	0.81			114	96		30			38	31	
10.0	69		56	21	36.8	1.00	1.25	22.3	0.80			113	96		30			37	29	
10.5	77		56	19	38.7	1.05	1.23	22.1	0.85			115	95		30			37	31	
11.0	84		58	21	45.1	1.15	1.29	22.0	0.90			118	95		28			39	35	
11.5	91	156/62	67	20	44.0	1.22	1.41	21.0	0.87			115	96		30			36	31	
12.0	99		72	23	52.5	1.40	1.56	21.7	0.90			117	95		29			37	34	
12.5	106		74	19	47.3	1.34	1.54	20.8	0.87			113	96		32			35	31	
13.0	114		77	22	54.3	1.52	1.68	21.8	0.90			116	96		30			36	32	
13.5	122		82	25	58.4	1.66	1.90	23.0	0.88			113	96		32			35	31	
14.0	129		79	24	64.8	1.81	1.91	24.1	0.95			117	94		31			36	34	
14.5	137	175/66	83	25	66.1	1.89	2.02	24.3	0.93			116	94		31			35	33	
15.0	144		83	26	69.9	1.95	2.04	24.6	0.96			118	94		30			36	34	
15.5	152		85	25	69.9	2.00	2.16	25.5	0.93			116	93		32			35	32	
16.0	159		90	28	73.0	2.12	2.20	24.6	0.96			116	94		32			34	33	
16.5	167	188/68	91	28	81.8	2.31	2.35	25.9	0.98			118	94		31			35	35	
17.0	174		94	27	79.5	2.29	2.30	24.4	1.00			118	94		31			35	35	
17.5	Recovery		97	27	78.8	2.22	2.20	22.7	1.00			118	93		32			36	36	
18.0	Recovery	190/68	98	27	79.3	2.00	1.63	16.7	1.23			125	93		27			40	49	
18.5	Recovery		87	25	66.1	1.52	1.11	12.8	1.37			128	94		26			43	59	
19.0	Recovery		81	24	51.6	1.16	0.88	10.9	1.31			128	95		25			45	58	

Abbreviations: BP, blood pressure; BTPS, body temperature pressure saturated; f, frequency; HCO_3^-, bicarbonate; HR, heart rate; $P(A-a)O_2$, alveolar-arterial P_{O_2} difference; $P(a-ET)CO_2$, arterial-end-tidal P_{CO_2} difference; P_{ETCO_2}, end-tidal P_{CO_2}; P_{ETO_2}, end-tidal P_{O_2}; R, respiratory exchange ratio; Sp_{O_2}, oxygen saturation as measured by pulse oximetry; STPD, standard temperature pressure dry; $\dot{V}_{CO_2}$, carbon dioxide output; V_D/V_T, physiological dead space-tidal volume ratio; $\dot{V}_E$, minute ventilation; $\dot{V}_E/\dot{V}_{CO_2}$, ventilatory equivalent for carbon dioxide; $\dot{V}_E/\dot{V}_{O_2}$, ventilatory equivalent for oxygen; $\dot{V}_{O_2}$, oxygen uptake.

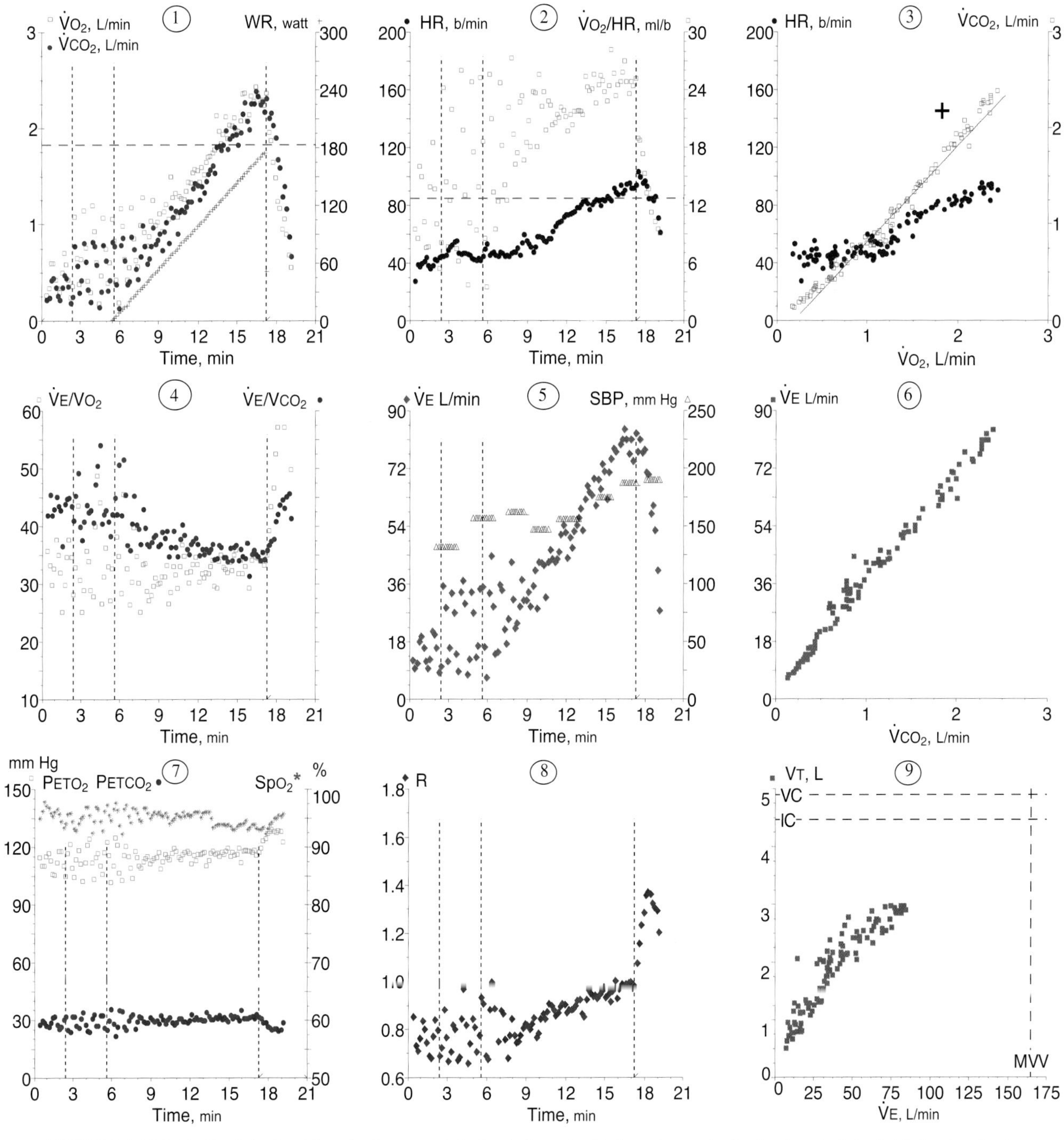

FIGURE 10.44.1. Vertical dashed lines in the panels in the left and middle columns indicate, from left to right, the beginning of unloaded cycling, start of increasing work rate (WR) at 15 W/min, and start of recovery. In **panel 1**, the increase in WR (right y-axis) is plotted with a scale of 100 W to 1 L of oxygen uptake ($\dot{V}O_2$) (left y-axis) such that WR is plotted parallel to a $\dot{V}O_2$ slope of 10 mL/min/W. Predicted peak $\dot{V}O_2$ is shown as a dashed horizontal line. In **panel 3**, carbon dioxide output ($\dot{V}CO_2$) (right y-axis) is plotted as a function of $\dot{V}O_2$ (x-axis) with identical scales so that the diagonal blue line has a slope of 1 (45°). The $\dot{V}CO_2$ increasing more steeply than $\dot{V}O_2$ defines carbon dioxide CO_2 derived from bicarbonate buffer, as long as ventilatory equivalent for CO_2 ($\dot{V}E/\dot{V}CO_2$) (**panel 4**) is not increasing and end-tidal P_{CO_2} (P_{ETCO_2}) (**panel 7**) is not decreasing, simultaneously. The black + symbol in **panel 3** indicates predicted peak values of heart rate (HR) (left y-axis) and $\dot{V}O_2$ for this individual. Abbreviations: IC, inspiratory capacity; MVV, maximum voluntary ventilation; P_{ETO_2}, end-tidal P_{O_2}; R, respiratory exchange ratio; SBP, systolic blood pressure; Sp_{O_2}, oxygen saturation as measured by pulse oximetry; VC, vital capacity; $\dot{V}E$, minute ventilation; $\dot{V}E/\dot{V}O_2$, ventilatory equivalent for oxygen; V_T, tidal volume.

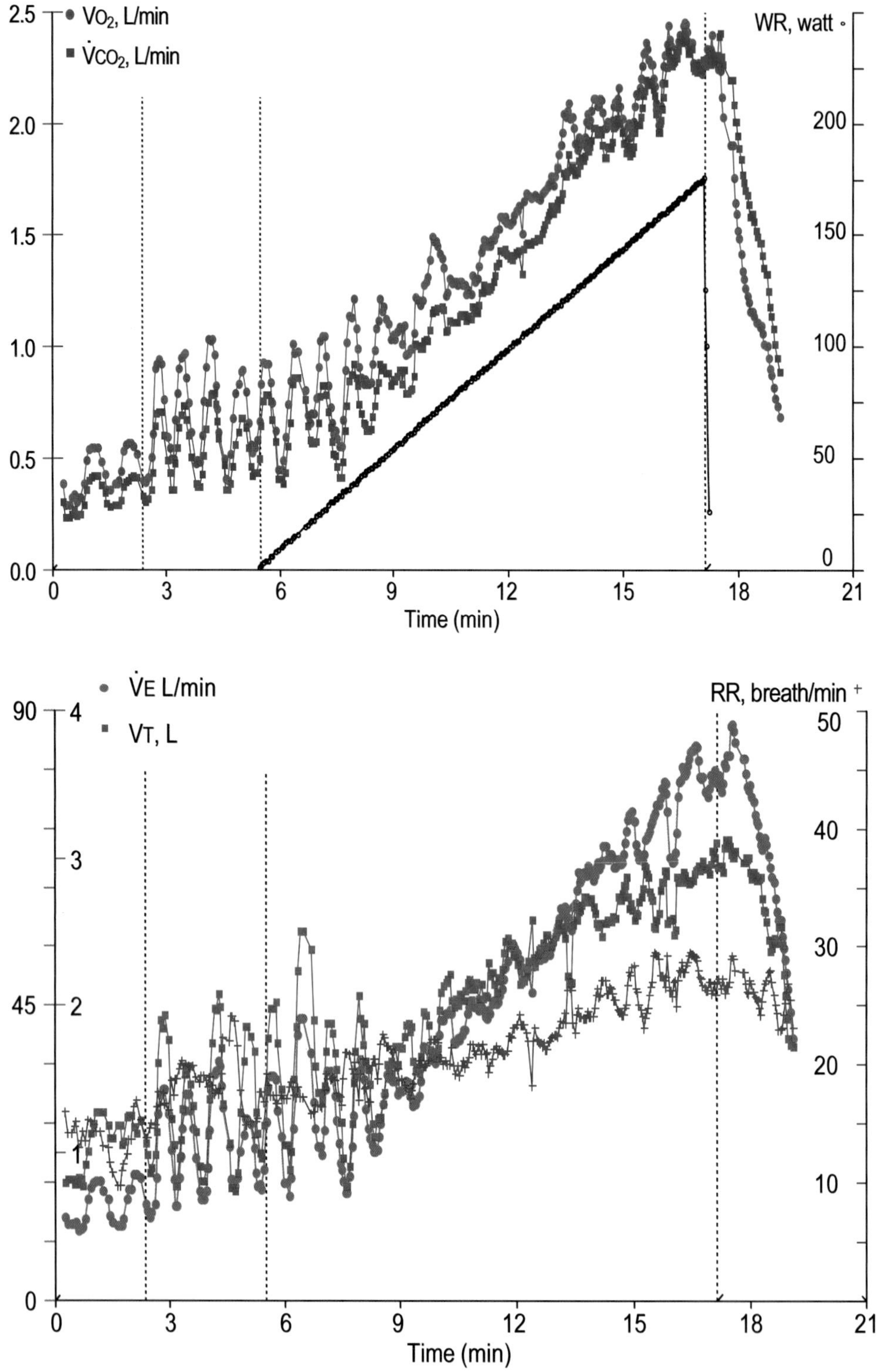

FIGURE 10.44.2. Exercise gas exchange and ventilation variables are displayed as rolling, or moving, averages in which each plotted point represents the average of a set of consecutive breathes, with the data set shifted by one breath for each point. In this case, the plotted points are averages of values for 5 of each set of 7 consecutive breathes, the highest and lowest value in each set being discarded. This dampens extreme variations in the measures but emphasizes the temporal oscillatory trend. The top panel shows oxygen uptake ($\dot{V}O_2$) and carbon dioxide output ($\dot{V}CO_2$) and the bottom panel minute ventilation ($\dot{V}E$), tidal volume (VT), and breathing frequency (RR), all plotted as a function of time over the course of the incremental test. Vertical dashed lines indicate the start of unloaded cycling, the start of incremental work and the start of recovery. Abbreviations: RR, respiratory frequency; WR, work rate.

Cardiovascular and metabolic responses: The peak oxygen uptake ($\dot{V}O_2$) was above predicted, and anaerobic threshold (*AT*) was a high percentage of the peak $\dot{V}O_2$. The heart rate response was highly attenuated, especially during the early minutes of the test. As noted earlier, it appeared that the sinus rate did not increase appreciably and the increase in heart rate resulted from an alternative pacemaker site. The O_2 pulse was higher than predicted, although individual calculated values were distorted by the oscillations in $\dot{V}O_2$; averaging over longer periods of time showed that peak O_2 pulse was approximately double the predicted value. This implies a much higher than average exercise stroke volume. The *AT* was also difficult to identify precisely but, based on the V-slope graph in panel 3 of **Figure 10.44.1**, appeared to be around 1.75 L/min. The ventilatory equivalents and end-tidal gas tensions (panels 4 and 7) were not particularly helpful in confirming this but do not suggest a different value. The very slow rise of the R (panel 8) to a value of only around 1.0 at peak exercise suggests that exercise ended with symptoms prior to his getting very far into the high-intensity (ie, above *AT*) range.

Ventilatory responses: There was a large breathing reserve and no appearance of respiratory compensation for metabolic acidosis, consistent with exercise ending not long after the *AT*.

Gas exchange efficiency: The $\dot{V}E/\dot{V}CO_2$ values decline throughout the test, but the lowest value remained near the upper limit of normal and the slope of $\dot{V}E/\dot{V}CO_2$ is also near the upper limit of normal. This suggests some increase in effective V_D/V_T. Oxygenation remained normal.

Conclusion

The primary findings on cardiopulmonary exercise testing were related to a highly attenuated heart rate response. There were conduction system defects, which had likely been slowly progressive and were manifest symptomatically as a reduction in his normally excellent exercise tolerance, rather than light-headedness or syncope. Peak exercise $\dot{V}O_2$, the *AT*, and O_2 pulse were well above the reference values, undoubtedly reflecting his exercise conditioning and the ability of his heart to compensate for reduced rate with an increase in stroke volume. The oscillatory breathing pattern and elevated ventilatory equivalents are characteristic of heart failure, and it is not unreasonable to consider that his rate impairment constituted a form of heart failure despite evidence for excellent systolic and diastolic ventricular function. He was referred to his cardiologist for follow up.

CASE 45

Early Onset of Exercise Lactic Acidosis: Differentiating Circulatory From Muscular Impairment

CLINICAL FINDINGS

This 29-year-old male executive presented with about a 1-year history of exercise intolerance due to fatigue, dyspnea, and light-headedness associated with exertion. He had a history of incompletely reversible asthma, but evaluation by his pulmonologist, allergist, and cardiologist, including an unremarkable echocardiogram, failed to identify the cause of his symptoms. He was referred for cardiopulmonary exercise testing to better define the pathophysiology of his symptoms.

All together, three tests were performed by this patient. His initial exercise test was performed without blood sampling. This showed that peak $\dot{V}O_2$, anaerobic threshold (*AT*), $\Delta\dot{V}O_2/\Delta WR$, and O_2 pulse were all reduced, but the basis for this was unclear. A second test was done with arterial blood gas sampling. This showed similar results to the noninvasive test and confirmed that the noninvasively determined *AT* represented early onset of lactic acidosis. Although this test also demonstrated abnormal V_D/V_T, consistent with his known airway disease, he did not appear clearly ventilatory limited, and this seemed unlikely to account for the degree of reduction in the peak $\dot{V}O_2$ and *AT*. Also, there were no ischemic electrocardiogram (ECG) changes or arrhythmia to account for his impairment. He was thus suspected to have either a circulatory problem with a reduced stroke volume or, less likely, a skeletal muscle myopathy in which the muscles could not consume O_2 normally.

To distinguish between a cardiovascular disorder and a muscle bioenergetic problem, a third exercise test was performed. On this occasion, testing was conducted with brachial arterial, pulmonary arterial, and femoral venous catheters (the latter directed caudally) in place. Cardiac output and stroke volume were determined by the direct Fick method using arterial and central venous O_2 measurements to assess the adequacy of O_2 delivery, and critical capillary P_{O_2} was determined from the femoral venous O_2 saturation, content, and P_{O_2} to assess the ability of the muscles to extract and use O_2. In addition, direct arterial blood pressure was recorded. This test is presented in detail here.

EXERCISE FINDINGS

After catheter placement, the patient performed exercise on a cycle ergometer while breathing through a mouthpiece, with nose occluded, for breath-by-breath measurements of gas exchange. Heart rate and rhythm were continuously monitored. The protocol consisted of 3 minutes of rest and 3 minutes of unloaded pedaling at 60 rpm, followed by a progressive increase in work rate of 20 W/min until the patient became too symptomatic to continue. Blood was sampled from the three sites for blood gases, pH, and lactate at rest, at the end of 3 minutes of unloaded cycling, periodically during the incremental exercise period, and at 6 minutes of recovery. Twelve-lead ECG recordings were obtained during rest, exercise, and recovery. The patient performed the exercise test with good effort. His resting and exercise ECGs were normal, and there was no cardiac ectopy.

The patient had a near-syncopal event during preexercise spirometry and again in the immediate recovery period. During these events, he complained of dizziness and was diaphoretic. Similar symptoms had occurred previously after exercise, including the two prior exercise tests performed in the laboratory. On this occasion, his blood pressure was noted to drop to 82/64 mm Hg soon after exercise ended, whereas his pulse remained around 90 beats/min. Lying flat with his legs raised helped him recover from these episodes. The typical cardiac slowing of a vasovagal event was not observed.

INTERPRETATION

Comments

Respiratory function tests showed moderate airflow obstruction with a normal D_{LCO} (**Table 10.45.1**).

Analysis

Peak $\dot{V}O_2$ was low, indicating abnormal maximum exercise. The *AT* was very low (<1 L/min), suggesting a problem (**Tables 10.45.2** and **10.45.3** and **Figure 10.45.1**) with O_2 delivery or, as noted earlier, a problem of O_2 uptake by the muscles. Notably, he had a very steep heart rate–$\dot{V}O_2$ response to exercise, low slope of $\Delta\dot{V}O_2/\Delta WR$, and low and nonchanging O_2 pulse when nearing peak $\dot{V}O_2$. He had normal breathing reserve despite a mildly elevated but abnormal $\dot{V}E/\dot{V}CO_2$ at its lowest point. These findings support either heart disease or myopathy, but as noted, these were found on the two earlier tests.

If using the flowcharts (Chapter 9), the low peak $\dot{V}O_2$ and *AT* leads to Flowchart 4, where the first branch point (Branch Point 4.1) is the normal breathing reserve. At the next branch point (Branch Point 4.3), the $\dot{V}E/\dot{V}CO_2$ is mildly but abnormally high, leading to consideration of heart disease or pulmonary vascular disease. There is little or no support

TABLE 10.45.1 Selected Respiratory Function Data

Measurement	Predicted	Measured
Age (y)		29
Sex		Male
Height (cm)		180
Weight (kg)	81	86
Hematocrit (%)		47
VC (L)	4.95	4.29
IC (L)	3.30	2.94
FEV_1 (L)	4.13	2.74
FEV_1/VC (%)	83	64
MVV (L/min)	163	110
D_{LCO} (mL/mm Hg/min)[a]	34.6	31.6

Abbreviations: D_{LCO}, diffusing capacity of the lung for carbon monoxide; FEV_1, forced expiratory volume in 1 second; IC, inspiratory capacity; MVV, maximum voluntary ventilation; VC, vital capacity.

[a]Measured on a separate occasion.

TABLE 10.45.2 Selected Exercise Data

Measurement	Predicted	Measured
Peak $\dot{V}O_2$ (L/min)	3.28	1.69
Maximum heart rate (beats/min)	192	178
Maximum O_2 pulse (mL/beat)	17.2	9.8
$\Delta\dot{V}O_2/\Delta WR$ (mL/min/W)	10.3	7.9
AT (L/min)	<1.41	0.90
Blood pressure (mm Hg [rest, max])		155/85, 160/90
Maximum $\dot{V}_E$ (L/min)		90
Exercise breathing reserve (L/min)	>15	20
$\dot{V}_E/\dot{V}CO_2$ @ *AT* or lowest	23.6	32.6
PaO_2 (mm Hg [rest, max ex])		86, 105
$P(A - a)O_2$ (mm Hg [rest, max ex])		11, 17
$PaCO_2$ (mm Hg [rest, max ex])		41, 38
$P(a - ET)CO_2$ (mm Hg [rest, max ex])		4, 7
V_D/V_T (rest, sub max, max ex)		0.47, 0.31, 0.41
HCO_3^- (mEq/L [rest, recov])		26, 17
Lactate (mEq/L [recov])		13.7

Abbreviations: *AT*, anaerobic threshold; $\Delta\dot{V}O_2/\Delta WR$, change in $\dot{V}O_2$/change in work rate; ex, exercise; HCO_3^-, bicarbonate; O_2, oxygen; $P(A - a)O_2$, alveolar-arterial PO_2 difference; $P(a - ET)CO_2$, arterial–end-tidal PCO_2 difference; recov, recovery; V_D/V_T, physiological dead space–tidal volume ratio; $\dot{V}_E$, minute ventilation; $\dot{V}_E/\dot{V}CO_2$, ventilatory equivalent for carbon dioxide; $\dot{V}O_2$, oxygen uptake.

for the latter, so heart disease is more likely. If, however, the $\dot{V}_E/\dot{V}CO_2$ is considered to be normal, then subsequent branch points lead to an O_2 flow problem of nonpulmonary origin such as anemia (not present), peripheral arterial disease, or heart failure. The last is more strongly supported.

However, the invasive measurements with hemodynamics are important in this case (**Table 10.45.4**). Cardiac output, calculated by the Fick method, increased at the expected rate relative to the increase in $\dot{V}O_2$ during exercise (normally 5-6 L/min of cardiac output for each L/min increase in $\dot{V}O_2$), but the absolute value was lower than expected at rest and at all levels of $\dot{V}O_2$, with a peak cardiac output of only 10 L/min. Accordingly, the calculated stroke volume was abnormally low, starting at 44 mL at rest and increasing to only about 65 mL/beat during exercise. These findings identified inadequate blood flow as the basis for the low peak $\dot{V}O_2$ and steep heart rate–$\dot{V}O_2$ relationship, whereas O_2 extraction was normal both across the leg (normal critical capillary PO_2) and across the entire systemic circulation. The maximum O_2 extraction (75%-80%) was reached at a lower $\dot{V}O_2$ than expected due to the reduced cardiac output.

The key finding in this case was thus the low stroke volume. The basis for this was not evident from the prior echocardiogram, which excluded systolic dysfunction or structural heart disease. Although diastolic dysfunction could account for the exercise response, he did not have recognized risk factors for this condition, nor any echocardiographic findings in support of it. A restrictive cardiomyopathy or pericardial process would also be compatible with the exercise responses but were not supported by data from the right heart catheterization (data not shown). Normal extraction of O_2 across the leg excluded a skeletal muscle myopathy with impaired O_2 use as the cause of the limited peak $\dot{V}O_2$ and O_2 pulse. Had exercise capacity been limited by a defect in oxidative function of the skeletal muscle, O_2 extraction would have been less than normal and cardiac output would probably have been higher, rather than lower, than normal for a given $\dot{V}O_2$. Autonomic dysfunction with impaired distribution of blood flow to the exercising muscles, on the other hand, would be associated with normal O_2 extraction across the leg but low extraction across the circulation as a whole, so this too was excluded by the data. Dynamic hyperinflation of the lungs resulting from obstructive airways disease can limit venous return and, therefore, cardiac stroke volume due to development of high intrathoracic pressures. This condition should be considered in light of the patient's obstructive lung disease but was thought unlikely to account for the low cardiac output at rest and early stages of exercise. It was speculated that the findings may reflect low cardiac preload, limiting diastolic filling of the heart, and, consequently, reduced cardiac output. This could result from an abnormally low blood volume and be exacerbated with exercise by peripheral vascular dilatation due to high-grade lactic acidosis. The low venous return would predispose to hypotension after exercise with a tachycardia, in contrast to the bradycardia that would characterize a vasovagal event. A condition of low venous

TABLE 10.45.3 Air Breathing

												P_{O_2}, mm Hg			P_{CO_2}, mm Hg					
Time (min)	Work rate (W)	BP (mm Hg)	HR (min^{-1})	f (min^{-1})	$\dot{V}_E$ (L/min BTPS)	$\dot{V}CO_2$ (L/min STPD)	$\dot{V}O_2$ (L/min STPD)	$\frac{\dot{V}O_2}{HR}$ (mL/beat)	R	pH	HCO_3^- (mEq/L)	ET	a	(A − a)	ET	a	(a − ET)	$\frac{\dot{V}_E}{\dot{V}CO_2}$	$\frac{\dot{V}_E}{\dot{V}O_2}$	$\frac{V_D}{V_T}$
0.5	Rest		74	17	12.0	0.26	0.34	4.6	0.76			105			36			39	30	
1.0	Rest		72	15	9.7	0.20	0.27	3.8	0.74			104			37			41	30	
1.5	Rest		70	16	9.2	0.16	0.21	3.0	0.76			106			37			47	36	
2.0	Rest		71	15	9.0	0.17	0.22	3.1	0.77			105			37			44	34	
2.5	Rest	155/85	69	15	8.9	0.15	0.19	2.8	0.79	7.40	25	107	86	14	37	41	4	49	39	0.47
3.0	Rest		71	16	10.9	0.21	0.26	3.7	0.81			107			37			44	35	
3.5	Unloaded		82	16	13.3	0.31	0.37	4.5	0.84			106			37			37	31	
4.0	Unloaded		85	19	16.7	0.40	0.49	5.8	0.82			107			37			37	30	
4.5	Unloaded		87	17	17.1	0.42	0.51	5.9	0.82			106			37			36	30	
5.0	Unloaded		88	19	17.8	0.44	0.54	6.1	0.81			105			37			36	29	
5.5	Unloaded		85	20	18.2	0.43	0.52	6.1	0.83			108			36			37	31	
6.0	Unloaded	145/85	83	22	19.4	0.45	0.55	6.6	0.82	7.41	25	107	90	13	36	40	4	38	31	0.38
6.5	4		84	20	18.1	0.43	0.52	6.2	0.83			107			37			37	31	
7.0	14		87	23	21.4	0.52	0.63	7.2	0.83			108			36			37	30	
7.5	24		82	21	20.3	0.48	0.58	7.1	0.83			106			37			38	31	
8.0	34		89	21	23.1	0.59	0.69	7.8	0.86			107			37			35	30	
8.5	44	155/85	98	23	25.0	0.66	0.75	7.7	0.88	7.40	24	108	92	14	37	40	3	34	30	0.33
9.0	54		99	22	26.8	0.77	0.84	8.5	0.92			107			39			32	29	
9.5	64		103	27	30.5	0.84	0.86	8.3	0.98			110			38			33	32	
10.0	79		117	26	34.4	1.02	0.96	8.2	1.06			109			40			31	33	
10.5	85	175/90	124	28	39.2	1.14	1.05	8.5	1.09	7.38	24	111	95	17	39	41	2	32	35	0.31
11.0	94		130	30	46.2	1.30	1.13	8.7	1.15			115			37			33	38	
11.5	104		136	31	49.7	1.39	1.21	8.9	1.15			115			37			33	38	
12.0	114		144	28	51.7	1.49	1.31	9.1	1.14			114			38			33	37	
12.5	124	160/90	152	30	57.5	1.61	1.38	9.1	1.17	7.39	23	116	102	14	37	38	1	34	39	0.31
13.0	134		160	28	58.7	1.74	1.50	9.4	1.16			115			37			32	37	
13.5	144		166	31	64.7	1.87	1.62	9.8	1.15			115			37			33	38	
14.0	154		171	36	74.1	2.02	1.67	9.8	1.21			118			35			35	42	
14.5	164		178	48	89.3	2.11	1.69	9.5	1.25	7.35	21	123	106	12	31	38	7	40	50	0.41
15.0	152		178	54	90.2	2.08	1.64	9.2	1.27			124			31			41	52	
15.5	Recovery		164	37	69.2	1.53	1.23	7.5	1.24	7.32	17	124	105	16	30	34	4	43	53	0.38
16.0	Recovery		136	36	56.1	1.15	0.90	6.6	1.28			126			28			45	58	

Abbreviations: BP, blood pressure; BTPS, body temperature pressure saturated; f, frequency; HCO_3^-, bicarbonate; HR, heart rate; $P(A-a)O_2$, alveolar-arterial P_{O_2} difference; $P(a-ET)CO_2$, arterial-end-tidal P_{CO_2} difference; P_{ETCO_2}, end-tidal P_{CO_2}; P_{ETO_2}, end-tidal P_{O_2}; R, respiratory exchange ratio; STPD, standard temperature pressure dry; $\dot{V}CO_2$, carbon dioxide output; V_D/V_T, physiological dead space-tidal volume ratio; $\dot{V}_E$, minute ventilation; $\dot{V}_E/\dot{V}CO_2$, ventilatory equivalent for carbon dioxide; $\dot{V}_E/\dot{V}O_2$, ventilatory equivalent for oxygen; $\dot{V}O_2$, oxygen uptake.

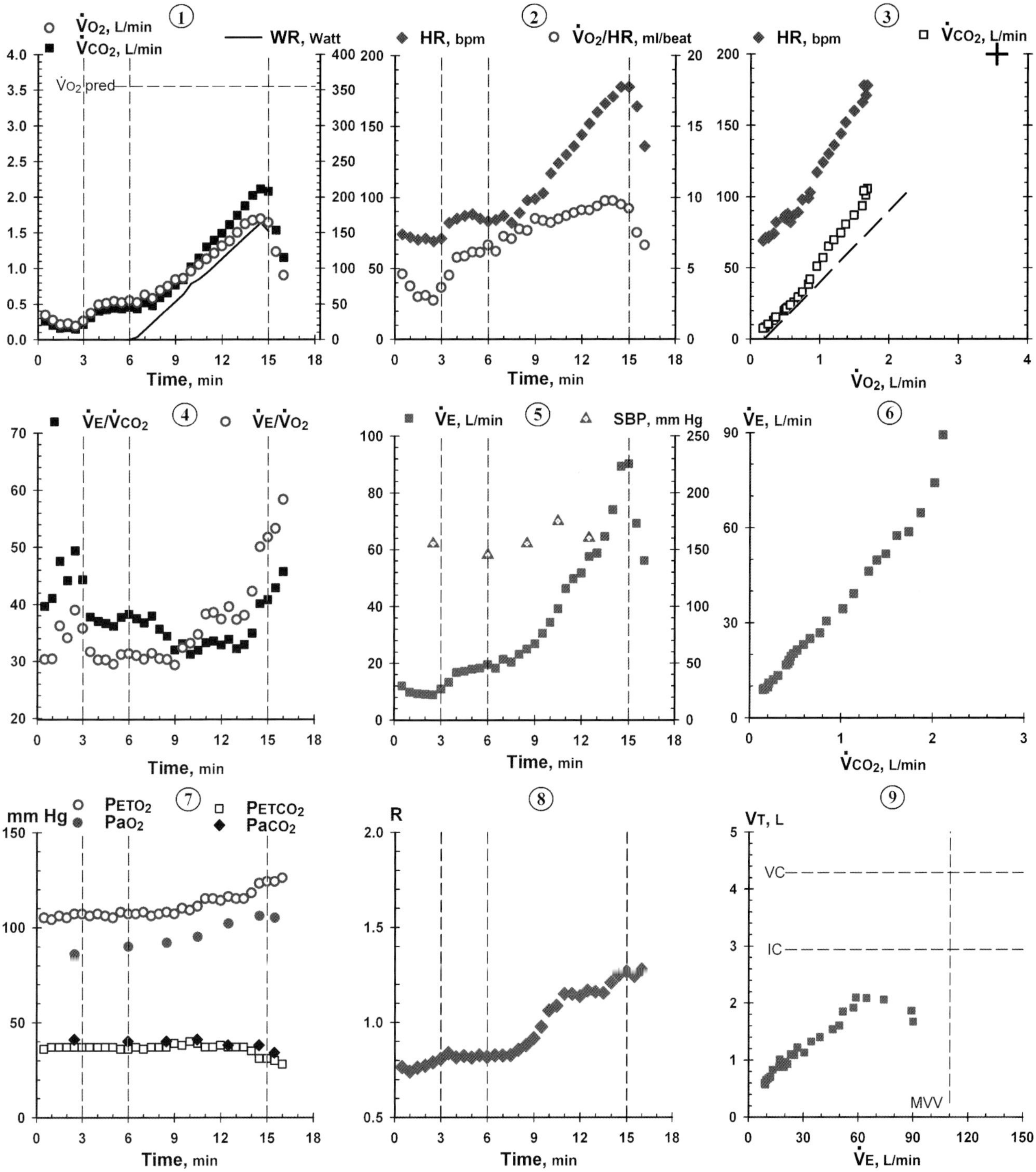

FIGURE 10.45.1. Vertical dashed lines in the panels in the left and middle columns indicate, from left to right, the beginning of unloaded cycling, start of increasing work rate (WR) at 20 W/min, and start of recovery. In **panel 1**, the increase in WR (right y-axis) is plotted with a scale of 100 W to 1 L of oxygen uptake ($\dot{V}O_2$) (left y-axis) such that WR is plotted parallel to a $\dot{V}O_2$ slope of 10 mL/min/W. In **panel 3**, carbon dioxide output ($\dot{V}CO_2$) (right y-axis) is plotted as a function of $\dot{V}O_2$ (x-axis) with identical scales so that the diagonal dashed line has a slope of 1 (45°). The $\dot{V}CO_2$ increasing more steeply than $\dot{V}O_2$ defines carbon dioxide (CO_2) derived from bicarbonate buffer, as long as ventilatory equivalent for CO_2 ($\dot{V}E/\dot{V}CO_2$) (**panel 4**) is not increasing and end-tidal PCO_2 ($PETCO_2$) (**panel 7**) is not decreasing, simultaneously. The black + symbol in **panel 3** indicates predicted peak values of heart rate (HR) (left y-axis) and $\dot{V}O_2$ for this individual. Abbreviations: IC, inspiratory capacity; MVV, maximum voluntary ventilation; $PETO_2$, end-tidal PO_2; R, respiratory exchange ratio; SBP, systolic blood pressure; VC, vital capacity; $\dot{V}E$, minute ventilation; $\dot{V}E/\dot{V}O_2$, ventilatory equivalent for oxygen; V_T, tidal volume.

TABLE 10.45.4 Hemodynamic Responses to Exercise

			Systemic artery			Pulmonary artery			Femoral vein					
Status	$\dot{V}O_2$ (mL/min)	Heart rate (beats/min)	O_2 cont (mL/100 mL)	PO_2 (mm Hg)	O_2 sat (%)	O_2 cont (mL/100 mL)	PO_2 (mm Hg)	O_2 sat (%)	O_2 cont (mL/100 mL)	PO_2 (mm Hg)	O_2 sat (%)	$C(a-\bar{v})O_2$ (mL/100 mL)	S.V. (mL)	C.O. (L/min)
Rest	250	71	20.0	86	97	12.1	33	60	6.0	20	32	7.9	44	3.1
0 load	520	83	21.0	90	97	8.7	26	47	5.0	18	25	12.3	51	4.2
44 W	720	98	21.0	92	97	8.6	26	44	4.9	18	25	12.4	59	5.8
85 W	1000	124	21.0	95	97	8.2	25	39	5.8	21	29	12.8	63	7.8
124 W	1340	152	21.5	102	97	7.9	25	37	7.4	26	35	13.6	65	9.8
164 W	1680	176	22.0	106	97	6.1	23	29	6.7	25	31	15.9	60	10
(Max ex)	1640	164	22.0	105	97	4.8	20	22	5.1	23	24	17.2	58	9.5
6 min rec			21.0	99	97	14.5	45	69	17.0	55	80	6.5		

Abbreviations: $C(a-\bar{v})O_2$, arterial-mixed venous O_2 content difference; C.O., cardiac output; ex, exercise; O_2 cont, O_2 content; O_2 sat, O_2 saturation; rec, recovery; S.V., stroke volume; $\dot{V}O_2$, oxygen uptake.

return could account for the prominent symptom of syncope or near-syncope with exercise.

Conclusion

This was a very challenging case. It is presented here as an illustration of one of the relatively uncommon instances in which measurement of cardiac output is critical for distinguishing between circulatory problems versus muscle disease as the cause of abnormalities in exercise $\dot{V}O_2$. In metabolic myopathy with impaired O_2 use by the muscle, the relationship of cardiac output to $\dot{V}O_2$ is higher than normal and O_2 extraction is low. Thus, the ability to confirm normal O_2 extraction across the exercising muscles was a key finding excluding a myopathic condition.

CASE 46

Early Onset of Exercise Lactic Acidosis Suggesting Circulatory Impairment

CLINICAL FINDINGS

This 26-year-old man was referred for exercise testing after approximately 6 years of progressive exercise intolerance. He was active in competitive sports through high school and continued with recreational sports in college but at some point noted that he was becoming unable to keep up with his peers. This progressed to feeling fatigued, light-headed, near syncopal, and sometimes nauseated during or after vigorous exercise. He progressively scaled back his exercise activities to avoid these symptoms. At the time of referral, he had already undergone a number of diagnostic evaluations including tilt table test and Holter monitoring of his cardiac rhythm, which were normal, and an echocardiogram with normal findings except for mild mitral prolapse without mitral regurgitation. A cardiopulmonary exercise test by his referring physician had been interpreted as showing a borderline low anaerobic threshold (*AT*) but normal peak oxygen uptake ($\dot{V}O_2$) and did not reproduce his symptoms. A muscle biopsy was reported to show normal histology and normal concentrations of key enzymes involved in oxidative metabolism. He was referred for repeat exercise testing to further characterize his problem and determine if his functional capacity was changing. His medical history was notable only for Lyme disease, which was treated 3 years previously. Physical examination was unremarkable, and the resting electrocardiogram was normal.

EXERCISE FINDINGS

This patient represented an unusual diagnostic challenge and underwent a number of exercise tests over a period of several years. One test will be presented in detail, and selected data from others are presented in tabular form for comparison. At the time of his initial referral to our laboratory, exercise testing was conducted without blood sampling and showed that *AT* was reduced and peak $\dot{V}O_2$ and O_2 pulse were low normal or mildly reduced. All of these measures were lower than on a test performed 2 years earlier by the referring physician. This suggested progression of his impairment and raised the question of whether it was a circulatory or metabolic problem. Repeat testing was therefore planned with sampling of arterial, mixed venous, and femoral venous blood for hemodynamic assessment. Results of the latter test are presented here.

Femoral venous (directed caudally), brachial artery, and pulmonary artery catheters were placed prior to exercise. Exercise testing was conducted on a cycle ergometer starting with 3 minutes of unloaded cycling, followed by a progressive increase in work rate by 25 W/min. The patient stopped exercise with symptoms of light-headedness and was noted to be pale in the postexercise period. He denied chest pain or symptoms of leg pain or fatigue. The brachial artery tracing demonstrated marked respiratory variation in blood pressure constituting a pulsus paradoxus of 40 to 50 mm Hg at peak exercise (150/110/70 mm Hg). At the end of exercise, systolic pressure dropped immediately to 98/70/50 and slowly recovered to 110/67 after 2 minutes of recovery. During this time, heart rate declined only from a peak of 190 to 140 beats/min; there was no ectopy.

INTERPRETATION

Comments

Pulmonary function tests were essentially normal (**Table 10.46.1**). Exercise data are summarized in **Table 10.46.2** and shown in **Table 10.46.3** and graphically in **Figure 10.46.1**.

Analysis

Peak $\dot{V}O_2$ was within the normal range, although below the average predicted value and lower than what had been reported 2 years earlier by his referring physician. The striking finding on this test was that the *AT* was lower than predicted

TABLE 10.46.1 Selected Respiratory Function Data

Measurement	Predicted	Measured
Age (y)		26
Sex		Male
Height (cm)		180
Weight (kg)		78
Hemoglobin (g/dL)		16.4
VC (L)	5.69	6.06
IC (L)	3.80	4.48
FEV_1 (L)	4.75	5.05
FEV_1/VC (%)	83	83
MVV (L/min)	188	188
D_{LCO} (mL/mm Hg/min)[a]	36.9	37.1

Abbreviations: D_{LCO}, diffusing capacity of lung for carbon monoxide; FEV_1, forced expiratory volume in 1 second; IC, inspiratory capacity; MVV, maximum voluntary ventilation; VC, vital capacity.

[a]Measured on a separate occasion.

TABLE 10.46.2 Selected Exercise Data

Measurement	Predicted	Measured
Peak $\dot{V}O_2$ (L/min)	3.27	2.80
Maximum heart rate (beats/min)	194	192
Maximum O_2 pulse (mL/beat)	16.9	14.6
$\Delta\dot{V}O_2/\Delta WR$ (mL/min/W)	10.3	9.0
AT (L/min)	>1.4	1.1
Blood pressure (mm Hg [rest, max])		100/70, 158/80
Maximum $\dot{V}E$ (L/min)		161
Exercise breathing reserve (L/min)	>15	27
$\dot{V}E/\dot{V}CO_2$ @ *AT* or lowest	24.2	26.1
PaO_2 (mm Hg [rest, max ex])		89, 112
$P(A - a)O_2$ (mm Hg [rest, max ex])		8, 9
$PaCO_2$ (mm Hg [rest, max ex])		43, 34
$P(a - ET)CO_2$ (mm Hg [rest, max ex])		5, −3
VD/VT (rest, max ex)		0.47, 0.14
HCO_3^- (mEq/L [rest, recov])		27, 16

Abbreviations: *AT*, anaerobic threshold; $\Delta\dot{V}O_2/\Delta WR$, change in $\dot{V}O_2$/change in work rate; ex, exercise; HCO_3^-, bicarbonate; O_2, oxygen; $P(A - a)O_2$, alveolar-arterial PO_2 difference; $P(a - ET)CO_2$, arterial-end-tidal PCO_2 difference; recov, recovery; VD/VT, physiological dead space-tidal volume ratio; $\dot{V}E$, minute ventilation; $\dot{V}E/\dot{V}CO_2$, ventilatory equivalent for carbon dioxide; $\dot{V}O_2$, oxygen uptake.

and was a relatively low percentage of the patient's peak $\dot{V}O_2$. Indices of pulmonary gas exchange were normal and the hemoglobin was high normal, so the finding of a low *AT* suggests either a circulatory or metabolic problem. Hemodynamic data are shown in **Table 10.46.4**. At peak exercise, O_2 extraction across the leg was normal (74%) and was also normal across the entire systemic circulation (70%). Thus, the distribution of cardiac output to the working legs and extraction of O_2 by the muscle appeared intact. Cardiac output was measured at rest by thermodilution and at two points during exercise by the Fick method, with the highest value of 16.6 L/min measured at approximately 2 minutes prior to the end of exercise. From these measures, the slope of the increase in cardiac output was less than 4 L/min for each liter per minute increase in $\dot{V}O_2$, which is lower than expected (5-6 L/min per liter per minute $\dot{V}O_2$). So, in this case, as in the preceding Case 45 of this chapter, the cause of exercise intolerance appeared to be an inadequate increase in cardiac output despite imaging studies showing normal cardiac structure and function. In this case, the effect of limited blood flow was offset in part by a mild erythrocytosis, which increased the potential $C(a - \bar{v})O_2$ such that peak $\dot{V}O_2$ was within the normal range.

Over the following year, the patient continued to have reduced exercise tolerance and near-syncope with exertion and so returned for further evaluation. To test the possibility that the circulatory problem was due to relative intravascular volume deficit, he underwent a pair of exercise tests, the first performed as a baseline and the second the following day after intravenous volume loading with 750 mL of lactated Ringer solution and 150 mL of 25% albumin. Volume loading was associated with improved peak $\dot{V}O_2$ and *AT* (see **Table 10.46.4**) without significant difference in peak heart rate. No hematologic or endocrine basis for relative volume depletion was identified.

Conclusion

This perplexing patient had a near-normal peak exercise capacity with low *AT* but had exertional light-headedness (near-syncope), fatigue, and nausea. The findings of pulsus paradoxus during exercise and postexercise hypotension supported the impression that these symptoms might result from reduced cardiac output due to inadequate preload. Hemodynamic studies confirmed a marginally reduced cardiac output response to exercise, and an empiric challenge with intravenous loading was associated with acute improvement in exercise performance. The underlying cause of this condition was not clear. It is compatible with either a low blood volume or impaired venous return to the central circulation.

TABLE 10.46.3 Air Breathing

Time (min)	Work rate (W)	BP (mm Hg)	HR (min^{-1})	f (min^{-1})	$\dot{V}E$ (L/min BTPS)	$\dot{V}CO_2$ (L/min STPD)	$\dot{V}O_2$ (L/min STPD)	$\frac{\dot{V}O_2}{HR}$ (mL/beat)	R	pH	HCO_3^- (mEq/L)	PO_2, mm Hg ET	a	(A − a)	PCO_2, mm Hg ET	a	(a − ET)	$\frac{\dot{V}E}{\dot{V}CO_2}$	$\frac{\dot{V}E}{\dot{V}O_2}$	$\frac{VD}{VT}$
0.5	Rest		86	17	10.0	0.20	0.25	2.9	0.80			102			38			40	50	
1.0	Rest	100/70	88	17	10.0	0.17	0.23	2.6	0.74			101			39			43	59	
1.5	Rest		85	14	7.8	0.13	0.18	2.1	0.74			100			40			43	59	
2.0	Rest	94/70	88	16	10.9	0.22	0.30	3.4	0.74			102			39			36	49	
2.5	Rest		90	13	11.2	0.20	0.30	3.3	0.65	7.40	27	107	89	8	38	43	5.0	37	57	0.47
3.0	Rest	108/62	99	18	15.7	0.40	0.52	5.3	0.76			101			40			30	39	
3.5	Unloaded		102	18	14.2	0.34	0.46	4.5	0.75			100			40			31	41	
4.0	Unloaded		102	19	17.2	0.48	0.61	6.0	0.79			102			40			28	36	
4.5	Unloaded	121/72	103	17	17.9	0.54	0.69	6.7	0.78	7.40	26	102	101	−3	40	42	1.0	26	33	0.30
5.0	Unloaded		102	18	19.9	0.55	0.67	6.6	0.83			105			39			30	36	
5.5	Unloaded		102	17	15.6	0.43	0.55	5.4	0.79			101			41			28	36	
6.0	Unloaded	111/69	103	14	18.4	0.56	0.69	6.7	0.81			103			40			27	33	
6.5	−2		102	15	17.9	0.55	0.68	6.7	0.81	7.41	27	103	105	−5	40	41	1.0	26	32	0.32
7.0	1		104	16	17.9	0.55	0.66	6.3	0.83			103			40			27	33	
7.5	7		104	18	18.5	0.48	0.58	5.6	0.83			101			41			32	39	
8.0	33	115/70	112	20	23.8	0.80	1.03	9.2	0.78			100			42			23	30	
8.5	41		110	17	25.0	0.79	0.97	8.9	0.81	7.38	26	103	91	6	41	45	3.0	26	32	0.31
9.0	64		114	18	23.1	0.82	0.95	8.3	0.87			102			43			24	28	
9.5	66		118	19	28.7	1.01	1.10	9.3	0.92			103			43			26	28	
10.0	75	123/68	124	18	28.8	1.03	1.12	9.0	0.92			103			44			26	28	
10.5	94		131	19	33.1	1.22	1.24	9.5	0.98	7.37	27	105	98	3	45	46	2.0	27	27	0.28
11.0	101		139	17	35.1	1.37	1.40	10.1	0.98			105			46			25	26	
11.5	116		143	19	39.1	1.53	1.47	10.3	1.04			105			46			27	26	
12.0	132	134/98	149	20	44.2	1.72	1.55	10.4	1.11			108			45			29	26	
12.5	139		155	17	47.7	1.91	1.73	11.2	1.10	7.36	25	107	100	10	45	43	−1.0	28	25	0.21
13.0	156		162	16	55.7	2.17	1.90	11.7	1.14			110			44			29	26	
13.5	168		166	17	56.1	2.17	1.91	11.5	1.14			109			44			29	26	
14.0	183	158/74	171	18	64.3	2.42	2.10	12.3	1.15			111			43			31	27	
14.5	191		177	19	74.5	2.72	2.26	12.8	1.20	7.34	23	114	100	15	41	40	−2.0	33	27	0.19
15.0	203		181	21	80.5	2.84	2.32	12.8	1.22			116			40			[illegible]	[illegible]	
15.5	219		182	23	84.6	2.94	2.41	13.2	1.22			116			38			35	29	
16.0	231	148/70	188	23	93.0	3.19	2.55	13.6	1.25			118			38			36	29	
16.5	242		191	37	125.5	3.63	2.74	14.3	1.32	7.31	19	124	112	9	33	34	−3.0	46	35	0.14
17.0	251	158/80	192	52	161.0	3.71	2.80	14.6	1.33			130			26			58	43	
17.5	276		190	45	123.4	2.70	1.96	10.3	1.38			132			24			63	46	
18.0	Recovery		184	39	102.7	2.20	1.40	7.6	1.57			134			24			73	47	
18.5	Recovery	101/63	179	38	95.8	1.88	1.15	6.4	1.63			135			22			83	51	
19.0	Recovery		170	34	82.9	1.59	1.01	5.9	1.57			135			22			82	52	
19.5	Recovery		161	34	72.2	1.37	0.91	5.7	1.51	7.23	16	135	152	−17	22	21	0.0	79	53	0.21
20.0	Recovery		152	28	52.9	1.12	0.81	5.3	1.38			131			25			65	47	
20.5	Recovery		143	32	48.5	1.00	0.78	5.5	1.28			131			24			62	49	

Abbreviations: BP, blood pressure; BTPS, body temperature pressure saturated; f, frequency; HCO_3^-, bicarbonate; HR, heart rate; P(A − a)O_2, alveolar-arterial PO_2 difference; P(a − ET)CO_2, arterial-end-tidal PCO_2 difference; $PETCO_2$, end-tidal PCO_2; $PETO_2$, end-tidal PO_2; R, respiratory exchange ratio; STPD, standard temperature pressure dry; $\dot{V}CO_2$, carbon dioxide output; VD/VT, physiological dead space-tidal volume ratio; $\dot{V}E$, minute ventilation; $\dot{V}E/\dot{V}CO_2$, ventilatory equivalent for carbon dioxide; $\dot{V}E/\dot{V}O_2$, ventilatory equivalent for oxygen; $\dot{V}O_2$, oxygen uptake.

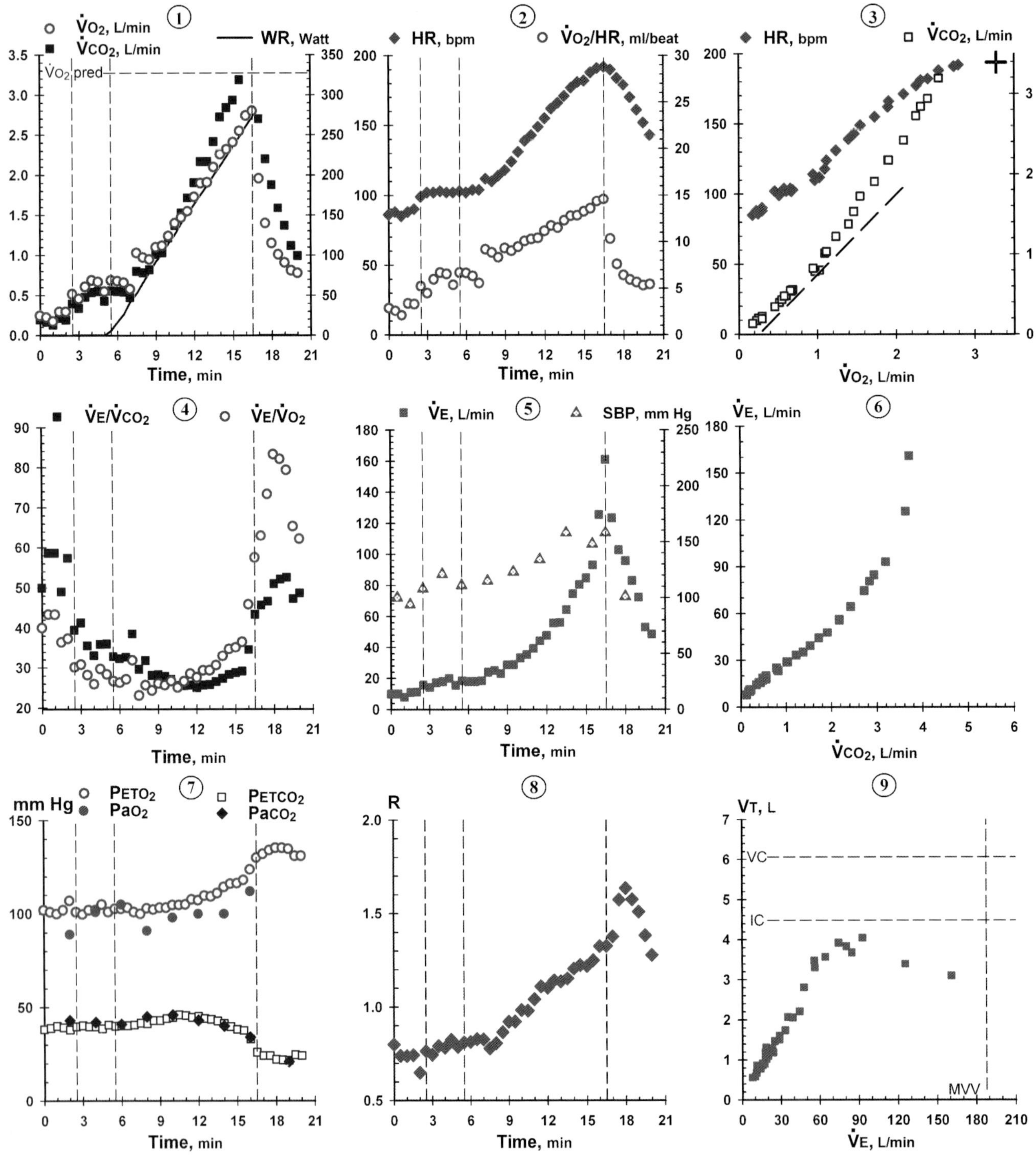

FIGURE 10.46.1. Vertical dashed lines in the panels in the left and middle columns indicate, from left to right, the beginning of unloaded cycling, start of increasing work rate (WR) at 25 W/min, and start of recovery. In **panel 1**, the increase in WR (right y-axis) is plotted with a scale of 100 W to 1 L of oxygen uptake ($\dot{V}O_2$) (left y-axis) such that WR is plotted parallel to a $\dot{V}O_2$ slope of 10 mL/min/W. In **panel 3**, carbon dioxide output ($\dot{V}CO_2$) (right y-axis) is plotted as a function of $\dot{V}O_2$ (x-axis) with identical scales so that the diagonal dashed line has a slope of 1 (45°). The $\dot{V}CO_2$ increasing more steeply than $\dot{V}O_2$ defines carbon dioxide (CO_2) derived from bicarbonate buffer, as long as ventilatory equivalent for CO_2 ($\dot{V}E/\dot{V}CO_2$) (**panel 4**) is not increasing and end-tidal PCO_2 ($PETCO_2$) (**panel 7**) is not decreasing, simultaneously. The black + symbol in **panel 3** indicates predicted peak values of heart rate (HR) (left y-axis) and $\dot{V}O_2$ for this individual. Abbreviations: IC, inspiratory capacity; MVV, maximum voluntary ventilation; $PETO_2$, end-tidal PO_2; R, respiratory exchange ratio; SBP, systolic blood pressure; VC, vital capacity; $\dot{V}E$, minute ventilation; $\dot{V}E/\dot{V}O_2$, ventilatory equivalent for oxygen; V_T, tidal volume.

TABLE 10.46.4 Selected Hemodynamic Variables

Work rate (W)	$\dot{V}O_2$ (L/min)	Cardiac output (L/min)	Stroke volume (mL)	Systemic		Leg	
				$C(a-\bar{v})O_2$ (mL/dL)	O_2 extraction (%)	$C(a-\bar{v})O_2$ (mL/dL)	O_2 extraction (%)
Rest (supine)	0.34	7.8	92	4.35	20	11.4	54
Unloaded	0.56					11.6	56
11	0.69					11.1	54
58	0.91					12.9	61
107	1.19	12.74	91	9.34	43	12.5	59
156	1.6					13.8	65
204	2.16					15.6	72
252	2.65	16.67	87	15.9	70	16.3	72
276	2.49					16.6	74
Recovery	0.97					5.9	27

Abbreviations: $C(a-\bar{v})O_2$, arterial-mixed venous O_2 content difference; O_2, oxygen; $\dot{V}O_2$, oxygen uptake.

TABLE 10.46.5 Selected Measures From Exercise Tests Conducted Over 4 Years

Time relative to presented test	Peak $\dot{V}O_2$ (L/min)	*AT* (L/min)	Peak HR (beats/min)	Peak O_2 pulse (mL/beat)	$\Delta\dot{V}O_2/\Delta WR$	(Hb), rest (g/dL)	Blood pressure (mm Hg)	
							Rest	Peak exercise
2 y earlier	3.57	1.37	192	18.6		17.2		
1 y earlier	2.66	1.3	193	13.8	8.6		127/81	156/86
1 d earlier	2.67	1.1	189	14.1	8.2		133/84	169/77
Present test	2.80	1.1	192	14.6	9.0	16.4	100/70	158/80
1 y later baseline	3.30	1.1	187	17.7	9.8	18.6	127/73	194/94
1 y later post-volume loading	3.73	1.4	185	20.5	10.7	16.5	113/70	167/56

Abbreviations: *AT*, anaerobic threshold; $\Delta\dot{V}O_2/\Delta WR$, change in $\dot{V}O_2$/change in work rate; Hb, hemoglobin; HR, heart rate; O_2, oxygen; $\dot{V}O_2$, oxygen uptake.

CASE 47

Mixed Connective Tissue Disease With Pulmonary Involvement

CLINICAL FINDINGS

This 38-year-old man with known mixed connective tissue disease and restrictive lung function was referred for exercise testing to determine his level of disability. He has had a productive cough for 3 years and had been dyspneic for over 2 years. He has never smoked but had been exposed to multiple chemical agents in a rubber factory. His medications at the time of testing were prednisone, theophylline, and cimetidine.

EXERCISE FINDINGS

The patient performed exercise on a cycle ergometer. He pedaled at 60 rpm without an added load for 3 minutes. The work rate was then increased 15 W/min to his symptom-limited maximum. Arterial blood was sampled every second minute, and intra-arterial blood pressure was recorded from a percutaneously inserted brachial artery catheter. Resting echocardiogram was normal except for occasional premature ectopic beats, which increased in frequency to a maximum of 12 per minute near peak exercise. No ST-segment or T-wave abnormalities occurred. Exercise was stopped because the patient seemed unsteady and indicated that he was light-headed. These symptoms cleared within a few minutes of ending exercise. He indicated that he was also out of breath but did not identify this as limiting at the time the test ended.

TABLE 10.47.1 Selected Respiratory Function Data

Measurement	Predicted	Measured
Age (y)		38
Sex		Male
Height (cm)		188
Weight (kg)	88	88
Hematocrit (%)		43
VC (L)	5.09	2.28
IC (L)	3.39	1.36
TLC (L)	7.14	3.43
FEV_1 (L)	4.09	1.99
FEV_1/VC (%)	81	87
MVV (L/min)		
Direct	163	107
Indirect	164	80
D_{LCO} (mL/mm Hg/min)	32.7	10.7

Abbreviations: D_{LCO}, diffusing capacity of the lung for carbon monoxide; FEV_1, forced expiratory volume in 1 second; IC, inspiratory capacity; MVV, maximum voluntary ventilation; VC, vital capacity; TLC, total lung capacity.

INTERPRETATION

Comments

The resting respiratory function studies show severe restriction with severe loss of effective pulmonary capillary bed (low diffusing capacity of the lung for carbon monoxide) (**Table 10.47.1**). Exercise data are summarized in **Table 10.47.2** and shown in **Table 10.47.3** and graphically in **Figure 10.47.1**.

Analysis

Exercise capacity was severely reduced (peak oxygen uptake [$\dot{V}O_2$] only 33% of predicted) along with a very low anaerobic threshold. With severe restriction on pulmonary function tests, it was not surprising that he had evidence for ventilatory limitation during exercise (low breathing reserve when compared to "indirect" maximum voluntary ventilation, tidal volume (V_T) close to inspiratory capacity, and high respiratory frequency). Other features of lung disease include progressively worse arterial hypoxemia, positive $P(a - ET)CO_2$, and elevated physiological dead space–tidal volume ratio (V_D/V_T) during exercise. In addition to these findings, the patient also had a high heart rate–$\dot{V}O_2$ slope, very low peak O_2 pulse, and very low anaerobic threshold; these findings would be characteristic of an O_2 flow problem that could be related to or separate from his interstitial lung disease. This is further manifest in the slow recovery of $\dot{V}O_2$ and O_2 pulse toward baseline during recovery, reflecting the need to reverse the consequences of the accumulated oxygen deficit in the tissues. Consistent with this, respiratory exchange ratio decreased rather than increased in early recovery (see **Fig. 10.47.1**, panel 8) due to $\dot{V}O_2$ decreasing more slowly than carbon dioxide output ($\dot{V}CO_2$). One way to characterize this constellation of

TABLE 10.47.2 Selected Exercise Data

Measurement	Predicted	Measured
Peak $\dot{V}O_2$ (L/min)	3.21	1.07
Maximum heart rate (beats/min)	182	128
Maximum O_2 pulse (mL/beat)	17.6	8.4
$\Delta\dot{V}O_2/\Delta WR$ (mL/min/W)	>10.3	7.3
AT (L/min)	>1.35	0.60
Blood pressure (mm Hg [rest, max ex])		141/90, 222/102
Maximum $\dot{V}E$ (L/min)		76
Exercise breathing reserve (L/min)		
Using direct MVV	>15	31
Using indirect MVV	>15	4
$\dot{V}E/\dot{V}CO_2$ @ *AT* or lowest	25.2	38.5
PaO_2 (mm Hg [rest, max ex])		79, 63
$P(A - a)O_2$ (mm Hg [rest, max ex])		16, 58
$PaCO_2$ (mm Hg [rest, max ex])		40, 39
$P(a - ET)CO_2$ (mm Hg [rest, max ex])		5, 9
VD/VT (rest, max ex)		0.46, 0.48
HCO_3^- (mEq/L [rest, recov])		25, 20

Abbreviations: *AT*, anaerobic threshold; $\Delta\dot{V}O_2/\Delta WR$, change in $\dot{V}O_2$/change in work rate; ex, exercise; HCO_3^-, bicarbonate; MVV, maximum voluntary ventilation; O_2, oxygen; $P(A - a)O_2$, alveolar-arterial PO_2 difference; $P(a - ET)CO_2$, arterial-end-tidal PCO_2 difference; recov, recovery; VD/VT, physiological dead space-tidal volume ratio; $\dot{V}E$, minute ventilation; $\dot{V}O_2$, oxygen uptake.

findings would be pulmonary vascular involvement related to his underlying mixed connective tissue disease that is already known to involve the lungs.

A flowchart approach (Chapter 9) to this study would lead to Flowchart 4 because of the low peak $\dot{V}O_2$ and low anaerobic threshold. The next branch point (Branch Point 4.1) is breathing reserve, which is judged to be low, indicating ventilatory limitation, and supported by the high respiratory rate, known restriction, and high VT/IC ratio. At Branch Point 4.3, the $\dot{V}E/\dot{V}CO_2$ at the anaerobic threshold is clearly high (abnormal) leading to a choice of left ventricular failure or pulmonary vascular disease, with the latter being well supported by gas exchange abnormalities. The coincidence of findings of restriction lung disease and pulmonary vascular disease would fit well with the clinical diagnosis of mixed connective tissue disease with features of pulmonary vascular disease.

Conclusion

Significant defects were demonstrated in breathing mechanics, pulmonary gas exchange, and cardiovascular responses, attributable to interstitial lung disease with secondary effects on the pulmonary vasculature. The increased carbon dioxide production resulting from bicarbonate buffering of early onset of lactic acidosis (due to cardiovascular impairment), together with high VD/VT, resulted in an exceptionally high ventilatory requirement. The increased VD/VT and arterial hypoxemia, accompanied by the reduced ventilatory capacity due to lung restriction, all likely contributed to his breathlessness with exercise.

TABLE 10.47.3 Air Breathing

Time (min)	Work rate (W)	BP (mm Hg)	HR (min^{-1})	f (min^{-1})	$\dot{V}E$ (L/min BTPS)	$\dot{V}CO_2$ (L/min STPD)	$\dot{V}O_2$ (L/min STPD)	$\frac{\dot{V}O_2}{HR}$ (mL/beat)	R	pH	HCO_3^- (mEq/L)	PO_2, mm Hg			PCO_2, mm Hg			$\frac{\dot{V}E}{\dot{V}CO_2}$	$\frac{\dot{V}E}{\dot{V}O_2}$	$\frac{V_D}{V_T}$
												ET	a	(A − a)	ET	a	(a − ET)			
	Rest	141/90								7.45	25		92			37				
0.5	Rest		86	20	10.5	0.18	0.29	3.4	0.62			100			34			49	30	
1.0	Rest		92	20	11.1	0.21	0.33	3.6	0.64			100			34			45	28	
1.5	Rest		87	21	12.4	0.23	0.34	3.9	0.68			102			34			46	31	
2.0	Rest	156/96	80	19	9.8	0.17	0.25	3.1	0.68	7.41	25	103	79	16	35	40	5	48	33	0.46
2.5	Rest		80	20	11.0	0.20	0.28	3.5	0.71			105			35			47	33	
3.0	Rest		87	20	11.1	0.20	0.30	3.4	0.67			103			36			47	31	
3.5	Unloaded		94	27	17.6	0.35	0.49	5.2	0.71			103			36			44	31	
4.0	Unloaded		97	27	17.3	0.37	0.55	5.7	0.67			101			36			41	27	
4.5	Unloaded		102	29	24.3	0.57	0.68	6.7	0.84			109			35			38	32	
5.0	Unloaded		100	31	26.6	0.63	0.69	6.9	0.91			111			36			38	35	
5.5	Unloaded		101	34	27.8	0.64	0.66	6.5	0.97			111			37			39	38	
6.0	Unloaded	192/99	103	32	29.2	0.70	0.72	7.0	0.97	7.38	26	114	66	39	36	44	8	38	37	0.44
6.5	15		109	37	31.6	0.72	0.73	6.7	0.99			114			36			40	39	
7.0	15		110	35	33.7	0.81	0.79	7.2	1.03			114			37			38	39	
7.5	30		112	39	38.5	0.89	0.82	7.3	1.09			117			36			40	43	
8.0	30	204/102	118	42	41.5	0.96	0.87	7.4	1.10	7.38	26	117	66	43	35	44	9	40	44	0.46
8.5	45		123	47	47.8	1.09	0.96	7.8	1.14			117			35			40	46	
9.0	45		127	48	50.8	1.16	0.97	7.6	1.20			120			35			40	48	
9.5	60		128	59	66.5	1.43	1.04	8.1	1.38			124			32			43	59	
10.0	60	222/102	128	64	76.1	1.55	1.07	8.4	1.45	7.38	23	126	63	58	30	39	9	46	66	0.48
10.5	Recovery		117	62	70.9	1.39	0.97	8.3	1.43			126			31			47	68	
11.0	Recovery		111	58	61.5	1.23	0.90	8.1	1.37			127			30			46	63	
11.5	Recovery		110	51	49.7	1.01	0.79	7.2	1.28			124			31			45	57	
12.0	Recovery		105	49	47.5	0.95	0.75	7.1	1.27			123			32			46	58	
12.5	Recovery	180/88	103	47	45.2	0.89	0.71	6.9	1.25	7.35	20	123	76	43	32	37	5	46	58	0.45

Abbreviations: BP, blood pressure; BTPS, body temperature pressure saturated; f, frequency; HCO_3^-, bicarbonate; HR, heart rate; $P(A - a)O_2$, alveolar-arterial PO_2 difference; $P(a - ET)CO_2$, arterial-end-tidal PCO_2 difference; $PETCO_2$, end-tidal PCO_2; $PETO_2$, end-tidal PO_2; R, respiratory exchange ratio; STPD, standard temperature pressure dry; V_D/V_T, physiological dead space-tidal volume ratio; $\dot{V}E$, minute ventilation; $\dot{V}CO_2$, carbon dioxide output; $\dot{V}E/\dot{V}CO_2$, ventilatory equivalent for carbon dioxide; $\dot{V}E/\dot{V}O_2$, ventilatory equivalent for carbon dioxide; $\dot{V}O_2$, oxygen output.

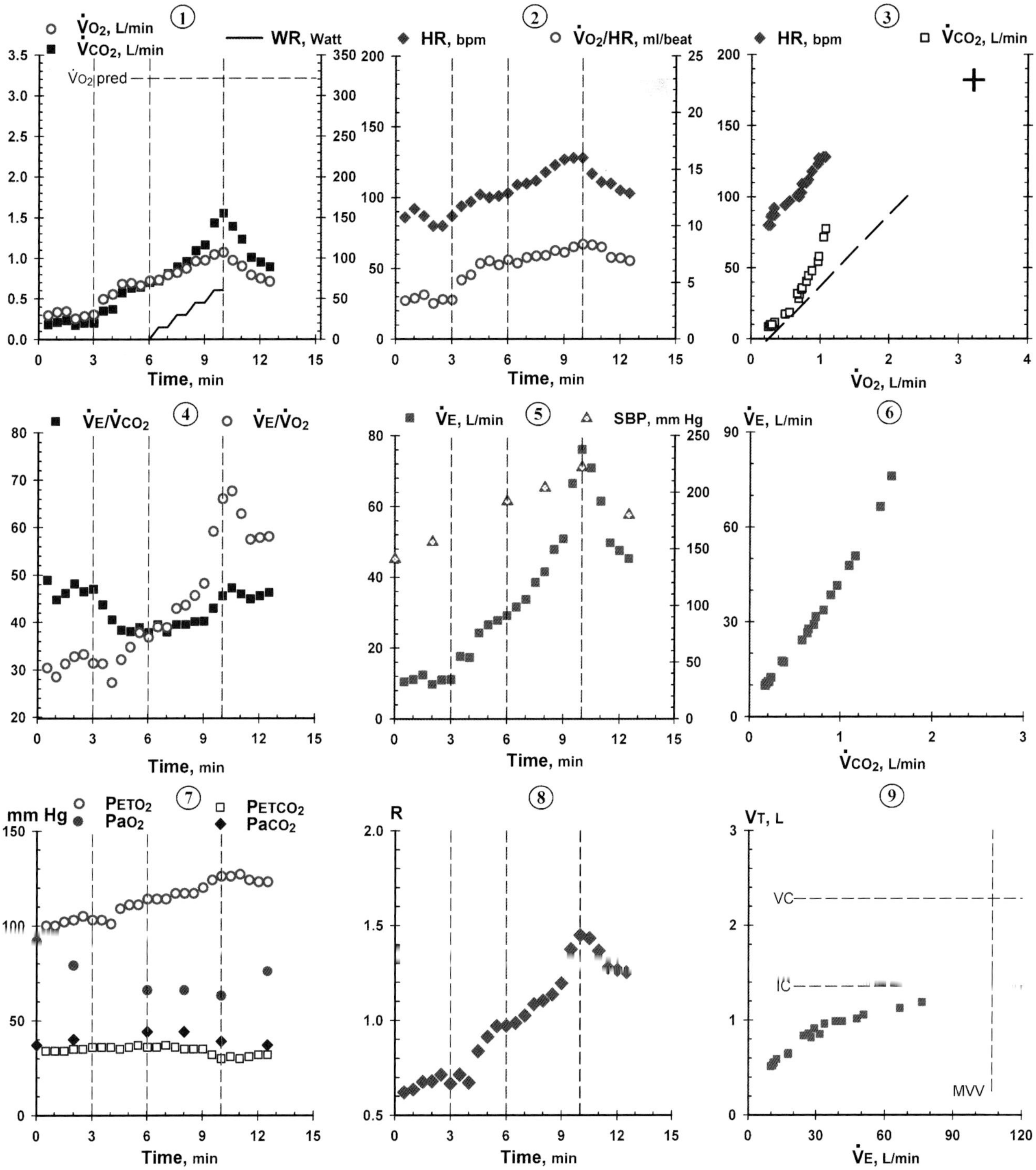

FIGURE 10.47.1. Vertical dashed lines in the panels in the left and middle columns indicate, from left to right, the beginning of unloaded cycling, start of increasing work rate (WR) at 15 W/min, and start of recovery. In **panel 1**, the increase in WR (right y-axis) is plotted with a scale of 100 W to 1 L of oxygen uptake ($\dot{V}O_2$) (left y-axis) such that WR is plotted parallel to a $\dot{V}O_2$ slope of 10 mL/min/W. In **panel 3**, carbon dioxide output ($\dot{V}CO_2$) (right y-axis) is plotted as a function of $\dot{V}O_2$ (x-axis) with identical scales so that the diagonal dashed line has a slope of 1 (45 degrees). The $\dot{V}CO_2$ increasing more steeply than $\dot{V}O_2$ defines carbon dioxide derived from bicarbonate buffer, as long as ventilatory equivalent for carbon dioxide $\dot{V}E/\dot{V}CO_2$ (**panel 4**) is not increasing and partial pressure of carbon dioxide in end-tidal gas (P_{ETCO_2}) (**panel 7**) is not decreasing, simultaneously. The black + symbol in **panel 3** indicates predicted peak values of heart rate (HR) (left y-axis) and $\dot{V}O_2$ for this individual. Abbreviations: HR, heart rate; IC, inspiratory capacity; MVV, maximum voluntary ventilation; P_{ETO_2}, end-tidal partial pressure of oxygen; R, respiratory exchange ratio; SBP, systolic blood pressure; VC, vital capacity; $\dot{V}E$, minute ventilation; $\dot{V}E/\dot{V}O_2$, ventilatory equivalent for oxygen; V_T, tidal volume.

CASE 48

Pulmonary and Systemic Vasculitis: Air and Oxygen Breathing Studies

To view this case please access the eBook bundled with this text. Instructions are located on the inside front cover.

CASE 49

Idiopathic Pulmonary Arterial Hypertension

CLINICAL FINDINGS

This 47-year-old woman had pulmonary hypertension associated with prior anorexigen use. Exercise testing was performed periodically to assess her functional capacity, which improved gradually over a period of several years of pharmacologic treatment. She was first treated with a calcium channel blocking agent and subsequently transitioned to other therapies. At the time that this test was conducted, she had been treated for pulmonary hypertension for 10 years and reported feeling "great." She performed all her normal daily activities without difficulty and walked for 20 to 30 minutes each day for exercise. Her medications included a prostacyclin analog and a phosphodiesterase inhibitor along with diuretics, warfarin, and a statin. On examination, she was flushed, had a prominent second heart sound, and had trace peripheral edema of the ankles. An electrocardiogram showed right ventricular hypertrophy with strain.

EXERCISE FINDINGS

Exercise was performed on a cycle ergometer. After 3 minutes of pedaling at 60 rpm without added load, work rate was continuously increased by 10 W/min until the patient stopped with symptoms of airway irritation and cough. There were no significant changes to the electrocardiogram.

TABLE 10.49.1 Selected Respiratory Function Data

Measurement	Predicted	Measured
Age (y)		47
Sex		Female
Height (cm)		160
Weight (kg)		74
VC (L)	3.12	2.68
IC (L)	2.08	2.40
FEV_1 (L)	2.6	1.87
FEV_1/VC (%)	83	70
MVV (L/min)	97	85
D_{LCO} (mL/mm Hg/min)	22.7	19.8

Abbreviations: D_{LCO}, diffusing capacity of the lung for carbon monoxide; FEV_1, forced expiratory volume in 1 second; IC, inspiratory capacity; MVV, maximum voluntary ventilation; VC, vital capacity.

TABLE 10.49.2 Selected Exercise Data

Measurement	Predicted	Measured
Peak $\dot{V}O_2$ (L/min)	1.61	0.89
Maximum heart rate (beats/min)	173	136
Maximum O_2 pulse (mL/beat)	9.3	7.0
$\Delta\dot{V}O_2/\Delta WR$ (mL/min/W)	10.3	5.4
AT (L/min)	>0.79	0.72
Blood pressure (mm Hg [rest, max])		107/76, 125/88
Maximum $\dot{V}_E$ (L/min)		40
Exercise breathing reserve (L/min)	>15	45
$\dot{V}_E/\dot{V}CO_2$ @ *AT* or lowest	28.2	42.2

Abbreviations: *AT*, anaerobic threshold; $\Delta\dot{V}O_2/\Delta WR$, change in $\dot{V}O_2$/change in work rate; O_2, oxygen; $\dot{V}_E$, minute ventilation; $\dot{V}_E/\dot{V}CO_2$, ventilatory equivalent for carbon dioxide; $\dot{V}O_2$, oxygen uptake.

TABLE 10.49.3 Air Breathing

Time (min)	Work rate (W)	BP (mm Hg)	HR (min^{-1})	f (min^{-1})	$\dot{V}E$ (L/min BTPS)	$\dot{V}CO_2$ (L/min STPD)	$\dot{V}O_2$ (L/min STPD)	$\frac{\dot{V}O_2}{HR}$ (mL/beat)	R	pH	HCO_3^- (mEq/L)	PO_2, mm Hg ET	a	(A − a)	PCO_2, mm Hg ET	a	(a − ET)	$\frac{\dot{V}E}{\dot{V}CO_2}$	$\frac{\dot{V}E}{\dot{V}O_2}$	$\frac{V_D}{V_T}$
0.5	Rest	107/76	89	16	16.8	0.37	0.42	4.7	0.87			120			24			46	40	
1.0	Rest		87	15	15.4	0.35	0.42	4.8	0.83			118			24			44	37	
1.5	Rest		86	15	13.0	0.29	0.36	4.2	0.81			115			25			45	36	
2.0	Rest		84	18	14.6	0.32	0.38	4.5	0.83			117			24			46	39	
2.5	Rest		86	15	14.3	0.32	0.40	4.6	0.80			116			25			45	36	
3.0	Rest		84	16	13.9	0.31	0.37	4.4	0.83			117			24			45	37	
3.5	Unloaded	107/76	88	22	14.8	0.31	0.39	4.4	0.81			115			25			47	38	
4.0	Unloaded		93	23	18.5	0.38	0.43	4.7	0.88			120			23			49	43	
4.5	Unloaded		94	22	18.2	0.39	0.44	4.7	0.88			120			23			47	41	
5.0	Unloaded		96	21	19.5	0.43	0.52	5.4	0.83			118			24			46	38	
5.5	Unloaded	113/73	98	22	20.1	0.44	0.53	5.4	0.83			118			24			46	38	
6.0	Unloaded		98	22	19.6	0.43	0.53	5.4	0.82			117			24			46	37	
6.5	3		100	22	20.5	0.45	0.55	5.5	0.81			117			25			46	37	
7.0	8		100	22	21.1	0.47	0.57	5.7	0.83			118			25			45	37	
7.5	12		100	21	20.3	0.46	0.56	5.6	0.81			116			25			44	36	
8.0	17		102	22	21.1	0.48	0.57	5.6	0.84			117			25			44	37	
8.5	22	125/79	102	22	21.2	0.48	0.58	5.7	0.83			117			25			44	36	
9.0	27		106	21	21.7	0.50	0.60	5.7	0.83			117			25			43	36	
9.5	32		107	22	22.7	0.53	0.63	5.8	0.84			117			25			43	36	
10.0	37		109	22	23.8	0.56	0.66	6.0	0.85			117			25			43	36	
10.5	42		110	22	24.2	0.58	0.67	6.1	0.86			117			26			42	36	
11.0	47		117	21	25.9	0.62	0.72	6.2	0.86			117			26			42	36	
11.5	52		119	23	28.1	0.68	0.75	6.3	0.90			118			26			42	37	
12.0	57		122	23	29.1	0.72	0.77	6.3	0.93			119			26			41	38	
12.5	62		130	25	33.1	0.81	0.82	6.3	0.98			120			26			41	40	
13.0	67		132	26	36.0	0.87	0.86	6.5	1.01			121			26			42	42	
13.5	70		136	28	39.6	0.95	0.89	6.6	1.06			123			25			42	44	
14.0	Recovery	125/88	119	29	37.9	0.92	0.83	7.0	1.10			123			25			41	45	
14.5	Recovery		110	26	31.8	0.79	0.69	6.1	1.14			123			25			40	46	
15.0	Recovery	121/88	104	28	29.0	0.67	0.54	5.2	1.23			126			24			44	54	
15.4	Recovery		100	24	24.7	0.55	0.46	4.6	1.22			126			24			45	54	

Abbreviations: BP, blood pressure; BTPS, body temperature pressure saturated; f, frequency; HCO_3^-, bicarbonate; HR, heart rate; $P(A - a)O_2$, alveolar-arterial PO_2 difference; $P(a - ET)CO_2$, arterial–end-tidal PCO_2 difference; $PETCO_2$, end-tidal PCO_2; $PETO_2$, end-tidal PO_2; R, respiratory exchange ratio; STPD, standard temperature pressure dry; $\dot{V}CO_2$, carbon dioxide output; V_D/V_T, physiological dead space–tidal volume ratio; $\dot{V}E$, minute ventilation; $\dot{V}E/\dot{V}CO_2$, ventilatory equivalent for carbon dioxide; $\dot{V}E/\dot{V}O_2$, ventilatory equivalent for oxygen; $\dot{V}O_2$, oxygen uptake.

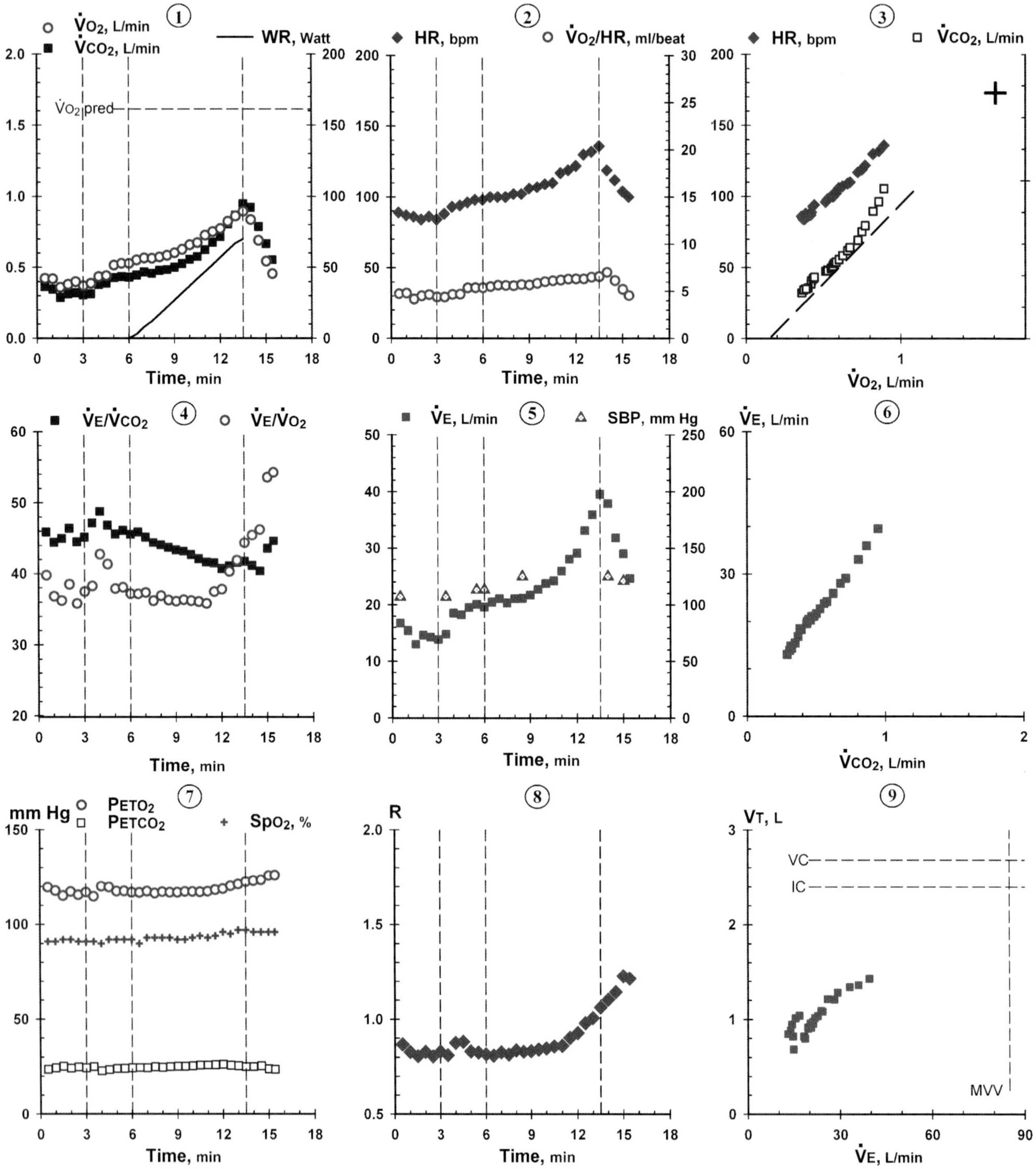

FIGURE 10.49.1. Vertical dashed lines in the panels in the left and middle columns indicate, from left to right, the beginning of unloaded cycling, start of increasing work rate (WR) at 10 W/min, and start of recovery. In **panel 1**, the increase in WR (right y-axis) is plotted with a scale of 100 W to 1 L of oxygen uptake ($\dot{V}O_2$) (left y-axis) such that WR is plotted parallel to a $\dot{V}O_2$ slope of 10 mL/min/W. In **panel 3**, carbon dioxide output ($\dot{V}CO_2$) (right y-axis) is plotted as a function of $\dot{V}O_2$ (x-axis) with identical scales so that the diagonal dashed line has a slope of 1 (45 degrees). The $\dot{V}CO_2$ increasing more steeply than $\dot{V}O_2$ defines carbon dioxide derived from bicarbonate buffer, as long as ventilatory equivalent for carbon dioxide ($\dot{V}E/\dot{V}CO_2$) (**panel 4**) is not increasing and partial pressure of carbon dioxide in end-tidal gas (P_{ETCO_2}) (**panel 7**) is not decreasing, simultaneously. The black + symbol in **panel 3** indicates predicted peak values of heart rate (HR) (left y-axis) and $\dot{V}O_2$ for this individual. Abbreviations: IC, inspiratory capacity; MVV, maximum voluntary ventilation; P_{ETO_2}, end-tidal partial pressure of oxygen; R, respiratory exchange ratio; SBP, systolic blood pressure; SpO_2, oxygen saturation as measured by pulse oximetry; VC, vital capacity; $\dot{V}E$, minute ventilation; $\dot{V}E/\dot{V}O_2$, ventilatory equivalent for oxygen; V_T, tidal volume.

INTERPRETATION

Comments

Pulmonary function tests (**Table 10.49.1**) showed a mild ventilatory defect and a low-normal diffusing capacity of the lung for carbon monoxide. The exercise test is presented to illustrate some common findings in patients on stable treatment for pulmonary arterial hypertension. Exercise data are summarized in **Table 10.49.2** and shown in **Table 10.49.3** and graphically in **Figure 10.49.1**.

Analysis

Peak oxygen uptake ($\dot{V}O_2$) and anaerobic threshold (*AT*) were both reduced. In addition, the change in $\dot{V}O_2$/change in work rate ($\Delta\dot{V}O_2/\Delta WR$) was less than normal, and the rate of increase of heart rate relative to $\dot{V}O_2$ was steeper than normal (panel 1 and 3 of **Figure 10.49.1**). The O_2 pulse increased very little during exercise and its peak value was low. These findings are all consistent with an impairment of O_2 flow. Because the patient reported that she stopped exercise due to airway irritation, rather than due to systemic symptoms, the peak values might underestimate her true maximal exercise capacity. Even if so, the low *AT*, low $\Delta\dot{V}O_2/\Delta WR$, and unchanging value of O_2 pulse indicate limitation of O_2 flow in response to the exercise stress. Similarly, ventilation was high relative to metabolic rate throughout exercise, as reflected in the ventilatory equivalent for carbon dioxide at the *AT* of 42, indicative of areas of high $\dot{V}A/\dot{Q}$ in the lung. Abnormal indices of oxygen flow and elevated ventilatory requirements are characteristic of pulmonary vascular disease. The typical findings of exercise-induced right-to-left shunt (illustrated in Case 53) are not evident in this patient. Indeed, although oxygen saturation, estimated by pulse oximeter, was around 90% at rest, it increased slightly during exercise, which is not a typical finding in pulmonary vascular disease, and does not negate the evidence for pulmonary vasculopathy as the primary cause of exercise intolerance.

Conclusion

This case is presented to illustrate findings typical of pulmonary vascular disease. The abnormal cardiorespiratory responses persist despite symptomatic improvement with pharmacologic therapy.

CASE 50

Severe Pulmonary Vascular Disease Secondary to Sarcoidosis: Air and Oxygen Breathing Studies

CLINICAL FINDINGS

This 29-year-old man with a 6-year history of sarcoidosis was referred for evaluation of worsening dyspnea and grading of his disease severity in consideration of lung transplantation. His condition was manifest in hilar lymphadenopathy; patchy interstitial infiltrates, which had improved with prior corticosteroid therapy; and severe pulmonary hypertension. He was on continuous oxygen (O_2) supplementation and an inhaled corticosteroid, but he was no longer taking systemic corticosteroids. His weight had decreased earlier in the course of his disease but was stable over the year prior to testing. He had a remote history of smoking cigarettes for 1 year.

EXERCISE FINDINGS

The patient performed exercise on a cycle ergometer while breathing room air. After a period of rest, the test was repeated while breathing 100% O_2. On both occasions, he pedaled at 60 rpm without an added load for 3 minutes. The work rate was then increased 10 W/min to tolerance. Arterial blood was sampled every second minute, and intra-arterial pressure was recorded from a percutaneously placed brachial artery catheter. The patient stopped exercise because of shortness of breath while breathing room air and because of leg fatigue while breathing O_2. The resting electrocardiogram showed right-axis deviation and inverted T waves anteriorly. The T waves became upright during exercise. No arrhythmias were noted.

INTERPRETATION

Comments

Resting respiratory function studies showed mild-to-moderate restrictive and obstructive defects in ventilatory mechanics, an extremely low DLCO, and severe arterial hypoxemia (**Table 10.50.1**).

Analysis

Peak oxygen uptake ($\dot{V}O_2$) was very severely reduced, compatible with severe exercise limitation, to less than 1 L/min, in conjunction with a very low peak heart rate (**Tables 10.50.2** and **10.50.3** and **Figure 10.50.1**). Of note is that despite anticipating ventilatory limitation, he had a relatively normal breathing reserve; however, his $\dot{V}E$ versus $\dot{V}CO_2$ slope and $\dot{V}E/\dot{V}CO_2$ were very high throughout exercise, and he had marked arterial hypoxemia. These likely limited his exercise performance, and also accounted for his very flat $\dot{V}O_2$ and O_2 pulse, and steep heart rate–$\dot{V}O_2$ relationship along with a very low anaerobic threshold (*AT*). Although low O_2 pulse implies a low stroke volume, for this patient with severe arterial hypoxemia, the low O_2 pulse may be due in part to low arterial-mixed venous O_2 content difference.

The test done on O_2 breathing (**Table 10.50.4** and **Fig. 10.50.2**) demonstrated that the patient's hypoxemia was due to $\dot{V}A/\dot{Q}$ mismatch rather than right-to-left shunt (PaO_2 was >550 mm Hg on breathing 100% O_2). The reversal of hypoxemia and reduction in ventilatory drive allowed the patient to tolerate a considerably higher work rate.

Using the flowcharts (Chapter 9), the peak $\dot{V}O_2$ and *AT* were severely reduced, leading to Flowchart 4. Through Branch Point 4.1, the breathing reserve was normal, but the high $\dot{V}E/\dot{V}CO_2$ at the *AT* (Branch Point 4.3) and high VD/VT (Branch Point 4.2) lead to the boxes representing lung disease with impaired oxygenation and abnormal pulmonary circulation.

Conclusion

This patient had only a mild-to-moderate disturbance in ventilatory mechanics but severe gas exchange abnormality and cardiovascular limitation attributable to pulmonary vascular disease. He had severe hypoxemia at rest and during exercise when breathing air, but although supplemental O_2 reversed his hypoxemia, exercise impairment remained severe.

TABLE 10.50.1 Selected Respiratory Function Data

Measurement	Predicted	Measured
Age (y)		29
Sex		Male
Height (cm)		171
Weight (kg)	73	58
Hematocrit (%)		45
VC (L)	4.28	3.11
IC (L)	2.85	1.59
TLC (L)	5.82	4.78
FEV_1 (L)	3.46	2.27
FEV_1/VC (%)	81	73
MVV (L/min)	138	91
DLCO (mL/mm Hg/min)	29.9	6.9

Abbreviations: DLCO, diffusing capacity of lung for carbon monoxide; FEV_1, forced expiratory volume in 1 second; FEV_1/VC, ratio of FEV_1 to VC; IC, inspiratory capacity; MVV, maximum voluntary ventilation; TLC, total lung capacity; VC, vital capacity.

TABLE 10.50.2 Selected Exercise Data

Measured	Predicted	Measurement: Air	Measurement: 100% O_2
Maximum work rate (W)		40	70
Peak $\dot{V}O_2$ (L/min)	2.64	0.8	
Maximum heart rate (beats/min)	191	149	150
Maximum O_2 pulse (mL/beat)	13.6	5.7	
AT (L/min)	>1.08	0.7	
Blood pressure (mm Hg [rest, max ex])		114/72, 135/78	111/69, 141/87
Maximum $\dot{V}E$ (L/min)		64	70
Exercise breathing reserve (L/min)	>15	27	21
$\dot{V}E/\dot{V}CO_2$ @ *AT* or lowest	24.9	61.8	63.5
PaO_2 (mm Hg [rest, max ex])		42, 35	585, 605
$P(A - a)O_2$ (mm Hg [rest, max ex])		52, 74	84, 57
$PaCO_2$ (mm Hg [rest, max ex])		46, 45	44, 51
$P(a - ET)CO_2$ (mm Hg [rest, max ex])		16, 22	19, 28
V_D/V_T (rest, max ex)		0.57, 0.67	0.63, 0.71
HCO_3^- (mEq/L [rest, 2-min recov])		27, 24	25, 24

Abbreviations: *AT*, anaerobic threshold; ex, exercise; HCO_3^-, bicarbonate; O_2, oxygen; $P(a - ET)CO_2$, arterial-end-tidal PCO_2 difference; $P(A - a)O_2$, alveolar-arterial PO_2 difference; recov, recovery; V_D/V_T, physiological dead space-tidal volume ratio; $\dot{V}E$, minute ventilation; $\dot{V}E/\dot{V}CO_2$, ventilatory equivalent for carbon dioxide; $\dot{V}O_2$, oxygen uptake.

TABLE 10.50.3 Air Breathing

Time (min)	Work rate (W)	BP (mm Hg)	HR (min^{-1})	f (min^{-1})	$\dot{V}E$ (L/min BTPS)	$\dot{V}CO_2$ (L/min STPD)	$\dot{V}O_2$ (L/min STPD)	$\frac{\dot{V}O_2}{HR}$ (mL/beat)	R	pH	HCO_3^- (mEq/L)	PO_2, mm Hg: ET	PO_2, mm Hg: a	PO_2, mm Hg: (A − a)	PCO_2, mm Hg: ET	PCO_2, mm Hg: a	PCO_2, mm Hg: (a − ET)	$\frac{\dot{V}E}{\dot{V}CO_2}$	$\frac{\dot{V}E}{\dot{V}O_2}$	$\frac{V_D}{V_T}$
	Rest	111/66								7.39	27		41			45				
0.5	Rest		96	18	15.6	0.27	0.34	3.5	0.79			113			30			52	41	
1.0	Rest		93	19	15.8	0.26	0.32	3.4	0.81			114			29			55	44	
1.5	Rest		95	19	16.1	0.26	0.31	3.3	0.84			116			28			56	47	
2.0	Rest		92	18	14.3	0.25	0.30	3.3	0.83			114			29			51	43	
2.5	Rest	[illegible]	[illegible]	[illegible]	16.3	0.28	0.36	3.9	0.78	7.38	27	111	42	52	30	46	16	52	41	0.57
3.0	Rest		94	23	20.6	0.41	0.34	[illegible]	[illegible]			112			30			45	35	
3.5	Unloaded		108	29	19.2	0.31	0.34	3.1	0.91			116			29			[illegible]	[illegible]	
4.0	Unloaded		114	31	31.0	0.50	0.57	5.0	0.88			119			26			57	50	
4.5	Unloaded		120	30	33.0	0.52	0.55	4.6	0.95			120			26			59	55	
5.0	Unloaded		122	32	36.5	0.56	0.60	4.9	0.93			119			28			60	56	
5.5	Unloaded		123	32	39.1	0.60	0.61	5.0	0.98			122			26			61	60	
6.0	Unloaded	116/72	123	35	42.5	0.65	0.66	5.4	0.98	7.38	26	122	37	67	26	45	19	61	60	0.64
6.5	10		125	36	45.1	0.68	0.69	5.5	0.99			123			25			62	61	
7.0	10		129	38	45.8	0.69	0.69	5.3	1.00			122			27			62	62	
7.5	20		130	39	54.4	0.81	0.78	6.0	1.04			125			24			63	65	
8.0	20	129/78	131	37	51.7	0.77	0.73	5.6	1.05	7.37	26	126	35	72	23	45	22	63	67	0.65
8.5	30		140	41	57.4	0.82	0.77	5.5	1.06			126			24			66	70	
9.0	30		140	44	63.3	0.88	0.80	5.7	1.10			127			24			68	74	
9.5	40	135/78	145	43	63.6	0.89	0.79	5.4	1.13	7.35	24	127	35	74	23	45	22	67	76	0.67
10.0	Recovery		149	48	63.0	0.89	0.80	5.4	1.11			129			22			66	74	
10.5	Recovery		140	39	56.3	0.81	0.72	5.1	1.13			126			25			65	74	
11.0	Recovery		140	36	50.5	0.80	0.79	5.6	1.01			122			26			59	60	
11.5	Recovery		138	34	50.1	0.75	0.70	5.1	1.07			123			25			63	67	
12.0	Recovery	114/69	133	39	52.5	0.77	0.74	5.6	1.04	7.33	24	122	35	70	28	46	18	64	66	0.66

Abbreviations: BP, blood pressure; BTPS, body temperature pressure saturated; f, frequency; HCO_3^-, bicarbonate; HR, heart rate; $P(A - a)O_2$, alveolar-arterial PO_2 difference; $P(a - ET)CO_2$, arterial-end-tidal PCO_2 difference; $PETCO_2$, end-tidal PCO_2; $PETO_2$, end-tidal PO_2; R, respiratory exchange ratio; STPD, standard temperature pressure dry; $\dot{V}CO_2$, carbon dioxide output; V_D/V_T, physiological dead space-tidal volume ratio; $\dot{V}E$, minute ventilation; $\dot{V}E/\dot{V}CO_2$, ventilatory equivalent for carbon dioxide; $\dot{V}E/\dot{V}O_2$, ventilatory equivalent for oxygen; $\dot{V}O_2$, oxygen uptake.

TABLE 10.50.4 Oxygen Breathing

Time (min)	Work rate (W)	BP (mm Hg)	HR (min^{-1})	f (min^{-1})	$\dot{V}E$ (L/min BTPS)	$\dot{V}CO_2$ (L/min STPD)	$\dot{V}O_2$ (L/min STPD)	$\frac{\dot{V}O_2}{HR}$ (mL/beat)	R	pH	HCO_3^- (mEq/L)	PO_2, mm Hg ET	PO_2, mm Hg a	PO_2, mm Hg (A − a)	PCO_2, mm Hg ET	PCO_2, mm Hg a	PCO_2, mm Hg (a − ET)	$\frac{\dot{V}E}{\dot{V}CO_2}$	$\frac{\dot{V}E}{\dot{V}O_2}$	$\frac{V_D}{V_T}$
	Rest									7.34	25		519			47				
0.5	Rest		67	21	20.6	0.29									24			65		
1.0	Rest		63	21	16.0	0.24									27			59		
1.5	Rest		58	19	17.2	0.23									25			68		
2.0	Rest	111/69	59	18	16.7	0.24				7.36	24		585	84	25	44	19	62		0.63
2.5	Rest		66	18	14.4	0.18									25			72		
3.0	Rest		64	20	17.1	0.23									25			67		
3.5	Unloaded		90	23	25.9	0.36									23			67		
4.0	Unloaded		93	28	26.0	0.37									25			64		
4.5	Unloaded		90	23	24.6	0.34									23			67		
5.0	Unloaded		95	25	28.4	0.40									25			66		
5.5	Unloaded		93	25	29.8	0.42									24			66		
6.0	Unloaded	116/75	94	24	28.6	0.41				7.35	25		615	52	25	46	21	65		0.66
6.5	10		92	26	33.1	0.46									25			67		
7.0	10		100	27	30.9	0.44									27			65		
7.5	20		103	29	35.8	0.52									26			64		
8.0	20	120/78	108	27	38.1	0.56				7.33	25		620	44	26	49	23	64		0.68
8.5	30		110	31	38.6	0.56									26			64		
9.0	30		114	28	40.6	0.60									26			64		
9.5	40		123	35	50.6	0.73									26			65		
10.0	40	132/81	125	34	50.8	0.75				7.31	25		612	51	26	50	24	64		0.69
10.5	50		132	34	52.5	0.79									27			63		
11.0	50		140	43	62.8	0.87									24			68		
11.5	60		150	40	63.5	0.91									25			66		
12.0	60	141/87	150	47	69.9	0.96				7.28	24		605	57	23	51	28	68		0.71
12.5	Recovery		133	40	57.6	0.83									25			65		
13.0	Recovery		112	31	42.1	0.82									31			48		

Abbreviations: BP, blood pressure; BTPS, body temperature pressure saturated; f, frequency; HCO_3^-, bicarbonate; HR, heart rate; $P(A-a)O_2$, alveolar-arterial PO_2 difference; $P(a-ET)CO_2$, arterial-end-tidal PCO_2 difference; P_{ETCO_2}, end-tidal PCO_2; P_{ETO_2}, end-tidal PO_2; R, respiratory exchange ratio; STPD, standard temperature pressure dry; $\dot{V}CO_2$, carbon dioxide output; V_D/V_T, physiological dead space-tidal volume ratio; $\dot{V}E$, minute ventilation; $\dot{V}E/\dot{V}CO_2$, ventilatory equivalent for carbon dioxide; $\dot{V}E/\dot{V}O_2$, ventilatory equivalent for oxygen; $\dot{V}O_2$, oxygen uptake.

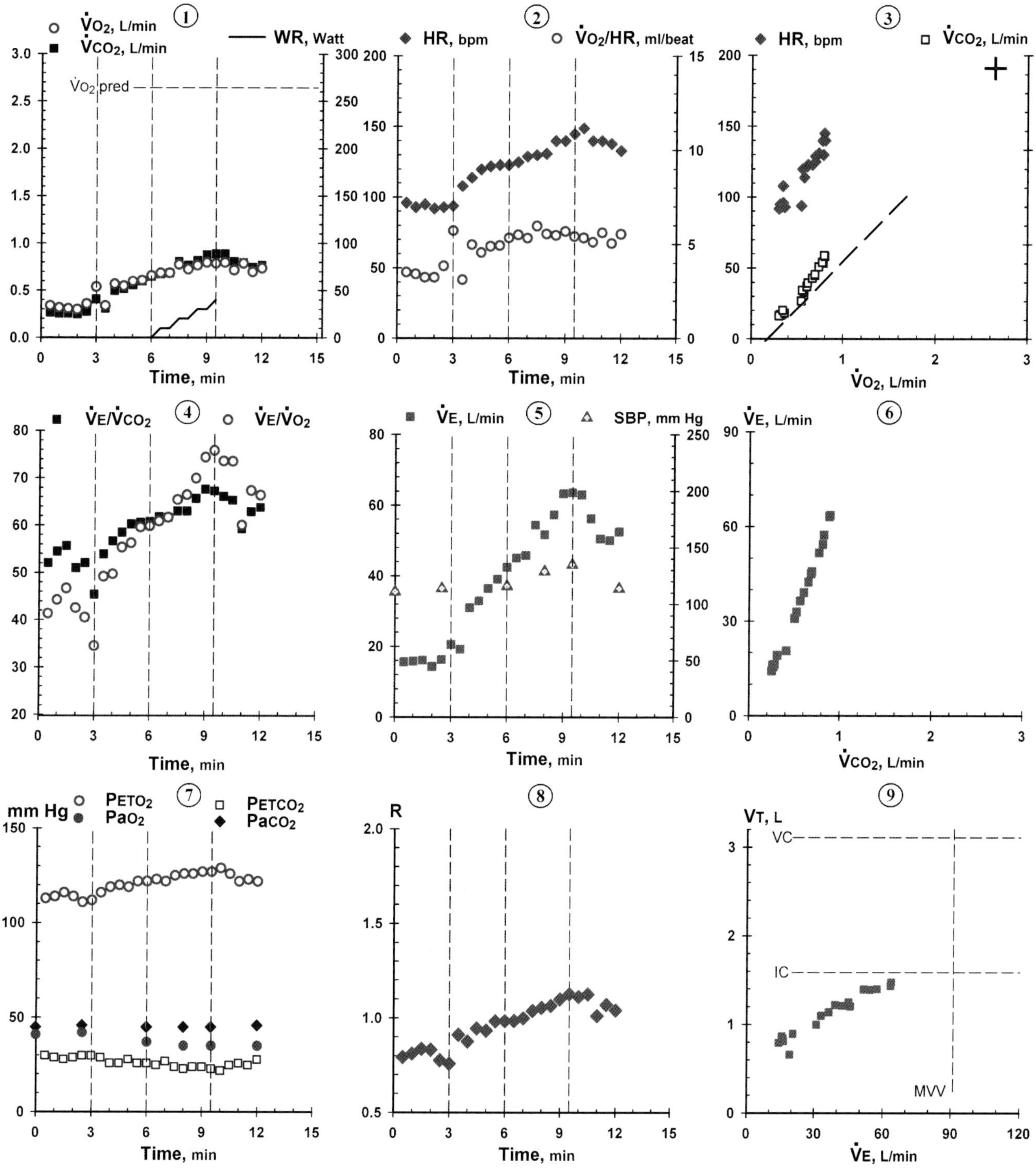

FIGURE 10.50.1. Air breathing. Vertical dashed lines in the panels in the left and middle columns indicate, from left to right, the beginning of unloaded cycling, start of increasing work rate (WR) at 10 W/min, and start of recovery. In **panel 1**, the increase in WR (right y-axis) is plotted with a scale of 100 W to 1 L of oxygen uptake ($\dot{V}O_2$) (left y-axis) such that WR is plotted parallel to a $\dot{V}O_2$ slope of 10 mL/min/W. In **panel 3**, carbon dioxide output ($\dot{V}CO_2$) (right y-axis) is plotted as a function of $\dot{V}O_2$ (x-axis) with identical scales so that the diagonal dashed line has a slope of 1 (45°). The $\dot{V}CO_2$ increasing more steeply than $\dot{V}O_2$ defines carbon dioxide CO_2 derived from bicarbonate buffer, as long as ventilatory equivalent for CO_2 ($\dot{V}E/\dot{V}CO_2$) (**panel 4**) is not increasing and end-tidal PCO_2 ($PETCO_2$) (**panel 7**) is not decreasing, simultaneously. The black + symbol in **panel 3** indicates predicted peak values of heart rate (HR) (left y-axis) and $\dot{V}O_2$ for this individual. Abbreviations: IC, inspiratory capacity; MVV, maximum voluntary ventilation; $PETO_2$, end-tidal PO_2; R, respiratory exchange ratio; SBP, systolic blood pressure; VC, vital capacity; $\dot{V}E$, minute ventilation; $\dot{V}E/\dot{V}O_2$, ventilatory equivalent for oxygen; V_T, tidal volume.

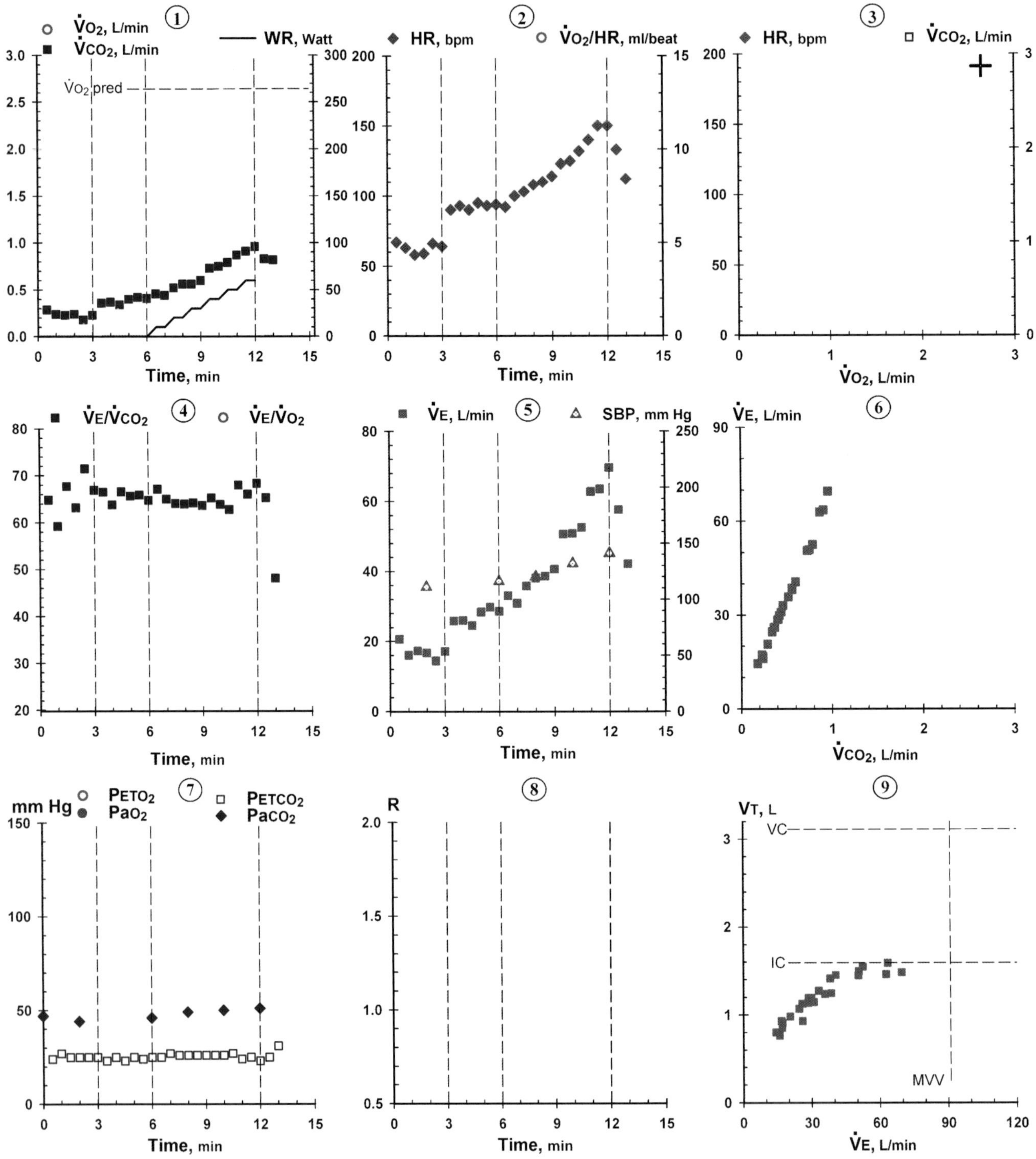

FIGURE 10.50.2. Oxygen breathing. Vertical dashed lines in the panels in the left and middle columns indicate the beginning of unloaded cycling, the start of increasing work rate (WR) at 10 W/min, and the start of recovery. Oxygen uptake ($\dot{V}O_2$) data are not shown because of technical limitations of calculation with very high inspired oxygen levels. Abbreviations: HR, heart rate; IC, inspiratory capacity; MVV, maximum voluntary ventilation; P_{ETCO_2}, end-tidal P_{CO_2}; P_{ETO_2}, end-tidal P_{O_2}; R, respiratory exchange ratio; SBP, systolic blood pressure; VC, vital capacity; $\dot{V}CO_2$, carbon dioxide output; $\dot{V}E$, minute ventilation; $\dot{V}E/\dot{V}CO_2$, ventilatory equivalent for carbon dioxide; $\dot{V}E/\dot{V}O_2$, ventilatory equivalent for oxygen; V_T, tidal volume.

CASE 51

Pulmonary Arterial Hypertension on Multidrug Therapy

CLINICAL FINDINGS

A 41-year-old woman with idiopathic pulmonary hypertension had serial exercise tests to monitor her condition. She had been treated since age 34 with a number of classes of pulmonary hypertension drugs. At age 40, she reported that she was able to do essential work and home activities but avoided strenuous activities and was short of breath on walking uphill or ascending stairs. She worked in an office. She had experienced hemoptysis in the year prior, which was treated with bronchial artery embolization. Her medications included sildenafil and ambrisentan for pulmonary hypertension and an angiotensin-converting enzyme inhibitor for systemic hypertension. When she returned for testing 1 year later, she was taking an inhaled investigational pulmonary hypertension drug as part of a clinical trial, along with continued use of medications she had been taking the prior year. She felt generally better and reported that she had been able to resume yoga classes, which she had discontinued years earlier. Physical examination on the occasion of both tests revealed clear breath sounds and a regular cardiac rhythm with a II/VI holosystolic murmur. There was no peripheral edema. Resting electrocardiograms showed sinus rhythm with T-wave inversions in inferior and lateral leads. Demographic and pulmonary function data are shown in **Table 10.51.1**.

TABLE 10.51.1 Selected Respiratory Function Data

Measurement	Predicted age 40	Measured	Measured
Age (y)		40	41
Sex		Female	Female
Height (cm)		150	150
Weight (kg)		42.7	44.5
VC (L)	2.5	2.09	2.07
IC (L)	1.95	1.44	1.41
ERV (L)	0.55	0.62	0.72
FEV_1 (L)	2.07	1.58	1.63
FEV_1/VC (%)	83	76	79
MVV (L/min)	92	76	78

Abbreviations: ERV, expiratory reserve volume; FEV_1, forced expiratory volume in 1 second; IC, inspiratory capacity; MVV, maximum voluntary ventilation; VC, vital capacity.

EXERCISE FINDINGS

For both tests the patient exercised on a cycle ergometer beginning with 3 minutes of unloaded pedaling at 60 rpm followed by continuous increase in work rate by 10 W/min. On both occasions, she ended exercise with symptoms of leg fatigue. Key variables from the two tests are shown in **Table 10.51.2**. Exercise data for tests at ages 40 and 41 are shown in **Tables 10.51.3** and **10.51.4** and in **Figures 10.51.1** and **10.51.2**, respectively.

INTERPRETATION

Comment

This case is presented because it illustrates the effect of shunting through a patent foramen ovale on the gas exchange measurements in a patient with pulmonary arterial hypertension. On the first test, monitoring of transcutaneous P_{CO_2} as an approximation of arterial P_{CO_2} showed the effect of the ventilatory responses in maintaining P_{CO_2} homeostasis. On the second test 1 year later, there were unusually marked improvements in exercise gas exchange variables, much of which is attributable to reduction or absence of exercise induced right-to-left shunt on the second test. This may have resulted from beneficial effects of a new medication, although there could be additional factors affecting right atrial pressures, and therefore the occurrence of shunting, at the time of testing.

Analysis

Test at Age 40 (see Fig. 10.51.1 and Table 10.51.3)

The cardiovascular and metabolic responses to exercise were very abnormal. Peak $\dot{V}O_2$ increased less than normal relative to work rate and peak $\dot{V}O_2$ was low (panel 1). The oxygen pulse increased very little between rest and exercise and remained lower than the predicted maximum throughout the test (panel 2). Although the peak heart rate was low, the slope of heart rate relative to $\dot{V}O_2$ (panel 3) was steeper than average. The anaerobic threshold was low (panel 3).

The ventilatory response to exercise was typical of the response to exercise-induced right-to-left shunt, with an abrupt increase in $\dot{V}E$, respiratory exchange ratio, the ventilatory equivalents, and P_{ETO_2} at the start of exercise. There was a simultaneous decrease in P_{ETCO_2}, but transcutaneous P_{CO_2} remained stable at resting values (see **Table 10.51.3**),

TABLE 10.51.2 Selected Exercise Data

Measurement	Predicted age 40	Measured age 40	Measured age 41
Peak $\dot{V}O_2$ (L/min)	1.46	0.58	0.76
Maximum heart rate (beats/min)	180	135	133
Maximum O_2 pulse (mL/beat)	8.1	4.4	5.7
$\Delta\dot{V}O_2/\Delta WR$ (mL/min/W)	10.3	5.1	8.4
AT (L/min)	>0.68	0.43	0.48
Blood pressure (mm Hg [rest, max])		130/83, 208/87	134/81, 174/88
Maximum $\dot{V}E$ (L/min)	76	45	38
Breathing reserve (L/min)	>15	31	38
$\dot{V}E/\dot{V}CO_2$ @ *AT* (L/min)	<32	54	38
SpO_2 (% [rest, max ex])		97, 80	97, 95

Abbreviations: *AT*, anaerobic threshold; $\Delta\dot{V}O_2/\Delta WR$, change in $\dot{V}O_2$/change in work rate; ex, exercise; O_2, oxygen; SpO_2, oxygen saturation as measured by pulse oximetry; $\dot{V}E$, minute ventilation; $\dot{V}E/\dot{V}CO_2$, ventilatory equivalent for carbon dioxide; $\dot{V}O_2$, oxygen uptake.

TABLE 10.51.3 Age 40[a]

Time (min)	Work rate (W)	BP (mm Hg)	HR (min^{-1})	f (min^{-1})	$\dot{V}E$ (L/min BTPS)	$\dot{V}CO_2$ (L/min STPD)	$\dot{V}O_2$ (L/min STPD)	$\frac{\dot{V}O_2}{HR}$ (mL/beat)	R	pH	HCO_3^- (mEq/L)	a ET	a SpO_2	a (A − a)	PCO_2, mm Hg ET	PCO_2, mm Hg tc	PCO_2, mm Hg (a − ET)	$\frac{\dot{V}E}{\dot{V}CO_2}$	$\frac{\dot{V}E}{\dot{V}O_2}$	$\frac{V_D}{V_T}$
0.5	Rest		95	17	10.0	0.20	0.22	2.3	0.89			120	96		25	24.8		50	45	0.25
1.0	Rest		98	18	11.4	0.22	0.24	2.5	0.92			121	96		25	24.9		52	47	0.28
1.5	Rest		94	22	11.6	0.21	0.21	2.2	1.01			124	97		24	25.3		55	55	0.32
2.0	Rest	130/83	93	21	10.2	0.19	0.22	2.3	0.90			119	97		26	25.3		52	47	0.29
2.5	Rest		93	21	10.5	0.20	0.20	2.1	0.99			123	96		25	25.4		53	52	0.28
3.0	Rest		93	22	9.8	0.18	0.19	2.1	0.94			121	97		26	25.7		54	50	0.29
3.5	Unloaded		100	28	16.6	0.31	0.28	2.8	1.08			126	97		23	25.8		54	59	0.32
4.0	Unloaded		104	28	19.0	0.35	0.30	2.9	1.15			128	95		22	25.8		55	63	0.34
4.5	Unloaded		103	29	18.5	0.35	0.31	3.0	1.13			127	94		23	25.5		54	60	0.31
5.0	Unloaded		103	28	18.1	0.33	0.29	2.9	1.11			127	94		23	25.3		55	61	0.33
5.5	Unloaded	166/91	103	26	16.4	0.30	0.29	2.8	1.04			125	93		23	25.3		54	57	0.32
6.0	Unloaded		106	31	18.6	0.34	0.33	3.1	1.04			126	93		23	25.2		54	56	0.32
6.5	3		106	27	18.6	0.35	0.34	3.2	1.04			125	93		23	25.3		52	54	0.31
7.0	8		109	27	19.1	0.37	0.35	3.2	1.05			126	92		23	25.3		52	54	0.30
7.5	13		113	30	23.0	0.42	0.38	3.4	1.12			128	91		22	25.3		54	61	0.34
8.0	18	170/94	115	29	22.4	0.41	0.37	3.2	1.12			128	90		22	25.2		54	60	0.34
8.5	23		117	28	23.8	0.45	0.41	3.5	1.11			127	90		23	24.9		53	58	0.32
9.0	28		118	26	26.1	0.52	0.45	3.8	1.15			128	89		23	24.9		51	58	0.29
9.5	33		123	29	31.5	0.61	0.48	3.9	1.26			130	88		22	25.1		52	65	0.32
10.0	38	208/87	126	31	34.8	0.66	0.50	4.0	1.31			131	87		22	25.2		53	69	0.34
10.5	43		129	31	38.0	0.71	0.53	4.1	1.34			132	85		21	25.1		53	71	0.35
11.0	48		132	30	37.7	0.73	0.56	4.3	1.30			131	83		22	25.2		51	67	0.33
11.5	53		135	38	44.6	0.80	0.57	4.3	1.40			133	81		20	25.2		56	78	0.37
12.0	Recovery		134	36	45.1	0.82	0.59	4.4	1.38			133	80		20	25.3		55	76	0.37
12.5	Recovery		127	33	43.2	0.81	0.60	4.8	1.35			132	77		21	25.3		53	71	0.35
13.0	Recovery		125	30	37.6	0.72	0.53	4.3	1.35			131	79		22	25.4		52	71	0.34
13.5	Recovery		122	31	36.3	0.68	0.49	4.0	1.37			132	84		22	25.4		54	74	0.35

Abbreviations: BP, blood pressure; BTPS, body temperature pressure saturated; f, frequency; HCO_3^-, bicarbonate; HR, heart rate; $P(A - a)O_2$, alveolar-arterial PO_2 difference; $P(a - ET)CO_2$, arterial-end-tidal PCO_2 difference; $PETCO_2$, end-tidal PCO_2; $PETO_2$, end-tidal PO_2; $PtcCO_2$, transcutaneous PCO_2; R, respiratory exchange ratio; SpO_2, oxygen saturation as measured by pulse oximetry; STPD, standard temperature pressure dry; $\dot{V}CO_2$, carbon dioxide output; V_D/V_T, physiological dead space-tidal volume ratio; $\dot{V}E$, minute ventilation; $\dot{V}E/\dot{V}CO_2$, ventilatory equivalent for carbon dioxide; $\dot{V}E/\dot{V}O_2$, ventilatory equivalent for oxygen; $\dot{V}O_2$, oxygen uptake.

[a]The V_D/V_T was calculated using $PtcCO_2$ as an estimate of arterial PCO_2.

TABLE 10.51.4 Age 41

Time (min)	Work rate (W)	BP (mm Hg)	HR (min^{-1})	f (min^{-1})	$\dot{V}E$ (L/min BTPS)	$\dot{V}CO_2$ (L/min STPD)	$\dot{V}O_2$ (L/min STPD)	$\frac{\dot{V}O_2}{HR}$ (mL/beat)	R	pH	HCO_3^- (mEq/L)	PO_2, mm Hg and SpO_2, % ET	SpO_2	(A − a)	PCO_2, mm Hg ET	a	(a − ET)	$\frac{\dot{V}E}{\dot{V}CO_2}$	$\frac{\dot{V}E}{\dot{V}O_2}$	$\frac{VD}{VT}$
0.5	Rest		65	18	7.4	0.16	0.20	3.1	0.81			112	98		32			46	37	
1.0	Rest		80	17	6.8	0.14	0.19	2.3	0.78			109	97		33			47	36	
1.5	Rest	134/81	74	20	7.7	0.16	0.20	2.7	0.79			111	97		32			48	38	
2.0	Unloaded		74	22	10.3	0.22	0.25	3.3	0.90			117	98		30			47	42	
2.5	Unloaded		81	26	11.7	0.25	0.28	3.5	0.88			116	98		30			47	41	
3.0	Unloaded		83	31	12.1	0.24	0.29	3.5	0.81			114	97		30			51	41	
3.5	Unloaded		84	27	12.6	0.28	0.34	4.0	0.83			114	97		30			46	38	
4.0	Unloaded		88	28	13.4	0.30	0.36	4.1	0.83			114	97		30			45	37	
4.5	Unloaded	136/85	88	26	13.7	0.31	0.35	4.0	0.87			116	97		30			44	39	
5.0	2		87	28	14.5	0.32	0.37	4.2	0.89			116	98		30			45	40	
5.5	7		92	27	13.5	0.30	0.35	3.8	0.87			115	98		30			44	38	
6.0	12		92	30	14.7	0.33	0.38	4.1	0.86			115	98		30			45	39	
6.5	17		95	29	15.1	0.35	0.40	4.2	0.89			115	98		31			43	38	
7.0	22	150/85	99	29	16.5	0.41	0.45	4.5	0.92			115	98		31			40	37	
7.5	27		104	27	18.4	0.48	0.48	4.6	0.99			117	97		32			39	38	
8.0	32		107	29	21.1	0.54	0.51	4.8	1.06			119	97		32			39	41	
8.5	37		113	29	24.0	0.63	0.56	5.0	1.13			120	97		31			38	43	
9.0	42	174/88	117	28	25.9	0.69	0.59	5.0	1.17			121	97		31			38	44	
9.5	47		123	29	28.8	0.77	0.65	5.2	1.19			122	96		31			38	45	
10.0	52		130	32	33.1	0.85	0.70	5.4	1.22			124	96		30			39	47	
10.5	57		133	38	38.3	0.93	0.76	5.7	1.23			125	95		28			41	50	
11.0	Recovery		129	29.	33.6	0.88	0.73	5.7	1.20			123	95		30			38	46	
11.5	Recovery	188/67	116	29	30.4	0.78	0.59	5.1	1.32			125	96		29			39	52	
12.0	Recovery		109	28	25.7	0.63	0.45	4.1	1.41			127	98		28			41	57	
12.5	Recovery		104	27	22.1	0.51	0.37	3.6	1.38			127	98		28			43	59	
13.0	Recovery		104	27	17.9	0.41	0.32	3.0	1.31			126	98		28			43	57	

Abbreviations: BP, blood pressure; BTPS, body temperature pressure saturated; f, frequency; HCO_3^-, bicarbonate; HR, heart rate; $P(A - a)O_2$, alveolar-arterial PO_2 difference; $P(a - ET)CO_2$, arterial-end-tidal PCO_2 difference; $PETCO_2$, end-tidal PCO_2; $PETO_2$, end-tidal PO_2; R, respiratory exchange ratio; SpO_2, oxygen saturation as measured by pulse oximetry; STPD, standard temperature pressure dry; $\dot{V}CO_2$, carbon dioxide output; VD/VT, physiological dead space–tidal volume ratio; $\dot{V}E$, minute ventilation; $\dot{V}E/\dot{V}CO_2$, ventilatory equivalent for carbon dioxide; $\dot{V}E/\dot{V}O_2$, ventilatory equivalent for oxygen; $\dot{V}O_2$, oxygen uptake.

supporting the interpretation that the augmented ventilatory response was compensation for the amount of shunted carbon dioxide. The pulse oximeter SpO_2 began to decline shortly thereafter, also consistent with central shunting.

Inefficiency of pulmonary gas exchange is reflected in the decrease in SpO_2, the steep slope of $\dot{V}E$ relative to $\dot{V}CO_2$, and associated high values for the ventilatory equivalents. These findings are expected consequences of right-to-left shunt.

Test at Age 41 (see Fig. 10.51.2 and Table 10.51.4)

This test also demonstrated gas exchange responses that are consistent with impaired cardiac output and stroke volume. Peak $\dot{V}O_2$, peak O_2 pulse, and anaerobic threshold were all low. A higher peak $\dot{V}O_2$ was attained and the $\Delta\dot{V}O_2/\Delta WR$ is less shallow than on the prior test. The R value increased at the start of recovery on the second test, in contrast to the previous study. This results from faster recovery dynamics of $\dot{V}O_2$ at the end of exercise because there was less accumulation of abnormal oxygen deficit during incremental work. In this test, the ventilatory equivalents decreased during exercise, end-tidal gas tensions were less changed, and SpO_2 was better maintained than on the prior test.

Conclusion

Both of these tests demonstrated impaired cardiovascular responses to exercise. The most striking difference between the two was the reduction or absence of findings reflecting augmentation of ventilation due to right-to-left shunting at the start of exercise on the second test.

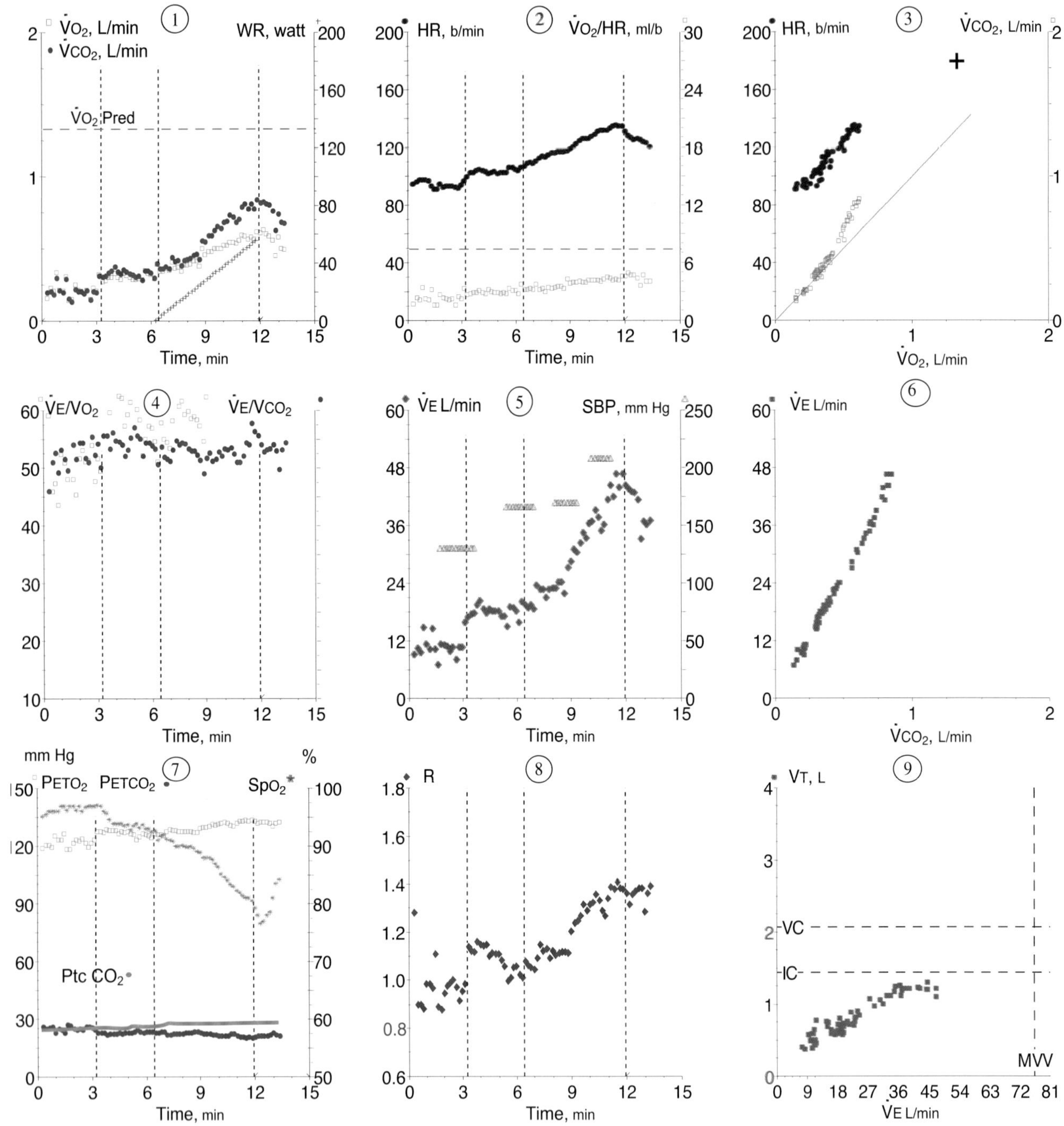

FIGURE 10.51.1. Age 40. Vertical dashed lines in the panels in the left and middle columns indicate, from left to right, the beginning of unloaded cycling, start of increasing work rate (WR) at 10 W/min, and start of recovery. In **panel 1**, the increase in WR (right y-axis) is plotted with a scale of 100 W to 1 L of oxygen uptake ($\dot{V}O_2$) (left y-axis) such that WR is plotted parallel to a $\dot{V}O_2$ slope of 10 mL/min/W. Predicted peak $\dot{V}O_2$ is shown as a dashed horizontal line. In **panel 3**, carbon dioxide output ($\dot{V}CO_2$) (right y-axis) is plotted as a function of $\dot{V}O_2$ (x-axis) with identical scales so that the diagonal blue line has a slope of 1 (45°). The $\dot{V}CO_2$ increasing more steeply than $\dot{V}O_2$ defines carbon dioxide (CO_2) derived from bicarbonate buffer, as long as ventilatory equivalent for CO_2 ($\dot{V}E/\dot{V}CO_2$) (**panel 4**) is not increasing and end-tidal PCO_2 ($PETCO_2$) (**panel 7**) is not decreasing, simultaneously. The black + symbol in **panel 3** indicates predicted peak values of heart rate (HR) (left y-axis) and $\dot{V}O_2$ for this individual. Abbreviations: IC, inspiratory capacity; MVV, maximum voluntary ventilation; $PETO_2$, end-tidal PO_2; PtcCO$_2$, transcutaneous PCO_2 R, respiratory exchange ratio; SBP, systolic blood pressure; SpO_2, oxygen saturation as measured by pulse oximetry; VC, vital capacity; $\dot{V}E$, minute ventilation; $\dot{V}E/\dot{V}O_2$, ventilatory equivalent for oxygen; V_T, tidal volume.

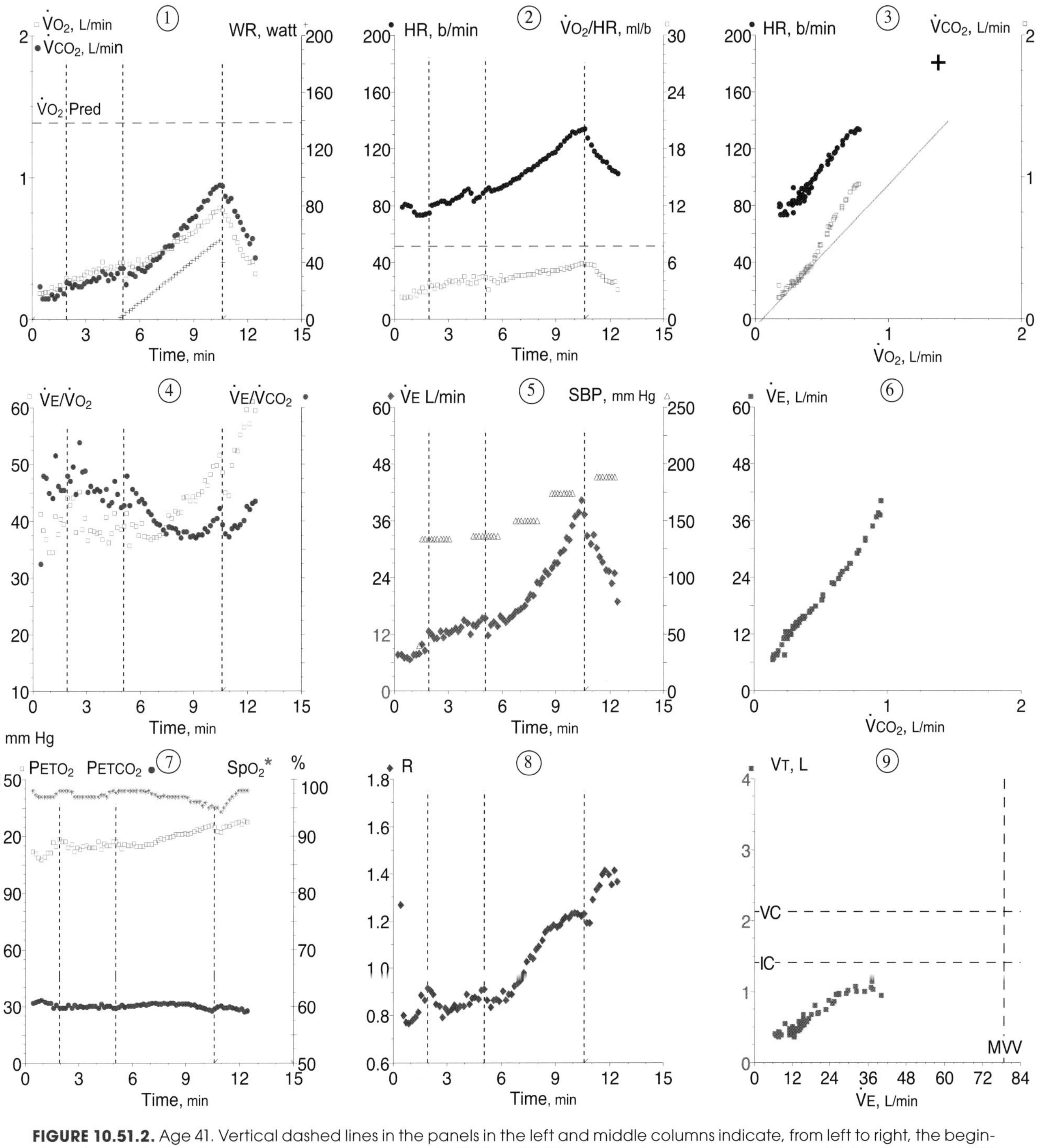

FIGURE 10.51.2. Age 41. Vertical dashed lines in the panels in the left and middle columns indicate, from left to right, the beginning of unloaded cycling, start of increasing work rate (WR) at 10 W/min, and start of recovery. In **panel 1**, the increase in WR (right y-axis) is plotted with a scale of 100 W to 1 L of oxygen uptake ($\dot{V}O_2$) (left y-axis) such that WR is plotted parallel to a $\dot{V}O_2$ slope of 10 mL/min/W. Predicted peak $\dot{V}O_2$ is shown as a dashed horizontal line. In **panel 3**, carbon dioxide output ($\dot{V}CO_2$) (right y-axis) is plotted as a function of $\dot{V}O_2$ (x-axis) with identical scales so that the diagonal blue line has a slope of 1 (45°). The $\dot{V}CO_2$ increasing more steeply than $\dot{V}O_2$ defines carbon dioxide (CO_2) derived from bicarbonate buffer, as long as ventilatory equivalent for CO_2 ($\dot{V}E/\dot{V}CO_2$) (**panel 4**) is not increasing and end-tidal PCO_2 ($PETCO_2$) (**panel 7**) is not decreasing, simultaneously. The black + symbol in **panel 3** indicates predicted peak values of heart rate (HR) (left y-axis) and $\dot{V}O_2$ for this individual. Abbreviations: IC, inspiratory capacity; MVV, maximum voluntary ventilation; $PETO_2$, end-tidal PO_2; R, respiratory exchange ratio; SBP, systolic blood pressure; SpO_2, oxygen saturation as measured by pulse oximetry; VC, vital capacity; $\dot{V}E$, minute ventilation; $\dot{V}E/\dot{V}O_2$, ventilatory equivalent for oxygen; V_T, tidal volume.

CASE 52

Pulmonary Hypertension, Patent Foramen Ovale, and Exercise-Induced Right-to-Left Shunt

CLINICAL FINDINGS

This 61-year-old woman had first noted mild exertional dyspnea 3 years prior to evaluation. Sometime later, she began to have recurring episodes of depression and confusion. She was evaluated in emergency departments for acute episodes of dyspnea, chest pain, and anxiety, which were interpreted as panic anxiety attacks. She was given a benzodiazepam for her mental symptoms and a β-blocker for systemic hypertension. She subsequently presented to the psychiatric emergency department with acute anxiety and suicidal ideation. Medical evaluation revealed findings of pulmonary hypertension including right ventricular hypertrophy on electrocardiogram, and hypoxemia on arterial blood gas analysis. With oxygen (O_2) therapy, her mental status improved. There was no history of cigarette smoking, exposure to other medications or drugs, environmental toxins, pulmonary emboli, or thrombophlebitis. Exercise testing was requested to evaluate her functional status and the mechanism of her hypoxemia. Examination at the time revealed mild obesity, hypertension, and a prominent S4 heart sound.

EXERCISE FINDINGS

The patient performed exercise on a cycle ergometer. She pedaled at 60 rpm without added load for 3 minutes. The work rate was then increased 5 W/min to her symptom-limited maximum. Arterial blood was sampled every second minute, and intra-arterial blood pressure was recorded from a percutaneously placed brachial artery catheter. She stopped exercise because of shortness of breath. There were no arrhythmias, ST-segment changes, or T-wave changes with exercise. Following a rest period of 30 minutes, the exercise study was repeated with the patient breathing 100% O_2.

INTERPRETATION

Comments

The results of this patient's resting respiratory function tests showed mild airway obstruction (**Table 10.52.1**). The electrocardiogram was compatible with right ventricular hypertrophy. The exercise test was repeated with the subject breathing 100% O_2 to evaluate the possible development of a right-to-left shunt through a foramen ovale when exercise-induced right atrial pressure rose due to increased venous return—a possible cause of activity-induced hypoxemia, which might contribute to this patient's symptoms. Data for the two exercise studies are summarized in **Table 10.52.2** and shown in **Tables 10.52.3** and **10.52.4** and graphically in **Figures 10.52.1** and **10.52.2**.

Analysis

On the room air study, peak oxygen uptake ($\dot{V}O_2$) was reduced and the anaerobic threshold was judged indeterminate but probably low. Notably, she had a very high heart rate reserve because she stopped exercising at a peak heart rate of only 87 beats/min. She had a very steep $\dot{V}E$ versus $\dot{V}CO_2$ slope (panel 6) and very high ventilatory equivalent for carbon dioxide ($\dot{V}E/\dot{V}CO_2$), which was due partly to hyperventilation (low $PaCO_2$). This was likely chronic because R was not elevated during the study. Despite this, her breathing reserve was normal. While a high $\dot{V}E/\dot{V}CO_2$ would be seen with hyperventilation, arterial blood gases allow calculation of physiological dead space–tidal volume ratio (V_D/V_T), which was abnormally high and increased during exercise. The rising V_D/V_T, positive $P(a - ET)CO_2$, and severely reduced PaO_2 during exercise highly suggest pulmonary vascular disease.

Using the flowcharts (Chapter 9), the low $\dot{V}O_2$ and likely low anaerobic threshold lead to Flowchart 4, where the breathing reserve was normal (Branch Point 4.1). The $\dot{V}E/\dot{V}CO_2$ during exercise was high (Branch Point 4.3), supporting the diagnosis of abnormal pulmonary circulation.

TABLE 10.52.1 Selected Respiratory Function Data

Measurement	Predicted	Measured
Age (y)		61
Sex		Female
Height (cm)		147
Weight (kg)	53	61
Hematocrit (%)		37
VC (L)	2.33	2.31
IC (L)	1.56	1.59
TLC (L)	3.66	4.53
FEV_1 (L)	1.90	1.59
FEV_1/VC (%)	81	69
MVV (L/min)	73	59
DLCO (mL/mm Hg/min)	17.6	17.3

Abbreviations: DLCO, diffusing capacity of lung for carbon monoxide; FEV_1, forced expiratory volume in 1 second; IC, inspiratory capacity; MVV, maximum voluntary ventilation; TLC, total lung capacity; VC, vital capacity.

TABLE 10.52.2 Selected Exercise Data

Measurement	Predicted	Room air	Oxygen
Maximum work rate (W)		20	25
Peak $\dot{V}O_2$ (L/min)	1.23	0.62	
Maximum heart rate (beats/min)	159	87	85
Maximum O_2 pulse (mL/beat)	7.8	7.1	
AT (L/min)	>0.61	Indeterminate	
Blood pressure (mm Hg [rest, max])		186/90, 204/90	172/84, 210/102
Maximum $\dot{V}E$ (L/min)		38	42
Exercise breathing reserve (L/min)	>15	21	17
$\dot{V}E/\dot{V}CO_2$ @ *AT* or lowest	30.1	46.3	50.4
PaO_2 (mm Hg [rest, max ex])		71, 40	550, 70
$P(A - a)O_2$ (mm Hg [rest, max ex])		42, 79	138, 612
$PaCO_2$ (mm Hg [rest, max ex])		28, 31	25, 31
$P(a - ET)CO_2$ (mm Hg [rest, max ex])		5, 12	4, 9
VD/VT (rest, heavy ex)		0.31, 0.47	0.34, 0.47
HCO_3^- (mEq/L [rest, 2-min recov])		22, 20	22, 18

Abbreviations: *AT*, anaerobic threshold; ex, exercise; HCO_3^-, bicarbonate; O_2, oxygen; $P(A - a)O_2$, alveolar-arterial PO_2 difference; $P(a - ET)CO_2$, arterial-end-tidal PCO_2 difference; recov, recovery; VD/VT, physiological dead space–tidal volume ratio; $\dot{V}E$, minute ventilation; $\dot{V}E/\dot{V}CO_2$, ventilatory equivalent for carbon dioxide; $\dot{V}O_2$, oxygen uptake.

The patient was hyperventilating (low $PaCO_2$) with a very high $\dot{V}E/\dot{V}CO_2$. However, based on the gas exchange ratio of 0.8 at rest and exercise, the reduced $PaCO_2$ was chronic. Furthermore, the VD/VT calculated using the $PaCO_2$ was increased, confirming that the elevated ventilatory response to exercise was due to elevated dead space, rather than hyperventilation alone. Branch Point 4.5 further distinguishes between abnormal pulmonary circulation due to moderate-to-severe left ventricular failure and that due to pulmonary vascular disease, in that the patient became very hypoxemic with exercise. These findings are supportive of the diagnosis of primary pulmonary vascular disease.

At the lowest work rate, PaO_2 abruptly decreased and continued to decrease as work rate increased. Moreover, $P(a - ET)CO_2$ continued to increase, and VD/VT becomes progressively more abnormal as the work rate increased (**Table 10.52.3**). These changes suggest the development of a right-to-left shunt during exercise. There was also clear evidence of O_2 flow limitation in that $\dot{V}O_2$ and O_2 pulse failed to increase with increasing work rate (panels 1 and 2, respectively, of **Fig 10.52.1**).

To verify whether a right-to-left shunt developed with exercise, PaO_2 was measured at rest and during exercise while the patient was breathing 100% O_2 (**Table 10.52.4**). At rest, PaO_2 was at the lower limit of normal (550 mm Hg); however, with mild exercise, it dropped to 70 mm Hg. This can only be explained by the development of a right-to-left shunt (in contrast, see Cases 48 and 50 in this chapter in which exercise hypoxemia results from $\dot{V}A/\dot{Q}$ mismatching, which is fully reversed with O_2 breathing).

The patient subsequently underwent right heart catheterization, which documented that pulmonary artery pressures were at systemic levels and the catheter slipped easily through a foramen ovale into the left atrium.

Conclusion

A diagnosis of pulmonary arterial hypertension with exercise-induced right-to-left shunt through a patent foramen ovale was made by the exercise studies and was later confirmed by a right heart catheterization. Etiologies of secondary pulmonary vascular disease were excluded, and she was diagnosed as having idiopathic pulmonary hypertension. We speculate that episodic anxiety may have been triggered by transient hypoxemia due to right-to-left shunting during exercise. Her depression and anxiety improved markedly once a physical basis for her symptoms was identified.

TABLE 10.52.3 Air Breathing

Time (min)	Work rate (W)	BP (mm Hg)	HR (min^{-1})	f (min^{-1})	$\dot{V}E$ (L/min BTPS)	$\dot{V}CO_2$ (L/min STPD)	$\dot{V}O_2$ (L/min STPD)	$\frac{\dot{V}O_2}{HR}$ (mL/beat)	R	pH	HCO_3^- (mEq/L)	PO_2, mm Hg ET	a	(A − a)	PCO_2, mm Hg ET	a	(a − ET)	$\frac{\dot{V}E}{\dot{V}CO_2}$	$\frac{\dot{V}E}{\dot{V}O_2}$	$\frac{VD}{VT}$
	Rest	186/90								7.56	21		77			24				
0.5	Rest		60	16	6.8	0.11	0.14	2.3	0.79			122			23			49	39	
1.0	Rest		60	11	6.7	0.12	0.16	2.7	0.75			120			23			48	36	
1.5	Rest		59	17	8.8	0.15	0.22	3.7	0.68			119			24			49	33	
2.0	Rest	206/114	61	14	8.4	0.15	0.21	3.4	0.71	7.52	22	120	71	42	23	28	5	48	34	0.31
2.5	Unloaded		66	22	11.7	0.19	0.25	3.8	0.76			122			23			52	39	
3.0	Unloaded		67	17	11.2	0.20	0.27	4.0	0.74			121			23			49	36	
3.5	Unloaded		71	19	13.7	0.25	0.32	4.5	0.78			121			23			48	38	
4.0	Unloaded	191/94	73	23	14.9	0.27	0.35	4.8	0.77	7.50	21	121	58	57	23	28	5	48	37	0.31
4.5	5		74	32	15.0	0.27	0.37	5.0	0.73			115			27			45	33	
5.0	5		76	23	15.3	0.30	0.39	5.1	0.77			119			25			44	34	
5.5	10		79	26	23.6	0.45	0.58	7.3	0.78			116			26			48	37	
6.0	10	202/96	81	27	25.3	0.46	0.52	6.4	0.88	7.47	23	125	43	72	22	32	10	50	44	0.42
6.5	15		81	25	23.9	0.47	0.57	7.0	0.82			120			25			46	38	
7.0	15		84	32	26.6	0.47	0.54	6.4	0.87			124			23			51	44	
7.5	20		87	36	27.8	0.47	0.58	6.7	0.81			126			22			53	43	
8.0	20	204/90	87	35	37.7	0.61	0.62	7.1	0.98	7.45	21	130	40	79	19	31	12	57	56	0.47
8.5	Recovery		82	33	33.3	0.57	0.61	7.4	0.93			127			21			54	50	
9.0	Recovery		80	28	29.1	0.51	0.55	6.9	0.93			127			21			52	49	
9.5	Recovery		79	23	21.9	0.41	0.46	5.8	0.89			122			24			49	43	
10.0	Recovery	198/87	79	27	24.8	0.43	0.48	6.1	0.90	7.45	20	126	50	67	22	30	8	52	47	0.41

Abbreviations: BP, blood pressure; BTPS, body temperature pressure saturated; f, frequency; HCO_3^-, bicarbonate; HR, heart rate; $P(A-a)O_2$, alveolar-arterial PO_2 difference; $P(a-ET)CO_2$, arterial-end-tidal PCO_2 difference; $PETCO_2$, end-tidal PCO_2; $PETO_2$, end-tidal PO_2; R, respiratory exchange ratio; STPD, standard temperature pressure dry; $\dot{V}CO_2$, carbon dioxide output; VD/VT, physiological dead space-tidal volume ratio; $\dot{V}E$, minute ventilation; $\dot{V}E/\dot{V}CO_2$, ventilatory equivalent for carbon dioxide; $\dot{V}E/\dot{V}O_2$, ventilatory equivalent for oxygen; $\dot{V}O_2$, oxygen uptake.

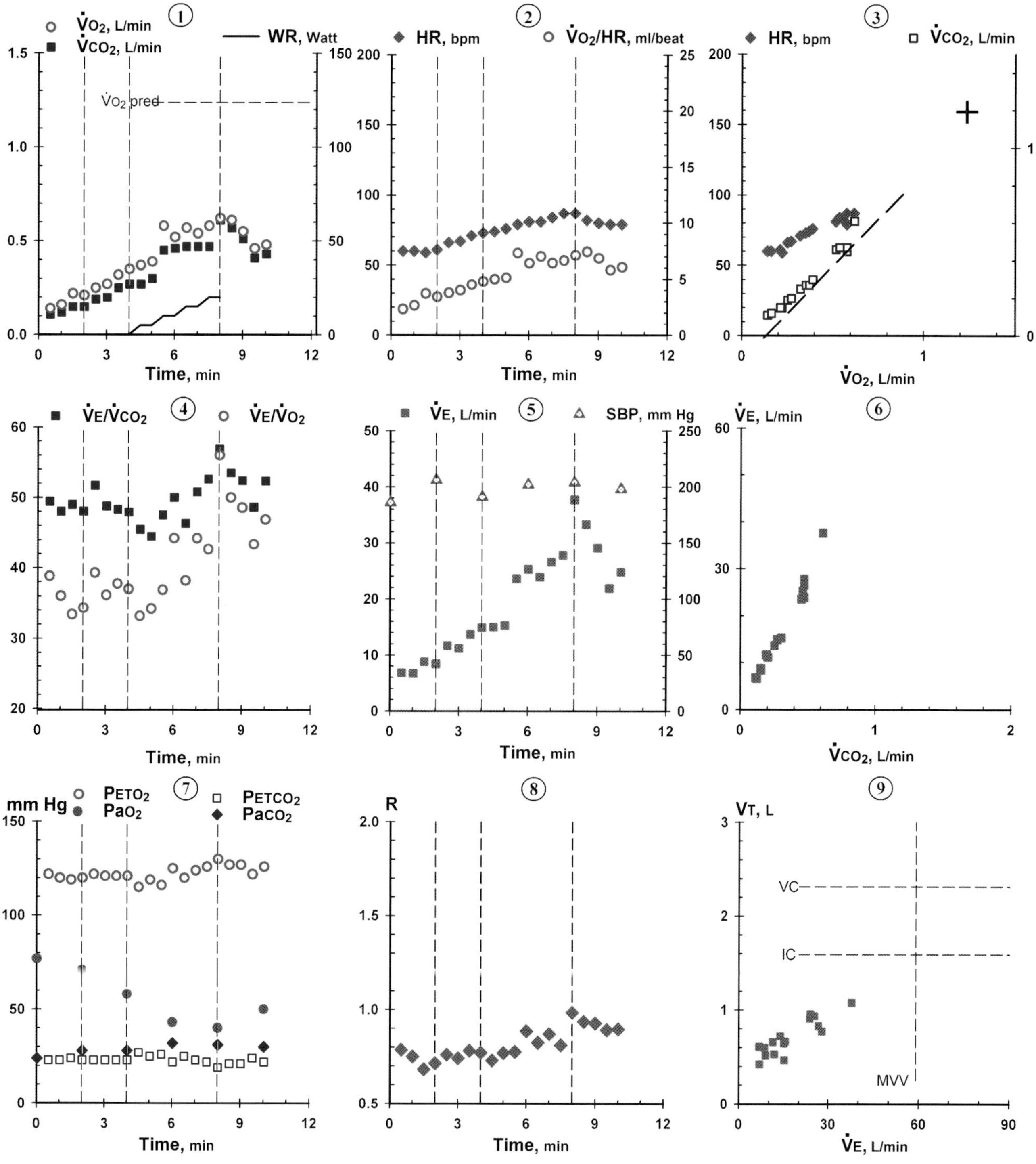

FIGURE 10.52.1. Air breathing. Vertical dashed lines in the panels in the left and middle columns indicate, from left to right, the beginning of unloaded cycling, start of increasing work rate (WR) at 5 W/min, and start of recovery. In **panel 1**, the increase in WR (right y-axis) is plotted with a scale of 100 W to 1 L of oxygen uptake ($\dot{V}O_2$) (left y-axis) such that WR is plotted parallel to a $\dot{V}O_2$ slope of 10 mL/min/W. In **panel 3**, carbon dioxide output ($\dot{V}CO_2$) (right y-axis) is plotted as a function of $\dot{V}O_2$ (x-axis) with identical scales so that the diagonal dashed line has a slope of 1 (45°). The $\dot{V}CO_2$ increasing more steeply than $\dot{V}O_2$ defines carbon dioxide (CO_2) derived from bicarbonate buffer, as long as ventilatory equivalent for CO_2 ($\dot{V}E/\dot{V}CO_2$) (**panel 4**) is not increasing and end-tidal PCO_2 ($PETCO_2$) (**panel 7**) is not decreasing, simultaneously. The black + symbol in **panel 3** indicates predicted peak values of heart rate (HR) (left y-axis) and $\dot{V}O_2$ for this individual. Abbreviations: IC, inspiratory capacity; MVV, maximum voluntary ventilation; $PETO_2$, end-tidal PO_2; R, respiratory exchange ratio; SBP, systolic blood pressure; VC, vital capacity; $\dot{V}E$, minute ventilation; $\dot{V}E/\dot{V}O_2$, ventilatory equivalent for oxygen; V_T, tidal volume.

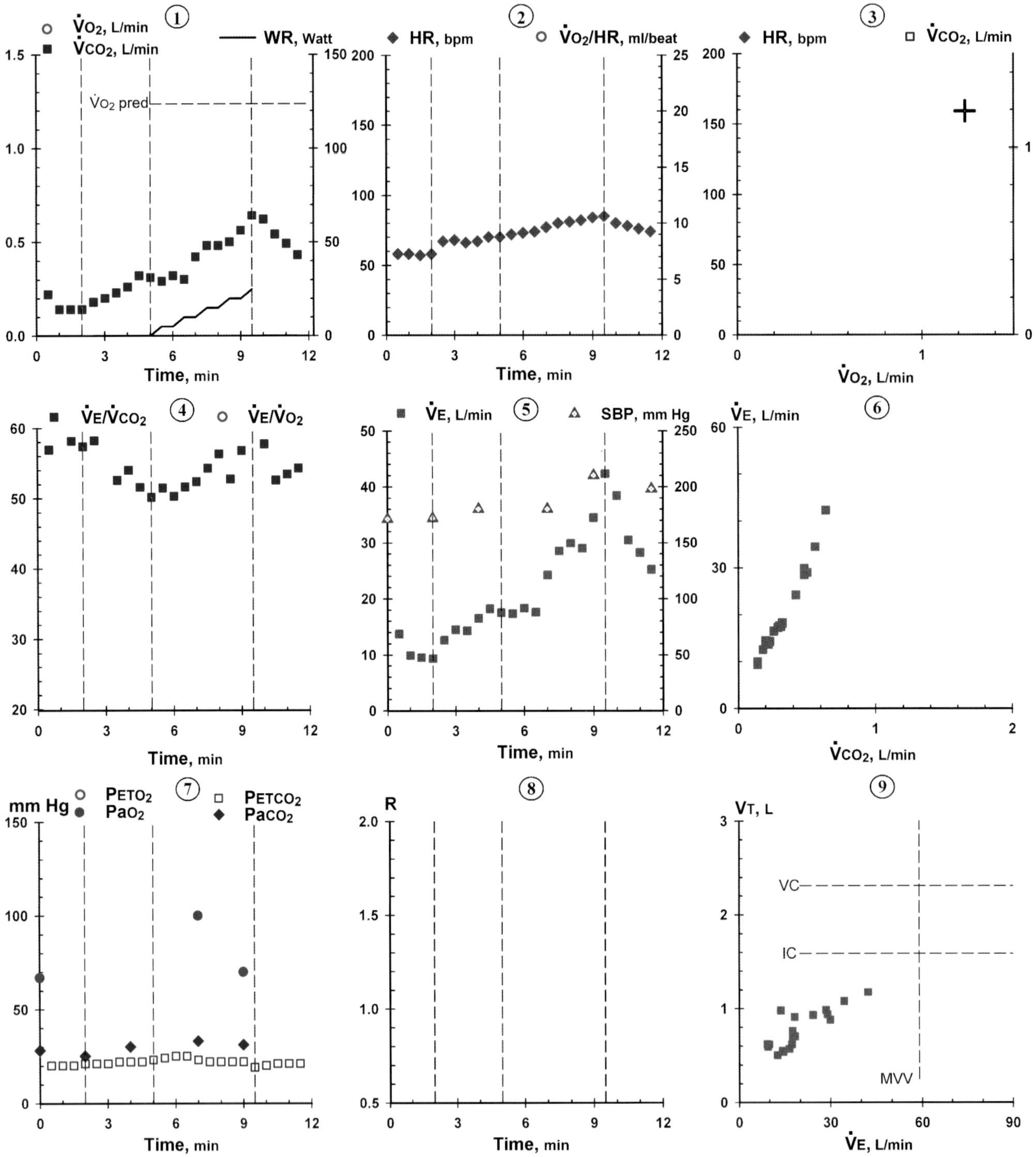

FIGURE 10.52.2. Oxygen breathing. Vertical dashed lines in the panels in the left and middle columns indicate, from left to right, the beginning of unloaded cycling, start of increasing work rate (WR) at 5 W/min, and start of recovery. Oxygen uptake ($\dot{V}O_2$) data are not shown because of technical limitations of calculation with very high-inspired oxygen levels. Abbreviations: HR, heart rate; IC, inspiratory capacity; MVV, maximum voluntary ventilation; P_{ETCO_2}, end-tidal P_{CO_2}; P_{ETO_2}, end-tidal P_{O_2}; R, respiratory exchange ratio; SBP, systolic blood pressure; VC, vital capacity; $\dot{V}CO_2$, carbon dioxide output; $\dot{V}E$, minute ventilation; $\dot{V}E/\dot{V}CO_2$, ventilatory equivalent for carbon dioxide; $\dot{V}E/\dot{V}O_2$, ventilatory equivalent for oxygen; V_T, tidal volume.

TABLE 10.52.4 Oxygen Breathing

Time (min)	Work rate (W)	BP (mm Hg)	HR (min^{-1})	f (min^{-1})	$\dot{V}_E$ (L/min BTPS)	$\dot{V}CO_2$ (L/min STPD)	$\dot{V}O_2$ (L/min STPD)	$\frac{\dot{V}O_2}{HR}$ (mL/beat)	R	pH	HCO_3^- (mEq/L)	PO_2, mm Hg ET	a	(A − a)	PCO_2, mm Hg ET	a	(a − ET)	$\frac{\dot{V}_E}{\dot{V}CO_2}$	$\frac{\dot{V}_E}{\dot{V}O_2}$	$\frac{V_D}{V_T}$
	Rest	171/78								7.50	21		67			28				
0.5	Rest		58	14	13.7	0.22									20			57		
1.0	Rest		58	16	9.9	0.14									20			61		
1.5	Rest		57	16	9.5	0.14									20			58		
2.0	Rest	172/84	58	15	9.3	0.14				7.53	21		550	138	21	25	4	57		0.34
2.5	Unloaded		67	25	12.6	0.18									21			58		
3.0	Unloaded		68	27	14.5	0.20									21			61		
3.5	Unloaded		66	26	14.3	0.23									22			53		
4.0	Unloaded	180/87	67	29	16.5	0.26				7.48	22		386	297	22	30	8	54		0.40
4.5	Unloaded		70	20	18.2	0.32									22			52		
5.0	Unloaded		70	23	17.5	0.31									23			50		
5.5	5		72	28	17.3	0.29									24			51		
6.0	5		73	26	18.3	0.32									25			50		
6.5	10		74	25	17.6	0.30									25			52		
7.0	10	180/84	77	26	24.2	0.42				7.44	22		100	580	23	33	10	52		0.45
7.5	15		80	29	28.5	0.48									22			54		
8.0	15		81	34	29.9	0.48									22			56		
8.5	20		82	31	29.0	0.50									22			53		
9.0	20	210/102	84	32	34.5	0.56				7.45	21		70	612	22	31	9	57		0.47
9.5	25		85	36	42.3	0.64									19			61		
10.0	Recovery		80	31	38.4	0.62									20			58		
10.5	Recovery		78	25	30.5	0.54									21			53		
11.0	Recovery		76	24	28.2	0.49									21			53		
11.5	Recovery	198/92	74	22	25.2	0.43									21			54		

Abbreviations: BP, blood pressure; BTPS, body temperature pressure saturated; f, frequency; HCO_3^-, bicarbonate; HR, heart rate; $P(A - a)O_2$, alveolar-arterial PO_2 difference; $P(A - ET)CO_2$, arterial-end-tidal PCO_2 difference; $PETCO_2$, end-tidal PCO_2; $PETO_2$, end-tidal PO_2; R, respiratory exchange ratio; STPD, standard temperature pressure dry; $\dot{V}CO_2$, carbon dioxide output; V_D/V_T, physiological dead space–tidal volume ratio; $\dot{V}_E$, minute ventilation; $\dot{V}_E/\dot{V}CO_2$, ventilatory equivalent for carbon dioxide; $\dot{V}_E/\dot{V}O_2$, ventilatory equivalent for oxygen; $\dot{V}O_2$, oxygen uptake.

CASE 53

Idiopathic Pulmonary Arterial Hypertension Before and After Treatment

To view this case please access the eBook bundled with this text. Instructions are located on the inside front cover.

CASE 54

Long-Standing Idiopathic Pulmonary Arterial Hypertension: Serial Tests Over 17 Years of Treatment

CLINICAL FINDINGS

At age 34, this man was found to have idiopathic pulmonary hypertension and was treated with a calcium channel blocker, the only medication available for this condition at the time. His condition deteriorated such that, by age 38, he was disabled from his work and placed on a waiting list for heart–lung transplant. At age 40, pulmonary artery pressures were at systemic levels, and he was largely nonambulatory with signs and symptoms of right heart failure. After initiation of investigational intravenous epoprostenol therapy, he had gradual improvement and progressively resumed activities. He first underwent exercise testing as part of a research protocol at age 41 soon after beginning epoprostenol. At age 47, he began to have annual exercise tests to track his functional capacity and response to changes in medications. Exercise tests performed at age 50 and at age 58 are presented here. At the time of both of these tests, he reported being physically active and doing construction projects around his home and property. He frequently experienced symptoms of light-headedness but did not have syncope, and identified fatigue and dyspnea as his major limiting symptoms. At age 50, his medications included intravenous epoprostenol, diuretics, warfarin, and digoxin. At the time of the test at age 58, epoprostenol had been replaced with subcutaneous treprostinil and oral sildenafil, and he was using supplemental oxygen (O_2) at night. On both occasions, he was noted to have a flushed appearance, consistent with his eicosanoid therapy. Cardiac examinations were notable for a prominent second heart sound; there was minimal ankle edema. The resting electrocardiograms showed right ventricular hypertrophy.

EXERCISE FINDINGS

Both tests were conducted on a cycle ergometer, beginning after a period of rest with 3 minutes of pedaling at 60 rpm without added load, followed by continuous increase in work rate until the patient reached symptom limitation. On the first test, work rate was incremented by 10 W/min, and on the subsequent test, the increment was 15 W/min. He ended both tests with leg fatigue. There were no significant ischemic changes on electrocardiogram during either test. Occasional ventricular ectopy was noted during the latter part of the second test.

INTERPRETATION

Comments

Pulmonary function tests showed low normal vital capacity and mild airflow obstruction with a reduction in DLCO at age 50. Airflow obstruction was of moderate severity at age 58 (**Table 10.54.1**).

TABLE 10.54.1 Selected Respiratory Function Data

	Age 50		Age 58	
Measurement	Predicted	Measured	Predicted	Measured
Age (y)		50		58
Sex		Male		Male
Height (cm)		183		183
Weight (kg)		88		90
VC (L)	5.16	4.59	5.17	3.83
IC (L)	3.44	3.46	3.53	3.27
FEV_1 (L)	4.19	3.02	3.93	2.12
FEV_1/VC (%)	81	66	76	55
MVV (L/min)	160	123	150	103
DLCO (mL/mm Hg/min)	31.6	23.8		

Abbreviations: DLCO, diffusing capacity of lung for carbon monoxide; FEV_1, forced expiratory volume in 1 second; IC, inspiratory capacity; MVV, maximum voluntary ventilation; VC, vital capacity.

Analysis

On the first test shown at age 50 (**Table 10.54.3** and **Figure 10.54.1**), peak oxygen uptake ($\dot{V}O_2$) was moderately reduced relative to predicted values, and the anaerobic threshold (*AT*) was low (**Table 10.54.2**). However, $\Delta\dot{V}O_2/\Delta WR$ was normal, and O_2 pulse was only mildly reduced. The ventilatory equivalents decreased early in exercise but remained higher than normal at the *AT* (panel 4, **Figure 10.54.1**), consistent with ventilation-perfusion ($\dot{V}A/\dot{Q}$) mismatching. The abnormalities are typical of pulmonary vascular disease limiting cardiac output and impairing normal $\dot{V}A/\dot{Q}$ matching in the lung. Findings at age 58 (**Tables 10.54.2** and **10.54.4** and **Fig. 10.54.2**) were qualitatively similar, but the abnormalities were more severe, with lower values for peak $\dot{V}O_2$ and *AT*, higher ventilatory equivalents, and lower O_2 saturation readings. Results of serial exercise tests spanning a period of 17 years are summarized in **Table 10.54.5**. During the first decade of treatment of his pulmonary hypertension, there were progressive increases in peak $\dot{V}O_2$, *AT*, and O_2 pulse and a decrease in the $\dot{V}E/\dot{V}CO_2$ value measured at the *AT*. Over subsequent years, there was a trend for reduction in peak $\dot{V}O_2$, O_2 pulse, and *AT*, indicative of deteriorating cardiovascular function, and increase in $\dot{V}E/\dot{V}CO_2$ at the *AT*, consistent with worsening $\dot{V}/\dot{Q}$ matching.

Conclusion

This patient is presented both as an example of typical exercise findings related to pulmonary vascular disease and as a unique longitudinal series over an extended period of observation. The first test shown reflects the patient near his best function; the decline in exercise capacity over the next 8 years is associated with worsening indices of pulmonary gas exchange, reflecting the functional effects of persistent pulmonary vascular disease.

TABLE 10.54.2 Selected Exercise Data

	Age 50		Age 58	
Measurement	Predicted	Measured	Predicted	Measured
Peak $\dot{V}O_2$ (L/min)	2.69	1.66	2.46	1.35
Maximum heart rate (beats/min)	170	133	162	150
Maximum O_2 pulse (mL/beat)	15.8	12.7	15.2	9.9
$\Delta\dot{V}O_2/\Delta WR$ (mL/min/W)	10.3	8.9	10.3	7.8
AT (L/min)	>1.21	0.89	>1.13	0.66
Blood pressure (mm Hg [rest, max])		110/64, 165/84		103/76, 192/118
Maximum $\dot{V}E$ (L/min)		81		78
Exercise breathing reserve (L/min)	>15	42	>15	25
$\dot{V}E/\dot{V}CO_2$ @ *AT* or lowest	26.7	40.7	27.5	45.7

Abbreviations: *AT*, anaerobic threshold; $\Delta\dot{V}O_2/\Delta WR$, change in $\dot{V}O_2$/change in work rate; O_2, oxygen; $\dot{V}E$, minute ventilation; $\dot{V}E/\dot{V}CO_2$, ventilatory equivalent for carbon dioxide; $\dot{V}O_2$, oxygen uptake.

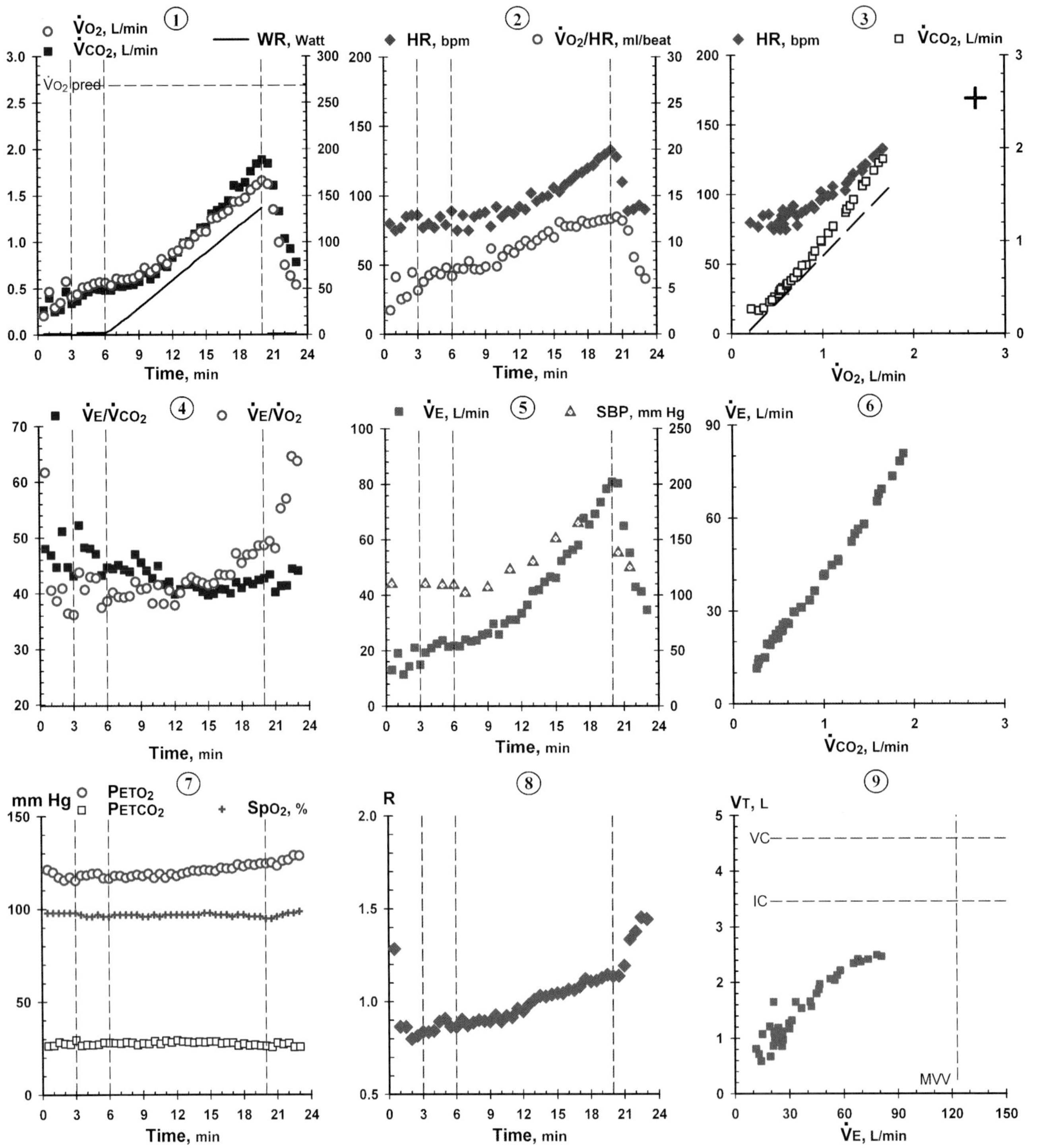

FIGURE 10.54.1. Test performed at age 50. Vertical dashed lines in the panels in the left and middle columns indicate, from left to right, the beginning of unloaded cycling, start of increasing work rate (WR) at 10 W/min, and start of recovery. In **panel 1**, the increase in WR (right y-axis) is plotted with a scale of 100 W to 1 L of oxygen uptake ($\dot{V}O_2$) (left y-axis) such that WR is plotted parallel to a $\dot{V}O_2$ slope of 10 mL/min/W. In **panel 3**, carbon dioxide output ($\dot{V}CO_2$) (right y-axis) is plotted as a function of $\dot{V}O_2$ (x-axis) with identical scales so that the diagonal dashed line has a slope of 1 (45°). The $\dot{V}CO_2$ increasing more steeply than $\dot{V}O_2$ defines carbon dioxide (CO_2) derived from bicarbonate buffer, as long as ventilatory equivalent for CO_2 ($\dot{V}E/\dot{V}CO_2$) (**panel 4**) is not increasing and end-tidal PCO_2 ($PETCO_2$) (**panel 7**) is not decreasing, simultaneously. The black + symbol in **panel 3** indicates predicted peak values of heart rate (HR) (left y-axis) and $\dot{V}O_2$ for this individual. Abbreviations: IC, inspiratory capacity; MVV, maximum voluntary ventilation; $PETO_2$, end-tidal PO_2; R, respiratory exchange ratio; SBP, systolic blood pressure; SpO_2, oxygen saturation as measured by pulse oximetry; VC, vital capacity; $\dot{V}E$, minute ventilation; $\dot{V}E/\dot{V}O_2$, ventilatory equivalent for oxygen; V_T, tidal volume.

TABLE 10.54.3 Air Breathing, Age 50

Time (min)	Work rate (W)	BP (mm Hg)	HR (min^{-1})	f (min^{-1})	$\dot{V}_E$ (L/min BTPS)	$\dot{V}CO_2$ (L/min STPD)	$\dot{V}O_2$ (L/min STPD)	$\frac{\dot{V}O_2}{HR}$ (mL/beat)	R	pH	HCO_3^- (mEq/L)	PO_2, mm Hg ET	PO_2, mm Hg a	PO_2, mm Hg (A – a)	PCO_2, mm Hg ET	PCO_2, mm Hg a	PCO_2, mm Hg (a – ET)	$\frac{\dot{V}_E}{\dot{V}CO_2}$	$\frac{\dot{V}_E}{\dot{V}O_2}$	$\frac{V_D}{V_T}$
0																				
0.5	Rest	110/64	80	18	13.0	0.27	0.21	2.6	1.28			121			26			48	62	
1.0	Rest		75	16	19.0	0.41	0.47	6.3	0.87			120			27			47	41	
1.5	Rest		77	14	11.5	0.26	0.30	3.8	0.86			117			28			45	39	
2.0	Rest		85	24	14.3	0.28	0.35	4.1	0.80			116			28			51	41	
2.5	Rest		86	13	21.2	0.47	0.58	6.7	0.82			117			27			45	36	
3.0	Rest		86	14	15.0	0.35	0.41	4.8	0.84			115			30			43	36	
3.5	Unloaded	110/64	77	29	19.4	0.37	0.44	5.7	0.84			118			27			52	44	
4.0	Unloaded		80	24	21.0	0.43	0.52	6.4	0.84			118			27			48	41	
4.5	Unloaded		77	24	22.6	0.47	0.53	6.8	0.89			119			27			48	43	
5.0	Unloaded	109/65	85	24	23.8	0.51	0.56	6.5	0.91			119			27			47	43	
5.5	Unloaded		79	19	21.4	0.50	0.57	7.2	0.87			117			28			43	37	
6.0	Unloaded		89	22	21.9	0.49	0.57	6.4	0.86			117			28			45	39	
6.5	5		75	20	21.6	0.49	0.54	7.2	0.90			118			28			44	40	
7.0	10	102/66	86	23	24.1	0.53	0.61	7.1	0.87			118			28			45	39	
7.5	15		75	20	23.4	0.53	0.60	7.9	0.89			117			28			44	39	
8.0	19		85	20	23.8	0.54	0.60	7.1	0.90			118			28			44	40	
8.5	24		87	30	25.8	0.55	0.61	7.0	0.90			119			27			47	42	
9.0	29	107/69	88	27	26.4	0.58	0.65	7.4	0.89			118			28			46	41	
9.5	34		78	23	29.7	0.67	0.73	9.3	0.93			119			28			44	41	
10.0	39		92	23	25.9	0.61	0.68	7.4	0.89			117			29			43	38	
10.5	44		85	25	29.9	0.66	0.72	8.5	0.92			119			28			45	42	
11.0	49	123/68	89	24	31.2	0.75	0.82	9.2	0.92			117			29			42	38	
11.5	54		87	24	31.2	0.74	0.77	8.9	0.96			119			29			42	41	
12.0	59		92	20	33.5	0.84	0.89	9.6	0.95			118			29			40	38	
12.5	64		90	24	36.5	0.90	0.91	10.1	0.98			119			29			41	40	
13.0	69	130/78	102	25	41.4	1.00	0.99	9.7	1.01			120			29			42	42	
13.5	73		96	27	42.0	1.01	0.98	10.2	1.03			121			28			42	43	
14.0	79		99	25	44.8	1.09	1.06	10.7	1.03			121			29			41	42	
14.5	84		100	24	46.7	1.16	1.11	11.1	1.04			121			28			40	42	
15.0	88	151/80	106	25	46.2	1.16	1.11	10.5	1.04			121			29			40	41	
15.5	93		103	25	52.4	1.31	1.25	12.2	1.04			121			29			40	42	
16.0	98		108	27	54.9	1.35	1.26	11.7	1.06			122			28			41	43	
16.5	103		111	26	56.3	1.38	1.30	11.7	1.06			122			28			41	43	
17.0	108	165/84	115	26	58.1	1.45	1.34	11.7	1.08			122			28			40	43	
17.5	113		117	28	67.8	1.61	1.44	12.3	1.12			124			27			42	47	
18.0	118		120	28	65.5	1.60	1.44	12.0	1.11			123			28			41	45	
18.5	122		122	29	69.4	1.65	1.48	12.1	1.11			124			27			42	47	
19.0	127		127	30	73.6	1.76	1.56	12.3	1.13			124			27			42	47	
19.5	132		130	31	78.4	1.85	1.62	12.4	1.14			125			27			42	49	
20.0	137		133	33	80.9	1.89	1.66	12.5	1.14			125			26			43	49	
20.5	Recovery	138/72	128	32	80.4	1.85	1.63	12.7	1.14			125			26			43	49	
21.0	Recovery		110	25	65.0	1.62	1.35	12.3	1.19			124			28			40	48	
21.5	Recovery	125/68	89	23	55.3	1.34	1.00	11.2	1.34			126			28			41	55	
22.0	Recovery		90	18	43.0	1.04	0.75	8.4	1.38			127			28			41	57	
22.5	Recovery		93	21	41.3	0.93	0.64	6.9	1.45			129			26			44	65	
23.0	Recovery		90	19	34.7	0.79	0.54	6.0	1.44			129			26			44	64	

Abbreviations: BP, blood pressure; BTPS, body temperature pressure saturated; f, frequency; HCO_3^-, bicarbonate; HR, heart rate; $P(A - a)O_2$, alveolar-arterial PO_2 difference; $P(a - ET)CO_2$, arterial-end-tidal PCO_2 difference; $PETCO_2$, end-tidal PCO_2; $PETO_2$, end-tidal PO_2; R, respiratory exchange ratio; STPD, standard temperature pressure dry; $\dot{V}CO_2$, carbon dioxide output; V_D/V_T, physiological dead space–tidal volume ratio; $\dot{V}_E$, minute ventilation; $\dot{V}_E/\dot{V}CO_2$, ventilatory equivalent for carbon dioxide; $\dot{V}_E/\dot{V}O_2$, ventilatory equivalent for oxygen; $\dot{V}O_2$, oxygen uptake.

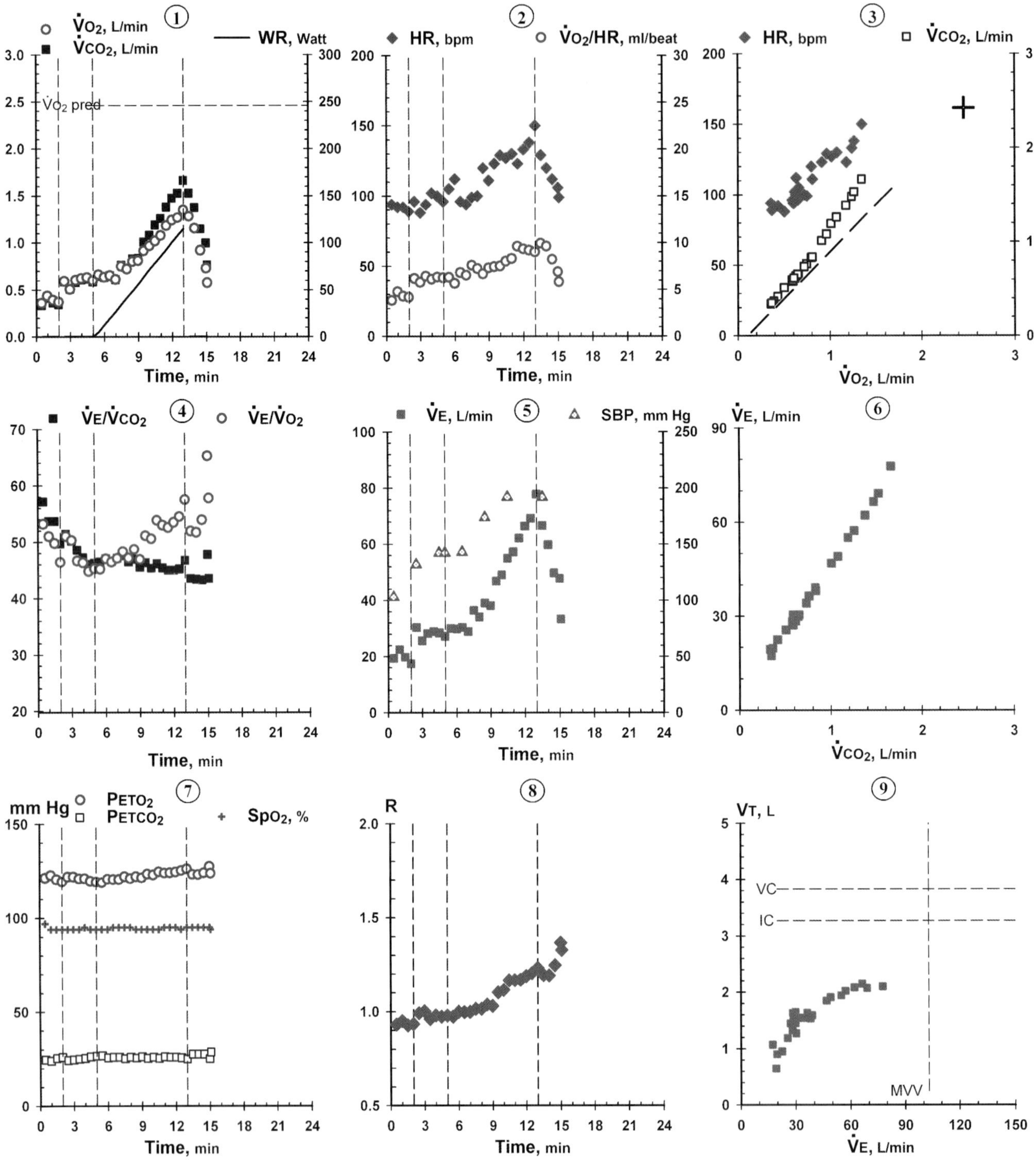

FIGURE 10.54.2. Test performed at age 58. Vertical dashed lines in the panels in the left and middle columns indicate, from left to right, the beginning of unloaded cycling, start of increasing work rate (WR) at 15 W/min, and start of recovery. In **panel 1**, the increase in WR (right y-axis) is plotted with a scale of 100 W to 1 L of oxygen uptake ($\dot{V}O_2$) (left y-axis) such that WR is plotted parallel to a $\dot{V}O_2$ slope of 10 mL/min/W. In **panel 3**, carbon dioxide output ($\dot{V}CO_2$) (right y-axis) is plotted as a function of $\dot{V}O_2$ (x-axis) with identical scales so that the diagonal dashed line has a slope of 1 (45°). The $\dot{V}CO_2$ increasing more steeply than $\dot{V}O_2$ defines carbon dioxide (CO_2) derived from bicarbonate buffer, as long as ventilatory equivalent for CO_2 ($\dot{V}E/\dot{V}CO_2$) (**panel 4**) is not increasing and end-tidal PCO_2 ($PETCO_2$) (**panel 7**) is not decreasing, simultaneously. The black + symbol in **panel 3** indicates predicted peak values of heart rate (HR) (left y-axis) and $\dot{V}O_2$ for this individual. Abbreviations: IC, inspiratory capacity; MVV, maximum voluntary ventilation; $PETO_2$, end-tidal PO_2; R, respiratory exchange ratio; SBP, systolic blood pressure; SpO_2, oxygen saturation as measured by pulse oximetry; VC, vital capacity; $\dot{V}E$, minute ventilation; $\dot{V}E/\dot{V}O_2$, ventilatory equivalent for oxygen; V_T, tidal volume.

TABLE 10.54.4 Air Breathing, Age 58

Time (min)	Work rate (W)	BP (mm Hg)	HR (min^{-1})	f (min^{-1})	$\dot{V}E$ (L/min BTPS)	$\dot{V}CO_2$ (L/min STPD)	$\dot{V}O_2$ (L/min STPD)	$\frac{\dot{V}O_2}{HR}$ (mL/beat)	R	pH	HCO_3^- (mEq/L)	PO_2, mm Hg ET	PO_2, mm Hg a	PO_2, mm Hg (A − a)	PCO_2, mm Hg ET	PCO_2, mm Hg a	PCO_2, mm Hg (a − ET)	$\frac{\dot{V}E}{\dot{V}CO_2}$	$\frac{\dot{V}E}{\dot{V}O_2}$	$\frac{VD}{VT}$
0.5	Rest	103/76	94	30	19.3	0.34	0.36	3.9	0.93			121			25			57	53	
1.0	Rest		92	24	22.5	0.42	0.44	4.8	0.95			123			24			54	51	
1.5	Rest		92	22	19.7	0.37	0.40	4.3	0.93			121			25			54	50	
2.0	Rest		89	16	17.4	0.35	0.37	4.2	0.93			119			26			50	46	
2.5	Unloaded	132/98	96	24	30.3	0.59	0.59	6.2	0.99			122			24			51	51	
3.0	Unloaded		88	22	25.6	0.51	0.51	5.8	1.00			122			25			50	50	
3.5	Unloaded		94	21	28.2	0.58	0.61	6.4	0.96			121			25			49	47	
4.0	Unloaded		102	19	28.9	0.61	0.62	6.1	0.98			121			25			47	46	
4.5	Unloaded	142/118	100	18	28.4	0.62	0.63	6.3	0.97			120			26			46	45	
5.0	Unloaded		96	19	27.2	0.59	0.60	6.3	0.98			119			27			46	45	
5.5	5	142/118	105	18	30.0	0.65	0.66	6.3	0.97			119			27			46	45	
6.0	13		112	21	29.9	0.63	0.64	5.7	1.00			121			26			47	47	
6.5	20	143/108	96	20	30.4	0.65	0.65	6.8	1.00			121			26			47	46	
7.0	27		94	20	28.9	0.61	0.61	6.5	1.00			121			26			47	47	
7.5	35		99	22	36.3	0.76	0.75	7.6	1.01			122			25			48	48	
8.0	42		100	22	34.1	0.73	0.72	7.2	1.02			121			26			46	47	
8.5	49	174/96	120	25	39.0	0.83	0.80	6.7	1.04			122			26			47	49	
9.0	56		111	25	38.1	0.84	0.81	7.3	1.03			122			26			46	47	
9.5	64		123	25	46.8	1.01	0.92	7.4	1.10			124			25			46	51	
10.0	72		129	26	49.0	1.08	0.97	7.5	1.12			123			26			45	51	
10.5	79	192/108	127	28	55.0	1.19	1.02	8.0	1.17			125			25			46	54	
11.0	86		130	28	57.2	1.26	1.08	8.3	1.17			124			26			45	53	
11.5	93		123	30	62.2	1.38	1.18	9.6	1.17			124			26			45	53	
12.0	101		133	31	66.5	1.48	1.24	9.3	1.19			125			26			45	54	
12.5	108		138	33	69.2	1.53	1.27	9.2	1.21			125			26			45	55	
13.0	115		150	37	77.8	1.67	1.35	9.0	1.23			126			25			47	58	
13.5	Recovery	192/108	129	29	66.6	1.53	1.28	9.9	1.19			123			28			44	52	
14.0	Recovery		120	27	59.8	1.38	1.16	9.6	1.19			123			28			43	52	
14.5	Recovery		112	23	49.7	1.15	0.92	8.2	1.25			124			28			43	54	
15.0	Recovery		106	28	47.7	1.00	0.73	6.9	1.37			128			25			48	65	
15.5	Recovery		99	16	33.4	0.77	0.58	5.8	1.33			124			29			44	58	

Abbreviations: BP, blood pressure; BTPS, body temperature pressure saturated; f, frequency; HCO_3^-, bicarbonate; HR, heart rate; $P(A - a)O_2$, alveolar-arterial PO_2 difference; $P(a - ET)CO_2$, arterial-end-tidal PCO_2 difference; $PETCO_2$, end-tidal PCO_2; $PETO_2$, end-tidal PO_2; R, respiratory exchange ratio; STPD, standard temperature pressure dry; $\dot{V}CO_2$, carbon dioxide output; VD/VT, physiological dead space–tidal volume ratio; $\dot{V}E$, minute ventilation; $\dot{V}E/\dot{V}CO_2$, ventilatory equivalent for carbon dioxide; $\dot{V}E/\dot{V}O_2$, ventilatory equivalent for oxygen; $\dot{V}O_2$, oxygen uptake.

TABLE 10.54.5 Selected Exercise Data Over 17 Years of Treatment for Pulmonary Hypertension

Age (y)	Peak $\dot{V}O_2$ (L/min)	*AT* (L/min)	Peak $\dot{V}O_2$/HR (mL/beat)	$\dot{V}E/\dot{V}CO_2$ at *AT*
41	1.10	0.80	8.5	50
47	1.46	0.95	11.4	42
48	1.55	0.90	12.2	40
49	1.60	0.75	11.3	40
50	1.66	0.89	12.7	41
51	1.68	1.0	13.0	42
52	1.75	0.90	11.5	40
53	1.74	1.10	10.8	43
54	1.64	0.84	10.6	46
55	1.46	0.96	9.6	44
56	1.43	0.95	9.4	41
57	1.45	0.95	9.6	45
58	1.35	0.66	9.9	46

Abbreviations: *AT*, anaerobic threshold; HR, heart rate; $\dot{V}E/\dot{V}CO_2$, ventilatory equivalent for carbon dioxide; $\dot{V}O_2$, oxygen output.

CASE 55

Intrapulmonary Right-to-Left Shunt Due to Pulmonary Arteriovenous Fistulae

CLINICAL FINDINGS

This 26-year-old man had multiple pulmonary arteriovenous malformations (AVMs) and recurrent brain abscesses. He was referred for exercise testing to assess his functional status before undergoing embolization of the pulmonary AVMs. He denied shortness of breath and, until recently, had worked as an aerobics instructor. The patient was normally developed and thin but muscular. He had no rales or murmurs on examination of the chest but had marked cyanosis and clubbing of the fingers. A recent study while the patient was seated at rest breathing oxygen (O_2) reported an estimated right-to-left shunt of 53%.

EXERCISE FINDINGS

The patient performed exercise on a cycle ergometer. He pedaled at 60 rpm without an added load for 3 minutes. The work rate was then increased continuously at a rate of 20 W/min to tolerance. Blood was sampled every second minute, and intra-arterial pressure was recorded from a percutaneously placed brachial artery catheter. Heart rate and rhythm were continuously monitored; 12-lead electrocardiograms were obtained during rest, exercise, and recovery. The patient appeared to give an excellent effort and stopped exercise because of general and leg fatigue without dyspnea or chest pain. No arrhythmias or ischemic changes were noted on electrocardiogram.

INTERPRETATION

Comments

Resting respiratory function studies showed a mild restrictive defect (**Table 10.55.1**). Hemoglobin concentration was elevated (21.8 g/100 mL) and resting arterial blood analysis showed hypoxemia and a chronic respiratory alkalosis. This case is presented both as an uncommon form of pulmonary vascular disease and to illustrate the effect of right-to-left shunt on the calculated value of V_D/V_T. Exercise data are summarized in **Table 10.55.2** and shown in **Table 10.55.3** and **Figure 10.55.1**.

Analysis

As expected, this patient had severe resting and exercise hypoxemia due to his known large right-to-left shunt from AVMs. What may be surprising is that he also had elevated V_D/V_T and positive $P(a - ET)CO_2$, usually attributed to increased high $\dot{V}_A/\dot{Q}$ regions that would not be seen with the "low" (zero) $\dot{V}_A/\dot{Q}$ of an AVM. In fact, high V_D/V_T and positive $P(a - ET)CO_2$ result from marked "alveolar" hyperventilation of perfused lung regions that is needed to compensate for venous carbon dioxide delivered through the right-to-left shunts to the systemic arterial circulation. The net result is a relatively normal Pa_{CO_2} but with a marked increase in alveolar and minute ventilation ($\dot{V}_E$), as well as $\dot{V}_E/\dot{V}_{CO_2}$. When the high $\dot{V}_E$ and normal Pa_{CO_2} are used to calculate V_D/V_T using the modified Bohr equation, the result is a high V_D/V_T. This phenomenon is also reflected in the large difference between P_{ETCO_2} and Pa_{CO_2}.

Interestingly, the combined effect of the patient's low saturation with secondary erythrocytosis resulted in an arterial O_2 content that was near-normal (**Table 10.55.3**). Although this might make normal convective delivery of O_2 to the periphery possible, the final step of O_2 delivery is diffusive and is dependent on the partial pressure of O_2 in the capillary. This, together with the symptom of breathlessness, likely contributed to the patient's low peak $\dot{V}O_2$ and anaerobic threshold and the termination of exercise prior to attaining predicted peak heart rate.

TABLE 10.55.1 Selected Respiratory Function Data

Measurement	Predicted	Measured
Age (y)		26
Sex		Male
Height (cm)		189
Weight (kg)	87	64
Hemoglobin (g/100 mL)		21.8
VC (L)	5.55	4.18
IC (L)	3.70	2.94
FEV_1 (L)	4.50	3.95
FEV_1/VC (%)	81	94
MVV (L/min)		
Direct	183	169
Indirect	180	158

Abbreviations: FEV_1, forced expiratory volume in 1 second; IC, inspiratory capacity; MVV, maximum voluntary ventilation; VC, vital capacity.

TABLE 10.55.2 Selected Exercise Data

Measurement	Predicted	Measured
Peak $\dot{V}O_2$ (L/min)	3.12	2.19
Maximum heart rate (beats/min)	194	160
Maximum O_2 pulse (mL/beat)	16.1	13.7
$\Delta\dot{V}O_2/\Delta WR$ (mL/min/W)	10.3	9.9
AT (L/min)	>1.28	1.1
Blood pressure (mm Hg [rest, max])		144/84, 180/90
Maximum $\dot{V}E$ (L/min)		123
Exercise breathing reserve (L/min)	>15	35
$\dot{V}E/\dot{V}CO_2$ @ *AT* or lowest	23.9	43.5
SaO_2 (% [rest, max ex])		76, 64
PaO_2 (mm Hg [rest, max ex])		39, 39
$P(A - a)O_2$ (mm Hg [rest, max ex])		74, 76
$PaCO_2$ (mm Hg [rest, max ex])		32, 38
$P(a - ET)CO_2$ (mm Hg [rest, max ex])		9, 15
VD/VT (rest, max ex)		0.42, 0.52
HCO_3^- (mEq/L [rest, 2-min recov])		22, 16

Abbreviations: *AT*, anaerobic threshold; $\Delta\dot{V}O_2/\Delta WR$, change in $\dot{V}O_2$/change in work rate; ex, exercise; HCO_3^-, bicarbonate; O_2, oxygen; $P(A - a)O_2$, alveolar-arterial PO_2 difference; $P(a - ET)CO_2$, arterial-end-tidal PCO_2 difference; recov, recovery; SaO_2, arterial oxygen saturation; VD/VT, physiological dead space-tidal volume ratio; $\dot{V}E$, minute ventilation; $\dot{V}E/\dot{V}CO_2$, ventilatory equivalent for carbon dioxide; $\dot{V}O_2$, oxygen uptake.

Conclusion

The patient had a large right-to-left shunt because of pulmonary AVMs. The high VD/VT and positive $P(a - ET)CO_2$ values reflect the relative inefficiency of ventilation for removing carbon dioxide from the blood, consistent with a portion of right ventricular output bypassing the alveolar capillaries. In this patient, the wide $P(A - a)O_2$, positive $P(a - ET)CO_2$, and high VD/VT reflect the effects of shunting rather than the pulmonary ventilation to perfusion mismatch typical of more common lung and pulmonary vascular diseases.

TABLE 10.55.3 Air Breathing

Time (min)	Work rate (W)	BP (mm Hg)	HR (min^{-1})	f (min^{-1})	$\dot{V}E$ (L/min BTPS)	$\dot{V}CO_2$ (L/min STPD)	$\dot{V}O_2$ (L/min STPD)	$\frac{\dot{V}O_2}{HR}$ (mL/beat)	R	pH	HCO_3^- (mEq/L)	PO_2, mm Hg			PCO_2, mm Hg			$\frac{\dot{V}E}{\dot{V}CO_2}$	$\frac{\dot{V}E}{\dot{V}O_2}$	$\frac{VD}{VT}$
												ET	a	(A − a)	ET	a	(a − ET)			
	Rest									7.43	22		51			33				
0.5	Rest		92	21	22.8	0.38	0.43	4.7	0.88			124			22			55	49	
1.0	Rest		92	21	22.8	0.38	0.43	4.7	0.88			121			22			55	49	
1.5	Rest		92	21	22.8	0.38	0.43	4.7	0.88			124			22			55	49	
2.0	Rest		78	28	18.5	0.31	0.37	4.7	0.84	7.45	22	121	39	74	23	32	9	52	44	0.42
2.5	Rest		83	21	18.6	0.31	0.35	4.2	0.89			123			22			54	48	
3.0	Rest		87	23	17.0	0.27	0.31	3.6	0.87			120			24			56	49	
3.5	Unloaded		88	23	19.1	0.31	0.35	4.0	0.89			124			21			55	49	
4.0	Unloaded		104	29	23.8	0.46	0.61	5.9	0.75			118			24			46	35	
4.5	Unloaded		90	31	30.1	0.59	0.76	8.4	0.78			118			25			47	36	
5.0	Unloaded		86	30	31.3	0.61	0.73	8.5	0.84			120			25			47	39	
5.5	Unloaded		90	30	36.0	0.68	0.80	8.9	0.85			120			25			49	42	
6.0	Unloaded	144/84	91	26	26.9	0.61	0.73	8.0	0.84	7.43	22	118	38	73	30	34	4	45	38	0.41
6.5	10		91	31	38.8	0.74	0.88	9.7	0.84			120			25			49	41	
7.0	20		92	27	32.4	0.66	0.78	8.5	0.85			119			25			46	39	
7.5	30		94	29	36.1	0.72	0.84	8.9	0.86			120			26			47	40	
8.0	40	150/90	96	27	37.2	0.81	0.95	9.9	0.85	7.42	22	118	39	72	25	34	9	43	37	0.39
8.5	50		97	30	40.4	0.85	0.98	10.1	0.87			121			24			45	39	
9.0	60		100	33	40.2	0.90	1.03	10.3	0.87			119			25			42	36	
9.5	70		103	32	40.6	0.94	1.06	10.3	0.89			120			26			40	36	
10.0	80	162/90	102	34	46.2	0.95	1.09	10.7	0.87	7.42	22	121	39	73	25	34	9	46	40	0.42
10.5	90		111	32	58.2	1.16	1.24	11.2	0.94			119			26			48	45	
11.0	100		111	36	63.6	1.25	1.28	11.5	0.98			123			24			48	47	
11.5	110		115	35	63.7	1.30	1.35	11.7	0.96			119			27			47	45	
12.0	120	174/96	122	38	69.0	1.42	1.44	11.8	0.99	7.38	20	124	39	76	24	35	11	46	46	0.45
12.5	130		127	39	73.7	1.54	1.53	12.0	1.01			124			25			46	46	
13.0	140		136	44	90.2	1.76	1.70	12.5	1.05			126			23			49	51	
13.5	150		161	43	92.9	1.90	1.80	11.2	1.06			126			24			47	50	
14.0	160	180/90	149	41	91.5	1.93	1.84	12.3	1.05	7.36	20	121	39	76	27	36	9	46	48	0.46
14.5	170		154	53	115.0	2.23	2.03	13.2	1.10			125			24			50	54	
15.0	180	180/96	160	53	123.3	2.42	2.19	13.7	1.11	7.31	19	127	39	76	23	38	15	49	54	0.52
15.5	Recovery		162	49	115.0	2.12	1.84	11.4	1.15			129			28			52	60	
16.0	Recovery		140	45	106.9	1.75	1.37	9.8	1.28			132			20			59	75	
16.5	Recovery		125	41	86.4	1.32	0.99	7.9	1.33			134			18			63	84	
17.0	Recovery	156/84	124	41	73.7	1.15	0.88	7.1	1.31	7.30	16	134	43	79	19	34	15	61	80	0.56

Abbreviations: BP, blood pressure; BTPS, body temperature pressure saturated; f, frequency; HCO_3^-, bicarbonate; HR, heart rate; $P(A - a)O_2$, alveolar-arterial PO_2 difference; $P(a - ET)CO_2$, arterial-end-tidal PCO_2 difference; $PETCO_2$, end-tidal PCO_2; $PETO_2$, end-tidal PO_2; R, respiratory exchange ratio; STPD, standard temperature pressure dry; $\dot{V}CO_2$, carbon dioxide output; VD/VT, physiological dead space–tidal volume ratio; $\dot{V}E$, minute ventilation; $\dot{V}E/\dot{V}CO_2$, ventilatory equivalent for carbon dioxide; $\dot{V}E/\dot{V}O_2$, ventilatory equivalent for oxygen; $\dot{V}O_2$, oxygen uptake.

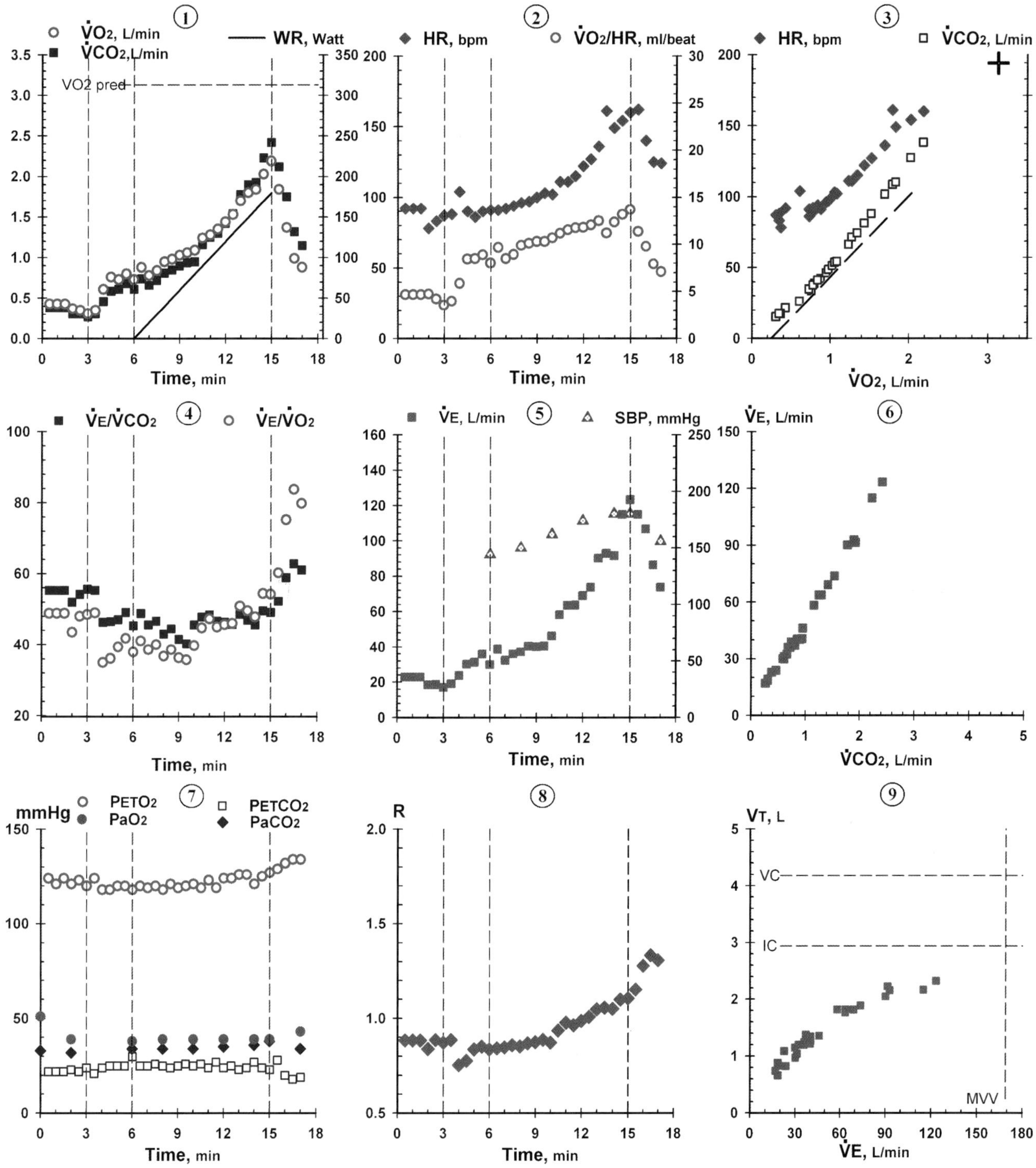

FIGURE 10.55.1. Vertical dashed lines in the panels in the left and middle columns indicate, from left to right, the beginning of unloaded cycling, start of increasing work rate (WR) at 20 W/min, and start of recovery. In **panel 1**, the increase in WR (right y-axis) is plotted with a scale of 100 W to 1 L of oxygen uptake ($\dot{V}O_2$) (left y-axis) such that WR is plotted parallel to a $\dot{V}O_2$ slope of 10 mL/min/W. In **panel 3**, carbon dioxide output ($\dot{V}CO_2$) (right y-axis) is plotted as a function of $\dot{V}O_2$ (x-axis) with identical scales so that the diagonal dashed line has a slope of 1 (45°). The $\dot{V}CO_2$ increasing more steeply than $\dot{V}O_2$ defines carbon dioxide (CO_2) derived from bicarbonate buffer, as long as ventilatory equivalent for CO_2 ($\dot{V}E/\dot{V}CO_2$) (**panel 4**) is not increasing and end-tidal P_{CO_2} (P_{ETCO_2}) (**panel 7**) is not decreasing, simultaneously. The black + symbol in **panel 3** indicates predicted peak values of heart rate (HR) (left y-axis) and $\dot{V}O_2$ for this individual. Abbreviations: IC, inspiratory capacity; MVV, maximum voluntary ventilation; P_{ETO_2}, end-tidal P_{O_2}; R, respiratory exchange ratio; SBP, systolic blood pressure; VC, vital capacity; $\dot{V}E$, minute ventilation; $\dot{V}E/\dot{V}O_2$, ventilatory equivalent for oxygen; V_T, tidal volume.

CASE 56

Severe Interstitial Lung Disease

CLINICAL FINDINGS

This 20-year-old man with prior exposure to agricultural work and crop dusting chemicals was found to have an interstitial pneumonitis with mica deposits on lung biopsy. The patient noted severe dyspnea with walking one block or climbing two flights of stairs. He denied cough, wheezing, orthopnea, chest pain, syncope, peripheral edema, or cyanosis. An exercise test was performed to evaluate his response to an empiric trial of prednisone. Demographic and respiratory function data are shown in **Table 10.56.1**.

EXERCISE FINDINGS

The patient performed exercise on a cycle ergometer. He pedaled at 60 rpm without an added load for 3 minutes. The work rate was then increased 10 W/min to tolerance. Arterial blood was sampled every second minute, and intra-arterial pressure was recorded from a percutaneously placed brachial artery catheter. The patient was well-motivated and cooperative and stopped exercise because of fatigue and shortness of breath. Exercise data are summarized in **Tables 10.56.2** and **10.56.3** and in **Figure 10.56.1**. No electrocardiogram abnormalities occurred at rest or during exercise, but a significant pulsus paradoxus (blood pressure variations with breathing) was noted during exercise.

INTERPRETATION

Comments

Resting respiratory function studies showed severe restrictive lung disease. Arterial blood gases revealed a chronic, compensated respiratory acidosis with mild hypoxemia.

TABLE 10.56.1 Selected Respiratory Function Data

Measurement	Predicted	Measured
Age (y)		20
Sex		Male
Height (cm)		160
Weight (kg)	66	48
Hematocrit (%)		51
VC (L)	3.52	1.21
IC (L)	2.37	0.74
FEV_1 (L)	2.99	1.21
FEV_1/VC (%)	85	97
MVV (L/min)	125	51

Abbreviations: FEV_1, forced expiratory volume in 1 second; IC, inspiratory capacity; MVV, maximum voluntary ventilation; VC, vital capacity.

Analysis

Peak $\dot{V}O_2$ and the anaerobic threshold were both markedly reduced, but it is interesting that he appeared to be ventilatory limited (low breathing reserve) while able to come very close to his maximum predicted heart rate for age. Ventilatory limitation was expected because of severely reduced lung function, but he also had a very steep heart rate–$\dot{V}O_2$ relationship and a very flat $\Delta\dot{V}O_2/\Delta WR$, resulting in a very low, nonrising oxygen (O_2) pulse throughout exercise. These findings imply impaired O_2 delivery with resultant low anaerobic threshold. Notably, the bicarbonate during recovery was 14 mmol/L, suggesting marked metabolic (lactic) acidosis. With all of these abnormalities, the evidence is that the patient made an excellent effort during the test.

The lack of severe hypoxemia is remarkable but could be explained by normal red cell transit time through the pulmonary circulation. The extremely low O_2 pulse implies that exercise stroke volume must be very low, and the cardiac

TABLE 10.56.2 Selected Exercise Data

Measurement	Predicted	Measured
Peak $\dot{V}O_2$ (L/min)	2.46	0.74
Maximum heart rate (beats/min)	200	182
Maximum O_2 pulse (mL/beat)	12.3	4.1
$\Delta\dot{V}O_2/\Delta WR$ (mL/min/W)	10.3	4.2
AT (L/min)	>0.98	<0.55
Blood pressure (mm Hg [rest, max])[a]		118/81, 165-126/ 102-63
Maximum $\dot{V}E$ (L/min)		47
Exercise breathing reserve (L/min)	>15	4
$\dot{V}E/\dot{V}CO_2$ @ *AT* or lowest	24.4	30.1
PaO_2 (mm Hg [rest, max ex])		73, 85
$P(A-a)O_2$ (mm Hg [rest, max ex])		15, 36
$PaCO_2$ (mm Hg [rest, max ex])		46, 42
$P(A-ET)CO_2$ (mm Hg [rest, max ex])		3, 4
VD/VT (rest, max ex)		0.37, 0.36
HCO_3^- (mEq/L [rest, 2-min recov])		28, 14

Abbreviations: *AT*, anaerobic threshold; $\Delta\dot{V}O_2/\Delta WR$, change in $\dot{V}O_2$/change in work rate; ex, exercise; HCO_3^-, bicarbonate; O_2, oxygen; $P(A-a)O_2$, alveolar-arterial PO_2 difference; $P(a-ET)CO_2$, arterial-end-tidal PCO_2 difference; recov, recovery; VD/VT, physiological dead space-tidal volume ratio; $\dot{V}E$, minute ventilation; $\dot{V}E/\dot{V}CO_2$, ventilatory equivalent for carbon dioxide; $\dot{V}O_2$, oxygen uptake.

[a]Ranges reflect pulsus paradox.

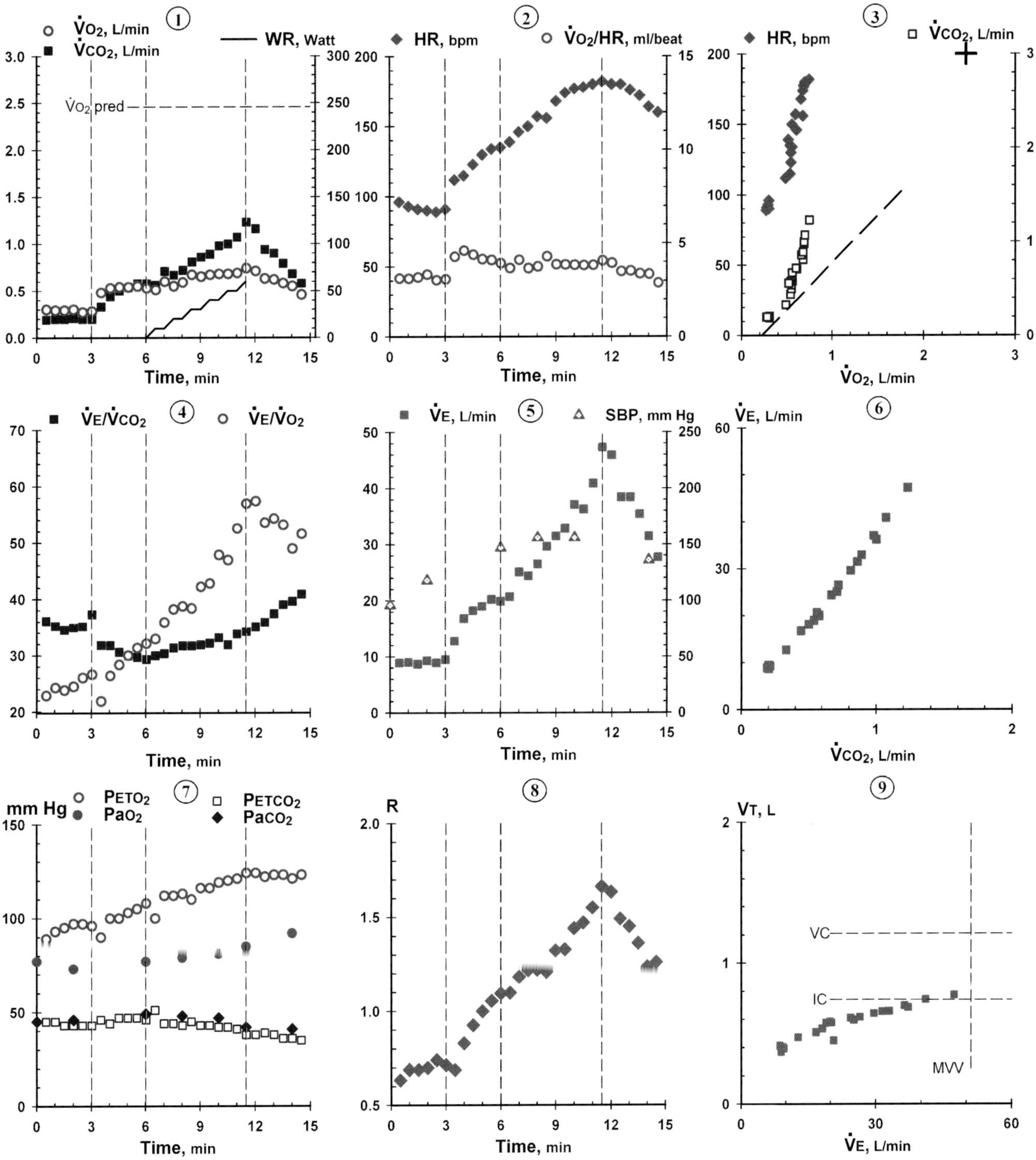

FIGURE 10.56.1. Vertical dashed lines in the panels in the left and middle columns indicate, from left to right, the beginning of unloaded cycling, start of increasing work rate (WR) at 10 W/min, and start of recovery. In **panel 1**, the increase in WR (right y-axis) is plotted with a scale of 100 W to 1 L of oxygen uptake ($\dot{V}O_2$) (left y-axis) such that WR is plotted parallel to a $\dot{V}O_2$ slope of 10 mL/min/W. In **panel 3**, carbon dioxide output ($\dot{V}CO_2$) (right y-axis) is plotted as a function of $\dot{V}O_2$ (x-axis) with identical scales so that the diagonal dashed line has a slope of 1 (45°). The $\dot{V}CO_2$ increasing more steeply than $\dot{V}O_2$ defines carbon dioxide (CO_2) derived from bicarbonate buffer, as long as ventilatory equivalent for CO_2 ($\dot{V}E/\dot{V}CO_2$) (**panel 4**) is not increasing and end-tidal PCO_2 ($PETCO_2$) (**panel 7**) is not decreasing, simultaneously. The black + symbol in **panel 3** indicates predicted peak values of heart rate (HR) (left y-axis) and $\dot{V}O_2$ for this individual. Abbreviations: IC, inspiratory capacity; MVV, maximum voluntary ventilation; $PETO_2$, end-tidal PO_2; R, respiratory exchange ratio; SBP, systolic blood pressure; VC, vital capacity; $\dot{V}E$, minute ventilation; $\dot{V}E/\dot{V}O_2$, ventilatory equivalent for oxygen; VT, tidal volume.

TABLE 10.56.3 Air Breathing

Time (min)	Work rate (W)	BP (mm Hg)	HR (min^{-1})	f (min^{-1})	$\dot{V}E$ (L/min BTPS)	$\dot{V}CO_2$ (L/min STPD)	$\dot{V}O_2$ (L/min STPD)	$\frac{\dot{V}O_2}{HR}$ (mL/beat)	R	pH	HCO_3^- (mEq/L)	PO_2, mm Hg ET	a	(A − a)	PCO_2, mm Hg ET	a	(a − ET)	$\frac{\dot{V}E}{\dot{V}CO_2}$	$\frac{\dot{V}E}{\dot{V}O_2}$	$\frac{VD}{VT}$
	Rest	96/68								7.40	27		77			45				
0.5	Rest		96	24	8.9	0.19	0.30	3.1	0.63			89			45			36	23	
1.0	Rest		93	23	9.0	0.20	0.29	3.1	0.69			93			45			35	24	
1.5	Rest		91	21	8.7	0.20	0.29	3.2	0.69			95			43			35	24	
2.0	Rest	118/81	90	23	9.3	0.21	0.30	3.3	0.70	7.40	28	97	73	15	43	46	3	35	24	0.37
2.5	Rest		89	22	8.9	0.20	0.27	3.0	0.74			97			43			35	26	
3.0	Rest		91	24	9.5	0.20	0.28	3.1	0.71			96			43			37	27	
3.5	Unloaded		112	27	12.8	0.33	0.48	4.3	0.69			90			46			32	22	
4.0	Unloaded		115	33	16.8	0.44	0.53	4.6	0.83			100			44			32	26	
4.5	Unloaded		123	34	18.2	0.50	0.54	4.4	0.93			100			47			31	28	
5.0	Unloaded		130	33	19.0	0.54	0.54	4.2	1.00			103			47			30	30	
5.5	Unloaded		134	35	20.2	0.58	0.55	4.1	1.05			105			47			30	31	
6.0	Unloaded	147/93	135	34	19.9	0.58	0.53	3.9	1.09	7.35	27	108	77	27	46	49	3	29	32	0.34
6.5	10		139	46	20.7	0.56	0.51	3.7	1.10			100			51			30	33	
7.0	10		146	42	25.1	0.71	0.60	4.1	1.18			112			44			30	36	
7.5	20		150	40	24.4	0.67	0.55	3.7	1.22			112			44			31	38	
8.0	20	156/96	157	43	26.5	0.72	0.59	3.8	1.22	7.33	25	113	79	30	43	48	5	32	39	0.37
8.5	30		156	46	29.6	0.81	0.67	4.3	1.21			110			45			32	38	
9.0	30		168	48	31.5	0.86	0.65	3.9	1.32			116			43			32	42	
9.5	40		174	50	32.9	0.89	0.67	3.9	1.33			116			43			32	43	
10.0	40	156/90	177	54	37.1	0.98	0.68	3.8	1.44	7.28	22	119	81	33	42	47	5	33	48	0.39
10.5	50		178	52	36.3	1.00	0.68	3.8	1.47			120			42			32	47	
11.0	50		180	55	40.9	1.07	0.69	3.8	1.55			121			41			34	53	
11.5	60	165-126/102-63	182	61	47.3	1.23	0.74	4.1	1.66	7.23	17	124	85	36	38	42	4	34	57	0.36
12.0	Recovery		180	61	45.9	1.16	0.71	3.9	1.63			124			38			35	57	
12.5	Recovery		180	55	38.4	0.94	0.63	3.5	1.49			122			39			36	54	
13.0	Recovery		176	56	38.4	0.90	0.62	3.5	1.45			123			38			37	54	
13.5	Recovery		172	54	35.4	0.79	0.58	3.4	1.36			123			36			39	53	
14.0	Recovery	136/69	164	54	31.5	0.68	0.55	3.4	1.24	7.15	14	121	92	23	36	41	5	40	49	0.40
14.5	Recovery		160	47	27.7	0.58	0.46	2.9	1.26			123			35			41	52	

Abbreviations: BP, blood pressure; BTPS, body temperature pressure saturated; f, frequency; HCO_3^-, bicarbonate; HR, heart rate; $P(A-a)O_2$, alveolar-arterial PO_2 difference; $P(a-ET)CO_2$, arterial-end-tidal PCO_2 difference; $PETCO_2$, end-tidal PCO_2; $PETO_2$, end-tidal PO_2; R, respiratory exchange ratio; STPD, standard temperature pressure dry; $\dot{V}CO_2$, carbon dioxide output; VD/VT, physiological dead space-tidal volume ratio; $\dot{V}E$, minute ventilation; $\dot{V}E/\dot{V}CO_2$, ventilatory equivalent for carbon dioxide; $\dot{V}E/\dot{V}O_2$, ventilatory equivalent for oxygen; $\dot{V}O_2$, oxygen uptake.

output appears to be relatively fixed, as indicated by the failure of $\dot{V}O_2$ to increase despite the increasing work rate. Failure to increase cardiac output during exercise means that red blood cell pulmonary residence time could remain at resting levels, allowing time for equilibration of alveolar PO_2 with pulmonary capillary PO_2. This may explain the absence of severe arterial hypoxemia, although $P(A-a)O_2$ increased to borderline high values. The VD/VT and $P(a-ET)CO_2$ were abnormal.

A flowchart analysis using flow charts in Chapter 9 would lead from Flowchart 1 to Flowchart 4 (low peak $\dot{V}O_2$ and anaerobic threshold). Branch Points 4.1 and 4.2 leads to lung disease with impaired peripheral oxygenation. We are prompted to verify other findings consistent with this in the pulmonary vascular disease box. The high breathing frequency, high VT/IC ratio, and low breathing reserve are all typical of severe restrictive lung disease. The elevated VD/VT and positive $P(a-ET)CO_2$ indicate inadequate perfusion of ventilated air spaces.

Conclusion

This young man had extremely severe restrictive lung disease and secondary pulmonary vascular disease. As a result, he had high dead space ventilation and extremely low stroke volume and cardiac output but little arterial hypoxemia.

CASE 57

Sarcoidosis

CLINICAL FINDINGS

This 39-year-old woman was referred for exercise testing with complaints of mild shortness of breath of 1 year's duration and diminished exercise tolerance of 18 months' duration. One year previously, she was found to have a thin-walled cystic lesion in the right lower lung field without infiltrates or adenopathy. On follow-up studies, the cyst was found to be enlarging and was therefore surgically resected. Preoperative exercise testing suggested cardiovascular limitation prompting monitoring during surgery of pulmonary artery pressures, which were normal. The resected lesion was found to contain noncaseating granulomata compatible with sarcoidosis; stains and cultures for organisms were negative. The patient had never smoked cigarettes and took no medications. The test presented here is a postoperative exercise test conducted with an intra-arterial catheter to follow up the prior findings in more detail. Demographic and respiratory function data are shown in **Table 10.57.1**.

TABLE 10.57.1 Selected Respiratory Function Data

Measurement	Predicted	Measured
Age (y)		39
Sex		Female
Height (cm)		162
Weight (kg)	63	68
Hematocrit (%)		41
VC (L)	3.38	2.89
IC (L)	2.25	1.80
TLC (L)	5.84	4.34
FEV_1 (L)	2.75	2.40
FEV_1/VC (%)	81	88
MVV (L/min)	105	98
D_{LCO} (mL/mm Hg/min)	24.2	17.9

Abbreviations: D_{LCO}, diffusing capacity of lung for carbon monoxide; FEV_1, forced expiratory volume in 1 second; IC, inspiratory capacity; MVV, maximum voluntary ventilation; TLC, total lung capacity; VC, vital capacity.

EXERCISE FINDINGS

The patient performed exercise on a cycle ergometer. She pedaled at 60 rpm without an added load for 3 minutes. The work rate was then increased 15 W/min to tolerance. Arterial blood was sampled every second minute, and intra-arterial pressure was recorded from a percutaneously placed brachial artery catheter. The patient stopped exercise because of light-headedness and shortness of breath. No electrocardiogram abnormalities occurred at rest or during exercise. Exercise data are summarized in **Tables 10.57.2** and **10.57.3** and **Figure 10.57.1**.

INTERPRETATION

Comments

The resting respiratory function studies were similar to her prelung resection values and showed mild restrictive lung disease.

Analysis

The patient was cooperative with the study and developed a significant lactic acidosis as reflected in the end-exercise R of 1.2. She had a low peak oxygen uptake ($\dot{V}O_2$) and low anaerobic threshold and somewhat steeper heart rate–oxygen uptake relationship with flat oxygen (O_2) pulse with a low peak value, although $\Delta\dot{V}O_2/\Delta WR$ appeared to be normal. She was not ventilatory limited given normal breathing reserve. Noninvasive indices of impaired pulmonary gas exchange were not abnormal ($\dot{V}E$ versus $\dot{V}CO_2$ slope and $\dot{V}E/\dot{V}CO_2$ at the anaerobic threshold), and because arterial blood gases were obtained, this was confirmed by normal PaO_2, $P(A - a)O_2$, $P(a - ET)CO_2$, and VD/VT. Therefore, despite known mild lung disease, exercise testing did not support a lung gas exchange problem. The low peak $\dot{V}O_2$ and low anaerobic threshold was better explained by a disorder resulting in low O_2 delivery. Because anemia was excluded, a tentative diagnosis of low stroke volume was considered. There were no electrocardiogram findings to suggest coronary disease, and pulmonary vascular pressures measured previously were normal. Therefore, the findings were felt to be most compatible with cardiac sarcoidosis. An alternative consideration would be sarcoidosis affecting skeletal muscle, which would give similar findings on exercise testing.

Using flowchart analysis outlined in Chapter 9, low peak $\dot{V}O_2$ and low anaerobic threshold were both decreased lead-

TABLE 10.57.2 Selected Exercise Data

Measurement	Predicted	Measured
Peak $\dot{V}O_2$ (L/min)	1.70	1.12
Maximum heart rate (beats/min)	181	173
Maximum O_2 pulse (mL/beat)	9.4	6.5
$\Delta\dot{V}O_2/\Delta WR$ (mL/min/W)	10.3	7.3
AT (L/min)	>0.81	<0.65
Blood pressure (mm Hg [rest, max])		146/88, 189/105
Maximum $\dot{V}E$ (L/min)		55
Exercise breathing reserve (L/min)	>15	43
$\dot{V}E/\dot{V}CO_2$ @ *AT* or lowest	27.3	31.5
PaO_2 (mm Hg [rest, max ex])		104, 119
$P(A - a)O_2$ (mm Hg [rest, max ex])		7, 7
$PaCO_2$ (mm Hg [rest, max ex])		32, 28
$P(a - ET)CO_2$ (mm Hg [rest, max ex])		0, −4
V_D/V_T (rest, max ex)		0.30, 0.19
HCO_3^- (mEq/L [rest, 2-min recov])		22, 13

Abbreviations: *AT*, anaerobic threshold; $\Delta\dot{V}O_2/\Delta WR$, change in $\dot{V}O_2$/change in work rate; ex, exercise; HCO_3^-, bicarbonate; O_2, oxygen; $P(A - a)O_2$, alveolar-arterial PO_2 difference; $P(a - ET)CO_2$, arterial-end-tidal PCO_2 difference; recov, recovery; V_D/V_T, physiological dead space–tidal volume ratio; $\dot{V}E$, minute ventilation; $\dot{V}E/\dot{V}CO_2$, ventilatory equivalent for carbon dioxide; $\dot{V}O_2$, oxygen uptake.

ing to Flowchart 4. The breathing reserve was high (Branch Point 4.1), and the mildly elevated ventilatory equivalents were accounted for by a low $PaCO_2$ as V_D/V_T and $P(a - ET)CO_2$ were normal. The $P(A - a)O_2$ values (Branch Point 4.3) were also normal, indicating uniform ventilation–perfusion ratios. These findings imply an O_2 flow problem of nonpulmonary origin. In the absence of anemia, consideration of low stroke volume remains.

Conclusion

Although resting pulmonary function tests demonstrated mild-to-moderate abnormalities due to pulmonary sarcoidosis, she was not limited by lung mechanics, nor were indices of pulmonary gas exchange abnormal. The exercise impairment instead reflected a pattern consistent with a defect in nonpulmonary O_2 transport, such as myocardial dysfunction or O_2 utilization at the muscle.

TABLE 10.57.3 Air Breathing

Time (min)	Work rate (W)	BP (mm Hg)	HR (min^{-1})	f (min^{-1})	$\dot{V}_E$ (L/min BTPS)	$\dot{V}CO_2$ (L/min STPD)	$\dot{V}O_2$ (L/min STPD)	$\frac{\dot{V}O_2}{HR}$ (mL/beat)	R	pH	HCO_3^- (mEq/L)	PO_2, mm Hg ET	a	(A − a)	PCO_2, mm Hg ET	a	(a − ET)	$\frac{\dot{V}_E}{\dot{V}CO_2}$	$\frac{\dot{V}_E}{\dot{V}O_2}$	$\frac{V_D}{V_T}$
	Rest	156/90								7.41	22		102			35				
0.5	Rest		105	23	11.4	0.23	0.25	2.4	0.92			116			31			41	38	
1.0	Rest		103	20	8.4	0.15	0.17	1.7	0.88			113			32			45	39	
1.5	Rest		108	23	9.2	0.17	0.22	2.0	0.77			112			32			43	33	
2.0	Rest	146/88	105	23	10.1	0.19	0.24	2.3	0.79	7.43	21	112	104	7	32	32	0	43	34	0.30
2.5	Rest		106	22	12.2	0.26	0.31	2.9	0.84			109			33			40	33	
3.0	Rest		106	24	8.1	0.14	0.17	1.6	0.82			111			33			43	36	
3.5	Unloaded		122	33	14.4	0.33	0.39	3.2	0.85			111			32			35	30	
4.0	Unloaded		129	21	15.4	0.42	0.55	4.3	0.76			104			35			32	25	
4.5	Unloaded		131	23	19.1	0.53	0.66	5.0	0.80			107			35			32	26	
5.0	Unloaded		131	23	19.8	0.55	0.61	4.7	0.90			112			35			32	29	
5.5	Unloaded		129	20	19.7	0.58	0.64	5.0	0.91			110			36			31	28	
6.0	Unloaded	165/99	135	18	21.3	0.64	0.65	4.8	0.98	7.39	20	112	108	8	36	34	−2	31	30	0.17
6.5	10		132	28	22.4	0.63	0.62	4.7	1.02			115			35			32	32	
7.0	10		139	29	25.2	0.68	0.68	4.9	1.00			113			35			33	33	
7.5	20		141	21	21.6	0.63	0.66	4.7	0.95			110			37			31	30	
8.0	20	168/97	143	24	22.2	0.66	0.66	4.6	1.00	7.38	20	112	115	1	37	34	−3	31	31	0.15
8.5	30		148	23	28.7	0.84	0.76	5.1	1.11			116			35			32	35	
9.0	30		149	28	26.5	0.76	0.73	4.9	1.04			113			37			32	33	
9.5	40		154	24	31.7	0.90	0.82	5.3	1.10			116			36			33	36	
10.0	40	189/105	160	29	33.7	0.93	0.81	51	1.15	7.37	19	117	117	3	35	33	−2	34	39	0.21
10.5	50		163	24	35.6	1.00	0.88	5.4	1.14			117			35			34	38	
11.0	50		164	25	36.7	1.02	0.89	5.4	1.15			118			35			34	39	
11.5	60		167	29	40.7	1.08	0.98	5.9	1.10			120			33			35	39	
12.0	60	189/105	169	31	45.8	1.18	1.02	6.0	1.16	7.35	16	119	120	3	33	30	−3	37	42	0.20
12.5	70		171	31	48.1	1.24	1.07	6.3	1.16			120			33			37	42	
13.0	70		173	32	45.2	1.20	1.05	6.1	1.14			115			36			35	40	
13.5	80	189/105	173	38	55.0	1.34	1.12	6.5	1.20	7.32	14	122	119	7	32	28	−4	39	46	0.19
14.0	Recovery		159	33	47.2	1.10	0.96	6.0	1.15			117			34			40	46	
14.5	Recovery	118/60	139	28	41.0	[illegible]	[illegible]	[illegible]	1.18			[illegible]			30			41	48	
15.0	Recovery		129	29	37.2	0.86	0.74	5.7	1.16			121			31			40	47	

Abbreviations: BP, blood pressure; BTPS, body temperature pressure saturated; f, frequency; HCO_3^-, bicarbonate; HR, heart rate; $P(A - a)O_2$, alveolar-arterial PO_2 difference; $P(a - ET)CO_2$, arterial–end-tidal PCO_2 difference; $P_{ET}CO_2$, end-tidal PCO_2; $P_{ET}O_2$, end-tidal PO_2; R, respiratory exchange ratio; STPD, standard temperature pressure dry; $\dot{V}CO_2$, carbon dioxide output; V_D/V_T, physiological dead space–tidal volume ratio; $\dot{V}_E$, minute ventilation; $\dot{V}_E/\dot{V}CO_2$, ventilatory equivalent for carbon dioxide; $\dot{V}_E/\dot{V}O_2$, ventilatory equivalent for oxygen; $\dot{V}O_2$, oxygen uptake.

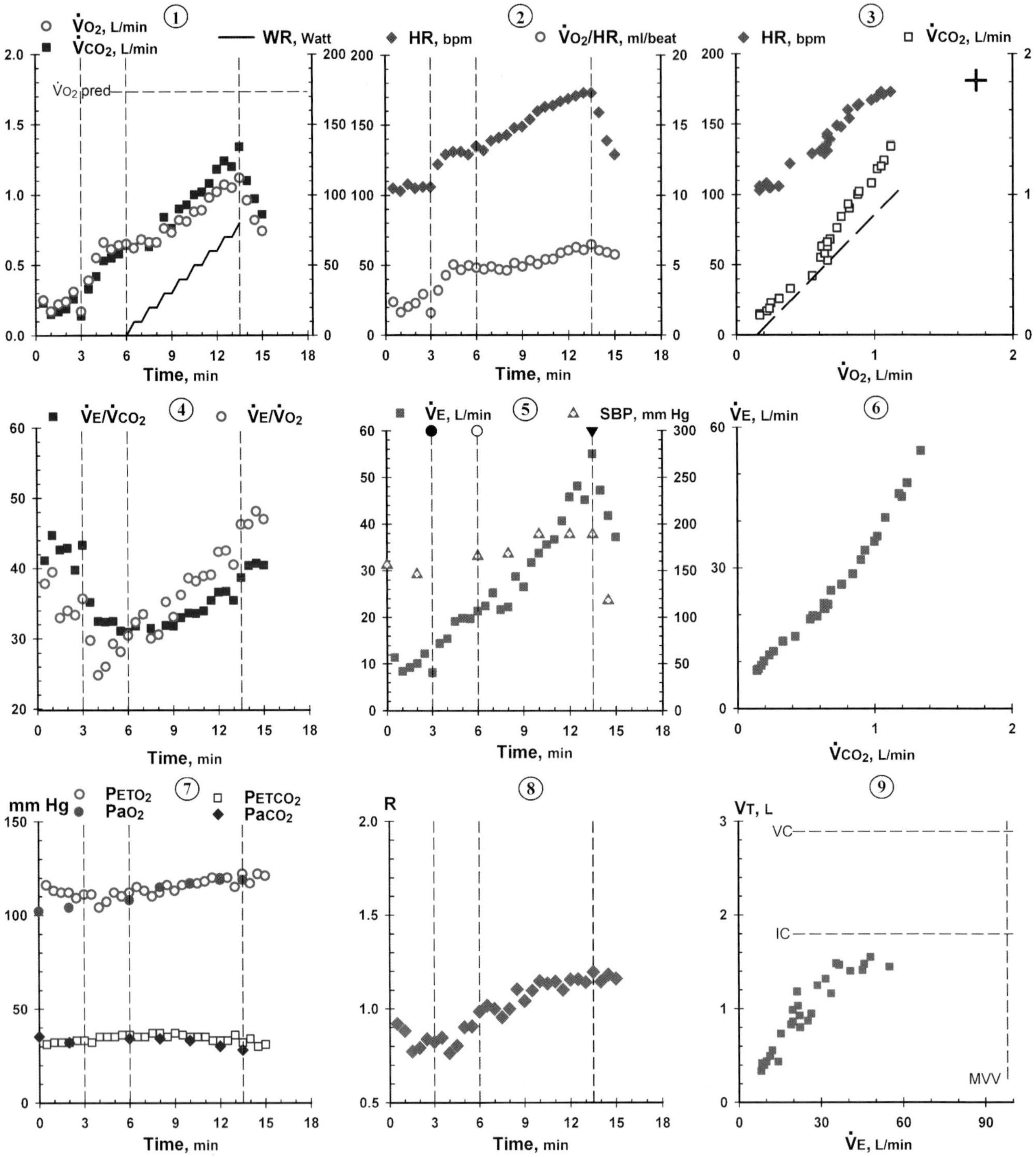

FIGURE 10.57.1. Vertical dashed lines in the panels in the left and middle columns indicate, from left to right, the beginning of unloaded cycling, start of increasing work rate (WR) at 15 W/min, and start of recovery. In **panel 1**, the increase in WR (right y-axis) is plotted with a scale of 100 W to 1 L of oxygen uptake ($\dot{V}O_2$) (left y-axis) such that WR is plotted parallel to a $\dot{V}O_2$ slope of 10 mL/min/W. In **panel 3**, carbon dioxide output ($\dot{V}CO_2$) (right y-axis) is plotted as a function of $\dot{V}O_2$ (x-axis) with identical scales so that the diagonal dashed line has a slope of 1 (45°). The $\dot{V}CO_2$ increasing more steeply than $\dot{V}O_2$ defines carbon dioxide (CO_2) derived from bicarbonate buffer, as long as ventilatory equivalent for CO_2 ($\dot{V}E/\dot{V}CO_2$) (**panel 4**) is not increasing and end-tidal PCO_2 ($PETCO_2$) (**panel 7**) is not decreasing, simultaneously. The black + symbol in **panel 3** indicates predicted peak values of heart rate (HR) (left y-axis) and $\dot{V}O_2$ for this individual. Abbreviations: IC, inspiratory capacity; MVV, maximum voluntary ventilation; $PETO_2$, end-tidal PO_2; R, respiratory exchange ratio; SBP, systolic blood pressure; VC, vital capacity; $\dot{V}E$, minute ventilation; $\dot{V}E/\dot{V}O_2$, ventilatory equivalent for oxygen; V_T, tidal volume.

CASE 58

Interstitial Pneumonitis: Before and After Empiric Corticosteroid Therapy

To view this case please access the eBook bundled with this text. Instructions are located on the inside front cover.

CASE 59

Severe Interstitial Lung Disease: Air and Oxygen Breathing Studies

To view this case please access the eBook bundled with this text. Instructions are located on the inside front cover.

CASE 60

Mild Pulmonary Asbestosis

CLINICAL FINDINGS

This 55-year-old male shipyard worker had a long history of asbestos exposure and was a former cigarette smoker. He had a daily cough productive of scant, yellow-tinged sputum but noted shortness of breath only after climbing three to four flights of stairs. He denied any other symptoms or illnesses. No rales were noted on examination. Chest radiograph revealed minimal, but definite, basilar fibrosis, typical of asbestosis. Exercise testing was requested to identify the presence and degree of physiologic impairment associated with the asbestosis. Demographic and respiratory function data are shown in **Table 10.60.1**.

EXERCISE FINDINGS

The patient performed exercise on a cycle ergometer. He pedaled at 60 rpm without an added load for 3 minutes. The work rate was then increased 10 W/min to tolerance. Arterial blood was sampled every second minute, and intra-arterial pressure was recorded from a percutaneously placed brachial artery catheter. The patient stopped exercise because of shortness of breath. The electrocardiogram showed nonspecific T-wave abnormalities and occasional premature ventricular contractions at rest and during exercise. Exercise data are summarized in **Tables 10.60.2** and **10.60.3** and **Figure 10.60.1**.

INTERPRETATION

Comments

Resting pulmonary function studies showed a mild restrictive defect with proportionate reduction in diffusing capacity of the lung for carbon monoxide, suggesting loss of pulmonary capillary bed (**Table 10.60.1**).

Analysis

Peak $\dot{V}O_2$ was mildly reduced and the patient nearly reached his predicted peak heart rate for age. He did have a borderline low breathing reserve suggesting possible ventilatory limitation during exercise. He did have elevated $\dot{V}E/\dot{V}CO_2$ and a mildly increased $\dot{V}E$ versus $\dot{V}CO_2$ slope. These findings would suggest potential abnormal lung gas exchange. Because arterial blood gases were obtained, this can be confirmed as showing borderline increases in V_D/V_T and

TABLE 10.60.1 Selected Respiratory Function Data

Measurement	Predicted	Measured
Age (y)		55
Sex		Male
Height (cm)		181
Weight (kg)	82	84
Hematocrit (%)		45
VC (L)	4.24	3.50
IC (L)	2.83	2.26
TLC (L)	6.32	5.15
FEV_1 (L)	3.35	2.94
FEV_1/VC (%)	79	84
MVV (L/min)	135	107
D_{LCO} (mL/mm Hg/min)	27.3	22.7

Abbreviations: D_{LCO}, diffusing capacity of the lung for carbon monoxide; FEV_1, forced expiratory volume in 1 second; IC, inspiratory capacity; MVV, maximum voluntary ventilation; TLC, total lung capacity; VC, vital capacity.

$P(a - ET)CO_2$ but normal $P(A - a)O_2$. These subtle abnormalities are likely due to interstitial lung disease.

Referring to the flowcharts in Chapter 9; using Flowchart 1, peak $\dot{V}O_2$ was decreased, but the anaerobic threshold was normal, leading to Flowchart 3. At Branch Point 3.1, the breathing reserve was borderline low. The flowchart prompts us to review the gas exchange abnormalities usually associated with lung diseases. Again, these were borderline, with V_D/V_T around the upper limit of normal at rest, and at or above the upper limit of normal at peak exercise as reflected in the last two exercise values, which averaged 0.30. At Branch Point 3.2, the high breathing frequency is characteristic of restrictive lung disease.

Conclusion

This patient with pulmonary asbestosis had mild restrictive lung disease at rest. Exercise testing revealed lower than normal peak $\dot{V}O_2$. The high breathing frequency and low breathing reserve in response to maximal exercise testing support the conclusion that exercise was limited by ventilatory restriction. Measurements of gas exchange confirmed mild $\dot{V}/\dot{Q}$ mismatching.

TABLE 10.60.2 Selected Exercise Data

Measurement	Predicted	Measured
Peak $\dot{V}O_2$ (L/min)	2.50	2.03
Maximum heart rate (beats/min)	165	154
Maximum O_2 pulse (mL/beat)	15.1	13.2
$\Delta\dot{V}O_2/\Delta WR$ (mL/min/W)	10.3	8.7
AT (L/min)	>1.08	1.3
Blood pressure (mm Hg [rest, max])		156/90, 216/99
Maximum $\dot{V}_E$ (L/min)		93
Exercise breathing reserve (L/min)	>15	14
$\dot{V}_E/\dot{V}CO_2$ @ *AT* or lowest	27.2	31.0
PaO_2 (mm Hg [rest, max ex])		88, 99
$P(A - a)O_2$ (mm Hg [rest, max ex])		14, 21
$PaCO_2$ (mm Hg [rest, max ex])		38, 32
$P(a - ET)CO_2$ (mm Hg [rest, max ex])		3, −2
V_D/V_T (rest, max ex)		0.37, 0.30
HCO_3^- (mEq/L [rest, 2-min recov])		25, 20

Abbreviations: *AT*, anaerobic threshold; $\Delta\dot{V}O_2/\Delta WR$, change in $\dot{V}O_2$/change in work rate; ex, exercise; HCO_3^-, bicarbonate; O_2, oxygen; $P(A - a)O_2$, alveolar-arterial PO_2 difference; $P(a - ET)CO_2$, arterial-end-tidal PCO_2 difference; recov, recovery; V_D/V_T, physiological dead space-tidal volume ratio; $\dot{V}_E$, minute ventilation; $\dot{V}_E/\dot{V}CO_2$, ventilatory equivalent for carbon dioxide; $\dot{V}O_2$, oxygen uptake.

TABLE 10.60.3 Air Breathing

Time (min)	Work rate (W)	BP (mm Hg)	HR (min^{-1})	f (min^{-1})	$\dot{V}_E$ (L/min BTPS)	$\dot{V}CO_2$ (L/min STPD)	$\dot{V}O_2$ (L/min STPD)	$\frac{\dot{V}O_2}{HR}$ (mL/beat)	R	Ph	HCO_3^- (mEq/L)	PO_2, mm Hg ET	a	(A − a)	PCO_2, mm Hg ET	a	(a − ET)	$\frac{\dot{V}_E}{\dot{V}CO_2}$	$\frac{\dot{V}_E}{\dot{V}O_2}$	$\frac{V_D}{V_T}$
0	Rest	156/90								7.43	25		79			38				
0.5	Rest		81	21	12.3	0.24	0.32	4.0	0.75			106			35			44	33	
1.0	Rest		83	23	11.8	0.23	0.31	3.7	0.74			106			35			43	32	
1.5	Rest		88	21	11.9	0.23	0.30	3.4	0.77			108			34			44	34	
2.0	Rest	162/96	80	22	11.2	0.23	0.31	3.9	0.74	7.42	24	105	88	14	35	38	3	41	30	0.37
2.5	Rest		84	18	11.4	0.23	0.31	3.7	0.74			104			36			43	32	
3.0	Rest		86	20	12.2	0.25	0.32	3.7	0.78			106			36			42	33	
3.5	Unloaded		97	21	16.3	0.40	0.50	5.2	0.80			105			37			36	29	
4.0	Unloaded		93	33	21.8	0.48	0.66	7.1	0.73			102			37			40	29	
4.5	Unloaded		93	32	23.8	0.52	0.64	6.9	0.81			109			34			41	33	
5.0	Unloaded		95	30	22.7	0.53	0.69	7.3	0.77			104			37			38	29	
5.5	Unloaded		94	36	22.3	0.51	0.67	7.1	0.76			100			38			38	29	
6.0	Unloaded	192/96	96	35	29.2	0.65	0.75	7.8	0.87	7.43	25	108	91	16	34	38	4	40	35	0.39
6.5	20		97	36	26.6	0.62	0.78	8.0	0.79			105			36			38	30	
7.0	20		98	39	28.3	0.62	0.78	8.0	0.79			108			35	38		40	32	
7.5	40		95	41	28.7	0.62	0.80	8.4	0.78			204			37			41	32	
8.0	40	192/90	103	26	27.7	0.75	0.98	9.5	0.77	7.43	25	101	87	16	38		0	34	26	0.31
8.5	60		104	31	28.3	0.73	0.91	8.8	0.80			104			37			35	28	
9.0	60		110	35	40.2	1.02	1.16	10.5	0.88			110			35	40		36	32	
9.5	80		113	36	39.6	1.06	1.29	11.4	0.82			104			38			34	28	
10.0	80	198/93	120	28	35.4	1.07	1.41	11.8	0.76	7.41	25	97	89	11	42		−2	31	23	0.28
10.5	100		128	37	47.4	1.26	1.39	10.9	0.91			110			37			35	32	
11.0	100		130	52	55.2	1.36	1.44	11.1	0.94			113			35	35		37	35	
11.5	120		130	49	60.6	1.50	1.50	11.5	1.00			113			35			38	38	
12.0	120	201/93	131	58	66.8	1.64	1.67	12.7	0.98	7.43	23	114	98	16	34		1	38	37	0.32
12.5	140		138	50	68.0	1.73	1.72	12.5	1.01			114			35			37	37	
13.0	140		140	50	73.4	1.87	1.78	12.7	1.05			115			35	33		37	39	
13.5	160		148	60	87.0	2.09	1.93	13.0	1.08			119			32	32		39	42	
14.0	160	198/99	149	59	92.9	2.24	2.03	13.6	1.10	7.43	22	119	99	20	32		1	39	43	0.32
14.5	180	216/99	154	55	89.3	2.21	2.02	13.1	1.09	7.42	20	117	99	21	34		−2	38	42	0.28
15.0	Recovery		146	32	61.5	1.73	1.64	11.2	1.05			115			35			34	36	
15.5	Recovery		132	32	53.4	1.37	1.14	8.6	1.20			118			35	33		37	44	
16.0	Recovery		128	28	37.8	0.96	0.76	5.9	1.26			121			33			37	47	
16.5	Recovery	189/93	125	27	30.1	0.75	0.63	5.0	1.19	7.39	20	119	114	7	34		−1	37	44	0.27

Abbreviations: BP, blood pressure; BTPS, body temperature pressure saturated; f, frequency; HCO_3^-, bicarbonate; HR, heart rate; P(A − a)O_2, alveolar-arterial PO_2 difference; P(a − ET)CO_2, arterial-end-tidal PCO_2 difference; $P_{ET}CO_2$, end-tidal PCO_2; $P_{ET}O_2$, end-tidal PO_2; R, respiratory exchange ratio; STPD, standard temperature pressure dry; $\dot{V}CO_2$, carbon dioxide output; V_D/V_T, physiological dead space-tidal volume ratio; $\dot{V}_E$, minute ventilation; $\dot{V}_E/\dot{V}CO_2$, ventilatory equivalent for carbon dioxide; $\dot{V}_E/\dot{V}O_2$, ventilatory equivalent for oxygen; $\dot{V}O_2$, oxygen uptake.

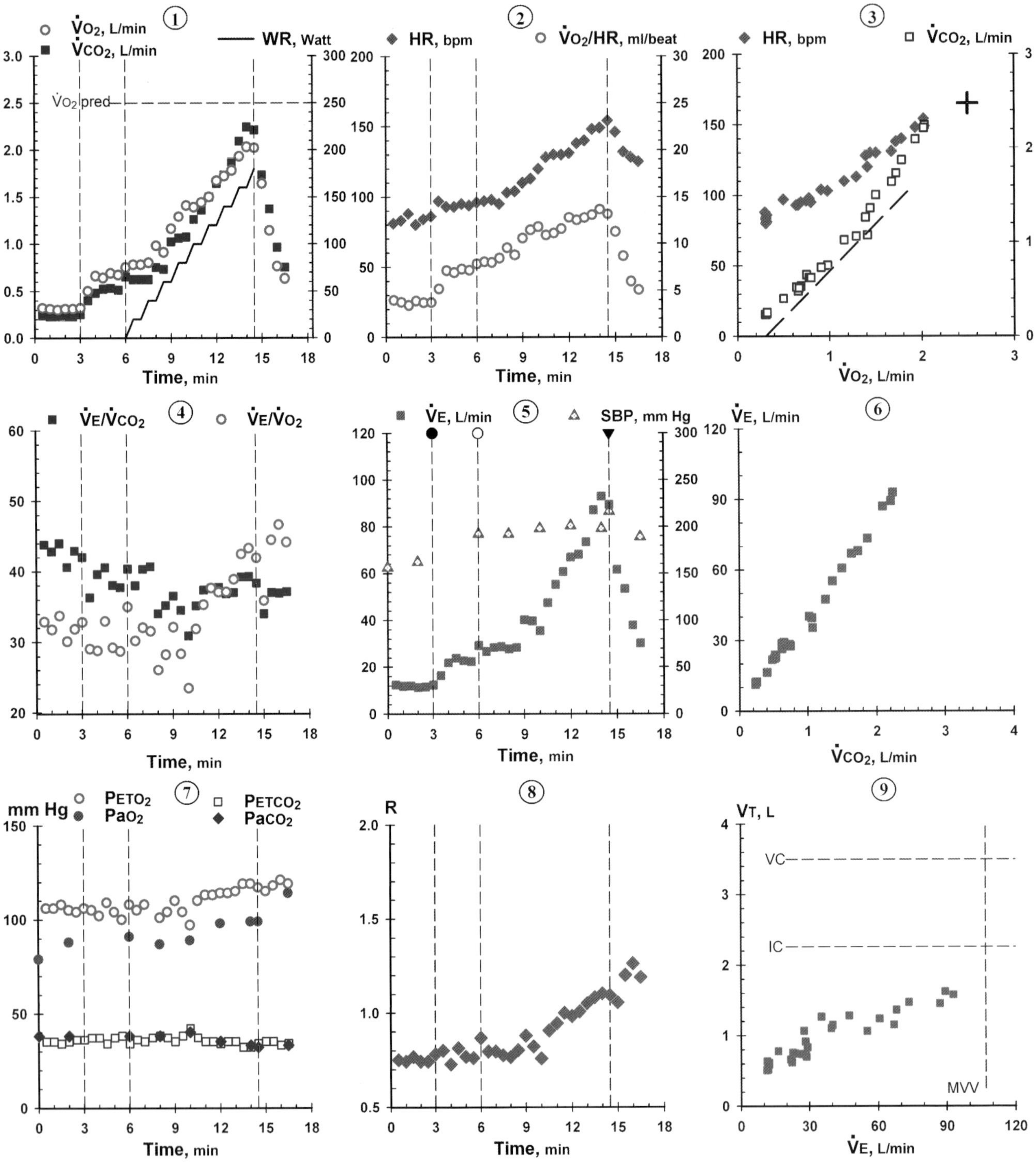

FIGURE 10.60.1. Vertical dashed lines in the panels in the left and middle columns indicate, from left to right, the beginning of unloaded cycling, start of increasing work rate (WR) at 10 W/min, and start of recovery. In **panel 1**, the increase in WR (right y-axis) is plotted with a scale of 100 W to 1 L of oxygen uptake ($\dot{V}O_2$) (left y-axis) such that WR is plotted parallel to a $\dot{V}O_2$ slope of 10 mL/min/W. In **panel 3**, carbon dioxide output ($\dot{V}CO_2$) (right y-axis) is plotted as a function of $\dot{V}O_2$ (x-axis) with identical scales so that the diagonal dashed line has a slope of 1 (45°). The $\dot{V}CO_2$ increasing more steeply than $\dot{V}O_2$ defines carbon dioxide (CO_2) derived from bicarbonate buffer, as long as ventilatory equivalent for CO_2 ($\dot{V}E/\dot{V}CO_2$) (**panel 4**) is not increasing and end-tidal P_{CO_2} (P_{ETCO_2}) (**panel 7**) is not decreasing, simultaneously. The black + symbol in **panel 3** indicates predicted peak values of heart rate (HR) (left y-axis) and $\dot{V}O_2$ for this individual. Abbreviations: IC, inspiratory capacity; MVV, maximum voluntary ventilation; P_{ETO_2}, end-tidal P_{O_2}; R, respiratory exchange ratio; SBP, systolic blood pressure; VC, vital capacity; $\dot{V}E$, minute ventilation; $\dot{V}E/\dot{V}O_2$, ventilatory equivalent for oxygen; V_T, tidal volume.

CASE 61

Severe Pulmonary Asbestosis

CLINICAL FINDINGS

This 67-year-old woman was referred for exercise testing for assessment of her functional capacity. She had been exposed to asbestos for 3 years while working in a shipyard approximately 40 years earlier. She had never smoked. Three years prior to this evaluation, she noted fatigability, clubbing of fingernails, and shortness of breath. She was unable to climb a flight of stairs or walk rapidly on level ground. A transbronchial lung biopsy was reported to show "fibrosis." Her symptoms improved significantly on treatment with prednisone, but this was discontinued after 1 year because of concern for side effects. Five months prior to this evaluation, she was started on oxygen therapy, but corticosteroids were not restarted. Examination revealed a thin woman with fine inspiratory rales in the lateral and inferior lung fields that did not clear with coughing. There was dramatic digital clubbing. Chest radiographs showed extensive interstitial infiltrates, compatible with pulmonary fibrosis. There was also a small patch of pleural calcification consistent with asbestos-related pleural disease. Given her history and findings, the clinical diagnosis of pulmonary asbestosis was made. A resting electrocardiogram was normal.

EXERCISE FINDINGS

The patient performed exercise on a cycle ergometer. She pedaled at 60 rpm without added load for 3 minutes. The work rate was then increased 10 W/min to her symptom-limited maximum. Arterial blood was sampled every second minute, and intra-arterial blood pressure was recorded from a percutaneously placed brachial artery catheter. The patient stopped exercising because of dyspnea. Premature atrial contractions occurred during exercise, but the electrocardiogram otherwise was not remarkable.

INTERPRETATION

Comments

Results of the respiratory function studies indicate a severe restrictive defect with a marked reduction in diffusing capacity (**Table 10.61.1**). Exercise data are summarized in **Table 10.61.2** and shown in **Table 10.61.3** and graphically in **Figure 10.61.1**.

Analysis

This woman was severely impaired with a very low peak oxygen uptake ($\dot{V}O_2$) (0.42 L/min), which would generally preclude nearly any physical activity, and was accompanied by a very low breathing reserve. In addition, noninvasive estimates of pulmonary gas exchange were very abnormal ($\dot{V}E$ versus $\dot{V}CO_2$ slope and $\dot{V}E/\dot{V}CO_2$), and these were confirmed by markedly abnormal V_D/V_T, $P(A - ET)CO_2$, and $P(A - a)O_2$ during exercise. In terms of oxygen delivery, she does have a very flat and low $\Delta\dot{V}O_2/\Delta WR$, but anaerobic threshold was indeterminant because of her very low peak $\dot{V}O_2$. Most likely, these findings were mostly due to arterial hypoxemia.

If using flowchart analysis (Chapter 9), the peak $\dot{V}O_2$ was reduced at less than half the predicted value, and the anaerobic threshold was indeterminate; this suggests using Flowchart 5. There, V_D/V_T, $P(a - ET)CO_2$, and $P(A - a)O_2$ during exercise were all markedly abnormal (Branch Point 5.1) and breathing reserve was low (Branch Point 5.3). The breathing frequency was high even at rest and remained

TABLE 10.61.1 Selected Respiratory Function Data

Measurement	Predicted	Measured
Age (y)		67
Sex		Female
Height (cm)		163
Weight (kg)	63	48
Hematocrit (%)		38
VC (L)	2.77	1.51
IC (L)	1.85	0.70
TLC (L)	4.82	2.65
FEV_1 (L)	2.19	1.24
FEV_1/VC (%)	79	82
MVV (L/min)	82	33
D_{LCO} (mL/mm Hg/min)	22.3	6.4

Abbreviations: D_{LCO}, diffusing capacity of lung for carbon monoxide; FEV_1, forced expiratory volume in 1 second; IC, inspiratory capacity; MVV, maximum voluntary ventilation; TLC, total lung capacity; VC, vital capacity.

TABLE 10.61.2 Selected Exercise Data

Measurement	Predicted	Measured
Peak $\dot{V}O_2$ (L/min)	1.12	0.42
Maximum heart rate (beats/min)	153	108
Maximum O_2 pulse (mL/beat)	7.3	4.1
AT (L/min)	>0.56	Indeterminate
Blood pressure (mm Hg [rest, max])		122/74, 140/80
Maximum $\dot{V}E$ (L/min)		29
Exercise breathing reserve (L/min)	>15	4
$\dot{V}E/\dot{V}CO_2$ @ *AT* or lowest	30.2	57.2
PaO_2 (mm Hg [rest, max ex])		58, 46
$P(A - a)O_2$ (mm Hg [rest, max ex])		41, 64
$PaCO_2$ (mm Hg [rest, max ex])		41, 41
$P(a - ET)CO_2$ (mm Hg [rest, max ex])		8, 10
V_D/V_T (rest, heavy ex)		0.56, 0.55
HCO_3^- (mEq/L [rest, 2-min recov])		25, 24

Abbreviations: *AT*, anaerobic threshold; ex, exercise; HCO_3^-, bicarbonate; O_2, oxygen; $P(A - a)O_2$, alveolar-arterial PO_2 difference; $P(a - ET)CO_2$, arterial-end-tidal PCO_2 difference; recov, recovery; V_D/V_T, physiological dead space-tidal volume ratio; $\dot{V}E$, minute ventilation; $\dot{V}E/\dot{V}CO_2$, ventilatory equivalent for carbon dioxide; $\dot{V}O_2$, oxygen uptake.

high at approximately 50 breaths/min through the incremental exercise period (Branch Point 5.7) with low V_T and low V_T/IC ratio. The maximum ventilation achieved approximated the patient's maximum ventilatory capacity. These findings indicate exercise limitation due to restrictive lung disease. Also consistent with this were the progressive decrease in PaO_2 and increase in $P(A - a)O_2$ as the work rate increased (**Table 10.61.3** and **Fig. 10.61.1**, panel 7).

Conclusion

This test demonstrates ventilatory limitation to exercise in a patient with severe interstitial lung disease. The findings are consistent with asbestosis but could also be seen in other interstitial processes. Both reduced ventilatory capacity, due to pulmonary restriction, and increased ventilatory requirements, due to marked ventilation–perfusion mismatching, contributed to exercise limitation.

TABLE 10.61.3 Air Breathing

Time (min)	Work rate (W)	BP (mm Hg)	HR (min^{-1})	f (min^{-1})	$\dot{V}E$ (L/min BTPS)	$\dot{V}CO_2$ (L/min STPD)	$\dot{V}O_2$ (L/min STPD)	$\frac{\dot{V}O_2}{HR}$ (mL/beat)	R	pH	HCO_3^- (mEq/L)	PO_2, mm Hg ET	a	(A − a)	PCO_2, mm Hg ET	a	(a − ET)	$\frac{\dot{V}E}{\dot{V}CO_2}$	$\frac{\dot{V}E}{\dot{V}O_2}$	$\frac{VD}{VT}$
	Rest	122/74								7.44	25		48			37				
0.5	Rest		86	38	14.3	0.14	0.19	2.2	0.74			111			32			79	58	
1.0	Rest		89	36	15.2	0.18	0.23	2.6	0.78			113			32			67	53	
1.5	Rest		87	37	13.4	0.12	0.16	1.8	0.75			110			32			85	64	
2.0	Rest	119/71	90	36	15.0	0.17	0.22	2.4	0.77	7.40	25	109	58	41	33	41	8	70	54	0.56
2.5	Rest		89	39	15.5	0.15	0.20	2.2	0.75			111			32			81	61	
3.0	Rest		92	37	15.1	0.16	0.20	2.2	0.80			113			32			75	60	
3.5	Unloaded		92	42	18.3	0.24	0.31	3.4	0.77			108			36			61	48	
4.0	Unloaded		90	46	21.0	0.26	0.30	3.3	0.87			114			32			66	57	
4.5	Unloaded		92	51	23.4	0.29	0.35	3.8	0.83			113			32			66	54	
5.0	Unloaded		92	49	24.0	0.32	0.36	3.9	0.89			114			33			62	55	
5.5	Unloaded	126/71	93	48	24.1	0.33	0.37	4.0	0.89	7.41	26	115	52	53	32	41	9	61	54	0.54
6.0	Unloaded		95	50	24.3	0.30	0.33	3.5	0.91			117			31			67	61	
6.5	10		99	50	24.7	0.32	0.36	3.6	0.89			114			33			64	57	
7.0	10		97	51	25.0	0.32	0.36	3.7	0.89			114			33			65	57	
7.5	20		100	47	26.0	0.37	0.40	4.0	0.93			115			32			59	55	
8.0	20	137/74	105	47	25.8	0.37	0.40	3.8	0.93	7.41	25	116	49	58	32	40	8	59	55	0.54
8.5	30		104	49	28.6	0.43	0.46	4.4	0.93			118			31			57	53	
9.0	30		106	45	27.6	0.42	0.43	4.1	0.98			118			31			57	55	
9.5	40	140/80	108	45	29.1	0.44	0.42	3.9	1.05	7.39	24	120	46	64	31	41	10	57	60	0.55
10.0	Recovery		101	39	24.8	0.41	0.40	4.0	1.03			116			34			52	54	
10.5	Recovery		94	41	21.7	0.32	0.33	3.5	0.97			115			35			57	55	
11.0	Recovery		92	40	20.8	0.30	0.30	3.3	1.00			115			34			58	58	
11.5	Recovery	134/68	91	43	22.4	0.32	0.30	3.3	1.07	7.36	24	118	53	56	33	43	10	59	62	0.55
12.0	Recovery		91	43	17.8	0.16	0.15	1.6	1.07			122			30			88	94	

Abbreviations: BP, blood pressure; BTPS, body temperature pressure saturated; f, frequency; HCO_3^-, bicarbonate; HR, heart rate; $P(A - a)O_2$, alveolar-arterial PO_2 difference; $P(a - ET)CO_2$, arterial-end-tidal PCO_2 difference; $PETCO_2$, end-tidal PCO_2; $PETO_2$, end-tidal PO_2; R, respiratory exchange ratio; STPD, standard temperature pressure dry; $\dot{V}CO_2$, carbon dioxide output; VD/VT, physiological dead space-tidal volume ratio; $\dot{V}E$, minute ventilation; $\dot{V}E/\dot{V}CO_2$, ventilatory equivalent for carbon dioxide; $\dot{V}E/\dot{V}O_2$, ventilatory equivalent for oxygen; $\dot{V}O_2$, oxygen uptake.

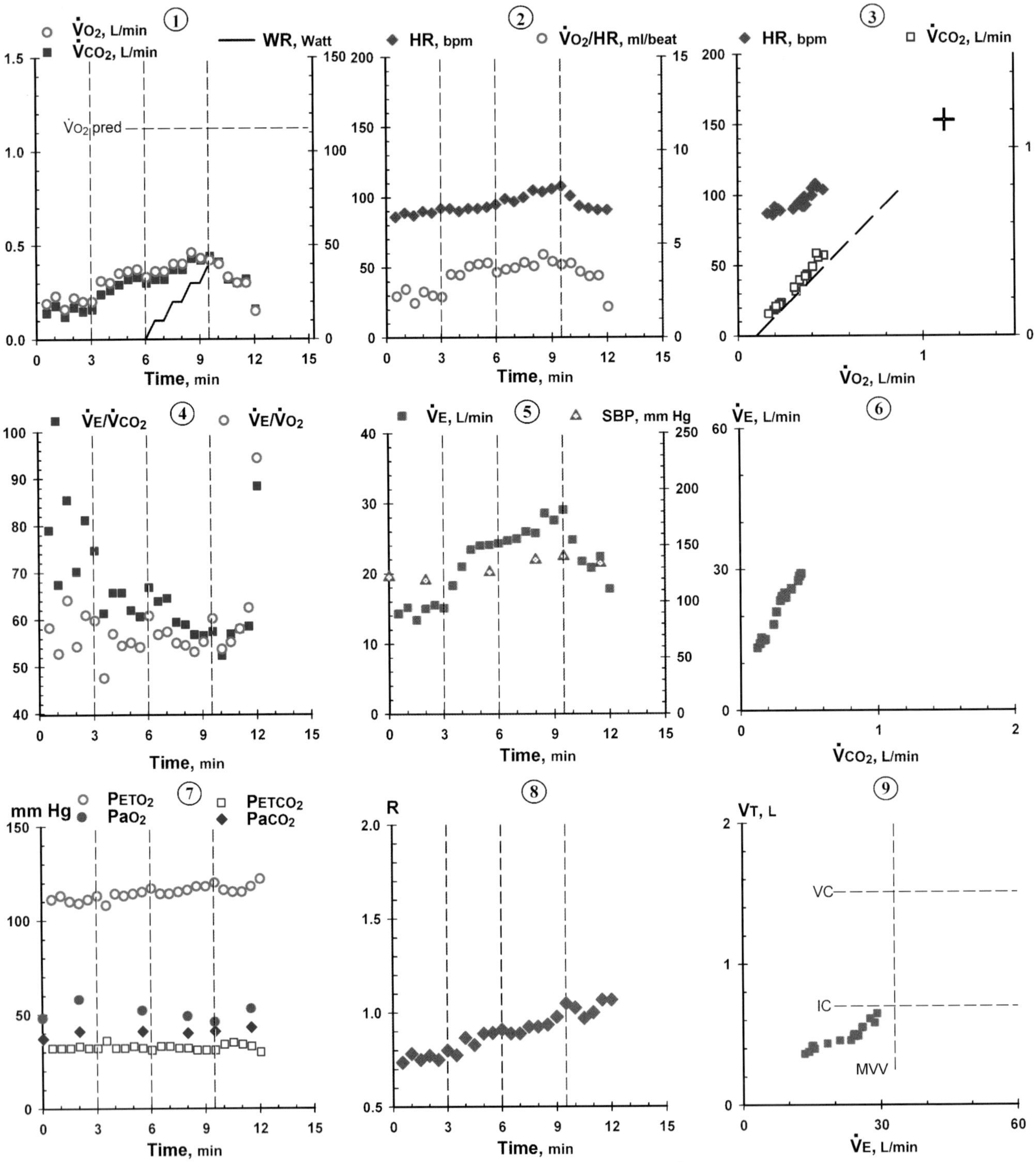

FIGURE 10.61.1. Vertical dashed lines in the panels in the left and middle columns indicate, from left to right, the beginning of unloaded cycling, start of increasing work rate (WR) at 5 W/min, and start of recovery. In **panel 1**, the increase in WR (right y-axis) is plotted with a scale of 100 W to 1 L of oxygen uptake ($\dot{V}O_2$) (left y-axis) such that WR is plotted parallel to a $\dot{V}O_2$ slope of 10 mL/min/W. In **panel 3**, carbon dioxide output ($\dot{V}CO_2$) (right y-axis) is plotted as a function of $\dot{V}O_2$ (x-axis) with identical scales so that the diagonal dashed line has a slope of 1 (45°). The $\dot{V}CO_2$ increasing more steeply than $\dot{V}O_2$ defines carbon dioxide (CO_2) derived from bicarbonate buffer, as long as ventilatory equivalent for CO_2 ($\dot{V}E/\dot{V}CO_2$) (**panel 4**) is not increasing and end-tidal PCO_2 ($PETCO_2$) (**panel 7**) is not decreasing, simultaneously. The black + symbol in **panel 3** indicates predicted peak values of heart rate (HR) (left y-axis) and $\dot{V}O_2$ for this individual. Abbreviations: IC, inspiratory capacity; MVV, maximum voluntary ventilation; $PETO_2$, end-tidal PO_2; R, respiratory exchange ratio; SBP, systolic blood pressure; VC, vital capacity; $\dot{V}E$, minute ventilation; $\dot{V}E/\dot{V}O_2$, ventilatory equivalent for oxygen; V_T, tidal volume.

CASE 62

Pleural and Pulmonary Asbestosis

CLINICAL FINDINGS

A 76-year-old man with asbestosis was referred for testing to assess his degree of impairment. He had been exposed to asbestos while working in a shipyard as a young man. Asbestos-related pleural disease was identified when he was in his 40s, and interstitial lung disease was identified sometime later. Measured lung volumes and flow rates at the time of diagnosis of asbestosis were all within the normal range, but over subsequent years, pulmonary function tests showed a progressive restrictive defect. Imaging of the chest also demonstrated progression of diffuse pleural thickening, and to a lesser extent, basilar interstitial fibrosis. His medical history was otherwise notable for diabetes, hypertension, hyperlipidemia, and benign prostatic hypertrophy. He reported dyspnea when walking up a slope or even with walking on level ground at more than a modest pace. Medications included a statin, an angiotensin-converting enzyme inhibitor, terazosin, metformin, and low-dose aspirin. Physical examination was notable for limited respiratory excursion and faint bibasilar crackles on lung auscultation. Heart tones were regular without murmur. There was no cyanosis, clubbing or peripheral edema. The resting electrocardiogram showed a sinus rhythm. Pulmonary function tests showed severe restrictive defect with a proportional reduction in diffusing capacity for carbon monoxide. Demographic and pulmonary function data are shown in **Table 10.62.1**.

TABLE 10.62.1 Selected Respiratory Function Data

Measurement	Predicted	Measured
Age (y)		76
Sex		Male
Height (cm)		168
Weight (kg)		85
VC (L)	3.14	1.84
IC (L)		0.64
TLC (L)	6.18	3.0
ERV (L)		1.50
FEV_1 (L)	2.33	1.47
FEV_1/VC (%)	73	80
MVV (L/min)		73
DLCO (mL/mm Hg/min)	21.3	9.1
DLCO/VA (mL/mm Hg/min/L)	3.45	3.98

Abbreviations: DLCO, diffusing capacity of lung for carbon monoxide; ERV, expiratory reserve volume; FEV_1, forced expiratory volume in 1 second; IC, inspiratory capacity; MVV, maximum voluntary ventilation; TLC, total lung capacity; VA, alveolar volume; VC, vital capacity.

EXERCISE FINDINGS

The patient exercised on a cycle ergometer beginning with 3 minutes of unloaded pedaling at 60 rpm followed by continuous increase in work rate by 10 W/min until the test ended with symptoms of shortness of breath. There were no ischemic changes or arrhythmias on exercise electrocardiogram. Exercise data are shown in **Tables 10.62.2** and **10.62.3** and in **Figure 10.62.1**.

INTERPRETATION

Comment

This case is presented as an example of combined pulmonary and extrapulmonary restriction. Based on the imaging studies, and the normal diffusing capacity of lung for carbon monoxide divided by alveolar volume on pulmonary function testing (DLCO/VA), it was thought that most of his restrictive pulmonary function defect was due to extensive

TABLE 10.62.2 Selected Exercise Data

Measurement	Predicted	Measured
Peak $\dot{V}O_2$ (L/min)	1.69	0.88
Maximum heart rate (beats/min)	144	103
Maximum O_2 pulse (mL/beat)	11.7	8.6
$\Delta\dot{V}O_2/\Delta WR$ (mL/min/W)	10.3	7.6
AT (L/min)	>0.81	0.59
Blood pressure (mm Hg [rest, max])		162/83, 212/89
Maximum $\dot{V}E$ (L/min)		35
Breathing reserve (L/min)	>15	38
$\dot{V}E/\dot{V}CO_2$ @ *AT*	<34	32
SpO_2 (% [rest, max ex])		95, 92

Abbreviations: *AT*, anaerobic threshold; $\Delta\dot{V}O_2/\Delta WR$, change in $\dot{V}O_2$/change in work rate; ex, exercise; O_2, oxygen; SpO_2, oxygen saturation as measured by pulse oximetry; $\dot{V}E/\dot{V}CO_2$, ventilatory equivalent for carbon dioxide; $\dot{V}O_2$, oxygen uptake.

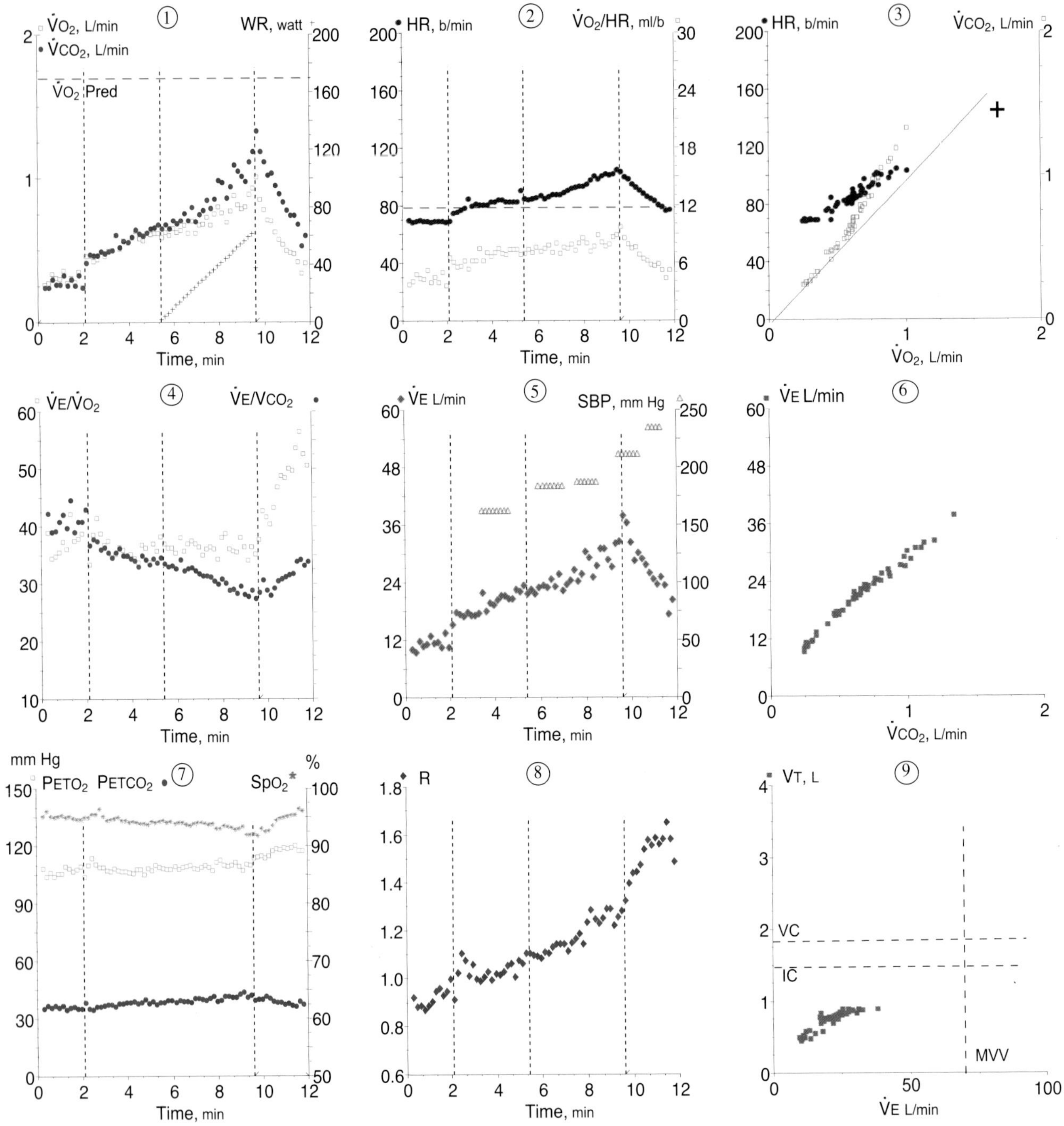

FIGURE 10.62.1. Vertical dashed lines in the panels in the left and middle columns indicate, from left to right, the beginning of unloaded cycling, start of increasing work rate (WR) at 10 W/min, and start of recovery. In **panel 1**, the increase in WR (right y-axis) is plotted with a scale of 100 W to 1 L of oxygen uptake ($\dot{V}O_2$) (left y-axis) such that WR is plotted parallel to a $\dot{V}O_2$ slope of 10 mL/min/W. Predicted peak $\dot{V}O_2$ is shown as a dashed horizontal line. In **panel 3**, carbon dioxide output ($\dot{V}CO_2$) (right y-axis) is plotted as a function of $\dot{V}O_2$ (x-axis) with identical scales so that the diagonal blue line has a slope of 1 (45°). The $\dot{V}CO_2$ increasing more steeply than $\dot{V}O_2$ defines carbon dioxide (CO_2) derived from bicarbonate buffer, as long as ventilatory equivalent for CO_2 ($\dot{V}E/\dot{V}CO_2$) (**panel 4**) is not increasing and end-tidal P_{CO_2} (P_{ETCO_2}) (**panel 7**) is not decreasing, simultaneously. The black + symbol in **panel 3** indicates predicted peak values of heart rate (HR) (left y-axis) and $\dot{V}O_2$ for this individual. Abbreviations: IC, inspiratory capacity; MVV, maximum voluntary ventilation; P_{ETO_2}, end-tidal P_{O_2}; R, respiratory exchange ratio; SBP, systolic blood pressure; Sp_{O_2}, oxygen saturation as measured by pulse oximetry; VC, vital capacity; $\dot{V}E$, minute ventilation; $\dot{V}E/\dot{V}O_2$, ventilatory equivalent for oxygen; V_T, tidal volume.

TABLE 10.62.3 Air Breathing

Time (min)	Work rate (W)	BP (mm Hg)	HR (min^{-1})	f (min^{-1})	$\dot{V}E$ (L/min BTPS)	$\dot{V}CO_2$ (L/min STPD)	$\dot{V}O_2$ (L/min STPD)	$\frac{\dot{V}O_2}{HR}$ (mL/beat)	R	pH	HCO_3^- (mEq/L)	PO_2, mm Hg and SpO_2, % ET	SpO_2	(A − a)	PCO_2, mm Hg ET	a	(a − ET)	$\frac{\dot{V}E}{\dot{V}CO_2}$	$\frac{\dot{V}E}{\dot{V}O_2}$	$\frac{VD}{VT}$
0.5	Rest		61	21	9.8	0.23	0.26	4.2	0.91			107	96		36			42	38	
1.0	Rest		69	21	11.0	0.27	0.31	4.5	0.88			105	95		36			41	36	
1.5	Rest		69	22	11.7	0.28	0.30	4.4	0.94			108	95		35			41	39	
2.0	Rest		69	24	11.4	0.27	0.29	4.2	0.96			108	95		35			42	40	
2.5	Unloaded		73	25	17.0	0.46	0.45	6.2	1.01			109	95		36			37	37	
3.0	Unloaded		80	24	17.2	0.48	0.45	5.7	1.05			109	96		36			36	38	
3.5	Unloaded	162/83	81	27	18.9	0.53	0.53	6.6	1.00			107	95		37			36	35	
4.0	Unloaded		81	25	18.9	0.55	0.54	6.6	1.01			106	95		38			35	35	
4.5	Unloaded		83	27	20.9	0.62	0.60	7.2	1.03			106	94		38			34	35	
5.0	Unloaded		83	27	21.2	0.62	0.60	7.2	1.05			107	94		39			34	36	
5.5	3		86	29	22.3	0.66	0.60	7.0	1.09			108	94		38			34	37	
6.0	11	184/83	85	29	22.4	0.68	0.62	7.3	1.09			108	94		39			33	36	
6.5	18		86	30	23.8	0.72	0.65	7.5	1.12			109	94		39			33	37	
7.0	25		88	30	23.7	0.73	0.64	7.3	1.14			109	94		39			32	37	
7.5	33	188/86	91	30	24.9	0.80	0.70	7.7	1.14			109	94		40			31	36	
8.0	41		93	32	26.9	0.89	0.74	8.0	1.19			109	93		40			30	36	
8.5	48		98	32	27.1	0.92	0.74	7.5	1.25			110	93		41			29	37	
9.0	55		100	34	30.3	1.06	0.83	8.3	1.27			110	93		42			29	37	
9.5	63	212/99	103	35	31.0	1.10	0.88	8.6	1.25			109	92		42			28	35	
10.0	Recovery		101	41	35.4	1.20	0.87	8.6	1.39			114	92		40			29	41	
10.5	Recovery		92	33	29.2	1.00	0.67	7.3	1.49			115	93		40			29	44	
11.0	Recovery	235/140	86	31	25.9	0.83	0.53	6.1	1.57			118	95		38			31	49	
11.5	Recovery		81	32	24.0	0.72	0.45	5.6	1.59			119	95		37			33	53	
12.0	Recovery	196/75	78	28	19.9	0.59	0.39	5.0	1.53			118	96		37			34	52	

Abbreviations: BP, blood pressure; BTPS, body temperature pressure saturated; f, frequency; HCO_3^-, bicarbonate; HR, heart rate; $P(A - a)O_2$, alveolar-arterial PO_2 difference; $P(a - ET)CO_2$, arterial-end-tidal PCO_2 difference; $PETCO_2$, end-tidal PCO_2; $PETO_2$, end-tidal PO_2; R, respiratory exchange ratio; SpO_2, oxygen saturation as measured by pulse oximetry; STPD, standard temperature pressure dry; $\dot{V}CO_2$, carbon dioxide output; VD/VT, physiological dead space-tidal volume ratio; $\dot{V}E$, minute ventilation; $\dot{V}E/\dot{V}CO_2$, ventilatory equivalent for carbon dioxide; $\dot{V}E/\dot{V}O_2$, ventilatory equivalent for oxygen; $\dot{V}O_2$, oxygen uptake.

pleural disease and that he would have ventilatory limitation to exercise. The exercise findings, however, were more characteristic of interstitial lung disease causing cardiovascular impairment.

Analysis

The change in $\Delta\dot{V}O_2/\Delta WR$ was shallow and peak $\dot{V}O_2$ was low. The anaerobic threshold was also low. Peak O_2 pulse was low and did not appear to be increasing appreciably over the final minutes of the test. These findings are characteristic of impaired cardiovascular response to exercise with low peak cardiac output and stroke volume.

Despite marked reduction in lung volumes and breathing capacity, there was an exercise breathing reserve, so it did not appear that the patient was overtly limited by breathing mechanics. He was limited symptomatically by dyspnea, however, and likely had increased work of breathing related to his restricted ventilatory mechanics.

Gas exchange efficiency was mildly abnormal with a reduction of oxygen saturation as measured by pulse oximetry to 92% at peak exercise. Ventilatory equivalents were above average but not above the upper limit of normal for his age.

Conclusion

Although this patient has severe impairment in lung mechanics related to extensive pleural fibrosis and interstitial asbestosis, his exercise function appeared proximally limited by the cardiovascular response. This is likely a secondary effect of his lung disease, although a co-existent primary cardiac impairment is not excluded..

CASE 63

Mild Chronic Bronchitis With Normal Exercise Performance

CLINICAL FINDINGS

This 54-year-old man complained of dyspnea after walking up one flight of stairs or a few blocks on a level surface. He had morning cough several months of each year and had noted occasional retrosternal pain unrelated to exertion or emotional upset. He had 35 pack-years of smoking until stopping 12 years ago. He exercised regularly. The physical examination was normal except for mild obesity. Chest radiographs showed bilateral pleural thickening in the midlung zones and areas of old granulomatous disease. Resting electrocardiogram (ECG) was normal.

EXERCISE FINDINGS

The patient performed exercise on a cycle ergometer. He first pedaled at 60 rpm without added load for 3 minutes. The work rate was then increased 20 W/min to his symptom-limited maximum. Arterial blood was sampled every second minute, and intra-arterial blood pressure was recorded from a percutaneously placed brachial artery catheter. The patient stopped exercise because of "exhaustion." The ECG remained normal throughout exercise.

TABLE 10.63.1 Selected Respiratory Function Data

Measurement	Predicted	Measured
Age (y)		54
Sex		Male
Height (cm)		174
Weight (kg)	77	88
Hematocrit (%)		45
VC (L)	4.28	3.59
IC (L)	2.86	3.12
TLC (L)	6.38	6.15
FEV_1 (L)	3.39	2.40
FEV_1/VC (%)	79	67
MVV (L/min)	142	112
D_{LCO} (mL/mm Hg/min)	28.8	29.8

Abbreviations: D_{LCO}, diffusing capacity of lung for carbon monoxide; FEV_1, forced expiratory volume in 1 second; IC, inspiratory capacity; MVV, maximum voluntary ventilation; TLC, total lung capacity; VC, vital capacity.

INTERPRETATION

Comments

Resting respiratory function was compatible with mild airflow obstruction (**Table 10.63.1**). The resting ECG was normal. Exercise data are summarized in **Table 10.63.2** and shown in **Table 10.63.3** and graphically in **Figure 10.63.1**.

Analysis

This was essentially a normal exercise test despite the patient's complaints of dyspnea on exertion and mildly reduced forced expiratory volume in 1 second. His peak oxygen uptake ($\dot{V}O_2$) and anaerobic threshold were normal, and he reached his expected peak heart rate. Importantly, there was no evidence of ventilatory limitation based on minute ventilation and maximum voluntary ventilation (normal breathing reserve). His exercise ECG was normal. While not obtained in every patient, arterial blood gases were normal, helping to confirm his normal status. The patient was

TABLE 10.63.2 Selected Exercise Data

Measurement	Predicted	Measured
Peak $\dot{V}O_2$ (L/min)	2.42	2.66
Maximum heart rate (beats/min)	166	169
Maximum O_2 pulse (mL/beat)	14.6	15.7
$\Delta\dot{V}O_2/\Delta WR$ (mL/min/W)	10.3	9.9
AT (L/min)	>1.04	1.3
Blood pressure (mm Hg [rest, max])		144/93, 225/117
Maximum $\dot{V}E$ (L/min)		86
Exercise breathing reserve (L/min)	>15	26
$\dot{V}E/\dot{V}CO_2$ @ *AT* or lowest	27.4	26.7
PaO_2 (mm Hg [rest, max ex])		81, 92
$P(A - a)O_2$ (mm Hg [rest, max ex])		18, 21
$PaCO_2$ (mm Hg [rest, max ex])		43, 40
$P(a - ET)CO_2$ (mm Hg [rest, max ex])		5, −3
V_D/V_T (rest, heavy ex)		0.41, 0.23
HCO_3^- (mEq/L [rest, 2-min recov])		26, 16

Abbreviations: *AT*, anaerobic threshold; $\Delta\dot{V}O_2/\Delta WR$, change in $\dot{V}O_2$/change in work rate; ex, exercise; HCO_3^-, bicarbonate; O_2, oxygen; $P(A - a)O_2$, alveolar-arterial PO_2 difference; $P(a - ET)CO_2$, arterial-end-tidal PCO_2 difference; recov, recovery; V_D/V_T, physiological dead space-tidal volume ratio; $\dot{V}E$, minute ventilation; $\dot{V}E/\dot{V}CO_2$, ventilatory equivalent for carbon dioxide; $\dot{V}O_2$, oxygen uptake.

overweight (body mass index 29.1), and his slightly higher $\dot{V}O_2$ during unloaded cycling (about 100 mL/min) reflects mildly increased metabolic cost of cycle exercise. The combination of mild obesity and mild obstruction may explain his symptoms despite having being in the "normal" range for peak $\dot{V}O_2$ and anaerobic threshold.

Using the flowcharts (Chapter 9), the normal peak $\dot{V}O_2$ and anaerobic threshold lead to Flowchart 2, where we are reassured by normal arterial blood gases and ECG at peak $\dot{V}O_2$. Therefore, this flowchart leads to tentative considerations of the effects of obesity.

Conclusion

This study illustrates normal exercise performance by a man with mild chronic obstructive pulmonary disease.

TABLE 10.63.3 Air Breathing

Time (min)	Work rate (W)	BP (mm Hg)	HR (min^{-1})	f (min^{-1})	$\dot{V}E$ (L/min BTPS)	$\dot{V}CO_2$ (L/min STPD)	$\dot{V}O_2$ (L/min STPD)	$\dot{V}O_2$/HR (mL/beat)	R	pH	HCO_3^- (mEq/L)	PO_2, mm Hg ET	a	(A − a)	PCO_2, mm Hg ET	a	(a − ET)	$\dot{V}E/\dot{V}CO_2$	$\dot{V}E/\dot{V}O_2$	VD/VT
0.5	Rest	141/93								7.42	26		77			41				
1.0	Rest		73	20	11.1	0.27	0.34	4.7	0.79			100			40			35	28	
1.5	Rest		76	20	10.5	0.23	0.27	3.6	0.85			107			38			38	33	
2.0	Rest		81	21	11.1	0.24	0.29	3.6	0.83			105			38			39	32	
2.5	Rest	144/90	78	19	10.2	0.22	0.27	3.5	0.81	7.40	26	104	81	18	38	43	5	39	32	0.41
3.0	Rest		81	18	11.8	0.28	0.34	4.2	0.82			101			39			37	30	
3.5	Rest		77	24	10.4	0.21	0.26	3.4	0.81			102			39			40	32	
4.0	Rest		77	22	10.8	0.22	0.28	3.6	0.79			105			37			41	32	
4.5	Rest		78	17	10.0	0.24	0.29	3.7	0.83			104			38			36	30	
5.0	Unloaded		94	16	15.5	0.46	0.60	6.4	0.77			98			40			31	24	
5.5	Unloaded		94	21	15.2	0.46	0.62	6.6	0.74			95			42			29	22	
6.0	Unloaded		93	21	18.5	0.54	0.70	7.5	0.77			98			41			31	24	
6.5	Unloaded		88	20	18.2	0.59	0.72	8.2	0.82			95			43			28	23	
7.0	Unloaded		88	18	17.6	0.56	0.70	8.0	0.80			98			41			29	23	
7.5	Unloaded	162/99	94	19	19.4	0.62	0.75	8.0	0.83	7.39	26	98	83	17	41	43	2	29	24	0.28
8.0	20		91	19	18.0	0.58	0.72	7.9	0.81			96			44			28	23	
8.5	20		98	22	19.6	0.63	0.81	8.3	0.78			93			43			28	22	
9.0	40		98	22	22.5	0.74	0.92	9.4	0.80			97			42			28	22	
9.5	40	174/96	102	20	24.3	0.82	1.02	10.0	0.80	7.37	26	97	91	5	42	45	3	28	22	0.28
10.0	60		104	20	23.8	0.82	1.03	9.9	0.80			94			44			27	21	
10.5	60		107	23	30.9	1.05	1.25	11.7	0.84			94			44			28	23	
11.0	80		108	25	31.8	1.10	1.27	11.8	0.87			91			48			27	23	
11.5	80	174/93	110	25	36.1	1.25	1.39	12.6	0.90	7.37	24	100	95	8	43	43	0	27	24	0.25
12.0	100		115	26	40.6	1.39	1.48	12.9	0.94			98			46			28	26	
12.5	100		117	26	40.1	1.39	1.46	12.5	0.95			98			46			27	26	
13.0	120		120	24	42.4	1.52	1.56	13.0	0.97			99			46			27	26	
13.5	120	204/99	127	25	48.7	1.76	1.80	14.2	0.98	7.36	24	94	92	14	49	43	−6	26	26	0.23
14.0	140		130	28	51.0	1.85	1.86	14.3	0.99			100			46			26	26	
14.5	140		132	29	55.4	2.00	1.92	14.5	1.04			103			46			26	28	
15.0	160		137	29	56.9	2.06	2.00	14.6	1.03			100			48			26	27	
15.5	160	210/105	143	32	63.7	2.24	2.09	14.6	1.07	7.35	23	105	93	16	45	43	−2	27	29	0.25
16.0	180		146	37	67.9	2.37	2.23	15.3	1.06			102			47			27	29	
16.5	180		152	33	68.8	2.52	2.35	15.5	1.07			104			47			26	28	
17.0	200		159	38	81.4	2.70	2.48	15.6	1.12			110			41			28	32	
17.5	200	228/114	164	38	85.7	2.89	2.55	15.5	1.13	7.33	21	108	91	22	43	41	−2	29	32	0.25
18.0	220	225/117	169	38	86.0	2.97	2.66	15.7	1.12	7.31	20	108	92	21	44	40	−4	28	31	0.22
18.5	Recovery		166	32	78.5	2.74	2.27	13.7	1.21			111			42			28	33	
19.0	Recovery		154	29	69.7	2.39	1.65	10.7	1.45			115			42			28	41	
19.5	Recovery		148	28	58.3	1.85	1.18	8.0	1.57			116			42			30	47	
20.0	Recovery	183/96	141	26	51.2	1.58	1.04	7.4	1.52	7.27	16	121	119	5	37	35	−2	31	47	0.20

Abbreviations: BP, blood pressure; BTPS, body temperature pressure saturated; f, frequency; HCO_3^-, bicarbonate; HR, heart rate; P(A − a)O_2, alveolar-arterial PO_2 difference; P(a − ET)CO_2, arterial-end-tidal PCO_2 difference; $PETCO_2$, end-tidal PCO_2; $PETO_2$, end-tidal PO_2; R, respiratory exchange ratio; STPD, standard temperature pressure dry; $\dot{V}CO_2$, carbon dioxide output; VD/VT, physiological dead space-tidal volume ratio; $\dot{V}E$, minute ventilation; $\dot{V}E/\dot{V}CO_2$, ventilatory equivalent for carbon dioxide; $\dot{V}E/\dot{V}O_2$, ventilatory equivalent for oxygen; $\dot{V}O_2$, oxygen uptake.

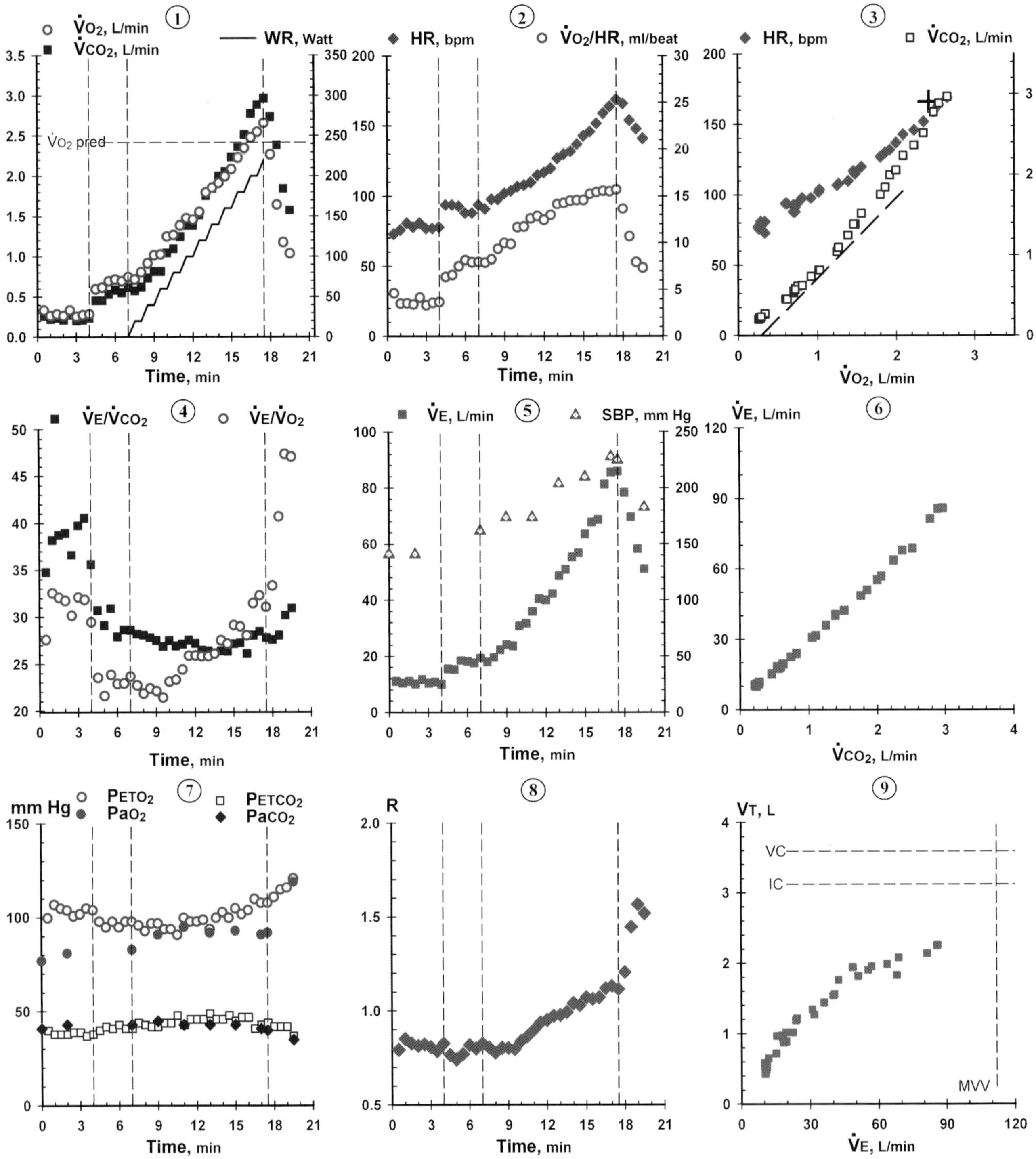

FIGURE 10.63.1. Vertical dashed lines in the panels in the left and middle columns indicate, from left to right, the beginning of unloaded cycling, start of increasing work rate (WR) at 20 W/min, and start of recovery. In **panel 1**, the increase in WR (right y-axis) is plotted with a scale of 100 W to 1 L of oxygen uptake ($\dot{V}O_2$) (left y-axis) such that WR is plotted parallel to a $\dot{V}O_2$ slope of 10 mL/min/W. In **panel 3**, carbon dioxide output ($\dot{V}CO_2$) (right y-axis) is plotted as a function of $\dot{V}O_2$ (x-axis) with identical scales so that the diagonal dashed line has a slope of 1 (45°). The $\dot{V}CO_2$ increasing more steeply than $\dot{V}O_2$ defines carbon dioxide (CO_2) derived from bicarbonate buffer, as long as ventilatory equivalent for CO_2 ($\dot{V}E/\dot{V}CO_2$) (**panel 4**) is not increasing and end-tidal P_{CO_2} (P_{ETCO_2}) (**panel 7**) is not decreasing, simultaneously. The black + symbol in **panel 3** indicates predicted peak values of heart rate (HR) (left y-axis) and $\dot{V}O_2$ for this individual. Abbreviations: IC, inspiratory capacity; MVV, maximum voluntary ventilation; P_{ETO_2}, end-tidal P_{O_2}; R, respiratory exchange ratio; SBP, systolic blood pressure; VC, vital capacity; $\dot{V}E$, minute ventilation; $\dot{V}E/\dot{V}O_2$, ventilatory equivalent for oxygen; V_T, tidal volume.

CASE 64

Emphysema With Mild Airway Obstruction

CLINICAL FINDINGS

This 50-year-old male, long-term smoker was referred for cardiopulmonary exercise testing for evaluation of his exertional dyspnea. He became symptomatic after walking one block. He had mild obstructive lung disease of long duration consistent with emphysema. His only medication was an inhaled β-agonist, which he used frequently.

EXERCISE FINDINGS

The patient performed exercise on a cycle ergometer. He pedaled at 60 rpm without an added load for 3 minutes. The work rate was then increased 15 W/min to tolerance. Heart rate (HR) and rhythm were continuously monitored; 12-lead electrocardiograms were obtained during rest, exercise, and recovery. Blood pressure was measured with a sphygmomanometer, and oxygen saturation was monitored with a pulse oximeter (data not plotted). The patient appeared to give an excellent effort and stopped exercise because of shortness of breath. He denied chest pain during or after the study. Resting, exercise, and recovery electrocardiograms were not remarkable except for occasional multifocal premature ventricular contractions during exercise and recovery.

INTERPRETATION

Comments

Resting respiratory function studies showed mild obstruction, an insignificant bronchodilator response to inhaled β-agonist, elevated total lung capacity, and a moderately reduced diffusing capacity of lung for carbon monoxide (**Table 10.64.1**). Exercise data are summarized in **Table 10.64.2** and shown in **Table 10.64.3** and graphically in **Figure 10.64.1**.

Analysis

This patient did not reach his predicted peak oxygen uptake ($\dot{V}O_2$) nor predicted peak HR, although his HR–$\dot{V}O_2$ relationship was normal. Noting that he stopped the symptom-limited test because of dyspnea and his peak minute ventilation reached his maximum voluntary ventilation (low breathing reserve), he was likely ventilatory limited. This was in fact due to a combination of a high ventilatory requirement, shown by steep minute ventilation versus carbon dioxide output slope and very high ventilatory equivalent for carbon dioxide, and low ventilatory capacity (low maximum voluntary ventilation). Two other factors would contribute to higher ventilatory requirement: low anaerobic threshold (*AT*) means additional carbon dioxide from lactic acid buffering must be eliminated, and hypoxemia (pulse oximeter 88% at peak exercise). Furthermore, his ventilatory capacity could also be reduced due to dynamic hyperinflation; the measurements during this test did not allow for examining this potential contribution.

TABLE 10.64.1 Selected Respiratory Function Data

Measurement	Predicted	Measured
Age (y)		50
Sex		Male
Height (cm)		168
Weight (kg)	72	66
Hematocrit (%)		46
VC (L)	4.06	4.10
IC (L)	2.71	3.30
TLC (L)	5.92	7.07
FEV_1 (L)	3.22	2.57
FEV_1/VC (%)	79	63
MVV (L/min)	141	91
D_{LCO} (mL/mm Hg/min)	25.4	14.7

Abbreviations: D_{LCO}, diffusing capacity of lung for carbon monoxide; FEV_1, forced expiratory volume in 1 second; IC, inspiratory capacity; MVV, maximum voluntary ventilation; TLC, total lung capacity; VC, vital capacity.

TABLE 10.64.2 Selected Exercise Data

Measurement	Predicted	Measured
Peak $\dot{V}O_2$ (L/min)	2.22	1.39
Maximum heart rate (beats/min)	170	126
Maximum O_2 pulse (mL/beat)	13.1	11.0
$\Delta\dot{V}O_2/\Delta WR$ (mL/min/W)	10.3	7.3
AT (L/min)	>0.95	0.9
Blood pressure (mm Hg [rest, max])		120/80, 160/100
Maximum $\dot{V}E$ (L/min)		89
Exercise breathing reserve (L/min)	>15	2
$\dot{V}E/\dot{V}CO_2$ @ *AT* or lowest	27.2	53.3
O_2 saturation (oximeter) (rest, max)		93, 88

Abbreviations: *AT*, anaerobic threshold; $\Delta\dot{V}O_2/\Delta WR$, change in $\dot{V}O_2$/change in work rate; O_2, oxygen; $\dot{V}E$, minute ventilation; $\dot{V}E/\dot{V}CO_2$, ventilatory equivalent for carbon dioxide; $\dot{V}O_2$, oxygen uptake.

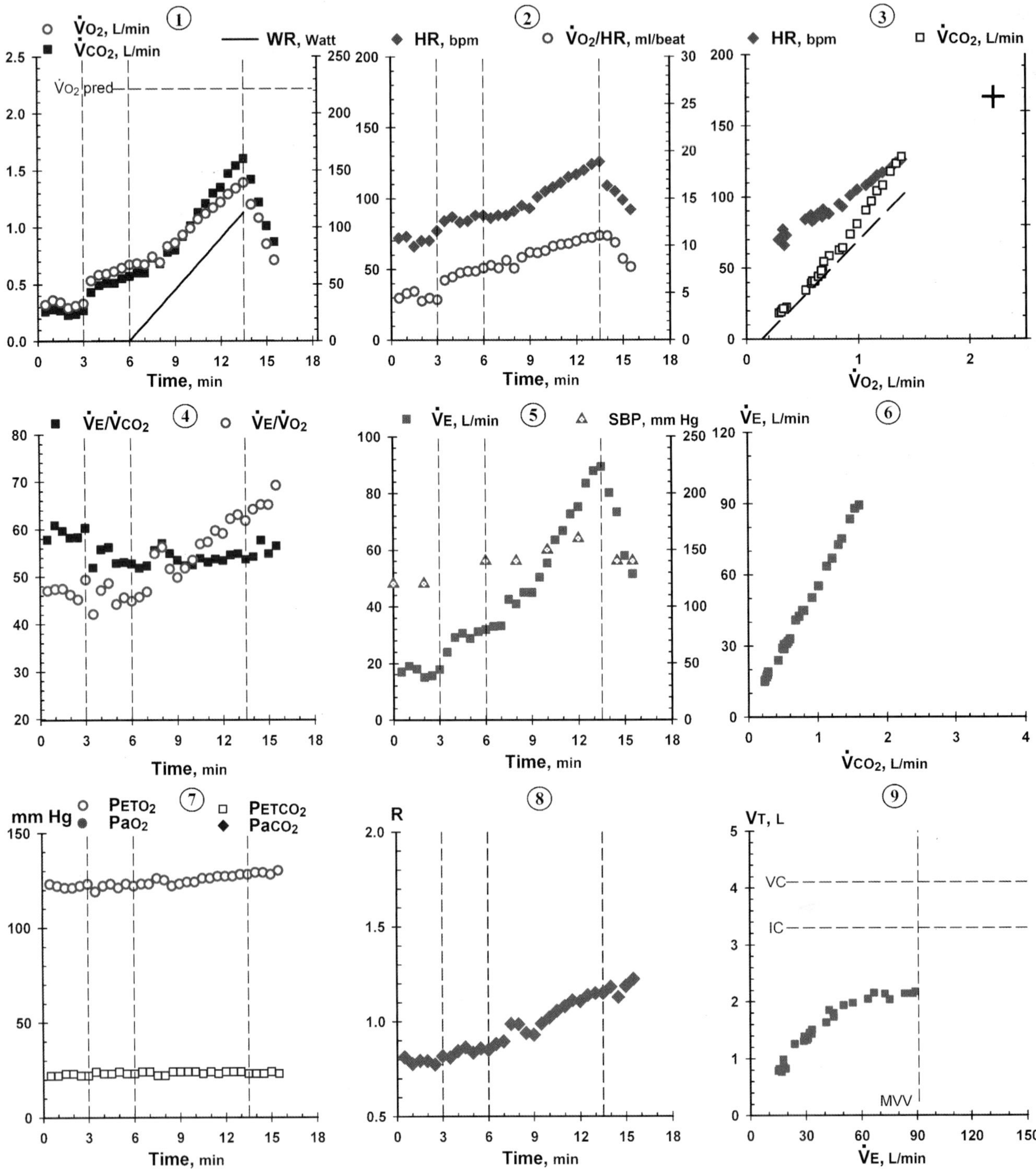

FIGURE 10.64.1. Vertical dashed lines in the panels in the left and middle columns indicate, from left to right, the beginning of unloaded cycling, start of increasing work rate (WR) at 15 W/min, and start of recovery. In **panel 1**, the increase in WR (right y-axis) is plotted with a scale of 100 W to 1 L of oxygen uptake ($\dot{V}O_2$) (left y-axis) such that WR is plotted parallel to a $\dot{V}O_2$ slope of 10 mL/min/W. In **panel 3**, carbon dioxide output ($\dot{V}CO_2$) (right y-axis) is plotted as a function of $\dot{V}O_2$ (x-axis) with identical scales so that the diagonal dashed line has a slope of 1 (45°). The $\dot{V}CO_2$ increasing more steeply than $\dot{V}O_2$ defines carbon dioxide (CO_2) derived from bicarbonate buffer, as long as ventilatory equivalent for CO_2 ($\dot{V}E/\dot{V}CO_2$) (**panel 4**) is not increasing and end-tidal PCO_2 ($PETCO_2$) (**panel 7**) is not decreasing, simultaneously. The black + symbol in **panel 3** indicates predicted peak values of heart rate (HR) (left y-axis) and $\dot{V}O_2$ for this individual. Abbreviations: IC, inspiratory capacity; MVV, maximum voluntary ventilation; $PETO_2$, end-tidal partial pressure of oxygen; R, respiratory exchange ratio; SBP, systolic blood pressure; VC, vital capacity; $\dot{V}E$, minute ventilation; $\dot{V}E/\dot{V}O_2$, ventilatory equivalent for oxygen; V_T, tidal volume.

The flow sheet approach (Chapter 9) would lead to Flowchart 4 because of the low peak $\dot{V}O_2$ and *AT*. On Flowchart 4, the breathing reserve (Branch Point 4.1) is very low, consistent with exercise limitation from lung disease. Although blood gases were not measured, the very high ventilatory equivalents, without a high respiratory exchange ratio that would indicate acute hyperventilation likely reflect increased dead space ventilation (Branch Point 4.2). The low *AT* further augmented ventilatory requirements at the higher work rates. As a result, the patient required an inordinately high level of ventilation for a given level of exercise. The arterial oxygen saturation estimated from oximetry decreased during exercise, which may also have contributed to ventilatory drive. The HR reserve was high, consistent with ventilation limiting exercise prior to attainment of maximal cardiovascular stress. The low change in $\Delta\dot{V}O_2/\Delta WR$ might be due to pulmonary vascular disease secondary to the patient's obstructive lung disease or to reduced venous return during exercise, resulting from high intrathoracic pressure consequent to air trapping and hyperinflation.

Conclusion

This patient had only mild-to-moderate obstructive lung disease on resting pulmonary function tests. He nevertheless demonstrated ventilatory limitation to exercise due to the increased ventilatory requirements resulting from ventilation–perfusion mismatching and low *AT*, while having reduced ventilatory capacity. Based on this patient's history, these findings were most likely attributable to his emphysema; comorbid pulmonary vascular disease of another cause could have similar findings.

TABLE 10.64.3 Air Breathing

Time (min)	Work rate (W)	BP (mm Hg)	HR (min^{-1})	f (min^{-1})	$\dot{V}E$ (L/min BTPS)	$\dot{V}CO_2$ (L/min STPD)	$\dot{V}O_2$ (L/min STPD)	$\dot{V}O_2$/HR (mL/beat)	R	pH	HCO_3^- (mEq/L)	PO_2, mm Hg ET	PO_2, mm Hg a	PO_2, mm Hg (A − a)	PCO_2, mm Hg ET	PCO_2, mm Hg a	PCO_2, mm Hg (a − ET)	$\dot{V}E/\dot{V}CO_2$	$\dot{V}E/\dot{V}O_2$	VD/VT
	Rest	120/80																		
0.5	Rest		72	22	16.9	0.26	0.32	4.4	0.81			123			22			58	47	
1.0	Rest		73	23	19.0	0.28	0.36	4.9	0.78			122			22			61	47	
1.5	Rest		66	21	17.9	0.27	0.34	5.2	0.79			121			23			60	47	
2.0	Rest	120/80	70	19	15.0	0.23	0.29	4.1	0.79			121			23			58	46	
2.5	Rest		70	19	15.6	0.24	0.31	4.4	0.77			122			22			58	45	
3.0	Rest		77	18	17.8	0.27	0.33	4.3	0.82			123			22			60	49	
3.5	Unloaded		84	19	23.9	0.43	0.53	6.3	0.81			119			24			52	42	
4.0	Unloaded		87	21	29.1	0.49	0.58	6.7	0.84			122			23			56	47	
4.5	Unloaded		83	23	30.6	0.51	0.59	7.1	0.86			123			23			56	49	
5.0	Unloaded		84	22	28.8	0.51	0.61	7.3	0.84			121			24			53	44	
5.5	Unloaded		88	23	31.1	0.55	0.64	7.3	0.86			123			23			53	46	
6.0	Unloaded	140/90	88	22	31.9	0.57	0.67	7.6	0.85			122			23			53	25	
6.5	8		86	23	33.0	0.60	0.68	7.9	0.88			123			24			52	46	
7.0	15		88	22	33.2	0.60	0.67	7.6	0.90			123			24			52	47	
7.5	23		88	23	42.5	0.73	0.74	8.4	0.99			126			22			56	55	
8.0	30	140/90	91	25	40.9	0.68	0.69	7.6	0.99			125			22			57	56	
8.5	38		95	26	45.0	0.78	0.83	8.7	0.94			122			24			55	52	
9.0	45		93	25	44.9	0.80	0.86	9.2	0.93			123			24			53	50	
9.5	53		101	26	50.3	0.92	0.93	9.2	0.99			124			24			52	52	
10.0	60	150/92	105	28	55.3	1.01	0.99	9.4	1.02			124			24			52	53	
10.5	68		108	31	63.5	1.13	1.07	9.9	1.06			126			23			54	57	
11.0	75		111	31	66.8	1.21	1.12	10.1	1.08			126			24			53	57	
11.5	83		115	34	72.7	1.30	1.17	10.2	1.11			127			23			54	60	
12.0	90	160/100	117	37	75.2	1.35	1.22	10.4	1.11			127			24			53	59	
12.5	98		120	39	83.5	1.47	1.29	10.8	1.14			127			24			55	62	
13.0	105		124	41	87.9	1.54	1.34	10.8	1.15			128			24			55	63	
13.5	113		126	41	89.3	1.60	1.39	11.0	1.15			128			23			54	62	
14.0	Recovery		109	37	80.1	1.42	1.20	11.0	1.18			129			23			54	64	
14.5	Recovery	140/90	105	36	73.4	1.22	1.08	10.3	1.13			129			23			58	65	
15.0	Recovery		99	30	57.9	1.01	0.85	8.6	1.19			128			24			55	65	
15.5	Recovery	140/80	92	28	51.5	0.87	0.71	7.7	1.23			130			23			56	69	

Abbreviations: BP, blood pressure; BTPS, body temperature pressure saturated; f, frequency; HCO_3^-, bicarbonate; HR, heart rate; P(A − a)O_2, alveolar-arterial PO_2 difference; P(a − ET)CO_2, arterial-end-tidal PCO_2 difference; $PETCO_2$, end-tidal PCO_2; $PETO_2$, end-tidal PO_2; R, respiratory exchange ratio; STPD, standard temperature pressure dry; $\dot{V}CO_2$, carbon dioxide output; VD/VT, physiological dead space–tidal volume ratio; $\dot{V}E$, minute ventilation; $\dot{V}E/\dot{V}CO_2$, ventilatory equivalent for carbon dioxide; $\dot{V}E/\dot{V}O_2$, ventilatory equivalent for oxygen; $\dot{V}O_2$, oxygen uptake.

CASE 65

Severe Combined Obstructive and Restrictive Lung Disease

CLINICAL FINDINGS

A 66-year-old woman was referred for exercise testing for evaluation of dyspnea. She reported having shortness of breath since her 20s. By early adulthood, she had had at least 12 episodes of pneumothorax and bilateral thoracotomies for pleurodesis. She had never smoked tobacco products but had been exposed to pesticides and cotton dust and reported sensitivity to common inhaled allergens. She had severe obstructive and restrictive defects on pulmonary function tests and was treated with inhalers. She could tolerate walking on level grade for 12 minutes before needing to stop to catch her breath. For exercise, she had a friend drive her up a hill each morning in her car so that she could walk down. Her medications included a combination corticosteroid and long-acting β-agonist inhaler, vitamins, and supplemental oxygen that she used at night only. Physical examination was notable for numerous healed thoracostomy scars. Breath sounds were diminished throughout, and the expiratory phase was prolonged on forced exhalation. Cardiac rhythm was regular. There was no cyanosis, clubbing, or edema. Resting electrocardiogram showed a sinus tachycardia. Demographic and respiratory function data are shown in **Table 10.65.1**.

EXERCISE FINDINGS

The patient exercised on a cycle ergometer beginning with 3 minutes of unloaded pedaling at 60 rpm followed by continuous increase in work rate by 10 W/min until the test ended with shortness of breath. She was too dyspneic to breathe through the mouthpiece once she stopped exercise, so no recovery data were recorded. Exercise electrocardiogram showed no ischemic changes or arrhythmia. Exercise data are summarized in **Tables 10.65.2** and **10.65.3** and in **Figures 10.65.1** and **10.65.2**.

TABLE 10.65.1 Selected Respiratory Function Data

Measurement	Predicted	Measured
Age (y)		66
Sex		Female
Height (cm)		166
Weight (kg)		65
VC (L)	3.28	1.72
IC (L)	2.25	1.55
ERV (L)	1.03	0.31
FEV_1 (L)	2.5	0.69
FEV_1/VC (%)	77	40
MVV (L/min)	91	28

Abbreviations: ERV, expiratory reserve volume; FEV_1, forced expiratory volume in 1 second; IC, inspiratory capacity; MVV, maximum voluntary ventilation; VC, vital capacity.

INTERPRETATION

Comment

Although this patient had mixed forms of lung disease, the case is included as an example of the development of hyperinflation during exercise, which was detected by measurement of inspiratory capacity (IC) during the test.

Analysis

Cardiovascular and metabolic responses: The peak $\dot{V}O_2$ is low, but it appears that she stopped exercise prior to developing lactic acidosis as there is no break in the slope of $\dot{V}CO_2$ versus $\dot{V}O_2$ (panel 3) and R value remained stable at

TABLE 10.65.2 Selected Exercise Data

Measurement	Predicted	Measured
Peak $\dot{V}O_2$ (L/min)	1.25	0.65
Maximum heart rate (beats/min)	154	125
Maximum O_2 pulse (mL/beat)	8.1	5.2
$\Delta\dot{V}O_2/\Delta WR$ (mL/min/W)	10.3	7.5
AT (L/min)	>0.66	NA
Blood pressure (mm Hg [rest, max])		123/80, 166/80
Maximum $\dot{V}E$ (L/min)		24
Breathing reserve (L/min)	>15	4
$\dot{V}E/\dot{V}CO_2$ @ *AT*	<33	NA
$\Delta\dot{V}E/\Delta\dot{V}CO_2$ slope	<33	40
VD/VT (rest, max ex)		0.40, 0.38
IC (L [rest, max ex])		1.55, 0.99
SpO_2 (% [rest, max ex])		94, 90

Abbreviations: *AT*, anaerobic threshold; $\Delta\dot{V}O_2/\Delta WR$, change in $\dot{V}O_2$/change in work rate; ex, exercise; IC, inspiratory capacity; NA, not applicable; O_2, oxygen; SpO_2, oxygen saturation as measured by pulse oximetry; $\dot{V}CO_2$, carbon dioxide output; VD/VT, physiological dead space–tidal volume ratio; $\dot{V}E$, minute ventilation; $\dot{V}E/\dot{V}CO_2$, ventilatory equivalent for carbon dioxide; $\dot{V}O_2$, oxygen uptake.

TABLE 10.65.3 Air Breathing

Time (min)	Work rate (W)	BP (mm Hg)	HR (min^{-1})	f (min^{-1})	$\dot{V}E$ (L/min BTPS)	$\dot{V}CO_2$ (L/min STPD)	$\dot{V}O_2$ (L/min STPD)	$\frac{\dot{V}O_2}{HR}$ (mL/beat)	R	pH	HCO_3^- (mEq/L)	PO_2, mm Hg and SpO_2, % ET	SpO_2	(A − a)	PCO_2, mm Hg ET	tc	(a − ET)	$\frac{\dot{V}E}{\dot{V}CO_2}$	$\frac{\dot{V}E}{\dot{V}O_2}$	IC, L	$\frac{VD}{VT}$
0.5	Rest		99	15	12.5	0.29	0.30	3.1	0.95			113	94		32	35		43	41		0.39
1.0	Rest		99	17	11.1	0.25	0.25	2.5	0.98			113	94		32	35.3		45	44	1.55	0.40
1.5	Rest	123/80	100	20	12.5	0.27	0.29	2.9	0.94			114	94		32	35.6		46	43		0.42
2.0	Rest		103	16	12.3	0.28	0.29	2.8	0.97			114	93		32	35.9		44	42		0.41
2.5	Rest		102	17	11.7	0.27	0.28	2.7	0.96			114	94		31	35.9		44	42		0.40
3.0	Unloaded		106	23	14.7	0.33	0.35	3.3	0.96			114	94		32	36		44	43		0.41
3.5	Unloaded		112	26	16.9	0.38	0.39	3.5	0.96			114	93		32	36.2		45	43		0.41
4.0	Unloaded		110	26	16.3	0.37	0.40	3.6	0.94			113	93		32	36.3		44	41		0.41
4.5	Unloaded	140/80	109	27	17.7	0.40	0.42	3.8	0.96			114	93		32	36.3		44	43	1.48	0.41
5.0	Unloaded		109	25	16.5	0.38	0.41	3.8	0.93			112	93		33	36.5		43	40		0.40
5.5	Unloaded		111	28	18.6	0.43	0.45	4.1	0.95			114	93		32	36.5		43	41		0.40
6.0	3		111	30	19.1	0.43	0.45	4.1	0.95			114	93		32	36.5		44	42		0.41
6.5	8		112	31	19.4	0.45	0.47	4.2	0.96			115	93		32	36.8		43	42	1.23	0.40
7.0	13		111	30	19.6	0.46	0.47	4.3	0.97			115	93		31	36.7		43	41		0.40
7.5	18	148/81	112	29	18.5	0.44	0.47	4.2	0.94			113	93		32	36.6		42	39		0.39
8.0	23		118	31	20.8	0.49	0.54	4.6	0.90			113	93		32	36.8		43	39		0.40
8.5	28		117	33	22.2	0.52	0.58	4.9	0.91			113	92		32	36.8		42	38	1.14	0.40
9.0	33		121	33	23.1	0.57	0.62	5.1	0.91			112	91		33	36.8		41	37		0.38
9.5	38	166/80	129	32	23.3	0.59	0.64	5.0	0.93			112	89		33	36.8		39	36		0.37
10.0	42		125	31	23.6	0.61	0.65	5.2	0.94			112	89		34	37.1		39	37	0.99	0.37

Abbreviations: BP, blood pressure; BTPS, body temperature pressure saturated; f, frequency; HCO_3^-, bicarbonate; HR, heart rate; IC, inspiratory capacity; $P(A-a)O_2$, alveolar-arterial PO_2 difference; $P(a-ET)CO_2$, arterial-end-tidal PCO_2 difference; $PETCO_2$, end-tidal PCO_2; $PETO_2$, end-tidal PO_2; R, respiratory exchange ratio; SpO_2, oxygen saturation as measured by pulse oximetry; STPD, standard temperature pressure dry; tc, transcutaneous; $\dot{V}CO_2$, carbon dioxide output; VD/VT, physiological dead space-tidal volume ratio; $\dot{V}E$, minute ventilation; $\dot{V}E/\dot{V}CO_2$, ventilatory equivalent for carbon dioxide; $\dot{V}E/\dot{V}O_2$, ventilatory equivalent for oxygen; $\dot{V}O_2$, oxygen uptake.

resting levels throughout the test. Although the latter could result from inability to increase ventilation sufficiently to clear metabolic carbon dioxide, this does not appear to be the case because there was no significant rise in the end-tidal PCO_2 or transcutaneous PCO_2 ($PtcCO_2$) values. It can be inferred that the anaerobic threshold was likely normal because the lower limit of normal was reached without evidence of having exceeding it.

Ventilatory responses: Breathing reserve was small with peak $\dot{V}E$ within 4 L/min of the calculated maximum voluntary ventilation (40 × FEV_1). Tidal volume (VT) remained relatively stable over the course of the test (panel 9). However, as the IC was decreasing, the VT was becoming a progressively higher proportion of IC. The decreasing IC from 1.55 L at rest to less than 1 L at peak exercise is evidence of dynamic hyperinflation. As a result, inspiratory reserve volume decreased progressively to only 150 mL by peak exercise. The progressive changes in IC and inspiratory reserve volume and their positions relative to the patient's maximal flow volume profile over the course of exercise are shown in **Figure 10.65.2**.[1]

Gas exchange efficiency. Ventilatory equivalents remained high up to the level of exercise attained and the $\dot{V}E/\dot{V}CO_2$ slope was steeper than normal, consistent with elevated VD/VT. While this could also result from low arterial PCO_2, this is unlikely, based on the transcutaneous PCO_2 values, which remained around 34 mm Hg throughout the study. The end-tidal PCO_2 values remained lower than transcutaneous, and VD/VT, calculated using the transcutaneous as an estimate of arterial PCO_2, was elevated at rest and did not decrease appreciably with exercise. Arterial saturation by oximetry decreased during the last several minutes of the test as well.

Conclusion

There is mechanical ventilatory limitation to exercise due to the combined effects of restrictive and obstructive defects in lung function and abnormal pulmonary gas exchange consistent with areas of both high and low $\dot{V}A/\dot{Q}$ regions. Dynamic hyperinflation was demonstrated and was undoubtedly a factor in her dyspnea.

REFERENCE

1. Guenette JA, Chin RC, Cory JM, Webb KA, O'Donnell DE. Inspiratory capacity during exercise: measurement, analysis, and interpretation. *Pulm Med.* 2013;2013:956081.

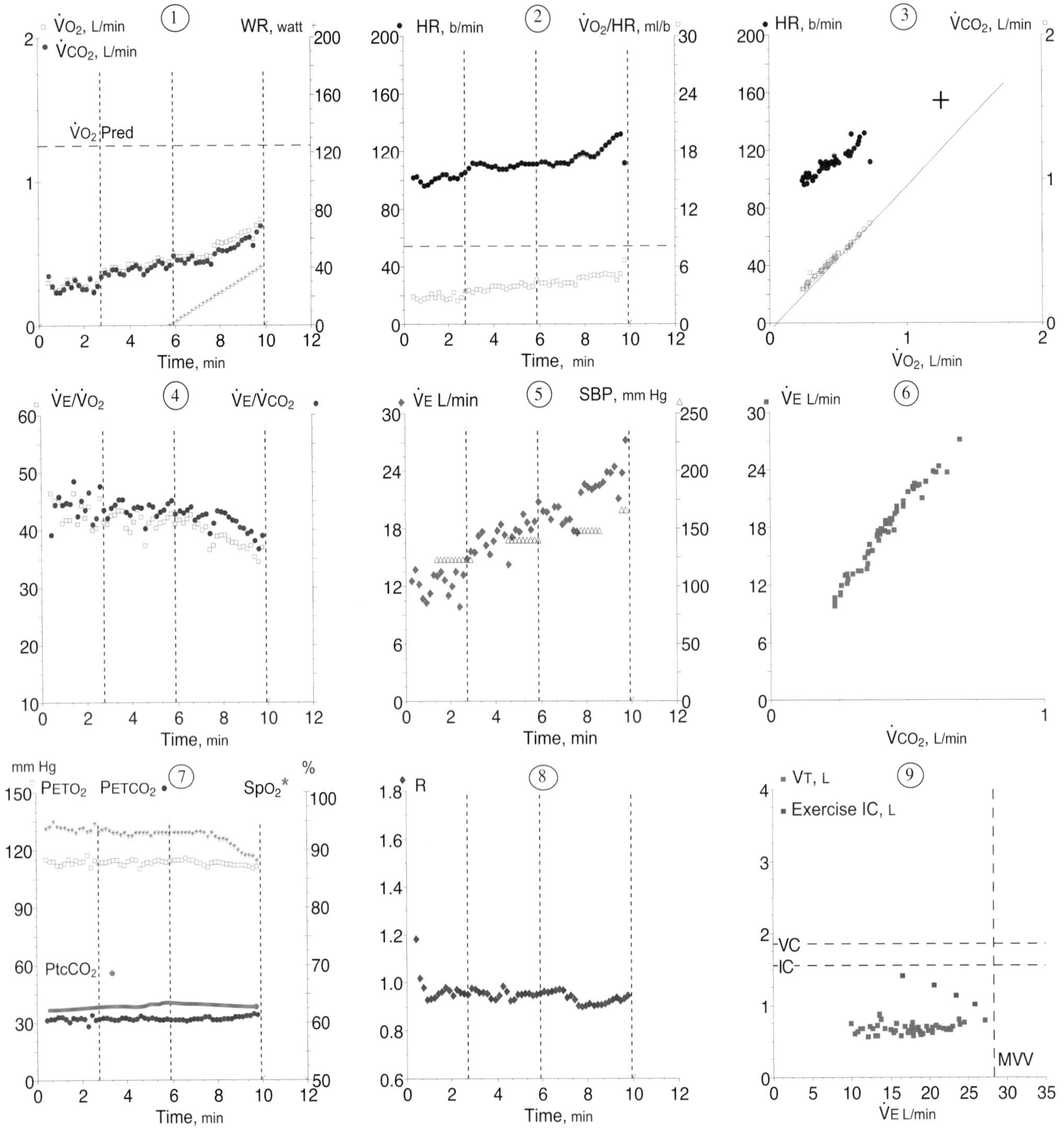

FIGURE 10.65.1. Vertical dashed lines in the panels in the left and middle columns indicate, from left to right, the beginning of unloaded cycling, start of increasing work rate (WR) at 10 W/min, and end exercise. In **panel 1**, the increase in WR (right y-axis) is plotted with a scale of 100 W to 1 L of oxygen uptake ($\dot{V}O_2$) (left y-axis) such that WR is plotted parallel to a $\dot{V}O_2$ slope of 10 mL/min/W. Predicted peak $\dot{V}O_2$ is shown as a dashed horizontal line. In **panel 3**, carbon dioxide output ($\dot{V}CO_2$) (right y-axis) is plotted as a function of $\dot{V}O_2$ (x-axis) with identical scales so that the diagonal blue line has a slope of 1 (45°). The $\dot{V}CO_2$ increasing more steeply than $\dot{V}O_2$ defines carbon dioxide (CO_2) derived from bicarbonate buffer, as long as ventilatory equivalent for CO_2 ($\dot{V}E/\dot{V}CO_2$) (**panel 4**) is not increasing and end-tidal P_{CO_2} (P_{ETCO_2}) (**panel 7**) is not decreasing, simultaneously. The black + symbol in **panel 3** indicates predicted peak values of heart rate (HR) (left y-axis) and $\dot{V}O_2$ for this individual. Abbreviations: IC, inspiratory capacity; MVV, maximum voluntary ventilation; P_{ETO_2}, end-tidal P_{O_2}; $PtcCO_2$, transcutaneous P_{CO_2}; R, respiratory exchange ratio; SBP, systolic blood pressure; Sp_{O_2}, oxygen saturation as measured by pulse oximetry; VC, vital capacity; $\dot{V}E$, minute ventilation; $\dot{V}E/\dot{V}O_2$, ventilatory equivalent for oxygen; V_T, tidal volume.

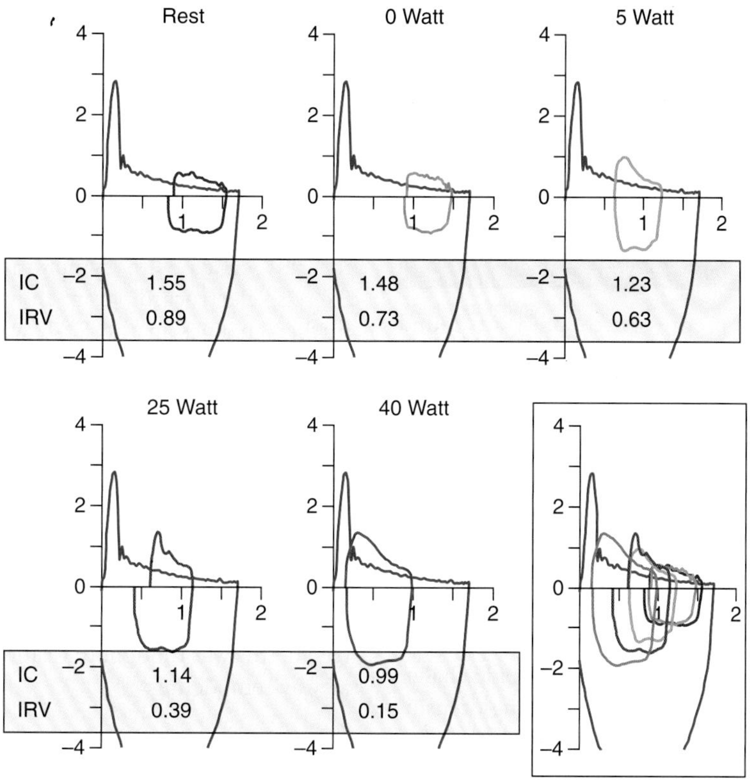

FIGURE 10.65.2. Spontaneous flow volume loops at rest and at four points in time during incremental exercise (at 0, 5, 25, and 40 W) are shown individually and superimposed (bottom right panel). Flow rates in L/sec are shown on the y-axis with expiratory flow above the x-axis and inspiratory flow below. Volume is shown in L on the x-axis. The horizontal positioning of the loops within the maximal flow volume loop measured prior to exercise (shown in red) was determined by remeasurement of the inspiratory capacity (IC). The IC and inspiratory reserve volume (IRV) are shown for each measurement point in liters. Progressive hyperinflation is implied by the progressive decrease in IC, depicted as leftward migration of the spontaneous breaths toward total lung capacity with increasing levels of exercise resulting in decreasing IRV.

CASE 66

Severe Chronic Obstructive Lung Disease

CLINICAL FINDINGS

A 72-year-old woman with progressive dyspnea was found to have elevated estimated pulmonary artery pressures by echocardiogram. Pulmonary function tests subsequently showed severe obstructive lung disease with only minimal reversibility. She had a history of asthma and recurrent bronchitis and a remote history of smoking in her 20s. She was able to walk on level grade but had to pace herself or stop periodically to catch her breath. Medical history was also notable for intermittent atrial fibrillation and systemic hypertension. She had Raynaud phenomenon but no diagnosis of a collagen vascular disorder. Medications included combined long-acting β-agonist and corticosteroid inhaler, long-acting muscarinic blocker by inhaler, an angiotensin-converting enzyme inhibitor, calcium channel blocker, flecainide, and supplemental oxygen for use at night. Physical examination was notable for prolonged expiratory phase. Cardiac tones were regular, and there was no clubbing or peripheral edema. Resting electrocardiogram showed a sinus rhythm with diffuse ST-T wave abnormalities. Demographic and respiratory function data are shown in **Table 10.66.1**.

EXERCISE FINDINGS

The patient exercised on a cycle ergometer beginning with 3 minutes of unloaded pedaling at 60 rpm followed by continuous increase in work rate by 10 W/min until the test ended with symptoms of shortness of breath. Exercise electrocardiogram showed no arrhythmia and no further changes in the ST-T wave morphology. Exercise data are summarized in **Tables 10.66.2** and **10.66.3** and in **Figure 10.66.1**.

INTERPRETATION

Comment

Spirometry showed severe obstructive lung disease with a forced expiratory volume in 1 second of approximately one-third the normal value. Because her smoking history was trivial, this was thought to result from chronic asthma with airway remodeling.

Analysis

Exercise capacity was severely reduced, as reflected in a peak $\dot{V}O_2$ of only 10 mL/min/kg. There were a number of findings indicating an impairment in delivery and/or use of oxygen. These include a shallow $\Delta\dot{V}O_2/\Delta WR$ slope and plateau of the oxygen pulse early in exercise at a level lower than the predicted maximum. The ventilatory response was characterized by a small breathing reserve indicating that the exercise was limited by breathing mechanics. There was little increase in tidal volume during exercise, so

TABLE 10.66.1 Selected Respiratory Function Data

Measurement	Predicted	Measured
Age (y)		72
Sex		Female
Height (cm)		161
Weight (kg)		61
VC (L)	2.85	1.41
IC (L)	2.85	1.46
ERV (L)	0.72	0.22
FEV_1 (L)	2.15	0.73
FEV_1/VC (%)	75	52
MVV (L/min)	83	33

Abbreviations: ERV, expiratory reserve volume; FEV_1, forced expiratory volume in 1 second; IC, inspiratory capacity; MVV, maximum voluntary ventilation; VC, vital capacity.

TABLE 10.66.2 Selected Exercise Data

Measurement	Predicted	Measured
Peak $\dot{V}O_2$ (L/min)	1.1	0.59
Maximum heart rate (beats/min)	148	91
Maximum O_2 pulse (mL/beat)	7.4	6.5
$\Delta\dot{V}O_2/\Delta WR$ (mL/min/W)	10.3	5.9
AT (L/min)	>0.60	0.425
Blood pressure (mm Hg [rest, max])		162/73, 191/76
Maximum $\dot{V}E$ (L/min)		27
Breathing reserve (L/min)	>15	9
$\dot{V}E/\dot{V}CO_2$ @ *AT* (L/min)	<35	40
SpO_2 (% [rest, max ex])		92, 89

Abbreviations: *AT*, anaerobic threshold; $\Delta\dot{V}O_2/\Delta WR$, change in $\dot{V}O_2$/change in work rate; ex, exercise; O_2, oxygen; SpO_2, oxygen saturation as measured by pulse oximetry; $\dot{V}E$, minute ventilation; $\dot{V}E/\dot{V}CO_2$, ventilatory equivalent for carbon dioxide; $\dot{V}O_2$, oxygen uptake.

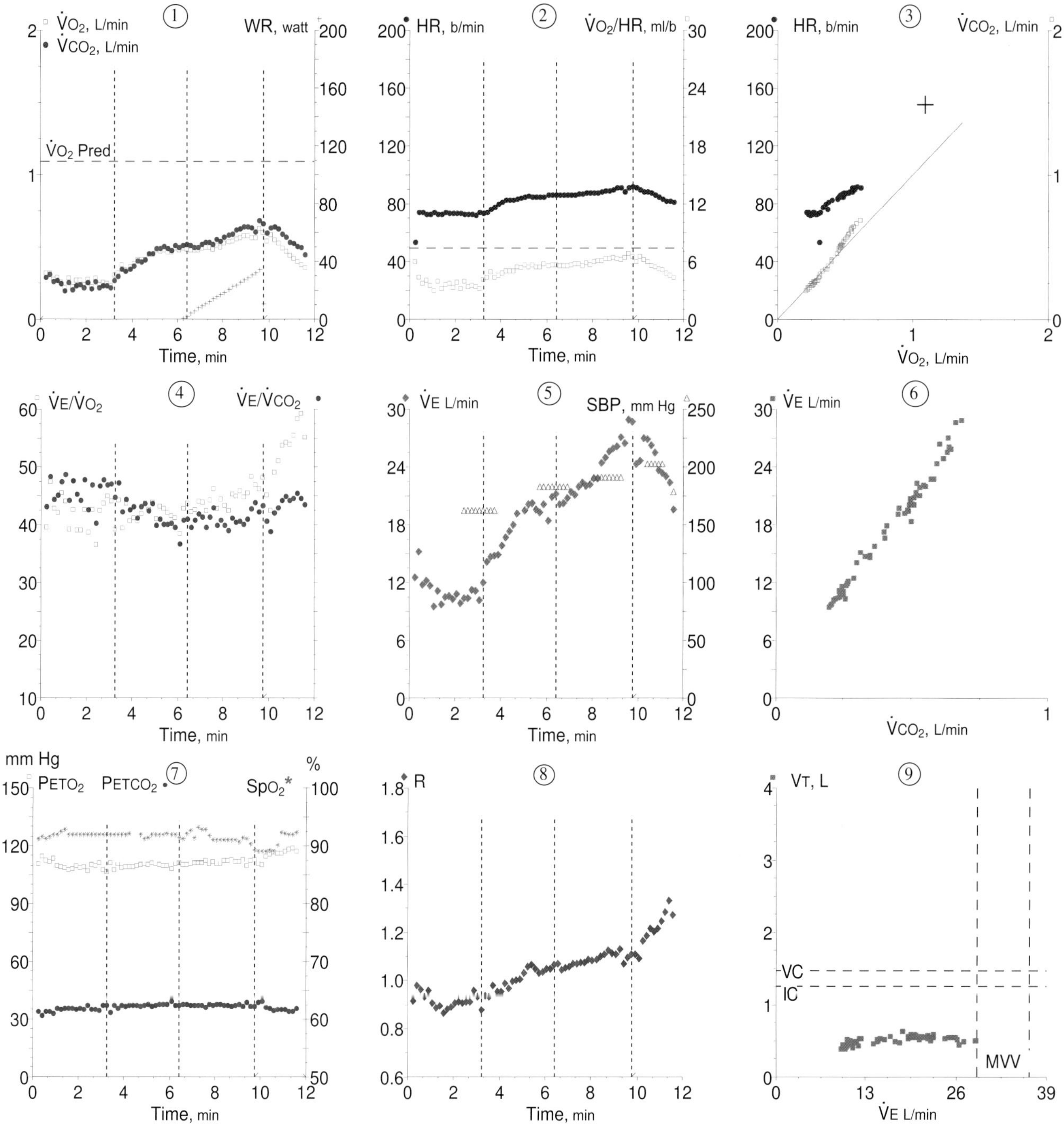

FIGURE 10.66.1. Vertical dashed lines in the panels in the left and middle columns indicate, from left to right, the beginning of unloaded cycling, start of increasing work rate (WR) at 10 W/min, and start of recovery. In **panel 1**, the increase in WR (right y-axis) is plotted with a scale of 100 W to 1 L of oxygen uptake ($\dot{V}O_2$) (left y-axis) such that WR is plotted parallel to a $\dot{V}O_2$ slope of 10 mL/min/W. Predicted peak $\dot{V}O_2$ is shown as a dashed horizontal line. In **panel 3**, carbon dioxide output ($\dot{V}CO_2$) (right y-axis) is plotted as a function of $\dot{V}O_2$ (x-axis) with identical scales so that the diagonal blue line has a slope of 1 (45°). The $\dot{V}CO_2$ increasing more steeply than $\dot{V}O_2$ defines carbon dioxide (CO_2) derived from bicarbonate buffer, as long as ventilatory equivalent for CO_2 ($\dot{V}E/\dot{V}CO_2$) (**panel 4**) is not increasing and end-tidal P_{CO_2} (P_{ETCO_2}) (**panel 7**) is not decreasing, simultaneously. The black + symbol in **panel 3** indicates predicted peak values of heart rate (HR) (left y-axis) and $\dot{V}O_2$ for this individual. Abbreviations: IC, inspiratory capacity; MVV, maximum voluntary ventilation; P_{ETO_2}, end-tidal P_{O_2}; R, respiratory exchange ratio; SBP, systolic blood pressure; Sp_{O_2}, oxygen saturation as measured by pulse oximetry; VC, vital capacity; $\dot{V}E$, minute ventilation; $\dot{V}E/\dot{V}O_2$, ventilatory capacity for oxygen; V_T, tidal volume.

TABLE 10.66.3 Air Breathing

Time (min)	Work rate (W)	BP (mm Hg)	HR (min^{-1})	f (min^{-1})	$\dot{V}_E$ (L/min BTPS)	$\dot{V}CO_2$ (L/min STPD)	$\dot{V}O_2$ (L/min STPD)	$\frac{\dot{V}O_2}{HR}$ (mL/beat)	R	pH	HCO_3^- (mEq/L)	PO_2, mm Hg and SpO_2, % ET	SpO_2	(A − a)	PCO_2, mm Hg ET	a	(a − ET)	$\frac{\dot{V}_E}{\dot{V}CO_2}$	$\frac{\dot{V}_E}{\dot{V}O_2}$	$\frac{V_D}{V_T}$
0.5	Rest		61	25	14.0	0.31	0.33	5.5	0.95			113	91		33			44	42	
1.0	Rest		73	24	11.8	0.26	0.27	3.7	0.95			113	92		34			46	43	
1.5	Rest		73	24	10.2	0.22	0.24	3.4	0.89			109	93		35			47	42	
2.0	Rest		73	24	10.4	0.23	0.26	3.5	0.88			109	92		36			46	40	
2.5	Rest	162/73	73	21	10.3	0.24	0.26	3.6	0.91			108	92		36			43	39	
3.0	Rest		72	26	11.0	0.23	0.25	3.4	0.93			110	92		35			48	44	
3.5	Unloaded		74	29	11.9	0.25	0.27	3.7	0.91			109	92		35			48	43	
4.0	Unloaded		78	29	14.7	0.34	0.35	4.5	0.96			109	92		37			43	42	
4.5	Unloaded		82	32	16.6	0.39	0.40	4.9	0.97			109	69		37			43	41	
5.0	Unloaded		84	36	19.0	0.44	0.44	5.2	1.00			110	61		37			43	43	
5.5	Unloaded		85	35	20.0	0.50	0.47	5.5	1.05			111	92		37			40	42	
6.0	Unloaded	183/75	85	35	19.6	0.49	0.47	5.5	1.04			110	92		38			40	42	
6.5	3		86	35	20.2	0.51	0.48	5.6	1.05			110	92		38			40	42	
7.0	8		86	37	20.4	0.50	0.47	5.5	1.06			111	92		38			41	43	
7.5	13		86	40	21.5	0.53	0.49	5.7	1.07			111	93		37			41	44	
8.0	18	191/76	88	41	22.3	0.54	0.50	5.7	1.08			112	92		37			41	45	
8.5	23		88	42	23.4	0.58	0.54	6.1	1.09			111	91		38			40	44	
9.0	28		89	46	25.5	0.63	0.56	6.3	1.12			112	91		37			41	45	
9.5	33		91	55	26.6	0.62	0.56	6.2	1.10			112	91		38			43	47	
10.0	38		91	55	27.4	0.65	0.59	6.5	1.10			112	90		38			42	47	
10.5	Recovery	203/75	89	48	26.3	0.63	0.55	6.2	1.15			114	89		37			41	48	
11.0	Recovery		86	50	25.1	0.56	0.46	5.4	1.22			116	91		35			45	54	
11.5	Recovery		82	44	22.8	0.51	0.39	4.8	1.29			118	92		34			45	58	
12.0	Recovery	173/63	81	38	19.6	0.44	0.35	4.3	1.27			117	93		35			44	56	

Abbreviations: BP, blood pressure; BTPS, body temperature pressure saturated; f, frequency; HCO_3^-, bicarbonate; HR, heart rate; $P(A-a)O_2$, alveolar-arterial PO_2 difference; $P(a-ET)CO_2$, arterial-end-tidal PCO_2 difference; $PETCO_2$, end-tidal PCO_2; $PETO_2$, end-tidal PO_2; R, respiratory exchange ratio; SpO_2, oxygen saturation as measured by pulse oximetry; STPD, standard temperature pressure dry; $\dot{V}CO_2$, carbon dioxide output; V_D/V_T, physiological dead space-tidal volume ratio; $\dot{V}_E$, minute ventilation; $\dot{V}_E/\dot{V}CO_2$, ventilatory equivalent for carbon dioxide; $\dot{V}_E/\dot{V}O_2$, ventilatory equivalent for oxygen; $\dot{V}O_2$, oxygen uptake.

that it remained a relatively small proportion of the resting inspiratory capacity. Inspiratory capacity was not remeasured during the test, so it cannot be known with certainty whether it decreased due to hyperinflation, but that would certainly account for the breathing pattern observed. There was also inefficiency of pulmonary gas exchange, reflected in the high values of $\dot{V}_E/\dot{V}CO_2$ and arterial oxygen desaturation by pulse oximetry. The low breathing reserve thus resulted both from a reduced breathing capacity and elevated breathing requirements.

Conclusion

This patient was initially referred for testing because of suspicion of a primary pulmonary vascular disease. Pulmonary function testing showed severe airflow obstruction, however, which is likely the basis of the pulmonary hypertension. Exercise testing demonstrates ventilatory limitation to exercise and evidence of abnormal oxygen flow, which could be secondary to the effects of chronic lung disease (with or without dynamic hyperinflation) or associated pulmonary vasculopathy, on cardiac output.

CASE 67

Emphysema, Untreated

CLINICAL FINDINGS

This 61-year-old man with bullous emphysema was referred for evaluation regarding the need for oxygen supplementation. He had a 35 pack-year history of cigarette smoking. He had not sought medical care until 4 months previously, when he was hospitalized for pneumonia, severe dyspnea, and hemoptysis. No specific cause was found for his hemoptysis, but he was found to have significant obstructive lung disease. A resting electrocardiogram showed poor R-wave progression.

EXERCISE FINDINGS

The patient performed exercise on a cycle ergometer. He pedaled at 60 rpm without an added load for 3 minutes. The work rate was then increased 10 W/min to tolerance. Arterial blood was sampled every second minute, and intra-arterial pressure was recorded from a percutaneously placed brachial artery catheter. The patient stopped exercise because of leg fatigue. The patient had no chest pain or further electrocardiogram abnormalities.

INTERPRETATION

Comments

The patient was relatively thin (body mass index 21). Resting pulmonary function tests showed a moderate obstructive ventilatory defect, increased total lung capacity, and low diffusing capacity of the lung for carbon monoxide (**Table 10.67.1**). Exercise data are summarized in **Table 10.67.2** and shown in **Table 10.67.3** and graphically in **Figure 10.67.1**.

Analysis

This patient had severely reduced maximum exercise capacity with low peak oxygen uptake ($\dot{V}O_2$) along with the anticipating finding of ventilatory limitation to exercise as shown by his low breathing reserve (maximum voluntary ventilation – peak minute ventilation), high tidal volume/inspiratory capacity ratio, and high heart rate reserve. As is not uncommon with obstructive lung disease, ventilatory limitation resulted from a combination of decreased ventilatory capacity (obstructive airways disease and exercise-related hyperinflation) and increased ventilatory requirement (hypoxemia, elevated physiological dead space–tidal volume

TABLE 10.67.1 Selected Respiratory Function Data

Measurement	Predicted	Measured
Age (y)		61
Sex		Male
Height (cm)		173
Weight (kg)	76	63
Hematocrit (%)		45
VC (L)	4.00	4.37
IC (L)	2.67	2.62
TLC (L)	6.15	9.11
FEV_1 (L)	3.13	2.11
FEV_1/VC (%)	78	48
MVV (L/min)	131	87
D_{LCO} (mL/mm Hg/min)	26.0	8.4

Abbreviations: D_{LCO}, diffusing capacity of the lung for carbon monoxide; FEV_1, forced expiratory volume in 1 second; IC, inspiratory capacity; MVV, maximum voluntary ventilation; TLC, total lung capacity; VC, vital capacity.

TABLE 10.67.2 Selected Exercise Data

Measurement	Predicted	Measured
Peak $\dot{V}O_2$ (L/min)	1.95	1.25
Maximum heart rate (beats/min)	159	149
Maximum O_2 pulse (mL/beat)	12.3	8.4
$\Delta\dot{V}O_2/\Delta WR$ (mL/min/W)	10.3	8.5
AT (L/min)	>0.86	0.7
Blood pressure (mm Hg [rest, max])		127/75, 190/96
[illegible]		[illegible]
Exercise breathing reserve (L/min)	>15	2
$\dot{V}E/\dot{V}CO_2$ @ *AT* or lowest	28.2	38.0
PaO_2 (mm Hg [rest, max ex])		83, 72
$P(A - a)O_2$ (mm Hg [rest, max ex])		32, 52
$PaCO_2$ (mm Hg [rest, max ex])		36, 34
$P(a - ET)CO_2$ (mm Hg [rest, max ex])		4, 8
V_D/V_T (rest, max ex)		0.28, 0.41
HCO_3^- (mEq/L [rest, 2-min recov])		22, 13

Abbreviations: *AT*, anaerobic threshold; $\Delta\dot{V}O_2/\Delta WR$, change in $\dot{V}O_2$/change in work rate; ex, exercise; HCO_3^-, bicarbonate; O_2, oxygen; $P(A - a)O_2$, alveolar-arterial PO_2 difference; $P(a - ET)CO_2$, arterial-end-tidal PCO_2 difference; recov, recovery; V_D/V_T, physiological dead space-tidal volume ratio; $\dot{V}E$, minute ventilation; $\dot{V}E/\dot{V}CO_2$, ventilatory equivalent for carbon dioxide; $\dot{V}O_2$, oxygen uptake.

TABLE 10.67.3 Air Breathing

Time (min)	Work rate (W)	BP (mm Hg)	HR (min^{-1})	f (min^{-1})	$\dot{V}E$ (L/min BTPS)	$\dot{V}CO_2$ (L/min STPD)	$\dot{V}O_2$ (L/min STPD)	$\frac{\dot{V}O_2}{HR}$ (mL/beat)	R	pH	HCO_3^- (mEq/L)	PO_2, mm Hg ET	PO_2, mm Hg a	PO_2, mm Hg (A − a)	PCO_2, mm Hg ET	PCO_2, mm Hg a	PCO_2, mm Hg (a − ET)	$\frac{\dot{V}E}{\dot{V}CO_2}$	$\frac{\dot{V}E}{\dot{V}O_2}$	$\frac{VD}{VT}$
	Rest	129/75								7.44	22		86			33				
0.5	Rest		77	15	13.9	0.30	0.28	3.6	1.07			122			30			42	45	
1.0	Rest		75	13	10.8	0.23	0.23	3.1	1.00			121			31			42	42	
1.5	Rest		76	14	9.9	0.21	0.21	2.8	1.00			118			32			41	41	
2.0	Rest	129/75	75	15	10.8	0.27	0.26	3.5	1.04	7.41	22	118	83	32	32	36	4	35	37	0.28
2.5	Rest		74	12	10.4	0.22	0.20	2.7	1.10			123			29			43	47	
3.0	Rest		75	11	10.4	0.25	0.24	3.2	1.04			120			31			38	39	
3.5	Unloaded		83	20	17.8	0.40	0.38	4.6	1.05			117			32			40	42	
4.0	Unloaded	138/41	86	19	18.6	0.43	0.41	4.8	1.05	7.41	22	121	91	25	30	35	5	40	41	0.34
4.5	Unloaded		89	16	19.6	0.48	0.46	5.2	1.04			120			30			38	40	
5.0	Unloaded		94	17	21.2	0.52	0.51	5.4	1.02			120			31			38	39	
5.5	Unloaded		94	18	24.4	0.59	0.57	6.1	1.04			121			30			39	40	
6.0	Unloaded	168/90	95	18	25.0	0.62	0.59	6.2	1.05	7.40	21	121	78	38	30	35	5	38	40	0.33
6.5	10		97	17	25.3	0.64	0.59	6.1	1.08			120			31			37	40	
7.0	10	168/90	98	20	29.0	0.71	0.65	6.6	1.09	7.41	22	122	77	40	29	35	6	38	42	0.34
7.5	20		101	22	28.5	0.70	0.64	6.3	1.09			119			32			38	42	
8.0	20	174/90	102	21	32.5	0.78	0.70	6.9	1.11	7.40	21	123	74	45	29	34	5	39	44	0.34
8.5	30		104	24	28.9	0.73	0.67	6.4	1.09			120			32			37	40	
9.0	30	174/40	110	21	40.1	0.96	0.83	7.5	1.16	7.40	21	124	71	48	28	35	7	40	46	0.37
9.5	40		115	20	38.7	0.97	0.84	7.3	1.15			122			30			38	44	
10.0	40	180/90	119	23	44.4	1.08	0.92	7.7	1.17	7.39	20	123	71	49	29	34	5	39	46	0.34
10.5	50		123	22	47.7	1.16	0.95	7.7	1.22			125			28			40	48	
11.0	50	182/88	126	25	51.7	1.22	0.97	7.7	1.26	7.38	19	125	70	52	28	33	5	41	51	0.34
11.5	60		130	25	56.9	1.35	1.05	8.1	1.29			126			28			41	52	
12.0	60	189/93	132	26	58.7	1.40	1.08	8.2	1.30	7.36	18	125	72	51	29	33	4	40	52	0.34
12.5	70		138	26	62.3	1.47	1.12	8.1	1.31			127			28			41	54	
13.0	70	190/90	140	31	68.1	1.54	1.14	8.1	1.35	7.32	17	128	72	51	27	34	7	43	57	0.39
13.5	80		144	32	71.4	1.62	1.19	8.3	1.36			127			28			42	58	
14.0	80	190/96	149	38	80.2	1.73	1.24	8.3	1.40	7.32	17	129	72	52	26	34	8	44	62	0.41
14.5	90		148	39	85.2	1.80	1.25	8.4	1.44			129			26			45	66	
15.0	Recovery		141	27	66.6	1.49	1.07	7.6	1.39			129			26			43	60	
15.5	Recovery		140	26	63.3	1.38	0.90	6.4	1.53			130			26			44	68	
16.0	Recovery		133	22	54.5	1.19	0.74	5.6	1.61			131			26			44	71	
16.5	Recovery	174/87	126	22	51.3	1.07	0.65	5.2	1.65	7.26	13	132	115	14	25	30	5	46	76	0.36
17.0	Recovery		120	24	45.5	0.88	0.54	4.5	1.63			133			24			49	80	

Abbreviations: BP, blood pressure; BTPS, body temperature pressure saturated; f, frequency; HCO_3^-, bicarbonate; HR, heart rate; $P(A-a)O_2$, alveolar-arterial PO_2 difference; $P(a-ET)CO_2$, arterial-end-tidal PCO_2 difference; $PETCO_2$, end-tidal PCO_2; $PETO_2$, end-tidal PO_2; R, respiratory exchange ratio; STPD, standard temperature pressure dry; $\dot{V}CO_2$, carbon dioxide output; VD/VT, physiological dead space-tidal volume ratio; $\dot{V}E$, minute ventilation; $\dot{V}E/\dot{V}CO_2$, ventilatory equivalent for carbon dioxide; $\dot{V}E/\dot{V}O_2$, ventilatory equivalent for oxygen; $\dot{V}O_2$, oxygen uptake.

ratio [VD/VT]). The patient also had low anaerobic threshold and a decrease in bicarbonate to 13 mmol/L, suggesting decreased oxygen (O_2) delivery to exercising muscles, ie, an O_2 flow problem that could represent hypoxemia, anemia (not present in this patient), or low stroke volume due to heart or pulmonary vascular disease. Furthermore, low O_2 flow due to low stroke volume may be seen in patients with obstructive lung disease who develop hyperinflation during exercise.

Using the flowcharts (Chapter 9) leads to at a similar interpretation. Because peak $\dot{V}O_2$ and anaerobic threshold are low, this branches to Flowchart 4, where a low breathing reserve (at Branch Point 4.1) directs to consideration of lung disease with impaired peripheral oxygenation (high VD/VT at Branch Point 4.2). Confirmatory findings include those that suggest pulmonary vascular disease, but, in this case, the major considerations are whether the patient has

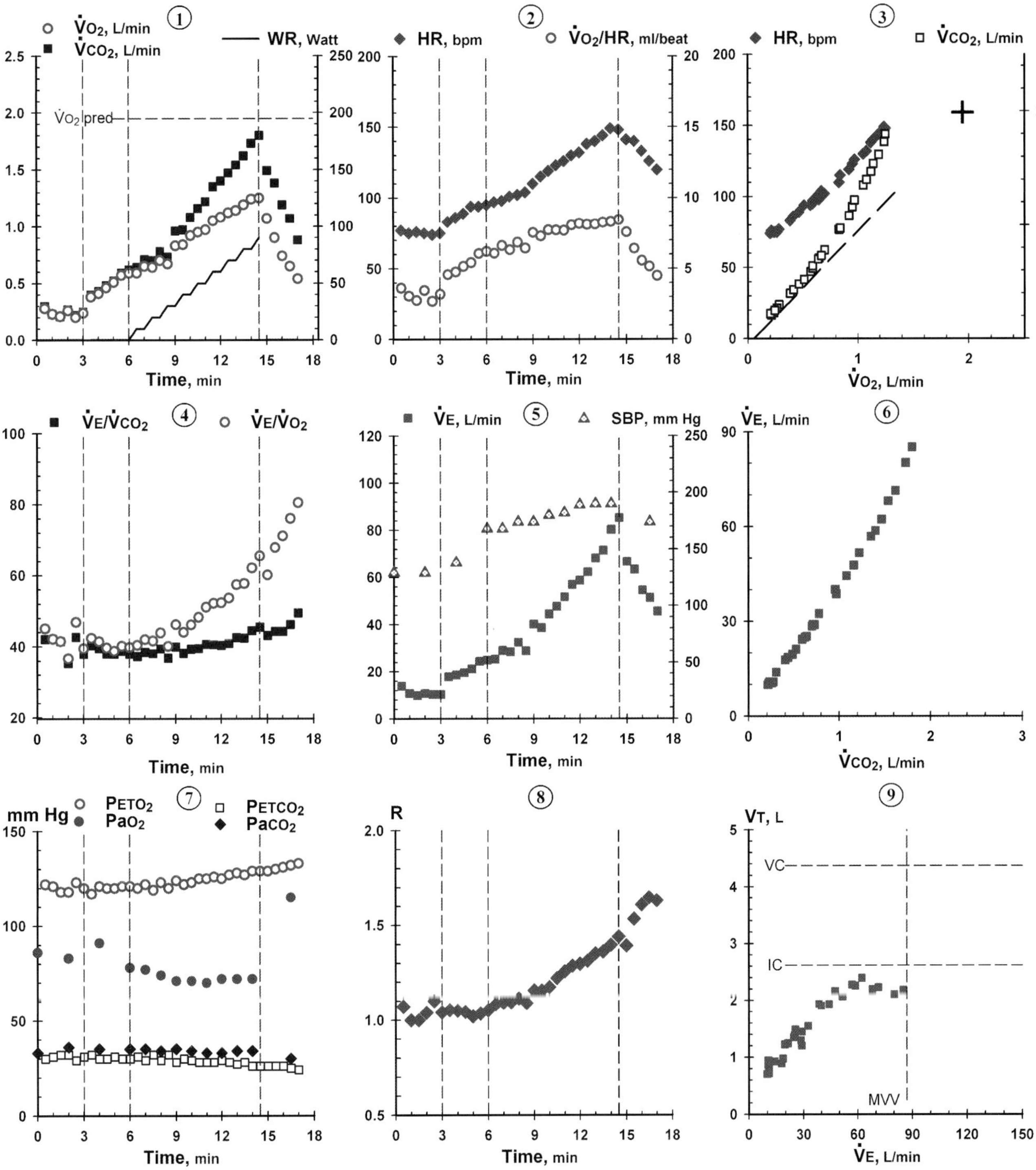

FIGURE 10.67.1. Vertical dashed lines in the panels in the left and middle columns indicate, from left to right, the beginning of unloaded cycling, start of increasing work rate (WR) at 10 W/min, and start of recovery. In **panel 1**, the increase in WR (right y-axis) is plotted with a scale of 100 W to 1 L of oxygen uptake ($\dot{V}O_2$) (left y-axis) such that WR is plotted parallel to a $\dot{V}O_2$ slope of 10 mL/min/W. In **panel 3**, carbon dioxide output ($\dot{V}CO_2$) (right y-axis) is plotted as a function of $\dot{V}O_2$ (x-axis) with identical scales so that the diagonal dashed line has a slope of 1 (45°). The $\dot{V}CO_2$ increasing more steeply than $\dot{V}O_2$ defines carbon dioxide (CO_2) derived from bicarbonate buffer, as long as ventilatory equivalent for CO_2 ($\dot{V}E/\dot{V}CO_2$) (**panel 4**) is not increasing and end-tidal PCO_2 ($PETCO_2$) (**panel 7**) is not decreasing, simultaneously. The black + symbol in **panel 3** indicates predicted peak values of heart rate (HR) (left y-axis) and $\dot{V}O_2$ for this individual. Abbreviations: IC, inspiratory capacity; MVV, maximum voluntary ventilation; $PETO_2$, end-tidal PO_2; R, respiratory exchange ratio; SBP, systolic blood pressure; VC, vital capacity; $\dot{V}E$, minute ventilation; $\dot{V}E/\dot{V}O_2$, ventilatory equivalent for oxygen; V_T, tidal volume.

pulmonary vascular disease entirely related to bullous emphysema or another primary disorder.

Conclusion

In addition to ventilatory limitation, this patient had evidence of abnormal oxygen flow, which may result from secondary pulmonary vascular disease, coexistent systemic vascular disease, or reduction in skeletal muscle capacity for oxygen utilization, all commonly associated with obstructive lung disease. The degree of exercise hypoxemia was mild and would not likely to account for this. This case is presented as an example of the effects of cardiovascular dysfunction in patients with chronic lung disease. Lung disease frequently causes secondary cardiovascular impairment, which in turn raises ventilatory requirements by causing lactic acidosis at low levels of exercise. As a result, ventilatory limitation may be reached earlier than might be expected from the degree of abnormality on pulmonary function testing.

CASE 68

Severe Emphysema and Bronchitis: Air and Oxygen Breathing Studies

CLINICAL FINDINGS

This 62-year-old retired accountant had a long history of heavy cigarette smoking, which he had stopped 4 years previously. He had a chronic cough and shortness of breath. He had gradually increased his activity by physical training and rode his bicycle many miles daily. There was no history of heart disease. He took oral theophylline but no other medications. He participated in a study evaluating the effects of oxygen (O_2) supplementation.

EXERCISE FINDINGS

The patient performed exercise on a cycle ergometer. He pedaled at 60 rpm without added load for 3 minutes while breathing humidified air. The work rate was then increased 10 W/min to his symptom-limited maximum. Blood was sampled every second minute, and intra-arterial blood pressure was recorded from a percutaneously placed brachial artery catheter. He stopped exercise complaining of shortness of breath. Following 30 minutes of rest, he was given humidified 100% O_2 to breathe while the exercise study was repeated. He again stopped exercise complaining of shortness of breath. The 12-lead electrocardiogram showed no ST-segment changes or arrhythmia. While breathing 100% O_2, the patient was able to exercise longer and attain a higher peak work rate.

INTERPRETATION

Comments

Resting respiratory function studies indicated severe obstructive lung disease (**Table 10.68.1**). He also had significant systemic hypertension at rest. This test is presented to illustrate the effect of carbon dioxide retention on the gas exchange and ventilatory response to exercise in a patient who has limited ventilatory capacity. Exercise data are summarized in **Table 10.68.2**. The air breathing exercise test is shown in **Table 10.68.3** and **Figure 10.68.1**, and the 100% O2 study is shown in **Table 10.68.4** and **Figure 10.68.2**.

Analysis

On the room air study, the patient's peak $\dot{V}O_2$ was moderately severely reduced and he demonstrated ventilatory limitation (low breathing reserve and high heart rate [HR] reserve). Of interest, ventilatory equivalent for carbon dioxide ($\dot{V}E/\dot{V}CO_2$) and slope of minute ventilation ($\dot{V}E$) versus carbon dioxide output ($\dot{V}CO_2$) were not elevated, as might be anticipated in a patient with severe lung disease, but arterial blood gases showed that, in fact, physiological dead space–tidal volume ratio (V_D/V_T), arterial–end-tidal P_{CO_2} difference ($P[a - ET]CO_2$), and alveolar-arterial P_{O_2} difference ($P[A - a]O_2$) were abnormal. The $\dot{V}E/\dot{V}CO_2$ was not elevated because the patient was unable to increase $\dot{V}E$ as needed for the increase $\dot{V}CO_2$. In fact, Pa_{CO_2} was elevated at rest and increased during the exercise protocol, causing respiratory acidosis with pH decreasing at peak exercise to 7.32.

Because peak $\dot{V}O_2$ was moderately to severely reduced and the anaerobic threshold was not reached, Flowchart 5 (Chapter 9) can be used to characterize the exercise response. At the first branch point, indices of ventilation–perfusion mismatching (V_D/V_T, $P[a - ET]CO_2$, and $P[A - a]O_2$) were abnormal (Branch Point 5.1). The breathing reserve was zero (Branch Point 5.3), indicating exercise limitation due to lung disease. The breathing frequency (f) is less than 50 at the maximum work rate (Branch Point 5.7), consistent with known obstructive lung disease. Other abnormal findings are an obstructive expiratory flow pattern (not shown), arterial oxygen saturation and $P(A - a)O_2$ that

TABLE 10.68.1 Selected Respiratory Function Data

Measurement	Predicted	Measured
Age (y)		62
Sex		Male
Height (cm)		173
Weight (kg)	76	78
Hematocrit (%)		51
VC (L)	4.30	1.67
IC (L)	2.87	1.22
TLC (L)	6.87	8.30
FEV_1 (L)	3.40	0.54
FEV_1/VC (%)	79	32
MVV (L/min)	131	32
D_{LCO} (mL/mm Hg/min)	30.9	18.5

Abbreviations: D_{LCO}, diffusing capacity of lung for carbon monoxide; FEV_1, forced expiratory volume in 1 second; IC, inspiratory capacity; MVV, maximum voluntary ventilation; TLC, total lung capacity; VC, vital capacity.

TABLE 10.68.2 Selected Exercise Data

Measurement	Predicted	Room air	100% O_2
Maximum work rate (W)		80	120
Peak $\dot{V}O_2$ (L/min)	2.11	0.96	
Maximum heart rate (beats/min)	158	140	165
Maximum O_2 pulse (mL/beat)	13.4	6.9	
$\Delta\dot{V}O_2/\Delta WR$ (mL/min/W)	10.3	8.3	
AT (L/min)	>0.93	Not reached	
Blood pressure (mm Hg [rest, max])		169/106, 250/125	144/94, 234/119
Maximum $\dot{V}E$ (L/min)		32	40
Exercise breathing reserve (L/min)	>15	0	−8
$\dot{V}E/\dot{V}CO_2$ @ *AT* or lowest	28.3	28.5	23.2
PaO_2 (mm Hg [rest, max ex])		78, 53	587, 583
$P(A - a)O_2$ (mm Hg [rest, max ex])		21, 51	77, 66
$PaCO_2$ (mm Hg [rest, max ex])		47, 53	49, 64
$P(a - ET)CO_2$ (mm Hg [rest, max ex])		6, 5	8, 3
VD/VT (rest, heavy ex)		0.42, 0.38	0.48, 0.37
HCO_3^- (mEq/L [rest, 2-min recov])		25, 24	27, 22

Abbreviations: *AT*, anaerobic threshold; $\Delta\dot{V}O_2/\Delta WR$, change in $\dot{V}O_2$/change in work rate; ex, exercise; HCO_3^-, bicarbonate; O_2, oxygen; $P(A - a)O_2$, alveolar-arterial PO_2 difference; $P(a - ET)CO_2$, arterial-end-tidal PCO_2 difference; recov, recovery; VD/VT, physiological dead space–tidal volume ratio; $\dot{V}E$, minute ventilation; $\dot{V}E/\dot{V}CO_2$, ventilatory equivalent for carbon dioxide; $\dot{V}O_2$, oxygen uptake.

were borderline at rest and became abnormal with exercise, a high HR reserve, and an acute respiratory acidosis at end exercise.

While breathing 100% O_2 (**Fig. 10.68.2** and **Table 10.68.4**), the patient attained a maximal work rate that was 40 W higher and a maximum HR that was 25 beats/min higher than during air breathing. These results confirm that the high HR reserve seen during the air breathing test resulted from his ventilatory limitation. Moreover, the maximum exercise ventilation increased from 32 L/min (similar to his measured maximum voluntary ventilation [MVV]) while breathing air to 40 L/min while breathing O_2.

The increased work rate achieved during O_2 breathing was due in part to further depression of the ventilatory response to exercise, as evidenced by a greater degree of respiratory acidosis on the O_2 breathing test (increase in $PaCO_2$ of 6 mm Hg above rest during air breathing, as compared with 15 mm Hg for O_2 breathing). The PaO_2 remained above 580 mm Hg when breathing O_2 (see **Table 10.68.4**), excluding a significant right-to-left shunt, and establishing that the exercise-associated hypoxemia on air breathing was due primarily to ventilation–perfusion mismatch. Bicarbonate did not decrease in either study until 2 minutes after the exercise was terminated because of the increase in $PaCO_2$ during exercise, which subsequently decreased in recovery.

Conclusion

Exercise performance was limited by severe obstructive lung disease. The O_2 breathing resulted in an increased work capacity despite the lack of hypoxemia at rest when breathing room air but at the expense of worsening hypercapnia during exercise.

TABLE 10.68.3 Air Breathing

Time (min)	Work rate (W)	BP (mm Hg)	HR (min^{-1})	f (min^{-1})	$\dot{V}E$ (L/min BTPS)	$\dot{V}CO_2$ (L/min STPD)	$\dot{V}O_2$ (L/min STPD)	$\frac{\dot{V}O_2}{HR}$ (mL/beat)	R	pH	HCO_3^- (mEq/L)	PO_2, mm Hg ET	a	(A − a)	PCO_2, mm Hg ET	a	(a − ET)	$\frac{\dot{V}E}{\dot{V}CO_2}$	$\frac{\dot{V}E}{\dot{V}O_2}$	$\frac{V_D}{V_T}$
	Rest		107	20	9.7	0.23	0.24	2.2	0.96			99			44			35	33	
0.5	Rest		109	21	8.7	0.17	0.19	1.7	0.89			94			46			41	36	
1.0	Rest		108	20	8.8	0.19	0.21	1.9	0.90			98			44			37	34	
1.5	Rest		110	20	9.8	0.22	0.24	2.2	0.92			102			42			37	34	
2.0	Rest		112	20	8.4	0.16	0.18	1.6	0.89			103			41			42	37	
2.5	Rest	169/106	108	19	9.1	0.20	0.22	2.0	0.91	7.35	25	102	78	21	42	47	6	37	34	0.42
3.0	Unloaded		109	23	10.9	0.22	0.25	2.3	0.88			96			45			41	36	
3.5	Unloaded		111	25	13.4	0.31	0.37	3.3	0.84			97			44			36	30	
4.0	Unloaded		114	24	13.6	0.32	0.36	3.2	0.89			97			44			36	32	
4.5	Unloaded		121	23	14.2	0.35	0.40	3.3	0.88			96			45			35	31	
5.0	Unloaded		119	25	13.1	0.30	0.34	2.9	0.88			98			44			37	32	
5.5	Unloaded	181/100	117	24	15.3	0.39	0.44	3.8	0.89	7.35	27	99	71	25	43	49	6	34	30	0.42
6.0	10		119	24	14.4	0.36	0.41	3.4	0.88			98			44			34	30	
6.5	10		121	25	14.8	0.38	0.42	3.5	0.90			99			43			33	30	
7.0	20		121	24	15.1	0.37	0.41	3.4	0.90			98			44			35	32	
7.5	20	187/106	124	25	16.3	0.42	0.48	3.9	0.88	7.35	27	97	68	27	44	49	6	34	30	0.42
8.0	30		125	29	16.4	0.40	0.46	3.7	0.87			97			44			35	30	
8.5	30		128	22	18.6	0.56	0.64	5.0	0.88	7.35	27	94			46			30	26	
9.0	40		131	27	18.9	0.52	0.58	4.4	0.90			95			46			32	29	
9.5	40	213/113	130	24	21.1	0.64	0.72	5.5	0.89	7.35	26	94	61	36	47	48	1	30	26	0.36
10.0	50		132	27	21.9	0.66	0.72	5.5	0.92			96			46			30	27	
10.5	50		136	28	23.9	0.72	0.77	5.7	0.94			96			46			30	28	
11.0	60		137	30	25.0	0.77	0.82	6.0	0.94			96			47			29	27	
11.5	60	225/119	135	28	25.6	0.81	0.86	6.4	0.94	7.35	27	96	57	42	48	49	1	29	27	0.35
12.0	70		138	31	25.4	0.80	0.84	6.1	0.95			95			49			28	27	
12.5	70		138	32	29.0	0.91	0.94	6.8	0.97			95			48			29	28	
13.0	80		140	32	29.2	0.94	0.96	6.9	0.98			98			48			28	28	
13.5	80	250/125	124	37	32.1	1.02	0.85	6.9	1.20	7.32	27	101	53	51	48	53	5	28	34	0.38
14.0	Recovery		104	32	30.7	0.99	0.95	9.1	1.04			99			48			28	29	
14.5	Recovery		102	26	26.0	0.83	0.79	7.7	1.06			98			50			28	29	
15.0	Recovery		114	24	21.3	0.66	0.61	5.4	1.08			101			48			29	32	
15.5	Recovery		102	22	17.8	0.52	0.47	4.6	1.11	7.30	24	103	89	15	47	50	3	31	34	0.39

Abbreviations: BP, blood pressure; BTPS, body temperature pressure saturated; f, frequency; HCO_3^-, bicarbonate; HR, heart rate; $P(A - a)O_2$, alveolar-arterial PO_2 difference; $P(a - ET)CO_2$, arterial-end-tidal PCO_2 difference; $PETCO_2$, end-tidal PCO_2; $PETO_2$, end-tidal PO_2; R, respiratory exchange ratio; STPD, standard temperature pressure dry; $\dot{V}CO_2$, carbon dioxide output; V_D/V_T, physiological dead space–tidal volume ratio; $\dot{V}E$, minute ventilation; $\dot{V}E/\dot{V}CO_2$, ventilatory equivalent for carbon dioxide; $\dot{V}E/\dot{V}O_2$, ventilatory equivalent for oxygen; $\dot{V}O_2$, oxygen uptake.

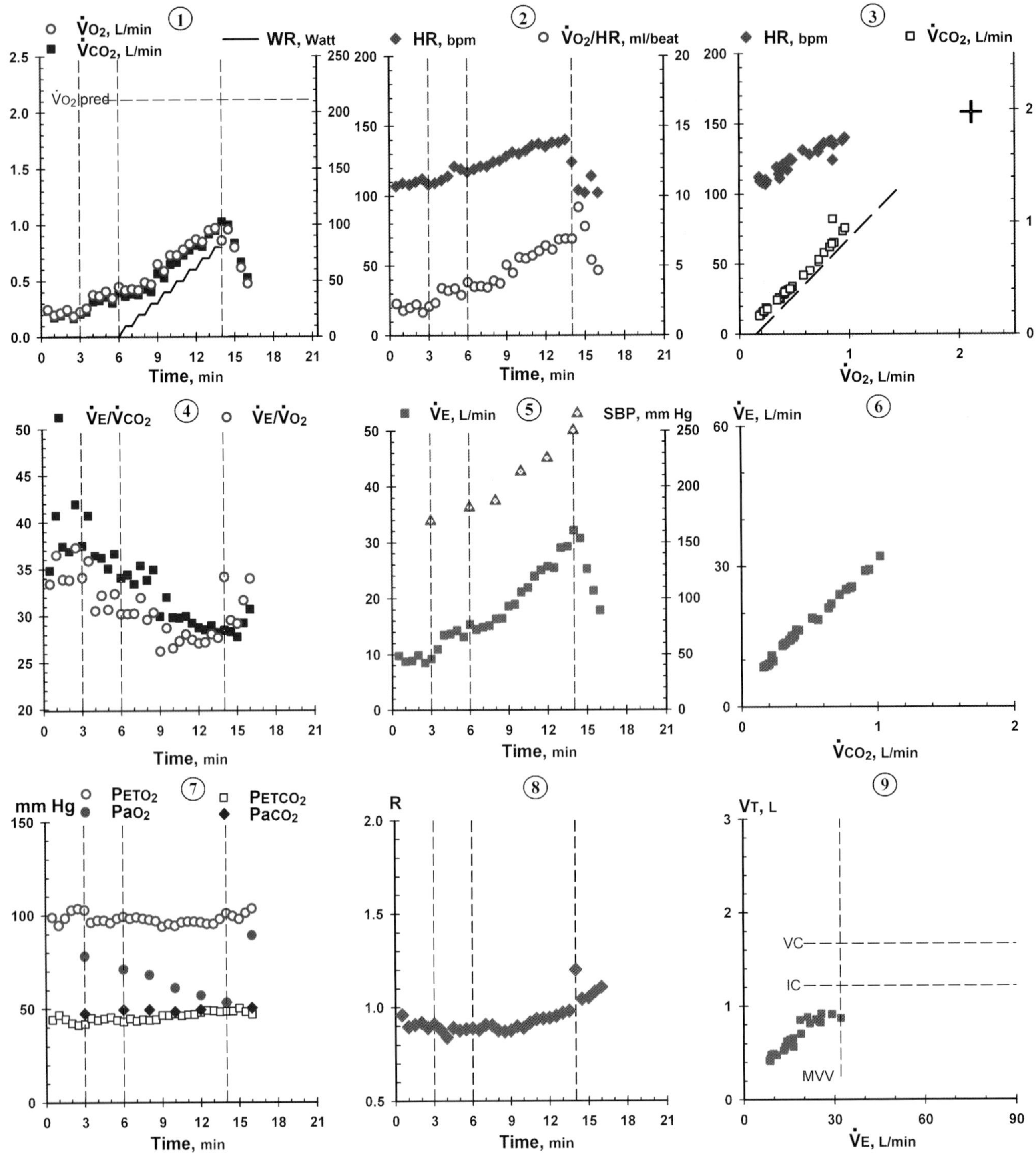

FIGURE 10.68.1. Air breathing. Vertical dashed lines in the panels in the left and middle columns indicate, from left to right, the beginning of unloaded cycling, start of increasing work rate (WR) at 10 W/min, and start of recovery. In **panel 1**, the increase in WR (right y-axis) is plotted with a scale of 100 W to 1 L of oxygen uptake ($\dot{V}O_2$) (left y-axis) such that WR is plotted parallel to a $\dot{V}O_2$ slope of 10 mL/min/W. In **panel 3**, carbon dioxide output ($\dot{V}CO_2$) (right y-axis) is plotted as a function of $\dot{V}O_2$ (x-axis) with identical scales so that the diagonal dashed line has a slope of 1 (45°). The $\dot{V}CO_2$ increasing more steeply than $\dot{V}O_2$ defines carbon dioxide (CO_2) derived from bicarbonate buffer, as long as ventilatory equivalent for CO_2 ($\dot{V}E/\dot{V}CO_2$) (**panel 4**) is not increasing and end-tidal PCO_2 ($PETCO_2$) (**panel 7**) is not decreasing, simultaneously. The black + symbol in **panel 3** indicates predicted peak values of heart rate (HR) (left y-axis) and $\dot{V}O_2$ for this individual. Abbreviations: IC, inspiratory capacity; MVV, maximum voluntary ventilation; $PETO_2$, end-tidal PO_2; R, respiratory exchange ratio; SBP, systolic blood pressure; VC, vital capacity; $\dot{V}E$, minute ventilation; $\dot{V}E/\dot{V}O_2$, ventilatory equivalent for oxygen; V_T, tidal volume.

TABLE 10.68.4 Oxygen Breathing

Time (min)	Work rate (W)	BP (mm Hg)	HR (min^{-1})	f (min^{-1})	$\dot{V}E$ (L/min BTPS)	$\dot{V}CO_2$ (L/min STPD)	$\dot{V}O_2$ (L/min STPD)	$\frac{\dot{V}O_2}{HR}$ (mL/beat)	R	pH	HCO_3^- (mEq/L)	PO_2, mm Hg ET	PO_2, mm Hg a	PO_2, mm Hg (A − a)	PCO_2, mm Hg ET	PCO_2, mm Hg a	PCO_2, mm Hg (a − ET)	$\frac{\dot{V}E}{\dot{V}CO_2}$	$\frac{\dot{V}E}{\dot{V}O_2}$	$\frac{V_D}{V_T}$
	Rest		111	23	12.3	0.23									37			45		
0.5	Rest		113	21	8.3	0.13									40			50		
1.0	Rest		111	23	11.8	0.23									39			43		
1.5	Rest		111	26	10.6	0.17									39			49		
2.0	Rest		113	22	8.7	0.14									39			49		
2.5	Rest	144/94	113	19	8.6	0.16				7.35	27		587	77	41	49	8	44		0.48
3.0	Unloaded		111	11											53					
3.5	Unloaded		114	22	7.9	0.14									49			43		
4.0	Unloaded		114	20	9.0	0.19									47			38		
4.5	Unloaded		108	20	9.6	0.22									49			36		
5.0	Unloaded		112	22	9.9	0.23									55			35		
5.5	Unloaded	181/106	114	21	10.5	0.24				7.29	28		587	67	50	59	9	36		0.50
6.0	10		113	21	12.8	0.35									50			31		
6.5	10		114	21	11.2	0.31									52			30		
7.0	20		113	21	12.6	0.36									55			30		
7.5	20	194/106	112	22	14.8	0.45				7.30	28		584	72	52	57	5	29		0.41
8.0	30		118	27	15.3	0.45									52			29		
8.5	30		119	23	18.1	0.57									53			28		
9.0	40		121	26	18.7	0.55									52			30		
9.5	40	200/106	123	24	19.9	0.65				7.29	28		580	74	54	59	5	27		0.42
10.0	50		127	24	20.8	0.68									54			28		
10.5	50		130	24	22.2	0.75									53			27		
11.0	60		132	25	22.8	0.76									54			27		
11.5	60	206/100	132	26	23.6	0.78				7.29	27		595	60	55	58	3	27		0.41
12.0	70		135	27	25.9	0.88									54			27		
12.5	70		138	29	25.8	0.91									57			26		
13.0	80		141	28	28.7	1.02									55			26		
13.5	80	213/106	144	29	29.8	1.07				7.27	28		601	50	57	62	5	26		0.42
14.0	90		149	26	30.0	1.14									57			24		
14.5	90		150	28	31.5	1.21									58			24		
15.0	100		153	30	33.8	1.28									58			24		
15.5	100	231/106	155	29	34.2	1.33				7.24	27		606	43	60	64	4	24		0.40
16.0	110		162	31	34.5	1.35									60			24		
16.5	110	234/119	159	39	35.4	1.40				7.23	26		583	66	62	64	2	23		0.37
17.0	120		165	34	37.3	1.52									64			23		
17.5	120		165	37	40.1	1.64									66			23		
18.0	Recovery		148	30	35.0	1.51									64			21		
18.5	Recovery		141	26	32.1	1.38									62			22		
19.0	Recovery		138	26	31.1	1.19									58			24		
19.5	Recovery	214/100	138	28	27.6	0.97				7.21	22		587	69	54	57	3	26		0.38

Abbreviations: BP, blood pressure; BTPS, body temperature pressure saturated; f, frequency; HCO_3^-, bicarbonate; HR, heart rate; $P(A - a)O_2$, alveolar-arterial PO_2 difference; $P(a - ET)CO_2$, arterial-end-tidal PCO_2 difference; $PETCO_2$, end-tidal PCO_2; $PETO_2$, end-tidal PO_2; R, respiratory exchange ratio; STPD, standard temperature pressure dry; $\dot{V}CO_2$, carbon dioxide output; V_D/V_T, physiological dead space-tidal volume ratio; $\dot{V}E$, minute ventilation; $\dot{V}E/\dot{V}CO_2$, ventilatory equivalent for carbon dioxide; $\dot{V}E/\dot{V}O_2$, ventilatory equivalent for oxygen; $\dot{V}O_2$, oxygen uptake.

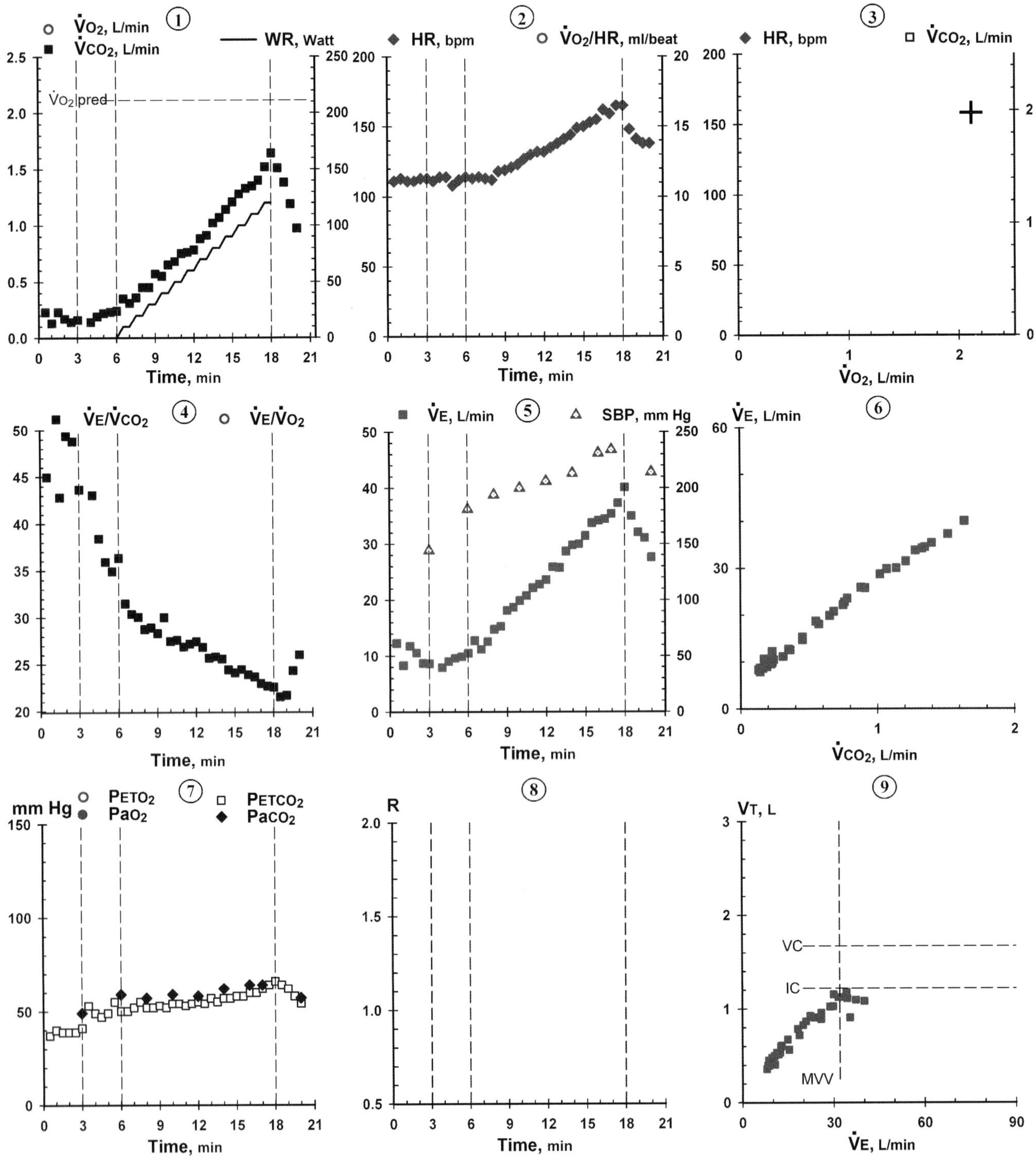

FIGURE 10.68.2. Oxygen breathing. Vertical dashed lines in the panels in the left and middle columns indicate, from left to right, the beginning of unloaded cycling, the start of increasing work rate (WR) at 10 W/min, and the start of recovery. Oxygen uptake ($\dot{V}O_2$) data are not shown because of technical limitations of calculations with very high-inspired oxygen levels. Abbreviations: HR, heart rate; IC, inspiratory capacity; MVV, maximum voluntary ventilation; P_{ETCO_2}, end-tidal P_{CO_2}; P_{ETO_2}, end-tidal P_{O_2}; R, respiratory exchange ratio; SBP, systolic blood pressure; VC, vital capacity; $\dot{V}CO_2$, carbon dioxide output; $\dot{V}_E$, minute ventilation; $\dot{V}_E/\dot{V}CO_2$, ventilatory equivalent for carbon dioxide; $\dot{V}_E/\dot{V}O_2$, ventilatory equivalent for oxygen; V_T, tidal volume.

CASE 69

Bullous Emphysema: Before and After Bullectomy

CLINICAL FINDINGS

This 50-year-old computer technician had retired approximately 10 years prior to initial evaluation because of progressive dyspnea. He was a heavy cigarette smoker. He denied cough, sputum production, wheezing, or chest pain. There was no family history of lung disease. Chest radiographs showed large bullae in the right middle and upper lung fields. Perfusion scan demonstrated no perfusion in these areas or at the left apex. α_1-Antitrypsin levels were normal. Exercise testing was performed to quantify his functional capacity in anticipation of surgical bullectomy. The patient subsequently underwent resection of the right upper lobe and affected portions of the right middle lobe. The resected lung showed bullous and centroacinar emphysema; a small squamous cell scar carcinoma was found in the upper lobe. Exercise testing was repeated 3 months after surgery.

EXERCISE FINDINGS

Preoperatively, the patient performed exercise on a cycle ergometer while breathing room air and, following a 90-minute rest, breathing 100% oxygen (not shown). At 3 months postoperatively, the air breathing study was repeated. On each occasion, he pedaled at 60 rpm on an unloaded cycle for 2 or 3 minutes. The work rate was then increased 20 W/min. Arterial blood was sampled every second minute, and the intra-arterial blood pressure was recorded from a percutaneous brachial artery catheter. Resting electrocardiograms were normal. On the preoperative studies, the patient stopped exercise because of dyspnea without an exercise-induced abnormality in the electrocardiogram. He stopped during the postoperative test because of dyspnea and pressure-like right-sided chest pain. There were multifocal, back-to-back, and salvos of premature ventricular contractions at the end of exercise and for 2 minutes of recovery without abnormal ST-segment changes.

INTERPRETATION

Comments

Resting respiratory function studies show moderate obstructive lung disease without reversibility and with marked reduction in diffusing capacity of lung for carbon monoxide (DLCO). Lung mechanics improved following the bullectomy (**Table 10.69.1**), but the DLCO remained disproportionately low relative to the severity of airflow obstruction. Despite the improvement in resting pulmonary function, exercise tolerance was only marginally improved postoperatively. Although in this case surgery was done with the goal of improving lung function and symptoms, coincident resection of stage I lung cancer was an unanticipated effect. The patient's peak oxygen uptake ($\dot{V}O_2$) of 14 mL/min/kg on the preoperative study identifies an intermediate risk for complications related to lung resection surgery. Exercise data for the two studies are summarized in **Table 10.69.2**. The preoperative test is shown in **Table 10.69.3** and **Figure 10.69.1**; the postoperative test is shown in **Table 10.69.4** and **Figure 10.69.2**.

Analysis

In both studies, peak $\dot{V}O_2$ and anaerobic threshold were severely reduced, and there was evidence of ventilatory limitation in the preoperative study (low breathing reserve, high heart rate reserve) that was not as apparent after bullectomy. Nevertheless, there was little objective improvement in maximum exercise capacity. In looking for other reasons for exercise limitation, it was notable that the patient's preoperative test showed evidence for severe ventilation-perfusion mismatching, including elevated alveolar-arterial PO_2 difference ($P[A - a]O_2$), physiological dead space–tidal

TABLE 10.69.1 Selected Respiratory Function Data

Measurement	Predicted	Preoperative	Postoperative
Age (y)		50	
Sex		Male	
Height (cm)		170	
Weight (kg)	74	71	
Hematocrit (%)		46	
VC (L)	3.89	3.01	3.57
IC (L)	2.59	2.03	2.46
TLC (L)	5.69	7.05	5.56
FEV_1 (L)	3.09	1.93	2.44
FEV_1/VC (%)	79	64	68
MVV (L/min)	131	90	110
DLCO (mL/mm Hg/min)	26.5	10.0	13.0

Abbreviations: DLCO, diffusing capacity of lung for carbon monoxide; FEV_1, forced expiratory volume in 1 second; IC, inspiratory capacity; MVV, maximum voluntary ventilation; TLC, total lung capacity; VC, vital capacity.

TABLE 10.69.2 Selected Exercise Data

Measurement	Predicted	Preoperative	Postoperative
Peak $\dot{V}O_2$ (L/min)	2.32	0.99	1.06
Maximum heart rate (beats/min)	170	144	144
Maximum O_2 pulse (mL/beat)	13.7	7.5	7.9
$\Delta\dot{V}O_2/\Delta WR$ (mL/min/W)	10.3	5.1	5.8
AT (L/min)	>1.00	0.6	0.75
Blood pressure (mm Hg [rest, max])		144/90, 187/100	144/88, 238/94
Maximum $\dot{V}E$ (L/min)		84	80
Exercise breathing reserve (L/min)	>15	6	30
$\dot{V}E/\dot{V}CO_2$ @ *AT* or lowest	27.1	56.0	44.5
PaO_2 (mm Hg [rest, max ex])		67, 54	74, 74
$P(A - a)O_2$ (mm Hg [rest, max ex])		47, 72	34, 52
$PaCO_2$ (mm Hg [rest, max ex])		30, 28	34, 31
$P(a - ET)CO_2$ (mm Hg [rest, max ex])		4, 8	4, 3
VD/VT (rest, heavy ex)		0.39, 0.47	0.41, 0.40
HCO_3^- (mEq/L [rest, 2-min recov])		21, 14	21, 14

Abbreviations: *AT*, anaerobic threshold; $\Delta\dot{V}O_2/\Delta WR$, change in $\dot{V}O_2$/change in work rate; ex, exercise; HCO_3^-, bicarbonate; O_2, oxygen; $P(A - a)O_2$, alveolar-arterial PO_2 difference; $P(a - ET)CO_2$, arterial-end-tidal PCO_2 difference; recov, recovery; VD/VT, physiological dead space-tidal volume ratio; $\dot{V}E$, minute ventilation; $\dot{V}E/\dot{V}CO_2$, ventilatory equivalent for carbon dioxide; $\dot{V}O_2$, oxygen uptake.

volume ratio (VD/VT), and arterial–end-tidal PCO_2 difference [$P(a - ET)CO_2$] and severe arterial hypoxemia, which also manifested as very high minute ventilation ($\dot{V}E$) requirement (high slope of $\dot{V}E$ versus carbon dioxide output [$\dot{V}CO_2$] and high $\dot{V}E/\dot{V}CO_2$). Although slightly improved, these gas exchange abnormalities likely continued to impair the patient despite improvement in lung mechanics after bullectomy.

Both studies, because of low peak $\dot{V}O_2$ and anaerobic threshold, would lead to Flowchart 4 (Chapter 9). Preoperatively, the exercise breathing reserve is low, but postoperatively, the breathing reserve is normal (Branch Point 4.1). Following the "low breathing reserve" branch of the flowchart with respect to the preoperative study, VD/VT was high, consistent with lung disease with impaired peripheral oxygenation (Branch Point 4.2). Postbullectomy, the breathing reserve was normal, although the patient ended exercise at a similar level of ventilation (maximum voluntary ventilation was higher). The ventilatory equivalent for carbon dioxide ($\dot{V}E/\dot{V}CO_2$) at the anaerobic threshold was lower than on the preoperative test but still higher than normal. Similarly, the indices of ventilation-perfusion mismatching ($P[A - a]O_2$, VD/VT, and $P[a - ET]O_2$) were less severely abnormal at peak exercise on the postoperative test but were not normal. This indicates that pulmonary ventilation-perfusion ($\dot{V}A/\dot{Q}$) abnormalities persisted and were classified by the flowchart as "abnormal pulmonary circulation" (at Branch Point 4.5) with low arterial oxygen saturation and normal vital capacity, further suggesting "pulmonary vascular disease" as the underlying pathophysiology. This is consistent with the patient's low resting $DLCO$. Other findings characteristic of abnormalities of the pulmonary circulation include (1) a steep heart rate response to the increase in $\dot{V}O_2$, becoming steeper as the peak $\dot{V}O_2$ was approached (panel 3); (2) a low oxygen pulse with a flat contour as the work rate was increased (panel 2); and (3) a decreasing change in $\dot{V}O_2$/change in work rate as the work rate was increased (panel 1). These findings were prominent in both the preoperative test and the postoperative test and suggest functionally important pulmonary vascular disease. Although the bullectomy improved ventilatory mechanics, it did not significantly improve the abnormalities in peak $\dot{V}O_2$.

Conclusion

Lung mechanics improved following resection of bullae in this patient with airflow obstruction and bullous lung disease. Postoperatively, he was no longer ventilatory limited, had less wasted ventilation, and less severe hypoxemia during exercise; however, maximal exercise capacity improved very little due to persistent cardiovascular (likely pulmonary vascular) impairment. Importantly, in this case, the patient also had unanticipated resection of an early-stage lung cancer. Results of the preoperative test have potential value for managing expectations with respect to postoperative exercise function, which was likely to remain impaired due to the finding of significant cardiovascular limitation. It is also valuable in gauging the risk associated with surgery; in this case, risk of perioperative complications would be graded as intermediate based on the preoperative peak $\dot{V}O_2$ of 14 mL/min/kg.

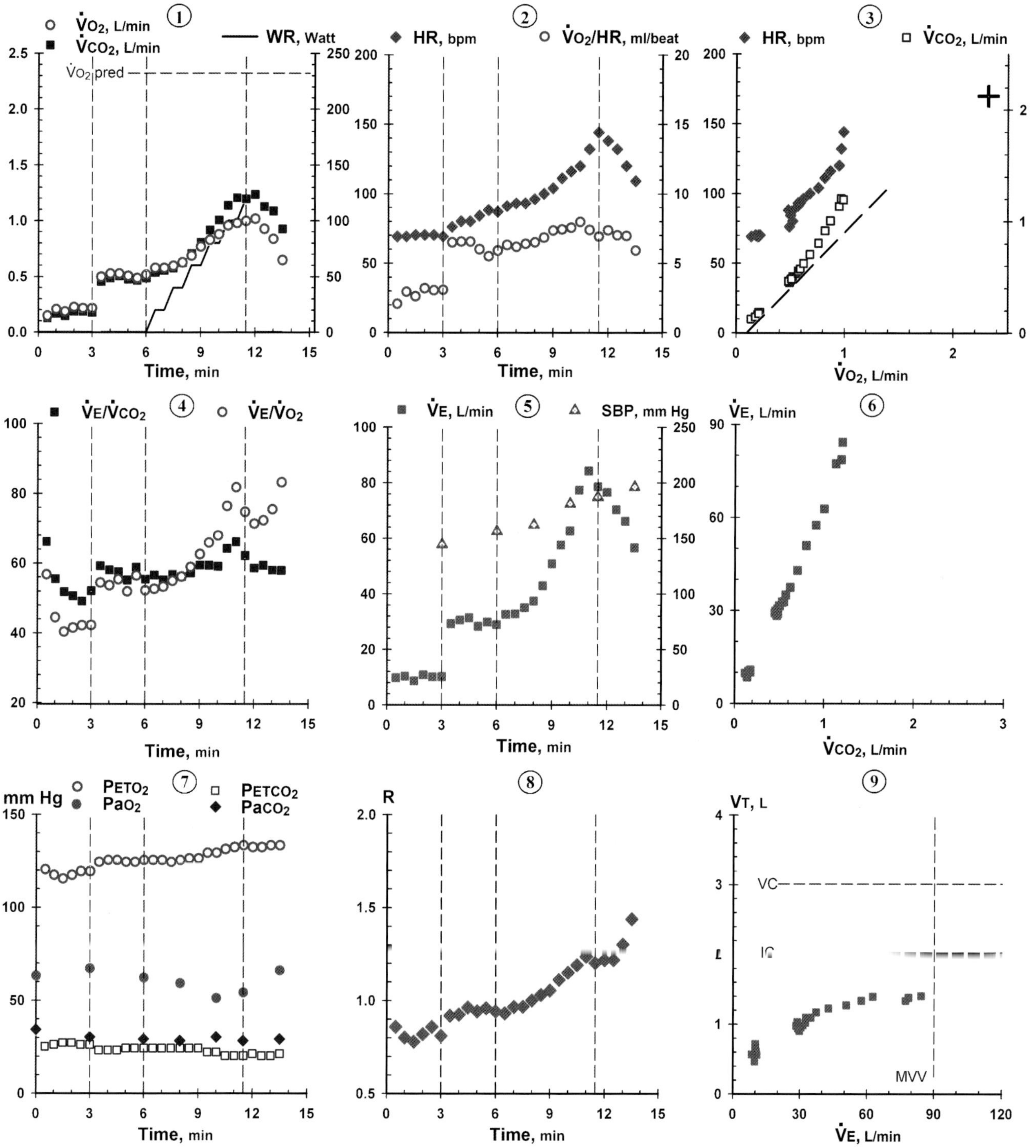

FIGURE 10.69.1. Preoperative. Vertical dashed lines in the panels in the left and middle columns indicate, from left to right, the beginning of unloaded cycling, start of increasing work rate (WR) at 20 W/min, and start of recovery. In **panel 1**, the increase in WR (right y-axis) is plotted with a scale of 100 W to 1 L of oxygen uptake ($\dot{V}O_2$) (left y-axis) such that WR is plotted parallel to a $\dot{V}O_2$ slope of 10 mL/min/W. In **panel 3**, carbon dioxide output ($\dot{V}CO_2$) (right y-axis) is plotted as a function of $\dot{V}O_2$ (x-axis) with identical scales so that the diagonal dashed line has a slope of 1 (45°). The $\dot{V}CO_2$ increasing more steeply than $\dot{V}O_2$ defines carbon dioxide (CO_2) derived from bicarbonate buffer, as long as ventilatory equivalent for CO_2 ($\dot{V}E/\dot{V}CO_2$) (**panel 4**) is not increasing and end-tidal PCO_2 (P_{ETCO_2}) (**panel 7**) is not decreasing, simultaneously. The black + symbol in **panel 3** indicates predicted peak values of heart rate (HR) (left y-axis) and $\dot{V}O_2$ for this individual. Abbreviations: IC, inspiratory capacity; MVV, maximum voluntary ventilation; P_{ETO_2}, end-tidal PO_2; R, respiratory exchange ratio; SBP, systolic blood pressure; VC, vital capacity; $\dot{V}E$, minute ventilation; $\dot{V}E/\dot{V}O_2$, ventilatory equivalent for oxygen; V_T, tidal volume.

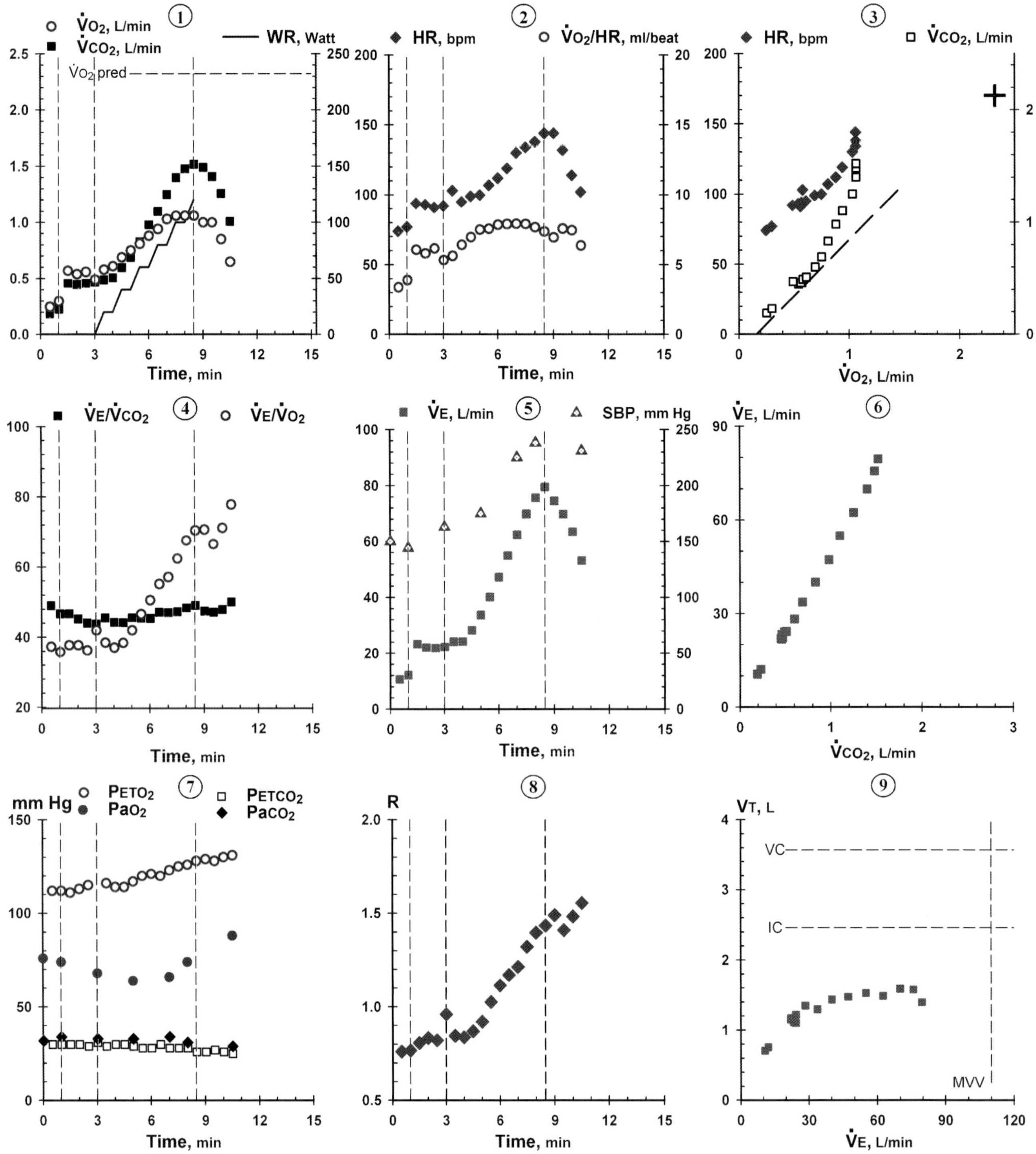

FIGURE 10.69.2. Postoperative. Vertical dashed lines in the panels in the left and middle columns indicate, from left to right, the beginning of unloaded cycling, start of increasing work rate (WR) at 20 W/min, and start of recovery. In **panel 1**, the increase in WR (right y-axis) is plotted with a scale of 100 W to 1 L of oxygen uptake ($\dot{V}O_2$) (left y-axis) such that WR is plotted parallel to a $\dot{V}O_2$ slope of 10 mL/min/W. In **panel 3**, carbon dioxide output ($\dot{V}CO_2$) (right y-axis) is plotted as a function of $\dot{V}O_2$ (x-axis) with identical scales so that the diagonal dashed line has a slope of 1 (45°). The $\dot{V}CO_2$ increasing more steeply than $\dot{V}O_2$ defines carbon dioxide (CO_2) derived from bicarbonate buffer, as long as ventilatory equivalent for CO_2 ($\dot{V}E/\dot{V}CO_2$) (**panel 4**) is not increasing and end-tidal PCO_2 ($PETCO_2$) (**panel 7**) is not decreasing, simultaneously. The black + symbol in **panel 3** indicates predicted peak values of heart rate (HR) (left y-axis) and $\dot{V}O_2$ for this individual. Abbreviations: IC, inspiratory capacity; MVV, maximum voluntary ventilation; $PETO_2$, end-tidal PO_2; R, respiratory exchange ratio; SBP, systolic blood pressure; VC, vital capacity; $\dot{V}E$, minute ventilation; $\dot{V}E/\dot{V}O_2$, ventilatory equivalent for oxygen; V_T, tidal volume.

TABLE 10.69.3 Prebullectomy Study

Time (min)	Work rate (W)	BP (mm Hg)	HR (min^{-1})	f (min^{-1})	$\dot{V}E$ (L/min BTPS)	$\dot{V}CO_2$ (L/min STPD)	$\dot{V}O_2$ (L/min STPD)	$\frac{\dot{V}O_2}{HR}$ (mL/beat)	R	pH	HCO_3^- (mEq/L)	PO_2, mm Hg ET	a	(A − a)	PCO_2, mm Hg ET	a	(a − ET)	$\frac{\dot{V}E}{\dot{V}CO_2}$	$\frac{\dot{V}E}{\dot{V}O_2}$	$\frac{V_D}{V_T}$
	Rest									7.41	21		63			34				
0.5	Rest		69	21	9.7	0.12	0.14	2.0	0.86			120			25			66	57	
1.0	Rest		69	17	10.3	0.16	0.20	2.9	0.80			117			26			55	44	
1.5	Rest		70	15	8.5	0.14	0.18	2.6	0.78			115			27			52	40	
2.0	Rest		70	19	10.7	0.18	0.22	3.1	0.82			117			27			50	41	
2.5	Rest		70	14	10.0	0.18	0.21	3.0	0.86			119			26			49	42	
3.0	Rest	144/90	69	15	10.1	0.17	0.21	3.0	0.81	7.41	19	119	67	47	26	30	4	52	42	0.39
3.5	Unloaded		76	31	29.2	0.45	0.49	6.4	0.92			124			23			59	54	
4.0	Unloaded		80	32	30.5	0.48	0.52	6.5	0.92			125			23			58	53	
4.5	Unloaded		80	32	31.4	0.50	0.52	6.5	0.96			125			23			57	55	
5.0	Unloaded		84	29	28.3	0.47	0.50	6.0	0.94			124			24			55	52	
5.5	Unloaded		88	33	29.8	0.46	0.48	5.5	0.96			124			24			59	56	
6.0	Unloaded	156/90	87	28	28.9	0.48	0.51	5.9	0.94	7.41	18	125	62	58	24	29	5	55	52	0.42
6.5	20		91	32	32.6	0.53	0.57	6.3	0.93			125			24			56	52	
7.0	20		93	30	32.8	0.55	0.57	6.1	0.96			125			24			55	53	
7.5	40		93	32	35.0	0.57	0.59	6.3	0.97			124			24			57	55	
8.0	40	162/94	96	32	37.4	0.62	0.62	6.5	1.00	7.40	17	125	59	63	24	28	4	56	56	0.42
8.5	60		100	35	42.9	0.70	0.68	6.8	1.03			126			24			57	59	
9.0	60		104	40	50.8	0.80	0.76	7.3	1.05			126			24			59	62	
9.5	80		111	43	57.5	0.91	0.82	7.4	1.11			129			22			59	66	
10.0	80	181/96	116	45	62.7	1.00	0.87	7.5	1.15	7.40	18	129	51	72	22	30	8	59	68	0.48
10.5	100		120	58	77.3	1.13	0.95	7.9	1.19			131			20			64	76	
11.0	100		132	60	84.2	1.20	0.97	7.3	1.24			132			20			66	82	
11.5	120	187/100	144	57	78.6	1.19	0.99	6.9	1.20	7.39	17	133	54	72	20	28	8	62	75	0.47
12.0	Recovery		138	55	76.5	1.23	1.01	7.3	1.22			132			21			58	71	
12.5	Recovery		132	47	70.3	1.12	0.92	7.0	1.22			132			20			59	72	
13.0	Recovery		120	44	66.2	1.08	0.83	6.9	1.30			133			20			58	75	
13.5	Recovery	196/99	109	40	56.5	0.92	0.64	5.9	1.44	7.31	14	133	66	62	21	29	8	58	83	0.46

Abbreviations: BP, blood pressure; BTPS, body temperature pressure saturated; f, frequency; HCO_3^-, bicarbonate; HR, heart rate; $P(A - a)O_2$, alveolar-arterial PO_2 difference; $P(a - ET)CO_2$, arterial-end-tidal PCO_2 difference; $PETCO_2$, end-tidal PCO_2; $PETO_2$, end-tidal PO_2; R, respiratory exchange ratio; STPD, standard temperature pressure dry; $\dot{V}CO_2$, carbon dioxide output; V_D/V_T, physiological dead space-tidal volume ratio; $\dot{V}E$, minute ventilation; $\dot{V}E/\dot{V}CO_2$, ventilatory equivalent for carbon dioxide; $\dot{V}E/\dot{V}O_2$, ventilatory equivalent for oxygen; $\dot{V}O_2$, oxygen uptake.

TABLE 10.69.4 Postbullectomy Study

Time (min)	Work rate (W)	BP (mm Hg)	HR (min^{-1})	f (min^{-1})	$\dot{V}E$ (L/min BTPS)	$\dot{V}CO_2$ (L/min STPD)	$\dot{V}O_2$ (L/min STPD)	$\frac{\dot{V}O_2}{HR}$ (mL/beat)	R	pH	HCO_3^- (mEq/L)	PO_2, mm Hg			PCO_2, mm Hg			$\frac{\dot{V}E}{\dot{V}CO_2}$	$\frac{\dot{V}E}{\dot{V}O_2}$	$\frac{VD}{VT}$
												ET	a	(A − a)	ET	a	(a − ET)			
	Rest	150/94								7.44	21		76			32				
0.5	Rest		74	15	10.6	0.19	0.25	3.4	0.76			112			30			49	37	
1.0	Rest	144/88	77	16	12.1	0.23	0.30	3.9	0.77	7.42	22	112	74	34	30	34		47	36	0.41
1.5	Unloaded		94	21	23.3	0.46	0.57	6.1	0.81			111			30			47	38	
2.0	Unloaded		93	19	22.0	0.45	0.54	5.8	0.83			113			30			45	38	
2.5	Unloaded		91	19	21.9	0.46	0.56	6.2	0.82			115			29			44	36	
3.0	Unloaded	163/38	92	19	22.2	0.47	0.49	5.3	0.96	7.42	21	115	68	48	31	33	2	44	42	0.37
3.5	20		103	22	24.2	0.49	0.58	5.6	0.84			116			29			46	39	
4.0	20		95	20	24.3	0.51	0.61	6.4	0.84			114			30			44	37	
4.5	40		99	21	28.3	0.60	0.69	7.0	0.87			114			30			44	38	
5.0	40	175/94	100	26	33.7	0.69	0.75	7.5	0.92	7.42	21	117	64	51	29	33	4	46	42	0.40
5.5	60		107	28	40.1	0.83	0.81	7.6	1.02			120			28			45	47	
6.0	60		112	32	47.2	0.98	0.88	7.9	1.11			121			28			45	51	
6.5	80		119	36	54.9	1.10	0.94	7.9	1.17			120			30			47	55	
7.0	80	225/94	130	42	62.4	1.25	1.03	7.9	1.21	7.39	20	123	66	55	28	34	6	47	57	0.43
7.5	100		134	44	69.9	1.40	1.06	7.9	1.32			125			28			47	62	
8.0	100	238/94	138	48	75.7	1.48	1.06	7.7	1.40	7.35	17	126	74	52	28	31	3	48	68	0.40
8.5	120		144	57	79.5	1.52	1.06	7.4	1.43			128			26			49	70	
9.0	Recovery		144	45	74.5	1.49	1.00	6.9	1.49			129			26			47	71	
9.5	Recovery		132	39	69.8	1.41	1.00	7.6	1.41			128			27			47	66	
10.0	Recovery		114	36	63.5	1.26	0.85	7.5	1.48			130			26			48	71	
10.5	Recovery	231/100	102	31	53.2	1.01	0.65	6.4	1.55	7.31	14	131	88	41	25	29	4	50	78	0.39

Abbreviations: BP, blood pressure; BTPS, body temperature pressure saturated; f, frequency; HCO_3^-, bicarbonate; HR, heart rate; $P(A - a)O_2$, alveolar-arterial PO_2 difference; $P(a - ET)CO_2$, arterial-end-tidal PCO_2 difference; $PETCO_2$, end-tidal PCO_2; $PETO_2$, end-tidal PO_2; R, respiratory exchange ratio; STPD, standard temperature pressure dry; $\dot{V}CO_2$, carbon dioxide output; VD/VT, physiological dead space-tidal volume ratio; $\dot{V}E$, minute ventilation; $\dot{V}E/\dot{V}CO_2$, ventilatory equivalent for carbon dioxide; $\dot{V}E/\dot{V}O_2$, ventilatory equivalent for oxygen; $\dot{V}O_2$, oxygen uptake.

CASE 70

A Runner With Obstructive Lung Disease

e To view this case please access the eBook bundled with this text. Instructions are located on the inside front cover.

CASE 71

Mild Obstructive Airway Disease With Disproportionate Exertional Dyspnea

CLINICAL FINDINGS

This 64-year-old retired shipyard worker was evaluated because of increasing shortness of breath that had begun 7 years previously and had progressed to become evident with walking two blocks or climbing a flight of stairs. He had smoked half a pack of cigarettes daily from age 40 to 60 years. He had also been treated for pulmonary tuberculosis two decades previously. Prostatic carcinoma had been found 8 months previously at the time of transurethral prostatectomy. He was treated with triamterene, hydrochlorothiazide, and methyldopa for systemic hypertension. The chest radiographs revealed a single small pleural plaque on the left, evidence of old granulomatous disease in the right apex, and flat diaphragms. Airflow obstruction was evident on pulmonary function tests. Exercise testing was requested, however, because the patient's symptoms seemed disproportionate to the degree of pulmonary function abnormality. Demographic and respiratory function data are shown in **Table 10.71.1**

EXERCISE FINDINGS

The patient performed exercise on a cycle ergometer. He pedaled at 60 rpm without added load for 3 minutes. The work rate was then increased 15 W/min to his symptom-limited maximum. Arterial blood was sampled every second minute, and intra-arterial blood pressure was recorded from a percutaneously placed brachial artery catheter. A resting electrocardiogram (ECG) showed some premature atrial and ventricular contractions, poor R-wave progression from leads V1 through V3, and left atrial enlargement. At 90 W, there were occasional pairs of premature ventricular contractions and two episodes of ventricular bigeminy. The patient stopped exercising because of shortness of breath. Under questioning, he also conceded that he had felt some substernal tightness at the highest work rate. Exercise data are summarized in **Tables 10.71.2** and **10.71.3**, and **Figure 10.71.1**.

INTERPRETATION

Comments

The results of the resting respiratory function studies showed hyperinflation and expiratory airflow obstruction. The FEV_1 was within the normal range, but FEV_1/VC was reduced (60%), and there was a moderately severe reduction of D_{LCO}. The resting ECG showed premature atrial and ventricular contractions and poor R-wave progression from V1

TABLE 10.71.1 Selected Respiratory Function Data

Measurement	Predicted	Measured	
Age (y)		64	
Sex		Male	
Height (cm)		178	
Weight (kg)	80	82	
Hematocrit (%)		47	
		Before bronchodilator	After bronchodilator
VC (L)	3.82	4.52	4.75
IC (L)	2.55	3.25	
TLC (L)	5.93	8.66	
FEV_1 (L)	2.98	2.69	2.78
FEV_1/VC (%)	78	60	58
MVV (L/min)	121	90	112
D_{LCO} (mL/mm Hg/min)	24.8	14.0	

Abbreviations: D_{LCO}, diffusing capacity of lung for carbon monoxide; FEV_1, forced expiratory volume in 1 second; IC, inspiratory capacity; MVV, maximum voluntary ventilation; TLC, total lung capacity; VC, vital capacity.

TABLE 10.71.2 Selected Exercise Data

Measurement	Predicted	Measured
Peak $\dot{V}O_2$ (L/min)	2.16	1.42
Maximum heart rate (beats/min)	156	159
Maximum O_2 pulse (mL/beat)	13.9	8.9
$\Delta\dot{V}O_2/\Delta WR$ (mL/min/W)	10.3	8.1
AT (L/min)	>0.95	Indeterminate
Blood pressure (mm Hg [rest, max])		186/116, 263/128
Maximum $\dot{V}E$ (L/min)		91
Exercise breathing reserve (L/min)	>15	91
$\dot{V}E/\dot{V}CO_2$ @ *AT* or lowest	28.3	42.4
PaO_2 (mm Hg [rest, max ex])		79, 57
$P(A - a)O_2$ (mm Hg [rest, max ex])		38, 65
$PaCO_2$ (mm Hg [rest, max ex])		32, 31
$P(a - ET)CO_2$ (mm Hg [rest, max ex])		4, 9
VD/VT (rest, heavy ex)		0.38, 0.47
HCO_3^- (mEq/L [rest, 2-min recov])		24, 17

Abbreviations: *AT*, anaerobic threshold; $\Delta\dot{V}O_2/\Delta WR$, change in $\dot{V}O_2$/change in work rate; ex, exercise; HCO_3^-, bicarbonate; O_2, oxygen; $P(A - a)O_2$, alveolar-arterial PO_2 difference; $P(a - ET)CO_2$, arterial–end-tidal PCO_2 difference; recov, recovery; VD/VT, physiological dead space–tidal volume ratio; $\dot{V}E$, minute ventilation; $\dot{V}E/\dot{V}CO_2$, ventilatory equivalent for carbon dioxide; $\dot{V}O_2$, oxygen uptake.

through V3. The arterial blood pressure was also elevated, even taking into consideration that the directly recorded intra-arterial pressures may exceed cuff measurements by 10 mm Hg. Given the degree of resting hypertension, testing might have been deferred pending control of blood pressure. In this case, exercise testing proceeded with caution.

Analysis

The peak oxygen uptake ($\dot{V}O_2$) was considerably reduced relative to predicted (66%). The anaerobic threshold was difficult to determine with certainty (**Fig. 10.71.1**, panel 3) but was likely low as well. The test ended as the patient's ventilation reached his maximum voluntary ventilation, indicating that he had reached his ventilatory capacity, despite relatively modest airflow obstruction on resting pulmonary function tests. The explanation appears to be the patient's high ventilatory requirements as manifested by high $\dot{V}E$ versus $\dot{V}CO_2$ slope and high $\dot{V}E/\dot{V}CO_2$. While he did have some hyperventilation, higher physiological dead space–tidal volume ratio (VD/VT) is the likely major contributor. The primary finding of this test, therefore, was that the patient had a greater exercise impairment than would be predicted by his FEV_1. This might be due entirely to mismatching of ventilation to perfusion, resulting in the very elevated VD/VT and low DLCO. However, the exercise-associated hypoxemia and the directional changes in ventilatory equivalents with exercise (see **Fig. 10.71.1**, panel 4) could reflect a development of right-to-left shunting through a patent foramen ovale, which sometimes occurs in patients with obstructive lung disease if there is sufficient pulmonary vascular disease to elevate right atrial pressures. Measurement of exercise blood gases while breathing 100% oxygen (O_2) would have clarified this. Alternatively, the patient's rapid breathing frequency may have led to dynamic hyperinflation, consistent with the relatively low VT/IC ratio throughout exercise (see **Fig. 10.71.1**, panel 9), which would tend to increase VD/VT. This test was done without measurements of inspiratory capacity that would confirm dynamic hyperinflation.

As in other cases of lung disease presented in this chapter, the test also included findings reflecting impaired O_2 flow, including a low $\Delta\dot{V}O_2/\Delta WR$ and steep increase in heart rate relative to $\dot{V}O_2$. These are consistent with the effect of hyperinflation on cardiac function or coexistent cardiac or pulmonary vascular pathophysiology. Although the patient experienced chest pressure at peak exercise, there were no ECG findings to indicate myocardial ischemia, nor was there a distinct change in the relationship of heart rate to $\dot{V}O_2$ at the time of symptoms.

Use of the flowcharts in Chapter 9 would lead from Flowchart 1 to Flowchart 4 (low peak $\dot{V}O_2$ and low anaerobic threshold). At Branch Points 4.1 and 4.2, low breathing reserve and high VD/VT fit well with a presumptive finding of lung disease with impaired O_2 delivery.

Conclusion

This case is presented to illustrate the considerable amount of gas exchange abnormality that can occur during exercise, even with only mild abnormalities in spirometry. Of particular interest are the various potential mechanisms for abnormal gas exchange, including secondary pulmonary vascular disease and the effects of dynamic hyperinflation.

TABLE 10.71.3 Air Breathing

Time (min)	Work rate (W)	BP (mm Hg)	HR (min^{-1})	f (min^{-1})	$\dot{V}_E$ (L/min BTPS)	$\dot{V}_{CO_2}$ (L/min STPD)	$\dot{V}_{O_2}$ (L/min STPD)	$\frac{\dot{V}_{O_2}}{HR}$ (mL/beat)	R	pH	HCO_3^- (mEq/L)	P_{O_2}, mm Hg ET	a	(A − a)	P_{CO_2}, mm Hg ET	a	(a − ET)	$\frac{\dot{V}_E}{\dot{V}_{CO_2}}$	$\frac{\dot{V}_E}{\dot{V}_{O_2}}$	$\frac{V_D}{V_T}$
	Rest	185/116								7.42	24		67			38				
0.5	Rest		103	16	13.6	0.27	0.30	2.9	0.90			116			30			45	41	
1.0	Rest		102	16	16.3	0.33	0.36	3.5	0.92			117			29			45	42	
1.5	Rest		102	22	18.3	0.33	0.35	3.4	0.94			121			26			50	47	
2.0	Rest		103	12	8.6	0.15	0.15	1.5	1.00			118			29			51	51	
2.5	Rest		105	15	14.2	0.26	0.28	2.7	0.93			119			27			50	46	
3.0	Rest	185/116	108	23	13.2	0.23	0.24	2.2	0.96	7.46	22	120	79	38	28	32	4	49	47	0.38
3.5	Unloaded		114	12	17.9	0.37	0.37	3.2	1.00			115			31			46	46	
4.0	Unloaded		115	21	22.9	0.50	0.55	4.8	0.91			116			30			42	38	
4.5	Unloaded		116	17	28.4	0.64	0.67	5.8	0.96			112			33			42	40	
5.0	Unloaded		117	19	28.5	0.64	0.65	5.6	0.98			117			30			42	41	
5.5	Unloaded		117	27	35.8	0.72	0.69	5.9	1.04			120			28			47	49	
6.0	Unloaded	236/126	119	27	35.6	0.74	0.71	6.0	1.04	7.43	22	122	72	46	28	33	5	45	47	0.39
6.5	15		121	23	38.1	0.78	0.73	6.0	1.07			118			30			46	50	
7.0	15		123	28	43.1	0.85	0.80	6.5	1.06			123			26			48	51	
7.5	30		128	29	44.5	0.85	0.79	6.2	1.08			125			25			49	53	
8.0	30	236/128	128	30	50.9	0.95	0.89	7.0	1.07	7.44	21	123	68	52	26	32	6	51	54	0.45
8.5	45		129	33	49.9	0.93	0.89	6.9	1.04			124			25			51	53	
9.0	45		133	38	49.8	0.91	0.92	6.9	0.99			121			27			51	51	
9.5	60		139	44	62.7	1.07	1.04	7.5	1.03			125			24			55	57	
10.0	60		143	39	63.2	1.12	1.08	7.6	1.04	7.44	21	126	61	59	24	31	7	53	55	0.45
10.5	75		146	40	62.7	1.15	1.13	7.7	1.02			123			26			52	52	
11.0	75		148	44	71.3	1.26	1.21	8.2	1.04			123			26			54	56	
11.5	90		153	50	86.6	1.46	1.35	8.8	1.08			127			23			56	61	
12.0	90		157	52	88.2	1.49	1.34	8.5	1.11	7.42	20	128	60	61	22	31	9	56	63	0.48
12.5	105	263/128	159	47	90.8	1.59	1.42	8.9	1.12	7.41	19	128	57	65	22	31	9	55	61	0.47
13.0	Recovery		161	43	84.4	1.54	1.25	7.8	1.23			128			23			52	65	
13.5	Recovery		160	41	78.6	1.39	1.22	7.6	1.14			127			23			54	62	
14.0	Recovery		161	44	75.2	1.31	1.14	7.1	1.15			122			29			55	63	
14.5	Recovery	233/139	138	35	60.3	1.12	0.95	6.9	1.18	7.39	17	127	73	51	24	29	5	51	60	0.40

Abbreviations: BP, blood pressure; BTPS, body temperature pressure saturated; f, frequency; HCO_3, bicarbonate; HR, heart rate; $P(A - a)_{O_2}$, alveolar arterial P_{O_2} difference; $P(a - ET)_{CO_2}$, arterial–end-tidal P_{CO_2} difference; P_{ETCO_2}, end-tidal P_{CO_2}; P_{ETO_2}, end-tidal P_{O_2}; R, respiratory exchange ratio; STPD, standard temperature pressure dry; $\dot{V}_{CO_2}$, carbon dioxide output; V_D/V_T, physiological dead space–tidal volume ratio; $\dot{V}_E$, minute ventilation; $\dot{V}_E/\dot{V}_{CO_2}$, ventilatory equivalent for carbon dioxide; $\dot{V}_E/\dot{V}_{O_2}$, ventilatory equivalent for oxygen; $\dot{V}_{O_2}$, oxygen uptake.

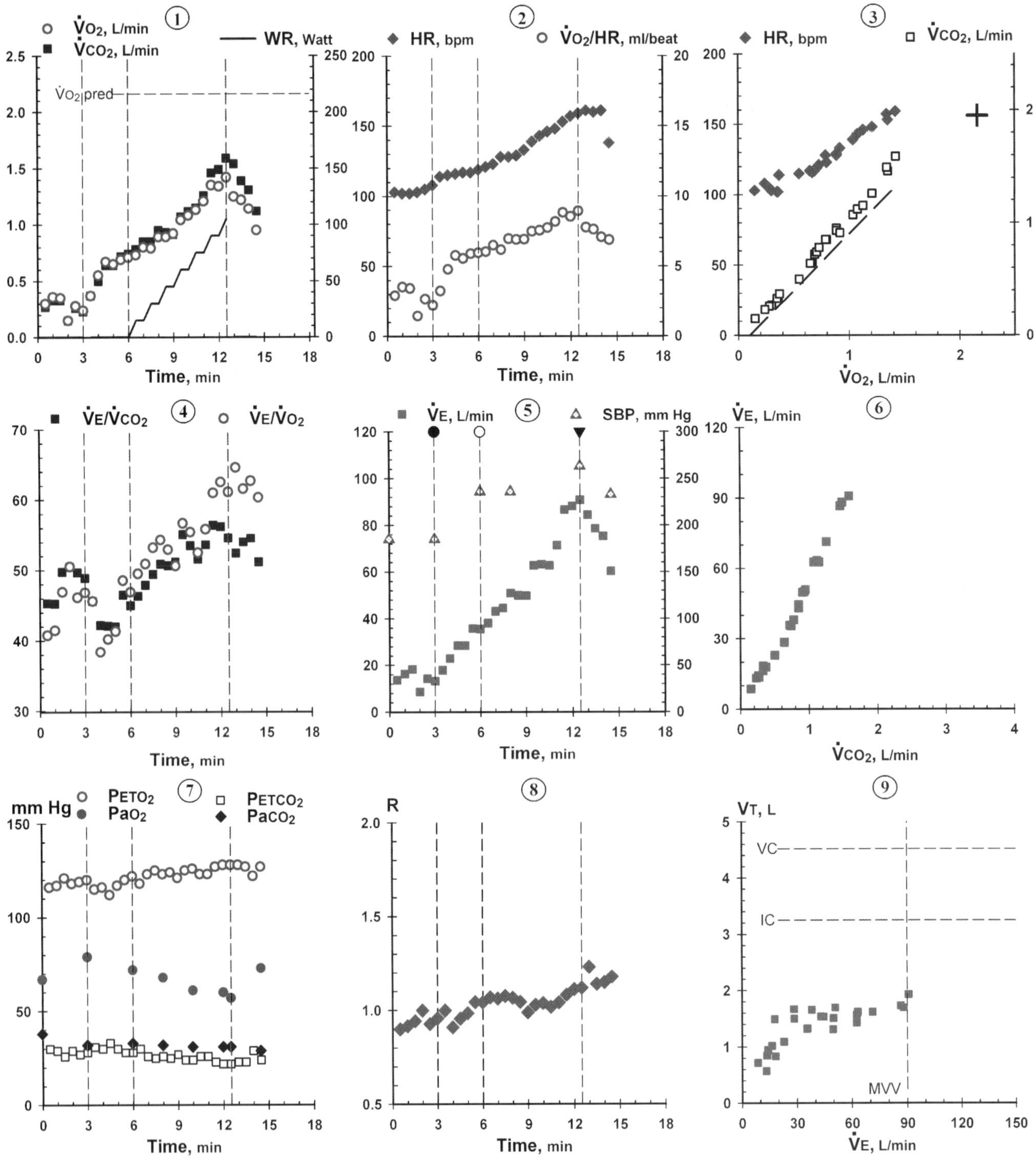

FIGURE 10.71.1. Vertical dashed lines in the panels in the left and middle columns indicate, from left to right, the beginning of unloaded cycling, start of increasing work rate (WR) at 15 W/min, and start of recovery. In **panel 1**, the increase in WR (right y-axis) is plotted with a scale of 100 W to 1 L of oxygen uptake ($\dot{V}O_2$) (left y-axis) such that WR is plotted parallel to a $\dot{V}O_2$ slope of 10 mL/min/W. In **panel 3**, carbon dioxide output ($\dot{V}CO_2$) (right y-axis) is plotted as a function of $\dot{V}O_2$ (x-axis) with identical scales so that the diagonal dashed line has a slope of 1 (45°). The $\dot{V}CO_2$ increasing more steeply than $\dot{V}O_2$ defines carbon dioxide (CO_2) derived from bicarbonate buffer, as long as ventilatory equivalent for CO_2 ($\dot{V}E/\dot{V}CO_2$) (**panel 4**) is not increasing and end-tidal PCO_2 ($PETCO_2$) (**panel 7**) is not decreasing, simultaneously. The black + symbol in **panel 3** indicates predicted peak values of heart rate (HR) (left y-axis) and $\dot{V}O_2$ for this individual. Abbreviations: IC, inspiratory capacity; MVV, maximum voluntary ventilation; $PETO_2$, end-tidal PO_2; R, respiratory exchange ratio; SBP, systolic blood pressure; VC, vital capacity; $\dot{V}CO_2$, carbon dioxide output; $\dot{V}E$, minute ventilation; $\dot{V}E/\dot{V}O_2$, ventilatory equivalent for oxygen; V_T, tidal volume.

CASE 72

Obesity Contributing to Ventilatory Limitation

To view this case please access the eBook bundled with this text. Instructions are located on the inside front cover.

CASE 73

Extrapulmonary Restriction: Ankylosing Spondylitis

CLINICAL FINDINGS

This 51-year-old airline employee had first developed symptoms of ankylosing spondylitis, primarily involving the neck and thoracic spine, approximately 6 years prior to evaluation. He was treated with nonsteroidal anti-inflammatory agents. He had stopped smoking more than 10 years previously. On the basis of apical pleural changes on chest radiographs, he had been treated empirically for tuberculosis several years previously, although the tuberculin skin test was negative. To maintain fitness, he had begun running approximately 3 miles a day. In the several months prior to testing, he felt as if he "could not get enough air" into his lungs and found himself taking gasping breaths. Physical examination revealed reduced neck movement and thoracic expansion. Chest radiograph revealed apical pleural thickening. The electrocardiogram (ECG) was normal. Demographic and respiratory function data are shown in **Table 10.73.1**.

TABLE 10.73.1 Selected Respiratory Function Data

Measurement	Predicted	Measured
Age (y)		51
Sex		Male
Height (cm)		178
Weight (kg)	80	79
Hematocrit (%)		39
VC (L)	4.62	3.61
IC (L)	3.08	2.60
FEV_1 (L)	3.67	2.76
FEV_1/VC (%)	79	76
MVV (L/min, direct)	151	132 at f = 80/min
MVV (L/min, indirect)	147	110

Abbreviations: f, frequency; FEV_1, forced expiratory volume in 1 second; IC, inspiratory capacity; MVV, maximum voluntary ventilation; VC, vital capacity.

EXERCISE FINDINGS

The patient performed exercise on a cycle ergometer. He pedaled at 60 rpm without added load for 3 minutes. The work rate was then increased 20 W/min to his symptom-limited maximum. He stopped exercise because of shortness of breath. Exercise ECGs were normal except for a single interpolated ventricular premature contraction. Exercise data are summerized in **Tables 10.73.2** and **10.73.3**, and **Figure 10.73.1**.

INTERPRETATION

Comments

Spirometry indicated mild restrictive disease (**Table 10.73.1**). This was reflected primarily in a reduction in the inspiratory capacity, due to impaired expansion of the chest wall.

TABLE 10.73.2 Selected Exercise Data

Measurement	Predicted	Measured
Peak $\dot{V}O_2$ (L/min)	2.52	2.54
Maximum heart rate (beats/min)	169	170
Maximum O_2 pulse (mL/beat)	14.9	14.9
$\Delta\dot{V}O_2/\Delta WR$ (mL/min/W)	10.3	9.4
AT (L/min)	>1.08	1.4
Blood pressure (mm Hg (rest, max))		126/86, 206/84
Maximum $\dot{V}E$ (L/min)		108
Exercise breathing reserve (L/min)	>15	2
$\dot{V}E/\dot{V}CO_2$ @ *AT* or lowest	26.9	24.3

Abbreviations: *AT*, anaerobic threshold; $\Delta\dot{V}O_2/\Delta WR$, change in $\dot{V}O_2$/change in work rate; O_2, oxygen; $\dot{V}E$, minute ventilation; $\dot{V}E/\dot{V}CO_2$, ventilatory equivalent for carbon dioxide; $\dot{V}O_2$, oxygen uptake.

TABLE 10.73.3 Air Breathing

Time (min)	Work rate (W)	BP (mm Hg)	HR (min^{-1})	f (min^{-1})	$\dot{V}E$ (L/min BTPS)	$\dot{V}CO_2$ (L/min STPD)	$\dot{V}O_2$ (L/min STPD)	$\frac{\dot{V}O_2}{HR}$ (mL/beat)	R	pH	HCO_3^- (mEq/L)	PO_2, mm Hg ET	PO_2, mm Hg a	PO_2, mm Hg (A − a)	PCO_2, mm Hg ET	PCO_2, mm Hg a	PCO_2, mm Hg (a − ET)	$\frac{\dot{V}E}{\dot{V}CO_2}$	$\frac{\dot{V}E}{\dot{V}O_2}$	$\frac{VD}{VT}$
0	Rest		72	15	8.3	0.20	0.26	3.6	0.77			97			39			35	27	
0.5	Rest		72	17	11.5	0.30	0.38	5.3	0.79			102			37			34	26	
1.0	Rest		74	14	12.1	0.33	0.40	5.4	0.83			102			37			33	27	
1.5	Rest		73	14	8.7	0.22	0.27	3.7	0.81			104			36			34	28	
2.0	Rest		69	15	6.3	0.13	0.18	2.6	0.72			95			39			39	28	
2.5	Rest	126/86	71	16	7.2	0.16	0.22	3.1	0.73			104			36			37	27	
3.0	Rest		69	22	7.0	0.16	0.23	3.3	0.70			96			39			32	22	
3.5	Rest		72	26	16.2	0.39	0.53	7.4	0.74			93			39			36	26	
4.0	Unloaded		78	19	9.1	0.24	0.37	4.7	0.65			84			43			31	20	
4.5	Unloaded		77	18	7.8	0.20	0.29	3.8	0.69			84			44			31	22	
5.0	Unloaded		81	21	9.7	0.28	0.45	5.6	0.62			83			44			28	18	
5.5	Unloaded		80	15	13.9	0.49	0.71	8.9	0.69			92			42			26	18	
6.0	Unloaded		76	19	17.7	0.56	0.76	10.0	0.74			86			45			29	21	
6.5	Unloaded		77	16	14.3	0.46	0.62	8.1	0.74			94			42			28	21	
7.0	20		78	17	14.0	0.46	0.63	8.1	0.73			95			41			27	20	
7.5	20	158/86	83	16	14.8	0.51	0.67	8.1	0.76			96			41			26	20	
8.0	40		82	19	17.7	0.59	0.78	9.5	0.76			95			41			27	21	
8.5	40	174/84	86	17	20.7	0.70	0.97	11.3	0.72			89			44			28	20	
9.0	60		91	17	21.4	0.76	1.00	11.0	0.76			93			43			26	20	
9.5	60		94	16	21.0	0.78	1.03	11.0	0.76			93			44			25	19	
10.0	80		99	18	23.5	0.88	1.15	11.6	0.77			90			45			25	19	
10.5	80	178/78	105	20	33.6	1.23	1.48	14.1	0.83			86			47			26	22	
11.0	100		107	20	28.9	1.14	1.37	12.8	0.83			94			46			24	20	
11.5	100		108	20	31.8	1.23	1.37	12.7	0.90			97			46			24	22	
12.0	120		119	20	38.0	1.46	1.58	13.3	0.92			94			46			25	23	
12.5	120	190/86	125	18	37.5	1.51	1.59	12.7	0.95			94			48			24	23	
13.0	140		128	25	38.8	1.53	1.58	12.3	0.97			95			50			24	23	
13.5	140		128	23	46.1	1.82	1.78	13.9	1.02			100			47			24	25	
14.0	160		137	25	48.3	1.88	1.82	13.3	1.03			95			51			25	25	
14.5	160	206/84	144	25	52.7	2.08	1.94	13.5	1.07			102			48			24	26	
15.0	180		148	30	55.1	2.17	1.98	13.4	1.10			104			46			24	27	
15.5	180		152	31	64.8	2.44	2.16	14.2	1.13			103			48			25	29	
16.0	200		161	34	73.6	2.71	2.24	13.9	1.21			110			44			26	32	
16.5	200		163	37	77.2	2.80	2.29	14.0	1.22			108			45			26	32	
17.0	220		169	39	97.2	3.20	2.50	14.8	1.28			111			43			29	38	
17.5	220		170	47	108.3	3.34	2.54	14.9	1.31			115			40			31	41	
18.0	Recovery		159	32	78.9	2.35	1.91	12.0	1.23			117			36			32	40	
18.5	Recovery		145	30	67.9	2.00	1.35	9.3	1.48			120			37			33	48	
19.0	Recovery	160/78	133	27	49.1	1.50	1.06	8.0	1.42			118			39			31	44	
19.5	Recovery		129	30	48.8	1.37	0.93	7.2	1.47			124			34			34	50	

Abbreviations: BP, blood pressure; BTPS, body temperature pressure saturated; f, frequency; HCO_3^-, bicarbonate; HR, heart rate; $P(A - a)O_2$, alveolar-arterial PO_2 difference; $P(a - ET)CO_2$, arterial-end-tidal PCO_2 difference; $PETCO_2$, end-tidal PCO_2; $PETO_2$, end-tidal PO_2; R, respiratory exchange ratio; STPD, standard temperature pressure dry; $\dot{V}CO_2$, carbon dioxide output; VD/VT, physiological dead space-tidal volume ratio; $\dot{V}E$, minute ventilation; $\dot{V}E/\dot{V}CO_2$, ventilatory equivalent for carbon dioxide; $\dot{V}E/\dot{V}O_2$, ventilatory equivalent for oxygen; $\dot{V}O_2$, oxygen uptake.

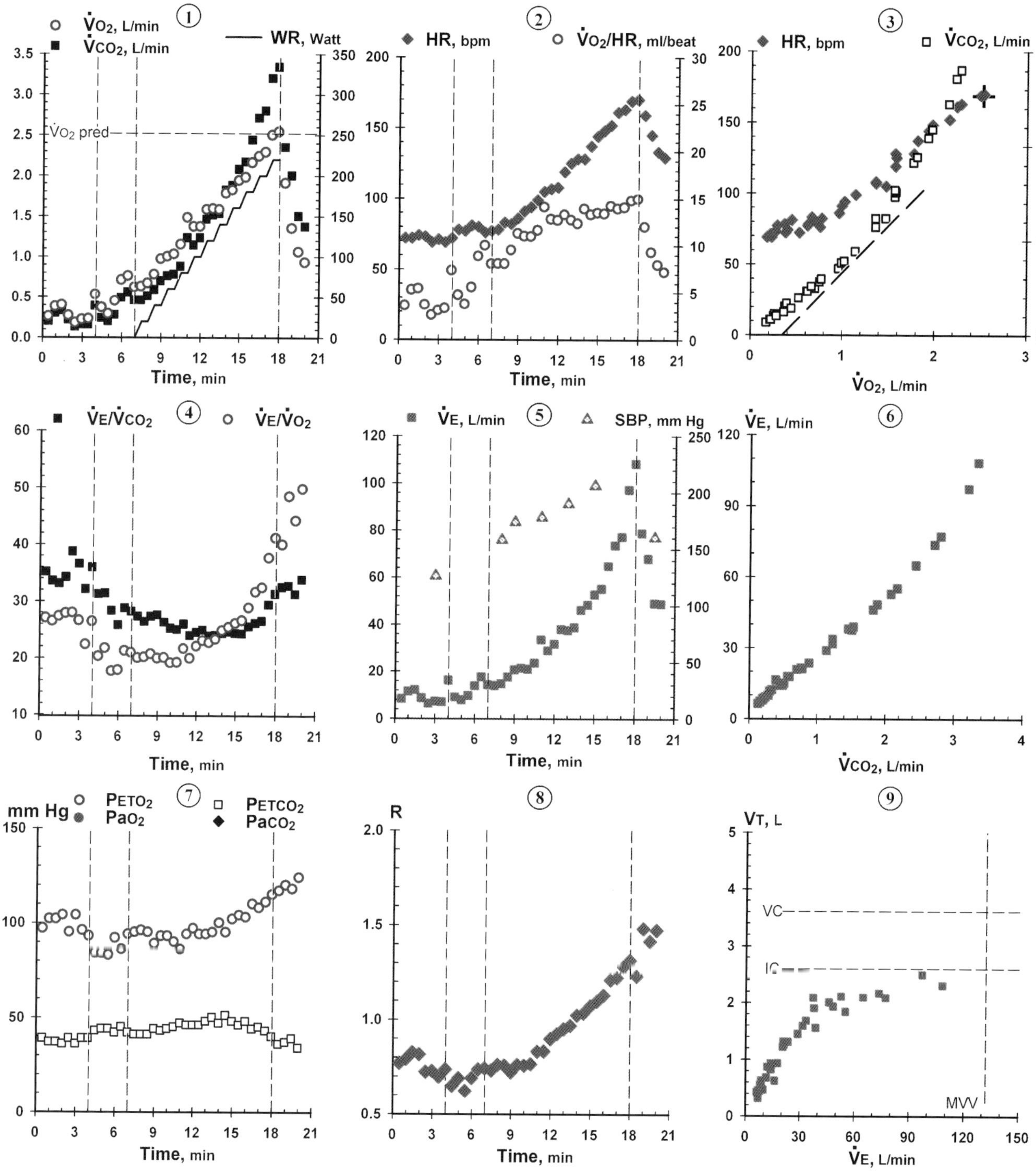

FIGURE 10.73.1. Vertical dashed lines in the panels in the left and middle columns indicate, from left to right, the beginning of unloaded cycling, start of increasing work rate (WR) at 20 W/min, and start of recovery. In **panel 1**, the increase in WR (right y-axis) is plotted with a scale of 100 W to 1 L of oxygen uptake ($\dot{V}O_2$) (left y-axis) such that WR is plotted parallel to a $\dot{V}O_2$ slope of 10 mL/min/W. In **panel 3**, carbon dioxide output ($\dot{V}CO_2$) (right y-axis) is plotted as a function of $\dot{V}O_2$ (x-axis) with identical scales so that the diagonal dashed line has a slope of 1 (45°). The $\dot{V}CO_2$ increasing more steeply than $\dot{V}O_2$ defines carbon dioxide (CO_2) derived from bicarbonate buffer, as long as ventilatory equivalent for CO_2 ($\dot{V}E/\dot{V}CO_2$) (**panel 4**) is not increasing and end-tidal PCO_2 ($PETCO_2$) (**panel 7**) is not decreasing, simultaneously. The black + symbol in **panel 3** indicates predicted peak values of heart rate (HR) (left y-axis) and $\dot{V}O_2$ for this individual. Abbreviations: IC, inspiratory capacity; MVV, maximum voluntary ventilation; $PETO_2$, end-tidal PO_2; R, respiratory exchange ratio; SBP, systolic blood pressure; VC, vital capacity; $\dot{V}E$, minute ventilation; $\dot{V}E/\dot{V}O_2$, ventilatory equivalent for oxygen; VT, tidal volume.

Analysis

Peak oxygen uptake ($\dot{V}O_2$) and anaerobic threshold were normal, as were the ECG and oxygen pulse at peak $\dot{V}O_2$. However, breathing reserve was abnormally low, notably when compared to the "indirect" maximum voluntary ventilation (MVV). In this case, derived MVV (from forced expiratory volume in 1 second) was preferred because the measured MVV during pulmonary function testing was performed a respiratory rate of 80 breaths/min, which is considered nonphysiologic. The low breathing reserve was also associated with a high VT/IC ratio characteristic of restrictive pulmonary disease, while normal $\dot{V}E/\dot{V}CO_2$ at the anaerobic threshold supports the restriction as due to chest wall impairment rather than lung parenchymal disease.

Using the flowcharts in Chapter 9, normal peak $\dot{V}O_2$ and the anaerobic threshold lead to Flowchart 2, where the normal ECG and peak oxygen pulse and lack of obesity suggest the diagnostic categories of normal/anxiety. However, the diagnosis of ankylosing spondylitis and finding of restriction on pulmonary function testing should lead to consideration of chest wall expansion limiting breathing during exercise.

Conclusion

The subject had exertional dyspnea and ventilatory limitation resulting from extrapulmonary restriction of the chest wall consequent to ankylosing spondylitis.

CASE 74

Extrapulmonary Restriction: Scoliosis

To view this case please access the eBook bundled with this text. Instructions are located on the inside front cover.

CASE 75

Interstitial Lung Disease and Hemidiaphragm Paralysis

CLINICAL FINDINGS

A 74-year-old man underwent exercise testing for follow up of his restrictive lung disease. He was a retired truck driver who had worked in construction many years earlier. He was known to have paralyzed right hemidiaphragm and interstitial lung disease, both of which had been present for at least 5 years. By imaging, the interstitial disease was predominantly subpleural and lower lobe in distribution and judged consistent with either asbestosis or idiopathic pulmonary fibrosis, but not pathognomonic for either. He had declined a lung biopsy and his pulmonary function had declined very little over 5 years. Despite significant pulmonary function abnormalities, he was not limited in his normal activities of gardening and household work by shortness of breath. He avoided vigorous activities. Medical history included systemic hypertension. He had no known cardiac disease. His regular medications were hydrochlorothiazide and candesartan. Physical examination was notable for fine inspiratory crackles in the lower half of both lung fields. Cardiac rhythm was regular without murmur and there was no clubbing, cyanosis, or edema. The resting electrocardiogram (ECG) showed normal sinus rhythm. Demographic and respiratory function data are shown in **Table 10.75.1**.

TABLE 10.75.1 Selected Respiratory Function Data

Measurement	Predicted	Measured
Age (y)		74
Sex		Male
Height (cm)		180
Weight (kg)		91.6
VC (L)	4.23	1.87
IC (L)	2.82	1.84
ERV (L)	1.41	0.37
TLC (L)	6.67	3.76
FEV_1 (L)	3.32	1.57
FEV_1/VC (%)	78	84
MVV (L/min)	126	70 (direct) 62 (indirect)
DLCO (mL/mm Hg/min)	25.64	16.37
DLCO/VA (mL/mm Hg/min/L)	3.84	4.81

Abbreviations: DLCO, diffusing capacity of lung for carbon monoxide; DLCO/VA, ; ERV, ; FEV_1, forced expiratory volume in 1 second; IC, inspiratory capacity; MVV, maximum voluntary ventilation; TLC, total lung capacity; VC, vital capacity.

EXERCISE FINDINGS

The patient exercised on a cycle ergometer beginning with 3 minutes of unloaded pedaling at 60 rpm followed by continuous increase in work rate by 15 W/min until the test ended with symptoms of shortness of breath. Exercise ECG showed a maximum of 2 mm upsloping ST-segment depression in the lateral leads. Exercise data are summarized in **Tables 10.75.2** and **10.75.3** and in **Figure 10.75.1**.

INTERPRETATION

Comment

On resting studies, this man had both extrapulmonary and pulmonary processes restricting lung mechanics. Based on the above-average diffusing capacity indexed to alveolar volume (DLCO/VA) (see **Table 10.75.1**), it was thought that restriction was primarily attributable to the hemidiaphragm paralysis. The exercise findings suggested more significance for the interstitial process.

Analysis

Exercise capacity was reduced relative to normal and was limited by dyspnea.

Cardiovascular and metabolic responses: The change in $\dot{V}O_2$/change in work rate ($\Delta\dot{V}O_2/\Delta WR$) was more shallow than normal, and peak oxygen uptake ($\dot{V}O_2$) was low. Anaerobic threshold was also below the lower limit of normal.

TABLE 10.75.2 Selected Exercise Data

Measurement	Predicted	Measured
Peak $\dot{V}O_2$ (L/min)	1.95	1.31
Maximum heart rate (beats/min)	146	134
Maximum O_2 pulse (mL/beat)	13.4	9.8
$\Delta\dot{V}O_2/\Delta WR$ (mL/min/W)	10.3	7.1
AT (L/min)	>0.93	0.9
Blood pressure (mm Hg [rest, peak ex])		170/93, 213/79
Maximum $\dot{V}E$ (L/min)		50
Breathing reserve (L/min)	>15	20, 12
$\dot{V}E/\dot{V}CO_2$ at the *AT*	<34	32
$\dot{V}E$-$\dot{V}CO_2$ slope	<30	31
SpO_2 (% [rest, Maximum ex])		96, 91

Abbreviations: *AT*, anaerobic threshold; $\Delta\dot{V}O_2/\Delta WR$, change in $\dot{V}O_2$/change in work rate; ex, exercise; O_2, oxygen; SpO_2, estimated arterial oxygen saturation by pulse oximeter; $\dot{V}CO_2$, carbon dioxide output; $\dot{V}E$, minute ventilation; $\dot{V}E/\dot{V}CO_2$, ventilatory equivalent for CO_2; $\dot{V}O_2$, oxygen uptake.

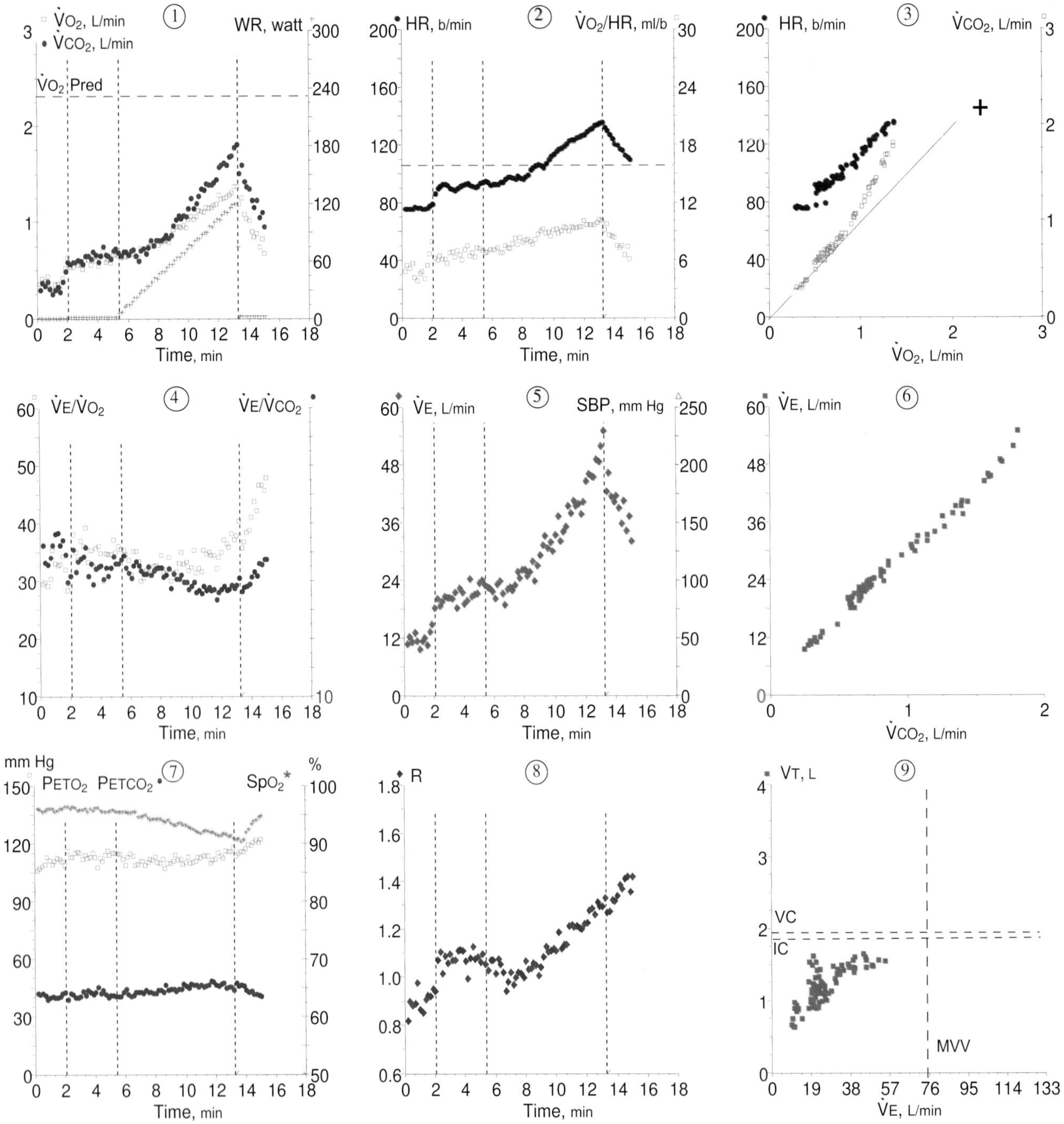

FIGURE 10.75.1. Vertical dashed lines in the panels in the left and middle columns indicate, from left to right, the beginning of unloaded cycling, start of increasing work rate at (WR) 15 W/min, and start of recovery. In **panel 1**, the increase in WR (right y-axis) is plotted with a scale of 100 W to 1 L of oxygen uptake ($\dot{V}O_2$) (left y-axis) such that WR is plotted parallel to a $\dot{V}O_2$ slope of 10 mL/min/W. Predicted peak $\dot{V}O_2$ is shown as a dashed horizontal line. In **panel 3**, carbon dioxide output ($\dot{V}CO_2$) (right y-axis) is plotted as a function of $\dot{V}O_2$ (x-axis) with identical scales so that the diagonal blue line has a slope of 1 (45°). The $\dot{V}CO_2$ increasing more steeply than $\dot{V}O_2$ defines carbon dioxide (CO_2) derived from bicarbonate buffer, as long as ventilatory equivalent for CO_2 ($\dot{V}E/\dot{V}CO_2$) (**panel 4**) is not increasing and partial pressure of CO_2 in end-tidal gas (P_{ETCO_2}) (**panel 7**) is not decreasing, simultaneously. The black + symbol in **panel 3** indicates predicted peak values of heart rate (HR) (left y-axis) and $\dot{V}O_2$ for this individual. Abbreviations: IC, inspiratory capacity; MVV, maximum voluntary ventilation; P_{ETO_2}, end-tidal partial pressure of oxygen; R, respiratory exchange ratio; SBP, systolic blood pressure; Sp_{O_2}, arterial O_2 saturation as estimated by pulse oximetry; VC, vital capacity; $\dot{V}E$, minute ventilation; $\dot{V}E/\dot{V}O_2$, ventilatory equivalent for O_2; $\dot{V}O_2$/HR, oxygen pulses; V_T, tidal volume.

TABLE 10.75.3 Air Breathing

Time (min)	Work rate (W)	BP (mm Hg)	HR (min^{-1})	f (min^{-1})	$\dot{V}E$ (L/min BTPS)	$\dot{V}CO_2$ (L/min STPD)	$\dot{V}O_2$ (L/min STPD)	$\frac{\dot{V}O_2}{HR}$ (mL/beat)	R	pH	HCO_3^- (mEq/L)	PO_2, mm Hg and SpO_2%: ET	SpO_2	(A − a)	PCO_2, mm Hg: ET	a	(a − ET)	$\frac{\dot{V}E}{\dot{V}CO_2}$	$\frac{\dot{V}E}{\dot{V}O_2}$	$\frac{VD}{VT}$
0.5	Rest		75	15	10.8	0.31	0.36	4.8	0.85			107	96		42			35	30	
1.0	Rest		76	13	11.3	0.33	0.36	4.7	0.91			110	96		41			35	32	
1.5	Rest	170/93	76	16	11.2	0.29	0.34	4.5	0.86			110	96		40			38	33	
2.0	Unloaded		76	15	11.7	0.33	0.35	4.6	0.93			112	96		40			36	34	
2.5	Unloaded		83	18	18.9	0.59	0.57	6.9	1.03			112	96		41			32	33	
3.0	Unloaded		92	18	20.1	0.60	0.57	6.2	1.05			115	96		41			34	35	
3.5	Unloaded		90	19	20.8	0.62	0.57	6.4	1.08			114	96		41			33	36	
4.0	Unloaded		90	16	20.6	0.66	0.60	6.6	1.10			113	96		43			31	35	
4.5	Unloaded	168/90	93	18	21.3	0.67	0.64	6.9	1.05			111	96		43			32	33	
5.0	Unloaded		91	16	20.7	0.64	0.58	6.4	1.09			114	96		41			33	36	
5.5	8		93	22	23.2	0.70	0.65	7.0	1.07			115	96		41			33	36	
6.0	15		94	20	22.3	0.68	0.64	6.8	1.06			114	96		41			33	35	
6.5	23		93	17	22.0	0.69	0.66	7.1	1.04			112	95		42			32	34	
7.0	30	173/94	95	19	20.8	0.65	0.66	7.0	0.98			111	95		42			32	31	
7.5	34		98	21	22.4	0.71	0.72	7.4	0.99			110	95		43			31	31	
8.0	41		97	25	25.5	0.79	0.79	8.1	1.01			111	94		42			32	33	
8.5	49		98	22	25.6	0.81	0.78	8.0	1.04			111	94		43			31	33	
9.0	56		104	23	26.1	0.85	0.83	7.9	1.03			110	94		44			31	32	
9.5	64		105	25	31.1	1.02	0.94	8.9	1.08			112	93		44			31	33	
10.0	75	185/98	109	22	31.0	1.06	0.95	8.7	1.11			111	93		45			29	33	
10.5	82		115	23	34.3	1.19	1.04	9.0	1.14			111	93		46			29	33	
11.0	89		119	25	36.3	1.28	1.10	9.2	1.16			111	92		46			28	33	
11.5	96		123	26	39.4	1.38	1.14	9.2	1.21			113	92		46			29	35	
12.0	104		125	26	39.3	1.42	1.18	9.4	1.21			111	92		48			28	33	
12.5	111	213/79	129	30	46.0	1.60	1.26	9.8	1.27			114	91		46			29	36	
13.0	119		133	31	47.6	1.65	1.28	9.6	1.29			115	91		46			29	37	
13.5	126		134	32	49.9	1.70	1.31	9.8	1.30			116	91		45			29	38	
14.0	Recovery		127	28	42.6	1.47	1.13	8.9	1.30			115	91		46			29	38	
14.5	Recovery	179/87	119	28	38.7	1.24	0.91	7.7	1.36			119	93		43			31	42	
15.0	Recovery		113	31	37.6	1.13	0.81	7.1	1.39			121	94		41			33	46	
15.5	Recovery		109	26	30.3	0.90	0.65	6.0	1.38			122	95		41			34	46	

Abbreviations: BP, blood pressure; BTPS, body temperature pressure saturated; f, frequency; HCO_3, bicarbonate; HR, heart rate; R, respiratory exchange ratio; SpO_2, arterial O2 saturation as estimated by pulse oximetry; STPD, standard temperature pressure dry; $\dot{V}CO_2$, carbon dioxide output; VD/VT, physiological dead space-tidal volume ratio; $\dot{V}E$, minute ventilation; $\dot{V}E/\dot{V}CO_2$, ventilatory equivalent for carbon dioxide; $\dot{V}E/\dot{V}O_2$, ventilatory equivalent for oxygen; $\dot{V}O_2$, oxygen uptake.

The heart rate increased steeply relative to $\dot{V}O_2$ (panel 3), and the peak oxygen pulse was lower than predicted. These findings are characteristic of impaired oxygen delivery due to cardiovascular factors. The systemic blood pressure was elevated. The ECG changes were minor and nonspecific and not suggestive of high likelihood of myocardial ischemia.

Ventilatory responses: The breathing reserve was either normal or low depending on whether the measured or calculated maximum voluntary ventilation were used for comparison of exercise minute ventilation ($\dot{V}E$).

Efficiency of pulmonary gas exchange: There was abnormal decline in oxygen saturation as estimated by pulse oximetry (SpO_2) over the course of exercise. The ventilatory equivalent for carbon dioxide at the anaerobic threshold and the slope of $\dot{V}E$ relative to carbon dioxide output were both near the upper limits of normal. There were thus borderline findings with respect to efficiency of CO_2 elimination.

Conclusion

The most distinct abnormalities in this test were related to the $\dot{V}O_2$ response to exercise and arterial desaturation. This pattern of findings is typical of pulmonary vascular disease, which was most likely attributable to the pulmonary vascular effects of interstitial lung disease. Cardiac dysfunction from an undiagnosed coexisting disorder cannot be excluded based on these data alone. Although the breathing reserve was borderline, the patient was subjectively limited by dyspnea and was approaching his maximal ventilatory capacity at a relatively low level of $\dot{V}O_2$.

CASE 76

Active Man With Paralyzed Hemidiaphragm

CLINICAL FINDINGS

A 72-year-old man was referred for testing because of a history of abrupt change in exercise capacity. He played soccer regularly 1 or 2 times per week and was accustomed to playing for 90 minutes without respiratory discomfort. Beginning 7 months previously, however, he had been experiencing dyspnea soon after beginning to play and had to stop frequently to catch his breath. He was also short of breath on ascending two flights of stairs. He described transient dyspnea on lying down, which resolved within a half hour and did not recur. Coronary artery disease had been diagnosed 8 years earlier at which time he had also experienced exertional dyspnea, but symptoms had resolved after a coronary stenting procedure. Coronary angiography was repeated and demonstrated patent stents and no obstructing lesions. Imaging studies showed an elevated hemidiaphragm, however, and a sniff test was consistent with right diaphragm paralysis. There were no pulmonary parenchymal or mediastinal abnormalities noted. Medical history included hypertension, hyperlipidemia, and prostate cancer treated over a decade earlier. Medications at the time of testing were amlodipine, hydrochlorothiazide/triamterene, carvedilol, aspirin, tamsulosin, and bicalutamide. Physical examination found lack of breath sounds in the right base. Heart tones were regular, and there was a II/VI systolic murmur at the left sternal border. There was no peripheral edema. Resting electrocardiogram showed a sinus rhythm. Demographic and respiratory function data are shown in **Table 10.76.1**.

TABLE 10.76.1 Selected Respiratory Function Data

Measurement	Predicted	Measured
Age (y)		72
Sex		Male
Height (cm)		168
Weight (kg)		82
VC (L)	3.7	2.3
IC (L)	2.97	2.0
ERV (L)	0.73	0.49
FEV_1 (L)	2.68	1.64
FEV_1/VC (%)	72	71
MVV (L/min)	111	71

Abbreviations: ERV, expiratory reserve volume; FEV_1, forced expiratory volume in 1 second; IC, inspiratory capacity; MVV, maximum voluntary ventilation; VC, vital capacity.

EXERCISE FINDINGS

The patient exercised on a cycle ergometer beginning with 3 minutes of unloaded pedaling at 60 rpm followed by continuous increase in work rate by 15 W/min until the test ended with symptoms of shortness of breath. Exercise electrocardiogram showed no ischemic changes or arrhythmia. Exercise data are summarized in **Tables 10.76.2** and **10.76.3** and in **Figure 10.76.1**.

INTERPRETATION

Comment

This case is presented as an example of an extrapulmonary process that does not impair the efficiency of pulmonary gas exchange, but reduced breathing capacity, and likely increased the energetic cost of breathing, such that ventilation became the limiting factor to exercise.

Analysis

Exercise capacity was in the normal range, with a peak oxygen uptake ($\dot{V}O_2$) over 90% of the normal reference value. The change in $\dot{V}O_2$/change in work rate ($\Delta\dot{V}O_2/\Delta WR$) and anaerobic threshold were also normal. The heart rate increase relative to $\dot{V}O_2$ was more shallow than average (see panel 3 of the figure), and peak heart rate was slightly below the lower limit of

TABLE 10.76.2 Selected Exercise Data

Measurement	Predicted	Measured
Peak $\dot{V}O_2$ (L/min)	1.78	1.65
Maximum heart rate (beats/min)	148	128
Maximum O_2 pulse (mL/beat)	12.1	12.9
$\Delta\dot{V}O_2/\Delta WR$ (mL/min/W)	10.3	11.0
AT (L/min)	>0.84	0.85
Blood pressure (mm Hg [rest, peak ex])		144/81, 203/76
Maximum $\dot{V}E$ (L/min)		62
Breathing reserve (L/min)	>15	9
$\dot{V}E/\dot{V}CO_2$ @ *AT*	<34	30
$\dot{V}E$-$\dot{V}CO_2$ slope	<33	29
SpO_2 (% [rest, peak ex])		97, 95

Abbreviations: *AT*, anaerobic threshold; ex, exercise; O_2, oxygen; SpO_2, oxygen saturation as measured by pulse oximetry; $\dot{V}CO_2$, carbon dioxide output; $\dot{V}E$, minute ventilation; $\dot{V}E/\dot{V}CO_2$, ventilatory equivalent for CO_2; $\dot{V}O_2$, oxygen uptake; $\Delta\dot{V}O_2/\Delta WR$, change in $\dot{V}O_2$/change in work rate.

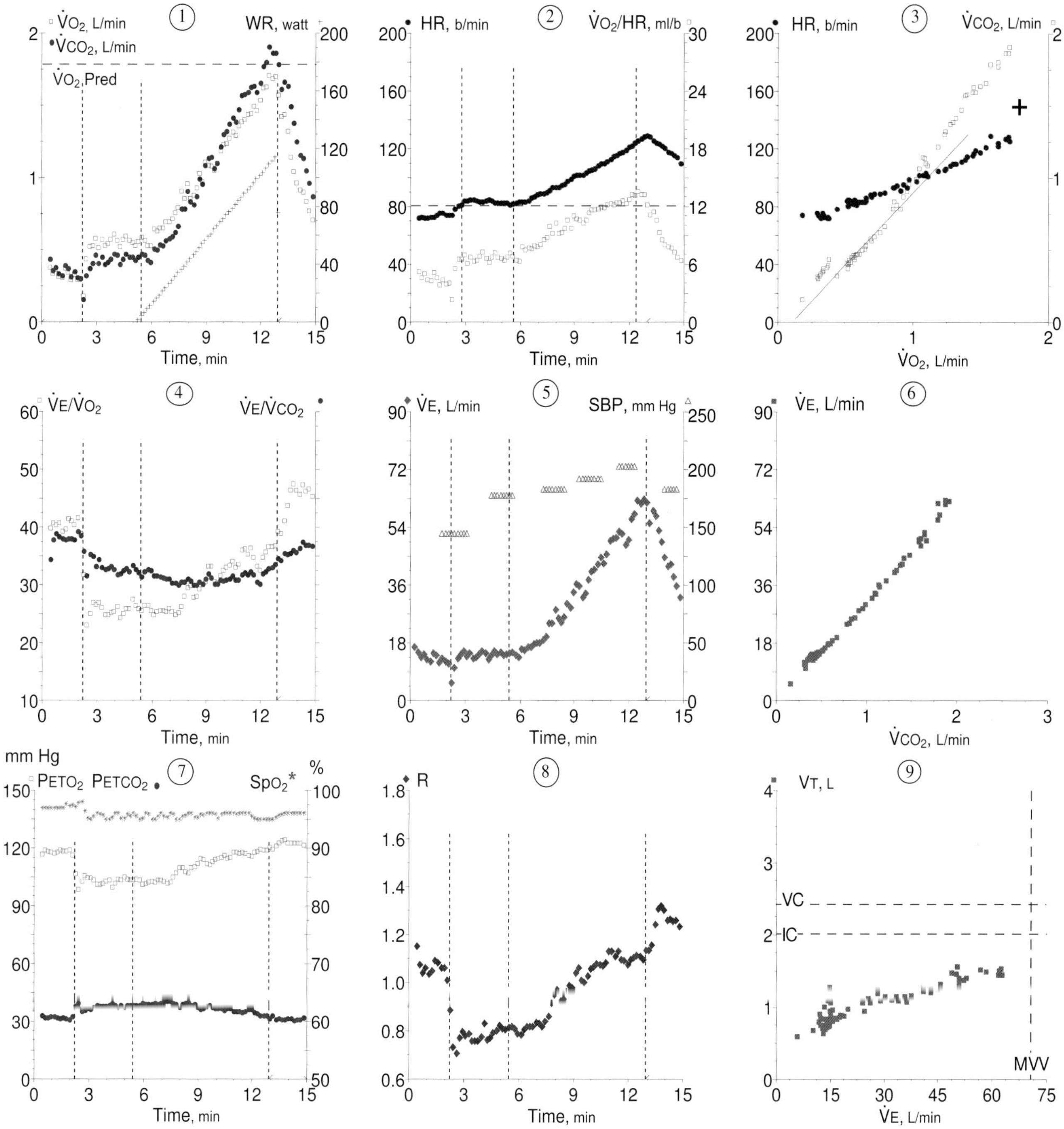

FIGURE 10.76.1. Vertical dashed lines in the panels in the left and middle columns indicate, from left to right, the beginning of unloaded cycling, start of increasing work rate (WR) at 15 W/min, and start of recovery. In **panel 1**, the increase in WR (right y-axis) is plotted with a scale of 100 W to 1 L of oxygen uptake ($\dot{V}O_2$) (left y-axis) such that WR is plotted parallel to a $\dot{V}O_2$ slope of 10 mL/min/W. Predicted peak $\dot{V}O_2$ is shown as a dashed horizontal line. In **panel 3**, carbon dioxide output ($\dot{V}CO_2$) (right y-axis) is plotted as a function of $\dot{V}O_2$ (x-axis) with identical scales so that the diagonal blue line has a slope of 1 (45°). The $\dot{V}CO_2$ increasing more steeply than $\dot{V}O_2$ defines carbon dioxide (CO_2) derived from bicarbonate buffer, as long as ventilatory equivalent for CO_2 ($\dot{V}E/\dot{V}CO_2$) (**panel 4**) is not increasing and end-tidal PCO_2 ($PETCO_2$) (**panel 7**) is not decreasing, simultaneously. The black + symbol in **panel 3** indicates predicted peak values of heart rate (HR) (left y-axis) and $\dot{V}O_2$ for this individual. Abbreviations: IC, inspiratory capacity; MVV, maximum voluntary ventilation; $PETO_2$, end-tidal PO_2; R, respiratory exchange ratio; SBP, systolic blood pressure; SpO_2, oxygen saturation as measured by pulse oximetry; VC, vital capacity; $\dot{V}E$, minute ventilation; $\dot{V}E/\dot{V}O_2$, ventilatory equivalent for oxygen; V_T, tidal volume.

TABLE 10.76.3 Air Breathing

Time (min)	Work rate (W)	BP (mm Hg)	HR (min^{-1})	f (min^{-1})	$\dot{V}E$ (L/min BTPS)	$\dot{V}CO_2$ (L/min STPD)	$\dot{V}O_2$ (L/min STPD)	$\frac{\dot{V}O_2}{HR}$ (mL/beat)	R	pH	HCO_3^- (mEq/L)	PO_2, mm Hg and SpO_2, %			PCO_2, mm Hg			$\frac{\dot{V}E}{\dot{V}CO_2}$	$\frac{\dot{V}E}{\dot{V}O_2}$	$\frac{V_D}{V_T}$
												ET	SpO_2	(A − a)	ET	a	(a − ET)			
0.5	Rest		54	14	15.6	0.43	0.41	7.6	1.04			116	97		33			37	38	
1.0	Rest		72	17	13.4	0.35	0.33	4.6	1.06			118	97		32			38	41	
1.5	Rest		73	15	13.7	0.36	0.34	4.7	1.06			118	97		32			38	40	
2.0	Rest	144/81	75	14	12.2	0.32	0.30	4.0	1.07			119	97		31			39	41	
2.5	Unloaded		76	13	8.8	0.25	0.30	4.0	0.84			107	98		37			35	30	
3.0	Unloaded		82	18	13.8	0.40	0.53	6.5	0.75			104	97		36			35	26	
3.5	Unloaded		84	17	13.9	0.42	0.54	6.4	0.78			103	95		37			33	26	
4.0	Unloaded		83	19	14.0	0.42	0.56	6.7	0.76			102	96		38			33	25	
4.5	Unloaded	178/80	84	16	13.7	0.43	0.54	6.4	0.79			101	96		39			32	25	
5.0	Unloaded		83	18	14.9	0.45	0.57	6.8	0.80			104	96		38			33	26	
5.5	4		82	18	14.3	0.45	0.55	6.8	0.81			103	96		38			32	26	
6.0	13		83	19	14.1	0.43	0.54	6.5	0.80			103	95		39			32	26	
6.5	20		84	19	16.2	0.51	0.64	7.7	0.80			102	96		39			31	25	
7.0	27		87	20	17.2	0.55	0.67	7.7	0.82			103	96		39			31	26	
7.5	35	183/79	89	21	19.0	0.63	0.76	8.5	0.83			102	96		40			30	25	
8.0	42		93	23	25.5	0.83	0.90	9.8	0.92			108	95		38			31	28	
8.5	50		94	24	25.2	0.84	0.89	9.4	0.94			108	96		40			30	28	
9.0	57		99	28	30.9	1.01	1.03	10.4	0.98			111	96		38			31	30	
9.5	65	192/77	102	31	34.5	1.11	1.07	10.5	1.04			114	96		37			31	32	
10.0	72		105	31	37.1	1.21	1.18	11.3	1.03			113	96		38			31	31	
10.5	80		108	34	42.7	1.37	1.27	11.8	1.07			115	96		36			31	34	
11.0	88		111	35	46.1	1.48	1.35	12.1	1.10			116	96		36			31	34	
11.5	95	203/76	116	37	51.3	1.60	1.43	12.3	1.12			118	96		35			32	36	
12.0	103		119	34	50.1	1.63	1.50	12.6	1.09			116	96		36			31	33	
12.5	110		124	39	59.0	1.83	1.65	13.3	1.11			118	95		34			32	36	
13.0	117		128	42	61.9	1.83	1.65	12.9	1.11			120	95		32			34	38	
13.5	Recovery		126	39	57.3	1.64	1.39	11.0	1.18			121	95		32			35	41	
14.0	Recovery	183/67	122	33	48.9	1.37	1.04	8.5	1.31			124	96		31			36	47	
14.5	Recovery		117	31	41.0	1.11	0.88	7.6	1.26			123	96		31			37	46	
15.0	Recovery		110	28	33.9	0.92	0.74	6.8	1.23			122	96		31			37	46	

Abbreviations: BP, blood pressure; BTPS, body temperature pressure saturated; f, frequency; HCO_3^-, bicarbonate; HR, heart rate; $P(A - a)O_2$, alveolar-arterial PO_2 difference; $P(a - ET)CO_2$, arterial–end-tidal PCO_2 difference; $PETCO_2$, end-tidal PCO_2; $PETO_2$, end-tidal PO_2; R, respiratory exchange ratio; SpO_2, oxygen saturation as measured by pulse oximetry; STPD, standard temperature pressure dry; $\dot{V}CO_2$, carbon dioxide output; V_D/V_T, physiological dead space–tidal volume ratio; $\dot{V}E$, minute ventilation; $\dot{V}E/\dot{V}CO_2$, ventilatory equivalent for carbon dioxide; $\dot{V}E/\dot{V}O_2$, ventilatory equivalent for oxygen; $\dot{V}O_2$, oxygen uptake.

the predicted normal range; these findings are consistent with β-blocker therapy. The shallow heart rate slope would also be consistent with cardiovascular fitness. The peak oxygen pulse had reached the normal predicted value at end exercise without having plateaued at the point when exercise ended, so it is not clear that the patient had attained the maximal possible levels of either heart rate or $C(a - \bar{v})O_2$ when exercise was terminated.

The breathing reserve was small, indicating that the patient was at or approaching his maximal ventilatory capacity.

Pulmonary gas exchange efficiency appeared normal, with normal SpO_2 and normal relationship of minute ventilation ($\dot{V}E$) to carbon dioxide output ($\dot{V}CO_2$).

Conclusion

Exercise ended when the patient reached the limits of his breathing capacity; however, this may have been at a $\dot{V}O_2$ lower than his true cardiovascular capacity. Furthermore, although the peak $\dot{V}O_2$ was in the normal range, it required a near maximal breathing effort to attain, which is not normal. Not directly measured was the work of breathing, which was likely higher than normal at any given level of ventilation due to both the higher percentage of maximum voluntary ventilation that it represented and the abnormal breathing mechanics associated with the diaphragm dysfunction.

CASE 77

McArdle Disease

CLINICAL FINDINGS

This 60-year-old elementary school teacher was referred for exercise testing by her pulmonologist for evaluation of long-standing exertional dyspnea of unclear cause. She recounted lifelong exercise intolerance to which she had adapted by taking a slow pace during prolonged activities and avoiding strenuous activities or performing them in a "stop and go" mode. As a girl, she hid her exercise intolerance in gym classes by stopping to tie her shoes frequently. She was able to be a cheerleader because each cheer lasted no longer than 3 minutes, which was within her tolerance. As an adult, she could walk at a slow pace for extended distances but inclines or increases in speed caused the abrupt onset of dyspnea and fatigue, which then resolved quickly with rest. She denied muscle pain or dark urine. One of the patient's brothers had a similar degree of exercise limitation due to muscle pain and rhabdomyolysis, which had been diagnosed as McArdle disease (muscle phosphorylase deficiency). A third sibling was healthy with no exercise limitation. Because she had no pain or pigmenturia, the patient had never equated her exercise intolerance to her brother's and had not mentioned this family history to her treating physicians. Her medications included hydrochlorothiazide and lisinopril for hypertension. Her physical examination was normal. Demographic and respiratory function data are shown in **Table 10.77.1**.

EXERCISE FINDINGS

Exercise testing was performed initially on a cycle ergometer. The patient ended this test with shortness of breath and leg fatigue after only a few minutes of incremental work but recovered promptly after several minutes of rest. In an attempt to obtain a longer test, testing was repeated with a treadmill walking protocol as a more familiar form of exercise. The patient initially walked at a self-selected pace of 1.7 mph and zero grade for 3 minutes, after which the grade was increased by 0.5% each minute. She was able to exercise for a little over 7 minutes on this test, which was stopped due to symptoms of leg fatigue and the patient's inability to keep up with the moving belt without handrail support.

Comments

Spirometry showed mild airflow obstruction. Results of the two exercise tests were qualitatively similar, but the treadmill test contained more data and is presented in **Figure 10.77.1** and **Tables 10.77.2** and **10.77.3**.

Analysis

Peak oxygen uptake ($\dot{V}O_2$) was low although heart rate increased to within the low end of the range of predicted maximum. There was no evidence of ventilatory limitation. There was an increase in carbon dioxide output ($\dot{V}CO_2$) relative to the increase in $\dot{V}O_2$ (panel 3) that may have been identified as the anaerobic threshold, but as discussed below, this is more likely due to acute hyperventilation.

TABLE 10.77.1 Selected Respiratory Function Data

Measurement	Predicted	Measured
Age (y)		60
Sex		Female
Height (cm)		166
Weight (kg)		63
VC (L)	3.49	3.00
IC (L)	2.29	2.38
FEV_1 (L)	2.7	2.07
FEV_1/VC (%)	78	69
MVV (L/min)	95	86

Abbreviations: FEV_1, forced expiratory volume in 1 second; IC, inspiratory capacity; MVV, maximum voluntary ventilation; VC, vital capacity.

TABLE 10.77.2 Selected Exercise Data

Measurement	Predicted	Measured
Peak $\dot{V}O_2$ (L/min)	1.48	0.91
Maximum heart rate (beats/min)	160	140
Maximum O_2 pulse(mL/beat)	9.3	7.6
$\Delta\dot{V}O_2/\Delta WR$ (mL/min/W)	10.3	NA
AT (L/min)	>0.79	Indeterminate
Blood pressure (mm Hg [rest, max ex])		124/85, 149/89
Maximum $\dot{V}E$ (L/min)		50
Exercise breathing reserve (L/min)	>15	36
$\dot{V}E/\dot{V}CO_2$ @ *AT* or lowest	29.4	36.2

Abbreviations: *AT*, anaerobic threshold; O_2, oxygen; $\dot{V}E$, minute ventilation; $\dot{V}E/\dot{V}CO_2$, ventilatory equivalent for CO_2; $\dot{V}O_2$, oxygen uptake; $\Delta\dot{V}O_2/\Delta WR$, change in $\dot{V}O_2$/change in work rate.

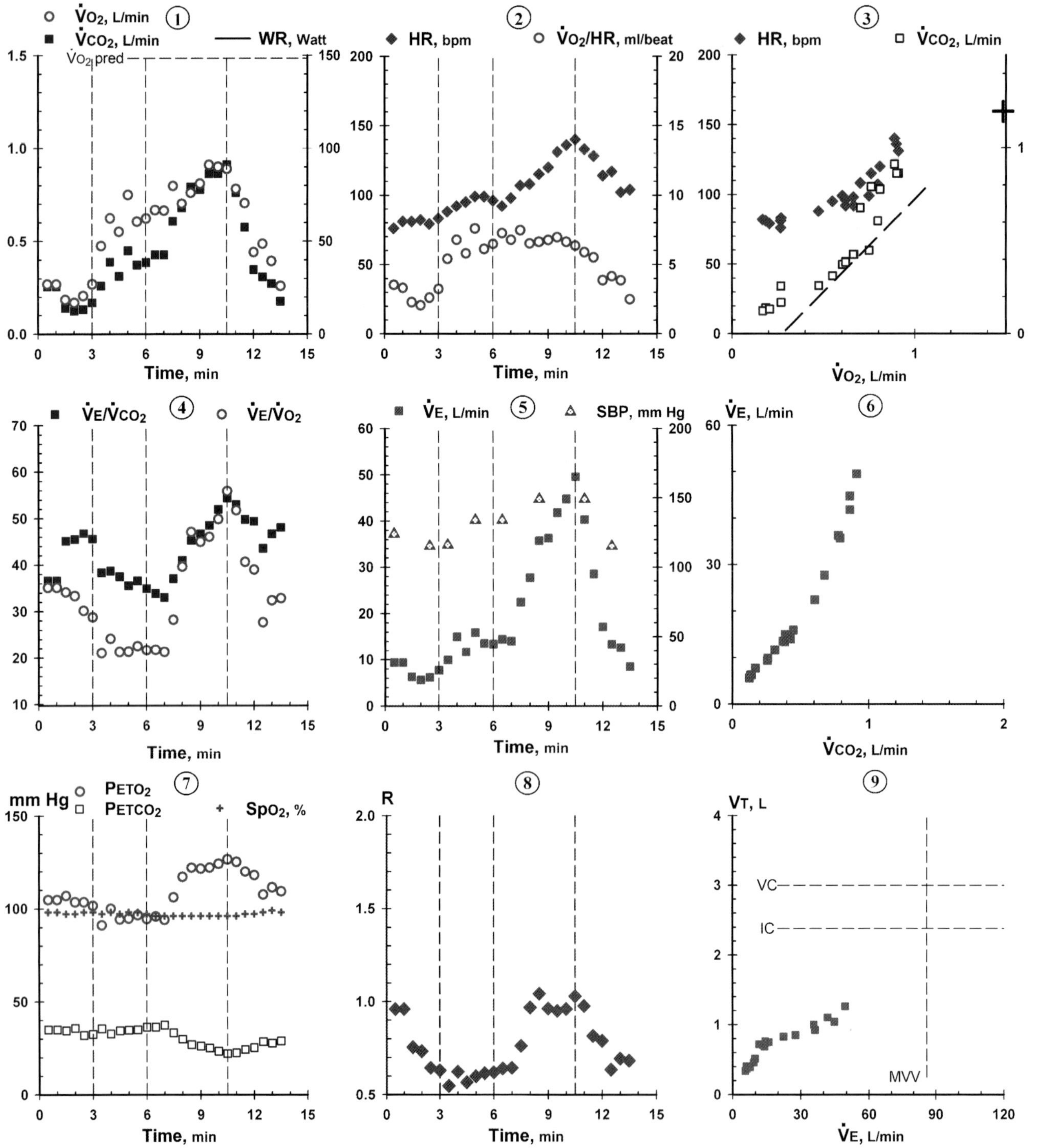

FIGURE 10.77.1. Vertical dashed lines in the panels in the left and middle columns indicate, from left to right, the beginning of treadmill walking at a speed of 1.7 mph at zero grade, the start of increasing grade by 0.5% per minute, and the start of recovery. In **panel 3**, carbon dioxide output ($\dot{V}CO_2$) (right y-axis) is plotted as a function of oxygen uptake ($\dot{V}O_2$) (x-axis) with identical scales so that the diagonal dashed line has a slope of 1 (45°). The $\dot{V}CO_2$ increasing more steeply than $\dot{V}O_2$ defines carbon dioxide (CO_2) derived from bicarbonate buffer, as long as ventilatory equivalent for CO_2 ($\dot{V}E/\dot{V}CO_2$) (**panel 4**) is not increasing and end-tidal PCO_2 ($PETCO_2$) (**panel 7**) is not decreasing, simultaneously. The black + symbol in **panel 3** indicates predicted peak values of heart rate (HR) (left y-axis) and $\dot{V}O_2$ for this individual. Abbreviations: IC, inspiratory capacity; MVV, maximum voluntary ventilation; $PETO_2$, end-tidal PO_2; R, respiratory exchange ratio; SBP, systolic blood pressure; SpO_2, oxygen saturation as measured by pulse oximetry; VC, vital capacity; $\dot{V}E$, minute ventilation; $\dot{V}E/\dot{V}O_2$, ventilatory equivalent for oxygen; V_T, tidal volume; WR, work rate.

TABLE 10.77.3 Air Breathing

Time (min)	Treadmill grade (%)*	BP (mm Hg)	HR (min^{-1})	f (min^{-1})	$\dot{V}E$ (L/min BTPS)	$\dot{V}CO_2$ (L/min STPD)	$\dot{V}O_2$ (L/min STPD)	$\frac{\dot{V}O_2}{HR}$ (mL/beat)	R	pH	HCO_3^- (mEq/L)	PO_2, mm Hg ET	a	(A − a)	PCO_2, mm Hg ET	a	(a − ET)	$\frac{\dot{V}E}{\dot{V}CO_2}$	$\frac{\dot{V}E}{\dot{V}O_2}$	$\frac{V_D}{V_T}$
0.5	Rest	124/85	76	20	9.4	0.26	0.27	3.5	0.96			105			35			37	35	
1.0	Rest		81	20	9.4	0.26	0.27	3.3	0.96			105			35			37	35	
1.5	Rest		81	17	6.3	0.14	0.18	2.3	0.76			107			34			45	34	
2.0	Rest		82	17	5.6	0.12	0.17	2.0	0.73			103			36			45	33	
2.5	Rest	115/77	79	15	6.2	0.13	0.21	2.6	0.64			103			32			47	30	
3.0	Rest		83	20	7.7	0.17	0.27	3.2	0.63			102			32			46	29	
3.5	0	116/76	88	19	9.9	0.26	0.47	5.4	0.55			91			35			38	21	
4.0	0		92	20	15.0	0.39	0.62	6.8	0.62			100			33			39	24	
4.5	0		95	16	11.7	0.31	0.55	5.8	0.57			94			34			37	21	
5.0	0	134/89	99	21	15.9	0.45	0.75	7.6	0.60			95			35			36	21	
5.5	0		99	19	13.6	0.37	0.60	6.1	0.62			97			35			37	22	
6.0	0		96	19	13.4	0.38	0.62	6.5	0.62			94			36			35	22	
6.5	0.5	134/89	92	19	14.4	0.43	0.67	7.2	0.64			96			36			34	22	
7.0	0.5		98	20	14.1	0.43	0.66	6.8	0.64			94			37			33	21	
7.5	1.0		107	27	22.4	0.61	0.80	7.4	0.76			106			33			37	28	
8.0	1.0		108	33	27.7	0.68	0.70	6.5	0.97			117			30			41	40	
8.5	1.5	149/89	115	36	35.7	0.79	0.76	6.6	1.04			122			27			45	47	
9.0	1.5		120	39	36.3	0.78	0.81	6.7	0.96			121			26			47	45	
9.5	2.0		131	38	41.8	0.86	0.91	6.9	0.95			122			25			49	46	
10.0	2.0		136	43	44.8	0.86	0.90	6.6	0.96			124			23			52	50	
10.5	2.5		140	39	49.5	0.91	0.89	6.3	1.03			127			22			54	56	
11.0	2.5		133	34	40.3	0.76	0.78	5.9	0.98			125			22			53	52	
11.5	Recovery		128	27	28.5	0.57	0.70	5.5	0.82			120			24			50	41	
12.0	Recovery		114	24	17.1	0.35	0.44	3.9	0.79			118			25			49	39	
12.5	Recovery	115/79	117	18	13.4	0.31	0.48	4.1	0.63			108			28			44	28	
13.0	Recovery		102	22	12.6	0.27	0.39	3.8	0.69			111			28			47	32	
13.5	Recovery		104	19	8.5	0.18	0.26	2.5	0.68			109			29			48	33	

*Throughout the exercise period treadmill speed was 1.7 mph.

Abbreviations: BP, blood pressure; BTPS, body temperature pressure saturated; f, frequency; HCO_3^-, bicarbonate; HR, heart rate; $P(A - a)O_2$, alveolar-arterial PO_2 difference; $P(a - ET)CO_2$, arterial-end-tidal PCO_2 difference; $PETCO_2$, end-tidal PCO_2; $PETO_2$, end-tidal PO_2; R, respiratory exchange ratio; STPD, standard temperature pressure dry; [illegible] physiological dead space–tidal volume ratio; $\dot{V}E$, minute ventilation; $\dot{V}E/\dot{V}CO_2$, ventilatory equivalent for carbon dioxide; $\dot{V}E/\dot{V}O_2$, ventilatory equivalent for oxygen; $\dot{V}O_2$, oxygen uptake.

The most unique finding on this test is the relationship of $\dot{V}O_2$ and $\dot{V}CO_2$. The initial 3 minutes of walking at 1.7 mph was associated with an increase of $\dot{V}O_2$ to around 650 mL per minute and with subsequent increase in grade, $\dot{V}O_2$ increased to a peak value that was around 60% of the predicted maximum value. Looking at panel 3 of **Figure 10.77.1**, there is a sharp break point in the V slope at a $\dot{V}O_2$ of 0.80 L per minute, at which $\dot{V}CO_2$ increases abruptly to 0.9 L per minute. Although this might appear to represent the anaerobic threshold, review of other plots show that this break point corresponds to the abrupt onset of hyperventilation. The slope of the increase of $\dot{V}CO_2$ relative to $\dot{V}O_2$ prior to this break point was 0.7, suggesting that fat was the predominant substrate of the exercising muscle early in the test. (This was also true during the cycle test.) This is in marked contrast to the usual finding that during a short-duration exercise test, the slope of $\dot{V}CO_2$ versus $\dot{V}O_2$ below the anaerobic threshold is around 1.0, reflecting carbohydrates as the preferred muscle substrate. Consistent with this, the patient's respiratory exchange ratio (R) value at rest during the 2 minutes prior to exercise was around 0.7, and it remained at this low level through the first 4 minutes of exercise. At the end of the test, the R value decreased back to the resting level within 1 or 2 minutes. This, too, is unusual, as R normally increases in recovery. (Note: Caution is warranted in the interpretation of the exercise R values. The R value reflects substrate mix under steady state conditions but is affected by numerous factors under the nonsteady state conditions of an exercise test. A period of hyperventilation preceding the test, eg, could also result in a low R value as carbon dioxide stores are reestablished [see Case 12 of this chapter for discussion]. In this case, the findings related to R have been interpreted in the context of the other exercise responses and the clinical and family history.)

At minute 7, as has been alluded to, when the treadmill grade was increased from 0.5% to 1.0%, there was an abrupt increase in ventilation with a marked decrease in end-tidal P_{CO_2}, and increases in end-tidal P_{O_2}, ventilatory equivalents, and R (see **Fig. 10.77.1**, panels 5, 7, 4, and 8, respectively). The coincident and abrupt increase in $\dot{V}_{CO_2}$ with very little increase in $\dot{V}_{O_2}$ on the V-slope plot is atypical and supports the impression of acute hyperventilation. Soon after the onset of incremental work, there was a steepening of the heart rate relative to $\dot{V}_{O_2}$ (see **Fig. 10.77.1**, panel 3) associated with an unchanging oxygen pulse, which remained below the predicted maximal value. This implies either a low exercise stroke volume or inability to widen $C(a - \bar{v})_{O_2}$.

Many features of this test, including hyperventilation, are quite nonspecific. However, the shallow slope of $\dot{V}_{CO_2}$ relative to $\dot{V}_{O_2}$ and the failure to demonstrate an anaerobic threshold are uniquely suggestive of the condition pointed to by her family history. McArdle disease results from a deficiency of skeletal muscle phosphorylase, which prevents utilization of glycogen as a substrate. Exercising muscle is thus dependent on fatty acids and circulating glucose as substrate for energy production. Because of the limited carbohydrate metabolism, little or no lactic acid is produced, which is consistent with the failure to identify a clear anaerobic threshold in this case. It has also been suggested that the low peak $\dot{V}_{O_2}$ in this condition results from a lack of local acidification of the muscle by lactic acid, resulting in failure to shift the oxyhemoglobin curve to the right to facilitate oxygen unloading (Bohr effect). This would limit $C(a - \bar{v})_{O_2}$, which can account for the low oxygen pulse of this patient. The steep increase in heart rate relative to $\dot{V}_{O_2}$ is characteristic in McArdle disease and reflects a hyperdynamic circulatory response. If cardiac output had been measured, the slope of cardiac output relative to $\dot{V}_{O_2}$ would be steeper than normal. Exercise hyperventilation, such as occurred in this case, is not uncommon in McArdle disease, but the basis for it is not well defined.

Conclusion

This patient's successful adaptation of exercise behavior to fit her limited capabilities delayed identification of a heritable muscle disease despite her family history. Her exercise responses reflected the metabolic consequences of this condition, although the occurrence of hyperventilation could easily distract one from the key findings.

CASE 78

Myopathy With Exertional Rhabdomyolysis

CLINICAL FINDINGS

This 53-year-old man was referred for exercise testing to characterize his impairment due to an unspecified myopathy. He was normally active as a child and young adult. In his early 30s, he had consulted a rheumatologist for vague muscle symptoms, but no specific diagnosis was made. At age 47 years, he had an episode of rhabdomyolysis complicated by acute renal failure after a day of river rafting and over the next 5 years had several more documented episodes of rhabdomyolysis. Laboratory evaluation, including electrolytes, thyroid function tests, and autoimmune studies, had been normal, and electromyography showed nonspecific abnormalities. At the time of testing, he reported easy fatigability and delayed muscle soreness after modest levels of exertion. He worked part-time as a nurse and did minimal exercise. Medical history included hypertension and prior back surgeries with residual chronic pain. He had undergone general anesthesia without adverse reactions. His family history was not contributory. His medications included metoprolol, lisinopril, and methadone. Examination demonstrated a normal body habitus without obvious skeletal muscle hypertrophy or wasting. The resting electrocardiogram was normal.

A muscle biopsy had been performed several years prior to this test, and the patient was screened for the most commonly recognized enzyme deficiencies associated with rhabdomyolysis. The report indicated no specific structural abnormalities and normal staining for phosphorylase a and b, myoadenylate deaminase, [illegible] phosphoglycerate mutase, lactate dehydrogenase, and carnitine palmitoyltransferase. The basis of his myopathy, therefore, was not defined. Selected demographic data are shown in **Table 10.78.1**.

TABLE 10.78.1 Selected Demographic Data

Measurement	Predicted	Measured
Age (y)		53
Sex		Male
Height (cm)		181
Weight (kg)		86
Hematocrit (%)		43

EXERCISE FINDINGS

The patient performed exercise on a cycle ergometer. After 3 minutes of rest, he pedaled at 60 rpm as work rate was increased by 20 W/min. He stopped exercise due to shortness of breath and "burning" in his leg muscles. There were no significant electrocardiogram changes. Exercise data are summarized in **Tables 10.78.2** and **10.78.3** and in **Figure 10.78.1**.

Comments

Pulmonary function tests were not available.

Analysis

The test appears to reflect good effort based on the high peak heart rate and end-exercise respiratory exchange ratio value of close to 1.4, indicating substantial carbon dioxide (CO_2) from buffering of lactic acid. Oxygen uptake ($\dot{V}O_2$) increased appropriately with work rate, but peak $\dot{V}O_2$ and anaerobic threshold were both low. The increase in heart rate was steep relative to $\dot{V}O_2$. The oxygen pulse increased during the first few minutes of exercise but failed to increase further and remained lower than the predicted maximum for the remainder of the test. These findings are consistent with either impairment in oxygen delivery (low stroke vol-

TABLE 10.78.2 Selected Exercise Data

Measurement	Predicted	Measured
Peak $\dot{V}O_2$ (L/min)	2.57	1.64
Maximum heart rate (beats/min)	167	150
Maximum O_2 pulse (mL/beat)	15.4	11.2
$\Delta\dot{V}O_2/\Delta WR$ (mL/min/W)	10.3	10.0
AT (L/min)	>1.16	0.89
Blood pressure (mm Hg [rest, max])		148/79, 198/89
Maximum $\dot{V}E$ (L/min)		63
$\dot{V}E/\dot{V}CO_2$ @ *AT* or lowest	27.0	24.9

Abbreviations: *AT*, anaerobic threshold; $\Delta\dot{V}O_2/\Delta WR$, change in $\dot{V}O_2$/change in work rate; O_2, oxygen; $\dot{V}E$, minute ventilation; $\dot{V}E/\dot{V}CO_2$, ventilatory equivalent for CO_2; $\dot{V}O_2$, oxygen uptake.

TABLE 10.78.3 Air Breathing

Time (min)	Work rate (W)	BP (mm Hg)	HR (min^{-1})	f (min^{-1})	$\dot{V}E$ (L/min BTPS)	$\dot{V}CO_2$ (L/min STPD)	$\dot{V}O_2$ (L/min STPD)	$\frac{\dot{V}O_2}{HR}$ (mL/beat)	R	pH	HCO_3^- (mEq/L)	PO_2, mm Hg ET	PO_2, mm Hg a	PO_2, mm Hg (A − a)	PCO_2, mm Hg ET	PCO_2, mm Hg a	PCO_2, mm Hg (a − ET)	$\frac{\dot{V}E}{\dot{V}CO_2}$	$\frac{\dot{V}E}{\dot{V}O_2}$	$\frac{V_D}{V_T}$
0																				
0.5	Rest	148/79	66	12	8.2	0.26	0.32	4.8	0.82			96			46			31	26	
1.0	Rest		76	10	8.7	0.28	0.31	4.1	0.88			99			45			32	28	
1.5	Rest		69	11	6.7	0.22	0.26	3.8	0.84			96			48			30	25	
2.0	Rest		71	12	10.2	0.38	0.43	6.1	0.87			97			47			27	24	
2.5	Rest		70	12	7.4	0.24	0.25	3.6	0.97			103			46			31	30	
3.0	Rest		69	10	6.5	0.20	0.21	3.1	0.93			101			46			33	30	
3.5	20		82	16	15.5	0.57	0.62	7.5	0.93			100			46			27	25	
4.0	20		79	14	12.9	0.49	0.54	6.9	0.90			97			47			26	24	
4.5	39		81	14	20.2	0.74	0.79	9.7	0.93			100			45			27	26	
5.0	39		83	16	18.3	0.72	0.80	9.6	0.90			95			49			25	23	
5.5	59		87	17	20.6	0.83	0.89	10.3	0.93			97			48			25	23	
6.0	59		94	14	22.7	0.95	0.96	10.2	0.99			97			50			24	24	
6.5	78		99	17	27.4	1.12	1.11	11.2	1.01			100			49			24	25	
7.0	78		104	18	30.4	1.24	1.17	11.2	1.07			102			48			25	26	
7.5	97		119	16	33.5	1.40	1.25	10.5	1.12			102			49			24	27	
8.0	97		125	19	39.5	1.59	1.38	11.0	1.15			104			48			25	29	
8.5	117	198/89	136	21	46.2	1.78	1.47	10.8	1.21			108			45			26	32	
9.0	117		145	21	51.7	1.96	1.57	10.8	1.25			110			44			26	33	
9.5	117		150	26	62.9	2.19	1.64	10.9	1.34			115			40			29	38	
10.0	Recovery		142	24	55.2	1.87	1.31	9.2	1.43			118			39			30	42	
10.5	Recovery	136/87	133	22	38.9	1.33	0.94	7.0	1.42			118			40			29	42	
11.0	Recovery		120	19	28.2	0.99	0.76	6.3	1.31			115			41			28	37	
11.4	Recovery		109	17	20.3	0.68	0.53	4.8	1.30			115			41			30	39	

Abbreviations: BP, blood pressure; BTPS, body temperature pressure saturated; f, frequency; HCO_3^-, bicarbonate; HR, heart rate; P(A − a)O_2, alveolar-arterial PO_2 difference; P(a − ET)CO_2, arterial-end-tidal PCO_2 difference; $PETCO_2$, end-tidal PCO_2; $PETO_2$, end-tidal PO_2; R, respiratory exchange ratio; STPD, standard temperature pressure dry; $\dot{V}CO_2$, carbon dioxide output; V_D/V_T, physiological dead space-tidal volume ratio; $\dot{V}E$, minute ventilation; $\dot{V}E/\dot{V}CO_2$, ventilatory equivalent for carbon dioxide; $\dot{V}E/\dot{V}O_2$, ventilatory equivalent for oxygen; $\dot{V}O_2$, oxygen uptake.

ume) or impaired oxygen extraction at the muscle level [low $C(a - \bar{v})O_2$]. The latter explanation is most consistent with the clinical history. Reduction in the capacity for oxidation of substrate in the muscle with early lactic acidosis, as occurred in this patient, would be associated with an abnormally low $C(a - \bar{v})O_2$, reflecting failure to utilize and extract oxygen normally in the muscle. This would be consistent with impaired mitochondrial oxidative metabolism. A hyperdynamic circulatory response, suggested by the heart rate pattern, is characteristic of defects in skeletal muscle oxidation. The test showed typical gas exchange changes associated with lactic acidosis, making McArdle disease (myophosphorylase deficiency) unlikely.

Conclusion

Although a specific metabolic defect was not identified on this patient's muscle biopsy, the exercise findings are suggestive of a deficiency in mitochondrial oxidative metabolism.

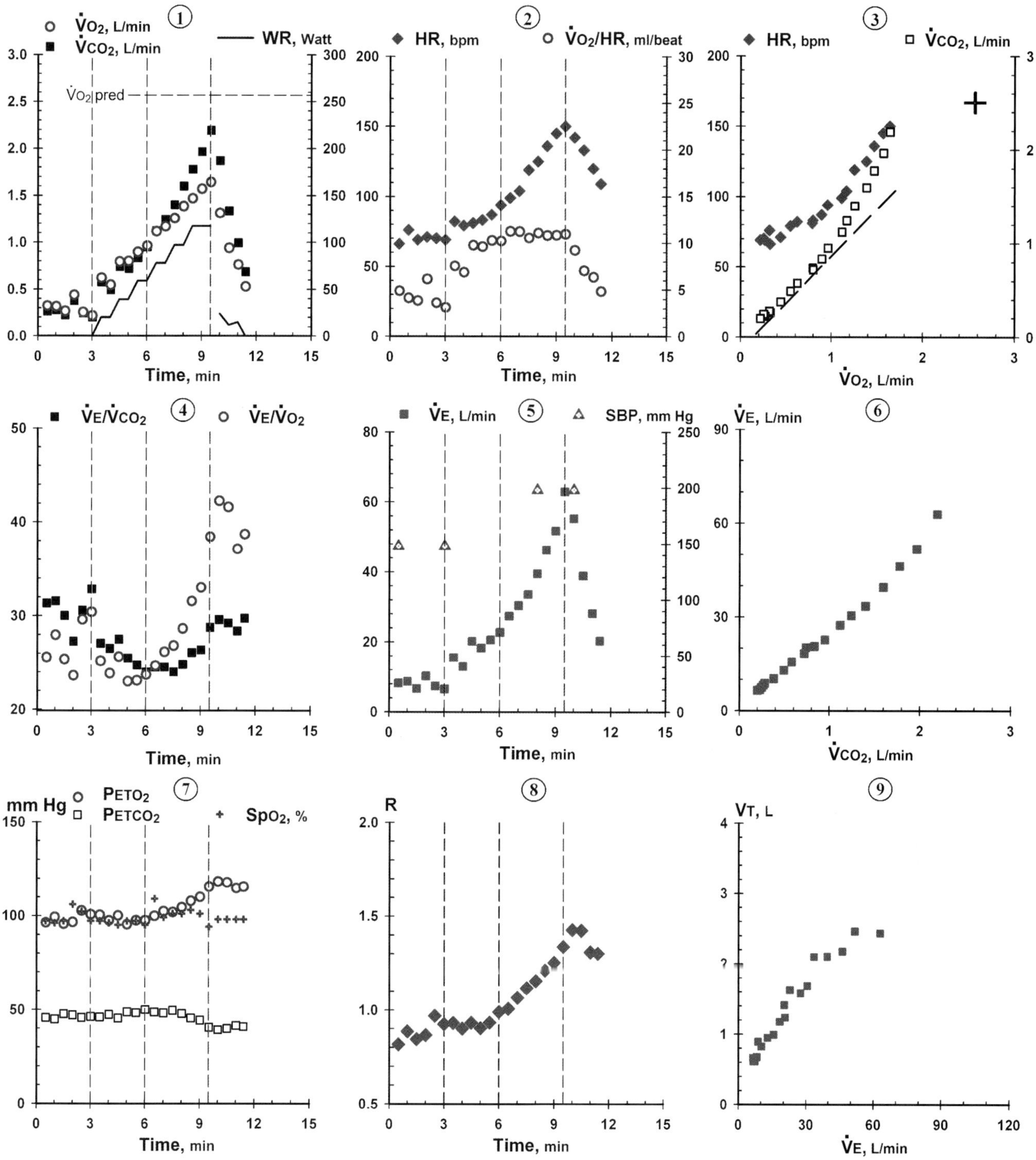

FIGURE 10.78.1. Vertical dashed lines in the panels in the left and middle columns indicate, from left to right, the beginning of exercise with increasing work rate (WR) at 20 W/min, and the start of recovery. In **panel 1**, the increase in WR (right y-axis) is plotted with a scale of 100 W to 1 L of oxygen uptake ($\dot{V}O_2$) (left y-axis) such that WR is plotted parallel to a $\dot{V}O_2$ slope of 10 mL/min/W. In **panel 3**, carbon dioxide output ($\dot{V}CO_2$) (right y-axis) is plotted as a function of $\dot{V}O_2$ (x-axis) with identical scales so that the diagonal dashed line has a slope of 1 (45°). The $\dot{V}CO_2$ increasing more steeply than $\dot{V}O_2$ defines carbon dioxide (CO_2) derived from bicarbonate buffer, as long as ventilatory equivalent for CO_2 ($\dot{V}E/\dot{V}CO_2$) (**panel 4**) is not increasing and partial pressure of CO_2 in end-tidal gas ($PETCO_2$) (**panel 7**) is not decreasing, simultaneously. The black + symbol in **panel 3** indicates predicted peak values of heart rate (HR) (left y-axis) and $\dot{V}O_2$ for this individual. Abbreviations: $PETCO_2$, partial pressure of CO_2 in end-tidal gas; $PETO_2$, end-tidal partial pressure of oxygen; R, respiratory exchange ratio; SBP, systolic blood pressure; SpO_2, oxygen saturation by pulse oximetry; $\dot{V}CO_2$, carbon dioxide output; $\dot{V}E$, minute ventilation; $\dot{V}E/\dot{V}CO_2$, ventilatory equivalent for CO_2; $\dot{V}E/\dot{V}O_2$, ventilatory equivalent for oxygen; $\dot{V}O_2$/HR, O_2 uptake per heart beat or O_2 pulse; VT, tidal volume.

CASE 79

Congenital Mitochondrial Myopathy

CLINICAL FINDINGS

This 37-year-old man was referred for exercise testing to quantify the functional effects of his recently identified mitochondrial myopathy. A mitochondrial DNA mutation had been identified in his sister, leading to testing of the patient. The abnormality was a point mutation (base pair m3302 A>G), affecting a gene that codes for a transfer RNA, resulting in a defect in the function of complex I of the electron transport chain. The patient reported being normally active as a child and initially denied any functional impairment. However, he admitted to having diffuse muscle pain and stiffness, along with generalized fatigue, at the end of a day working as a busboy in a restaurant. On several occasions this was severe enough to require assistance to stand and walk. He was characterized as having mild cognitive impairment but denied other features associated with mitochondrial mutation syndromes such as seizures, stroke, diabetes, or hearing or visual problems. An echocardiogram had shown mild left ventricular hypertrophy with normal systolic function. He was taking no medications. On examination, he was normally developed but had low muscle bulk. Heart and lung examination were unremarkable. The resting electrocardiogram (ECG) showed findings consistent with left ventricular hypertrophy. Demographic and respiratory function data are shown in **Table 10.79.1**.

EXERCISE FINDINGS

Exercise testing was performed on a cycle ergometer beginning with 3 minutes of cycling at 60 rpm without added load, followed by a continuous increase in work rate by 15 W/min. The patient had difficulty adjusting to breathing through the mouthpiece, and the test was interrupted briefly at the end of the unloaded cycling period to adjust the breathing apparatus. With some encouragement, he was able to complete the test and ended exercise with leg fatigue as his sole symptom. There were no significant ECG changes. Exercise data are summarized in **Tables 10.79.2** and **10.79.3** and in **Figure 10.79.1**.

Comments

Pulmonary function testing showed moderate lung restriction without evidence of airflow obstruction. The diffusing capacity of the lung for carbon monoxide was also mildly reduced, but when indexed to alveolar volume, it was within normal limits.

Analysis

Although the patient initially had some difficulty with test procedures, he clearly achieved high intensity exercise and reached an respiratory exchange ratio of 1.2 and a heart rate of 156 beats/min at end exercise, indicating that this test represents at least a near-maximal effort. Peak oxygen uptake ($\dot{V}O_2$), anaerobic threshold, and change in $\dot{V}O_2$/change in work rate

TABLE 10.79.1 Selected Respiratory Function Data

Measurement	Predicted	Measured
Age (y)		37
Sex		Male
Height (cm)		165
Weight (kg)		57
VC (L)	3.82	3.10
TLC (L)	6.26	4.57
FEV_1 (L)	3.17	2.96
FEV_1/VC (%)	82	95
MVV (L/min)	127	118
D_{LCO} (mL/mm Hg/min)	25.5	15.8

Abbreviations: D_{LCO}, diffusing capacity of the lung for carbon monoxide; FEV_1, forced expiratory volume in 1 second; MVV, maximum voluntary ventilation; VC, vital capacity; TLC, total lung capacity.

TABLE 10.79.2 Selected Exercise Data

Measurement	Predicted	Measured
Peak $\dot{V}O_2$ (L/min)	2.33	0.78
Maximum heart rate (beats/min)	183	156
Maximum O_2 pulse (mL/beat)	12.7	5.0
$\Delta\dot{V}O_2/\Delta WR$ (mL/min/W)	10.3	6.2
AT (L/min)	>1.02	0.60
Blood pressure (mm Hg [rest, max])		110/76, 172/108
Maximum $\dot{V}E$ (L/min)		32
Exercise breathing reserve (L/min)	>15	76
$\dot{V}E/\dot{V}CO_2$ @ *AT* or lowest	26.0	32.5

Abbreviations: *AT*, anaerobic threshold; $\Delta\dot{V}O_2/\Delta WR$, change in $\dot{V}O_2$/change in work rate; O_2, oxygen; $\dot{V}E$, minute ventilation; $\dot{V}E/\dot{V}CO_2$, ventilatory equivalent for carbon dioxide; $\dot{V}O_2$, oxygen uptake.

($\Delta\dot{V}O_2/\Delta WR$) slope were all lower than normal. Oxygen (O_2) pulse was low and remained flat over the period of incremental work with a low peak value. Consistent with this, heart rate increased steeply relative to $\dot{V}O_2$ (see **Fig. 10.79.1**, panel 3). These findings indicate impairment in oxygen delivery and/or utilization. Cardiac involvement by his mitochondrial disorder had been postulated due to the presence of left ventricular hypertrophy, but as there were no clinical or echocardiographic findings to suggest heart failure, it seemed likely that impairment in peripheral muscle oxygen utilization was the dominant cause of O_2 flow impairment. Indeed, the ventricular hypertrophy could have resulted from a chronic hyperdynamic state due to the peripheral muscle dysfunction. There also were no significant ECG changes with exercise.

With respect to the ventilatory response to exercise, there was an adequate breathing reserve and no evidence of arterial desaturation. The ventilatory equivalents are at the upper limit of normal, raising the possibility of pulmonary $\dot{V}/\dot{Q}$ mismatch. On review of panels 4 and 7, however, it appears that ventilatory equivalent for oxygen ($\dot{V}E/\dot{V}O_2$) and end-tidal partial pressure of oxygen (P_{ETO_2}) both began to increase systematically as soon as unloaded cycling began, suggesting that lactate was accumulating at the lowest level of exercise and that the high ventilatory equivalents simply result from the test being entirely above the lactate "threshold."

Conclusion

This case is presented as an illustration of findings of abnormal oxygen uptake in a patient with a mitochondrial myopathy. It is also a reminder that a low O_2 pulse is not synonymous with low stroke volume, as impaired O_2 uptake by the exercising muscles also results in a low O_2 pulse.

TABLE 10.79.3 Air Breathing

Time (min)	Work rate (W)	BP (mm Hg)	HR (min^{-1})	f (min^{-1})	$\dot{V}E$ (L/min BTPS)	$\dot{V}CO_2$ (L/min STPD)	$\dot{V}O_2$ (L/min STPD)	$\dot{V}O_2$/HR (mL/beat)	R	pH	HCO_3^- (mEq/L)	PO_2, mm Hg ET	PO_2 a	PO_2 (A − a)	PCO_2, mm Hg ET	PCO_2 a	PCO_2 (a − ET)	$\dot{V}E/\dot{V}CO_2$	$\dot{V}E/\dot{V}O_2$	VD/VT
0.5	Rest	110/76	81	15	8.7	0.26	0.39	4.9	0.64			91			41			34	22	
1.0	Rest		80	20	7.9	0.18	0.28	3.6	0.65			92			40			43	28	
1.5	Rest	132/91	76	15	6.1	0.15	0.22	2.8	0.68			95			40			41	28	
2.0	Rest		80	18	8.6	0.22	0.32	4.0	0.70			95			41			39	27	
2.5	Rest		84	20	7.8	0.18	0.25	3.0	0.69			93			42			45	31	
3.0	Rest		84	21	9.1	0.21	0.28	3.3	0.75			97			41			44	33	
3.5	Unloaded		104	23	12.8	0.37	0.47	4.5	0.79			97			43			35	27	
4.0	Unloaded		99	17	11.8	0.36	0.42	4.2	0.86			101			42			33	28	
4.5	Unloaded		102	13	8.8	0.28	0.31	3.1	0.88			102			43			32	28	
5.0	Unloaded		107	24	13.0	0.37	0.42	3.9	0.87			101			42			35	31	
5.5	Unloaded		113	28	14.7	0.41	0.44	3.9	0.94			104			41			36	34	
6.0	Unloaded	164/98	107	24	12.9	0.37	0.36	3.4	1.04			107			41			35	36	
6.5	2		119	17	14.7	0.45	0.48	4.0	0.93			108			39			33	30	
7.0	9		125	22	18.3	0.56	0.59	4.7	0.95			108			39			33	31	
7.5	17		123	22	16.0	0.48	0.55	4.4	0.88			105			[illegible]			33	29	
8.0	24		125	23	17.5	0.52	0.56	4.5	0.93			108			38			34	31	
8.5	32		133	27	19.0	0.57	0.60	4.5	0.95			108			39			33	32	
9.0	39		137	29	22.2	0.67	0.66	4.8	1.02			110			39			33	34	
9.5	46		145	27	24.6	0.77	0.70	4.8	1.09			113			39			32	35	
10.0	54		151	33	27.2	0.83	0.76	5.0	1.09			113			38			33	36	
10.5	61	172/108	154	36	24.7	0.72	0.62	4.0	1.17			115			37			34	40	
11.0	68		156	35	32.4	0.94	0.78	5.0	1.21			118			35			34	42	
11.5	Recovery		148	37	28.8	0.82	0.68	4.6	1.20			118			35			35	42	
12.0	Recovery	138/89	141	35	22.0	0.63	0.57	4.1	1.09			115			37			35	38	
12.5	Recovery		138	29	23.6	0.68	0.58	4.2	1.17			117			35			35	41	
13.0	Recovery		135	32	22.7	0.64	0.62	4.6	1.02			113			36			36	36	
13.5	Recovery		132	31	20.0	0.56	0.56	4.2	1.01			112			37			36	36	
14.0	Recovery		135	31	22.5	0.64	0.64	4.7	1.00			113			36			35	35	

Abbreviations: BP, blood pressure; BTPS, body temperature pressure saturated; f, frequency; HCO_3^-, bicarbonate; HR, heart rate; $P(A-a)O_2$, alveolar-arterial PO_2 difference; $P(a-ET)CO_2$, arterial-end-tidal PCO_2 difference; P_{ETCO_2}, end-tidal PCO_2; P_{ETO_2}, end-tidal PO_2; R, respiratory exchange ratio; STPD, standard temperature pressure dry; $\dot{V}CO_2$, carbon dioxide output; VD/VT, physiological dead space-tidal volume ratio; $\dot{V}E$, minute ventilation; $\dot{V}E/\dot{V}CO_2$, ventilatory equivalent for carbon dioxide; $\dot{V}E/\dot{V}O_2$, ventilatory equivalent for oxygen; $\dot{V}O_2$, oxygen uptake; $\dot{V}O_2$/HR, oxygen pulse in mL/beat.

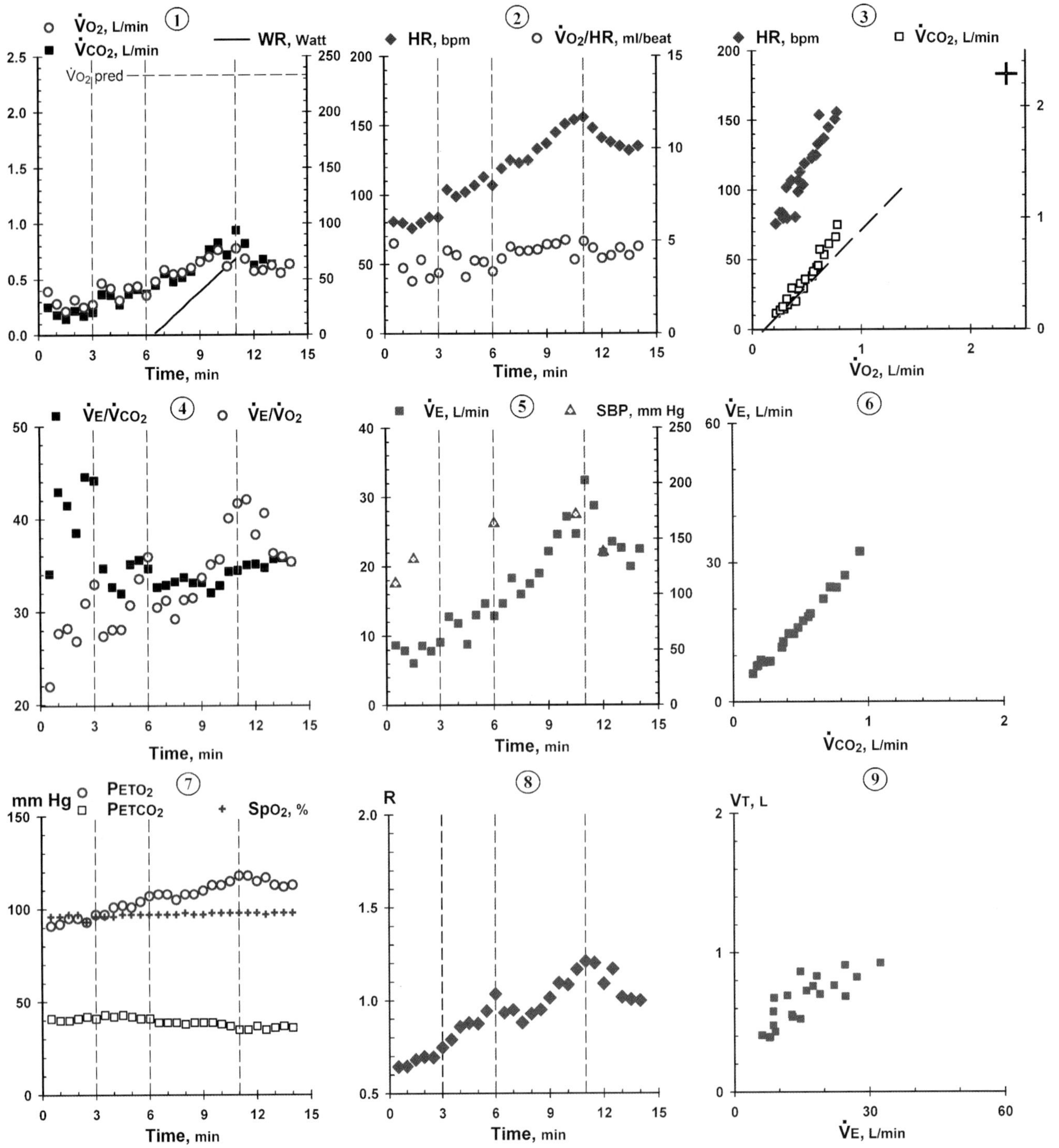

FIGURE 10.79.1. Vertical dashed lines in the panels in the left and middle columns indicate, from left to right, the beginning of unloaded cycling, start of increasing work rate (WR) at 15 W/min, and start of recovery. In **panel 1**, the increase in WR (right y-axis) is plotted with a scale of 100 W to 1 L of oxygen uptake ($\dot{V}O_2$) (left y-axis) such that WR is plotted parallel to a $\dot{V}O_2$ slope of 10 mL/min/W. In **panel 3**, carbon dioxide output ($\dot{V}CO_2$) (right y-axis) is plotted as a function of $\dot{V}O_2$ (x-axis) with identical scales so that the diagonal dashed line has a slope of 1 (45°). The $\dot{V}CO_2$ increasing more steeply than $\dot{V}O_2$ defines carbon dioxide (CO_2) derived from bicarbonate buffer, as long as ventilatory equivalent for carbon dioxide ($\dot{V}E/\dot{V}CO_2$) (**panel 4**) is not increasing and end-tidal P_{CO_2} (P_{ETCO_2}) (**panel 7**) is not decreasing, simultaneously. The black + symbol in **panel 3** indicates predicted peak values of heart rate (HR) (left y-axis) and $\dot{V}O_2$ for this individual. Abbreviations: IC, inspiratory capacity; MVV, maximum voluntary ventilation; P_{ETO_2}, end-tidal partial pressure of oxygen; R, respiratory exchange ratio; SBP, systolic blood pressure; Sp_{O_2}, oxygen saturation by pulse oximetry; VC, vital capacity; $\dot{V}E$, minute ventilation; $\dot{V}E/\dot{V}O_2$, ventilatory equivalent for oxygen; V_T, tidal volume.

CASE 80

Mitochondrial Myopathy

CLINICAL FINDINGS

This 52-year-old woman was referred for testing because of progressive exercise intolerance over many years. She had been athletic through young adulthood, but in her mid-30s, she began to experience the abrupt onset of severe fatigue and weakness with heavy exertion, especially swimming. At one time, she was suspected of having hypokalemic periodic paralysis (a defect in muscle potassium channels), but this diagnosis was excluded. Her activity tolerance progressively decreased, and at the time of referral, she reported fatigue, dyspnea, and weakness on ascending a flight of stairs or walking in a store. No family members had similar problems. An echocardiogram showed normal cardiac structure and function. Cardiac catheterization had shown normal coronary arteries. Her history was otherwise notable for several episodes of transient ischemic events or strokes in her 40s with minimal neurologic residua. She had a curative resection of a bronchoalveolar cell lung cancer and remote optic nerve tumor. Examination was notable only for a thin body habitus.

EXERCISE FINDINGS

Exercise was performed on a cycle ergometer. After cycling at 60 rpm for 3 minutes without added load, work rate was increased continuously by 10 W/min to her maximal tolerance. She ended exercise with symptoms of leg weakness and an inability to maintain the pedaling cadence, along with generalized weakness and shortness of breath. She required assistance in dismounting the ergometer and 10 minutes of seated recovery before she felt able to stand independently. Demographic and respiratory function data are shown in **Table 10.80.1**.

TABLE 10.80.1 Selected Respiratory Function Data

Measurement	Predicted	Measured
Age (y)		52
Sex		Female
Height (cm)		178
Weight (kg)		64
VC (L)	4.31	4.27
IC (L)	2.59	2.02
FEV_1 (L)	3.39	2.98
FEV_1/VC (%)	80	70
MVV (L/min)	109	102

Abbreviations: FEV_1, forced expiratory volume in 1 second; IC, inspiratory capacity; MVV, maximum voluntary ventilation; VC, vital capacity.

Comment

The spirometry results were normal.

Analysis

The peak oxygen uptake ($\dot{V}O_2$) was very low and the change in $\dot{V}O_2$/change in work rate ($\Delta\dot{V}O_2/\Delta WR$) was markedly reduced. The anaerobic threshold from the V-slope plot was also reduced. The progressive rise in respiratory exchange ratio throughout exercise is consistent with early onset of lactic acidosis. The oxygen (O_2) pulse increased initially at the start of exercise but failed to increase further over the next 6 minutes of exercise (see **Fig. 10.80.1**, panel 2). The low peak O_2 pulse implies either low stroke volume or low $C(a - \bar{v})O_2$. The ventilatory equivalent for carbon dioxide ($\dot{V}E/\dot{V}CO_2$) was high and end-tidal PCO_2 was low throughout the test, consistent with respiratory compensation for lactic acidosis, primary hyperventilation, or high pulmonary $\dot{V}/\dot{Q}$. Based on the V-slope in panel 3, it appears that she exceeded the anaerobic threshold during the initial period of unloaded cycling, so the high $\dot{V}E/\dot{V}CO_2$ is most likely due

TABLE 10.80.2 Selected Exercise Data

Measurement	Predicted	Measured
Peak $\dot{V}O_2$ (L/min)	1.54	0.62
Maximum heart rate (beats/min)	168	108
Maximum O_2 pulse (mL/beat)	9.1	6.0
$\Delta\dot{V}O_2/\Delta WR$ (mL/min/W)	10.3	2.0
AT (L/min)	>0.78	0.49
Blood pressure (mm Hg [rest, max])		103/63, 139/95
Maximum $\dot{V}E$ (L/min)		37
Exercise breathing reserve (L/min)	>15	65
$\dot{V}E/\dot{V}CO_2$ @ *AT* or lowest	28.1	40.6

Abbreviations: *AT*, anaerobic threshold; O_2, oxygen; $\dot{V}E$, minute ventilation; $\dot{V}E/\dot{V}CO_2$, ventilatory equivalent for carbon dioxide; $\dot{V}O_2$, oxygen uptake; $\Delta\dot{V}O_2/\Delta WR$, change in $\dot{V}O_2$/change in work rate.

to early onset of lactic acidosis. Furthermore, the abnormalities of O_2 pulse and reduced $\Delta\dot{V}O_2/\Delta WR$ were striking and indicative of severe abnormalities in O_2 delivery and/or muscle O_2 extraction. Given these findings, the history of weakness, and lack of evidence for a cardiovascular disorder, impaired skeletal muscle oxygen utilization was suspected. Evaluation for a muscle disorder was thus recommended and a muscle biopsy was subsequently performed at another facility. The findings were interpreted as indicative of a mitochondrial myopathy. The specific metabolic defect was not reported, but the patient's history of prior neurologic events suggested a variant of the MELAS (mitochondrial encephalopathy with myopathy, lactic acidosis, and stroke-like episodes) syndrome.

Conclusion

This was a challenging test to interpret, but the exercise findings and clinical history provided sufficient evidence to recommend focusing the subsequent workup on a muscle oxidative disorder. Impairment of oxygen utilization by the muscle results in inadequate adenosine triphosphate regeneration to meet the increased demands of exercise, with early onset of lactic acidosis and low O_2 pulse due to failure of the $C(a - \bar{v})O_2$ to increase.

TABLE 10.80.3 Air Breathing

Time (min)	Work rate (W)	BP (mm Hg)	HR (min⁻¹)	f (min⁻¹)	$\dot{V}E$ (L/min BTPS)	$\dot{V}CO_2$ (L/min STPD)	$\dot{V}O_2$ (L/min STPD)	$\dot{V}O_2$/HR (mL/beat)	R	pH	HCO_3^- (mEq/L)	PO_2, mm Hg ET	PO_2 a	PO_2 (A − a)	PCO_2, mm Hg ET	PCO_2 a	PCO_2 (a − ET)	$\dot{V}E/\dot{V}CO_2$	$\dot{V}E/\dot{V}O_2$	VD/VT
0.5	Rest	103/63	80	16	13.6	0.32	0.35	4.3	0.92			117			29			42	39	
1.0	Rest		84	18	14.2	0.33	0.35	4.2	0.93			118			28			44	41	
1.5	Rest		79	23	16.4	0.34	0.35	4.4	0.99			121			26			48	47	
2.0	Rest		77	15	13.3	0.30	0.29	3.8	1.01			120			28			45	46	
2.5	Rest		87	16	13.0	0.28	0.29	3.4	0.96			119			28			46	44	
3.0	Rest		85	20	13.3	0.28	0.30	3.5	0.92			118			27			48	44	
3.5	Unloaded	103/63	90	24	15.7	0.35	0.41	4.5	0.87			115			29			45	39	
4.0	Unloaded		90	24	18.2	0.43	0.49	5.5	0.87			115			29			43	37	
4.5	Unloaded		95	23	21.0	0.50	0.53	5.6	0.94			117			28			42	40	
5.0	Unloaded		93	21	21.7	0.53	0.53	5.7	0.99			119			28			41	41	
5.5	Unloaded	131/60	95	20	19.2	0.48	0.51	5.4	0.94			116			30			40	38	
6.0	Unloaded		95	25	22.0	0.53	0.57	6.0	0.94			116			29			41	39	
6.5	3	131/80	98	19	21.1	0.52	0.52	5.3	1.01			118			29			41	41	
7.0	8		94	22	23.2	0.55	0.55	5.8	1.01			119			28			42	43	
7.5	13		98	24	26.4	0.60	0.57	5.8	1.05			122			27			44	46	
8.0	17		99	23	31.6	0.69	0.58	5.9	1.19			125			25			46	54	
8.5	23	130/85	102	20	27.9	0.63	0.56	5.5	1.13			124			25			44	50	
9.0	28		101	20	31.5	0.69	0.61	6.0	1.13			125			25			46	52	
9.5	32		107	22	34.9	0.71	0.60	5.6	1.18			127			23			49	58	
10.0	37	138/95	108	24	36.5	0.73	0.62	5.7	1.19			128			22			50	59	
10.5	Recovery	139/78	99	28	37.4	0.68	0.56	5.6	1.22			130			21			55	67	
11.0	Recovery		94	26	28.3	0.53	0.47	5.0	1.13			127			22			54	61	
11.5	Recovery		94	25	26.9	0.50	0.48	5.1	1.05			126			22			54	56	
12.0	Recovery		97	25	24.8	0.45	0.43	4.4	1.05			126			22			55	58	
12.5	Recovery	124/74	95	28	27.3	0.48	0.45	4.7	1.07			128			21			57	61	
13.0	Recovery		98	25	29.1	0.49	0.43	4.4	1.15			130			20			59	68	

Abbreviations: BP, blood pressure; BTPS, body temperature pressure saturated; f, frequency; HCO_3^-, bicarbonate; HR, heart rate; R, respiratory exchange ratio; STPD, standard temperature pressure dry; $\dot{V}CO_2$, carbon dioxide output; VD/VT, physiological dead space-tidal volume ratio; $\dot{V}E$, minute ventilation; $\dot{V}E/\dot{V}CO_2$, ventilatory equivalent for carbon dioxide; $\dot{V}E/\dot{V}O_2$, ventilatory equivalent for oxygen; $\dot{V}O_2$, oxygen uptake.

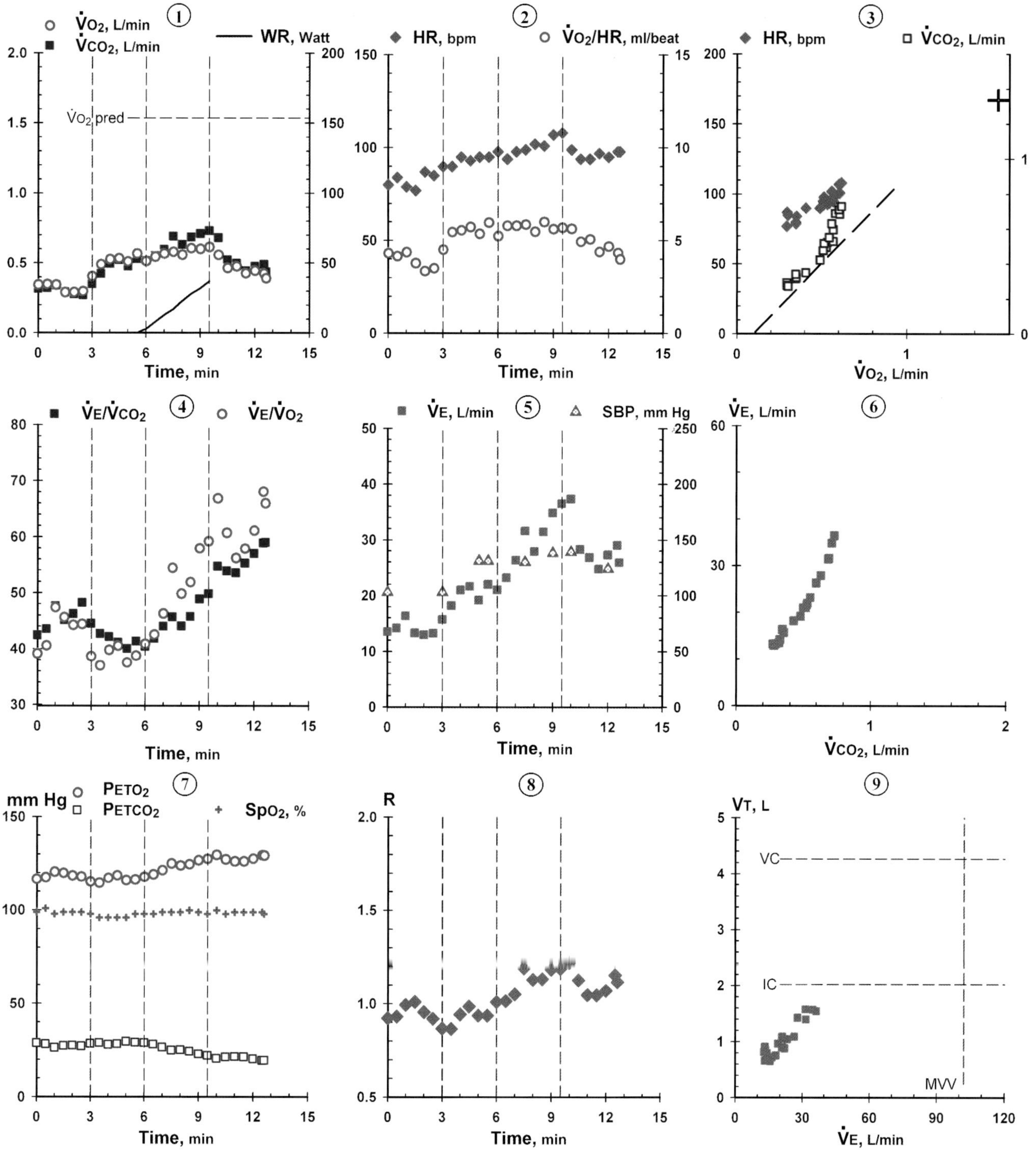

FIGURE 10.80.1. Vertical dashed lines in the panels in the left and middle columns indicate, from left to right, the beginning of unloaded cycling, start of increasing work rate (WR) at 10 W/min, and start of recovery. In **panel 1**, the increase in WR (right y-axis) is plotted with a scale of 100 W to 1 L of oxygen uptake ($\dot{V}O_2$) (left y-axis) such that WR is plotted parallel to a $\dot{V}O_2$ slope of 10 mL/min/W. In **panel 3**, carbon dioxide output ($\dot{V}CO_2$) (right y-axis) is plotted as a function of $\dot{V}O_2$ (x-axis) with identical scales so that the diagonal dashed line has a slope of 1 (45°). The $\dot{V}CO_2$ increasing more steeply than $\dot{V}O_2$ defines carbon dioxide (CO_2) derived from bicarbonate buffer, as long as ventilatory equivalent for CO_2 ($\dot{V}E/\dot{V}CO_2$) (**panel 4**) is not increasing and end-tidal P_{CO_2} (P_{ETCO_2}) (**panel 7**) is not decreasing, simultaneously. The black + symbol in **panel 3** indicates predicted peak values of heart rate (HR) (left y-axis) and $\dot{V}O_2$ for this individual. Abbreviations: IC, inspiratory capacity; MVV, maximum voluntary ventilation; P_{ETO_2}, end-tidal P_{O_2}; R, respiratory exchange ratio; SBP, systolic blood pressure; Sp_{O_2}, oxygen saturation as measured by pulse oximetry; VC, vital capacity; $\dot{V}E$, minute ventilation; $\dot{V}E/\dot{V}O_2$, ventilatory equivalent for O_2; V_T, tidal volume.

CASE 81

Woman With Multiple Sclerosis and Dyspnea

CLINICAL FINDINGS

A 57-year-old woman with relapsing-remitting multiple sclerosis (MS) had exertional dyspnea over the preceding year and a half. She had historically been active, exercising at a gym and doing sports such as skiing and horseback riding, but in recent years, her activities have been curtailed, and at the time of testing, she reported shortness of breath with ascending a flight of stairs or walking on level grade. She reported her MS symptoms to be primarily fatigue, visual changes, and headache. Over the preceding year or so, she also had light-headedness, and often needed to steady herself for support when standing or walking. She had frequent episodes of needing to lie down due to her vision "going black" but had never lost consciousness. She did not have orthopnea. She denied anxiety attacks and had undergone numerous magnetic resonance imaging scans without panic or claustrophobia. The MS had been diagnosed 20 years earlier. A number of disease modifying medications had been prescribed but discontinued due to adverse effects, so she was treated for episodic relapses with systemic corticosteroids. The last steroid course was a month earlier and was associated with improvement in dyspnea as well as her other symptoms. At the time of testing, her medication included transdermal estrogen and an antihistamine. Physical examination revealed normal heart and breath sounds. Motor strength was grossly intact. Resting electrocardiogram (ECG) showed normal sinus rhythm and diffuse ST-T wave abnormalities. Spirometric volumes were mildly reduced. Demographic and respiratory function data are shown in **Table 10.81.1**.

TABLE 10.81.1 Selected Respiratory Function Data

Measurement	Predicted	Measured
Age (y)		57
Sex		Female
Height (cm)		166
Weight (kg)		61
VC (L)	3.55	2.98
IC (L)	2.29	2.61
ERV (L)	1.26	0.40
FEV_1 (L)	2.76	2.24
FEV_1/VC (%)	79	75
MVV (L/min)	96	84

Abbreviations: ERV, expiratory reserve volume; FEV_1, forced expiratory volume in 1 second; IC, inspiratory capacity; MVV, maximum voluntary ventilation; VC, vital capacity.

EXERCISE FINDINGS

The patient exercised on a cycle ergometer beginning with 3 minutes of unloaded pedaling at 60 rpm followed by continuous increase in work rate by 10 W/min until the test was ended by examiners due to signs of progressive hyperventilation and a decrease in her degree of interaction. She later reported that she had felt short of breath and was dizzy but not presyncopal. On exercise, ECG right bundle branch block developed at heart rates above 80 beats/min. Exercise data are summarized in **Tables 10.81.2** and **10.81.3** and in **Figure 10.81.1**.

INTERPRETATION

Comment

A number of reports indicate that ambulatory patients with MS often have reduced exercise capacity on objective testing. The range of proposed mechanisms responsible for this is wide, including subclinical cardiac dysfunction, cardiovascular autonomic dysfunction, increased metabolic cost of exercise due to gait or other issues, or neuromuscular weakness. This case presents a puzzling set of findings that could thus have a number of different explanations. It is

TABLE 10.81.2 Selected Exercise Data

Measurement	Predicted	Measured
Peak $\dot{V}O_2$ (L/min)	1.39	0.69
Maximum heart rate (beats/min)	163	115
Maximum O_2 pulse (mL/beat)	8.5	6.4
$\Delta\dot{V}O_2/\Delta WR$ (mL/min/W)	10.3	~9.0
AT (L/min)	>0.71	NA
Blood pressure (mm Hg [rest, peak ex])		130/75, 134/79
Maximum $\dot{V}E$ (L/min)		44
Breathing reserve (L/min)	>15	40
$\dot{V}E/\dot{V}CO_2$ @ *AT* (L/min)	<33	NA
$\dot{V}E$-$\dot{V}CO_2$ slope	<32	36
SpO_2 (% [rest, max ex])		98, 99
V_D/V_T (rest, max ex)[a]		0.41, 0.37

Abbreviations: *AT*, anaerobic threshold; $\Delta\dot{V}O_2/\Delta WR$, change in $\dot{V}O_2$/change in work rate; ex, exercise; NA, not applicable; O_2, oxygen; $\dot{V}CO_2$, carbon dioxide output; V_D/V_T, physiological dead space-tidal volume ratio; $\dot{V}E$, minute ventilation; $\dot{V}O_2$, oxygen uptake.

[a] V_D/V_T was calculated using $PtcCO_2$ as an estimate of arterial PCO_2.

TABLE 10.81.3 Air Breathing

Time (min)	Work rate (W)	BP (mm Hg)	HR (min^{-1})	f (min^{-1})	$\dot{V}E$ (L/min BTPS)	$\dot{V}CO_2$ (L/min STPD)	$\dot{V}O_2$ (L/min STPD)	$\frac{\dot{V}O_2}{HR}$ (mL/beat)	R	pH	HCO_3^- (mEq/L)	PO_2, mm Hg and SpO_2, % ET	SpO_2	(A − a)	PCO_2, mm Hg ET	tc	(a − ET)	$\frac{\dot{V}E}{\dot{V}CO_2}$	$\frac{\dot{V}E}{\dot{V}O_2}$	$\frac{V_D}{V_T}$
0.5	Rest		69	12	11.5	0.29	0.34	4.9	0.85			111	98		32	35.9		40	34	0.41
1.0	Rest		73	17	8.4	0.20	0.25	3.3	0.82			113	98		31	35.9		42	34	0.45
1.5	Rest		75	9	7.8	0.19	0.22	2.9	0.89			111	98		33	35.8		41	36	0.43
2.0	Rest	130/75	69	17	8.7	0.22	0.25	3.6	0.88			108	98		33	35.6		40	35	0.41
2.5	Unloaded		77	18	10.1	0.27	0.34	4.5	0.80			109	98		34	35.9		37	29	0.38
3.0	Unloaded		79	19	15.6	0.40	0.45	5.7	0.89			114	98		31	36.1		39	34	0.41
3.5	Unloaded		84	11	16.4	0.44	0.43	5.2	1.01			116	98		32	35.6		38	38	0.37
4.0	Unloaded		90	14	17.1	0.48	0.47	5.2	1.01			117	98		32	34.4		36	36	0.32
4.5	Unloaded		87	13	23.1	0.57	0.50	5.7	1.15			121	98		30	33.4		40	46	0.39
5.0	Unloaded	139/79	91	12	19.9	0.48	0.40	4.4	1.19			121	99		29	32.3		41	49	0.38
5.5	3		87	11	18.9	0.48	0.46	5.3	1.04			119	99		30	30.8		39	41	0.31
6.0	8		86	9	16.6	0.43	0.46	5.3	0.95			113	98		32	30.4		38	36	0.29
6.5	13		77	15	20.2	0.49	0.48	6.2	1.04			121	98		28	30.5		41	42	0.34
7.0	18		86	16	26.0	0.60	0.56	6.4	1.08			121	98		28	30.4		43	47	0.37
7.5	24	134/79	94	18	30.4	0.65	0.55	5.8	1.19			126	99		25	29.3		46	55	0.39
8.0	28		99	19	27.4	0.60	0.55	5.5	1.09			125	99		25	27.9		46	50	0.35
8.5	33		102	24	35.6	0.72	0.64	6.3	1.13			127	99		24	26.8		49	56	0.37
9.0	38		108	34	43.7	0.81	0.69	6.4	1.17			131	99		21	25.9		54	64	0.41
9.5	Recovery		112	40	48.7	0.82	0.67	6.0	1.22			133	99		19	24.6		60	73	0.43
10.0	Recovery	145/78	103	39	39.9	0.67	0.59	5.7	1.13			132	99		20	23.3		59	67	0.40
10.5	Recovery		93	36	31.3	0.54	0.51	5.5	1.07			130	99		21	22.5		58	62	0.36
11.0	Recovery		87	41	41.4	0.61	0.52	6.0	1.17			134	99		18	22.1		68	79	0.45
11.5	Recovery		84	34	22.7	0.27	0.21	2.6	1.27			135	99		16	22.1		83	106	0.55

Abbreviations: BP, blood pressure; BTPS, body temperature pressure saturated; f, frequency; HCO_3^-, bicarbonate; HR, heart rate; $P(A - a)O_2$, alveolar-arterial PO_2 difference; $P(a - ET)CO_2$, arterial–end-tidal PCO_2 difference; $PETCO_2$, end-tidal PCO_2; $PETO_2$, end-tidal PO_2; $PtcCO_2$, transcutaneous PCO_2; R, respiratory exchange ratio; STPD, standard temperature pressure dry; $\dot{V}CO_2$, carbon dioxide output; V_D/V_T, physiological dead space–tidal volume ratio; $\dot{V}E$, minute ventilation; $\dot{V}E/\dot{V}CO_2$, ventilatory equivalent for carbon dioxide; $\dot{V}E/\dot{V}O_2$, ventilatory equivalent for oxygen; $\dot{V}O_2$, oxygen uptake.

[a]$PtcCO_2$, transcutaneous PCO_2; V_D/V_T was calculated using $PtcCO_2$ as an estimate of arterial PCO_2.

presented to acknowledge that the basis of impairment is sometimes poorly understood and also to identify the autonomic nervous system as a key component of normal exercise performance.

Analysis

The test was ended at a oxygen uptake ($\dot{V}O_2$) of half the predicted value at a time when the patient was symptomatic, although not volitionally limited, suggesting significant impairment.

Cardiovascular responses: There were nonspecific ECG abnormalities including a rate dependent right bundle branch block. Blood pressure did not increase appreciably with exercise, although the range of exercise was limited. The $\dot{V}O_2$ during unloaded cycling was approximately double the resting value, which is the expected magnitude of increase. The subsequent change in $\dot{V}O_2$/change in work rate ($\Delta\dot{V}O_2/\Delta WR$) during incremental work also appeared normal, although given the limited range of data it was difficult to quantify. Postexercise recovery of $\dot{V}O_2$ appeared slow, which implies a less than normal increase in $\dot{V}O_2$ during the test. The anaerobic threshold could not be identified. The oxygen pulse reached a stable plateau value at a level below the predicted normal maximal value. This pattern of findings suggests impaired delivery and/or utilization of oxygen, even in the limited range of exercise performed.

Ventilatory responses: The most notable finding was hyperventilation that appeared after the onset of exercise. Initially at rest, the respiratory exchange ratio was a normal resting value, and end-tidal PCO_2 and transcutaneous PCO_2 were around 35 mm Hg, which are low normal. With exercise, there was a progressive rise of respiratory exchange ratio and decrease in both end-tidal and transcutaneous PCO_2 values. This appeared to be due to hyperventilation, rather than a response to a normal exercise-induced metabolic acidosis, as there was no period of isocapnic buffering.

Gas exchange efficiency: Pulse oximetry was normal. Elevated values for ventilatory equivalents and minute ventilation ($\dot{V}E$) relative to carbon dioxide output ($\dot{V}CO_2$) slope can result purely from hyperventilation. However, using

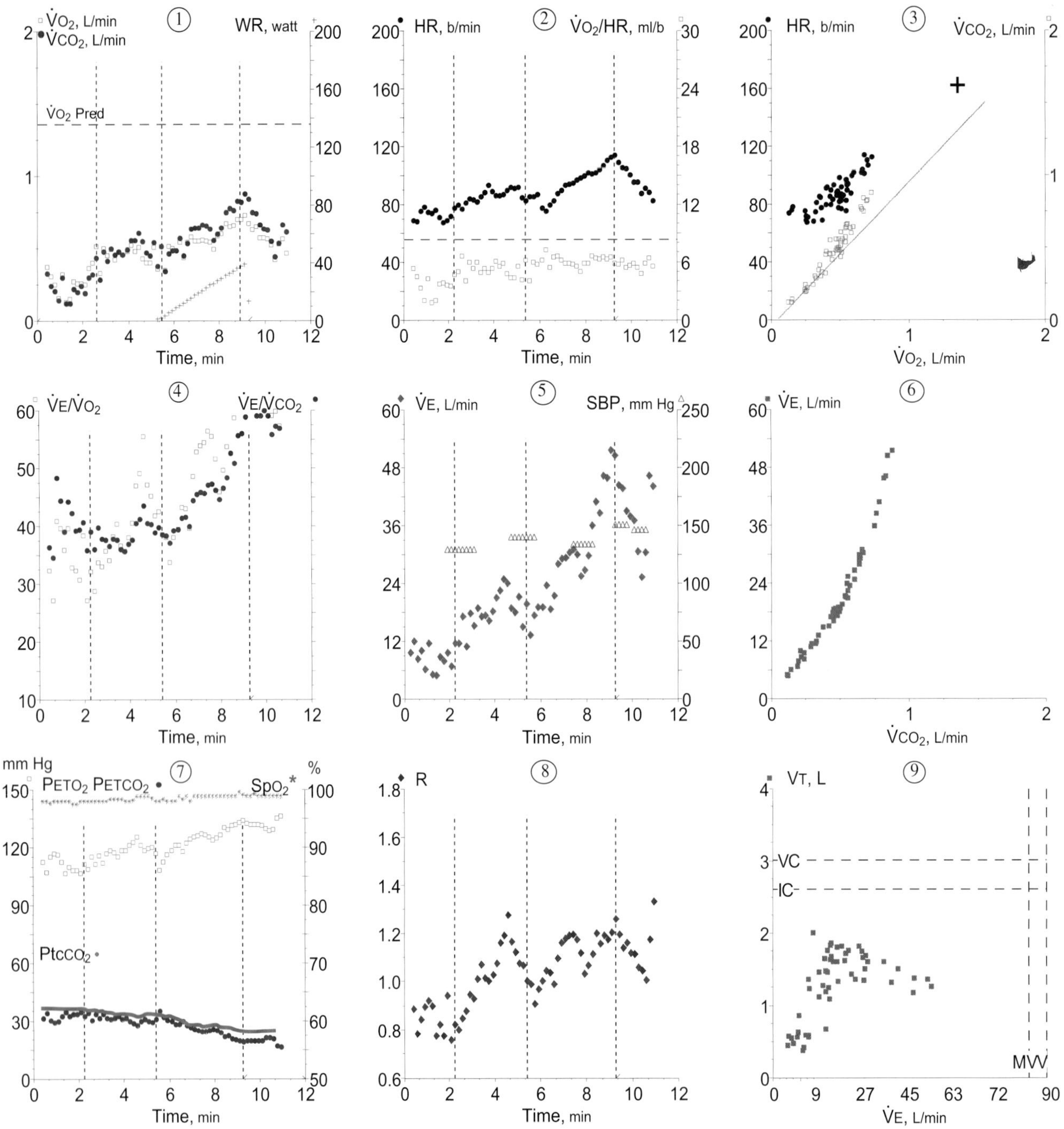

FIGURE 10.81.1. Vertical dashed lines in the panels in the left and middle columns indicate, from left to right, the beginning of unloaded cycling, start of increasing work rate (WR) at 10 W/min, and start of recovery. In **panel 1**, the increase in WR (right y-axis) is plotted with a scale of 100 W to 1 L of oxygen uptake ($\dot{V}O_2$) (left y-axis) such that work rate is plotted parallel to a $\dot{V}O_2$ slope of 10 mL/min/W. Predicted peak $\dot{V}O_2$ is shown as a dashed horizontal line. In **panel 3**, carbon dioxide output ($\dot{V}CO_2$) (right y-axis) is plotted as a function of $\dot{V}O_2$ (x-axis) with identical scales so that the diagonal blue line has a slope of 1 (45°). The $\dot{V}CO_2$ increasing more steeply than $\dot{V}O_2$ defines carbon dioxide (CO_2) derived from bicarbonate buffer, as long as ventilatory equivalent for carbon dioxide ($\dot{V}E/\dot{V}CO_2$) (**panel 4**) is not increasing and end-tidal P_{CO_2} (P_{ETCO_2}) (**panel 7**) is not decreasing, simultaneously. The black + symbol in **panel 3** indicates predicted peak values of heart rate (HR) (left y-axis) and $\dot{V}O_2$ for this individual. Abbreviations: IC, inspiratory capacity; MVV, maximum voluntary ventilation; P_{ETO_2}, end-tidal partial pressure of oxygen; R, respiratory exchange ratio; SBP, systolic blood pressure; VC, vital capacity; $\dot{V}E$, minute ventilation; $\dot{V}E/\dot{V}O_2$, ventilatory equivalent for oxygen; V_T, tidal volume.

transcutaneous P_{CO_2} as an estimate of arterial P_{CO_2}, the calculated physiological dead space–tidal volume ratio (V_D/V_T) was higher during exercise than at rest, which indicates that there were also areas of high pulmonary $\dot{V}/\dot{Q}$.

Conclusion

Hyperventilation is not a specific finding and could reflect idiopathic hyperventilation unrelated to the patient's neurologic condition. However, hyperventilation itself would not account for all of the abnormalities identified. Hyperventilation and dyspnea may alternatively be associated with autonomic dysfunction in conditions such as postural orthostatic tachycardia syndrome, and MS frequently affects the autonomic nervous system. We postulate that the abnormal cardiovascular, ventilatory, and gas exchange responses could all result from autonomic dysfunction related to the patient's MS, which would be consistent with the history that dyspnea improved during recent treatment of relapse with corticosteroids. From this perspective, the flat patterns of oxygen pulse and blood pressure responses would reflect inadequate peripheral vascular control, limiting oxygen extraction, and the marginal V_D/V_T values could represent failure of autonomic contributions to control of $\dot{V}/\dot{Q}$ matching within the lung. Given the abnormalities in $\dot{V}O_2$ variables and the ECG, a cardiac evaluation would be appropriate, as would specific assessment of autonomic function.

CASE 82

Congenital Myotonia

CLINICAL FINDINGS

A father and son were both referred for exercise testing by their neurologist following diagnosis of congenital myotonia.[1] The father was diagnosed at 46 years of age after his 18- and 20-year-old sons had both been given this diagnosis on evaluation for muscle stiffness. The father had always been aware of delayed muscle relaxation after forceful contraction, such as shaking hands or turning his head quickly when driving, but had not identified it as abnormal. He had occasional spasms of back muscles with changes in position and of extraocular muscles with changes in gaze. All muscle groups were affected. He could sustain moderate activities such as walking and cycling; however, he fatigued quickly with more vigorous activities. He described himself as the slowest and least athletic of his peers in his youth and had never participated in sports. He denied fixed muscle weakness or episodes of hematuria. His mother had always complained of muscle cramps.

The 20-year-old son reported more prominent symptoms than his father including overt muscle hypertrophy. He was amused that people often described him as "buff," despite his being very sedentary. Like his father, he was comfortable with walking, but had impaired muscle relaxation and cramping with sudden movements. In school, he had participated in gym class but described himself as "a horrible runner" and did not do any regular sports. Over the preceding year, he had experienced multiple episodes of general weakness and light-headedness with exertion but had not had syncope.

Physical examination of heart and lungs were normal in both father and son. The son appeared muscular. Limited testing suggested that muscle strength was grossly intact and symmetrical. Resting electrocardiograms showed sinus rhythm. Demographic and pulmonary function data for both father and son are shown in **Table 10.82.1**.

EXERCISE FINDINGS

Both patients exercised on a cycle ergometer beginning with 3 minutes of unloaded pedaling at 60 rpm followed by continuous increase in work rate by either 15 W/min (father) or 20 W/min (son). Both ended exercise with symptoms of leg fatigue. The son reported light-headedness but not to the degree he had experienced in the past. Exercise electrocardiograms did not show arrhythmias or ischemic changes. Exercise data for both father and son are summarized in **Table 10.82.2**, and individual responses for father and son are shown in **Tables 10.82.3** and **10.82.4**, respectively, and in **Figures 10.82.1** and **10.82.2**, respectively.

TABLE 10.82.1 Selected Respiratory Function Data

	Father		Son	
Measurement	Predicted	Measured	Predicted	Measured
Age (y)		46		20
Sex		Male		Male
Height (cm)		178		175
Weight (kg)		79		74
VC (L)	5.13	4.54	5.44	4.53
IC (L)	3.42	3.42	3.50	3.16
ERV (L)	1.14	1.71	1.94	1.15
FEV_1 (L)	3.68	4.02	4.55	3.78
FEV_1/VC (%)	81	79	84	84
MVV (L/min)	157	165	187	135

Abbreviations: ERV, expiratory reserve volume; FEV_1, forced expiratory volume in 1 second; IC, inspiratory capacity; MVV, maximum voluntary ventilation; VC, vital capacity.

TABLE 10.82.2 Selected Exercise Test Data

	Father		Son	
Measurement	Predicted	Measured	Predicted	Measured
Peak $\dot{V}O_2$ (L/min)	2.67	1.74	3.0	1.99
Maximum heart rate (beats/min)	174	153	200	168
Maximum O_2 pulse (mL/beat)	15.3	11.4	15.0	12.9
$\Delta\dot{V}O_2/\Delta WR$ (mL/min/W)	10.3	10.0	10.3	10.0
AT (L/min)	>1.07	0.95	>1.29	1.3
Blood pressure (mmHg [rest, peak ex])		127/71, 191/101		116/70, 143/84
Maximum $\dot{V}E$ (L/min)	165	68	135	60
Breathing reserve (L/min)	>15	97	>15	75
$\dot{V}E/\dot{V}CO_2$ at the *AT*	<30	28	<29	25
SpO_2 (% [rest, max ex])		97, 97		98, 96

Abbreviations: *AT*, anaerobic threshold; $\Delta\dot{V}O_2/\Delta WR$, change in $\dot{V}O_2$/change in work rate; ex, exercise; O_2, oxygen; SpO_2, oxygen saturation as measured by pulse oximetry; $\dot{V}E$, minute ventilation; $\dot{V}E/\dot{V}CO_2$, ventilatory equivalent for CO_2; $\dot{V}O_2$, oxygen uptake.

INTERPRETATION

Comment

Congenital myotonia results from a defect in the chloride channel and is said to be the most common inherited skeletal muscle channelopathy.[1] These cases are presented as examples of a neuromuscular disease that is a defect in skeletal muscle contractile function without known abnormality in muscle metabolic pathways. Little has been reported about aerobic exercise function in this condition.

Analysis

Findings in the tests of this father and son were similar and presented together. In both cases, peak oxygen uptake ($\dot{V}O_2$) was low but $\dot{V}O_2$ increased appropriately relative to work rate up to the level of work attained. The anaerobic threshold was slightly below normal for the father and at the lower limit of normal for the son. For both, heart rate increased more steeply than average relative to $\dot{V}O_2$ and the oxygen pulse was lower than the predicted average value at peak exercise. Ventilation, breathing reserve, and measures of the efficiency of pulmonary gas exchange all appeared normal in both tests.

Conclusion

Exercise capacities of this father and son were reduced relative to normal reference values but without findings of clearly pathologic responses in gas exchange. It is difficult to say whether the low exercise capacity resulted from lifelong avoidance of exercise due to unpleasant muscle symptoms, or is related to early muscle fatigue due to the abnormality in contractile function.

REFERENCE

1. Statland JM, Barohn RJ. Muscle channelopathies: the nondystrophic myotonias and periodic paralyses. *Continuum (Minneap Minn)*. 2013;19(6 Muscle Disease):1598-1614.

TABLE 10.82.3 Father

Time (min)	Work rate (W)	BP (mm Hg)	HR (min^{-1})	f (min^{-1})	$\dot{V}E$ (L/min BTPS)	$\dot{V}CO_2$ (L/min STPD)	$\dot{V}O_2$ (L/min STPD)	$\frac{\dot{V}O_2}{HR}$ (mL/beat)	R	pH	HCO_3^- (mEq/L)	PO_2, mm Hg and SpO_2, %: ET	SpO_2	(A − a)	PCO_2, mm Hg: ET	a	(a − ET)	$\frac{\dot{V}E}{\dot{V}CO_2}$	$\frac{\dot{V}E}{\dot{V}O_2}$	$\frac{VD}{VT}$
0.5	Rest		78	17	18.2	0.47	0.45	5.7	1.05			121	97		30			39	41	
1.0	Rest	127/71	76	19	14.1	0.31	0.29	3.9	1.07			122	98		29			45	48	
1.5	Rest		77	17	13.2	0.31	0.31	4.0	1.00			119	97		30			43	43	
2.0	Rest		81	16	13.5	0.32	0.32	3.9	1.00			119	97		29			43	43	
2.5	Rest		80	19	12.7	0.28	0.29	3.6	0.96			119	97		30			46	44	
3.0	Rest		81	19	13.7	0.31	0.32	4.0	0.94			119	97		29			45	42	
3.5	Unloaded		91	20	18.7	0.51	0.56	6.2	0.91			115	96		32			37	33	
4.0	Unloaded		92	21	19.2	0.51	0.54	5.8	0.95			115	97		33			38	36	
4.5	Unloaded		86	19	15.5	0.43	0.48	5.6	0.88			111	97		35			36	32	
5.0	Unloaded		87	19	18.0	0.50	0.54	6.2	0.92			113	97		34			36	33	
5.5	Unloaded	128/76	89	21	18.3	0.50	0.54	6.1	0.92			113	98		34			37	34	
6.0	Unloaded		87	22	18.4	0.51	0.61	7.1	0.84			108	97		36			36	30	
6.5	5		86	22	17.1	0.46	0.51	5.9	0.91			112	97		35			37	34	
7.0	12		86	23	19.6	0.55	0.62	7.2	0.89			111	97		35			36	32	
7.5	20		87	23	17.8	0.50	0.56	6.5	0.88			110	97		36			36	32	
8.0	27		93	24	20.1	0.58	0.67	7.2	0.87			109	97		36			34	30	
8.5	35		94	20	18.5	0.56	0.64	6.8	0.89			108	98		38			33	29	
9.0	41		96	19	21.1	0.66	0.70	7.3	0.94			110	97		37			32	30	
9.5	48		101	20	19.1	0.61	0.68	6.7	0.91			108	97		38			31	28	
10.0	56	147/74	103	20	25.2	0.83	0.88	8.6	0.94			109	97		39			30	28	
10.5	63		105	20	24.7	0.82	0.85	8.1	0.97			108	97		39			30	29	
11.0	71		114	21	27.3	0.92	0.92	8.0	1.00			110	97		39			30	30	
11.5	78		116	23	30.1	1.05	1.05	9.1	0.99			109	97		40			29	29	
12.0	86	178/84	121	25	37.9	1.27	1.16	9.6	1.09			114	97		38			30	33	
12.5	92		125	27	39.7	1.31	1.20	9.6	1.10			114	96		38			30	33	
13.0	100		129	25	40.9	1.39	1.23	9.5	1.13			115	97		38			29	33	
13.5	107		132	28	40.9	1.42	1.30	9.8	1.09			113	96		39			29	32	
14.0	115	191/101	138	31	50.5	1.68	1.47	10.7	1.14			115	97		37			30	34	
14.5	122		143	26	48.8	1.73	1.51	10.5	1.15			114	97		39			28	32	
15.0	129		147	27	54.6	1.90	1.58	10.7	1.21			116	97		38			29	35	
15.5	137		151	29	61.9	2.08	1.63	10.8	1.27			119	97		37			30	38	
16.0	144	211/96	153	32	67.7	2.18	1.74	11.4	1.25			120	97		35			31	39	
16.5	Recovery		159	32	71.3	2.26	1.79	11.3	1.26			120	96		35			32	40	
17.0	Recovery		153	30	61.1	1.95	1.58	10.3	1.24			119	99		35			31	39	
17.5	Recovery		144	28	56.6	1.74	1.21	8.5	1.43			123	96		34			33	47	
18.0	Recovery		135	31	55.2	1.53	1.01	7.5	1.51			127	97		31			36	55	
18.5	Recovery		127	28	44.3	1.20	0.89	7.0	1.35			125	96		31			37	50	
19.0	Recovery	155/90	125	28	43.1	1.11	0.83	6.7	1.34			125	96		30			39	52	
19.5	Recovery		120	27	36.4	0.91	0.74	6.1	1.23			124	96		30			40	49	

Abbreviations: BP, blood pressure; BTPS, body temperature pressure saturated; f, frequency; HCO_3^-, bicarbonate; P(A − a)O_2, alveolar-arterial PO_2 difference; P(a − ET) CO_2, arterial-end-tidal PCO_2 difference; $PETCO_2$, end-tidal PCO_2; $PETO_2$, end-tidal PO_2; HR, heart rate; R, respiratory exchange ratio; SpO_2, oxygen saturation by pulse oximetry; STPD, standard temperature pressure dry; $\dot{V}CO_2$, carbon dioxide output; VD/VT, physiological dead space-tidal volume ratio; $\dot{V}E$, minute ventilation; $\dot{V}E/\dot{V}CO_2$, ventilatory equivalent for carbon dioxide; $\dot{V}E/\dot{V}O_2$, ventilatory equivalent for oxygen; $\dot{V}O_2$, oxygen uptake.

TABLE 10.82.4 Son

Time (min)	Work rate (W)	BP (mm Hg)	HR (min^{-1})	f (min^{-1})	$\dot{V}E$ (L/min BTPS)	$\dot{V}CO_2$ (L/min STPD)	$\dot{V}O_2$ (L/min STPD)	$\frac{\dot{V}O_2}{HR}$ (mL/beat)	R	pH	HCO_3^- (mEq/L)	PO_2, mm Hg and SpO_2, % ET	SpO_2	(A − a)	PCO_2, mm Hg ET	a	(a − ET)	$\frac{\dot{V}E}{\dot{V}CO_2}$	$\frac{\dot{V}E}{\dot{V}O_2}$	$\frac{VD}{VT}$
0.5	Rest		82	21	11.3	0.30	0.33	4.0	0.93			109	97		37			37	34	
1.0	Rest	116/70	82	21	10.4	0.26	0.29	3.5	0.92			110	98		36			39	36	
1.5	Rest		84	21	11.1	0.30	0.32	3.8	0.94			110	98		36			37	35	
2.0	Rest		84	19	12.2	0.31	0.31	3.7	1.01			113	97		34			39	40	
2.5	Unloaded		93	28	13.8	0.39	0.47	5.0	0.84			105	97		38			35	30	
3.0	Unloaded		95	21	15.0	0.47	0.54	5.7	0.87			106	98		38			32	28	
3.5	Unloaded		91	20	12.2	0.39	0.45	4.9	0.87			104	97		40			32	27	
4.0	Unloaded		91	22	16.9	0.53	0.57	6.3	0.93			108	97		39			32	29	
4.5	Unloaded		92	21	15.1	0.47	0.51	5.5	0.92			107	97		40			32	30	
5.0	Unloaded		92	22	15.6	0.48	0.52	5.7	0.92			107	97		39			33	30	
5.5	Unloaded		90	23	15.9	0.49	0.53	5.9	0.92			107	98		40			32	30	
6.0	17		91	21	15.2	0.47	0.51	5.6	0.94			108	97		39			32	30	
6.5	26		96	22	15.0	0.47	0.52	5.4	0.89			106	97		40			32	29	
7.0	37	114/65	99	22	16.9	0.55	0.62	6.3	0.89			105	97		41			31	27	
7.5	46		101	22	16.9	0.56	0.63	6.2	0.89			105	97		41			30	27	
8.0	56		106	22	18.6	0.64	0.74	7.0	0.86			103	97		42			29	25	
8.5	66		108	21	19.7	0.70	0.77	7.1	0.91			104	97		42			28	26	
9.0	75	145/60	115	24	24.7	0.89	0.95	8.3	0.93			105	97		42			28	26	
9.5	86		120	25	26.4	0.96	1.00	8.3	0.96			106	97		43			27	26	
10.0	95		125	25	27.0	1.02	1.07	8.5	0.95			105	97		44			27	25	
10.5	105		131	26	32.0	1.22	1.24	9.4	0.98			106	97		44			26	26	
11.0	114	153/69	136	29	34.7	1.29	1.27	9.4	1.01			108	97		44			27	27	
11.5	124		142	28	36.2	1.39	1.36	9.6	1.02			107	97		44			26	27	
12.0	134		150	25	40.0	1.60	1.55	10.3	1.03			107	97		45			25	26	
12.5	143		152	30	41.8	1.65	1.59	10.4	1.04			107	97		45			25	26	
13.0	154	148/64	159	32	47.4	1.82	1.67	10.5	1.09			110	97		44			26	28	
13.5	163		158	33	49.3	1.91	1.74	11.0	1.10			110	97		45			26	28	
14.0	173		168	34	54.0	2.10	1.87	11.2	1.12			111	96		45			26	29	
14.5	183		155	32	59.5	2.35	1.90	12.0	1.19			112	96		45			25	30	
15.0	Recovery		166	32	63.1	2.38	1.83	11.0	1.31			117	95		43			26	35	
15.5	Recovery	143/100	151	31	51.3	1.96	1.30	8.6	1.50			120	97		43			26	39	
16.0	Recovery		152	32	43.6	1.55	0.96	6.3	1.62			124	97		41			28	46	
16.5	Recovery	162/77	140	35	43.1	1.37	0.84	6.0	1.63			127	97		37			31	51	
17.0	Recovery		136	33	38.3	1.17	0.76	5.6	1.55			127	98		36			33	50	

Abbreviations: BP, blood pressure; BTPS, body temperature pressure saturated; f, frequency; HCO_3^-, bicarbonate; HR, heart rate; $P(A - a)O_2$, alveolar-arterial PO_2 difference; $P(a - ET)CO_2$, arterial-end-tidal PCO_2 difference; $PETCO_2$, end-tidal PCO_2; $PETO_2$, end-tidal PO_2; R, respiratory exchange ratio; SpO_2, oxygen saturation by pulse oximetry; STPD, standard temperature pressure dry; $\dot{V}CO_2$, carbon dioxide output; VD/VT, physiological dead space-tidal volume ratio; $\dot{V}E$, minute ventilation; $\dot{V}E/\dot{V}CO_2$, ventilatory equivalent for carbon dioxide; $\dot{V}E/\dot{V}O_2$, ventilatory equivalent for oxygen; $\dot{V}O_2$, oxygen uptake.

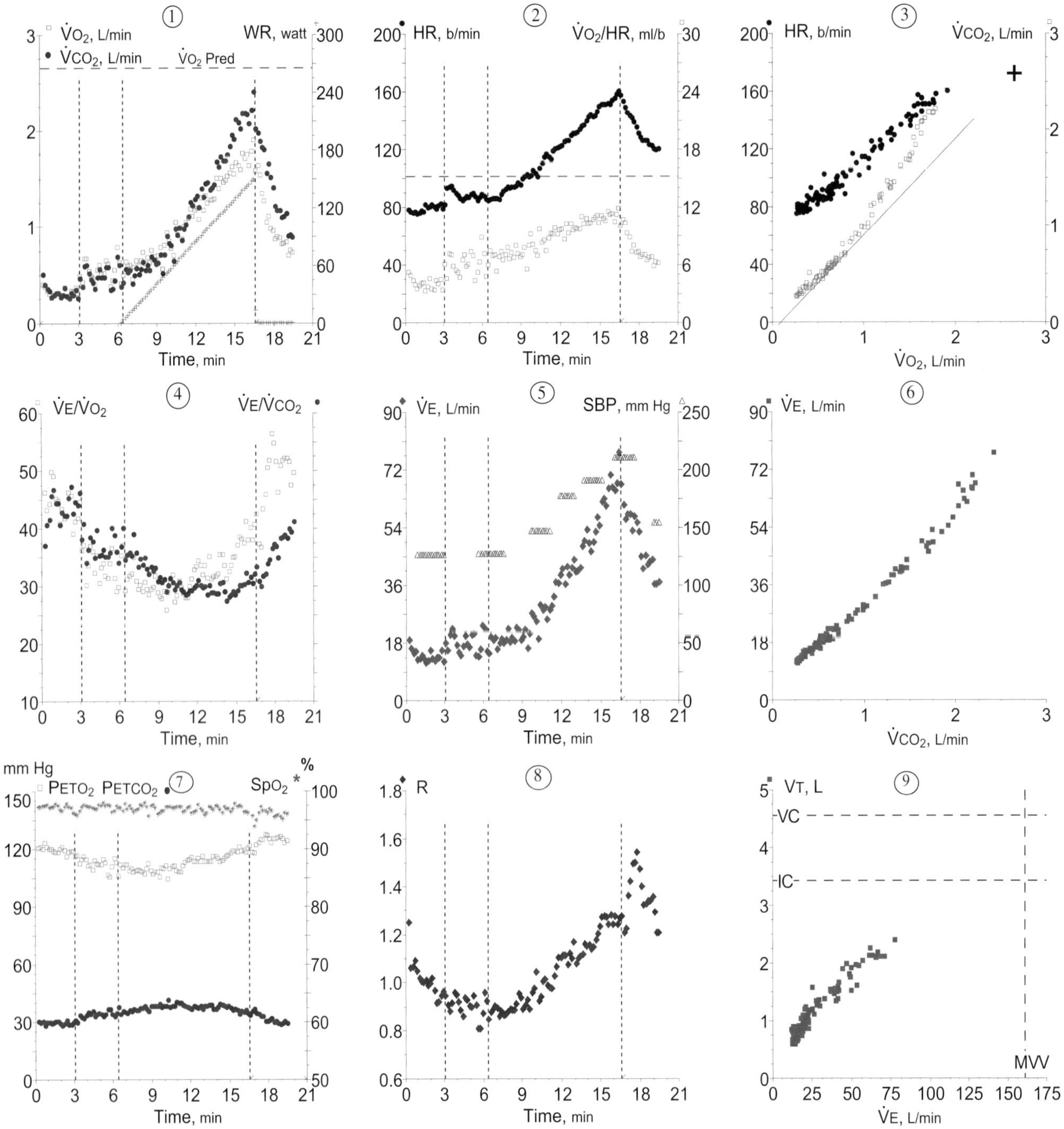

FIGURE 10.82.1. Father. Vertical dashed lines in the panels in the left and middle columns indicate, from left to right, the beginning of unloaded cycling, start of increasing work rate (WR) at 15 W/min, and start of recovery. In **panel 1**, the increase in WR (right y-axis) is plotted with a scale of 100 W to 1 L of oxygen uptake ($\dot{V}O_2$) (left y-axis) such that WR is plotted parallel to a $\dot{V}O_2$ slope of 10 mL/min/W. Predicted peak $\dot{V}O_2$ is shown as a dashed horizontal line. In **panel 3**, carbon dioxide output ($\dot{V}CO_2$) (right y-axis) is plotted as a function of $\dot{V}O_2$ (x-axis) with identical scales so that the diagonal blue line has a slope of 1 (45°). The $\dot{V}CO_2$ increasing more steeply than $\dot{V}O_2$ defines carbon dioxide (CO_2) derived from bicarbonate buffer, as long as ventilatory equivalent for CO_2 ($\dot{V}E/\dot{V}CO_2$) (**panel 4**) is not increasing and partial pressure of CO_2 in end-tidal gas (P_{ETCO_2}) (**panel 7**) is not decreasing, simultaneously. The black + symbol in **panel 3** indicates predicted peak values of heart rate (HR) (left y-axis) and $\dot{V}O_2$ for this individual. Abbreviations: IC, inspiratory capacity; MVV, maximum voluntary ventilation; P_{ETO_2}, end-tidal P_{O_2}; R, respiratory exchange ratio; SBP, systolic blood pressure; Sp_{O_2}, oxygen saturation by pulse oximetry; VC, vital capacity; $\dot{V}E$, minute ventilation; $\dot{V}E/\dot{V}CO_2$, ventilatory equivalent for carbon dioxide; $\dot{V}E/\dot{V}O_2$, ventilatory equivalent for oxygen; V_T, tidal volume.

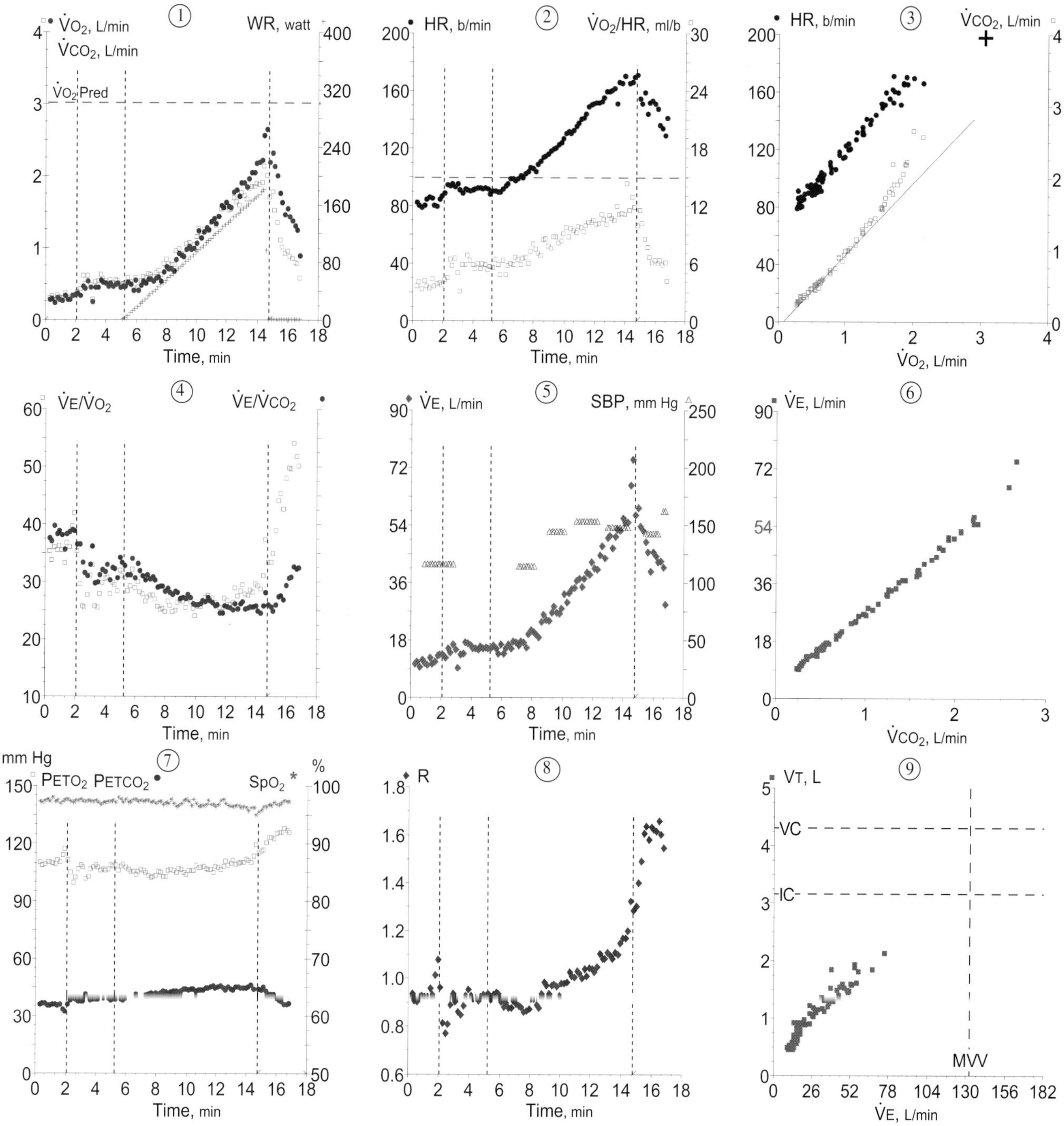

FIGURE 10.82.2. Son. Vertical dashed lines in the panels in the left and middle columns indicate, from left to right, the beginning of unloaded cycling, start of increasing work rate (WR) at 20 W/min, and start of recovery. In **panel 1**, the increase in WR (right y-axis) is plotted with a scale of 100 W to 1 L of oxygen uptake ($\dot{V}O_2$) (left y-axis) such that WR is plotted parallel to a $\dot{V}O_2$ slope of 10 mL/min/W. Predicted peak $\dot{V}O_2$ is shown as a dashed horizontal line. In **panel 3**, carbon dioxide output ($\dot{V}CO_2$) (right y-axis) is plotted as a function of $\dot{V}O_2$ (x-axis) with identical scales so that the diagonal blue line has a slope of 1 (45°). The $\dot{V}CO_2$ increasing more steeply than $\dot{V}O_2$ defines carbon dioxide (CO_2) derived from bicarbonate buffer, as long as ventilatory equivalent for CO_2 ($\dot{V}E/\dot{V}CO_2$) (**panel 4**) is not increasing and partial pressure of CO_2 in end-tidal gas ($PETCO_2$) (**panel 7**) is not decreasing, simultaneously. The black + symbol in **panel 3** indicates predicted peak values of heart rate (HR) (left y-axis) and $\dot{V}O_2$ for this individual. Abbreviations: IC, inspiratory capacity; MVV, maximum voluntary ventilation; $PETO_2$, end-tidal partial pressure of oxygen; R, respiratory exchange ratio; SBP, systolic blood pressure; SpO_2, oxygen saturation by pulse oximetry; VC, vital capacity; $\dot{V}E$, minute ventilation; $\dot{V}E/\dot{V}O_2$, ventilatory equivalent for oxygen; VT, tidal volume.

CASE 83

Mixed Disorder: Chronic Bronchitis and Obesity

To view this case please access the eBook bundled with this text. Instructions are located on the inside front cover.

CASE 84

Mixed Disorder: Peripheral Arterial Disease, Anemia, Carboxyhemoglobinemia, and Cardiac Dysfunction

CLINICAL FINDINGS

This 54-year-old bartender was referred for preoperative study to evaluate his exercise capacity. He had smoked at least 60 pack-years but denied cardiac or respiratory symptoms. He had not had regular medical care but presented with calf pain after walking one block and occasionally also at rest. Lower extremity angiography had shown obstructive arterial disease in the left iliac and superficial femoral arteries. He was also found to be mildly anemic (hematocrit = 34), with occult blood in the stool. Demographic and respiratory function data are shown in **Table 10.84.1**.

TABLE 10.84.1 Selected Respiratory Function Data

Measurement	Predicted	Measured
Age (years)		54
Sex		Male
Height (cm)		168
Weight (kg)	72	60
Hematocrit (%)		34
VC (L)	3.94	3.84
IC (L)	2.63	3.64
TLC (L)	5.86	7.16
FEV_1 (L)	3.12	3.07
FEV_1/VC (%)	79	80
MVV (L/min)	136	110
DLCO (mL/mm Hg/min)	23.0	22.9

Abbreviations: DLCO, diffusing capacity of the lung for carbon monoxide; FEV_1, forced expiratory volume in 1 second; IC, inspiratory capacity; MVV, maximum voluntary ventilation; VC, vital capacity; TLC, total lung capacity.

EXERCISE FINDINGS

The patient performed exercise on a cycle ergometer. He pedaled at 60 rpm without added load for 3 minutes. The work rate was then increased 15 W/min to his symptom-limited maximum. Blood was sampled every second minute, and intra-arterial blood pressure was recorded from a percutaneously placed brachial artery catheter. Resting and exercise electrocardiograms were normal. He stopped exercise because of severe leg pain, which was more prominent on the left. Exercise data are summarized in **Tables 10.84.2** and **10.84.3** and in **Figure 10.84.1**.

INTERPRETATION

Comments

The resting respiratory function is normal, including the diffusing capacity. Carboxyhemoglobin was 5.6% on an arterial blood sample prior to exercise.

Analysis

The patient had a history of claudication and ended exercise with this symptom, consistent with peripheral arterial disease, at a very low peak oxygen uptake ($\dot{V}O_2$). Anaerobic threshold was also low. There was no suggestion of ventilatory limitation. In contrast, there was flattening of the oxygen (O_2)-pulse response and shallow change in $\dot{V}O_2$/change in work rate ($\Delta\dot{V}O_2/\Delta WR$); these are consistent with an O_2-flow problem that could be attributed to peripheral arterial disease. However, a clear feature of this test was the very high minute ventilation ($\dot{V}E$) versus carbon dioxide output ($\dot{V}CO_2$) slope and very high ventilatory equivalent for carbon dioxide ($\dot{V}E/\dot{V}CO_2$) at the anaerobic threshold, highly suggestive of abnormal lung gas exchange in this range. Although hyperventilation could contribute to this finding, respiratory exchange ratio was not elevated, and the physiological dead space–tidal volume ratio (VD/VT) calculated

TABLE 10.84.2 Selected Exercise Data

Measurement	Predicted	Measured
Peak $\dot{V}O_2$ (L/min)	1.90	0.82
Maximum heart rate (beats/min)	161	141
Maximum O_2 pulse (mL/beat)	11.8	5.8
$\Delta\dot{V}O_2/\Delta WR$ (mL/min/W)	10.3	6.2
AT (L/min)	>0.84	0.7
Blood pressure (mm Hg [rest, max])		168/72, 255/114
Maximum $\dot{V}E$ (L/min)		60
Exercise breathing reserve (L/min)	<15	50
$\dot{V}E/\dot{V}CO_2$ @ *AT* or lowest	28.1	44.8
PaO_2 (mm Hg [rest, max ex])		94, 117
$P(A - a)O_2$ (mm Hg [rest, max ex])		20, 11
$PaCO_2$ (mm Hg [rest, max ex])		31, 26
$P(a - ET)CO_2$ (mm Hg [rest, max ex])		3, 2
VD/VT (rest, heavy ex)		0.45, 0.38
HCO_3^- (mEq/L [rest, 2-min recov])		20, 16

Abbreviations: *AT*, anaerobic threshold; $\Delta\dot{V}O_2/\Delta WR$, change in $\dot{V}O_2$/change in work rate; HCO_3^-, bicarbonate; ex, exercise; max, maximum; O_2, oxygen; $P(A - a)O_2$, alveolar-arterial PO_2 difference; $P(a - ET)CO_2$, arterial-end-tidal PCO_2 difference; recov, recovery; VD/VT, physiological dead space-tidal volume ratio; $\dot{V}E$, minute ventilation; $\dot{V}E/\dot{V}CO_2$, ventilatory equivalent for carbon dioxide; $\dot{V}O_2$, oxygen uptake.

from arterial blood gases was high. This is a feature of either lung disease or chronic heart failure but not of uncomplicated peripheral arterial disease. Given the normal resting pulmonary function studies, heart failure is likely in this patient, although a primary pulmonary vascular process could also cause this finding and should be considered if cardiac dysfunction is not confirmed. Blood pressure was high at rest and increased further with exercise. Finally, the patient's elevated carboxyhemoglobin level, together with anemia, further reduced O_2 flow. Therefore, several problems contributed to limiting O_2 delivery in this patient, including peripheral arterial disease, low arterial O_2 content, and probably low stroke volume.

Referring to the end of Flowchart 1 in Chapter 9, the category of peripheral arterial disease is characterized by several findings demonstrated in this case including leg pain, hypertension, mildly elevated heart rate reserve, and shallow $\Delta\dot{V}O_2/\Delta WR$ (**Table 10.84.2**).

Conclusion

This patient's exercise limitation due to peripheral arterial disease was compounded by reduction in arterial O_2 content. Although he stopped exercise due to the local symptoms of claudication and showed characteristic features of that condition, the gas exchange analyses also identified findings pointing to an additional undiagnosed impairment of central hemodynamics.

TABLE 10.84.3 Air Breathing

Time (min)	Work rate (W)	BP (mm Hg)	HR (min^{-1})	f (min^{-1})	$\dot{V}E$ (L/min BTPS)	$\dot{V}CO_2$ (L/min STPD)	$\dot{V}O_2$ (L/min STPD)	$\frac{\dot{V}O_2}{HR}$ (mL/beat)	R	pH	HCO_3^- (mEq/L)	PO_2, mm Hg ET	a	(A − a)	PCO_2, mm Hg ET	a	(a − ET)	$\frac{\dot{V}E}{\dot{V}CO_2}$	$\frac{\dot{V}E}{\dot{V}O_2}$	$\frac{VD}{VT}$
0	Rest	168/72								7.43	20		90			31				
0.5	Rest		93	18	12.0	0.20	0.24	2.6	0.83			116			27			52	44	
1.0	Rest		94	15	14.0	0.25	0.29	3.1	0.86			117			28			51	44	
1.5	Rest		92	16	14.3	0.19	0.23	2.5	0.83			116			28			68	56	
2.0	Rest	168/72	95	14	11.7	0.19	0.23	2.4	0.83	7.42	20	116	94	20	28	31	3	55	46	0.45
2.5	Rest		93	16	12.6	0.22	0.29	3.1	0.76			113			29			51	39	
3.0	Rest		92	16	11.1	0.19	0.23	2.5	0.83			115			29			51	42	
3.5	Unloaded		100	19	15.7	0.27	0.32	3.2	0.84			117			28			52	44	
4.0	Unloaded		108	20	17.9	0.31	0.35	3.2	0.89			119			27			52	46	
4.5	Unloaded		109	20	19.1	0.34	0.39	3.6	0.87			118			27			51	45	
5.0	Unloaded		110	20	20.5	0.38	0.43	3.9	0.88			117			28			49	44	
5.5	Unloaded		110	22	22.5	0.45	0.50	4.5	0.90			118			28			46	41	
6.0	Unloaded	231/93	111	21	22.3	0.46	0.52	4.7	0.88	7.43	20	117	97	20	28	30	2	45	39	0.33
6.5	15		114	22	25.2	0.54	0.59	5.2	0.92			118			28			43	40	
7.0	15		116	24	27.1	0.57	0.61	5.3	0.93			120			27			44	41	
7.5	30		118	24	26.8	0.56	0.59	5.0	0.95			119			28			44	42	
8.0	30	245/102	121	24	32.3	0.68	0.69	5.7	0.99	7.43	19	121	106	15	27	29	2	45	44	0.31
8.5	45		127	28	37.4	0.74	0.69	5.4	1.07			124			25			47	51	
9.0	45		128	31	40.1	0.78	0.72	5.6	1.08			124			26			48	52	
9.5	60		134	36	48.6	0.86	0.72	5.4	1.19			129			23			53	63	
10.0	60	255/114	141	38	59.7	1.02	0.82	5.8	1.24	7.44	17	128	117	11	24	26	2	55	69	0.38
10.5	Recovery		123	30	43.9	0.83	0.72	5.9	1.15			137			25			50	57	
11.0	Recovery		113	25	38.6	0.74	0.61	5.4	1.21			127			25			49	60	
11.5	Recovery		110	28	35.9	0.66	0.52	4.7	1.27			128			25			51	64	
12.0	Recovery	258/102	107	26	31.7	0.59	0.46	4.3	1.28	7.39	16	127	117	11	26	27	1	50	64	0.34

Abbreviations: BP, blood pressure; BTPS, body temperature pressure saturated; f, frequency; HCO_3^-, bicarbonate; HR, heart rate; $P(A - a)O_2$, alveolar-arterial PO_2 difference; $P(a - ET)CO_2$, arterial-end-tidal PCO_2 difference; $PETCO_2$, end-tidal PCO_2; $PETO_2$, end-tidal PO_2; R, respiratory exchange ratio; STPD, standard temperature pressure dry; $\dot{V}CO_2$, carbon dioxide output; VD/VT, physiological dead space–tidal volume ratio; $\dot{V}E$, minute ventilation; $\dot{V}E/\dot{V}CO_2$, ventilatory equivalent for carbon dioxide; $\dot{V}E/\dot{V}O_2$, ventilatory equivalent for oxygen; $\dot{V}O_2$, oxygen uptake.

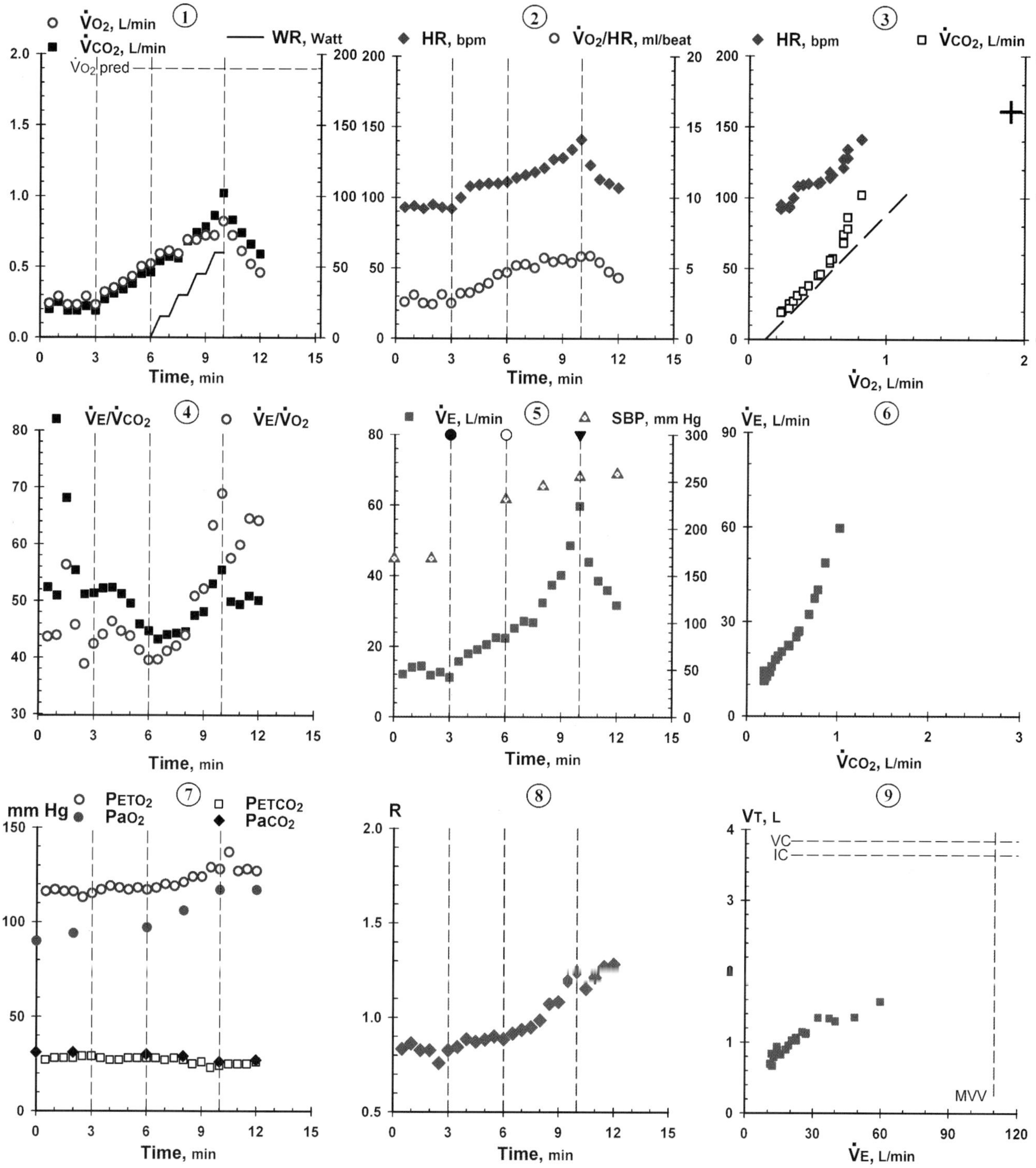

FIGURE 10.84.1. Vertical dashed lines in the panels in the left and middle columns indicate, from left to right, the beginning of unloaded cycling, start of increasing work rate (WR) at 15 W/min, and start of recovery. In **panel 1**, the increase in WR (right y-axis) is plotted with a scale of 100 W to 1 L of $\dot{V}O_2$ (left y-axis) such that WR is plotted parallel to a oxygen uptake ($\dot{V}O_2$) slope of 10 mL/min/W. In **panel 3**, carbon dioxide output ($\dot{V}CO_2$) (right y-axis) is plotted as a function of $\dot{V}O_2$ (x-axis) with identical scales so that the diagonal dashed line has a slope of 1 (45°). The $\dot{V}CO_2$ increasing more steeply than $\dot{V}O_2$ defines carbon dioxide derived from bicarbonate buffer, as long as ventilatory equivalent for carbon dioxide ($\dot{V}E/\dot{V}CO_2$) (**panel 4**) is not increasing and end-tidal PCO_2 ($PETCO_2$) (**panel 7**) is not decreasing, simultaneously. The black + symbol in **panel 3** indicates predicted peak values of heart rate (left y-axis) and $\dot{V}O_2$ for this individual. Abbreviations: HR, heart rate; IC, inspiratory capacity; MVV, maximum voluntary ventilation; $PETO_2$, end-tidal PO_2; R, respiratory exchange ratio; SBP, systolic blood pressure; VC, vital capacity; $\dot{V}E$, minute ventilation; $\dot{V}E/\dot{V}O_2$, ventilatory equivalent for oxygen; V_T, tidal volume.

CASE 85

Mixed Disorder: Mild Interstitial Lung Disease, Obstructive Airway Disease, and Myocardial Ischemia

CLINICAL FINDINGS

This 54-year-old man was referred for cardiopulmonary exercise testing because of his work exposure to asbestos of 15 years. He was a former smoker with a 30 pack-year history of cigarette use. He denied dyspnea, cough, chest pain, weight change, or ankle edema. He got little exercise and felt numbness in his legs after 20 minutes of walking. He was treated for borderline hypertension and dyslipidemia. There were crackles at the left lung base, and a chest roentgenogram showed linear interstitial changes in that area. Heart sounds and the resting electrocardiogram (ECG) were normal. Demographic and respiratory function data are shown in **Table 10.85.1**.

EXERCISE FINDINGS

The patient performed exercise on a cycle ergometer. He pedaled at 60 rpm without an added load for 3 minutes. The work rate was then increased 15 W/min to tolerance. Heart rate (HR) and rhythm were continuously monitored; 12-lead ECGs were obtained during rest, exercise, and recovery. Blood pressure was measured with a sphygmomanometer, and arterial oxygen (O_2) saturation was estimated with a pulse oximeter. The patient appeared to give a good effort and stopped exercise because of leg fatigue; he denied chest pain or dyspnea during or after the study. Significant ST-segment depression in leads II, III, aVF, and V3 to V6 was noted beginning at the 120-W work rate, with a maximum of 2.5-mm depression at end of exercise. The ST-segment abnormalities resolved after 9 minutes of recovery. No ectopy was present. Saturation as estimated by oximetry remained normal.

INTERPRETATION

Comments

Resting studies showed a mild ventilatory defect, which is at least in part due to airflow obstruction; the DLCO was normal.

Analysis

Peak oxygen uptake ($\dot{V}O_2$) was mildly decreased, but the anaerobic threshold was normal. Despite mildly abnormal pulmonary function at rest, the patient did not appear to be ventilatory limited during exercise with a high breathing reserve and noninvasive estimates of lung gas exchange were normal (ventilatory equivalent for carbon dioxide [$\dot{V}E/\dot{V}CO_2$] at the anaerobic threshold). The HR-$\dot{V}O_2$ relationship was normal (panel 3) until about the time the ECG showed evidence of myocardial ischemia at which point the HR increased more rapidly. This is also shown as a marked flattening of the O_2 pulse during the last minutes of exercise. The plateau in the O_2 pulse for the last 4 minutes of exercise at a level below the predicted maximum suggests that either both stroke volume and $C(a - \bar{v})O_2$ difference had reached

TABLE 10.85.1 Selected Respiratory Function Data

Measurement	Predicted	Measured
Age (y)		54
Sex		Male
Height (cm)		191
Weight (kg)	90	98
Hematocrit (%)		47
VC (L)	5.36	4.79
IC (L)	3.58	3.78
FEV_1 (L)	4.25	3.05
FEV_1/VC (%)	79	64
MVV (L/min)	164	126
DLCO (mL/mm Hg/min)	29.5	27.7

Abbreviations: DLCO, diffusing capacity of lung for carbon monoxide; FEV_1, forced expiratory volume in 1 second; IC, inspiratory capacity; MVV, maximum voluntary ventilation; VC, vital capacity.

TABLE 10.85.2 Selected Exercise Data

Measurement	Predicted	Measured
Peak $\dot{V}O_2$ (L/min)	2.81	2.09
Maximum heart rate (beats/min)	166	142
Maximum O_2 pulse (mL/beat)	16.9	14.8
$\Delta\dot{V}O_2/\Delta WR$ (mL/min/W)	10.3	8.9
AT (L/min)	>1.21	1.4
Blood pressure (mm Hg [rest, max])		154/90, 198/78
Maximum $\dot{V}E$ (L/min)		72
Exercise breathing reserve (L/min)	>15	54
$\dot{V}E/\dot{V}CO_2$ @ *AT* or lowest	26.8	28.4

Abbreviations: *AT*, anaerobic threshold; O_2, oxygen; $\dot{V}E$, minute ventilation; $\dot{V}E/\dot{V}CO_2$, ventilatory equivalent for CO_2; $\dot{V}O_2$, oxygen uptake; $\Delta\dot{V}O_2/\Delta WR$, change in $\dot{V}O_2$/change in work rate.

TABLE 10.85.3 Air Breathing

Time (min)	Work rate (W)	BP (mm Hg)	HR (min^{-1})	f (min^{-1})	$\dot{V}E$ (L/min BTPS)	$\dot{V}CO_2$ (L/min STPD)	$\dot{V}O_2$ (L/min STPD)	$\frac{\dot{V}O_2}{HR}$ (mL/beat)	R	pH	HCO_3^- (mEq/L)	PO_2, mm Hg ET	PO_2, mm Hg a	PO_2, mm Hg (A – a)	PCO_2, mm Hg ET	PCO_2, mm Hg a	PCO_2, mm Hg (a – ET)	$\frac{\dot{V}E}{\dot{V}CO_2}$	$\frac{\dot{V}E}{\dot{V}O_2}$	$\frac{VD}{VT}$
0	Rest	154/90																		
0.5	Rest		77	5	16.6	0.45	0.53	6.9	0.85			106			35			36	31	
1.0	Rest		78	10	14.9	0.44	0.50	6.4	0.88			112			33			32	28	
1.5	Rest		80	6	12.4	0.37	0.43	5.4	0.86			109			34			32	28	
2.0	Rest	150/96	79	5	9.9	0.32	0.40	5.1	0.80			107			34			30	24	
2.5	Rest		77	9	13.5	0.38	0.48	6.2	0.79			107			34			34	27	
3.0	Rest		79	10	9.4	0.27	0.32	4.1	0.84			107			35			32	27	
3.5	Unloaded		83	16	18.1	0.52	0.70	8.4	0.74			102			36			32	24	
4.0	Unloaded		82	13	16.4	0.50	0.64	7.8	0.78			104			36			31	24	
4.5	Unloaded		84	14	18.5	0.58	0.74	8.8	0.78			103			37			30	23	
5.0	Unloaded		86	15	16.7	0.52	0.66	7.7	0.79			100			39			30	23	
5.5	Unloaded		88	13	21.0	0.67	0.80	9.1	0.84			104			37			30	25	
6.0	Unloaded	148/88	85	13	26.1	0.82	0.93	10.9	0.88			105			37			30	27	
6.5	15		87	15	22.6	0.74	0.85	9.8	0.87			103			39			29	25	
7.0	15		87	15	24.7	0.77	0.88	10.1	0.88			107			37			30	27	
7.5	30		88	12	19.9	0.65	0.75	8.5	0.87			106			37			29	25	
8.0	30	152/90	90	16	27.5	0.85	0.98	10.9	0.87			107			36			31	27	
8.5	45		92	12	22.5	0.74	0.86	9.3	0.86			100			41			29	25	
9.0	45		94	13	28.3	0.94	1.06	11.3	0.89			105			39			29	26	
9.5	60		98	16	30.9	1.02	1.17	11.9	0.87			105			39			29	25	
10.0	60	148/84	98	16	33.9	1.12	1.25	12.8	0.90			104			39			29	26	
10.5	75		99	15	35.6	1.21	1.34	13.5	0.90			103			41			28	26	
11.0	75		103	17	37.7	1.27	1.36	13.2	0.93			105			40			29	27	
11.5	90		102	18	38.3	1.31	1.39	13.6	0.94			105			41			28	26	
12.0	90	178/86	108	18	43.4	1.49	1.54	14.3	0.97			105			41			28	27	
12.5	105		112	21	49.4	1.62	1.57	14.0	1.03			110			39			29	30	
13.0	105		109	20	49.6	1.71	1.71	15.7	1.00			103			44			28	28	
13.5	120		115	22	55.1	1.83	1.69	14.7	1.08			110			40			29	31	
14.0	120	170/88	120	23	51.4	1.79	1.72	14.3	1.04			108			41			28	29	
14.5	135		128	24	60.8	2.04	1.87	14.6	1.09			111			39			29	31	
15.0	135		132	25	64.8	2.15	1.95	14.8	1.10			110			41			29	32	
15.5	150		139	27	64.4	2.17	1.98	14.2	1.10			108			43			29	31	
16.0	150	198/78	142	30	71.9	2.34	2.09	14.7	1.12			113			39			30	33	
16.5	Recovery		137	23	68.4	2.33	2.02	14.7	1.15			113			40			29	33	
17.0	Recovery		122	23	55.4	1.95	1.52	12.5	1.28			114			42			27	35	
17.5	Recovery		119	22	60.1	2.02	1.29	10.8	1.57			119			40			29	45	
18.0	Recovery		127	20	58.5	1.81	1.04	8.2	1.74			124			37			31	55	

Abbreviations: BP, blood pressure; BTPS, body temperature pressure saturated; f, frequency; HCO_3^-, bicarbonate; HR, heart rate; $P(A - a)O_2$, alveolar-arterial PO_2 difference; $P(a - ET)CO_2$, arterial-end-tidal PCO_2 difference; $PETCO_2$, end-tidal PCO_2; $PETO_2$, end-tidal PO_2; R, respiratory exchange ratio; STPD, standard temperature pressure dry; $\dot{V}CO_2$, carbon dioxide output; VD/VT, physiological dead space-tidal volume ratio; $\dot{V}E$, minute ventilation; $\dot{V}E/\dot{V}CO_2$, ventilatory equivalent for CO_2; $\dot{V}E/\dot{V}O_2$, ventilatory equivalent for O_2; $\dot{V}O_2$, oxygen uptake.

their maximal values, or that stroke volume was decreasing as $C(a - \bar{v})O_2$ difference was increasing. Therefore, instead of the expected findings from lung disease, he was limited more by myocardial ischemia and its effects on O_2 delivery.

The flowchart method outlined in Chapter 9 results in a similar conclusion. Peak $\dot{V}O_2$ was mildly decreased, but the anaerobic threshold was normal leading to Flowchart 3. Subsequently, high breathing reserve and abnormal exercise ECG suggest a diagnosis of myocardial ischemia, although the patient had no chest pain or distress.

Conclusion

This patient was evaluated because of findings of chronic lung disease but the primary limitation to exercise appeared to be previously undiagnosed exercise-induced myocardial ischemia, most likely due to coronary artery disease. The ECG findings of myocardial ischemia were associated with concurrent gas exchange evidence of myocardial dysfunction. The normal ventilatory equivalents indicate essentially normal $\dot{V}/\dot{Q}$ matching despite the mild obstructive and interstitial lung disease.

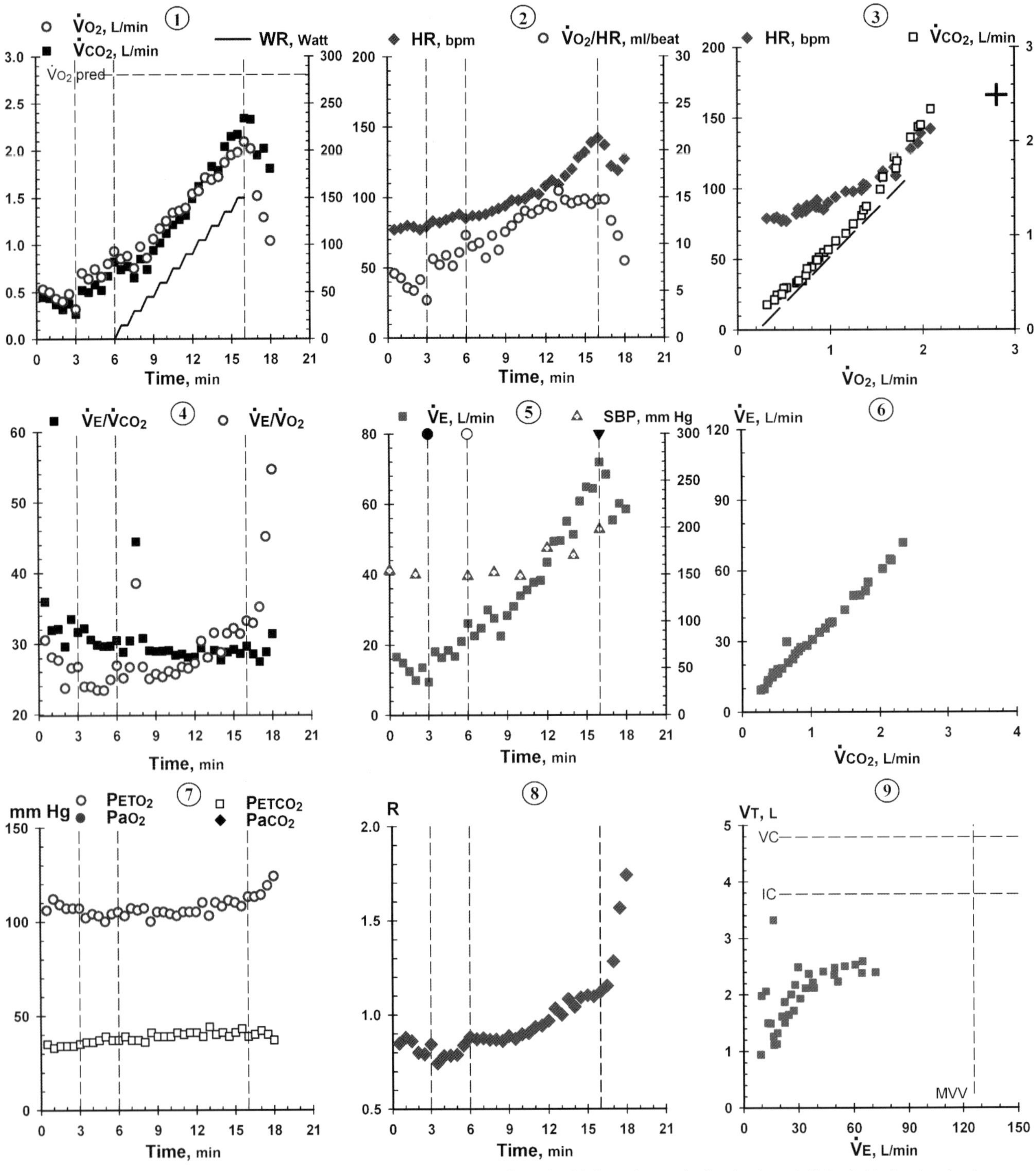

FIGURE 10.85.1. Vertical dashed lines in the panels in the left and middle columns indicate, from left to right, the beginning of unloaded cycling, start of increasing work rate (WR) at 15 W/min, and start of recovery. In **panel 1**, the increase in WR (right y-axis) is plotted with a scale of 100 W to 1 L of oxygen uptake ($\dot{V}O_2$) (left y-axis) such that WR is plotted parallel to a $\dot{V}O_2$ slope of 10 mL/min/W. In **panel 3**, carbon dioxide output ($\dot{V}CO_2$) (right y-axis) is plotted as a function of $\dot{V}O_2$ (x-axis) with identical scales so that the diagonal dashed line has a slope of 1 (45°). The $\dot{V}CO_2$ increasing more steeply than $\dot{V}O_2$ defines carbon dioxide (CO_2) derived from bicarbonate buffer, as long as ventilatory equivalent for CO_2 ($\dot{V}E/\dot{V}CO_2$) (**panel 4**) is not increasing and end-tidal PCO_2 ($PETCO_2$) (**panel 7**) is not decreasing, simultaneously. The black + symbol in **panel 3** indicates predicted peak values of heart rate (HR) (left y-axis) and $\dot{V}O_2$ for this individual. Abbreviations: IC, inspiratory capacity; MVV, maximum voluntary ventilation; $PETO_2$, end-tidal PO_2; R, respiratory exchange ratio; SBP, systolic blood pressure; VC, vital capacity; $\dot{V}E$, minute ventilation; $\dot{V}E/\dot{V}O_2$, ventilatory equivalent for oxygen; V_T, tidal volume.

CASE 86

Chronic Heart Failure With Preserved Ejection Fraction and Obesity Hypoventilation Syndrome

CLINICAL FINDINGS

A 65-year-old man with heart failure with preserved ejection fraction had a screening exercise test for enrollment in a clinical trial. Comorbid medical problems included diabetes, hyperlipidemia, hypertension, obesity, and obesity hypoventilation syndrome. He had been hospitalized twice for heart failure exacerbation, once complicated by respiratory failure requiring mechanical ventilation. At the time of testing, he reported his baseline walking tolerance of one or two blocks before stopping with fatigue and dyspnea. Medications included carvedilol, metformin, lisinopril, pravastatin, furosemide, and famotidine as well as continuous positive airway pressure at night for sleep disordered breathing. Physical examination was notable for morbid obesity. Breath sounds were clear. There were regular heart tones and an S_4 but no murmur. There was mild edema of the ankles bilaterally. A recent echocardiogram showed concentric left ventricular hypertrophy with ejection fraction of 55% to 60% and dilated right ventricle without other valvular or structural abnormalities. Resting electrocardiogram showed sinus rhythm. Demographic data are shown in **Table 10.86.1**.

EXERCISE FINDINGS

The patient exercised on a cycle ergometer beginning with 3 minutes of unloaded pedaling at 60 rpm followed by continuous increase in work rate by 10 W/min until the test ended with symptoms of leg fatigue. There were no ischemic changes on the electrocardiogram. Exercise data are summarized in **Tables 10.86.2** and **10.86.3** and in **Figure 10.86.1**.

TABLE 10.86.1 Demographic Data

Measurement	Predicted	Measured
Age (y)		65
Sex		M
Height (cm)		175
Weight (kg)		155
Body mass index (kg/m^2)		50.5
Hb (g/dL)		15.2

Abbreviation: Hb, hemoglobin.

INTERPRETATION

Comment

This test was conducted to characterize his heart failure for a clinical research protocol. It is presented to highlight how coexisting factors can confound the interpretation of cardiopulmonary exercise testing variables used to grade the severity of heart failure. In particular, hypoventilation (hypercapnia) associated with this patient's obesity hypoventilation syndrome resulted in lower values for ventilatory equivalents and the minute ventilation ($\dot{V}_E$) to carbon dioxide output ($\dot{V}CO_2$) slope than would be characteristic of chronic heart failure. He had a blunted ventilatory response to exercise, which made it difficult to identify the anaerobic threshold (*AT*) from gas exchange. Finally, arterial desaturation complicated interpretation of the limited rise of oxygen (O_2) pulse.

TABLE 10.86.2 Selected Exercise Data

Measurement	Predicted	Measured
Peak $\dot{V}O_2$ (L/min)	2.52	1.67
Peak $\dot{V}O_2$ (mL/min/kg)		10.8
Maximum heart rate (beats/min)	155	118
Maximum O_2 pulse (mL/beat)	16.3	14.1
$\Delta\dot{V}O_2/\Delta WR$ (mL/min/W)	10.3	10.0
AT (L/min)	>1.17	1.0
Blood pressure (mm Hg [rest, peak ex])		144/84, 184/90
Maximum $\dot{V}_E$ (L/min)		38
Breathing reserve (L/min)		NA
$\dot{V}_E/\dot{V}CO_2$ @ *AT* (L/min)	<32	23
$\dot{V}_E$-$\dot{V}CO_2$ slope	<32	20
V_D/V_T (rest, peak)[a]		0.45, 0.32
SpO_2 (% [rest, peak ex])		89, 75

Abbreviations: *AT*, anaerobic threshold; $\Delta\dot{V}O_2/\Delta WR$, change in $\dot{V}O_2$/change in work rate; ex, exercise; NA, not applicable; O_2, oxygen; V_D/V_T, physiological dead space–tidal volume ratio; $\dot{V}_E$, minute ventilation; $\dot{V}O_2$, oxygen uptake.

[a]Calculated using $PtcCO_2$.

TABLE 10.86.3 Cycle Exercise

Time (min)	Work rate (W)	BP (mm Hg)	HR (min^{-1})	f (min^{-1})	$\dot{V}E$ (L/min BTPS)	$\dot{V}CO_2$ (L/min STPD)	$\dot{V}O_2$ (L/min STPD)	$\frac{\dot{V}O_2}{HR}$ (mL/beat)	R	pH	HCO_3^- (mEq/L)	PO_2, mm Hg and SpO_2, % ET	SpO_2	(A − a)	PCO_2, mm Hg ET	tc	(a − ET)	$\frac{\dot{V}E}{\dot{V}CO_2}$	$\frac{\dot{V}E}{\dot{V}O_2}$	$\frac{V_D}{V_T}$
1.0	Rest	144/84	80	20	15.1	0.56	0.54	6.8	1.04			94	87		54	53.3		27	28	0.42
1.5	Rest		80	22	14.4	0.55	0.58	7.2	0.96			89	89		56	55.1		26	25	0.42
2.0	Rest		89	23	21.4	0.87	0.85	9.6	1.02			93	82		54	56.6		25	25	0.40
2.5	Rest		85	23	18.7	0.73	0.74	8.8	0.98			91	50		54	57.3		26	25	0.43
3.0	Rest		83	24	17.0	0.62	0.64	7.7	0.97			91	84		55	57.6		28	27	0.47
3.5	Rest		81	22	16.2	0.60	0.62	7.6	0.97			90	85		55	58.1		27	26	0.47
4.0	Rest		79	19	14.8	0.57	0.53	6.7	1.06			94	87		54	58.2		26	28	0.45
4.5	Rest	140/82	80	22	15.5	0.56	0.54	6.7	1.04			96	88		53	57.8		27	29	0.48
5.0	Rest		80	18	14.0	0.53	0.52	6.5	1.02			93	88		54	57.6		26	27	0.45
5.5	Unloaded		82	25	18.0	0.65	0.64	7.9	1.02			94	88		53	57.3		28	28	0.48
6.0	Unloaded		85	24	22.8	0.90	0.86	10.1	1.05			96	87		53	57.3		25	27	0.43
6.5	Unloaded		87	19	20.0	0.85	0.83	9.6	1.02			92	88		55	57		24	24	0.38
7.0	Unloaded		90	22	25.5	1.12	1.08	12.0	1.03			93	86		55	56.6		23	24	0.36
7.5	Unloaded		91	24	24.2	1.05	0.99	10.9	1.06			93	86		56	56.6		23	24	0.36
8.0	Unloaded	152/86	94	25	26.6	1.14	1.08	11.5	1.05			93	86		56	56.6		23	25	0.37
8.5	4		95	26	26.9	1.17	1.11	11.6	1.06			92	85		57	57.3		23	24	0.37
9.0	9		95	25	26.2	1.14	1.09	11.4	1.04			90	84		57	57.6		23	24	0.37
9.5	14		97	28	29.2	1.28	1.17	12.0	1.09			92	84		57	58.1		23	25	0.37
10.0	19		99	27	29.2	1.32	1.26	12.8	1.05			90	82		58	58.4		22	23	0.36
10.5	24	164/86	101	28	31.0	1.40	1.31	13.0	1.06			91	81		58	59		22	24	0.36
11.0	29		101	24	29.3	1.36	1.27	12.5	1.07			90	80		59	59.3		22	23	0.35
11.5	34		102	28	33.3	1.54	1.44	14.1	1.07			91	79		58	59.5		22	23	0.36
12.0	39		106	26	30.5	1.44	1.36	12.8	1.06			89	80		60	59.6		21	22	0.34
12.5	44		109	28	34.4	1.62	1.50	13.8	1.08			91	78		59	59.9		21	23	0.35
13.0	49	174/90	111	29	35.7	1.69	1.53	13.8	1.10			91	78		59	59.9		21	23	0.34
13.5	53		114	28	35.7	1.75	1.59	13.9	1.10			91	78		60	59.9		20	22	0.32
14.0	58		116	28	36.7	1.80	1.62	13.9	1.11			90	77		60	59.9		20	23	0.32
14.5	63		118	30	38.1	1.89	1.67	14.1	1.13			90	76		61	60.2		20	23	0.32
15.0	Recovery	184/90	119	29	35.8	1.79	1.59	13.4	1.12			89	75		63	60.6		20	22	0.32
15.5	Recovery		114	27	36.7	1.88	1.65	14.4	1.14			89	75		63	61.4		20	22	0.31
16.0	Recovery		113	27	33.2	1.67	1.49	13.2	1.12			87	75		64	61.8		20	22	0.32
16.5	Recovery		110	25	29.4	1.47	1.35	12.3	1.09			85	75		64	62.1		20	22	0.33
17.0	Recovery		108	28	31.5	1.51	1.35	12.5	1.12			88	75		62	62.9		21	23	0.37
17.5	Recovery	170/88	106	27	30.1	1.42	1.28	12.1	1.11			88	78		62	62.9		21	23	0.38
18.0	Recovery		104	28	29.9	1.38	1.24	12.0	1.11			89	78		61	62.6		22	24	0.39
18.5	Recovery		102	27	29.5	1.36	1.23	12.1	1.11			89	80		61	62.3		22	24	0.39
19.0	Recovery		99	27	26.9	1.21	1.10	11.1	1.10			88	80		61	62		22	24	0.40
19.5	Recovery	154/84	97	24	24.2	1.07	1.00	10.3	1.07			88	81		60	61.8		22	24	0.41
20.0	Recovery		96	24	25.2	1.11	0.96	10.0	1.16			92	81		59	61.8		23	26	0.4

Abbreviations: BP, blood pressure; BTPS, body temperature pressure saturated; f, frequency; HCO_3^-, bicarbonate; HR, heart rate; $P(A - a)O_2$, alveolar-arterial PO_2 difference; $P(a - ET)CO_2$, arterial-end-tidal PCO_2 difference; $PETCO_2$, end-tidal PCO_2; $PETO_2$, end-tidal PO_2; tc, transcutaneous; R, respiratory exchange ratio; STPD, standard temperature pressure dry; $\dot{V}CO_2$, carbon dioxide output; V_D/V_T, physiological dead space-tidal volume ratio; $\dot{V}E$, minute ventilation; $\dot{V}E/\dot{V}CO_2$, ventilatory equivalent for carbon dioxide; $\dot{V}E/\dot{V}O_2$, ventilatory equivalent for oxygen; $\dot{V}O_2$, oxygen uptake.

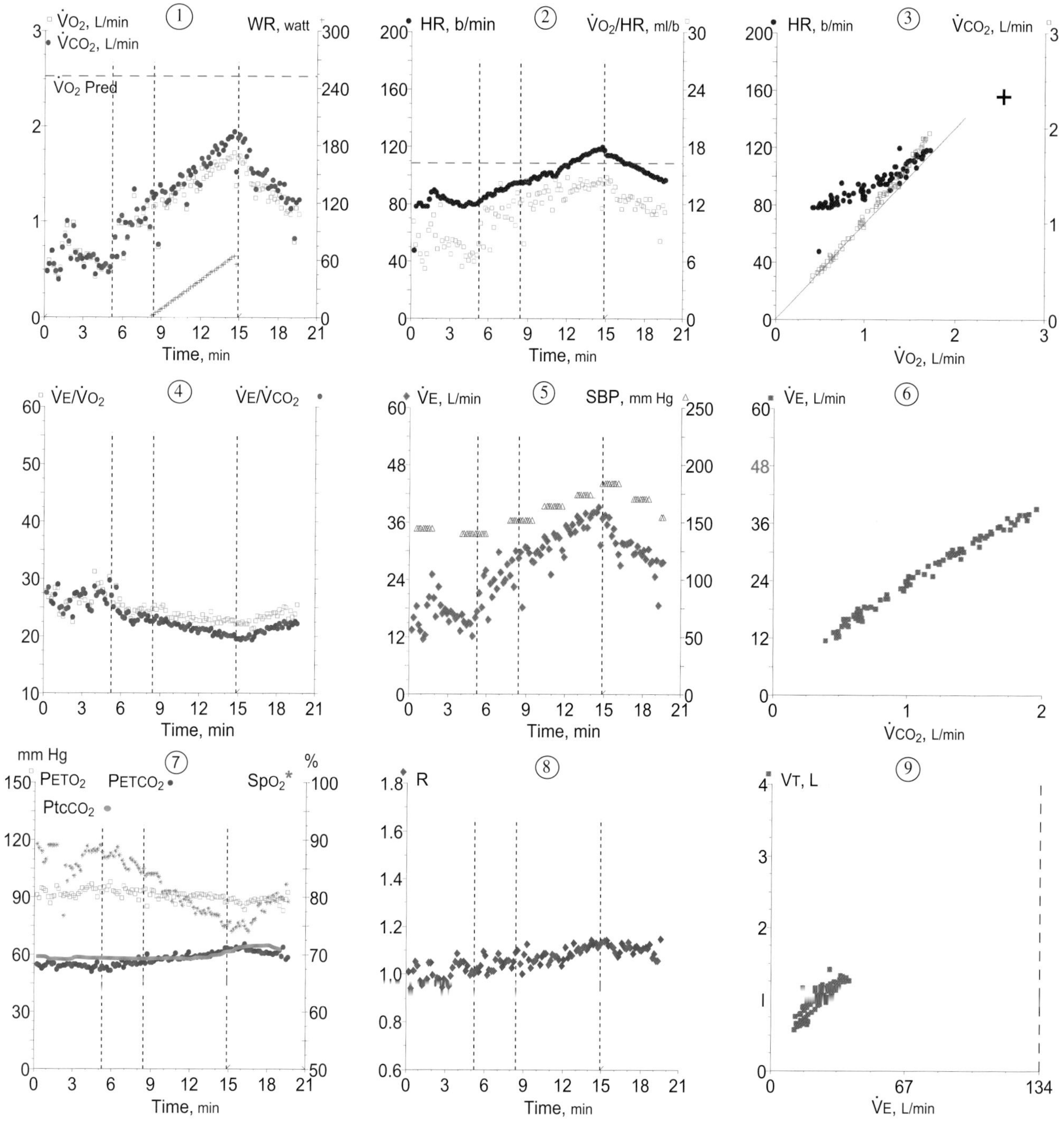

FIGURE 10.86.1. Vertical dashed lines in the panels in the left and middle columns indicate, from left to right, the beginning of unloaded cycling, start of increasing work rate (WR) at 10 W/min, and start of recovery. In **panel 1**, the increase in WR (right y-axis) is plotted with a scale of 100 W to 1 L of oxygen uptake ($\dot{V}O_2$) (left y-axis) such that WR is plotted parallel to a $\dot{V}O_2$ slope of 10 mL/min/W. Predicted peak $\dot{V}O_2$ is shown as a dashed horizontal line. In **panel 3**, carbon dioxide output ($\dot{V}CO_2$) (right y-axis) is plotted as a function of $\dot{V}O_2$ (x-axis) with identical scales so that the diagonal blue line has a slope of 1 (45°). The $\dot{V}CO_2$ increasing more steeply than $\dot{V}O_2$ defines carbon dioxide derived from bicarbonate buffer, as long as ventilatory equivalent for carbon dioxide ($\dot{V}E/\dot{V}CO_2$) (**panel 4**) is not increasing and end-tidal PCO_2 ($PETCO_2$) (**panel 7**) is not decreasing, simultaneously. The black + symbol in **panel 3** indicates predicted peak values of heart rate (HR) (left y-axis) and $\dot{V}O_2$ for this individual. Abbreviations: IC, inspiratory capacity; MVV, maximum voluntary ventilation; $PETO_2$, end-tidal partial pressure of oxygen; $PtcCO_2$, transcutaneous PCO_2; R, respiratory exchange ratio; SBP, systolic blood pressure; SpO_2, oxygen saturation as measured by pulse oximeter; VC, vital capacity; $\dot{V}E$, minute ventilation; $\dot{V}E/\dot{V}O_2$, ventilatory equivalent for oxygen; VT, tidal volume.

Analysis

Aerobic capacity was reduced (peak $\dot{V}O_2$ 67% predicted or approximately 22 mL/min/kg ideal weight), and capacity for ambulatory work was even more severely reduced (peak $\dot{V}O_2$ of 10.1 mL/min/kg actual weight).

Cardiovascular and metabolic responses: The $\dot{V}O_2$ was over 0.5 L/min at rest and exceeded 1 L/min during unloaded cycling, reflecting the elevated metabolic cost of supporting this patient's weight and lifting the legs against gravity. Peak $\dot{V}O_2$ was low and *AT* was at the lower limit of normal. The *AT* was somewhat difficult to identify because the normal ventilatory response to carbon dioxide was blunted and P_{CO_2} values rose over the course of the test. Consistent with the effects of β-blocker therapy, the rate of increase of heart rate relative to $\dot{V}O_2$ was shallow (panel 3 of **Fig. 10.86.1**) and the peak heart rate was lower than predicted maximum. The O_2 pulse nevertheless reached a plateau value that was lower than the predicted maximum, whereas it would be expected to be elevated if the only abnormality was constraint of heart rate. There are several potential factors that could account for low O_2 pulse. Stroke volume could be constrained either by left ventricular diastolic impairment or right ventricular failure. In addition, the Sp_{O_2}, and therefore arterial O_2 content, was low at rest and decreased progressively; this limits the potential to widen $C(a - \bar{v})_{O_2}$. There were additional findings in the early recovery period also implying impaired O_2 delivery and utilization. At the start of recovery, R values remained at end-exercise levels rather than increasing, consistent with an abnormally large O_2 deficit. Heart rate recovery was also slow, decreasing by only 6 beats/min at 1 minute into recovery.

Ventilatory responses: There is evidence of hypercapnia at rest with both end-tidal and transcutaneous P_{CO_2} values (mm Hg) in the mid-50s. Both of these measures climbed to the low 60s over the course of the test, and there was no evident respiratory compensation point.

Gas exchange efficiency: As noted earlier, there was both hypercapnia and hypoxemia at rest, which worsened with exercise. The ventilatory equivalents were normal, and even lower than average, but this cannot be interpreted to mean that physiological dead space–tidal volume ratio (V_D/V_T) is normal without taking into account the presence of hypercapnia. Using transcutaneous P_{CO_2} values as a surrogate for arterial P_{CO_2}, the V_D/V_T was indeed high at rest and remained above 0.30 throughout the test (see **Table 10.86.3**). The pulse oximeter readings suggest a degree of hypoxemia greater than would be expected due to the patient's hypoventilation alone. Hypoxemia is not characteristic of uncomplicated left heart failure but could be due to intrapulmonary shunting through atelectatic lung due to his body habitus or could result from another pulmonary process.

Conclusion

This patient had a clinical diagnosis of heart failure with preserved ejection fraction, but the exercise findings were complicated by coexistent chronic ventilatory failure. Two valuable observations can be made from this case. First, abnormal ventilatory responses had significant effects on variables commonly used to grade severity or estimate prognosis of heart failure, making ventilatory equivalent for carbon dioxide ($\dot{V}E/\dot{V}CO_2$) appear normal despite the fact that V_D/V_T was actually elevated. Second, although the test was not conducted for diagnostic purposes, but as a means of quantifying a known condition, thorough review of the data revealed findings that significantly changed the interpretation of the test values, and the differential diagnosis of the patient's condition.

CASE 87

Mixed Disease: Aortic Stenosis, Mitral Stenosis, and Obstructive Airway Disease

e To view this case please access the eBook bundled with this text. Instructions are located on the inside front cover.

CASE 88

Mixed Disorder: Obstructive Airway Disease, Talc Pneumoconiosis, and Pulmonary Vascular Disease

To view this case please access the eBook bundled with this text. Instructions are located on the inside front cover.

CASE 89

Mixed Disorder: Peripheral Arterial Disease and Obstructive Lung Disease: Cycle and Treadmill Exercise

CLINICAL FINDINGS

This 67-year-old man volunteered as a research subject for a study of chronic obstructive lung disease but was excluded from the research protocol because he identified calf pain, rather than dyspnea, as the limiting factor in his daily activities. He had an extensive smoking history. His only medications were inhaled bronchodilators and a statin. Examination of the lungs was notable for prolonged expiratory phase and scattered wheezes. Pulses were diminished in the right ankle. An electrocardiogram was unremarkable. Demographic and respiratory function data are shown in **Table 10.89.1**.

EXERCISE FINDINGS

Exercise tests were conducted on both a cycle ergometer and treadmill with an intervening rest period. On the cycle, after 2 minutes of rest, the patient pedaled at 60 rpm for 3 minutes without added resistance, after which the work rate was increased continuously by 20 W/min until he stopped with primary symptoms of right calf pain and lesser symptoms of dyspnea. For the treadmill, after 2 minutes of standing rest, the patient walked on the treadmill at 2 mph and zero grade for 3 minutes, after which the grade was increased by 2% each minute. The patient discontinued the test with the same symptoms as on the cycle. Pulse oximeter readings were 89% at rest and decreased to 86% during cycling and to 84% during treadmill walking. An electrocardiogram showed no significant changes. Exercise data for both tests are summarized in **Table 10.89.2**. Data for the cycle test are shown in **Table 10.89.3** and **Figure 10.89.1**, and for the treadmill test in **Table 10.89.4** and **Figure 10.89.2**.

TABLE 10.89.1 Selected Respiratory Function Data

Measurement	Predicted	Measured
Age (y)		67
Sex		Male
Height (cm)		180
Weight (kg)		72
VC (L)	4.70	4.68
FEV_1 (L)	3.49	1.20
FEV_1/VC (%)	74	26
MVV (L/min)	135	48

Abbreviations: FEV_1, forced expiratory volume in 1 second; MVV, maximum voluntary ventilation; VC, vital capacity.

Comment

Spirometry demonstrated very severe expiratory airflow obstruction. Based on measures of systolic blood pressures in upper and lower extremities, the ankle brachial index was calculated as 0.97 on the left (near-normal) but 0.54 on the right, indicative of peripheral arterial disease.

Analysis

The two tests were similar with peak $\dot{V}O_2$ reduced to around 60% of the modality-specific predicted value and the anaerobic threshold just below the lower limit of normal with either type of exercise. Consistent with termination of exercise prior to reaching maximal cardiac stress, the heart reserve was high. By the patient's report, he stopped due to claudication, so peripheral arterial disease was the proximal cause of limitation. Although symptoms were localized to the right calf and the ankle brachial index was near-normal in the left

TABLE 10.89.2 Selected Exercise Data

	Cycle		Treadmill	
Measurement	Predicted	Measured	Predicted	Measured
Peak $\dot{V}O_2$ (L/min)	1.96	1.17	2.18	1.25
Maximum heart rate (beats/min)	153	106	153	116
Maximum O_2 pulse (mL/beat)	12.8	10.8	14.2	11.1
$\Delta\dot{V}O_2/\Delta WR$ (mL/min/W)	10.3	6.8	10.3	—
AT (L/min)	>0.92	0.86	>1.02	0.92
Blood pressure (mm Hg [rest, max ex])		135/73, 190/134		126/80, 181/119
Maximum $\dot{V}E$ (L/min)		40		40
Exercise breathing reserve (L/min)	>15	8	>15	8
$\dot{V}E/\dot{V}CO_2$ @ *AT* or lowest	28.6	32.7	28.6	33.4
SpO_2 (% [rest, max ex])		89, 86		89, 84

Abbreviations: *AT*, anaerobic threshold; $\Delta\dot{V}O_2/\Delta WR$, change in $\dot{V}O_2$/change in work rate; ex, exercise; O_2, oxygen; SpO_2, oxygen saturation as measured by pulse oximetry; $\dot{V}E$, minute ventilation; $\dot{V}E/\dot{V}CO_2$, ventilatory equivalent for carbon dioxide; $\dot{V}O_2$, oxygen uptake.

TABLE 10.89.3 Air Breathing: Cycle Ergometer Test

Time (min)	Work rate (W)	BP (mm Hg)	HR (min^{-1})	f (min^{-1})	$\dot{V}E$ (L/min BTPS)	$\dot{V}CO_2$ (L/min STPD)	$\dot{V}O_2$ (L/min STPD)	$\dot{V}O_2$/HR (mL/beat)	R	pH	HCO_3^- (mEq/L)	PO_2, mm Hg ET	PO_2, mm Hg a	PO_2, mm Hg (A − a)	PCO_2, mm Hg ET	PCO_2, mm Hg a	PCO_2, mm Hg (a − ET)	$\dot{V}E/\dot{V}CO_2$	$\dot{V}E/\dot{V}O_2$	V_D/V_T
0.5	Rest	135/73	80	20	12.4	0.23	0.27	3.3	0.86			114			31			54	47	
1.0	Rest		81	20	12.3	0.22	0.26	3.3	0.85			114			30			55	47	
1.5	Rest		84	18	12.2	0.26	0.31	3.7	0.83			111			33			48	40	
2.0	Rest		84	18	11.4	0.22	0.26	3.1	0.84			113			32			52	44	
2.5	Unloaded	135/73	89	21	17.4	0.38	0.45	5.1	0.85			110			33			45	39	
3.0	Unloaded		88	20	16.4	0.36	0.44	5.0	0.83			110			34			45	38	
3.5	Unloaded		90	17	17.0	0.40	0.48	5.3	0.84			109			35			42	36	
4.0	Unloaded	144/71	86	17	17.4	0.41	0.49	5.7	0.84			108			35			42	36	
4.5	Unloaded		82	18	18.6	0.48	0.58	7.0	0.83			107			36			39	32	
5.0	Unloaded		86	17	17.7	0.43	0.50	5.8	0.85			108			35			41	35	
5.5	8	144/71	86	17	19.1	0.48	0.57	6.6	0.85			107			36			40	34	
6.0	19		88	14	16.5	0.43	0.51	5.8	0.85			105			38			38	32	
6.5	30	147/76	89	14	18.1	0.49	0.57	6.4	0.86			105			38			37	32	
7.0	38		92	17	21.2	0.55	0.63	6.9	0.87			107			37			39	34	
7.5	48		93	17	21.7	0.57	0.65	7.0	0.88			107			37			38	34	
8.0	57		94	17	24.0	0.66	0.74	7.9	0.88			106			38			36	32	
8.5	67	169/74	97	19	24.7	0.67	0.75	7.7	0.89			106			38			37	33	
9.0	75		100	18	27.0	0.77	0.86	8.6	0.90			105			40			35	32	
9.5	85		101	17	28.2	0.85	0.90	9.0	0.94			105			41			33	31	
10.0	94		102	17	31.1	0.96	1.00	9.8	0.95			105			42			33	31	
10.5	105	190/134	104	20	32.6	1.01	1.02	9.8	0.99			106			42			32	32	
11.0	114		106	23	39.1	1.23	1.17	11.0	1.05			107			43			32	33	
11.5	Recovery		101	22	37.6	1.25	1.12	11.1	1.11			107			45			30	33	
12.0	Recovery		101	22	39.9	1.35	1.15	11.4	1.17			108			45			30	35	
12.5	Recovery		101	21	36.5	1.22	0.97	9.6	1.26			111			45			30	38	
13.0	Recovery		101	21	37.4	1.20	0.91	9.0	1.32			113			43			31	41	

Abbreviations: BP, blood pressure; BTPS, body temperature pressure saturated; f, frequency; HCO_3^-, bicarbonate; HR, heart rate; $P(A - a)O_2$, alveolar-arterial PO_2 difference; $P(a - ET)CO_2$, arterial-end-tidal PCO_2 difference; $PETCO_2$, end-tidal PCO_2; $PETO_2$, end-tidal PO_2; R, respiratory exchange ratio; STPD, standard temperature pressure dry; $\dot{V}CO_2$, carbon dioxide output; V_D/V_T, physiological dead space-tidal volume ratio; $\dot{V}E$, minute ventilation; $\dot{V}E/\dot{V}CO_2$, ventilatory equivalent for carbon dioxide; $\dot{V}E/\dot{V}O_2$, ventilatory equivalent for oxygen; $\dot{V}O_2$, oxygen uptake.

TABLE 10.89.4 Air Breathing: Treadmill Test

Time (min)	Treadmill grade (%)*	BP (mm Hg)	HR (min^{-1})	f (min^{-1})	$\dot{V}E$ (L/min BTPS)	$\dot{V}CO_2$ (L/min STPD)	$\dot{V}O_2$ (L/min STPD)	$\dot{V}O_2$/HR (mL/beat)	R	pH	HCO_3^- (mEq/L)	PO_2, mm Hg ET	PO_2, mm Hg a	PO_2, mm Hg (A − a)	PCO_2, mm Hg ET	PCO_2, mm Hg a	PCO_2, mm Hg (a − ET)	$\dot{V}E/\dot{V}CO_2$	$\dot{V}E/\dot{V}O_2$	V_D/V_T
0.5	Rest	126/80	97	15	13.3	0.30	0.39	4.1	0.77			109			32			44	34	
1.0	Rest		96	18	10.3	0.19	0.25	2.6	0.74			110			31			55	41	
1.5	Rest		96	17	11.8	0.23	0.31	3.2	0.74			108			32			51	38	
2.0	Rest		97	18	11.0	0.21	0.29	3.0	0.73			107			33			51	38	
2.5	0		100	19	20.4	0.50	0.69	6.9	0.73			102			36			40	29	
3.0	0		102	20	20.3	0.48	0.66	6.5	0.73			103			35			42	31	
3.5	0		104	19	22.8	0.57	0.78	7.5	0.73			102			36			40	29	
4.0	0		106	18	25.4	0.69	0.92	8.7	0.74			100			38			37	27	
4.5	0		106	18	26.3	0.74	0.96	9.1	0.77			101			38			36	27	
5.0	0		105	18	26.3	0.75	0.95	9.0	0.79			101			39			35	28	
5.5	2.0	126/78	107	19	31.1	0.87	1.06	9.9	0.82			103			38			36	29	
6.0	2.0		107	19	29.5	0.84	0.99	9.3	0.85			104			39			35	30	
6.5	4.0		108	18	29.7	0.89	1.05	9.7	0.85			103			40			33	28	
7.0	4.0		110	21	32.8	0.96	1.11	10.0	0.87			103			40			34	30	
7.5	6.0	181/119	113	24	38.5	1.12	1.25	11.1	0.90			105			40			34	31	
8.0	6.0		116	24	39.7	1.17	1.24	10.7	0.94			107			39			34	32	
8.5	8.0		111	24	39.7	1.18	1.24	11.1	0.96			107			40			34	32	
9.0	8.0		114	24	39.0	1.18	1.23	10.7	0.97			107			41			33	32	
9.5	Recovery		112	23	38.2	1.18	1.22	10.9	0.97			106			42			32	31	
10.0	Recovery		114	21	33.6	1.03	1.07	9.4	0.96			106			41			33	31	
10.5	Recovery		110	21	31.0	0.97	0.96	8.7	1.01			108			41			32	32	
11.0	Recovery		108	21	29.3	0.88	0.80	7.4	1.09			110			41			33	37	

*Treadmill speed remained at 2 miles/hour throughout the exercise period.

Abbreviations: BP, blood pressure; BTPS, body temperature pressure saturated; f, frequency; HCO_3^-, bicarbonate; HR, heart rate; $P(A-a)O_2$, alveolar-arterial PO_2 difference; $P(a-ET)CO_2$, arterial-end-tidal PCO_2 difference; $P_{ET}CO_2$, end-tidal PCO_2; $P_{ET}O_2$, end-tidal PO_2; R, respiratory exchange ratio; STPD, standard temperature pressure dry; $\dot{V}CO_2$, carbon dioxide output; V_D/V_T, physiological dead space–tidal volume ratio; $\dot{V}E$, minute ventilation; $\dot{V}E/\dot{V}CO_2$, ventilatory equivalent for carbon dioxide; $\dot{V}E/\dot{V}O_2$, ventilatory equivalent for oxygen; $\dot{V}O_2$, oxygen uptake.

leg, the low $\Delta\dot{V}O_2/\Delta WR$ and early anaerobic threshold suggest a more generalized impairment in oxygen delivery and utilization. This could be due to diffuse arterial disease or may reflect pulmonary vascular impairment due to his severe obstructive lung disease. Despite the findings of cardiovascular impairment and limitation, the low breathing reserve indicated that the patient was also approaching ventilatory limitation probably due to chronic obstructive pulmonary disease. It is likely that V_D/V_T was elevated as well, although $\dot{V}E/\dot{V}CO_2$ was not elevated; in this case, the patient might not have increased $\dot{V}E$ appropriately because of lung disease. Alternatively, a somewhat unusual finding that might be seen with peripheral arterial disease is a low $\Delta\dot{V}CO_2/\Delta WR$. This is possibly because carbon dioxide is only slowly being removed from the exercising muscle because of vascular disease, such that there is a low R through exercise and a falling $\dot{V}E/\dot{V}CO_2$ until recovery is reached.

Conclusion

This case illustrates exercise impairment in a patient with comorbid peripheral arterial and obstructive lung disease. Exercise was limited symptomatically by claudication. Clearly, however, his lung disease amplified his impairment because he had arterial hypoxemia exacerbating the vascular limitations to oxygen delivery and appeared to reach ventilatory limitation during exercise with increasing PCO_2. Of interest is the similarity between the two studies conducting on cycle and treadmill.

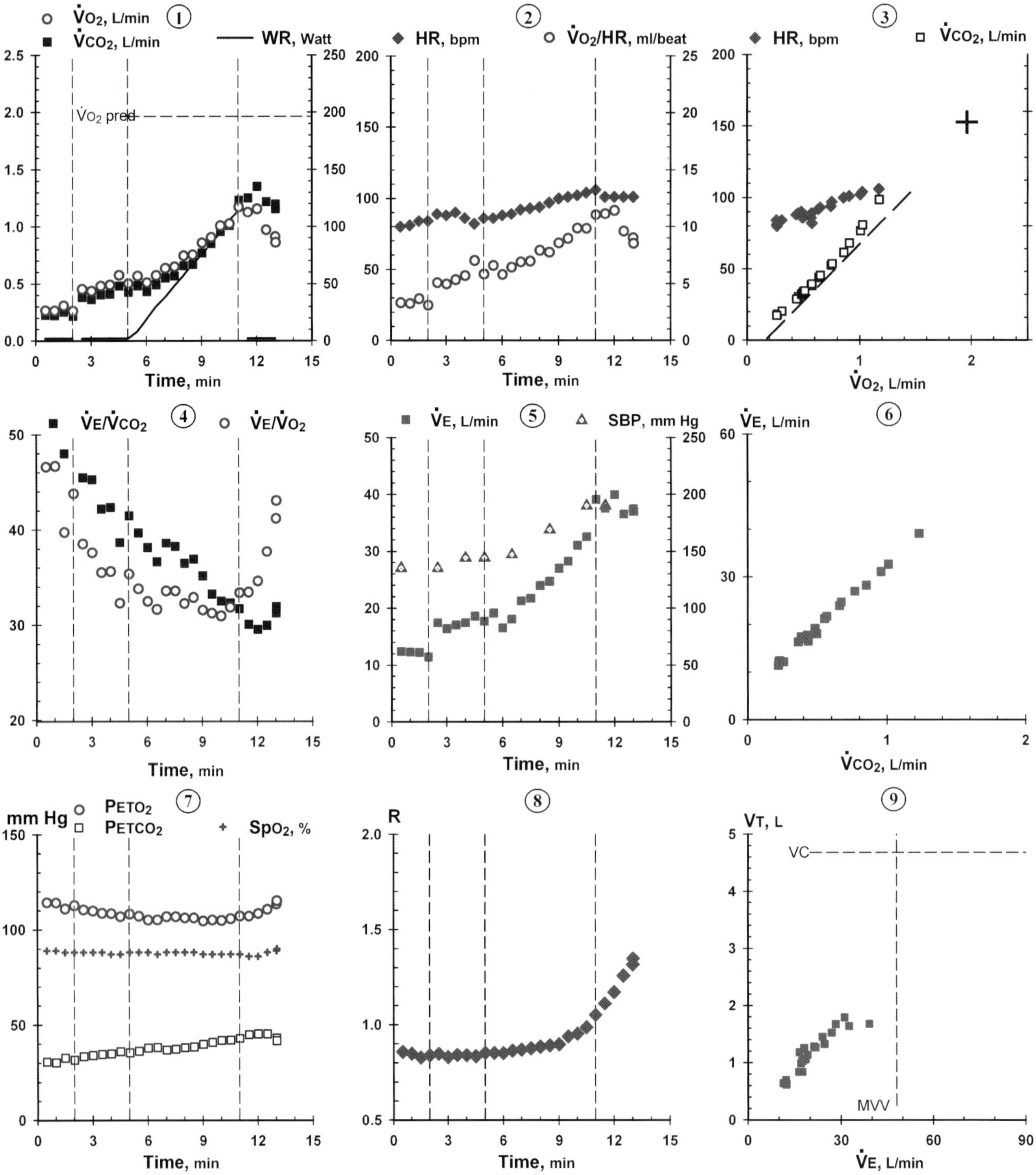

FIGURE 10.89.1. Cycle ergometer. Vertical dashed lines in the panels in the left and middle columns indicate, from left to right, the beginning of unloaded cycling, start of increasing work rate (WR) at 20 W/min, and start of recovery. In **panel 1**, the increase in WR (right y-axis) is plotted with a scale of 100 W to 1 L of oxygen uptake ($\dot{V}O_2$) (left y-axis) such that WR is plotted parallel to a $\dot{V}O_2$ slope of 10 mL/min/W. In **panel 3**, carbon dioxide output ($\dot{V}CO_2$) (right y-axis) is plotted as a function of $\dot{V}O_2$ (x-axis) with identical scales so that the diagonal dashed line has a slope of 1 (45°). The $\dot{V}CO_2$ increasing more steeply than $\dot{V}O_2$ defines carbon dioxide (CO_2) derived from bicarbonate buffer, as long as ventilatory equivalent for CO_2 ($\dot{V}E/\dot{V}CO_2$) (**panel 4**) is not increasing and end-tidal P_{CO_2} (P_{ETCO_2}) (**panel 7**) is not decreasing, simultaneously. The black + symbol in **panel 3** indicates predicted peak values of heart rate (HR) (left y-axis) and $\dot{V}O_2$ for this individual. Abbreviations: MVV, maximum voluntary ventilation; P_{ETO_2}, end-tidal P_{O_2}; R, respiratory exchange ratio; SBP, systolic blood pressure; Sp_{O_2}, oxygen saturation as measured by pulse oximetry; VC, vital capacity; $\dot{V}E$, minute ventilation; $\dot{V}E/\dot{V}O_2$, ventilatory equivalent for oxygen; V_T, tidal volume.

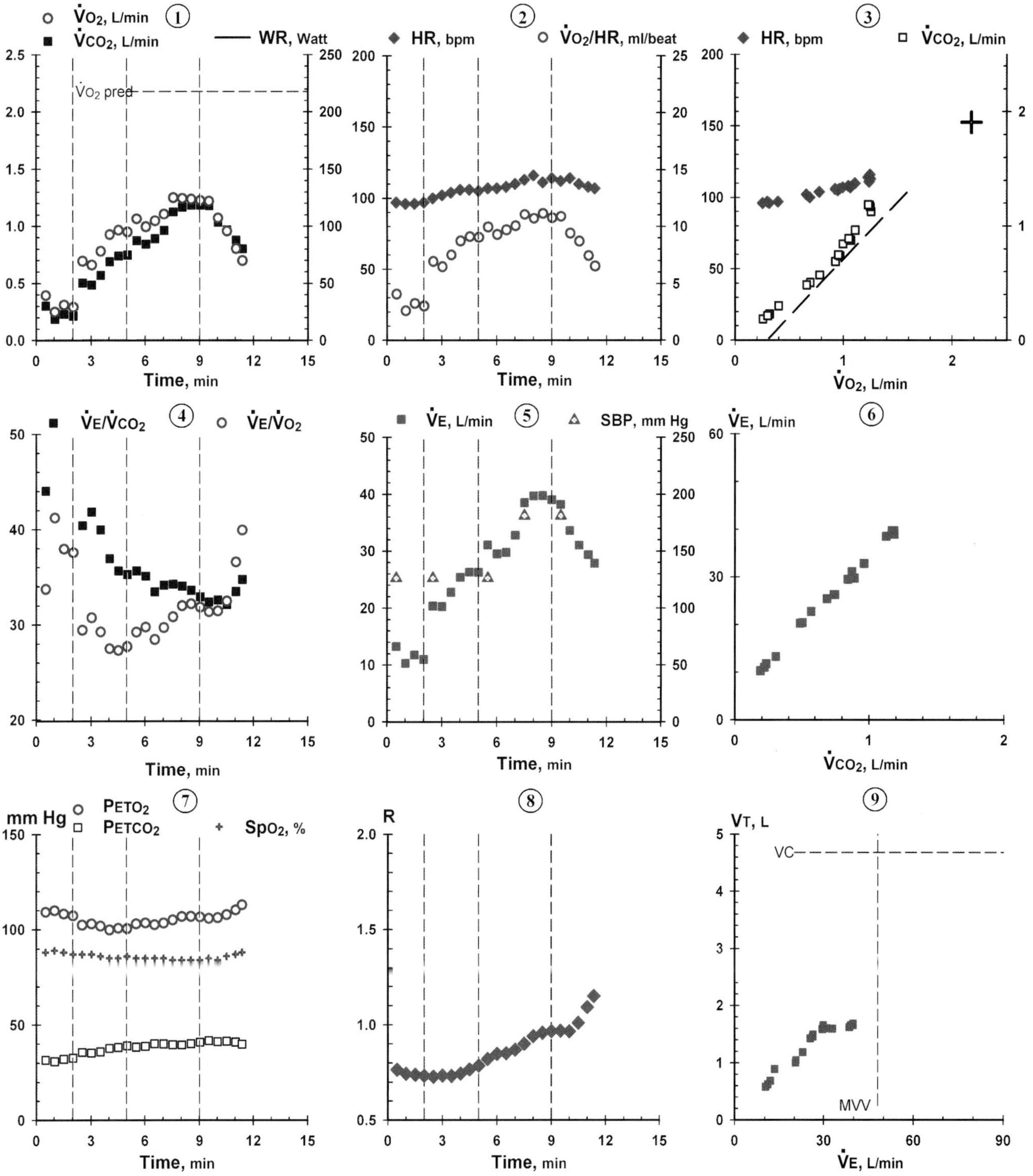

FIGURE 10.89.2. Treadmill. Vertical dashed lines in the panels in the left and middle columns indicate, from left to right, the beginning of treadmill walking at a speed of 2 mph at zero grade, the start of increasing grade by 2% per minute, and start of recovery. In **panel 3**, carbon dioxide output ($\dot{V}CO_2$) (right y-axis) is plotted as a function of oxygen uptake ($\dot{V}O_2$) (x-axis) with identical scales so that the diagonal dashed line has a slope of 1 (45°). The $\dot{V}CO_2$ increasing more steeply than $\dot{V}O_2$ defines carbon dioxide (CO_2) derived from bicarbonate buffer, as long as ventilatory equivalent for CO_2 ($\dot{V}E/\dot{V}CO_2$) (**panel 4**) is not increasing and end-tidal P_{CO_2} (P_{ETCO_2}) (**panel 7**) is not decreasing, simultaneously. The black + symbol in **panel 3** indicates predicted peak values of heart rate (HR) (left y-axis) and $\dot{V}O_2$ for this individual. Abbreviations: MVV, maximum voluntary ventilation; P_{ETO_2}, end-tidal P_{O_2}; R, respiratory exchange ratio; SBP, systolic blood pressure; SpO_2, oxygen saturation as measured by pulse oximetry; VC, vital capacity; $\dot{V}E$, minute ventilation; $\dot{V}E/\dot{V}O_2$, ventilatory equivalent for oxygen; V_T, tidal volume; WR, work rate.

CASE 90

Morbid Obesity and Aortic Valve Disease

CLINICAL FINDINGS

A 72-year-old man was referred for testing because of persistent exertional dyspnea following transcatheter aortic valve replacement. Aortic stenosis had been diagnosed after he presented with progressive fatigue, dyspnea, and other symptoms 18 months previously. Transcatheter aortic valve replacement had resulted in substantial improvement in symptoms; however, he felt that his breathing had not improved to his expected baseline. He was dyspneic with activities such as carrying groceries, walking uphill, or getting in and out of a golf cart. Medical history also included atrial flutter treated with an ablation procedure, gastroesophageal reflux, hypertension, obstructive lung disease, obstructive sleep apnea, and orthopedic issues including prior hip replacement and lumbar spine surgery. Medications at the time of testing included metoprolol, ipratropium and fluticasone nasal sprays, ranitidine, diltiazem, ezetimibe, atorvastatin, aspirin, and a combination long-acting β-agonist and muscarinic antagonist inhaler. He used bilevel positive airway pressure at night for sleep apnea and sildenafil as needed. Physical examination was notable for a regular cardiac rhythm and soft systolic murmur. Breath sounds were clear and there was no peripheral edema. Resting electrocardiogram showed a sinus rhythm with diffuse T wave inversions in leads V5 through V6. Demographic and respiratory function data are shown in **Table 10.90.1**.

TABLE 10.90.1 Selected Respiratory Function Data

Measurement	Predicted	Measured
Age (y)		72
Sex		Male
Height (cm)		187
Weight (kg)		141
Body mass index (kg/m^2)		40.3
VC (L)	4.92	3.36
IC (L)	3.56	2.21
ERV (L)	1.36	0.30
FEV_1 (L)	3.60	2.21
FEV_1/VC (%)	73	66
MVV (L/min)	136	89

Abbreviations: ERV, expiratory reserve volume; FEV_1, forced expiratory volume in 1 second; IC, inspiratory capacity; MVV, maximum voluntary ventilation; VC, vital capacity.

EXERCISE FINDINGS

The patient exercised on a cycle ergometer beginning with 3 minutes of unloaded pedaling at 60 rpm followed by continuous increase in work rate by 15 W/min. He had some difficulty with pedaling due to his body habitus relative to orientation of the pedals and the test ended due to muscle cramps in his legs. He was also short of breath but felt he might have exercised further if not for the cramps. Exercise electrocardiogram showed deepening of the T-wave inversions with downsloping ST-segment displacement of <2 mm in both leads. There was no chest pain. Exercise data are summarized in **Tables 10.90.2** and **10.90.3** and in **Figure 10.90.1**.

INTERPRETATION

Comment

This case is presented as an example of a test with multiple processes affecting exercise capacity. Although the primary diagnosis was cardiovascular, the exercise responses were significantly affected by morbid obesity.

TABLE 10.90.2 Selected Exercise Test Data

Measurement	Predicted	Measured
Peak $\dot{V}O_2$ (L/min)	2.41	2.01
Peak $\dot{V}O_2$ (mL/min/kg)		14.2
Maximum heart rate (beats/min)	148	118
Maximum O_2 pulse (mL/beat)	16.3	17.2
$\Delta\dot{V}O_2/\Delta WR$ (mL/min/W)	10.3	10.3
AT (L/min)	>1.14	1.45
Blood pressure (mm Hg [rest, peak])		140/78, 193/84
Maximum $\dot{V}E$ (L/min)		64
Breathing reserve (L/min)	>15	22
$\dot{V}E/\dot{V}CO_2$ @ *AT* (L/min)	<33	31
$\dot{V}E$-$\dot{V}CO_2$ slope	<32	30
SpO_2 (% [rest, max ex])		95, 95
VD/VT (rest, max ex)[a]		0.32, 0.29

Abbreviations: *AT*, anaerobic threshold; $\Delta\dot{V}O_2/\Delta WR$, change in $\dot{V}O_2$/change in work rate; ex, exercise; O_2, oxygen; SpO_2, oxygen saturation as measured by pulse oximetry; $\dot{V}CO_2$, carbon dioxide output; VD/VT, physiological dead space-tidal volume ratio; $\dot{V}E$, minute ventilation; $\dot{V}O_2$, oxygen uptake.

[a]Calculated using transcutaneous PCO_2.

TABLE 10.90.3 Cycle Exercise

Time (min)	Work rate (W)	BP (mm Hg)	HR (min^{-1})	f (min^{-1})	$\dot{V}_E$ (L/min BTPS)	$\dot{V}CO_2$ (L/min STPD)	$\dot{V}O_2$ (L/min STPD)	$\frac{\dot{V}O_2}{HR}$ (mL/beat)	R	pH	HCO_3^- (mEq/L)	PO_2, mm Hg and SpO_2, %: ET	SpO_2	(A − a)	PCO_2, mm Hg: ET	tc	(a − ET)	$\frac{\dot{V}_E}{\dot{V}CO_2}$	$\frac{\dot{V}_E}{\dot{V}O_2}$	$\frac{V_D}{V_T}$
0.5	Rest		68	11	16.8	0.50	0.58	8.4	0.88			110	95		35	37.5		33	29	0.34
1.0	Rest		71	10	14.3	0.44	0.52	7.3	0.86			108	94		36	37.3		32	28	0.31
1.5	Rest	140/78	69	11	16.3	0.49	0.56	8.0	0.88			109	94		36	37.3		33	29	0.33
2.0	Unloaded		71	12	16.8	0.51	0.61	8.6	0.84			106	93		36	37.2		33	28	0.32
2.5	Unloaded		82	16	22.6	0.69	0.85	10.3	0.81			106	92		36	37.2		33	27	0.32
3.0	Unloaded		85	23	27.8	0.83	1.07	12.6	0.78			105	92		36	37.2		33	26	0.33
3.5	Unloaded		89	23	33.7	1.05	1.24	13.9	0.84			107	93		36	37.3		32	27	0.31
4.0	Unloaded	174/79	90	23	34.3	1.08	1.24	13.8	0.87			108	93		37	37.3		32	28	0.30
4.5	Unloaded		90	23	35.0	1.10	1.24	13.8	0.89			109	93		37	37.3		32	28	0.30
5.0	4		88	21	31.8	1.02	1.16	13.2	0.88			107	93		38	37.2		31	27	0.29
5.5	11		88	24	34.6	1.08	1.22	13.9	0.88			109	93		36	37.3		32	28	0.31
6.0	19		87	24	33.3	1.04	1.18	13.5	0.89			109	93		36	37.3		32	28	0.31
6.5	26		89	24	33.9	1.06	1.19	13.4	0.89			109	93		36	37.3		32	28	0.31
7.0	34	185/82	92	28	37.2	1.14	1.33	14.5	0.86			106	93		37	37.3		33	28	0.32
7.5	41		95	25	40.2	1.29	1.40	14.8	0.92			109	93		37	37.3		31	29	0.29
8.0	49		97	28	42.4	1.35	1.50	15.5	0.90			108	93		37	37.3		31	28	0.29
8.5	56		98	28	45.0	1.44	1.55	15.8	0.93			109	93		37	37.3		31	29	0.29
9.0	64		101	28	46.0	1.48	1.63	16.1	0.91			108	93		37	37.3		31	28	0.29
9.5	71		104	29	53.7	1.70	1.73	16.7	0.98			112	92		36	37.4		32	31	0.30
10.0	79	193/84	109	30	53.4	1.73	1.80	16.5	0.96			110	92		37	37.3		31	30	0.28
10.5	86		112	31	60.4	1.94	1.92	17.2	1.01			112	93		37	37.3		31	31	0.29
11.0	Recovery		115	35	63.5	2.01	1.98	17.2	1.01			113	95		36	37.3		32	32	0.30
11.5	Recovery	208/84	110	33	59.0	1.87	1.75	15.9	1.07			114	94		37	37		31	34	0.29
12.0	Recovery		103	29	50.4	1.60	1.51	14.7	1.06			114	94		36	37		32	33	0.29
12.5	Recovery		96	29	46.4	1.42	1.30	13.5	1.09			115	95		36	36.8		33	36	0.31
13.0	Recovery		93	29	43.2	1.29	1.18	12.7	1.09			116	95		35	36.8		34	37	0.33

Abbreviations: BP, blood pressure; BTPS, body temperature pressure saturated; f, frequency; HCO_3^-, bicarbonate; HR, heart rate; $P(A-a)O_2$, alveolar-arterial PO_2 difference; $P(a-ET)CO_2$, arterial–end-tidal PCO_2 difference; $P_{ET}CO_2$, end-tidal PCO_2; $P_{ET}O_2$, end-tidal PO_2; $PtcCO_2$, transcutaneous PCO_2; R, respiratory exchange ratio; SpO_2, oxygen saturation as measured by pulse oximetry; STPD, $\dot{V}CO_2$, carbon dioxide output; V_D/V_T, physiological dead space–tidal volume ratio; $\dot{V}_E$, minute ventilation; $\dot{V}_E/\dot{V}CO_2$, ventilatory equivalent for carbon dioxide; $\dot{V}_E/\dot{V}O_2$, ventilatory equivalent for oxygen; $\dot{V}O_2$, oxygen uptake.

[a]The V_D/V_T was calculated using $PtcCO_2$ as an [illegible]

Analysis

Exercise capacity may be underestimated as the test ended with noncardiorespiratory symptoms without the patient having clearly reached a limiting capacity. Peak $\dot{V}O_2$ was lower than predicted, but submaximal responses, including the $\Delta\dot{V}O_2/\Delta WR$ and anaerobic threshold, were normal. The heart rate slope relative to $\dot{V}O_2$ was lower than average and the peak oxygen pulse higher than average, consistent with β-blocker usage. The $\dot{V}O_2$ values during the initial unloaded cycling period were high, consistent with obesity and/or suboptimal cycling ergonomics related to his body habitus.

The breathing reserve was normal, although not large, due to reduced breathing capacity on spirometry.

Gas exchange efficiency was mostly normal. The SpO_2 and ventilatory equivalents were normal. The exercise V_D/V_T decreased into the normal exercise range.

Conclusion

Cardiorespiratory responses were normal up to the level of work achieved. Effects of obesity are seen in the initial $\dot{V}O_2$ cost of unloaded cycling and the restriction of breathing capacity. Although these did not appear to be limiting to performance, they may be important in his experience of dyspnea during ambulatory activities.

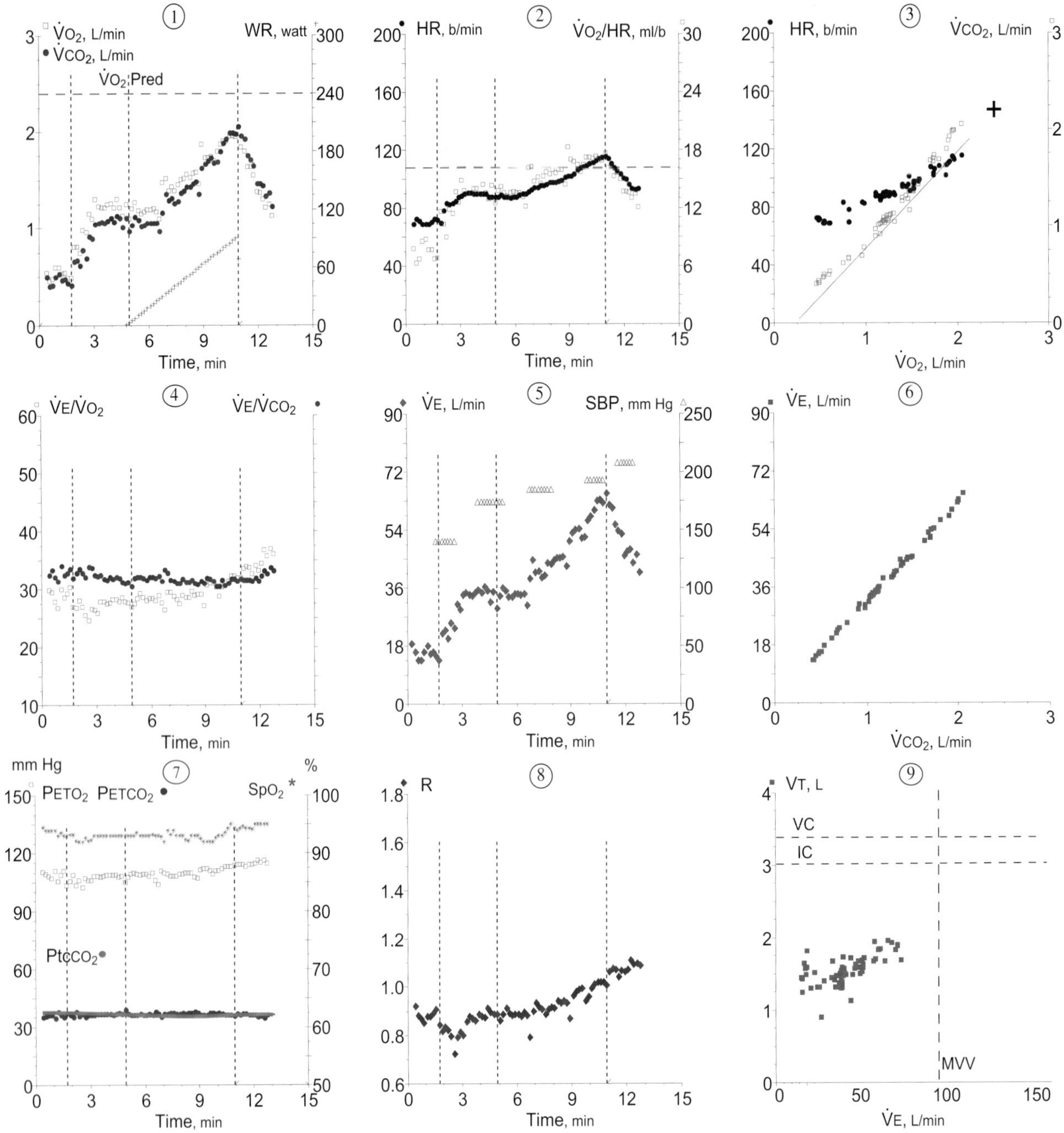

FIGURE 10.90.1. Vertical dashed lines in the panels in the left and middle columns indicate, from left to right, the beginning of unloaded cycling, start of increasing work rate (WR) at 15 W/min, and start of recovery. In **panel 1**, the increase in WR (right y-axis) is plotted with a scale of 100 W to 1 L of oxygen uptake ($\dot{V}O_2$) (left y-axis) such that WR is plotted parallel to a $\dot{V}O_2$ slope of 10 mL/min/W. Predicted peak $\dot{V}O_2$ is shown as a dashed horizontal line. In **panel 3**, carbon dioxide output ($\dot{V}CO_2$) (right y-axis) is plotted as a function of $\dot{V}O_2$ (x-axis) with identical scales so that the diagonal blue line has a slope of 1 (45°). The $\dot{V}CO_2$ increasing more steeply than $\dot{V}O_2$ defines carbon dioxide (CO_2) derived from bicarbonate buffer, as long as ventilatory equivalent for CO_2 ($\dot{V}E/\dot{V}CO_2$) (**panel 4**) is not increasing and end-tidal PCO_2 ($PETCO_2$) (**panel 7**) is not decreasing, simultaneously. The black + symbol in **panel 3** indicates predicted peak values of heart rate (HR) (left y-axis) and $\dot{V}O_2$ for this individual. Abbreviations: IC, inspiratory capacity; MVV, maximum voluntary ventilation; $PETO_2$, end-tidal PO_2; $PtcCO_2$, transcutaneous PCO_2; R, respiratory exchange ratio; SBP, systolic blood pressure; SpO_2, oxygen saturation as measured by pulse oximetry; VC, vital capacity; $\dot{V}E$, minute ventilation; $\dot{V}E/\dot{V}O_2$, ventilatory equivalent for oxygen; VT, tidal volume.

CASE 91

Morbid Obesity

CLINICAL FINDINGS

A 37-year-old woman was referred for exercise testing to evaluate dyspnea and fatigue with walking. Medical history was notable for morbid obesity without known heart or lung disease. Medical history also included obstructive sleep apnea, carpal tunnel syndrome, cholelithiasis, endometriosis, migraine, insomnia, and depression. She worked as an aide in adult day care. Medications were reported as citalopram, omeprazole, ibuprofen, and a combination inhaled long-acting β-agonist and corticosteroid. She used a continuous positive airway pressure device while sleeping. Physical examination was notable for obesity with body mass index of 57.6. Heart rate was regular, breath sounds were clear, and there was mild symmetric edema of the ankles. The electrocardiogram showed a sinus rhythm. Spirometry showed a mild reduction in spirometric volumes without significant airflow obstruction. Demographic and respiratory function data are shown in **Table 10.91.1**.

EXERCISE FINDINGS

The patient exercised on a cycle ergometer beginning with 3 minutes of unloaded pedaling at 60 rpm followed by continuous increase in work rate by 10 W/min until the test ended with symptoms of shortness of breath, which was similar to her daily symptoms. Exercise electrocardiogram showed no arrhythmia or ischemic changes.

TABLE 10.91.1 Selected Respiratory Function Data

Measurement	Predicted	Measured
Age (y)		37
Sex		Female
Height (cm)		161
Weight (kg)		149
Body mass index (kg/m²)		57.6
VC (L)	3.63	2.55
IC (L)	2.22	2.71
ERV (L)	1.41	0.09
FEV_1 (L)	2.99	2.19
FEV_1/VC (%)	83	86
MVV (L/min)	103	80

Abbreviations: ERV, expiratory reserve volume; FEV_1, forced expiratory volume in 1 second; IC, inspiratory capacity; MVV, maximum voluntary ventilation; VC, vital capacity.

Exercise data are summarized in **Tables 10.91.2** and **10.91.3** and **Figure 10.91.1**.

INTERPRETATION

Comment

This case was chosen as an example of morbid obesity, which is a common coexisting condition to consider in test interpretation but in this case appeared relatively uncomplicated by other disease that would alter exercise responses.

Analysis

Peak values for both oxygen uptake ($\dot{V}O_2$) and heart rate were slightly below the lower limit of their predicted ranges. The anaerobic threshold was normal, but a high percentage of the peak $\dot{V}O_2$ measured, which along with the high heart rate reserve, suggests that the test might have been less than maximal cardiovascular stress. Up to the level of exercise performed, both change in $\dot{V}O_2$/change in work rate and the slope of heart rate relative to $\dot{V}O_2$ were normal (see panels 1 and 3 of **Fig. 10.91.1**). The $\dot{V}O_2$ at rest prior to exercise was around 0.4 L/min

TABLE 10.91.2 Selected Exercise Test Data

Measurement	Predicted	Measured
Peak $\dot{V}O_2$ (L/min)	2.25	1.83
Peak $\dot{V}O_2$ (mL/min/kg actual weight)	~35	12.3
[illegible] (beats/min)	[illegible]	[illegible]
Maximum O_2 pulse (mL/beat)	12.3	11.6
$\Delta\dot{V}O_2/\Delta WR$ (mL/min/W)	10.3	10.3
AT (L/min)	>1.03	1.35
Blood pressure (mm Hg [rest, peak])		113/61, 189/62
Maximum $\dot{V}_E$ (L/min)		57
Breathing reserve (L/min)		23
$\dot{V}_E/\dot{V}CO_2$ @ *AT* (L/min)	<31	27
SpO_2 (% [rest, max ex])	<31	96, 93
V_D/V_T (rest, max ex)		0.20, 0.16

Abbreviations: *AT*, anaerobic threshold; $\Delta\dot{V}O_2/\Delta WR$, change in $\dot{V}O_2$/change in work rate; ex, exercise; O_2, oxygen; SpO_2, oxygen saturation as measured by pulse oximetry; V_D/V_T, physiological dead space-tidal volume ratio; $\dot{V}_E$, minute ventilation; $\dot{V}_E/\dot{V}CO_2$, ventilatory equivalent for carbon dioxide; $\dot{V}O_2$, oxygen uptake.

TABLE 10.91.3 Air Breathing

Time (min)	Work rate (W)	BP (mm Hg)	HR (min^{-1})	f (min^{-1})	$\dot{V}E$ (L/min BTPS)	$\dot{V}CO_2$ (L/min STPD)	$\dot{V}O_2$ (L/min STPD)	$\dot{V}O_2$/HR (mL/beat)	R	pH	HCO_3^- (mEq/L)	PO_2, mm Hg and SpO_2, % ET	SpO_2	(A − a)	PCO_2, mm Hg ET	tc	(a − ET)	$\dot{V}E/\dot{V}CO_2$	$\dot{V}E/\dot{V}O_2$	VD/VT
0.5	Rest		90	14	14.5	0.44	0.47	5.3	0.92			108	96		38	35.7		33	30	0.25
1.0	Rest		90	19	12.8	0.40	0.43	4.8	0.92			109	95		38	35.7		32	30	0.20
1.5	Rest	113/61	89	19	12.1	0.38	0.42	4.7	0.90			106	97		39	35.5		32	29	0.19
2.0	Rest		93	18	14.1	0.44	0.46	5.0	0.96			108	96		39	35.7		32	30	0.21
2.5	Unloaded		96	24	16.8	0.54	0.59	6.1	0.93			108	96		39	35.7		31	29	0.19
3.0	Unloaded		106	26	21.4	0.70	0.79	7.5	0.89			106	95		39	35.8		30	27	0.19
3.5	Unloaded		118	28	25.1	0.84	1.01	8.5	0.84			102	95		40	36		30	25	0.18
4.0	Unloaded		121	28	28.8	0.97	1.10	9.1	0.88			104	94		40	36.2		30	26	0.18
4.5	Unloaded		124	27	28.4	0.98	1.09	8.7	0.90			103	94		41	36.3		29	26	0.17
5.0	Unloaded	160/67	130	28	31.6	1.09	1.16	9.0	0.93			105	94		41	36.5		29	27	0.18
5.5	4		130	30	33.2	1.15	1.22	9.4	0.94			105	94		41	36.5		29	27	0.17
6.0	9		129	29	35.3	1.22	1.23	9.6	0.98			107	94		40	36.4		29	29	0.18
6.5	14		126	29	31.3	1.11	1.17	9.3	0.95			105	94		41	36.3		28	27	0.15
7.0	19		126	30	33.7	1.16	1.22	9.6	0.95			106	94		41	36.5		29	28	0.18
7.5	24		132	29	34.9	1.22	1.25	9.5	0.97			106	95		41	36.5		29	28	0.17
8.0	29	147/66	130	30	33.9	1.18	1.24	9.5	0.95			105	95		41	36.5		29	27	0.17
8.5	34		129	33	36.0	1.22	1.28	10.0	0.95			107	95		40	36.5		29	28	0.19
9.0	39		131	29	35.5	1.24	1.35	10.3	0.92			104	94		41	36.5		29	26	0.17
9.5	44	157/65	136	30	36.9	1.30	1.37	10.1	0.95			104	93		42	36.8		28	27	0.17
10.0	49		137	30	38.0	1.36	1.45	10.6	0.94			104	93		42	36.8		28	26	0.16
10.5	54		137	30	40.1	1.44	1.48	10.8	0.97			105	93		42	37.1		28	27	0.16
11.0	59		143	32	42.3	1.53	1.55	10.9	0.99			106	93		42	37.1		28	27	0.16
11.5	64	171/65	145	32	44.1	1.61	1.61	11.1	1.00			106	94		42	37.1		27	27	0.15
12.0	69		144	32	43.3	1.60	1.58	11.0	1.01			105	93		43	37.2		27	27	0.14
12.5	74		146	32	45.9	1.68	1.65	11.3	1.02			106	92		43	37.4		27	28	0.16
13.0	79		149	33	48.1	1.76	1.67	11.2	1.05			107	93		43	37.5		27	29	0.16
13.5	84	189/62	152	35	51.3	1.89	1.76	11.6	1.07			107	93		43	37.5		27	29	0.16
14.0	89		155	36	54.4	1.98	1.79	11.6	1.11			109	93		43	37.5		27	30	0.17
14.5	70		157	36	57.3	2.05	1.83	11.6	1.12			110	93		42	37.4		28	31	0.18
15.0	Recovery		151	30	50.0	1.92	1.72	11.3	1.12			107	94		45	37.4		26	29	0.12
15.5	Recovery	182/61	141	28	44.4	1.68	1.43	10.1	1.18			109	94		44	37.4		26	31	0.13

Abbreviations: BP, blood pressure; BTPS, body temperature pressure saturated; f, frequency; HCO_3^-, bicarbonate; HR, heart rate; P(A − a)O_2, alveolar-arterial PO_2 difference; P(a − ET)CO_2, arterial-end-tidal PCO_2 difference; $PETCO_2$, end-tidal PCO_2; $PETO_2$, end-tidal PO_2; R, respiratory exchange ratio; SpO_2, oxygen saturation as measured by pulse oximetry; STPD, standard temperature pressure dry; $\dot{V}CO_2$, carbon dioxide output; VD/VT, physiological dead space–tidal volume ratio; $\dot{V}E$, minute ventilation; $\dot{V}E/\dot{V}CO_2$, ventilatory equivalent for carbon dioxide; $\dot{V}E/\dot{V}O_2$, ventilatory equivalent for oxygen; $\dot{V}O_2$, oxygen uptake.

and tripled during the initial unloaded pedaling. The latter reflects a higher than average metabolic cost of moving heavy legs and/or unfavorable cycling ergonomics due to body habitus.

Ventilation: In **Table 10.91.1** and panel 9 of **Figure 10.91.1**, it is evident that the resting inspiratory capacity and vital capacity are very close, meaning expiratory reserve volume was small, a typical spirometric finding in obesity. The mild restrictive defect on resting spirometry and relatively large inspiratory reserve volume maintained during exercise were likely also due to extrapulmonary restriction due to obesity. There was a breathing reserve but no evidence of respiratory compensation for metabolic acidosis either in the graphical data (panels 4 and 6) or in the end-tidal and transcutaneous PCO_2 values (see **Table 10.91.3** and panel 7 of **Fig. 10.91.1**). This may simply reflect the test ending not long after exceeding the anaerobic threshold or could be a result of the increased work of breathing related to the obese body habitus.

Indices of gas exchange efficiency were within normal limits, with normal nadir value of ventilatory equivalent for carbon dioxide (panel 4 of **Fig.10.91.1**) and end-tidal PCO_2 values exceeding the transcutaneous values

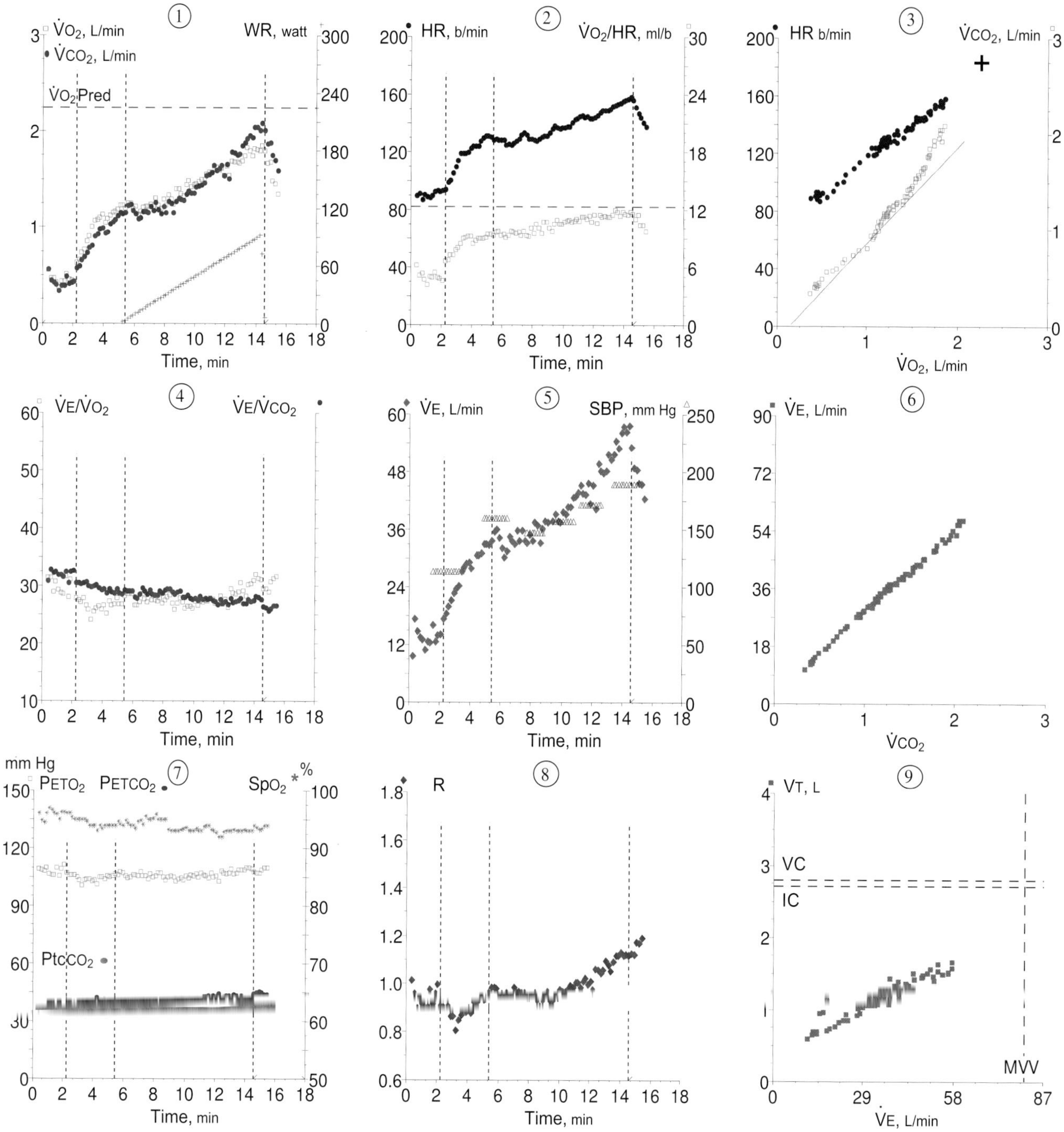

FIGURE 10.91.1. Vertical dashed lines in the panels in the left and middle columns indicate, from left to right, the beginning of unloaded cycling, start of increasing work rate (WR) at 10 W/min, and start of recovery. In **panel 1**, the increase in WR (right y-axis) is plotted with a scale of 100 W to 1 L of oxygen uptake ($\dot{V}O_2$) (left y-axis) such that WR is plotted parallel to a $\dot{V}O_2$ slope of 10 mL/min/W. Predicted peak $\dot{V}O_2$ is shown as a dashed horizontal line. In **panel 3**, carbon dioxide output ($\dot{V}CO_2$) (right y-axis) is plotted as a function of $\dot{V}O_2$ (x-axis) with identical scales so that the diagonal blue line has a slope of 1 (45 degrees). The $\dot{V}CO_2$ increasing more steeply than $\dot{V}O_2$ defines carbon dioxide (CO_2) derived from bicarbonate buffer, as long as ventilatory equivalent for CO_2 ($\dot{V}E/\dot{V}CO_2$) (**panel 4**) is not increasing and end-tidal P_{CO_2} (P_{ETCO_2}) (**panel 7**) is not decreasing, simultaneously. The black + symbol in **panel 3** indicates predicted peak values of heart rate (HR) (left y-axis) and $\dot{V}O_2$ for this individual. Abbreviations: IC, inspiratory capacity; MVV, maximum voluntary ventilation; P_{ETO_2}, end-tidal P_{O_2}; R, respiratory exchange ratio; SBP, systolic blood pressure; SpO_2, oxygen saturation as measured by pulse oximetry; VC, vital capacity; $\dot{V}E$, minute ventilation; $\dot{V}E/\dot{V}O_2$, ventilatory equivalent for oxygen; V_T, tidal volume.

(see panel 7 of **Fig.10.91.1** and **Table 10.91.3**). The ventilatory equivalents did not change very much between rest and exercise (panel 4). This is not because the nadir values were abnormally high, but because the resting values were relatively low. Consistent with this, the calculated physiological dead space–tidal volume ratio was only 20% at rest. This is not a consistent finding in obesity but could result from decreased thoracic compliance reducing both ventilation and perfusion to the lower lung zones, with capillary recruitment in the better aerated upper regions of the lung at rest, such that perfusion distribution did not change as much as usual during exercise. Oxygenation was normal at rest and declined slightly with exercise. This is in contrast to some obese individuals who have lower oxygen saturation as measured by pulse oximetry at rest due to dependent atelectasis, which improves with increasing tidal volumes during exercise.

Conclusion

Findings in this test were primarily related to obesity. The aerobic capacity (peak $\dot{V}O_2$) was lower than predicted, although this may reflect the test ending due to dyspnea prior to a maximal cardiovascular response. The weight-indexed peak $\dot{V}O_2$ (mL/min/kg actual weight) was severely reduced, in contrast, reflecting the impairment for ambulatory activities, for which a high proportion of the aerobic capacity would be obligated to support body weight. There was evidence of ventilatory restriction, likely due to the effect of obesity on respiratory mechanics, but efficiency of pulmonary gas exchange was essentially normal.

CASE 92

Exercise Testing for Staging and Prognosis in Chronic Heart Failure

e To view this case please access the eBook bundled with this text. Instructions are located on the inside front cover.

CASE 93

Exercise Testing for Preoperative Evaluation for Lung Cancer Resection

CLINICAL FINDINGS

A 62-year-old man with a long history of chronic obstructive pulmonary disease was referred for exercise testing to assess operative risk because of the finding of a malignant pulmonary nodule. The patient had quit smoking approximately 3 months earlier, and his obstructive lung disease was being treated aggressively with bronchodilators and oral corticosteroids. He had no known history of cardiovascular disease and stated he could walk 2 miles.

EXERCISE FINDINGS

The patient performed exercise on a cycle ergometer. He pedaled at 60 rpm without an added load for 3 minutes. The work rate was then increased 10 W/min to tolerance. Heart rate and rhythm were continuously monitored, and electrocardiograms (ECGs) were repeatedly obtained. Blood pressure was measured with a sphygmomanometer, and arterial saturation was estimated with an ear oximeter. The patient gave an excellent effort and stopped exercise because of shortness of breath and leg fatigue. Pulmonary function tests showed a moderately severe obstructive ventilatory defect with a normal diffusing capacity of lung for carbon monoxide (**Table 10.93.1**). Resting and exercise ECGs and pulse oximetry (not shown) were normal.

TABLE 10.93.1 Selected Respiratory Function Data

Measurement	Predicted	Measured
[illegible]		62
Sex		Male
Height (cm)		170
Weight (kg)	74	68
Hematocrit (%)		49
VC (L)	3.35	2.76
IC (L)	2.23	2.07
TLC (L)	5.20	5.46
FEV_1 (L)	2.62	1.28
FEV_1/VC (%)	78	46
MVV (L/min)	113	62
D_{LCO} (mL/mm Hg/min)	22.9	20.2

Abbreviations: D_{LCO}, diffusing capacity of lung for carbon monoxide; FEV_1, forced expiratory volume in 1 second; IC, inspiratory capacity; MVV, maximum voluntary ventilation; TLC, total lung capacity; VC, vital capacity.

INTERPRETATION

Comments

This case is presented as an example of exercise testing in the evaluation of the ability to tolerate lung resection surgery for lung cancer. Exercise data are summarized in **Table 10.93.2** and shown in **Table 10.93.3** and graphically in **Figure 10.93.1**.

Analysis

Although the patient had a low breathing reserve at the end of exercise and could be considered to be approaching ventilatory limitation as expected, the dominant findings were of cardiovascular impairment. Peak oxygen uptake ($\dot{V}O_2$) was reduced, and the anaerobic threshold was low. Of note is that respiratory exchange ratio rose to a value over 1.0 during unloaded cycling (without evidence of hyperventilation, ie, end-tidal P_{CO_2} did not decrease) and remained above 1.0 thereafter, indicating that the initial phase of exercise was above the patient's lactate threshold. The $\Delta\dot{V}O_2/\Delta WR$ slope was also lower than normal and became progressively more abnormal at the highest work rates. During the latter part of the test, heart rate increased

TABLE 10.93.2 Selected Exercise Data

Measurement	Predicted	Measured
Peak $\dot{V}O_2$ (L/min)	1.98	[illegible]
[illegible] $\dot{V}O_2$ (mL/min/kg)	26.8	17.9
Maximum heart rate (beats/min)	158	175
Maximum O_2 pulse (mL/beat)	12.5	7.1
$\Delta\dot{V}O_2/\Delta WR$ (mL/min/W)	10.3	6.7
AT (L/min)	>0.87	0.6
Blood pressure (mm Hg [rest, max])		130/80, 220/110
Maximum $\dot{V}E$ (L/min)		48
Exercise breathing reserve (L/min)	>15	14
$\dot{V}E/\dot{V}CO_2$ @ *AT* or lowest	28.4	28.2
O_2 saturation (oximeter [rest, max])		96, 96

Abbreviations: *AT*, anaerobic threshold; $\Delta\dot{V}O_2/\Delta WR$, change in $\dot{V}O_2$/change in work rate; O_2, oxygen; $\dot{V}E$, minute ventilation; $\dot{V}E/\dot{V}CO_2$, ventilatory equivalent for carbon dioxide; $\dot{V}O_2$, oxygen uptake.

TABLE 10.93.3 Air Breathing

Time (min)	Work rate (W)	BP (mm Hg)	HR (min^{-1})	f (min^{-1})	$\dot{V}E$ (L/min BTPS)	$\dot{V}CO_2$ (L/min STPD)	$\dot{V}O_2$ (L/min STPD)	$\frac{\dot{V}O_2}{HR}$ (mL/beat)	R	pH	HCO_3^- (mEq/L)	PO_2, mm Hg ET	a	(A − a)	PCO_2, mm Hg ET	a	(a − ET)	$\frac{\dot{V}E}{\dot{V}CO_2}$	$\frac{\dot{V}E}{\dot{V}O_2}$	$\frac{V_D}{V_T}$
0	Rest	130/80																		
0.5	Rest		108	15	9.7	0.26	0.28	2.6	0.93			108			37			32	30	
1.0	Rest		110	16	10.3	0.27	0.30	2.7	0.90			109			36			33	30	
1.5	Rest		110	13	10.1	0.27	0.29	2.6	0.93			109			36			33	31	
2.0	Rest	130/80	106	11	9.2	0.23	0.25	2.4	0.92			108			37			36	33	
2.5	Rest		108	9	9.7	0.26	0.29	2.7	0.90			108			37			34	31	
3.0	Rest		110	15	9.6	0.24	0.26	2.4	0.92			110			36			35	32	
3.5	Unloaded		118	13	14.8	0.41	0.43	3.6	0.95			109			37			33	32	
4.0	Unloaded		112	12	16.1	0.47	0.50	4.5	0.94			107			38			32	30	
4.5	Unloaded		118	10	15.3	0.51	0.56	4.7	0.91			103			41			28	26	
5.0	Unloaded		126	12	19.0	0.59	0.61	4.8	0.97			104			40			30	29	
5.5	Unloaded		128	13	18.3	0.59	0.57	4.5	1.04			109			40			29	30	
6.0	Unloaded	140/80	120	13	20.6	0.65	0.64	5.3	1.02			106			41			30	30	
6.5	10		120	15	20.9	0.65	0.64	5.3	1.02			108			39			30	31	
7.0	10	159/90	124	13	20.3	0.66	0.65	5.2	1.02			107			41			29	30	
7.5	20		124	15	22.5	0.72	0.70	5.6	1.03			108			39			29	30	
8.0	20		126	16	24.1	0.76	0.73	5.8	1.04			108			39			30	31	
8.5	30		124	15	23.5	0.77	0.74	6.0	1.04			105			42			29	30	
9.0	30		130	15	26.2	0.86	0.80	6.2	1.08			108			41			29	31	
9.5	40		132	16	27.4	0.93	0.87	6.6	1.07			107			41			28	30	
10.0	40	150/90	140	16	28.8	1.00	0.91	6.5	1.10			108			42			27	30	
10.5	50		139	18	32.1	1.06	0.93	6.7	1.14			108			42			29	33	
11.0	50		148	17	30.4	1.05	0.93	6.3	1.13			108			42			28	31	
11.5	60		150	19	34.0	1.14	1.01	6.7	1.13			110			41			28	32	
12.0	60	200/100	152	21	36.5	1.21	1.08	7.1	1.12			110			41			29	32	
12.5	70		160	23	39.3	1.29	1.16	7.3	1.11			110			40			29	32	
13.0	70		160	20	37.5	1.31	1.18	7.4	1.11			107			43			27	30	
13.5	80		170	24	41.6	1.39	1.19	7.0	1.17			109			42			28	33	
14.0	80	200/100	170	25	42.2	1.43	1.20	7.1	1.19			110			43			28	33	
14.5	90		175	28	46.5	1.52	1.22	7.0	1.25			112			42			29	36	
15.0	90		175	31	48.2	1.60	1.19	6.8	1.34			109			42			28	38	
15.5	Recovery		170	22	42.6	1.55	1.16	6.8	1.34			112			44			26	35	
16.0	Recovery		170	22	42.5	1.40	0.97	5.7	1.44			117			41			29	42	
16.5	Recovery		160	22	31.3	0.97	0.71	4.4	1.37			116			40			30	41	
17.0	Recovery	220/110	154	19	32.6	0.98	0.74	4.8	1.32			118			37			32	42	

Abbreviations: BP, blood pressure; BTPS, body temperature pressure saturated; f, frequency; HCO_3^-, bicarbonate; HR, heart rate; $P(A - a)O_2$, alveolar-arterial PO_2 difference; $P(a - ET)CO_2$, arterial-end-tidal PCO_2 difference; $PETCO_2$, end-tidal PCO_2; $PETO_2$, end-tidal PO_2; R, respiratory exchange ratio; STPD, standard temperature pressure dry; $\dot{V}CO_2$, carbon dioxide output; V_D/V_T, physiological dead space-tidal volume ratio; $\dot{V}E$, minute ventilation; $\dot{V}E/\dot{V}CO_2$, ventilatory equivalent for carbon dioxide; $\dot{V}E/\dot{V}O_2$, ventilatory equivalent for oxygen; $\dot{V}O_2$, oxygen uptake.

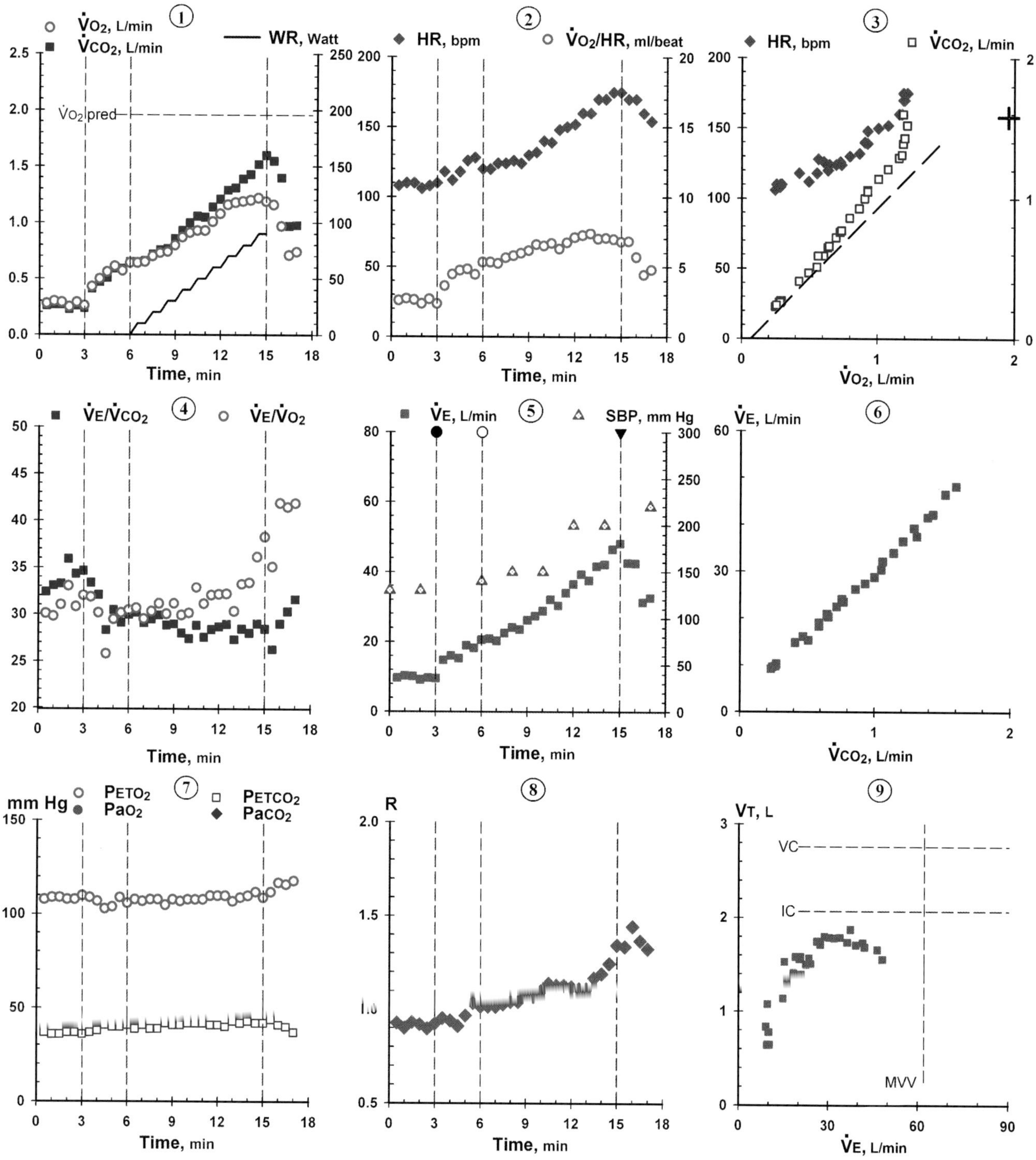

FIGURE 10.93.1. Vertical dashed lines in the panels in the left and middle columns indicate, from left to right, the beginning of unloaded cycling, start of increasing work rate (WR) at 10 W/min, and start of recovery. In **panel 1**, the increase in WR (right y-axis) is plotted with a scale of 100 W to 1 L of oxygen uptake ($\dot{V}O_2$) (left y-axis) such that WR is plotted parallel to a $\dot{V}O_2$ slope of 10 mL/min/W. In **panel 3**, carbon dioxide output ($\dot{V}CO_2$) (right y-axis) is plotted as a function of $\dot{V}O_2$ (x-axis) with identical scales so that the diagonal dashed line has a slope of 1 (45°). The $\dot{V}CO_2$ increasing more steeply than $\dot{V}O_2$ defines carbon dioxide (CO_2) derived from bicarbonate buffer, as long as ventilatory equivalent for CO_2 ($\dot{V}E/\dot{V}CO_2$) (**panel 4**) is not increasing and end-tidal PCO_2 (P_{ETCO_2}) (**panel 7**) is not decreasing, simultaneously. The black + symbol in **panel 3** indicates predicted peak values of heart rate (HR) (left y-axis) and $\dot{V}O_2$ for this individual. Abbreviations: IC, inspiratory capacity; MVV, maximum voluntary ventilation; P_{ETO_2}, end-tidal PO_2; R, respiratory exchange ratio; SBP, systolic blood pressure; VC, vital capacity; $\dot{V}E$, minute ventilation; $\dot{V}E/\dot{V}O_2$, ventilatory equivalent for oxygen; V_T, tidal volume.

steeply relative to $\dot{V}O_2$ such that the O_2 pulse reached its maximal value and remained stable over the last 2 minutes of exercise at a level well below the predicted peak value. These abnormalities of O_2 flow were not attributable to low arterial O_2 content (hematocrit and pulse oximeter values were normal), so imply a cardiovascular abnormality. The ventilatory equivalent for carbon dioxide relationship was normal, implying good pulmonary ventilation-perfusion matching. These findings, along with the normal diffusing capacity of lung for carbon monoxide, make it unlikely that the findings of cardiovascular impairment were attributable to pulmonary vascular disease complicating the patient's chronic lung disease. More likely, the patient had comorbid heart and lung diseases. There were no ECG findings to support exercise-induced ischemia, so chronic left ventricular dysfunction was suspected.

Despite the abnormal findings on this test, the peak $\dot{V}O_2$ value of 18 mL/min/kg predicted relatively little increased risk associated with resectional lung surgery. Peak $\dot{V}O_2$ values less than 15 mL/min/kg have been associated with increased risk of complications, and values of less than 10 mL/min/kg are generally regarded to carry such substantial risk of surgical morbidity and mortality that nonsurgical alternative are usually recommended.

Conclusion

This case is presented to illustrate the use of exercise testing in preoperative risk evaluations. Exercise testing is an established part of the assessment of physiologic resectability of patients with anatomically resectable lung lesions.[1,2] Test results do not necessarily represent absolute indications or contraindications to potentially lifesaving procedures but provide valuable information to inform the discussion of risks and benefits.

REFERENCES

1. Brunelli A, Charloux A, Bolliger CT, et al. ERS/ESTS clinical guidelines on fitness for radical therapy in lung cancer patients (surgery and chemoradiotherapy). *Eur Respir J*. 2009;34(1):17-41.
2. Brunelli A, Kim AW, Berger KI, Addrizzo-Harris DJ. Physiologic evaluation of the patient with lung cancer being considered for resectional surgery: Diagnosis and management of lung cancer, 3rd ed: American College of Chest Physicians evidence-based clinical practice guidelines. *Chest*. 2013;143(5 suppl):e166S-e190S.

CASE 94

Exercise Testing for Evaluation of Work Fitness: Morbid Obesity

CLINICAL FINDINGS

This 45-year-old man was referred by his attorney for an exercise study to evaluate his fitness for work as a security guard. Because of the employee's obesity, his employer was attempting to terminate him from his job on the belief that he would be unable to perform his duties, which could include running up stairs and chasing after intruders. The employee was a nonsmoker and denied any medical history, exercise limitation, or regular medications. The resting electrocardiogram was normal.

EXERCISE FINDINGS

The patient performed exercise on a treadmill using a modified Balke protocol because this was believed to be a better way to simulate his job functions than a cycle. After a short period of standing at rest, he walked on the treadmill belt at 3 mph (4.8 km/h) with no grade for 3 minutes; thereafter, the grade was increased 2% per minute to tolerance. The patient appeared to give an excellent effort and stopped exercise because of fatigue; he denied chest pain or dyspnea during or after the study. No ectopy or abnormal electrocardiogram changes occurred during or after exercise.

INTERPRETATION

Comments

Resting lung function studies are typical of extreme obesity, with reduction of the expiratory reserve volume and preservation of inspiratory capacity (**Table 10.94.1**). His height was 168 cm and weight 157 kg, giving him a body mass index of 49.6.

Analysis

The choice of an appropriate predicted peak oxygen uptake ($\dot{V}O_2$) determines if this patient is physiologically impaired. Using a peak $\dot{V}O_2$ predicted from height (ie, based on ideal weight), peak $\dot{V}O_2$ was well above predicted, as was his anaerobic threshold (**Table 10.94.2**). He was close to reaching ventilatory limitation with a low breathing reserve, but there was no evidence of increased minute ventilation ($\dot{V}E$) versus carbon dioxide output ($\dot{V}CO_2$) slope or of elevated ventilatory equivalent at the anaerobic threshold, markers of lung gas exchange abnormalities.

However, what is apparent is a large "step-up" in $\dot{V}O_2$ when he began walking on level grade at 3 mph. In fact, $\dot{V}O_2$ increased from about 0.70 to about 2.60 L/min, much more than anticipated for a nonoverweight individual. This reflects the high metabolic cost ($\dot{V}O_2$) of carrying the body weight while walking, even at a modest pace. The initial level grade walking required a large proportion of his total $\dot{V}O_2$ at maximum exercise, thereby limiting his capacity for "external work" beyond that of moving his larger body mass.

TABLE 10.94.1 Selected Respiratory Function Data

Measurement	Predicted	Measured
Age (y)		45
Sex		Male
Height (cm)		168
Weight (kg)	72	157
Hematocrit (%)		47
VC (L)	4.11	3.67
IC (L)	2.74	3.63
ERV (L)	1.37	0.04
FEV_1 (L)	3.31	3.19
FEV_1/VC (%)	81	87
MVV (L/min)	132	140

Abbreviations: ERV, expiratory reserve volume; FEV_1, forced expiratory volume in 1 second; IC, inspiratory capacity; MVV, maximum voluntary ventilation; VC, vital capacity.

TABLE 10.94.2 Selected Exercise Data

Measurement	Predicted	Measured
Peak $\dot{V}O_2$ (L/min)	3.28	4.14
Peak $\dot{V}O_2$ (mL/min/kg)	45.6	26.4
Maximum heart rate (beats/min)	175	191
Maximum O_2 pulse (mL/beat)	18.7	21.8
AT (L/min)	>1.39	3.25
Blood pressure (mm Hg [rest, max])		160/90, 225/100
Maximum $\dot{V}E$ (L/min)		128
Exercise breathing reserve (L/min)	>15	12
$\dot{V}E/\dot{V}CO_2$ @ *AT* or lowest	26.7	23.2

Abbreviations: *AT*, anaerobic threshold; O_2, oxygen; $\dot{V}E$, minute ventilation; $\dot{V}E/\dot{V}CO_2$, ventilatory equivalent for carbon dioxide; $\dot{V}O_2$, oxygen uptake.

TABLE 10.94.3 Air Breathing; Treadmill Test

Time (min)	Treadmill grade[a] (%)	BP (mm Hg)	HR (min^{-1})	f (min^{-1})	$\dot{V}E$ (L/min BTPS)	$\dot{V}CO_2$ (L/min STPD)	$\dot{V}O_2$ (L/min STPD)	$\frac{\dot{V}O_2}{HR}$ (mL/beat)	R	pH	HCO_3^- (mEq/L)	PO_2, mm Hg			PCO_2, mm Hg			$\frac{\dot{V}E}{\dot{V}CO_2}$	$\frac{\dot{V}E}{\dot{V}O_2}$	$\frac{V_D}{V_T}$
												ET	a	(A − a)	ET	a	(a − ET)			
0	Rest	160/90																		
0.5	Rest		106	20	15.2	0.45	0.60	5.7	0.75			94			42			30	23	
1.0	Rest		108	25	19.8	0.63	0.76	7.0	0.83			93			43			28	23	
1.5	Rest		113	29	16.0	0.50	0.64	5.7	0.78			89			46			27	21	
2.0	Rest	150/100	108	17	14.8	0.45	0.55	5.1	0.82			100			42			30	24	
2.5	Rest		107	20	17.7	0.55	0.69	6.4	0.80			94			42			29	23	
3.0	Rest		115	20	17.5	0.52	0.63	5.5	0.83			100			41			30	25	
3.5	0		128	35	27.1	0.81	1.20	9.4	0.68			84			44			30	20	
4.0	0		135	31	38.1	1.40	2.11	15.6	0.66			79			47			25	17	
4.5	0		141	31	51.1	1.96	2.54	18.0	0.77			81			49			25	19	
5.0	0		142	30	52.0	2.07	2.55	18.0	0.81			77			54			24	19	
5.5	0		145	33	49.2	2.01	2.43	16.8	0.83			82			53			23	19	
6.0	0	210/100	149	32	57.0	2.34	2.77	18.6	0.84			86			52			23	20	
6.5	2		152	33	59.5	2.42	2.80	18.4	0.86			74			57			23	20	
7.0	2		153	34	60.6	2.53	2.85	18.6	0.89			84			54			23	20	
7.5	4		156	34	64.6	2.66	2.96	19.0	0.90			90			51			23	21	
8.0	4	210/90	162	36	68.6	2.83	3.08	19.0	0.92			92			51			23	21	
8.5	6		162	36	72.7	2.92	3.12	19.3	0.94			88			53			24	22	
9.0	6		165	36	72.8	2.97	3.22	19.5	0.92			87			53			23	22	
9.5	8		168	40	81.1	3.28	3.43	20.4	0.96			92			52			24	23	
10.0	8	210/90	170	38	83.4	3.34	3.41	20.1	0.98			83			57			24	24	
10.5	10		175	42	88.7	3.56	3.63	20.7	0.98			90			53			24	23	
11.0	10		175	40	86.3	3.61	3.56	20.3	1.01			93			53			23	23	
11.5	12		180	43	93.6	3.79	3.64	20.2	1.04			97			51			24	25	
12.0	12	220/90	182	45	101.8	4.07	3.78	20.8	1.08			99			50			24	26	
12.5	14		186	46	106.3	4.28	3.92	21.1	1.09			99			51			24	26	
13.0	14		186	48	111.0	4.77	3.88	20.9	1.23			91			57			22	28	
13.5	16		187	52	123.5	4.75	4.08	21.8	1.16			103			49			25	29	
14.0	16	225/100	191	53	128.4	4.96	4.14	21.7	1.20			106			48			25	30	
14.5	Recovery		179	50	120.1	4.80	4.10	22.9	1.17			103			49			24	28	
15.0	Recovery	200/80	169	39	96.4	4.13	3.53	20.9	1.17			99			54			23	26	
15.5	Recovery		161	34	83.2	3.34	2.65	16.5	1.26			101			53			24	30	
16.0	Recovery	180/80	150	33	73.6	2.85	2.21	14.7	1.29			105			49			25	32	

Abbreviations: BP, blood pressure; BTPS, body temperature pressure saturated; f, frequency; HCO_3^-, bicarbonate; HR, heart rate; $P(A - a)O_2$, alveolar-arterial PO_2 difference; $P(a - ET)CO_2$, arterial–end-tidal PCO_2 difference; $PETCO_2$, end-tidal PCO_2; $PETO_2$, end-tidal PO_2; R, respiratory exchange ratio; STPD, standard temperature pressure dry; $\dot{V}CO_2$, carbon dioxide output; V_D/V_T, physiological dead space–tidal volume ratio; $\dot{V}E$, minute ventilation; $\dot{V}E/\dot{V}CO_2$, ventilatory equivalent for carbon dioxide; $\dot{V}E/\dot{V}O_2$, ventilatory equivalent for oxygen; $\dot{V}O_2$, oxygen uptake.

[a]Treadmill speed was 3 miles/hour throughout the exercise period.

Exercise capacity can be expressed in a number of ways; the most meaningful depends on the question being addressed by the test. Physiologically, he exceeds the predicted capacity of his lungs, heart, circulation, and exercising muscles to take up and consume oxygen; that is, he is not impaired from a cardiovascular or respiratory standpoint (normal peak $\dot{V}O_2$ for his age and ideal weight). When his peak $\dot{V}O_2$ is expressed as $\dot{V}O_2$/kg actual weight, however, the resultant value is low and reflects a limited capacity to do external work. This expression of peak $\dot{V}O_2$ would be in the domain of functional rather than physiological assessment.

Conclusion

This individual's exercise test demonstrated excellent physiologic capacity, but maximum work capacity that was compromised by the metabolic effects of obesity. The suggestion of carbon dioxide retention with exercise presumably reflects the increased metabolic cost of exercise and disproportionate high work of breathing. The question of whether his weight disqualifies him from his employment is more of a legal than medical issue. The test results suggest he would likely be capable of pursuing intruders but perhaps not of apprehending them.

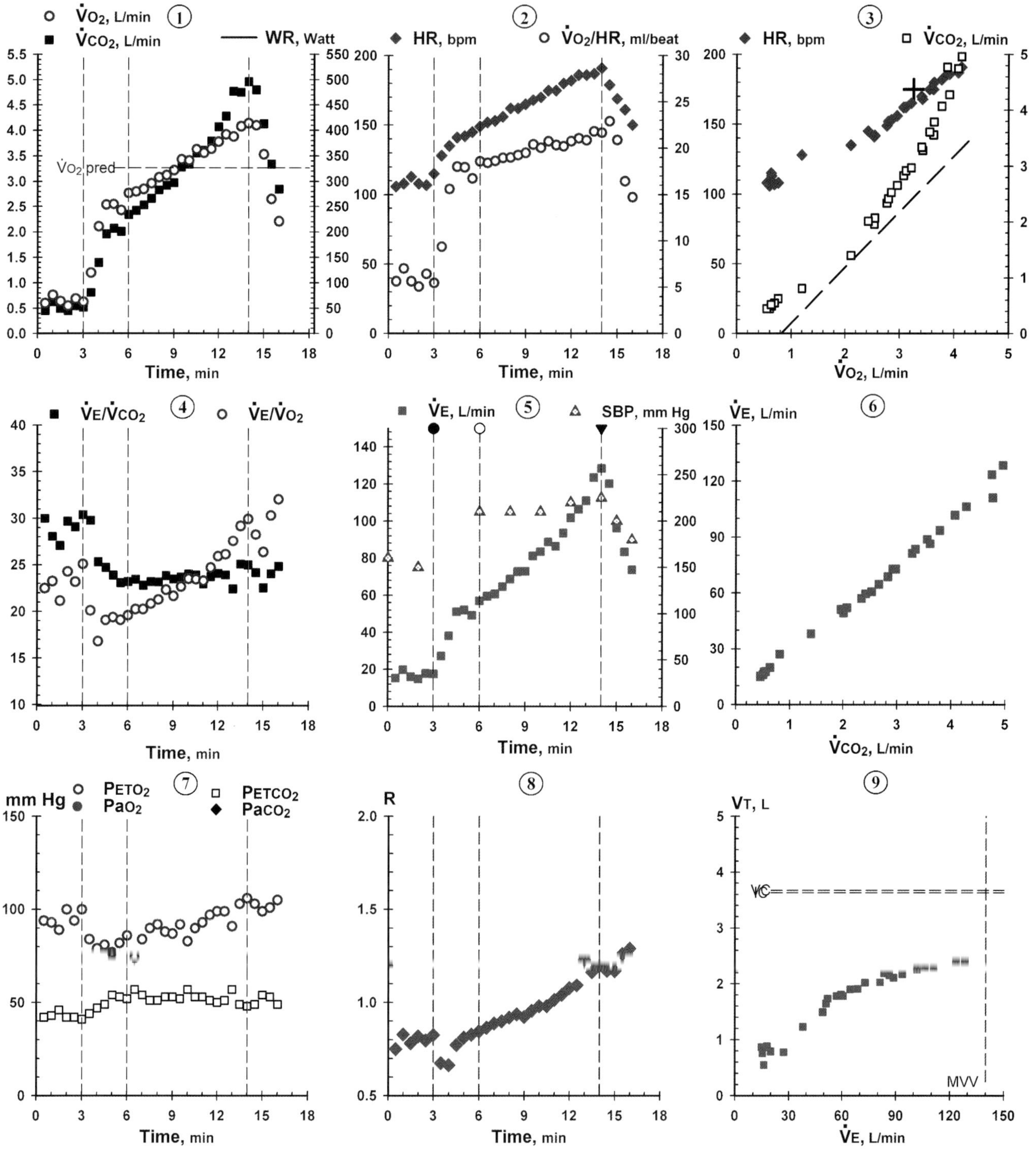

FIGURE 10.94.1. Vertical dashed lines in the panels in the left and middle columns indicate, from left to right, the beginning of treadmill walking at a speed of 3 mph at zero grade, the start of increasing grade by 2% per minute, and start of recovery. In **panel 3**, carbon dioxide output ($\dot{V}CO_2$) (right y-axis) is plotted as a function of oxygen uptake ($\dot{V}O_2$) (x-axis) with identical scales so that the diagonal dashed line has a slope of 1 (45°). The $\dot{V}CO_2$ increasing more steeply than $\dot{V}O_2$ defines carbon dioxide (CO_2) derived from bicarbonate buffer, as long as ventilatory equivalent for CO_2 ($\dot{V}E/\dot{V}CO_2$) (**panel 4**) is not increasing and end-tidal PCO_2 ($PETCO_2$) (**panel 7**) is not decreasing, simultaneously. The black + symbol in **panel 3** indicates predicted peak values of heart rate (HR) (left y-axis) and $\dot{V}O_2$ for this individual. Abbreviations: IC, inspiratory capacity; MVV, maximum voluntary ventilation; $PETO_2$, end-tidal PO_2; R, respiratory exchange ratio; SBP, systolic blood pressure; VC, vital capacity; $\dot{V}E$, minute ventilation; $\dot{V}E/\dot{V}O_2$, ventilatory equivalent for oxygen; V_T, tidal volume; WR, work rate.

CASE 95

Exercise Testing for Assessment Before and After Pulmonary Rehabilitation for Chronic Obstructive Pulmonary Disease

To view this case please access the eBook bundled with this text. Instructions are located on the inside front cover.

CASE 96

Evaluation of Unexplained Dyspnea: A Morbidly Obese Asthmatic

CLINICAL FINDINGS

This 55-year-old man was referred for cardiopulmonary exercise testing for evaluation of unexplained dyspnea that had not improved with escalation of his asthma therapy. Although he initially described symptoms over the preceding 12 months, he also indicated that his weight had increased by 80 lb several years previously, which he attributed to curtailing his activities due to exertional dyspnea. He was morbidly obese and was treated for hypertension, adult-onset diabetes, and obstructive sleep apnea. He had an episode of deep vein thrombosis several years previously without known pulmonary embolism. He worked in an office and was short of breath even with sustained walking indoors; he did no recreational activities. His medications included a diuretic, an angiotensin-converting enzyme inhibitor, oral hypoglycemic agents, inhaled corticosteroids and long-acting β-agonist, a leukotriene modifier, warfarin, and nocturnal continuous positive airway pressure. His examination was notable only for obesity with a body mass index of 45. The electrocardiogram showed a sinus rhythm and was normal.

TABLE 10.96.1 Selected Respiratory Function Data

Measurement	Predicted	Measured
Age (y)		55
Sex		Male
Height (cm)		185
Weight (kg)		169
VC (L)	5.44	4.26
IC (L)	3.62	3.98
FEV_1 (L)	4.16	3.01
FEV_1/VC (%)	77	71
MVV (L/min)	157	120

Abbreviations: FEV_1, forced expiratory volume in 1 second; IC, inspiratory capacity; MVV, maximum voluntary ventilation; VC, vital capacity.

EXERCISE FINDINGS

The patient exercised on a cycle ergometer beginning with 3 minutes of pedaling without an added load, followed by an increase in work rate by 15 W/min to tolerance. He cooperated well with the study and ended the test with

TABLE 10.96.2 Selected Exercise Data

Measurement	Predicted	Measured
Peak $\dot{V}O_2$ (L/min)	3.04	2.17
Peak $\dot{V}O_2$ (mL/min/kg)	40.5	12.8
Maximum heart rate (beats/min)	165	96
Maximum O_2 pulse (mL/beat)	18.5	23.1
$\Delta\dot{V}O_2/\Delta WR$ (mL/min/W)	10.3	9.2
AT (L/min)	>1.39	1.28
Blood pressure (mm Hg [rest, max])		132/83, 195/84
Maximum $\dot{V}E$ (L/min)		72
Exercise breathing reserve (L/min)	>15	48
$\dot{V}E/\dot{V}CO_2$ @ *AT* or lowest	27.2	27.4

Abbreviations: *AT*, anaerobic threshold; $\Delta\dot{V}O_2/\Delta WR$, change in $\dot{V}O_2$/change in work rate; O_2, oxygen; $\dot{V}E$, minute ventilation; $\dot{V}E/\dot{V}CO_2$, ventilatory equivalent for carbon dioxide; $\dot{V}O_2$, oxygen uptake.

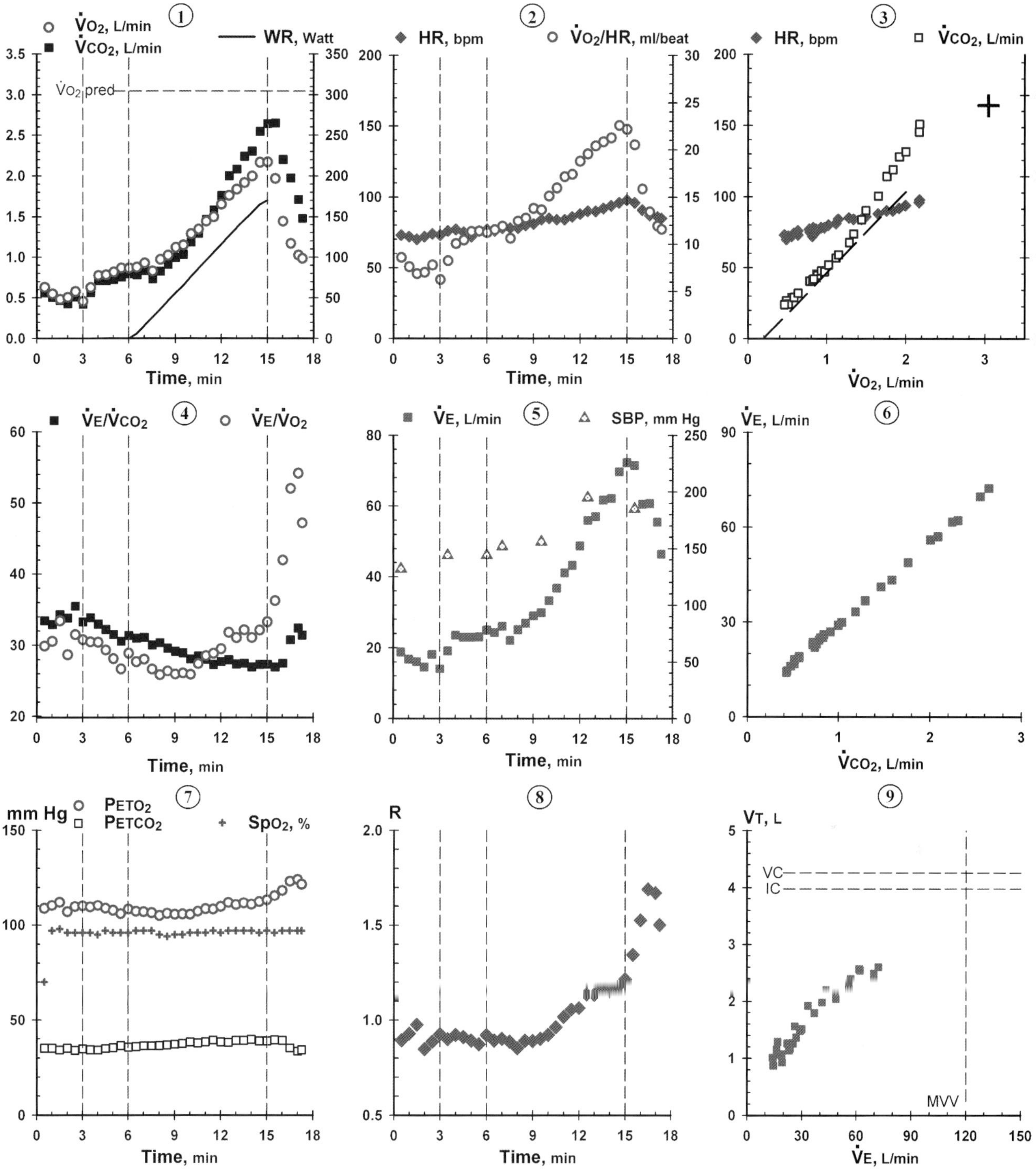

FIGURE 10.96.1. Vertical dashed lines in the panels in the left and middle columns indicate, from left to right, the beginning of unloaded cycling, start of increasing work rate (WR) at 20 W/min, and start of recovery. In **panel 1**, the increase in WR (right y-axis) is plotted with a scale of 100 W to 1 L of oxygen uptake ($\dot{V}O_2$) (left y-axis) such that WR is plotted parallel to a $\dot{V}O_2$ slope of 10 mL/min/W. In **panel 3**, carbon dioxide output ($\dot{V}CO_2$) (right y-axis) is plotted as a function of $\dot{V}O_2$ (x-axis) with identical scales so that the diagonal dashed line has a slope of 1 (45°). The $\dot{V}CO_2$ increasing more steeply than $\dot{V}O_2$ defines carbon dioxide (CO_2) derived from bicarbonate buffer, as long as ventilatory equivalent for carbon dioxide ($\dot{V}E/\dot{V}CO_2$) (**panel 4**) is not increasing and end-tidal PCO_2 ($PETCO_2$) (**panel 7**) is not decreasing, simultaneously. The black + symbol in **panel 3** indicates predicted peak values of heart rate (HR) (left y-axis) and $\dot{V}O_2$ this individual. Abbreviations: IC, inspiratory capacity; MVV, maximum voluntary ventilation; $PETO_2$, end-tidal partial pressure of oxygen; R, respiratory exchange ratio; SBP, systolic blood pressure; SpO_2, oxygen saturation as measured by pulse oximetry; VC, vital capacity; $\dot{V}E$, minute ventilation; $\dot{V}E/\dot{V}O_2$, ventilatory equivalent for oxygen; $\dot{V}O_2$/HR, O_2 uptake/heart beat or O_2 pulse; V_T, tidal volume.

TABLE 10.96.3 Air Breathing

Time (min)	Work rate (W)	BP (mm Hg)	HR (min^{-1})	f (min^{-1})	$\dot{V}E$ (L/min BTPS)	$\dot{V}CO_2$ (L/min STPD)	$\dot{V}O_2$ (L/min STPD)	$\dot{V}O_2$/HR (mL/beat)	R	pH	HCO_3^- (mEq/L)	PO_2, mm Hg			PCO_2, mm Hg			$\dot{V}E/\dot{V}CO_2$	$\dot{V}E/\dot{V}O_2$	V_D/V_T
												ET	a	(A − a)	ET	a	(a − ET)			
0.5	Rest	132/83	73	18	18.8	0.56	0.63	8.6	0.89			109			35			33	30	
1.0	Rest		72	13	16.8	0.51	0.55	7.6	0.93			110			35			33	31	
1.5	Rest		70	14	16.1	0.47	0.48	6.9	0.98			112			34			34	33	
2.0	Rest		72	17	14.5	0.43	0.51	7.0	0.85			107			35			34	29	
2.5	Rest		74	17	18.1	0.51	0.58	7.8	0.89			110			34			35	31	
3.0	Rest		73	14	14.0	0.42	0.46	6.2	0.93			110			35			33	31	
3.5	Unloaded	144/79	76	21	19.1	0.56	0.63	8.3	0.90			110			34			34	30	
4.0	Unloaded		77	20	23.6	0.71	0.77	10.1	0.92			110			34			33	30	
4.5	Unloaded		75	20	22.9	0.71	0.78	10.4	0.91			109			35			32	29	
5.0	Unloaded		72	19	22.9	0.73	0.82	11.3	0.89			108			36			32	28	
5.5	Unloaded		76	18	23.1	0.76	0.87	11.4	0.87			106			36			31	27	
6.0	Unloaded		77	20	25.0	0.80	0.86	11.2	0.92			108			36			31	29	
6.5	6	152/73	76	19	24.3	0.78	0.88	11.5	0.89			107			36			31	28	
7.0	16		78	17	26.0	0.84	0.93	11.9	0.90			107			36			31	28	
7.5	26		78	18	22.1	0.73	0.83	10.6	0.89			107			36			30	27	
8.0	36		78	20	25.1	0.83	0.97	12.4	0.85			105			37			30	26	
8.5	46		80	20	26.9	0.91	1.02	12.8	0.89			106			37			30	26	
9.0	56		81	20	29.0	1.00	1.12	13.8	0.89			106			37			29	26	
9.5	65	156/79	84	20	29.9	1.03	1.15	13.7	0.90			106			38			29	26	
10.0	76		85	17	33.3	1.18	1.28	15.1	0.92			106			38			28	26	
10.5	86		84	21	36.8	1.29	1.34	16.0	0.96			107			38			28	27	
11.0	96		84	21	41.1	1.47	1.44	17.2	1.02			109			38			28	29	
11.5	106		86	20	43.2	1.58	1.50	17.4	1.06			108			39			27	29	
12.0	116		88	24	48.8	1.76	1.65	18.8	1.06			110			39			28	30	
12.5	126	195/68	90	25	56.0	2.00	1.76	19.6	1.14			112			38			28	32	
13.0	136		90	24	57.1	2.08	1.84	20.4	1.13			111			39			27	31	
13.5	146		92	24	61.7	2.24	1.92	20.8	1.17			112			39			28	32	
14.0	155		94	24	62.1	2.30	2.00	21.2	1.15			111			40			27	31	
14.5	165		94	28	69.6	2.55	2.17	20.1	1.18			112			39			27	32	
15.0	170		94	28	72.3	2.64	2.17	23.1	1.22			113			39			27	33	
15.5	Recovery	185/84	96	27	71.4	2.65	1.97	20.5	1.34			116			40			27	36	
16.0	Recovery		91	21	60.5	2.20	1.44	15.8	1.53			118			39			27	42	
16.5	Recovery		87	23	60.8	1.97	1.17	13.4	1.69			123			35			31	52	
17.0	Recovery		86	21	55.5	1.71	1.02	11.9	1.67			124			34			32	54	

Abbreviations: BP, blood pressure; BTPS, body temperature pressure saturated; f, frequency; HCO_3^-, bicarbonate; HR, heart rate; $P(A - a)O_2$, alveolar-arterial PO_2 difference; $P(a - ET)CO_2$, arterial-end-tidal PCO_2 difference; $PETCO_2$, end-tidal PCO_2; $PETO_2$, end-tidal PO_2; R, respiratory exchange ratio; STPD, standard temperature pressure dry; V_D/V_T, physiological dead space-tidal volume ratio; $\dot{V}E$, minute ventilation; $\dot{V}CO_2$, carbon dioxide output; $\dot{V}E/\dot{V}CO_2$, ventilatory equivalent for carbon dioxide; $\dot{V}E/\dot{V}O_2$, ventilatory equivalent for carbon dioxide; $\dot{V}O_2$, oxygen uptake; $\dot{V}O_2$/HR, O_2 uptake per heart beat or O_2 pulse.

symptoms of leg fatigue and dyspnea. Because of the history of airflow obstruction, spirometry was repeated serially for 20 minutes after exercise. Spontaneous flow-volume loops were monitored on a breath-by-breath basis during exercise, and inspiratory capacity was measured periodically to identify the occurrence of dynamic hyperinflation.

Comments

On the day of testing, pulmonary function tests showed a mild restrictive defect, but no evident obstruction, and a normal diffusing capacity of the lung for carbon monoxide. The restrictive defect was characteristic of obesity; expiratory reserve volume was markedly reduced and inspiratory capacity was elevated (**Table 10.96.1**). Exercise data are summarized in **Table 10.96.2** and shown in **Table 10.96.3** and **Figure 10.96.1**.

Analysis

Peak oxygen uptake ($\dot{V}O_2$) and anaerobic threshold were mildly reduced relative to predicted. Expressed as L/min/kg, peak $\dot{V}O_2$ was even lower, due to the excess weight. However, ventilatory and gas exchange responses to exercise were normal, including a large breathing reserve, normal oximetry, and normal ventilatory equivalent for carbon dioxide ($\dot{V}E/\dot{V}CO_2$) at the anaerobic threshold. In addition, the inspiratory capacity remained stable during exercise, and postexercise spirometry was unchanged from rest (data not shown). These findings argue against occult pulmonary vascular disease or poorly controlled asthma as the cause of his symptoms.

The one abnormal finding in this test was the patient's strikingly reduced heart rate (HR) response to exercise, with decreased slope of HR versus $\dot{V}O_2$ in panel 3 and HR versus WR in panel 2. The cardiac rhythm remained sinus, and no ischemic changes in electrocardiogram developed. The attenuated HR response was not the result of poor effort, as the patient exercised considerably past his anaerobic threshold as shown by the V slope and reflected in an end-exercise respiratory exchange ratio of over 1.2, and the HR response was shallow relative to $\dot{V}O_2$ across the entire test (panel 3 of **Figure 10.96.1**). The peak O_2 pulse was much higher than predicted, implying a compensatory increase in stroke volume, which partially offsets the effect of the low HR on oxygen delivery and indicates excellent systolic function (consistent with the normal slope of minute ventilation ($\dot{V}E$) versus carbon dioxide output ($\dot{V}CO_2$) and $\dot{V}E/\dot{V}CO_2$). The patient's medication history was again reviewed in detail to confirm that he was not taking a β-blocker or other agent that would affect HR. It was concluded that he had intrinsic chronotropic insufficiency due to sinus node disease.

Conclusion

This test is presented as an example of a specific diagnosis being identified by exercise testing for evaluation of unexplained dyspnea. The potential causes of dyspnea in this case were diverse, including obesity, deconditioning, reactive airway disease, or unrecognized thromboembolism, as well as cardiovascular disease. If the testing had been performed without gas exchange measurements, the low peak HR might have been interpreted as an inadequate effort. The relationship of HR and $\dot{V}O_2$ allowed confident identification of chronotropic insufficiency as the cause of exercise intolerance.

CASE 97

Evaluation of Unexplained Dyspnea: Chronic Thromboembolic Pulmonary Vascular Disease

CLINICAL FINDINGS

This 50-year-old man was referred for evaluation of unexplained dyspnea. He had felt well until 1 year prior to evaluation, when he noted the insidious but progressive development of shortness of breath and easy fatigability. Six months prior to evaluation, he had an episode of acute severe substernal chest pain and dyspnea, which resulted in hospitalization and treatment for a suspected myocardial infarction. Following discharge from the hospital, he had lost 25 to 30 lb by watching his diet but remained somewhat dyspneic. He had no history of hypertension or diabetes mellitus. He had smoked three to four cigarettes daily until 2 years earlier. Physical examination was normal, with no signs of heart failure. Chest radiograph was unremarkable. Resting electrocardiogram showed normal QRS complexes and negative T waves in V_1 through V_3, suggesting right ventricular strain but no Q waves.

EXERCISE FINDINGS

The patient performed exercise on a cycle ergometer. He pedaled at 60 rpm without added load for 1 minute. The work rate was then increased 20 W/min. Arterial blood was sampled every second minute, and intra-arterial blood pressure was recorded from a percutaneously placed brachial artery catheter. The patient stopped exercise because of overall fatigue and exhaustion; he denied having chest pain or dyspnea. There was a maximum of 0.5-mm ST-segment depression in leads II, V_5, and V_6 that resolved by 3 minutes of recovery.

INTERPRETATION

Comments

The resting respiratory function studies showed normal lung mechanics but a significant reduction in diffusing capacity (**Table 10.97.1**). The electrocardiogram was suggestive of right ventricular strain. Exercise data are summarized in **Table 10.97.2** and shown in **Table 10.97.3** and **Figure 10.97.1**.

Analysis

Peak oxygen uptake ($\dot{V}O_2$) was reduced and the anaerobic threshold was borderline low. He did not have evidence of ventilatory limitation from with low breathing reserve; his heart rate–$\dot{V}O_2$ relationship was steeper than normal with low maximum O_2 pulse. The most interesting feature was the finding of noninvasive suggestion of pulmonary gas exchange abnormality with high minute ventilation ($\dot{V}E$) versus carbon dioxide output ($\dot{V}CO_2$) slope and high ventilatory equivalent for carbon dioxide ($\dot{V}E/\dot{V}CO_2$) at the anaerobic threshold. Because arterial blood gases were available, this finding was confirmed with elevated physiological dead space-tidal volume ratio (VD/VT), alveolar-arterial PO_2 difference (P[A − a]O_2), and arterial–end-tidal PCO_2 difference (P[a − ET]CO_2). The steep heart rate–$\dot{V}O_2$ relationship and low, relatively nonchanging O_2 pulse together with abnormal lung gas exchange suggested pulmonary vascular disease. A radionuclide ventilation-perfusion scan later demonstrated large unmatched perfusion defects, diagnostic of chronic pulmonary thromboembolic disease.

Using the flowcharts (Chapter 9), the low peak $\dot{V}O_2$ and borderline low anaerobic threshold lead to Flowchart 4. Because breathing reserve is normal (Branch Point 4.1) and $\dot{V}E/\dot{V}CO_2$ at the anaerobic threshold is high (Branch Point 4.3), VD/VT is evaluated, and when there is arterial hypoxemia especially marked in this patient, a tentative diagnosis of pulmonary vascular disease can be entertained.

Conclusion

This case is presented as an example of exercise testing providing direction to the diagnostic evaluation of a patient with unexplained dyspnea. The patient's physicians had attributed his acute symptoms to myocardial infarction, a diagnosis that was not well corroborated, and did not in itself explain his continued symptoms. Exercise findings were suggestive of a pulmonary vascular process, which directed testing to studies that established a diagnosis of chronic thromboembolic pulmonary vascular disease.

TABLE 10.97.1 Selected Respiratory Function Data

Measurement	Predicted	Measured
Age (y)		50
Sex		Male
Height (cm)		185
Weight (kg)	86	92
Hematocrit (%)		46
VC (L)	5.10	4.68
IC (L)	3.40	2.94
TLC (L)	7.45	5.94
FEV_1 (L)	4.06	3.62
FEV_1/VC (%)	80	77
MVV (L/min)	161	152
DLCO (mL/mm Hg/min)	32.3	21.2

Abbreviations: DLCO, diffusing capacity of the lung for carbon monoxide; FEV_1, forced expiratory volume in 1 second; IC, inspiratory capacity; MVV, maximum voluntary ventilation; TLC, total lung capacity; VC, vital capacity.

TABLE 10.97.2 Selected Exercise Data

Measurement	Predicted	Measured
Peak $\dot{V}O_2$ (L/min)	2.78	1.92
Maximum heart rate (beats/min)	170	164
Maximum O_2 pulse (mL/beat)	16.4	11.7
$\Delta\dot{V}O_2/\Delta WR$ (mL/min/W)	10.3	8.9
AT (L/min)	>1.25	1.25
Blood pressure (mm Hg [rest, max])		125/80, 161/92
Maximum $\dot{V}E$ (L/min)		104
Exercise breathing reserve (L/min)	>15	48
$\dot{V}E/\dot{V}CO_2$ @ *AT* or lowest	26.6	42.9
PaO_2 (mm Hg [rest, max ex])		83, 56
$P(A-a)O_2$ (mm Hg [rest, max ex])		26, 63
$PaCO_2$ (mm Hg [rest, max ex])		34, 33
$P(a-ET)CO_2$ (mm Hg [rest, max ex])		5, 9
V_D/V_T (rest, heavy ex)		0.40, 0.45
HCO_3^- (mEq/L [rest, 2-min recov])		22, 19

Abbreviations: *AT*, anaerobic threshold; $\Delta\dot{V}O_2/\Delta WR$, change in $\dot{V}O_2$/change in work rate; HCO_3^-, bicarbonate; $P(A-a)O_2$, alveolar-arterial PO_2 difference; $P(a-ET)CO_2$, arterial-end-tidal PCO_2 difference; O_2, oxygen; V_D/V_T, physiological dead space–tidal volume ratio; $\dot{V}E$, minute ventilation; $\dot{V}E/\dot{V}CO_2$, ventilatory equivalent for carbon dioxide; $\dot{V}O_2$, oxygen uptake.

TABLE 10.97.3 Air Breathing

Time (min)	Work rate (W)	BP (mm Hg)	HR (min^{-1})	f (min^{-1})	$\dot{V}E$ (L/min BTPS)	$\dot{V}CO_2$ (L/min STPD)	$\dot{V}O_2$ (L/min STPD)	$\dot{V}O_2$/HR (mL/beat)	R	pH	HCO_3^- (mEq/L)	PO_2, mm Hg ET	PO_2 a	PO_2 (A − a)	PCO_2, mm Hg ET	PCO_2 a	PCO_2 (a − ET)	$\dot{V}E/\dot{V}CO_2$	$\dot{V}E/\dot{V}O_2$	V_D/V_T
0	Rest	125/80								7.41	21		73			34				
0.5	Rest		82	24	12.9	0.22	0.25	3.0	0.88			116			28			49	43	
1.0	Rest		82	22	14.7	0.28	0.35	4.3	0.80			112			29			46	37	
1.5	Rest		81	21	14.8	0.28	0.35	4.3	0.80			110			30			46	37	
2.0	Rest	119/83	81	16	12.0	0.23	0.29	3.6	0.79	7.42	22	112	83	26	29	34	5	46	37	0.40
2.5	Unloaded		94	23	26.8	0.56	0.66	7.0	0.85			109			30			44	38	
3.0	Unloaded	140/86	92	26	26.1	0.55	0.63	6.8	0.87	7.42	22	116	69	42	28	35	7	43	38	0.40
3.5	20		100	25	28.9	0.64	0.77	7.7	0.83			113			29			42	35	
4.0	20		100	22	32.8	0.72	0.86	8.6	0.84			115			28			43	36	
4.5	40		104	20	34.2	0.77	0.91	8.8	0.85			115			28			42	36	
5.0	40		108	22	37.1	0.84	0.99	9.2	0.85			115			28			42	36	
[illegible]	[illegible]		[illegible]	[illegible]	[illegible]	[illegible]	1.10	[illegible]	0.88			110			27			44	39	
6.0	60	146/86	115	25	47.2	1.02	1.16	10.1	0.88	7.42	22	116	64	47	28	35	7	44	39	0.42
6.5	80		121	27	52.5	1.16	1.31	10.8	0.89			116			28			43	38	
7.0	80		125	29	56.5	1.21	1.31	10.5	0.92			120			25			45	41	
7.5	100		132	27	60.8	1.32	1.41	10.7	0.94			120			26			44	41	
8.0	100	155/89	137	28	63.9	1.39	1.47	10.7	0.95	7.43	22	121	60	55	25	33	8	44	42	0.39
8.5	120		143	27	69.1	1.52	1.58	11.0	0.96			122			25			44	42	
9.0	120		147	28	72.8	1.62	1.66	11.3	0.98			123			25			43	42	
9.5	140		152	33	87.8	1.80	1.74	11.4	1.03			124			24			47	49	
10.0	140	161/92	156	31	89.7	1.88	1.79	11.5	1.05	7.40	20	124	58	60	24	33	9	46	49	0.42
10.5	160		160	34	94.8	1.97	1.88	11.8	1.05			125			24			47	49	
11.0	160	155/86	164	37	104.5	2.07	1.92	11.7	1.08	7.40	20	126	56	63	24	33	9	49	53	0.45
11.5	Recovery		144	29	85.2	1.86	1.80	12.5	1.03			123			25			44	46	
12.0	Recovery		127	27	73.4	1.62	1.52	12.0	1.07			122			26			44	47	
12.5	Recovery		116	23	54.5	1.23	1.14	9.8	1.08			122			27			43	46	
13.0	Recovery	152/86	109	20	35.7	0.84	0.72	7.2	1.06	7.37	19	119	73	45	30	34	4	40	43	0.36

Abbreviations: BP, blood pressure; BTPS, body temperature pressure saturated; f, frequency; HCO_3^-, bicarbonate; HR, heart rate; $P(A-a)O_2$, alveolar-arterial PO_2 difference; $P(a-ET)CO_2$, arterial-end-tidal PCO_2 difference; $PETCO_2$, end-tidal PCO_2; $PETO_2$, end-tidal PO_2; R, respiratory exchange ratio; STPD, standard temperature pressure dry; $\dot{V}CO_2$, carbon dioxide output; V_D/V_T, physiological dead space–tidal volume ratio; $\dot{V}E$, minute ventilation; $\dot{V}E/\dot{V}CO_2$, ventilatory equivalent for carbon dioxide; $\dot{V}E/\dot{V}O_2$, ventilatory equivalent for oxygen; $\dot{V}O_2$, oxygen uptake; $\dot{V}O_2$/HR, O_2 uptake per heart beat or O_2 pulse.

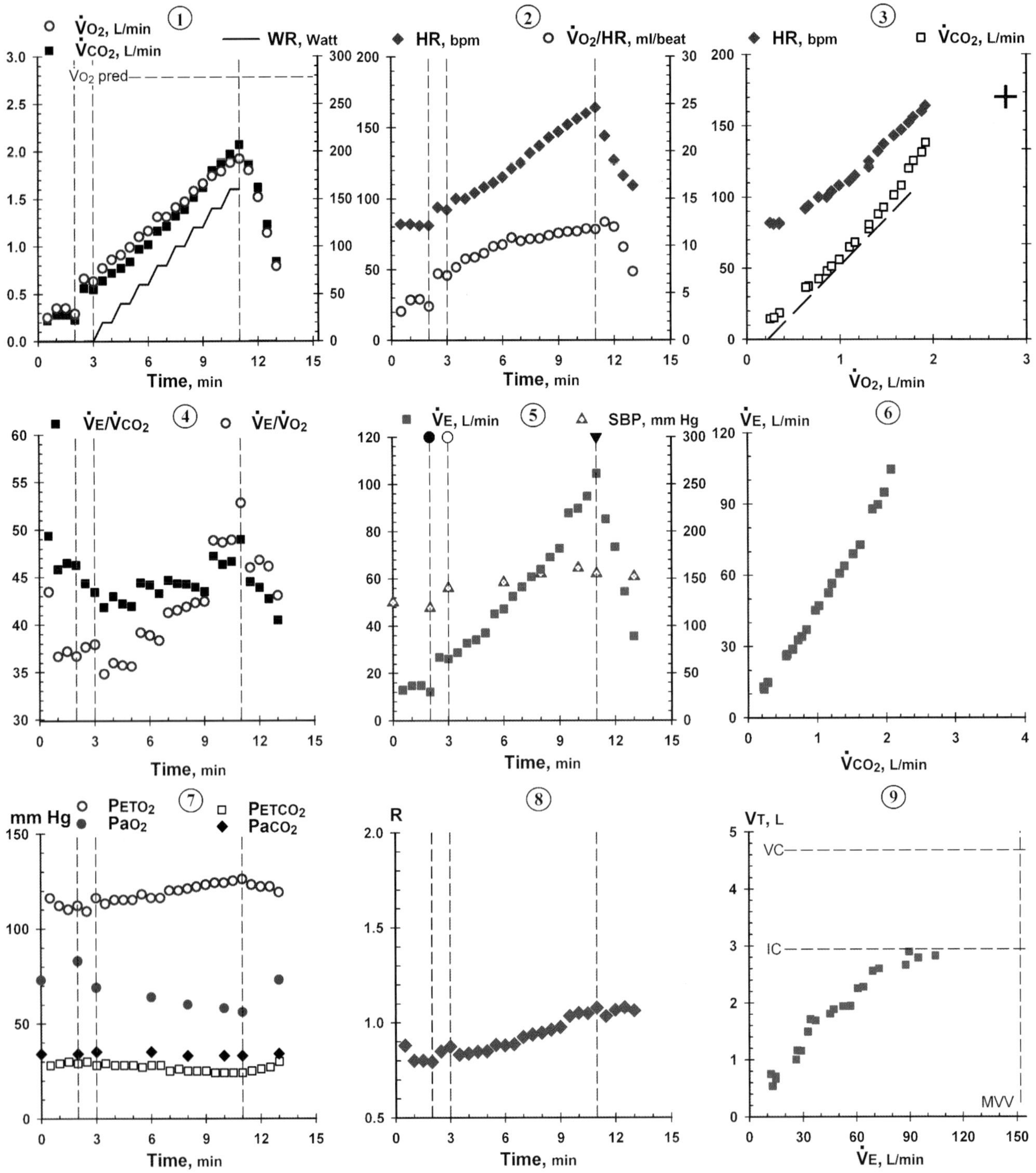

FIGURE 10.97.1. Vertical dashed lines in the panels in the left and middle columns indicate, from left to right, the beginning of unloaded cycling, start of increasing work rate(WR) at 20 W/min, and start of recovery. In **panel 1**, the increase in WR (right y-axis) is plotted with a scale of 100 W to 1 L of $\dot{V}O_2$ (left y-axis) such that WR is plotted parallel to a $\dot{V}O_2$ slope of 10 mL/min/W. In **panel 3**, carbon dioxide output ($\dot{V}CO_2$) (right y-axis) is plotted as a function of $\dot{V}O_2$ (x-axis) with identical scales so that the diagonal dashed line has a slope of 1 (45°). The $\dot{V}CO_2$ increasing more steeply than $\dot{V}O_2$ defines carbon dioxide (CO_2) derived from bicarbonate buffer, as long as ventilatory equivalent for CO_2 ($\dot{V}E/\dot{V}CO_2$) (**panel 4**) is not increasing and end-tidal PCO_2 ($PETCO_2$) (**panel 7**) is not decreasing, simultaneously. The black + symbol in **panel 3** indicates predicted peak values of heart rate (HR) (left y-axis) and $\dot{V}O_2$ for this individual. Abbreviations: IC, inspiratory capacity; MVV, maximum voluntary ventilation; $PETO_2$, end-tidal partial pressure of oxygen; R, respiratory exchange ratio; SBP, systolic blood pressure; VC, vital capacity; $\dot{V}E$, minute ventilation; $\dot{V}E/\dot{V}O_2$, ventilatory equivalent for oxygen; $\dot{V}O_2$/HR, O_2 uptake per heart beat or O_2 pulse; V_T, tidal volume.

CASE 98

Evaluation of Unexplained Dyspnea: An Obese Woman at Risk for Pulmonary Hypertension

CLINICAL FINDINGS

This 49-year-old woman was referred for exercise testing to screen for possible pulmonary vascular disease. Her sister had a diagnosis of idiopathic pulmonary hypertension, and the patient herself had used anorexigens for weight control in the past. She was sedentary and reported chronic exercise intolerance, limited by dyspnea after walking several blocks on level terrain. Echocardiogram showed normal left ventricular function, but assessment of the right-sided chambers was limited by her obese body habitus. She was treated for obstructive sleep apnea with continuous positive airway pressure and for systemic hypertension with an angiotensin-converting enzyme inhibitor and a diuretic. Physical examination was notable for obesity and mild peripheral edema. The electrocardiogram was normal.

EXERCISE FINDINGS

The patient performed exercise on a cycle ergometer beginning with 3 minutes of pedaling at 60 rpm without resistance, followed by continuous increase in work rate at a rate of 15 W/min. She ended exercise with symptoms of leg fatigue. There were no significant electrocardiogram changes.

Comments

Resting pulmonary function tests demonstrated a mild ventilatory defect and spirometric findings typical of obesity. The diffusing capacity of the lung for carbon monoxide was normal (**Table 10.98.1**). Exercise data are summarized in **Table 10.98.2** and shown in **Table 10.98.3** and graphically in **Figure 10.98.1**.

Analysis

The peak oxygen uptake ($\dot{V}O_2$) was within normal limits when compared to height-based (ideal weight) predicted values, indicating normal physiological cardiovascular capacity. The weight-indexed (mL/min/kg actual weight) peak $\dot{V}O_2$ was low, however, indicating reduced capacity for ambulatory work. Consistent with this, at the start of unloaded cycling exercise, $\dot{V}O_2$ increased to almost 1 L/min, reflecting the exaggerated metabolic cost of lifting heavy legs (**Fig. 10.98.1**, panel 1). Subsequently, the increase in $\dot{V}O_2$ relative to work rate was normal. The anaerobic threshold was normal and heart rate increased normally relative to $\dot{V}O_2$ with attainment of a normal peak oxygen pulse. Ventilatory responses were normal, including normal values for pulse oximetry and ventilatory equivalent for carbon dioxide $\dot{V}E/\dot{V}CO_2$ at the anaerobic threshold and a large breathing reserve.

The findings of normal cardiovascular capacity and pulmonary gas exchange were reassuring, as they argue against the presence of hemodynamically significant pulmonary vascular disease. The test also provided an alternative explanation for the patient's exertional dyspnea, which could be attributable to the higher energetic cost of ambulatory work related to obesity, rather than cardiovascular dysfunction. Although the test does not necessarily exclude early pulmonary vascular disease, it was helpful in supporting the decision to defer additional invasive diagnostic studies and provided a baseline against which to compare future measures.

Conclusion

This case demonstrates the effects of obesity on resting lung function and exercise gas exchange. It is presented as an illustration of how a normal exercise test can be useful in the evaluation of a patient with complaints of exertional dyspnea.

TABLE 10.98.1 Selected Respiratory Function Data

Measurement	Predicted	Measured
Age (y)		49
Sex		Female
Height (cm)		164
Weight (kg)	64	124
VC (L)	3.25	2.85
IC (L)	2.17	2.82
ERV (L)	1.08	0.03
FEV_1 (L)	2.69	2.05
FEV_1/VC (%)	83	72
MVV (L/min)	99	87
D_{LCO} (mL/mm Hg/min)	23.3	23.1

Abbreviations: D_{LCO}, diffusing capacity of the lung for carbon monoxide; ERV, expiratory reserve volume; FEV_1, forced expiratory volume in 1 second; IC, inspiratory capacity; MVV, maximum voluntary ventilation; VC, vital capacity.

TABLE 10.98.2 Selected Exercise Data

Measurement	Predicted	Measured
Peak $\dot{V}O_2$ (L/min)	1.88	1.69
Peak $\dot{V}O_2$ (mL/min/kg)	29.4	13.6
Maximum heart rate (beats/min)	171	150
Maximum O_2 pulse (mL/beat)	11.0	11.3
$\Delta\dot{V}O_2/\Delta WR$ (mL/min/W)	10.3	8.9
AT (L/min)	>0.94	1.12
Blood pressure (mm Hg [rest, max])		131/81, 237/99
Maximum $\dot{V}E$ (L/min)		46
Exercise breathing reserve (L/min)	>15	41
$\dot{V}E/\dot{V}CO_2$ @ *AT* or lowest	28.3	23.1

Abbreviations: *AT*, anaerobic threshold; $\Delta\dot{V}O_2/\Delta WR$, change in $\dot{V}O_2$/change in work rate; O_2, oxygen; $\dot{V}CO_2$, carbon dioxide output; $\dot{V}E$, minute ventilation; $\dot{V}E/\dot{V}CO_2$, ventilatory equivalent for carbon dioxide; $\dot{V}O_2$, oxygen uptake.

TABLE 10.98.3 Air Breathing

Time (min)	Work rate (W)	BP (mm Hg)	HR (min⁻¹)	f (min⁻¹)	$\dot{V}E$ (L/min BTPS)	$\dot{V}CO_2$ (L/min STPD)	$\dot{V}O_2$ (L/min STPD)	$\frac{\dot{V}O_2}{HR}$ (mL/beat)	R	pH	HCO_3^- (mEq/L)	PO_2, mm Hg ET	PO_2, mm Hg a	PO_2, mm Hg (A − a)	PCO_2, mm Hg ET	PCO_2, mm Hg a	PCO_2, mm Hg (a − ET)	$\frac{\dot{V}E}{\dot{V}CO_2}$	$\frac{\dot{V}E}{\dot{V}O_2}$	$\frac{V_D}{V_T}$
0.5	Rest	131/81	89	15	8.4	0.28	0.34	3.8	0.81			97			43			30	25	
1.0	Rest		91	15	8.9	0.30	0.36	4.0	0.83			99			42			30	25	
1.5	Rest		90	16	8.6	0.27	0.33	3.6	0.83			99			42			32	26	
2.0	Rest		96	20	10.6	0.32	0.38	4.0	0.84			100			41			33	27	
2.5	Rest		89	20	9.8	0.29	0.34	3.8	0.86			101			42			33	29	
3.0	Rest		88	17	9.7	0.32	0.35	4.0	0.90			102			41			31	28	
3.5	Unloaded	131/81	101	12	9.5	0.33	0.46	4.5	0.73			92			43			28	21	
4.0	Unloaded		107	27	17.8	0.60	0.71	6.6	0.85			98			42			30	25	
4.5	Unloaded		107	28	17.2	0.60	0.73	6.8	0.82			94			44			29	24	
5.0	Unloaded		108	22	15.8	0.61	0.76	7.1	0.80			89			47			26	21	
5.5	Unloaded		110	21	16.1	0.64	0.81	7.3	0.80			88			48			25	20	
6.0	Unloaded		113	22	17.5	0.71	0.88	7.8	0.80			87			49			25	20	
6.5	7		113	23	18.4	0.73	0.85	7.5	0.87			92			48			25	22	
7.0	15		116	23	18.5	0.76	0.89	7.7	0.85			90			49			24	21	
7.5	22		117	22	19.5	0.81	0.92	7.8	0.88			91			49			24	21	
8.0	30		120	24	22.2	0.91	1.01	8.5	0.89			93			48			25	22	
8.5	37		121	21	19.3	0.82	0.94	7.8	0.87			91			50			24	20	
9.0	45		122	20	19.9	0.87	1.03	8.5	0.84			88			51			23	19	
9.5	52		126	21	22.0	0.97	1.12	8.9	0.87			89			51			23	20	
10.0	60		127	25	25.0	1.07	1.19	9.4	0.90			91			50			23	21	
10.5	67		133	24	28.1	1.23	1.31	9.9	0.94			92			50			23	21	
11.0	75	237/99	135	28	30.5	1.31	1.33	9.8	0.99			95			50			23	23	
11.5	82		139	30	34.7	1.48	1.45	10.4	1.02			97			49			23	24	
12.0	90		141	31	39.2	1.63	1.48	10.5	1.10			102			47			24	26	
12.5	97		143	27	37.1	1.63	1.56	10.9	1.05			98			49			23	24	
13.0	105		150	29	43.3	1.87	1.69	11.3	1.11			101			49			23	26	
13.5	Recovery	237/99	149	28	45.8	1.90	1.62	10.8	1.17			104			47			24	28	
14.0	Recovery		137	24	37.7	1.58	1.17	8.5	1.35			109			47			24	32	
14.5	Recovery		133	26	34.4	1.34	0.89	6.7	1.51			113			45			26	39	
15.0	Recovery		127	22	27.7	1.01	0.66	5.2	1.54			117			42			27	42	
15.5	Recovery		126	23	22.0	0.78	0.52	4.1	1.50			117			42			28	42	

Abbreviations: BP, blood pressure; BTPS, body temperature pressure saturated; f, frequency; HCO_3^-, bicarbonate; HR, heart rate; $P(A - a)O_2$, alveolar-arterial PO_2 difference; $P(a - ET)CO_2$, arterial-end-tidal PCO_2 difference; $PETCO_2$, end-tidal PCO_2; $PETO_2$, end-tidal PO_2; R, respiratory exchange ratio; STPD, standard temperature pressure dry; V_D/V_T, physiological dead space-tidal volume ratio; $\dot{V}E$, minute ventilation; $\dot{V}CO_2$, carbon dioxide output; $\dot{V}E/\dot{V}CO_2$, ventilatory equivalent for carbon dioxide; $\dot{V}E/\dot{V}O_2$, ventilatory equivalent for oxygen; $\dot{V}O_2$, oxygen uptake; $\dot{V}O_2$/HR, O_2 uptake per heart beat or O_2 pulse.

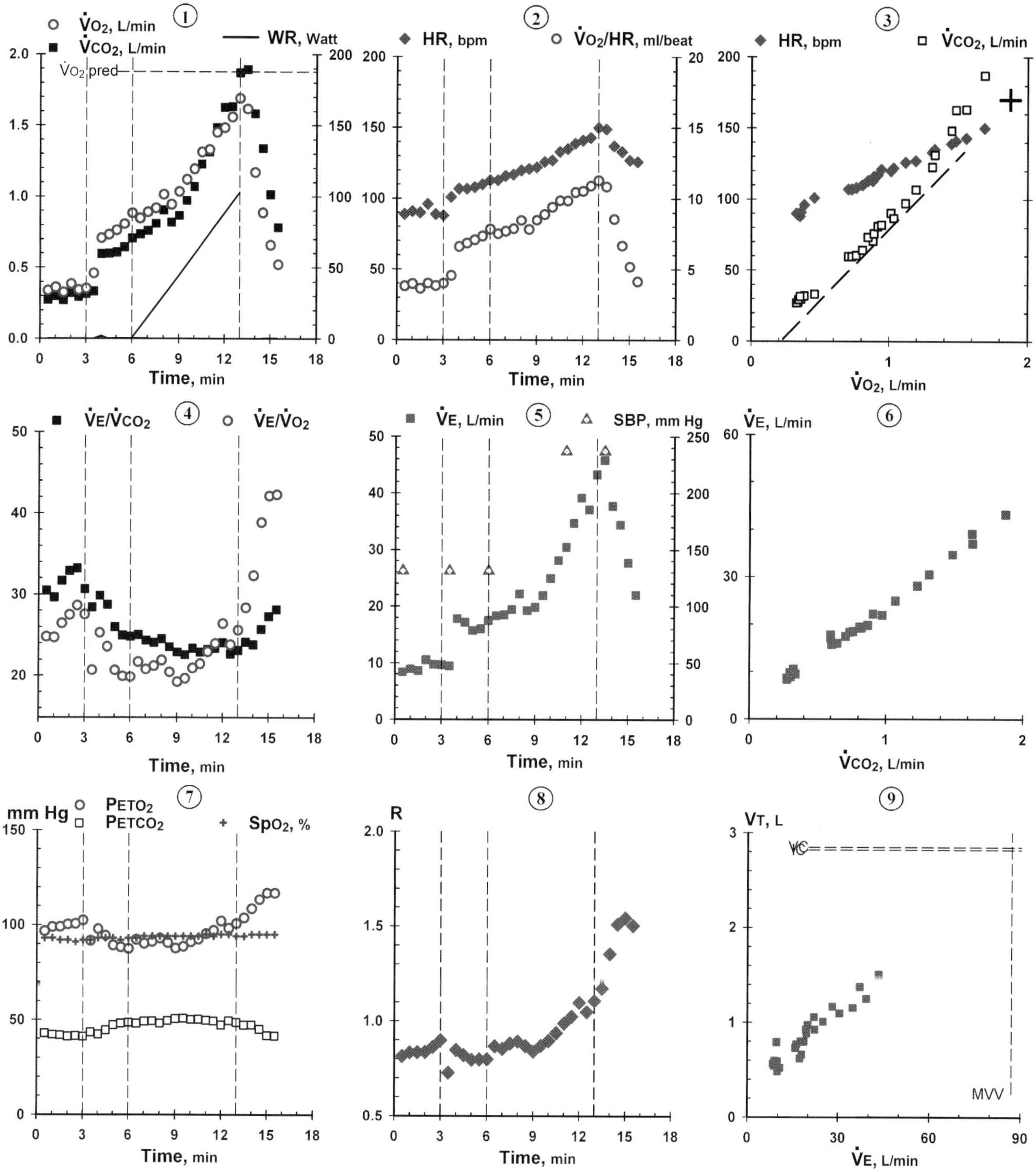

FIGURE 10.98.1. Vertical dashed lines in the panels in the left and middle columns indicate, from left to right, the beginning of unloaded cycling, start of increasing work rate (WR) at 15 W/min, and start of recovery. In **panel 1**, the increase in WR (right y-axis) is plotted with a scale of 100 W to 1 L of oxygen uptake ($\dot{V}O_2$) (left y-axis) such that WR is plotted parallel to a $\dot{V}O_2$ slope of 10 mL/min/W. In **panel 3**, carbon dioxide output ($\dot{V}CO_2$) (right y-axis) is plotted as a function of $\dot{V}O_2$ (x-axis) with identical scales so that the diagonal dashed line has a slope of 1 (45°). The $\dot{V}CO_2$ increasing more steeply than $\dot{V}O_2$ defines carbon dioxide (CO_2) derived from bicarbonate buffer, as long as ventilatory equivalent for carbon dioxide ($\dot{V}E/\dot{V}CO_2$) (**panel 4**) is not increasing and end-tidal P_{CO_2} (P_{ETCO_2}) (**panel 7**) is not decreasing, simultaneously. The black + symbol in **panel 3** indicates predicted peak values of heart rate (HR) (left y-axis) and $\dot{V}O_2$ for this individual. Abbreviations: IC, inspiratory capacity; MVV, maximum voluntary ventilation; P_{ETO_2}, end-tidal partial pressure of oxygen; R, respiratory exchange ratio; SBP, systolic blood pressure; Sp_{O_2}, O_2 saturation measured by pulse oximetry; VC, vital capacity; $\dot{V}E$, minute ventilation; $\dot{V}E/\dot{V}O_2$, ventilatory equivalent for oxygen; $\dot{V}O_2$/HR, O_2 uptake per heart beat or O_2 pulse; V_T, tidal volume.

CASE 99

Serial Tests: Active Man With CREST Syndrome

CLINICAL FINDINGS

A man underwent exercise testing as part of monitoring for development of pulmonary vascular disease. He had history of CREST syndrome (calcinosis, Raynaud phenomenon, esophageal dysmotility, sclerodactyly, and telangiectasia). His first exercise test was at age 67, at which time he had no exertional symptoms, and pulmonary function tests and echocardiogram were normal. He was a recreational cyclist with good exercise tolerance, riding his bicycle 50 to 75 miles/wk. Testing was performed again 2 years later when his pulmonary function tests showed decrements in lung volumes and diffusing capacity, without reported changes on echocardiogram. At that time, however, he was recovering from a bicycling accident in which he had suffered multiple fractures, and he had only recently resumed riding around 20 miles/wk. Changes in pulmonary function and exercise tolerance were considered likely related to healing rib fractures and deconditioning. Two years later, although his injuries were healed and he had resumed his prior mileage and working out in a gym, he had developed symptoms of exertional dyspnea. Repeat echocardiogram reported only grade 1 diastolic dysfunction. Over the period of testing his medications included tadalafil (for digital ulcers), omeprazole, pregabalin, aspirin, atorvastatin, and metoclopramide. Physical examinations were notable for marked sclerodactyly of the hands bilaterally. On each occasion breath sounds were clear, heart tones were regular, and there was no lower extremity edema. Demographics and respiratory function data are shown in **Table 10.99.1**.

TABLE 10.99.1 Selected Respiratory Function Data

Measurement	Predicted	Measured		
Age (y)	67	67	69	71
Sex		Male		
Height (cm)		175		
Weight (kg)		72.3		
VC (L)	4.23	3.80	3.29	3.70
IC (L)	3.16	3.23	2.25	3.0
ERV (L)	1.07	0.76	0.80	0.85
FEV_1 (L)	3.13	2.89	2.43	2.65
FEV_1/VC (%)	74	76	74	72
MVV (L/min)	125	135	97	128
D_{LCO} (mL /mm Hg/min)	25.6	20.7	14.1	16.5

Abbreviations: D_{LCO}, diffusing capacity of the lung for carbon monoxide; ERV, expiratory reserve volume; FEV_1, forced expiratory volume in 1 second; IC, inspiratory capacity; MVV, maximum voluntary ventilation; VC, vital capacity.

EXERCISE FINDINGS

On each of the three occasions, the patient exercised on a cycle ergometer beginning with 3 minutes of unloaded pedaling at 60 rpm followed by continuous increase in work rate by 20 W/min. All tests ended with symptoms of dyspnea. Exercise electrocardiogram did not show any evidence of ischemia or arrhythmia on any of the tests. Exercise data for all three tests are summarized in **Table 10.99.2.** Exercise data for the first and last tests are presented in **Tables 10.99.3** and **10.99.4** and **Figures 10.99.1** and **10.99.2.**

INTERPRETATION

Comment

These tests are presented as an example of serial testing. On the second testing occasion, there were changes in pulmonary function and exercise capacity that were reasonably suspected to reflect the patient's injuries and deconditioning, respectively. On the third set of tests, pulmonary function had improved, but differences in the exercise responses persisted, suggesting an underlying impairment in cardiovascular function.

Analysis

At age 67, the cardiovascular responses to exercise were normal with normal peak oxygen uptake ($\dot{V}O_2$), normal change in $\dot{V}O_2$/change in work rate ($\Delta\dot{V}O_2/\Delta WR$), and normal anaerobic threshold (*AT*). There was adequate breathing reserve and the ventilatory equivalents decreased normally. The end-tidal P_{CO_2} values were lower than average, but it is not possible to know whether this indicated elevated physiological dead space–tidal volume ratio (V_D/V_T) or a low arterial P_{CO_2}. The Sp_{O_2} was normal during rest and recovery, although the oximeter signal was inadequate during exercise due to sclerodactyly.

At age 71, the peak $\dot{V}O_2$ was lower than at age 67. The $\Delta\dot{V}O_2/\Delta WR$ initially appeared normal, but during the last few minutes of exercise, the slope decreased, with $\dot{V}O_2$ reaching a clear maximal value at the end of the test. The O_2 pulse reached a plateau value early in the test. The *AT* was near the lower limit of normal and lower than on the initial test at age 67. Although the values of these variables were within the normal ranges, the normal val-

TABLE 10.99.2 Selected Exercise Data

Measurement	Predicted Age 67, 71	Measured Age 67	Measured Age 69	Measured Age 71
Peak $\dot{V}O_2$ (L/min)	1.93, 1.82	1.82	1.56	1.57
Maximum heart rate (beats/min)	153, 151	161	147	159
Maximum O_2 pulse (mL/beat)	12.6, 12.2	11.4	10.4	10.2
$\Delta\dot{V}O_2/\Delta WR$ (mL/min/W)	10.3	11.3	8.7	8.7
AT (L/min)	>0.90, >0.86	1.07	0.9	0.9
Blood pressure (mmHg [rest, max ex])		113/69, 216/82	140/77, 167/68	144/71, 217/60
Maximum V_E (L/min)		67	81	78
Breathing reserve (L/min)		68	16	50
$\dot{V}_E/\dot{V}CO_2$ @ *AT* (L/min)	<33	30	33	31
SpO_2 (% [rest, max exercise])		98, NA	98, 98	98, 98
V_D/V_T (rest, lowest exercise)				0.45, 0.24

Abbreviations: *AT*, anaerobic threshold; $\Delta\dot{V}O_2/\Delta WR$, change in $\dot{V}O_2$/change in work rate; ex, exercise; NA, not applicable; O_2, oxygen; SpO_2, O_2 saturation measured by pulse oximetry; V_D/V_T, physiological dead space–tidal volume ratio; $\dot{V}_E/\dot{V}CO_2$, ventilatory equivalent for carbon dioxide; $\dot{V}O_2$, oxygen uptake.

TABLE 10.99.3 Air Breathing

Time (min)	Work rate (W)	BP (mm Hg)	HR (min^{-1})	f (min^{-1})	$\dot{V}_E$ (L/min BTPS)	$\dot{V}CO_2$ (L/min STPD)	$\dot{V}O_2$ (L/min STPD)	$\frac{\dot{V}O_2}{HR}$ (mL/beat)	R	pH	HCO_3^- (mEq/L)	PO_2, mm Hg and SpO_2, % ET	SpO_2	(A − a)	PCO_2, mm Hg ET	a	(a − ET)	$\frac{\dot{V}_E}{\dot{V}CO_2}$	$\frac{\dot{V}_E}{\dot{V}O_2}$	$\frac{V_D}{V_T}$
0.5	Rest		60	16	8.4	0.16	0.22	3.7	0.73			115	98		27			52	38	
1.0	Rest		94	22	13.8	0.26	0.34	3.6	0.78			120	98		23			52	41	
1.5	Rest	113/69	89	20	11.1	0.21	0.26	2.9	0.80			119	97		25			53	42	
2.0	Rest		91	17	8.3	0.17	0.23	2.6	0.71			112	98		29			50	36	
2.5	Unloaded		97	30	18.0	0.38	0.54	5.6	0.70			113	98		27			47	33	
3.0	Unloaded		96	24	17.6	0.40	0.55	5.7	0.73			114	97		28			44	32	
3.5	Unloaded		94	28	15.7	0.34	0.47	5.0	0.72			112	95		28			46	33	
4.0	Unloaded		96	22	17.2	0.42	0.57	6.0	0.72			112	94		29			41	30	
4.5	Unloaded	126/66	90	26	15.4	0.32	0.43	4.8	0.74			112	97		29			48	35	
5.0	Unloaded		91	26	15.1	0.33	0.48	5.2	0.69			109	97		30			46	32	
5.5	6		94	27	14.6	0.32	0.48	5.1	0.67			107	98		31			46	31	
6.0	17		96	23	14.6	0.35	0.54	5.6	0.66			104	97		32			41	27	
6.5	27		97	28	16.0	0.38	0.55	5.7	0.68			105	97		32			42	29	
7.0	[illegible]	[illegible]	102	[illegible]	[illegible]	[illegible]	[illegible]	[illegible]	[illegible]			[illegible]	[illegible]		[illegible]			[illegible]	[illegible]	
7.5	46		107	30	21.4	0.54	0.79	7.4	0.69			105	94		33			39	27	
8.0	56		111	27	21.9	0.60	0.88	7.9	0.69			103	96		34			36	25	
8.5	67		116	24	25.0	0.74	1.03	8.9	0.72			103	96		36			34	24	
9.0	77		123	24	28.5	0.88	1.11	9.1	0.79			105	96		36			32	26	
9.5	86	182/69	128	23	31.7	1.00	1.20	9.4	0.83			107	95		37			32	26	
10.0	97		133	25	35.7	1.15	1.31	9.8	0.88			108	94		37			31	27	
10.5	106		139	29	44.0	1.37	1.43	10.3	0.96			111	93		36			32	31	
11.0	116	216/82	145	30	46.6	1.47	1.49	10.3	0.99			113	91		36			32	31	
11.5	126		150	31	51.6	1.62	1.59	10.6	1.02			114	60		35			32	32	
12.0	136		155	34	57.4	1.78	1.69	10.9	1.05			116			35			32	34	
12.5	146		161	40	67.2	1.99	1.82	11.4	1.09			118			33			34	37	
13.0	Recovery		158	36	62.0	1.82	1.59	10.0	1.15			119			33			34	39	
13.5	Recovery		136	32	51.7	1.46	1.17	8.6	1.25			122			32			35	44	
14.0	Recovery	184/55	138	28	41.2	1.12	0.85	6.1	1.32			124			31			37	49	
14.5	Recovery		129	26	33.8	0.89	0.71	5.5	1.26			123	76		31			38	48	

Abbreviations: BP, blood pressure; BTPS, body temperature pressure saturated; f, frequency; HCO_3^-, bicarbonate; HR, heart rate; $P(A-a)O_2$, alveolar-arterial PO_2 difference; $P(a-ET)CO_2$, arterial-end-tidal PCO_2 difference; $PETCO_2$, end-tidal PCO_2; $PETO_2$, end-tidal PO_2; R, respiratory exchange ratio; SpO_2, O_2 saturation measured by pulse oximetry; STPD, standard temperature pressure dry; $\dot{V}CO_2$, carbon dioxide output V_D/V_T, physiological dead space–tidal volume ratio; $\dot{V}_E$, minute ventilation; $\dot{V}_E/\dot{V}CO_2$, ventilatory equivalent for carbon dioxide; $\dot{V}_E/\dot{V}O_2$, ventilatory equivalent for oxygen; $\dot{V}O_2$, oxygen uptake; $\dot{V}O_2$/HR, O_2 uptake per heart beat or O_2 pulse.

TABLE 10.99.4 Air Breathing

Time (min)	Work rate (W)	BP (mm Hg)	HR (min^{-1})	f (min^{-1})	$\dot{V}E$ (L/min BTPS)	$\dot{V}CO_2$ (L/min STPD)	$\dot{V}O_2$ (L/min STPD)	$\frac{\dot{V}O_2}{HR}$ (mL/beat)	R	pH	HCO_3^- (mEq/L)	PO_2, mm Hg and SpO_2, % ET	SpO_2	(A − a)	PCO_2, mm Hg ET	tc	(a − ET)	$\frac{\dot{V}E}{\dot{V}CO_2}$	$\frac{\dot{V}E}{\dot{V}O_2}$	$\frac{VD}{VT}$
0.5	Rest		58	23	12.6	0.25	0.37	6.5	0.68			110	98		28	30.2		50	34	0.41
1.0	Rest		70	21	11.7	0.22	0.31	4.4	0.72			114	98		27	31.3		52	38	0.46
1.5	Rest	144/71	68	27	12.1	0.21	0.30	4.5	0.70			111	98		28	31.7		57	40	0.50
2.0	Rest		71	23	9.9	0.18	0.26	3.6	0.70			110	98		29	32.5		56	39	0.49
2.5	Unloaded		62	30	14.2	0.27	0.41	6.6	0.67			109	98		29	32.9		52	35	0.47
3.0	Unloaded		77	22	14.5	0.33	0.47	6.1	0.71			109	98		29	33.5		44	31	0.39
3.5	Unloaded		77	20	13.7	0.32	0.49	6.4	0.66			105	98		31	33.5		43	28	0.38
4.0	Unloaded		81	24	15.9	0.38	0.56	6.9	0.68			107	98		30	34.1		42	29	0.37
4.5	Unloaded		78	30	16.4	0.36	0.49	6.3	0.72			109	98		30	34.1		46	33	0.42
5.0	Unloaded		76	26	13.0	0.29	0.44	5.8	0.67			104	98		32	34.4		44	29	0.42
5.5	4	151/72	78	30	15.5	0.36	0.56	7.2	0.64			101	98		33	35		43	27	0.40
6.0	13		79	38	24.3	0.52	0.65	8.2	0.80			114	98		28	36.1		47	37	0.46
6.5	24		77	28	15.0	0.35	0.45	5.8	0.77			109	98		32	35.5		43	34	0.41
7.0	34		81	33	16.3	0.39	0.59	7.3	0.66			102	98		33	35.3		42	28	0.39
7.5	44		88	32	21.6	0.55	0.80	9.1	0.69			105	98		33	36.2		39	27	0.37
8.0	53	151/78	91	27	20.6	0.57	0.81	8.9	0.71			103	98		35	36.6		36	26	0.33
8.5	63		98	20	21.6	0.67	0.91	9.3	0.74			102	98		36	37.1		32	24	0.26
9.0	73		107	25	30.0	0.91	1.10	10.3	0.83			107	98		35	37.4		33	27	0.28
9.5	83		113	25	32.0	1.00	1.14	10.1	0.88			109	98		36	37.4		32	28	0.26
10.0	93		120	24	35.4	1.15	1.23	10.3	0.93			110	98		36	37.4		31	29	0.23
10.5	104		130	28	42.6	1.36	1.34	10.3	1.01			113	98		36	37.3		31	32	0.24
11.0	114		137	32	49.4	1.53	1.42	10.4	1.08			115	98		35	37.1		32	35	0.26
11.5	124		144	36	58.9	1.75	1.51	10.5	1.16			118	98		34	36.8		34	39	0.28
12.0	133		148	38	63.6	1.85	1.50	10.1	1.23			120	98		34	36.1		34	42	0.29
12.5	66		155	48	77.5	2.04	1.57	10.2	1.30			124	98		31	35		38	49	0.33
13.0	Recovery		159	43	74.9	2.04	1.57	9.9	1.30			123	98		32	33.8		37	48	0.29
13.5	Recovery	217/60	144	40	63.1	1.70	1.18	8.2	1.44			125	98		31	33.1		37	53	0.28
14.0	Recovery		130	39	52.1	1.33	0.88	6.8	1.51			127	98		30	32.6		39	59	0.30
14.5	Recovery		118	38	42.4	1.03	0.70	5.9	1.48			127	98		29	31.7		41	61	0.32
15.0	Recovery		108	40	40.0	0.89	0.59	5.5	1.51			129	98		28	31.3		45	68	0.36
15.5	Recovery	197/66	96	40	30.7	0.68	0.55	5.7	1.25			125	98		29	30.4		45	56	0.35

Abbreviations: BP, blood pressure; BTPS, body temperature pressure saturated; f, frequency; HCO_3^-, bicarbonate; HR, heart rate; $P(A-a)O_2$, alveolar-arterial PO_2 difference; $P(a-ET)CO_2$, arterial-end-tidal PCO_2 difference; $PETCO_2$, end-tidal PCO_2; $PETO_2$, end-tidal PO_2; R, respiratory exchange ratio; SpO_2, O_2 saturation measured by pulse oximetry; STPD, standard temperature pressure dry; tc, transcutaneous; $\dot{V}CO_2$, carbon dioxide output VD/VT, physiological dead space-tidal volume ratio; $\dot{V}E$, minute ventilation; $\dot{V}E/\dot{V}CO_2$, ventilatory equivalent for carbon dioxide; $\dot{V}E/\dot{V}O_2$, ventilatory equivalent for oxygen; $\dot{V}O_2$, oxygen uptake; $\dot{V}O_2$/HR, O_2 uptake per heart beat or O_2 pulse.

ues reflect averages for healthy nonathletic individuals. For this patient, exercising regularly on a cycle, it would be expected that values would normally be above these averages.

The ventilatory equivalent for carbon dioxide ($\dot{V}E/\dot{V}CO_2$) values at *AT* were high normal and end-tidal PCO_2 remained lower than the transcutaneous estimate of arterial PCO_2 throughout most of the test; calculated VD/VT was normal, however. Finger pulse oximeter SpO_2 values could not be measured, but earlobe values were normal (see **Table 10.99.2**, not graphed). Pulmonary gas exchange efficiency thus appeared normal.

Conclusion

Over 4 years, there was a decrease in exercise capacity exceeding what would be predicted on the basis of aging alone. Although there was concern for pulmonary vascular disease, gas exchange efficiency remained essentially normal and the primary findings were more consistent with reduction in the exercise stroke volume response, such as resulting from ventricular systolic or diastolic dysfunction. The assessments on the second test were complicated by the intervening accident, which likely accounted for his change in pulmonary function but would be unlikely to explain persistent reduction in exercise oxygen pulse.

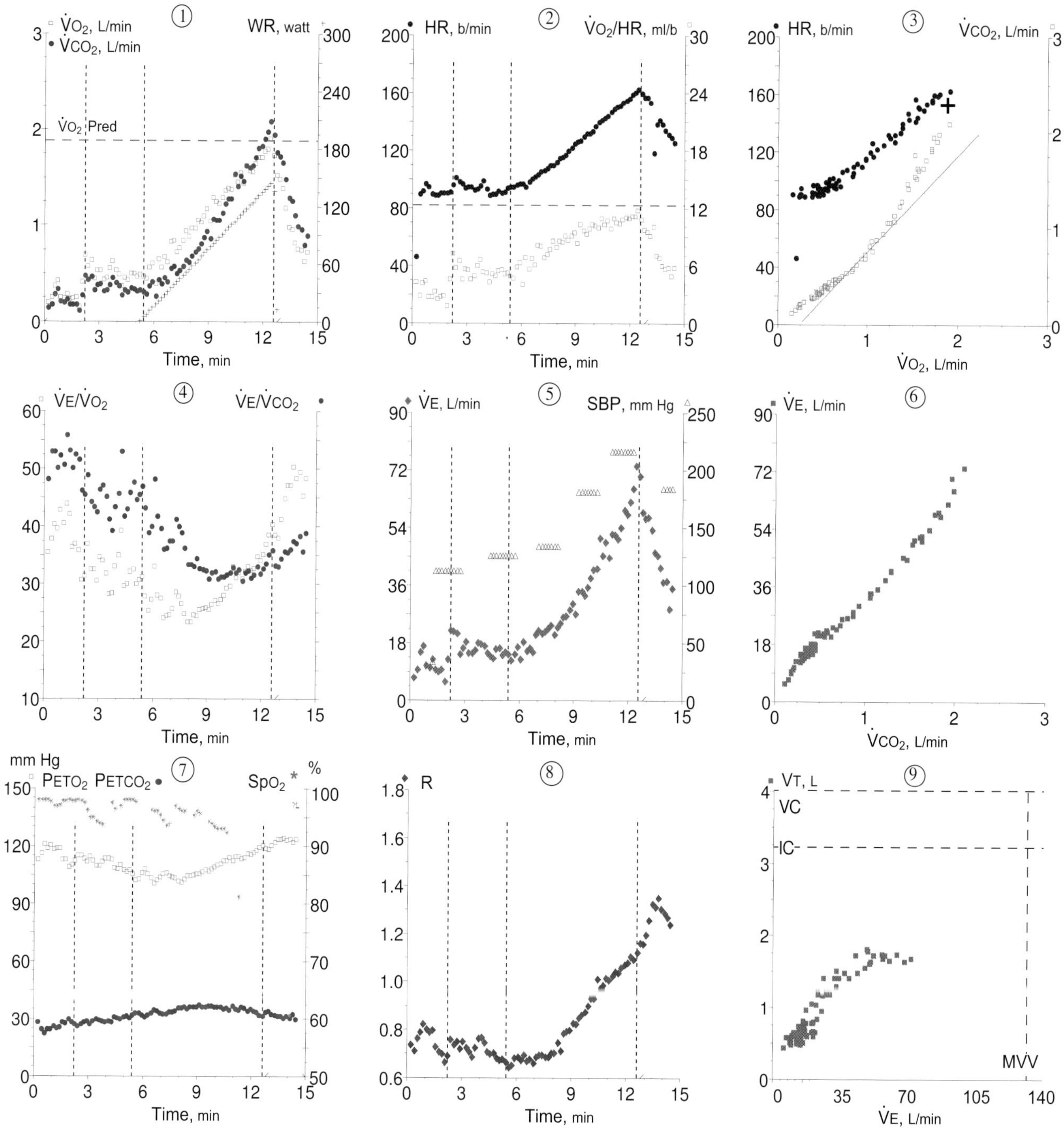

FIGURE 10.99.1. Age 67. Vertical dashed lines in the panels in the left and middle columns indicate, from left to right, the beginning of unloaded cycling, start of increasing work rate (WR) at 20 W/min, and start of recovery. In **panel 1**, the increase in WR (right y-axis) is plotted with a scale of 100 W to 1 L of oxygen uptake ($\dot{V}O_2$) (left y-axis) such that WR is plotted parallel to a $\dot{V}O_2$ slope of 10 mL/min/W. Predicted peak $\dot{V}O_2$ is shown as a dashed horizontal line. In **panel 3**, carbon dioxide output ($\dot{V}CO_2$) (right y-axis) is plotted as a function of $\dot{V}O_2$ (x-axis) with identical scales so that the diagonal blue line has a slope of 1 (45°). The $\dot{V}CO_2$ increasing more steeply than $\dot{V}O_2$ defines carbon dioxide (CO_2) derived from bicarbonate buffer, as long as ventilatory equivalent for carbon dioxide ($\dot{V}E/\dot{V}CO_2$) (**panel 4**) is not increasing and end-tidal PCO_2 ($PETCO_2$) (**panel 7**) is not decreasing, simultaneously. The black + symbol in **panel 3** indicates predicted peak values of heart rate (HR) (left y-axis) and $\dot{V}O_2$ for this individual. Abbreviations: IC, inspiratory capacity; MVV, maximum voluntary ventilation; $PETO_2$, end-tidal partial pressure of oxygen; R, respiratory exchange ratio; SBP, systolic blood pressure; SpO_2, O_2 saturation measured by pulse oximetry; VC, vital capacity; $\dot{V}E$, minute ventilation; $\dot{V}E/\dot{V}O_2$, ventilatory equivalent for oxygen; $\dot{V}O_2$/HR, O_2 uptake per heart beat or O_2 pulse; VT, tidal volume.

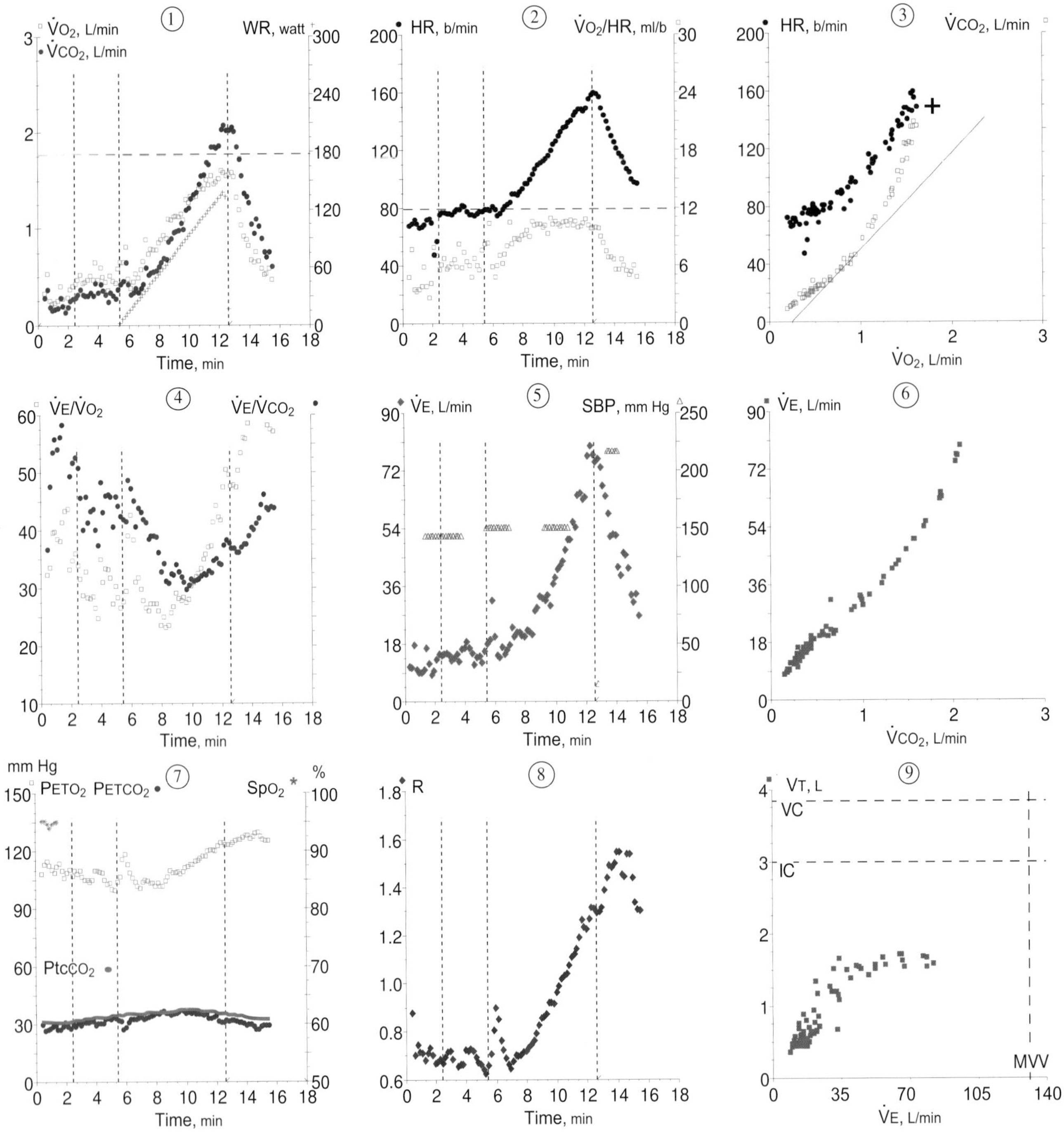

FIGURE 10.99.2. Age 71. Vertical dashed lines in the panels in the left and middle columns indicate, from left to right, the beginning of unloaded cycling, start of increasing work rate (WR) at 20 W/min, and start of recovery. In **panel 1**, the increase in WR (right y-axis) is plotted with a scale of 100 W to 1 L of oxygen uptake ($\dot{V}O_2$) (left y-axis) such that WR is plotted parallel to a $\dot{V}O_2$ slope of 10 mL/min/W. Predicted peak $\dot{V}O_2$ is shown as a dashed horizontal line. In **panel 3**, carbon dioxide output ($\dot{V}CO_2$) (right y-axis) is plotted as a function of $\dot{V}O_2$ (x-axis) with identical scales so that the diagonal blue line has a slope of 1 (45°).The $\dot{V}CO_2$ increasing more steeply than $\dot{V}O_2$ defines carbon dioxide (CO_2) derived from bicarbonate buffer, as long as ventilatory equivalent for carbon dioxide ($\dot{V}E/\dot{V}CO_2$) (**panel 4**) is not increasing and end-tidal PCO_2 $PETCO_2$ (**panel 7**) is not decreasing, simultaneously. The black + symbol in **panel 3** indicates predicted peak values of heart rate (HR) (left y-axis) and $\dot{V}O_2$ for this individual. Abbreviations: IC, inspiratory capacity; MVV, maximum voluntary ventilation; $PETO_2$, end-tidal partial pressure of oxygen; R, respiratory exchange ratio; SBP, systolic blood pressure; SpO_2, O_2 saturation measured by pulse oximetry; VC, vital capacity; $\dot{V}E$, minute ventilation; $PTCCO_2$, transcutaneous partial pressure of CO_2; $\dot{V}E/\dot{V}O_2$, ventilatory equivalent for oxygen; $\dot{V}O_2$/HR, O_2 uptake per heart beat or O_2 pulse; VT, tidal volume.

CASE 100

Serial Tests: Delayed Cardiotoxicity From Chemotherapy

CLINICAL FINDINGS

A 29-year-old man underwent a cardiopulmonary exercise test to monitor cardiovascular function. As a young child he had surgery and chemotherapy for treatment of a soft tissue sarcoma of the upper extremity. His treatment had included adriamycin, and he had periodic echocardiograms and exercise tests to screen for the development of delayed cardiotoxicity from that agent.[1] At the time of this test, he had no symptoms but reported having been seen in an emergency room for an episode of palpitations and light-headedness 2 months earlier, which had resolved spontaneously after 15 minutes without documentation of the rhythm. An echocardiogram following that event was reported as unchanged from prior images. He worked in an office and did no regular exercise other than walking. His only medication was lisinopril. Physical examination was notable for asymmetry of muscle mass and strength of the upper extremities related to his remote surgery. Resting electrocardiogram showed sinus rhythm with frequent premature atrial and ventricular contractions. Demographic and pulmonary function data are shown in **Table 10.100.1**.

The patient had performed three prior exercise tests at ages 22, 27, and 28 years. On the most recent of these, at age 28, peak oxygen uptake ($\dot{V}O_2$) was noted to be lower than earlier measurements. Because he had also decreased his activity levels in that interim, having finished school and taken a sedentary job, it was thought that this change might be due to a decrease in conditioning.

TABLE 10.100.1 Selected Respiratory Function Data

Measurement	Predicted	Measured
Age (y)		29
Sex		Male
Height (cm)		185
Weight (kg)		72.3
VC (L)	6.06	5.66
FEV_1 (L)	4.99	4.93
FEV_1/VC (%)	88	82
MVV (L/min)		204

Abbreviations: FEV_1, forced expiratory volume in 1 second; MVV, maximum voluntary ventilation; VC, vital capacity.

EXERCISE FINDINGS

The patient exercised on a cycle ergometer beginning with 3 minutes of unloaded pedaling at 60 rpm followed by continuous increase in work rate by 25 W/min and ended exercise with symptoms of leg fatigue. Ectopy decreased during exercise, and there were no ST segment changes; however, there were frequent premature ventricular beats including multiple couplets during the first 2 minutes of recovery, which were asymptomatic. Exercise data are summarized in **Table 10.100.2** and **Figure 10.100.1**. **Table 10.100.3**. **Figure 10.100.2** show selected exercise data in comparison with prior tests.

INTERPRETATION

Comment

This case is presented as an example of serial testing performed to detect change in functional status and also to comment on the value of comparing submaximal responses to exercise over time.

Analysis

At age 29, peak $\dot{V}O_2$ was lower than normal at 67% of the predicted value. This does not appear to be due to poor effort, as the peak heart rate was similar to that measured on prior tests (see **Table 10.100.3**). In addition, exercise was continued well beyond the anaerobic threshold, which was lower than normal, and end-exercise respiratory exchange ratio was over 1.3 (panel 8 in **Fig. 10.100.1**), consistent with substantial lactic acidosis. The change in $\dot{V}O_2$/change in work rate ($\Delta\dot{V}O_2/\Delta WR$) was normal, but the rate of increase of heart rate relative to $\dot{V}O_2$ was steeper than average and nonlinear, becoming steeper during the second half of the test (panel 3 of **Figs. 10.100.1** and **10.100.2**). Corresponding to this, the O_2 pulse plateaued several minutes prior to the end of exercise at a value lower than the predicted maximum; this was a change from prior tests. The ectopy noted at rest and in the early recovery period was also new. Blood pressure was normal at rest but increased less during exercise than on prior tests (see **Table 10.100.3**).

Ventilatory and pulmonary gas exchange responses: There was a normal breathing reserve. The efficiency of gas exchange appeared normal based on normal relationship between minute ventilation ($\dot{V}E$) and carbon dioxide output ($\dot{V}CO_2$), the normal decrease in the calculated physiological dead space-tidal volume ratio (VD/VT), and the normal pulse oximetry, similar to prior tests.

TABLE 10.100.2 Age 29[a]

Time (min)	Work rate (W)	BP (mm Hg)	HR (min^{-1})	f (min^{-1})	$\dot{V}E$ (L/min BTPS)	$\dot{V}CO_2$ (L/min STPD)	$\dot{V}O_2$ (L/min STPD)	$\frac{\dot{V}O_2}{HR}$ (mL/beat)	R	pH	HCO_3^- (mEq/L)	PO_2, mm Hg and SpO_2, %: *ET*	*SpO_2*	(*A* − *a*)	PCO_2, mm Hg: *ET*	*TC*	(*a* − *ET*)	$\frac{\dot{V}E}{\dot{V}CO_2}$	$\frac{\dot{V}E}{\dot{V}O_2}$	$\frac{VD}{VT}$
0.5	Rest		51	18	14.1	0.38	0.40	7.8	0.97			112	98		37	42.4		37	36	0.47
1.0	Rest		68	17	11.7	0.31	0.34	5.0	0.91			109	98		38	41.4		38	34	0.47
1.5	Rest		75	20	11.8	0.29	0.32	4.4	0.88			109	98		37	40.9		41	36	0.50
2.0	Rest	122/65	79	19	13.7	0.34	0.36	4.6	0.95			112	98		36	40.7		40	38	0.49
2.5	Unloaded		86	20	15.9	0.48	0.54	6.3	0.88			106	98		39	40.3		33	29	0.38
3.0	Unloaded		90	16	17.1	0.57	0.64	7.1	0.90			107	98		40	40.4		30	27	0.31
3.5	Unloaded		83	26	17.3	0.47	0.48	5.8	0.98			111	98		38	40.9		37	36	0.45
4.0	Unloaded		79	19	15.2	0.45	0.48	6.1	0.94			108	98		40	40.9		34	32	0.40
4.5	Unloaded		83	21	17.6	0.55	0.57	6.9	0.96			109	98		39	41.3		32	31	0.37
5.0	Unloaded	108/65	81	21	14.7	0.42	0.43	5.3	0.96			110	98		38	41.0		35	34	0.42
5.5	8		78	19	16.4	0.50	0.54	6.9	0.94			108	99		40	41.0		33	31	0.38
6.0	21		82	18	15.1	0.46	0.48	5.9	0.95			108	98		39	41.0		33	31	0.38
6.5	34		88	20	17.4	0.55	0.63	7.2	0.88			104	98		41	40.8		31	28	0.36
7.0	46	117/65	89	17	17.7	0.61	0.71	7.9	0.86			103	98		41	40.9		29	25	0.30
7.5	59		93	17	20.2	0.71	0.83	8.9	0.85			100	98		42	41.2		29	24	0.29
8.0	71		100	19	21.0	0.77	0.96	9.7	0.80			97	99		44	41.4		27	22	0.27
8.5	84		107	19	26.7	1.02	1.21	11.3	0.85			98	99		45	42.1		26	22	0.25
9.0	96	122/64	113	20	30.3	1.18	1.24	11.0	0.95			103	99		45	42.4		26	24	0.24
9.5	108		121	20	32.5	1.31	1.30	10.7	1.01			104	99		46	42.8		25	25	0.22
10.0	122		132	23	39.1	1.57	1.47	11.1	1.07			106	99		46	42.9		25	27	0.22
10.5	134		140	23	44.6	1.79	1.53	10.9	1.17			110	98		45	42.9		25	29	0.22
11.0	147	137/66	146	24	50.6	1.99	1.70	11.6	1.17			110	99		45	42.4		25	30	0.23
11.5	159		156	25	55.5	2.19	1.79	11.5	1.22			112	98		44	41.9		25	31	0.22
12.0	172		166	28	61.7	2.35	1.89	11.4	1.24			113	98		43	41.3		26	33	0.24
12.5	133		177	33	73.7	2.66	2.03	11.5	1.31			117	98		41	40.4		28	36	0.26
13.0	Recovery		174	30	63.0	2.30	1.65	9.5	1.39			118	99		41	39.4		27	38	0.23
13.5	Recovery	123/60	161	29	53.6	1.78	1.04	6.5	1.71			124	99		38	38.6		30	52	0.29
14.0	Recovery		143	31	41.0	1.25	0.73	5.1	1.71			126	99		36	37.4		33	56	0.32
14.5	Recovery		127	31	33.7	0.97	0.63	5.0	1.52			124	99		35	36.2		35	53	0.34
15.0	Recovery		129	29	27.5	0.79	0.60	4.6	1.33			121	99		36	35.3		35	46	0.32
15.5	Recovery		124	24	24.5	0.73	0.64	5.1	1.15			116	98		38	35.2		33	38	0.30
16.0	Recovery		127	30	27.6	0.74	0.67	5.3	1.11			117	99		36	35.6		37	41	0.38

Abbreviations: BP, blood pressure; BTPS, body temperature pressure saturated; f, frequency; HCO_3^-, bicarbonate; HR, heart rate; $P(A - a)O_2$, alveolar-arterial PO_2 difference; $P(a - ET)CO_2$, arterial-end-tidal PCO_2 difference; $PETCO_2$, end-tidal PCO_2; $PETO_2$, end-tidal PO_2; $PTCCO_2$, transcutaneous PCO_2; $P(A - a)O_2$, alveolar-arterial PO_2 difference; $P(a - ET)CO_2$, arterial-end-tidal PCO_2 difference; $PETCO_2$, end-tidal PCO_2; $PETO_2$, end-tidal PO_2; R, respiratory exchange ratio; SpO_2, O_2 saturation measured by pulse oximetry; STPD, standard temperature pressure dry; VD/VT, physiological dead space–tidal volume ratio; $\dot{V}E$, minute ventilation; $\dot{V}CO_2$, carbon dioxide output; $\dot{V}E/\dot{V}CO_2$, ventilatory equivalent for carbon dioxide; $\dot{V}E/\dot{V}O_2$, ventilatory equivalent for oxygen; $\dot{V}O_2$, oxygen uptake; $\dot{V}O_2$/HR, O_2 uptake per heart beat or O_2 pulse.

[a]The VD/VT values were calculated using $PtcCO_2$ as an estimate of arterial PCO_2.

TABLE 10.100.3 Selected Exercise Test Data From the Test at Age 29 in Comparison With Prior Tests

Measurement	Predicted[a]	Measured: Age 22	Age 27	Age 28	Age 29
Peak $\dot{V}O_2$ (L/min)	3.15	2.92	2.79	2.34	2.03
Maximum heart rate (beats/min)	190	178	178	174	177
Maximum O_2 pulse (mL/beat)	16.6	16.2	15.5	13.6	11.5
$\Delta\dot{V}O_2/\Delta WR$ (mL/min/W)	10.3	10.8	10.9	10.0	9.1
AT (L/min)	>1.35	1.5	1.4	1.21	1.17
Blood pressure (mm Hg [rest, max ex])		115/69, 165/65	110/50, 159/69	120/65, 149/70	122/65, 137/66
Maximum $\dot{V}E$ (L/min)	204	84	85	89	74
Breathing reserve (L/min)		120	119	115	130
$\dot{V}E/\dot{V}CO_2$ @ *AT* (L/min)	<28	24	22	24	25
SpO_2 (% [rest, max ex])		98, 99	99, 99	99, 98	98, 98

Abbreviations: *AT*, anaerobic threshold; $\Delta\dot{V}O_2/\Delta WR$, change in $\dot{V}O_2$/change in work rate; ex, exercise; O_2, oxygen; SpO_2, O_2 saturation measured by pulse oximetry; $\dot{V}E/\dot{V}CO_2$, ventilatory equivalent for carbon dioxide; $\dot{V}E$, minute ventilation; $\dot{V}O_2$, oxygen uptake.

[a]Predicted values were similar over the period of time these tests were conducted. Predicted $\dot{V}O_2$ was calculated using the age of 30, as recommended in Chapter 7 for subjects in their 20s, and height and weight had been stable.

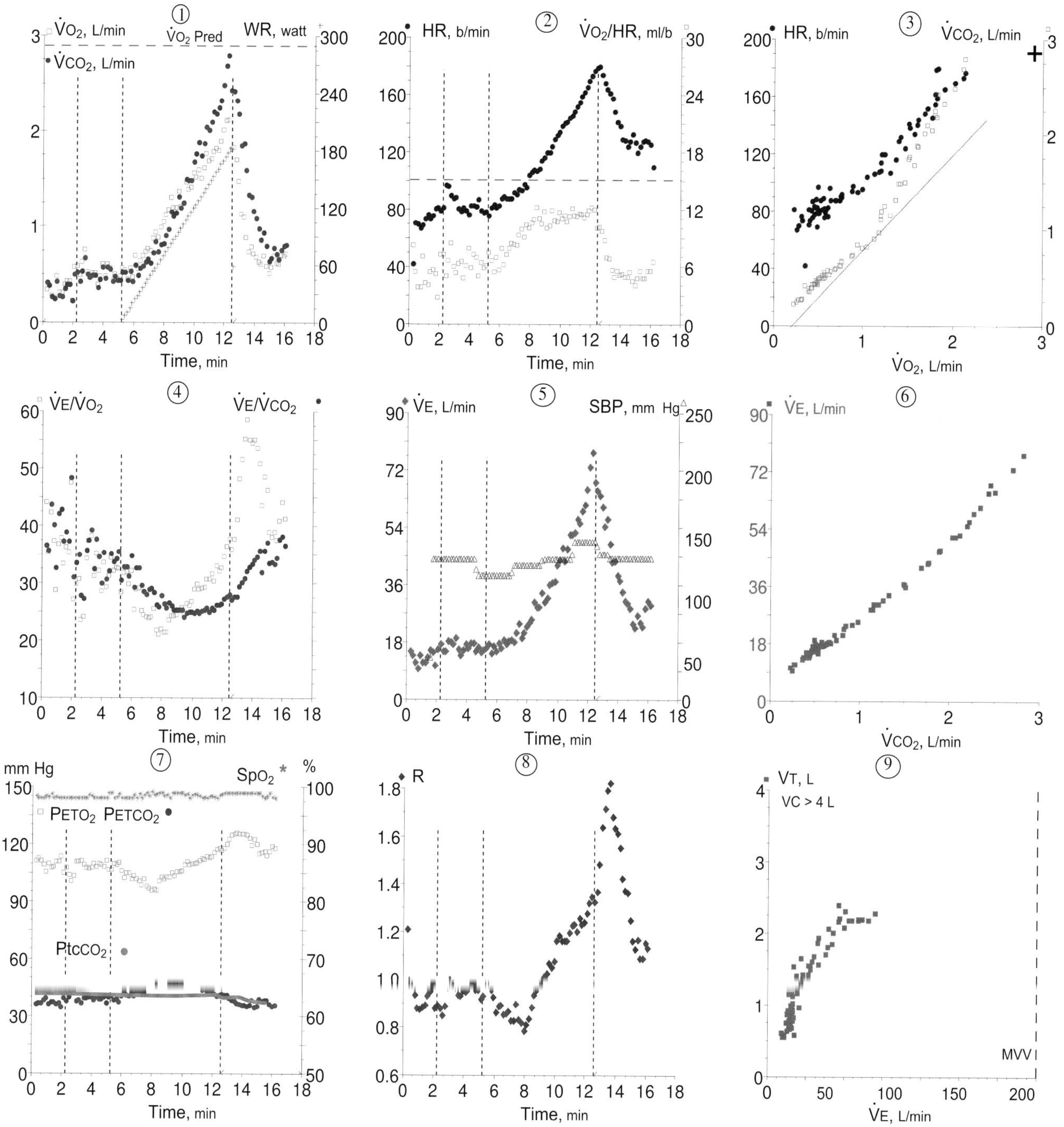

FIGURE 10.100.1. Age 29. Vertical dashed lines in the panels in the left and middle columns indicate, from left to right, the beginning of unloaded cycling, start of increasing work rate (WR) at 10 W/min, and start of recovery. In **panel 1**, the increase in WR (right y-axis) is plotted with a scale of 100 W to 1 L of oxygen uptake ($\dot{V}O_2$) (left y-axis) such that WR is plotted parallel to a $\dot{V}O_2$ slope of 10 mL/min/W. Predicted peak $\dot{V}O_2$ is shown as a dashed horizontal line. In **panel 3**, carbon dioxide output ($\dot{V}CO_2$) (right y-axis) is plotted as a function of $\dot{V}O_2$ (x-axis) with identical scales so that the diagonal blue line has a slope of 1 (45°). The $\dot{V}CO_2$ increasing more steeply than $\dot{V}O_2$ defines carbon dioxide derived from bicarbonate buffer, as long as ventilatory equivalent for carbon dioxide ($\dot{V}E/\dot{V}CO_2$) (**panel 4**) is not increasing and end-tidal PCO_2 ($PETCO_2$) (**panel 7**) is not decreasing, simultaneously. The black + symbol in **panel 3** indicates predicted peak values of heart rate (HR) (left y-axis) and $\dot{V}O_2$ for this individual. Abbreviations: IC, inspiratory capacity; MVV, maximum voluntary ventilation; $PETO_2$, end-tidal PO_2; $PtcCO_2$, transcutaneous PCO_2; R, respiratory exchange ratio; SBP, systolic blood pressure; SpO_2, O_2 saturation measured by pulse oximetry; VC, vital capacity; $\dot{V}E$, minute ventilation; $\dot{V}E/\dot{V}O_2$, ventilatory equivalent for oxygen; $\dot{V}O_2$/HR, O_2 uptake per heart beat or O_2 pulse; VT, tidal volume.

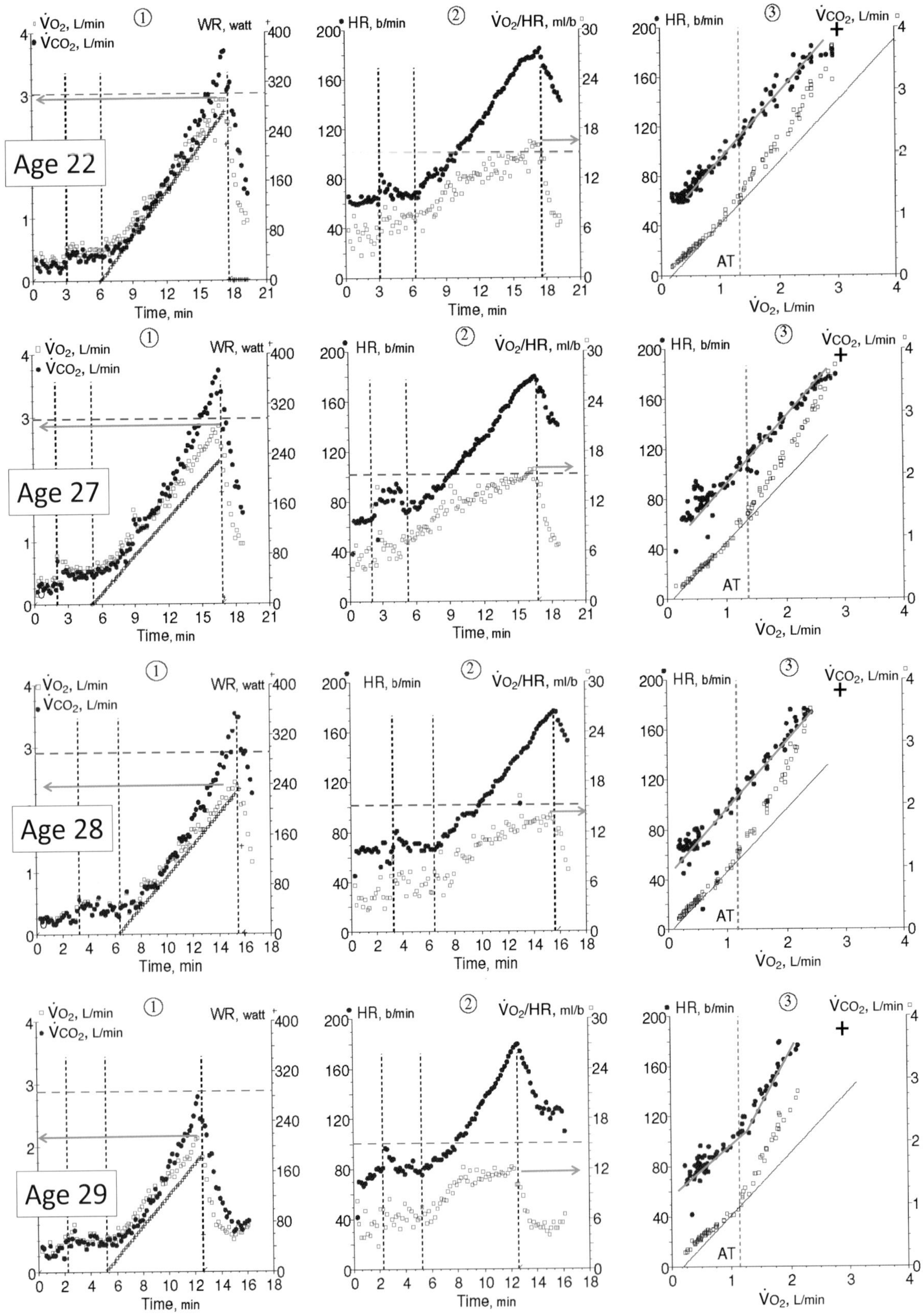

FIGURE 10.100.2. Graphical data for oxygen uptake ($\dot{V}O_2$) and heart rate responses for tests performed at ages 22, 27, 28, and 29 are plotted with the same scaling on the y-axis highlighting changes over time. Solid green lines in the left hand panels show peak $\dot{V}O_2$ and in the middle panel peak oxygen pulse. Horizontal dashed lines on **panel 1** and **panel 2** show predicted values for peak $\dot{V}O_2$ and oxygen pulse, respectively. In the right-hand panels (panel 3), the slope of heart rate (HR) relative to $\dot{V}O_2$ is shown by a solid line and the anaerobic threshold (*AT*) by a vertical dashed line. $\dot{V}CO_2$ (right y-axis) is plotted as a function of $\dot{V}O_2$ (x-axis) with identical scales so that the diagonal line has a slope of 1 (45°) Abbreviations are identical to Figure 10.100.1.

Conclusion

This test demonstrated impaired cardiovascular function reflected in low peak exercise capacity and abnormal relationship of heart rate to $\dot{V}O_2$. Although this could result from changes in peripheral blood flow distribution or oxygen extraction, in the context of this test, it was most suggestive of an abnormal exercise stroke volume. Data from prior tests were helpful in confirming that these findings represented a decrement in function in the face of a similar level of effort. Blood pressure response and electrocardiogram findings also differed from what had previously been observed. The findings supported the clinical concern of cardiotoxicity from prior drug exposure.

REFERENCE

1. Oeffinger KC, Mertens AC, Sklar CA, et al; for Childhood Cancer Survivor Study. Chronic health conditions in adult survivors of childhood cancer. *N Engl J Med*. 2006;355:1572-1582.

APPENDIX A

Symbols and Abbreviations

A bar above any symbol indicates a mean value.
A dot above any symbol indicates a time derivative.

TABLE A.1 Gases

Primary symbols		Examples	
V	Gas volume	V_A	Volume of alveolar gas
$\dot{V}$	Gas volume per unit time	$\dot{V}_{O_2}$	O_2 uptake per minute
P	Gas pressure	P_{AO_2}	Partial pressure of O_2 in alveolar gas
F	Fractional concentration of a gas	F_{IO_2}	Fractional concentration of O_2 in inspired gas
f	Respiratory frequency		
D	Diffusing capacity	D_{LCO}	Diffusing capacity of lung for carbon monoxide
R	Respiratory exchange ratio		
RQ	Respiratory quotient		
Q	Gas quantity		
$\dot{Q}$	Gas quantity per unit time (gas flow)	$\dot{Q}_{O_2}$	O_2 consumed per minute (O_2 consumption)
STPD	Standard temperature and pressure (0°C, 760 mm Hg), dry		
BTPS	Body temperature and pressure, saturated with water vapor		
Secondary symbols		**Examples**	
I	Inspired gas	F_{IO_2}	Fractional concentration of O_2 in inspired gas
E	Expired gas	V_E	Volume of expired gas
A	Alveolar gas	$\dot{V}_A$	Alveolar ventilation per minute
ET	End tidal	P_{ETCO_2}	Partial pressure of CO_2 in end-tidal gas
T	Tidal gas	V_T	Tidal volume
D	Dead space gas	V_D	Physiological dead space volume
B	Barometric	P_B	Barometric pressure

TABLE A.2 Blood

Primary symbols		Examples	
$\dot{Q}$	Volume flow of blood per unit time	$\dot{Q}_c$	Blood flow through pulmonary capillaries per minute
C	Concentration or content of gas in blood phase	Ca_{O_2}	Content of O_2 in arterial blood
S	Percentage saturation of Hb with O_2	$S\bar{v}_{O_2}$	Saturation of Hb with O_2 in mixed venous blood
Secondary symbols		**Examples**	
a	Arterial blood	Pa_{CO_2}	Partial pressure of CO_2 in arterial blood
v	Venous blood	$P\bar{v}_{O_2}$	Partial pressure of O_2 in mixed venous blood
c	Capillary blood	Pc_{CO_2}	Partial pressure of CO_2 in pulmonary capillary blood

TABLE A.3 Lung Volumes and Flows

V_T	Tidal volume = volume of air inhaled or exhaled with each breath
VC	Vital capacity = maximal volume that can be expired after a maximal inspiration
IC	Inspiratory capacity = maximal volume that can be inspired from the resting end-expiratory level
ERV	Expiratory reserve volume = maximal volume that can be expired from the resting end-expiratory level
FRC	Functional residual capacity = volume of gas in lungs at end of a relaxed expiration
RV	Residual volume = volume of gas in lungs after maximal expiration
TLC	Total lung capacity = volume of gas in lungs after a maximal inspiration
FEV_x	Forced expired volume in *x* seconds (eg, FEV_1 = forced expiratory volume in 1 second)
MVV	Maximal voluntary ventilation

TABLE A.4 Variables and Parameters

$\dot{V}O_2$	O_2 uptake	$\dot{V}E/\dot{V}O_2$	Ventilatory equivalent for O_2
$\dot{V}O_2max$	Maximal O_2 uptake	$\dot{V}E/\dot{V}CO_2$	Ventilatory equivalent for CO_2
$\dot{V}CO_2$	CO_2 output	V_D/V_T	Physiological dead space/tidal volume ratio
$\dot{Q}O_2$	O_2 consumption	V_D	Physiological dead space
$\dot{Q}CO_2$	CO_2 production	BR	Breathing reserve
AT	Anaerobic threshold	HR	Heart rate
LT	Lactate threshold	HRR	Heart rate reserve
LAT	Lactic acidosis threshold	WR	Work rate
R	Respiratory exchange ratio	$\Delta\dot{V}O_2/\Delta WR$	Change in $\dot{V}O_2$/change in WR
RQ	Respiratory quotient		

APPENDIX B

Glossary

Aerobic: Having molecular O_2 present; describes a metabolic process using O_2.

Alveolar to arterial P_{O_2} difference [$P(A - a)_{O_2}$]: The difference between the ideal alveolar P_{O_2} (estimated) and the arterial P_{O_2}. A larger difference reflects an increase in the lungs' inefficiency with respect to O_2 exchange.

Alveolar ventilation ($\dot{V}_A$): The theoretic alveolar ventilation necessary to eliminate the metabolic CO_2 being produced at the current arterial CO_2 partial pressure. It assumes that $\dot{V}_A/\dot{Q}$ is uniform in all the acini so that their mean alveolar P_{CO_2} is equal to the arterial P_{CO_2}.

Anaerobic: Lacking molecular O_2; describes any metabolic process that does not use molecular O_2.

Anaerobic threshold (*AT*): The exercise $\dot{V}_{O_2}$ above which anaerobic high-energy phosphate (ie, ATP) production supplements aerobic high-energy phosphate production, with the consequent lower redox state, increase in lactate-to-pyruvate (L/P) ratio, and net increase in lactate production at the site of anaerobiosis. Exercise above the *AT* is reflected by an increase in lactate concentration and L/P ratio in the muscle effluent and arterial blood, and a metabolic acidosis. Gas exchange is also affected by an increase in CO_2 output over that produced from aerobic metabolism, resulting from HCO_3^- buffering of lactic acid.

Analog-to-digital converter: A device for transforming continuously changing information (analog signal) into discrete units over some small timeframe within which the value is considered to be relatively constant (digital value). This transforms continuous signals to a form that can be analyzed by a digital computer. The rate at which the analog signal is sampled has important implications for the fidelity of the digital value.

Arterial to end-tidal P_{CO_2} difference [$P(a - ET)_{CO_2}$]: The difference between the mean arterial P_{CO_2} and the end-tidal P_{CO_2}. This is positive when the arterial P_{CO_2} is higher than the end-tidal P_{CO_2}. An increased positive difference generally reflects increased inefficiency of lung CO_2 exchange.

Arterial–mixed venous O_2 content difference [$C(a - \bar{v})_{O_2}$]: The difference in the O_2 content of the arterial and venous blood, usually expressed in mL of O_2 per dL or L of blood.

ATPS (ambient temperature and pressure, saturation): A convention for expressing gas volume conditioned to the ambient (eg, room) temperature and pressure and saturated with water vapor at ambient temperature.

Breath-by-breath: The expression of a particular physiological value averaged over one entire respiratory cycle, usually expressed as the value that variable would have if maintained over an entire minute (eg, ventilation expressed as L/min). Breath-by-breath is also used to describe a method for measurement of respiratory gas exchange in a breath during which respired gas volume and simultaneously measured expired gas concentration are integrated and reported.

Breathing reserve (BR): The difference between the maximum voluntary ventilation (measured at rest or estimated from FEV_1) and the maximum exercise minute ventilation. Hence, this represents the body's potential for further increasing ventilation at maximum exercise. See ***Maximum voluntary ventilation***.

BTPS (body temperature, ambient pressure, saturated): A convention for expressing gas volume conditioned to body temperature and the ambient atmospheric pressure and fully saturated with water vapor at the subject's body temperature.

Carbon dioxide output ($\dot{V}_{CO_2}$): The amount of CO_2 exhaled from the body into the atmosphere per unit time, expressed in mL or L/min, STPD. This differs from CO_2 production rate under conditions in which additional CO_2 may be evolved from the body's stores (ie, $\dot{V}_{CO_2}$ is higher than CO_2 production rate) or CO_2 is added to the body's stores (ie, $\dot{V}_{CO_2}$ is lower than CO_2 production rate). In the steady state, CO_2 output equals CO_2 production rate. In rare circumstances, appreciable quantities of CO_2 can be eliminated from the body as bicarbonate via the gastrointestinal tract or by hemodialysis.

Carbon dioxide production ($\dot{Q}_{CO_2}$): The amount of CO_2 produced metabolically by the body expressed in mL or L/min, STPD.

Cardiac output ($\dot{Q}$): The flow of blood from the heart in a particular period, usually expressed as L/min. It is the product of the average stroke volume per beat and the heart rate (ie, number of beats per minute).

Constant work rate test: An exercise test in which a constant power output or work rate is required of the subject, either for a fixed period or to the limit of tolerance.

Critical power: The highest work rate that can be sustained above the anaerobic threshold in a constant work-rate exercise test without a continuing rise in O_2 uptake or rise in arterial lactate concentration as the test progresses.

Dead space, physiological (V_D): The theoretic volume of gas taken into the lung that is not involved in gas exchange, assuming that the remaining volume (ie, the alveolar volume) consists of acini having uniform $\dot{V}_A/\dot{Q}$ so that the mean acinar P_{CO_2} equals the mean P_{CO_2} of the pulmonary capillary blood. The physiological dead space is made up of the anatomic dead space (the volume of the upper airways, trachea, and bronchi) and the alveolar dead space (the theoretical volume of alveoli that are ventilated but are unperfused).

Dead space/tidal volume ratio, physiological (V_D/V_T): The proportion of the tidal volume that is made up of the physiological dead space. This is an index of the relative inefficiency of pulmonary gas exchange to eliminate CO_2.

Diffusing capacity (of the lungs): A measure of the rate of uptake of a particular gas across the alveolar–capillary bed for a specified driving pressure for that gas. It is measured, therefore, as the volume of gas per unit time per pressure difference (eg, mL/min/mm Hg). It is also referred to as the pulmonary gas transfer index (a term that more properly reflects the measurement). It is most practical to use carbon monoxide as the test gas for measurement of diffusing capacity of the lungs, in which case it is referred to as D_{LCO}.

Diffusion defect: A defect in the lungs' capacity for gas diffusion. This is typically caused either by an abnormally increased diffusion path length or by conditions in which the transit time of the red cell through the pulmonary capillary bed is so fast that insufficient time is available for complete diffusion equilibrium.

Disability: A legal term that considers the effect of a functional impairment on the patient's ability to perform a specific physical task, along with other factors such as age, sex, education, social environment, job availability, and the energy requirements of the occupation.

End-expiratory lung volume (EELV): The volume of gas left in the lungs at the end of a spontaneous exhalation. If the expiration is fully relaxed, EELV will equal the functional residual capacity (FRC).

End-tidal P_{CO_2} (P_{ETCO_2}): The P_{CO_2} of the respired gas determined at the end of a spontaneous exhalation. This is commonly the highest P_{CO_2} measured during the alveolar phase of the exhalation.

End-tidal P_{O_2} (P_{ETO_2}): The P_{O_2} determined in the respired gas at the end of a spontaneous exhalation. This is typically the lowest P_{O_2} determined during the alveolar portion of the exhalation.

Expiratory reserve volume (ERV): The maximal volume that can be exhaled from functional residual capacity (FRC).

Exponential: A process in which the instantaneous rate of change of a variable is proportional to the "distance" from a steady-state or required level; hence, the rate of change of the function under consideration is rapid when it is far from its steady-state value and slows progressively as the function approaches its steady state. If the process is known to be (or may be reasonably estimated to be) exponential, the time to reach 63% of the final value (ie, to approach within 37% of the final value) is termed the time constant (τ) of the response. If the process is exponential, this time constant is related to the half-time (the time to reach 50% of the final value) by the equation $t_{1/2} = 0.693 \times \tau$. See ***Half-time***.

Fick method for cardiac output estimation: A means of estimating cardiac output ($\dot{Q}$) from the pulmonary O_2 uptake and the arterial–mixed venous O_2 content difference, that is, $\dot{Q} = \dot{V}_{O_2}/C(a - \bar{v})_{O_2}$. When the same principle is used to measure cardiac output with CO_2 as the test gas, $\dot{Q} = \dot{V}_{CO_2}/C(\bar{v} - a)_{CO_2}$.

Flow/volume sensor: A device used to measure the flow or volume of air respired (flow may also be integrated over time to yield volume). For example, a pneumotachograph measures flow as the pressure drop across a low-resistance screen or bundle of capillary tubes. A Pitot tube flow meter measures flow as the pressure difference between the upstream orifices of a set of small tubes mounted in parallel to the flow stream and that at a similar set mounted perpendicularly to the stream. A mass flow meter (or hot wire anemometer) measures mass flow rather than volumetric flow, that is, the electrical current required to heat a wire suspended in the flow stream to a certain temperature being proportional to the number of contained molecules. In contrast, a turbine sensor measures volume via the number of interruptions of a light beam produced by the rotation of a low-resistance vane in the gas flow stream.

Gas analyzer: A device used to measure the concentration of particular gas species (eg, CO_2, O_2, N_2) in respired air. The "gold standard" is the mass spectrometer, which ionizes the sampled gas in a high-vacuum environment allowing each component gas species to be measured on the basis of mass-charge ratio essentially simultaneously. Most commercial CPET systems use discrete O_2 and CO_2 analyzers operating in series. The operation of CO_2 analyzers is typically based on infrared light absorption. For O_2, paramagnetic analyzers measure O_2 as the degree of rotation of a N_2-filled glass dumbbell suspended within a magnetic field, whereas electrochemical fuel-cell analyzers measure P_{O_2} in proportion to the current generated by high-temperature O_2-substrate reactions.

Half-time ($t_{1/2}$): Unlike the time constant, which requires evidence of exponentiality for its determination, the half-time of a response is a simple description of the time to reach half of the change to the final value, regardless of the function. It is, therefore, generally representative of the speed of approaching the steady state. See ***Exponential***.

Heart rate reserve (HRR): The difference between the predicted highest heart rate attainable during maximum exercise and the actual highest heart rate, usually during exercise testing involving large muscle masses, such as cycle or treadmill ergometry.

Ideal alveolar Po_2: The hypothetical alveolar Po_2 that would be obtained if the lung were an ideal gas exchanger, that is, with alveolar ventilation uniformly matched to perfusion.

Impairment: A medical term reflecting a physiological abnormality. For exercise, it could represent any defect in the ventilatory-circulatory-metabolic coupling of external to internal respiration.

Incremental exercise test: An exercise test designed to provide a graded stress to the subject. The work rate required by the subject is usually increased over uniform periods, for example, every 4 minutes, every minute, every 15 seconds, or continuously (eg, ramp pattern).

Inspiratory capacity (IC): The maximal volume that can be inspired from functional residual capacity (FRC).

Isocapnic buffering: The period extending from the anaerobic threshold to the ventilatory compensation point during a rapid incremental or ramp exercise test, over which ventilation increases in proportion to CO_2 output ensuring continued constancy of arterial PCO_2.

Lactate: The anion of lactic acid.

Lactate threshold (*LT*): The exercise $\dot{V}o_2$ above which a net increase in lactate production results in a sustained increase in arterial blood lactate concentration.

Lactic acid: A three-carbon carboxylic acid ($CH_3CHOHCOOH$) that is one of the potential end products of glucose oxidation. Another major product is pyruvic acid ($CH_3COCOOH$), which can undergo conversion to acetyl coenzyme A and can thereby be further oxidized. The relative amounts of lactic acid and pyruvic acid are determined by the cytosolic redox state; a low redox state, reflected by a high ratio of NADH to NAD^+, favors the generation of lactic acid, which, in turn, maintains the supply of NAD^+ necessary for glycolysis to continue. The presence of lactic acid is a marker of anaerobic metabolism.

Lactic acidosis threshold (*LAT*): The exercise $\dot{V}o_2$ above which arterial standard HCO_3^- concentration decreases because of a net increase in lactate production. This can be detected by an increase in CO_2 output (from dissociation of H_2CO_3 as HCO_3^- buffers lactic acid) above that which would be predicted from aerobic metabolism alone during an incremental exercise test.

Maximum exercise heart rate: The highest obtainable heart rate during a maximum exercise test.

Maximum exercise ventilation: The highest minute ventilation achieved during a maximum exercise test. This is usually determined by tests that tax large muscle masses, such as cycle or treadmill ergometry.

Maximum oxygen uptake ($\dot{V}o_2max$): The highest O_2 uptake obtainable for a given form of ergometry despite further work rate increases and effort by the subject. This is characterized by a plateau of O_2 uptake despite further increases in work rate. See ***Peak oxygen uptake***.

Maximum voluntary ventilation (MVV): The upper limit of the body's ability to ventilate the lungs. This is conventionally measured from maximal volitional effort for short periods (eg, 12 seconds) and expressed in units of L/min, BTPS. Alternatively, the MVV may be estimated as a multiple of the FEV_1 (eg, 35 or 40 × FEV_1) from various population-derived formulas.

Mean response time: For an exponential process, this is the sum of the time constant (τ) of the exponential component and its delay (δ). See ***Exponential***.

MET: A MET, or metabolic equivalent, is the multiple of the resting metabolic rate expressed as O_2 uptake per minute per kilogram. The resting metabolic rate used in this calculation is usually 3.5 mL/min/kg, which is the average for a 40-year-old, 70-kg male. The weakness in applying this concept is that the exercise $\dot{V}o_2$ may not be measured but assumed for a given treadmill grade and speed or cycle ergometer work rate. A further weakness is the assumption that the resting $\dot{V}o_2$ is 3.5 mL/min/kg for everyone.

Minute ventilation ($\dot{V}_I$ or $\dot{V}_E$): The volume of air taken into or exhaled from the body in 1 minute. This is conventionally expressed at body temperature, saturated with water at atmospheric pressure (BTPS).

Mixed expired O_2 or CO_2: During expiration, gas from physiological dead space is mixed with gas from the exchanging alveoli, in which $\dot{V}_A/\dot{Q}$ is assumed to be uniform. Therefore, gas concentrations sampled from mixed expired gas, when compared to "ideal alveolar" samples, reflect the degree of inefficiency of gas exchange. This is especially true for CO_2, for which the mixed expired Pco_2 compared to arterial Pco_2 is used in the calculation of V_D/V_T. Mixed expired O_2 and CO_2 are the average partial pressures or concentrations in mixed expired gas collected over a timed interval and ideally over an integral number of breaths.

Mixed venous blood: A sample of blood representative of the flow-weighted venous blood returning from all the organs of the body. Usually, blood obtained from the pulmonary artery is considered to be mixed venous blood.

Mixed venous O_2 or CO_2: The average partial pressure or content of O_2 or CO_2 of the blood returning from all the tissues of the body and, having been fully mixed in the right heart, normally represented by the concentration or partial pressure of that substance in the pulmonary arterial blood.

Mixing chamber: A device that mixes the dead space (physiological) gas and alveolar gas to produce a gas that is representative of the mixed expired gas. This is typically achieved by exhaling into a baffled chamber that mixes several breaths. The mixed expired concentration of a gas can be measured downstream from the chamber. See ***Mixed expired O_2 or CO_2***.

Oximeter: A device that uses light transmission or reflectance techniques to estimate the saturation of hemoglobin with O_2. Direct oximetry is done on blood samples.

For indirect oximetry, a site for measurement, such as the earlobe or finger, is selected because blood comes close to the skin and traverses the capillary bed with little loss of O_2; hence, the mean capillary value will reflect the arterial value. See ***Pulse oximeter.***

Oxygen consumption ($\dot{Q}O_2$): The amount of O_2 used by the body's metabolic processes in a given time, expressed in mL or L/min, STPD.

Oxygen content (CO_2): The volume of O_2 (STPD) in a given volume (L, dL, or mL) of blood. This includes the major component that is bound to hemoglobin and the amount physically dissolved in the blood.

Oxygen debt: The additional O_2 used in excess of the baseline needs of the body following a bout of exercise.

Oxygen deficit: The O_2 equivalent of the total energy used to perform the exercise that did not derive from reactions using atmospheric O_2 taken into the body after the start of the exercise. Consequently, for moderate-intensity exercise, this O_2 deficit represents the energy equivalent of the depletion of the high-energy phosphate stores (eg, phosphocreatine) and O_2 stored in the body prior to the start of the exercise. For heavy or severe exercise, the O_2 deficit also includes the energy equivalent of the anaerobic processes.

Oxygen delivery: The amount of O_2 delivered to a tissue per unit time. It is, therefore, the product of the O_2 content of arterial blood and the blood flow to that tissue.

Oxygen pulse: The O_2 uptake ($\dot{V}O_2$) divided by the heart rate. Hence, it is the amount of O_2 extracted by the tissues of the body from the O_2 carried in each stroke volume.

Oxygen uptake ($\dot{V}O_2$): The amount of O_2 extracted from the inspired gas in a given period, expressed in mL/min or L/min, STPD. This can differ from O_2 consumption under conditions in which O_2 is flowing into or being used from the body's stores. In the steady state, O_2 uptake equals O_2 consumption.

Oxygen uptake efficiency slope (OUES): Defined as the slope of O_2 uptake versus log $\dot{V}E$ during an incremental exercise test, OUES relates the O_2 uptake response relative to ventilation. Using submaximal data from an incremental exercise test, OUES correlates with peak $\dot{V}O_2$, suggesting that this variable may be useful in assessing patients with cardiovascular disease.

Peak oxygen uptake: The highest O_2 uptake obtainable for a given form of ergometry at the end of a maximum exercise test. This is only equal to the maximum O_2 uptake if a plateau of O_2 uptake can be demonstrated despite further increases in work rate. See ***Maximum oxygen uptake.***

Physiological dead space: See ***Dead space.***

Power: See ***Work rate.***

Power-duration relationship: Relationship between power (ie, work rate) and its tolerable duration for constant work-rate exercise performed at work rates above critical power. See ***Critical power.***

Pulse oximeter: A noninvasive device for estimating arterial blood O_2 saturation using a combination of spectrophotometry and pulse plethysmography. The pulse oximeter probe is designed to be placed on the earlobe, fingertip, or forehead. See ***Oximeter.***

Pulse pressure: The difference between the systolic and the diastolic blood pressure.

Pump calibrator: A device that simulates the airflow and gas concentration waveforms encountered during respiration. Because the "metabolic rate" of such a device can be precisely calculated, it is useful for calibration of an exercise gas exchange measurement system.

Ramp exercise test: An exercise testing protocol in which the work rate is continuously increased at a constant rate (eg, 10 W/min). See ***Incremental exercise test.***

Respiratory exchange ratio (R or RER): The ratio of the CO_2 output to the O_2 uptake. This ratio reflects not only tissue metabolic exchange of the gases but also the influence of transient change in gas storage of O_2, and especially of CO_2. For example, the gas exchange ratio exceeds the respiratory quotient during hyperventilation as additional CO_2 is evolved from the body's stores, whereas the gas exchange ratio is less than the respiratory quotient during transient hypoventilation when CO_2 is retained in the body's stores.

Respiratory quotient (RQ): The ratio of the CO_2 production to O_2 consumption. This ratio reflects the metabolic exchange of the gases in the body's tissues and is dictated by the percentage of substrate species (carbohydrates, fatty acids, and amino acids) used in energy production by the cells.

Response time: A means of characterizing the rate at which a device or system responds to a given signal. For example, in response to a sudden application of a constant level of input (ie, a step), how long does the output take to become constant? This can be characterized by the time constant, half-time, or the time to reach 90% of the final value.

Set point: A term used in control system theory that reflects the particular value of a variable that the output of the system regulates. For example, a CO_2 set point is considered to be the operating level of arterial PCO_2, which is maintained at its relatively constant (ie, set-point) value by changes in ventilation at a given level of CO_2 output.

Steady state: A characteristic of a physiological system in which its functional demands are being met such that its output per unit time becomes constant. The time to achieve a steady state commonly differs for different physiological systems. For example, following the onset of constant work-rate exercise, O_2 uptake rises to reach its steady state appreciably faster than CO_2 output or ventilation. A constant value attained by the system is not sufficient, however, to determine that the system is in a steady state. If the system reaches the limit of its output, and, as a result, its output becomes constant (as in the case of O_2 uptake reaching its maximum value), a steady state does not prevail. The system in this instance is in a limited state, not a steady state.

STPD (standard temperature and pressure, dry): A convention for expressing gas volume at standard conditions of temperature and pressure, free of water vapor. The standard conditions are 0°C, 760 mm Hg, and dry gas.

Stroke volume: The volume of blood ejected from either ventricle of the heart in a single beat.

Sustainable work rate: A relative term that reflects the extent to which a particular work rate may be sustained for sufficient time for the successful completion of a particular occupational, recreational, or laboratory-induced task. Therefore, at a sustainable work rate, the subject does not fatigue within the time constraints of the requirements of the test.

Thermodilution cardiac output measurement: A technique in which a measured bolus of physiological fluid of known temperature, usually at 0°C, is injected into a vascular stream, such as in the right atrium, and the temperature of the blood is measured at a mixed downstream point, such as in the pulmonary artery. The decrease in mean temperature reflects the volume of blood into which the injectate is diluted; this plus the time the cooled blood takes to pass the temperature sensor allows blood flow to be determined. Thermodilution cardiac output measurements are usually performed using a thermistor-tipped pulmonary artery catheter (Swan-Ganz type).

Tidal volume (V_T): The volume of air inhaled or exhaled during a breath.

Tidal volume to inspiratory capacity ratio (V_T/IC): The ratio of the volume of air exhaled during a breath (V_T) to the volume potentially available for that breath, the latter measured from the end-expiratory lung volume to the maximum inspiratory volume (IC). Hence, it reflects the proportion of the potential inspiratory volume excursion that is actually used for a particular breath.

Transcutaneous gas partial pressure: A technique for estimating the partial pressure of a gas in the capillary blood perfusing a region of skin with high blood flow and low metabolic rate. When the intent of this measurement is to estimate arterial blood gas partial pressures, it must be interpreted with caution, especially when partial pressures are changing rapidly.

Transducer: A device that transforms energy from one form to another. For example, a pressure transducer is a device that changes fluid pressure into an electrical signal that can be analyzed and used for display or recording.

V-slope method: A method for estimating the anaerobic, lactate, or lactic acidosis threshold by plotting CO_2 output against O_2 uptake on equal scales. The onset of lactic acidosis during an incremental exercise test is detected when CO_2 output starts to systematically increase relative to O_2 uptake, which is assumed to reflect the increased CO_2 generated from bicarbonate as it buffers lactic acid.

Ventilatory efficiency: A term used to describe ventilation relative to CO_2 output, although not strictly a measure of "ventilatory efficiency" because the value of Pa_{CO_2} is not considered. Often defined during an incremental exercise test as the $\dot{V}_E$-$\dot{V}_{CO_2}$ slope below the ventilatory compensation point or as the value of $\dot{V}_E/\dot{V}_{CO_2}$ at the anaerobic threshold or at its nadir.

Ventilatory equivalent for O_2 or CO_2: The ratio of ventilation to O_2 uptake ($\dot{V}_E/\dot{V}_{O_2}$) or CO_2 output ($\dot{V}_E/\dot{V}_{CO_2}$).

$\Delta\dot{V}_{O_2}(6 - 3)$: The difference in O_2 uptake between the sixth and the third minute of a constant-load exercise test. Normal subjects typically attain a steady state for constant-load exercise within 3 minutes during moderate exercise; hence, the $\Delta\dot{V}_{O_2}(6 - 3)$ is zero. A positive value for this index reflects a degree of continuing nonsteady state for the work and usually signals fatiguing exercise.

$\Delta\dot{V}_{O_2}/\Delta WR$: The increase in O_2 uptake in response to a simultaneous increase in work rate. Under appropriate conditions (eg, steady-state aerobic exercise), this may be used to estimate the efficiency for muscular exercise. See ***Work efficiency***.

Wasted ventilation ($\dot{V}_D$): The difference between the computed alveolar ventilation and the measured minute ventilation. Also known as the physiological dead space ventilation, this term is meant to reflect the volume of the respired air that did not participate in alveolar gas exchange; it is equal to $V_D \times f$.

Work: A physical quantification of the force operating on a mass that causes it to change its location. Under conditions in which force is applied and no movement results (eg, during an isometric contraction), no work is performed, despite increased metabolic energy expenditure. The unit of work is the joule (kg m^2/sec^2).

Work efficiency: The fraction of the chemical energy of the metabolic substrate used that is actually transformed into the mechanical energy of the task performance, calculated in the steady state between at least two work rates, that is, as the ratio of the increment in the work rate being performed to the increment in the energy utilization for the task, with the latter standardly established from the associated steady-state increment in O_2 uptake and the caloric equivalent of the substrate mixture being oxidized,

Work rate or power: This reflects the rate at which work is performed (ie, work per unit time). Work rate is usually measured in watts (kg-m^2/s^3 or joule/s) or in kilopond meters per minute (kp-m/min); 1 W is equivalent to 6.12 kp-m/min.

APPENDIX C

Calculations, Formulas, and Examples

This appendix presents the most essential formulas for calculating gas exchange and other related variables during exercise. An example accompanies the formula for each variable, using typical data acquired during exercise testing. Calculation of these variables uses well-defined and tested formulas, but several areas deserve particularly close attention. We address the specific problems of water vapor in the calculation of $\dot{V}O_2$, of making corrections for the dead space of the breathing valve, and of collecting data for breath-by-breath gas exchange analysis.

With computerized systems for collecting expired gas, measuring gas concentrations and ventilation, and calculating and displaying the relevant variables, some might be curious why one would need to understand how these calculations are made. It is important to understand how and how much variables can be affected by changes in the environment or by dysfunction of measurement devices. This understanding can be helpful in troubleshooting or deciding on the need to recalibrate the systems or obtain service for the equipment.

FORMULAS AND EXAMPLES OF GAS EXCHANGE CALCULATION

Although almost all exercise gas exchange measurements are made with computerized systems, for the example calculations, we assume that expired gas is collected for exactly 2 minutes into a sealed meteorological balloon or Douglas bag. This type of collection, of course, was the traditional method and still is used for validation and calibration purposes. The formula for calculating each variable takes into account the conditions under which each measurement is made as well as certain conventions. We assume that the gas volume is measured in a large spirometer or other suitable device, that fractional concentrations of oxygen (O_2) and carbon dioxide (CO_2) are measured to within 0.04% using gas analyzers or a mass spectrometer, and that these are fractions of total gas volume excluding water vapor. For some calculations, we assume that an arterial blood sample is obtained simultaneously with the collection of expired gas.

The measurements used for the example calculations are given in **Table C.1**.

TABLE C.1 Measurements Used for Example of Calculation of Gas Exchange

Measured volume: 54.2 L (ATPS)
Collection time: 2 min
Number of breaths: 41 in 2 min
Heart rate = 120 beats/min
Body temperature = 37°C
F_{IO_2} = 0.2093 (20.93%)
F_{ICO_2} = 0.0004 (0.04%)
F_{EO_2} = 0.162 (16.2%)
F_{ECO_2} = 0.041 (4.1%)
(Fractions of dry gas volume)
Hemoglobin = 15 g/100 mL
Valve dead space = 0.064 L
Ambient temperature (T) = 22°C
Barometric pressure (P_B) = 760 mm Hg
Partial pressure of water, saturated gas at 22°C (P_{H_2O}) = 19 mm Hg
Pa_{O_2} = 91 mm Hg
Pa_{CO_2} = 36 mm Hg
pH = 7.44
Sa_{O_2} = 95%
P_{ETCO_2} = 38 mm Hg
$P\bar{v}_{O_2}$ = 27 mm Hg
$S\bar{v}_{O_2}$ = 50%

Minute Ventilation

The volume of gas exhaled divided by the time of collection in minutes is minute ventilation ($\dot{V}_E$). Most commonly, ventilation is measured at ambient temperature and the gas is fully saturated with water vapor at ambient temperature (ATPS). Equation 1 is used to adjust volume from ATPS to BTPS (body temperature and pressure, saturated with water vapor) conditions, as by convention, $\dot{V}_E$ is reported under BTPS conditions. It may be necessary during calculation to obtain $\dot{V}_E$ at standard temperature and pressure (STPD) using Equation 2.

$$\dot{V}_E\ (\text{L/min, BTPS}) = \dot{V}_E\ (\text{L/min, ATPS}) \times \frac{(273 + 37)}{273 + T} \times \frac{P_B - P_{H_2O}\ (\text{at } T)}{P_B - 47} \quad (1)$$

where T is ambient temperature (°C), body temperature is 37°C, P_{H_2O} at 37°C is 47 mm Hg (fully saturated), and P_B is barometric pressure.

Alternatively, ventilation can be measured at STPD. From $\dot{V}_E$ (BTPS), $\dot{V}_E$ (STPD) can be obtained using Equation 2, which converts BTPS to STPD (at 273°K, barometric pressure = 760 mm Hg, and no water vapor present) for $\dot{V}CO_2$ and $\dot{V}CO_2$ calculations.

$$\dot{V}E\ (L/min, STPD) = \dot{V}E\ (L/min, BTPS) \times \frac{273}{(273 + 37)} \times \frac{PB - 47}{760}$$

which becomes

$$\dot{V}E\ (L/min, STPD) = \dot{V}E\ (L/min, BTPS) \times 0.826 \quad (2)$$

if PB = 760 mm Hg.

Example

$$\dot{V}E\ (L/min, ATPS) = \frac{\text{Total volume (ATPS)}}{\text{Total collection time}} = 54.2/2\ min = 27.1$$

Then, from Equation 1,

$$\dot{V}E\ (L/min, BTPS) = 27.1 \times \frac{310}{(273 + 22)} \times \frac{(760 - 19)}{(760 - 47)} = 29.6$$

and, from Equation 2,

$$\dot{V}E\ (L/min, STPD) = 29.6 \times 0.826 = 24.3$$

Respiratory Frequency (*f*)

$$f(min^{-1}) = \frac{\text{Number of complete breaths}}{\text{Total time for complete breaths}} \quad (3)$$

Example

$$f(min^{-1}) = \frac{41\ \text{breaths}}{2\ \text{min}} = 20.5$$

Tidal Volume (VT)

$$VT\ (L, BTPS) = \frac{\dot{V}E\ (L/min, BTPS)}{f} \quad (4)$$

Example

$$VT\ (L, BTPS) = \frac{29.6}{20.5} = 1.44$$

Carbon Dioxide Output ($\dot{V}CO_2$)

The CO_2 output is reported, by convention, under STPD conditions. If $\dot{V}E$ is measured at or converted to STPD conditions, $FECO_2$ is the fraction of CO_2 in the dry gas volume, and $FICO_2$ is zero or negligible, then

$$\dot{V}CO_2\ (L/min, STPD) = \dot{V}E\ (L/min, STPD) \times FECO_2 \quad (5)$$

or, for PB = 760 mm Hg,

$$\dot{V}CO_2\ (L/min, STPD) = \dot{V}E\ (L/min, BTPS) \times 0.826 \times FECO_2 \quad (6)$$

Example

Substituting $\dot{V}E$ and $FECO_2$ (see Table C.1) into Equation 5,

$$\dot{V}CO_2\ (L/min, STPD) = 24.3 \times 0.041 = 0.997$$

Oxygen Uptake ($\dot{V}O_2$)

For the derivation of the formula for $\dot{V}O_2$ and consideration of water vapor, see "Special Considerations for Calculation of Gas Exchange Variables" later in this appendix. Equation 7 should be used only for expired gas containing no water vapor (or measured as such).

The O_2 uptake is reported, by convention, under STPD conditions. If $\dot{V}E$ is measured at or converted to STPD, FIO_2 is 0.2093 (as a fraction of dry room air), $FECO_2$ and FEO_2 are fractions of CO_2 and O_2 in dry gas, respectively, and $FICO_2$ is 0, then

$$\dot{V}O_2\ (L/min, STPD) = \dot{V}E\ (L/min, STPD) \times (\Delta FO_2)\text{true, dry} \quad (7)$$

where (ΔFO_2)true, dry $= 0.265 - 1.265 \times FEO_2 - 0.265 \times FECO_2$ for a person breathing room air.

Example

Substituting from Table C.1 into Equation 7:

$$(\Delta FO_2)\text{true, dry} = 0.265 - 0.205 - 0.0108 - 0.049$$

$$\dot{V}O_2\ (L/min, STPD) = 24.3 \times 0.049 = 1.19$$

Gas Exchange Ratio (R)

$$R = \frac{\dot{V}CO_2\ (L, min\ STPD)}{\dot{V}O_2\ (L, min\ STPD)} \quad (8)$$

Example

$$R = \frac{0.997}{1.19} = 0.84$$

Ventilatory Equivalents for Carbon Dioxide and Oxygen ($\dot{V}E/\dot{V}CO_2$, $\dot{V}E/\dot{V}O_2$)

The ventilatory equivalents for CO_2 and O_2 are measurements of the ventilatory requirement for that metabolic rate. By convention, they are expressed as $\dot{V}E$ (L/min, BTPS) divided by $\dot{V}CO_2$ or $\dot{V}O_2$ (L/min, STPD). Because the portion of the ventilation wasted in clearing the breathing valve dead space is disregarded in determining the ventilatory requirement, the product of valve dead space (VD_m) and respiratory frequency (*f*) is subtracted from the total $\dot{V}E$:

$$\dot{V}E/\dot{V}CO_2 = \frac{\dot{V}E\ (L/min, BTPS) - [f\,min^{-1} \times VD_m\ (L)]}{\dot{V}CO_2\ (L/min, STPD)} \quad (9)$$

$$\dot{V}E/\dot{V}O_2 = \frac{\dot{V}E\ (L/min, BTPS) - [f\,min^{-1} \times VD_m\ (L)]}{\dot{V}O_2\ (L/min, STPD)} \quad (10)$$

Example

$$\dot{V}E/\dot{V}CO_2 = \frac{29.6 - [20.5 \times 0.064]}{0.997} = 28.4$$

$$\dot{V}E/\dot{V}O_2 = \frac{29.6 - [20.5 \times 0.064]}{1.19} = 23.8$$

Oxygen Pulse ($\dot{V}O_2$/HR)

$$\dot{V}O_2/HR\ (mL, STPD/beat) = \frac{\dot{V}O_2\ (L/min, STPD) \times 1000\ mL/L}{HR\ (beats/min)} \quad (11)$$

Example

$$\dot{V}O_2/HR\ (mL, STPD/beat) = \frac{1.19 \times 1000}{120} = 9.9$$

Alveolar P_{O_2} (P_{AO_2})

$$P_{AO_2}\ (\text{mm Hg})$$
$$= F_{IO_2} \times (P_B - 47) - \frac{P_{ACO_2}}{R}[1 - F_{IO_2}(1 - R)]\ (12)$$

where P(uc)b(sc) is in mm Hg; P_{ACO_2} is ideal alveolar P_{CO_2} in mm Hg; R is the gas exchange ratio; and F_{IO_2} is the fraction of inspired O_2, dry. Usually, the assumption that $P_{ACO_2} = Pa_{CO_2}$ is used, and the term $F_{IO_2} \times (1 - R)$ is dropped because it is so small that it has an insignificant effect on the calculated P_{AO_2}, especially during ambient air breathing. This simplifies the formula to the following:

$$P_{AO_2}\ (\text{mm Hg}) = F_{IO_2} \times (P_B - 47) - \frac{P_{ACO_2}}{R}\ (13)$$

Whereas R in the fasting state is often assumed to be approximately 0.8 at rest, R should always be calculated during an exercise test because it may range from 0.7 to 1.4 or more. This will have an appreciable effect on the alveolar P_{O_2} calculation.

Example

Substituting into Equation 13,

$$P_{AO_2}\ (\text{mm Hg}) = (0.2093 \times 713) - \frac{36}{0.84} = 106$$

Alveolar–Arterial P_{O_2} Difference [$P(A - a)_{O_2}$]

$$P(A - a)_{O_2}\ (\text{mm Hg}) = P_{AO_2} - Pa_{O_2}\ (14)$$

where P_{AO_2} is determined from equation 13 and Pa_{O_2} is arterial P_{O_2}.

Example

$$P(A - a)_{O_2}\ (\text{mm Hg}) = 106 - 91 = 15$$

Arterial End-Tidal P_{CO_2} Difference [$P(a - ET)_{CO_2}$]

$$P(a - ET)_{CO_2} = Pa_{CO_2} - P_{ETCO_2}\ (15)$$

where Pa_{CO_2} is arterial P_{CO_2} and P_{ETCO_2} is end-tidal P_{CO_2}.

Example

$$P(a - ET)_{CO_2} = 36 - 38 = -2\ \text{mm Hg}$$

Physiological Dead Space–Tidal Volume Ratio (V_D/V_T)

$$\frac{V_D}{V_T} = \frac{Pa_{CO_2} - P\bar{E}_{CO_2}}{Pa_{CO_2}}\ (16)$$

where $P\bar{E}_{CO_2}$ is mixed expired partial pressure of CO_2. However, this calculation must be corrected for any dead space added by a breathing valve (V_{Dm}). Because it is assumed that Pa_{CO_2} does not change, the only correction is for the $P\bar{E}_{CO_2}$. The $\dot{V}_{CO_2}$ must be adjusted to BTPS conditions to match $\dot{V}_E$ (BTPS), and *f* is respiratory frequency.

$$\frac{V_D}{V_T} = \frac{Pa_{CO_2} - P_B \times \dfrac{\dot{V}_{CO_2}}{\dot{V}_E - V_{Dm} \times f}}{Pa_{CO_2}}$$

Example

$$\frac{V_D}{V_T} = \frac{36 - \dfrac{0.997}{29.6 - 1.31}}{36} = 0.30$$

The V_D/V_T must be calculated using the arterial P_{CO_2}, and it cannot be calculated by substituting P_{ETCO_2} for Pa_{CO_2} in the foregoing formulae or by estimating Pa_{CO_2} from P_{ETCO_2} using a regression formula derived from normal subjects. As shown in Chapter 3, P_{ETCO_2} and Pa_{CO_2} are nearly equal only in normal subjects at rest. During exercise, $P(a - ET)_{CO_2}$ becomes negative in normal subjects, whereas it becomes larger and more positive in patients with lung disease or heart disease who have increased V_D/V_T. The relationship between Pa_{CO_2} and P_{ETCO_2} during exercise ranges widely and unpredictably.[1] Furthermore, even small errors in Pa_{CO_2} may result in clinically important differences in the calculated V_D/V_T.

Cardiac Output

The cardiac output ($\dot{Q}$) can be determined by thermal indicator dilution or by the Fick method using $\dot{V}_{O_2}$ and arterial–mixed venous O_2 content difference:

$$\dot{Q}\ (\text{L/min}) = \frac{\dot{V}_{O_2}\ (\text{mL/min, STPD})}{[Ca_{O_2} - C\bar{v}_{O_2}]\ (\text{mL } O_2/\text{L blood})}\ (17)$$

where Ca_{O_2} is O_2 content in arterial blood and $C\bar{v}_{O_2}$ is O_2 content in mixed venous blood. These can be calculated as follows:

$$C_{O_2}\ (\text{mL } O_2/100\ \text{mL}) = (S_{O_2} \times 0.01 \times 1.34\ \text{mL } O_2/\text{g Hb} \times [\text{Hb}]) + (0.003\ \text{mL } O_2/\text{mm Hg}/100\ \text{mL} \times P_{O_2})\ (18)$$

where [Hb] is hemoglobin concentration in g/100 mL blood and S_{O_2} is the percentage of oxyhemoglobin saturation. Note that this calculation gives O_2 content in mL O_2/100 mL of blood and is converted to mL O_2/L blood by multiplying by 10.

Example

$$Ca_{O_2}(\text{mL } O_2/100\ \text{mL}) = (95\% \times 0.01 \times 1.34 \times 15) + (0.003 \times 91) = 19.4$$

$$C\bar{v}_{O_2}\ (\text{mL } O_2/100\ \text{mL}) = (50\% \times 0.01 \times 1.34 \times 15) + (0.003 \times 27) = 10.1$$

$$(Ca_{O_2} - C\bar{v}_{O_2}) = 19.4 - 10.1 = 9.3\ \text{mL } O_2/100\ \text{mL} = 93\ \text{mL } O_2/\text{L}$$

$$\dot{Q}\ (\text{L/min}) = \frac{1190\ (\text{mL/min, STPD})}{93\ \text{mL } O_2/\text{L blood}} = 12.8$$

A noninvasive determination of $\dot{Q}$ has been described using an analogous formula for CO_2 and an estimate of mixed venous CO_2 content ($C\bar{v}_{CO_2}$) (indirect Fick method) from a single-exhalation method[2] or a rebreathing method.[3] With the rebreathing method, as a mixture of CO_2 and high-inspired O_2 is rebreathed, the P_{CO_2} of the rebreathed gas rapidly approaches that of mixed venous blood. This value is then referred to a CO_2 dissociation curve to determine CO_2 content. However, as shown in Chapter 3 (Measurements), estimating $C\bar{v}_{CO_2}$ has great pitfalls during exercise.

Sun et al,[4,5] using direct measurements of blood gases and pH, addressed the problem of indirectly determining CO_2 contents in arterial and mixed venous blood. The pH profoundly affects the CO_2 dissociation curve, making it impossible to get a reasonably reliable estimate of C_{CO_2}, particularly for $C\bar{v}_{CO_2}$. This study showed that $C\bar{v}_{CO_2}$ did not increase in proportion to mixed venous partial pressure of carbon dioxide ($P\bar{v}_{CO_2}$) during exercise. In fact, $C\bar{v}_{CO_2}$ actually decreased as $P\bar{v}_{CO_2}$ increased above the anaerobic threshold because of the downward shift of the CO_2 dissociation curve as pH decreased. Also, as discussed in reference to calculating V_D/V_T, it is invalid to derive Pa_{CO_2} and Ca_{CO_2} from P_{ETCO_2} because the difference between these two measures of P_{CO_2} is variable, particularly in patients, and is too large to obtain reliable estimates of CO_2 content with the precision required for valid measurements.

Using direct measures of arterial and mixed venous O_2 and CO_2 gas tensions, pH, and hemoglobin concentrations, Sun et al[4,5] compared the O_2 and CO_2 values determined by direct Fick $\dot{Q}$ measurements during exercise from rest to peak $\dot{V}_{O_2}$. They found that the two test gases gave the same results, but the variability was greater with CO_2. The reader is referred to the two papers by Sun et al[4,5] on this topic, where the problems of measuring $\dot{Q}$ by the indirect Fick method are thoroughly discussed.

CALCULATIONS AT MAXIMUM EXERCISE

Breathing Reserve (BR)

$$\text{BR (L/min)} = \text{MVV (L/min)} - \dot{V}_E \text{ (L/min) at maximum exercise} \quad (19)$$

$$\text{BR (\%)} = \frac{\text{MVV (L/min)} - \dot{V}_E \text{ (L/min) at maximum exercise}}{\text{MVV (L/min)}} \times 100 \quad (20)$$

where MVV is maximum voluntary ventilation at rest.

Example

If MVV is 82 L/min and $\dot{V}_E$ at maximum exercise is 65 L/min, then

$$\text{BR (L/min)} = 82 - 65 = 17 \text{ L/min}$$

$$\text{BR (\%)} = \frac{82 - 65}{82} \times 100 = 21\%$$

Heart Rate Reserve (HRR)

$$\text{HRR (beats/min)} = \text{Predicted maximum HR} - \text{HR at maximum exercise} \quad (21)$$

$$\text{HRR (\%)} = \frac{\text{Predicted maximum HR} - \text{HR at maximum exercise}}{\text{Predicted maximum HR}} \times 100 \quad (22)$$

where predicted maximum heart rate (HR) (adults) = 220 − age (years).

Example

For a 60-year-old man, predicted maximum HR = 220 − 60 = 160 beats/min. If HR at maximum exercise is 145 beats/min, then

$$\text{HRR (beats/min)} = 160 - 145 = 15$$

$$\text{HRR (\%)} = \frac{160 - 145}{160} \times 100 = 9\%$$

SPECIAL CONSIDERATIONS FOR CALCULATION OF GAS EXCHANGE VARIABLES

Water Vapor and Oxygen Uptake

The $\dot{V}_{O_2}$ is determined most often by collection and analysis of expired gas. The usual calculation method determines $\dot{V}_{O_2}$ from expired ventilation, expired CO_2 fraction, and expired O_2 fraction, and is based on the assumption that the inspired and expired volumes of nitrogen (and other inert gases) do not differ during the collection period. During rest and exercise, this method has been found to be satisfactory.[6,7] Nevertheless, errors may be introduced if careful attention is not paid to methods and calculations. This is especially true of how water vapor is handled because this variable can greatly affect the calculation of $\dot{V}_{O_2}$.

If a mass spectrometer is used to measure gas fractional concentration (a mass spectrometer does not measure water vapor), or water vapor is removed from the gas prior to measurement, then measured gas concentration is relative to total gas volume minus the volume of water vapor. Thus, the dilution of each gas by water vapor can be ignored and calculations are relatively simple:

$$\dot{V}_{O_2} \text{ (L/min, STPD)} = [F_{IO_2} \times \dot{V}_I \text{ (L/min, STPD)}] - [F_{EO_2} \times \dot{V}_E \text{ (L/min, STPD)}]$$

where F_{IO_2} and F_{EO_2} are the O_2 fractions of dry gas volumes. If the volumes of inspired and expired nitrogen (and other inert gases) are equal over the period of collection, then

$$\dot{V}_I \times F_{IN_2} = \dot{V}_E \times F_{EN_2}$$

and

$$\dot{V}_I = (F_{EN_2}/F_{IN_2}) \times \dot{V}_E$$

where F_{IN_2} and F_{EN_2} are the fractional concentrations of nitrogen and other inert gases.

Because $(F_{IN_2} + F_{IO_2} + F_{ICO_2}) = 1$ and $(F_{EN_2} + F_{EO_2} + F_{ECO_2}) = 1$, then

$$\dot{V}_I = \frac{(1 - F_{EO_2} - F_{ECO_2})}{(1 - F_{IO_2} - F_{ICO_2})} \times \dot{V}_E$$

and

$$\dot{V}_{O_2} \text{(L/min, STPD)} = \left[\frac{F_{IO_2} \times (1 - F_{EO_2} - F_{ECO_2})}{(1 - F_{IO_2} - F_{ICO_2})} - F_{EO_2}\right] \times \dot{V}_E \quad (23)$$

The quantity in brackets is called the true O_2 difference, (ΔF_{O_2})true.

If we assume that $F_{ICO_2} = 0$, or is negligible, then

$$(\Delta F_{O_2})\text{true} = \frac{(F_{IO_2} - F_{EO_2} - F_{IO_2} \times F_{ECO_2})}{(1 - F_{IO_2})}$$

and

$$\dot{V}_{O_2} \text{ (L/min, STPD)} = \dot{V}_E \text{ (L/min, STPD)} \times (\Delta F_{O_2})\text{true}$$

For room-air inspired gas, F_{IO_2} (dry) = 0.2093, and

$$\dot{V}_{O_2} \text{ (L/min, STPD)} = \dot{V}_E \text{ (L/min, STPD)} \times (0.265 - 1.265 \times F_{EO_2} - 0.265 \times F_{ECO_2}) \quad (24)$$

If water vapor is not removed from the gas and the method of gas analysis measures gas fraction of the total gas volume including water vapor, as is the case for most discrete O_2 analyzers, then the water vapor will reduce each dry gas fraction by the following factor:

$$\frac{(P_B - P_{H_2O})}{P_B} \text{ or } (1 - F_{H_2O})$$

In this case, the determination of $\dot{V}O_2$ is affected by water vapor as follows. First, $\dot{V}O_2$ can be expressed using $\dot{V}_I$ and $\dot{V}_E$ determined under the conditions of measurement (ie, at temperature T and containing water vapor):

$$\dot{V}O_2 \text{ (L/min, STPD)} = \frac{273}{273 + T} \times \frac{P_B}{760} \times (\dot{V}_I \times F_{IO_2} - \dot{V}_E \times F_{EO_2}) \quad (25)$$

where $\dot{V}_I$ and $\dot{V}_E$ are L/min at temperature T and F_{IO_2} and F_{EO_2} are fractions of $\dot{V}_I$ and $\dot{V}_E$, respectively, including the volume of water vapor.

Because $\dot{V}_I = (F_{EN_2}/F_{IN_2}) \times \dot{V}_E$, and $(F_{EN_2} + F_{EO_2} + F_{ECO_2} + F_{EH_2O}) = 1$ and $(F_{IN_2} + F_{IO_2} + F_{ICO_2} + F_{IH_2O}) = 1$, then substituting into Equation 25 gives

$$\dot{V}O_2 \text{ (L/min, STPD)} = \dot{V}_E \text{ (L/min at } T) \times k(T, P_{H_2O}) \times (\Delta F_{O_2})\text{true} \quad (26)$$

where

$$k(T, P_{H_2O}) = \frac{273}{273 + T} \times \frac{P_B}{760}$$

and

$$(\Delta F_{O_2})\text{true} = \frac{F_{IO_2} \times (1 - F_{ECO_2} - F_{EH_2O}) - F_{EO_2} \times (1 - F_{IH_2O})}{(1 - F_{IO_2} - F_{IH_2O})}$$

The calculation of $\dot{V}O_2$ is simpler if the expired gas is dried prior to analysis for O_2 and CO_2. However, Beaver[8] provides a nomogram for calculation of $\dot{V}O_2$ in the presence of water vapor that can be used to determine $\dot{V}O_2$ and R from a sample of mixed expired gas assumed to be fully saturated with water vapor at a known temperature. The subject is assumed to be breathing room air, and the O_2 and CO_2 analyzers display the fractions of total expired gas including water vapor. Substantial errors would result if water vapor were not taken into account.

Breath-by-breath gas exchange measurement systems must deal with the effect of water vapor on calculation of $\dot{V}O_2$. Although rarely used, a mass spectrometer "ignores" water vapor as the sum of ion voltages is made up of only those measuring N_2, O_2, CO_2, and argon, with water vapor ignored in both inspired and expired gases. If this method is used, then the volume to be multiplied by true O_2 fraction should be the dry gas volume.

Rapidly responding O_2 analyzers and infrared CO_2 analyzers used without drying the analyzed gas read fractions of total gas volume and therefore read lower concentrations than if the same gas were measured after being dried. As shown in Equation 26, the values can be used in a breath-by-breath system if F_{EH_2O} and F_{IH_2O} are known.[9] The assumption that expired gas is fully saturated at some known temperature is the starting point for several approaches to dealing with this in breath-by-breath systems.

First, the expired gas sample can be kept warm (at a known temperature) to prevent loss of water vapor by condensation. If gas is fully saturated at a known temperature, F_{EH_2O} can be estimated. A heated sampling tube is necessary, and the temperature must be accurately known. For example, assuming a value of 37°C when actual expired gas temperature is 32°C can result in a 7% to 8% error in $\dot{V}O_2$. During exercise, expired gas rapidly cools in the mouthpiece and breathing valve to as low as 32°C. Because gas for analysis is most often sampled at this location in breath-by-breath systems, then even if the gas is rewarmed, there will have been some unknown loss of water vapor to condensation. A second approach is to allow the sampled gas to cool to a known temperature. This avoids the problem of indeterminate loss of water vapor from cooling followed by rewarming.

Another approach used by some exercise systems employs conducting tubing that allows water vapor to pass out of the gas being conveyed to the gas analyzer until water vapor equilibrium is reached with the atmosphere. Thus, water vapor partial pressure in the gas analyzers is equal to the ambient P_{H_2O} rather than saturated at some imprecisely known temperature. This method avoids the need to know the precise temperature of the respired gas and does not adversely affect the response time.

Measurement of $\dot{V}O_2$ While Breathing Oxygen-Enriched Inspired Gas

The calculation of $\dot{V}O_2$ shown is intended only for measurement during room-air breathing. The use of the same equations during breathing of oxygen-enriched inspired gas mixtures is problematic. The relation of $\dot{V}_I$ to $\dot{V}_E$ is sensitive to small measurement errors when F_{IO_2} and F_{EO_2} are high and F_{IN_2} and F_{EN_2} are low. In addition, the assumption that $\dot{V}_I \times F_{IN_2} = \dot{V}_E \times F_{EN_2}$ is not valid during the transient wash-out period during which hyperoxic gas is inspired and more nitrogen is removed during expiration than is added during inspiration. Finally, if the subject is breathing 100% oxygen, the equations given previously cannot be used at all because there is no inspired or expired nitrogen.

Although calculation of $\dot{V}O_2$ during enriched oxygen breathing is theoretically possible, the accuracy of $\dot{V}O_2$ using conventional equations and measurements is almost certainly less than when the subject is breathing room air. The $\dot{V}O_2$ calculated with F_{IO_2} greater than 0.21 should be interpreted with caution. Some investigators have demonstrated that accurate determination of $\dot{V}O_2$ can be achieved with F_{IO_2} up to 0.30 to 0.50.

An alternative approach to testing subjects during oxygen breathing is to ignore or not make measurements of $\dot{V}O_2$. Often, a reason for exercise testing is to determine the need for supplemental oxygen in a particular patient. This question can usually be answered by comparison of maximum work rate, heart rate, respiratory frequency, minute ventilation, $\dot{V}_E/\dot{V}CO_2$, and exercise endurance between a maximum exercise test on room air with a similar test during oxygen breathing. An objective improvement in exercise capacity and decreased $\dot{V}_E$ and $\dot{V}_E/\dot{V}_{CO_2}$ are supportive evidence of a beneficial effect of supplemental O_2.

Valve Dead Space and Physiological Dead Space

The physiological dead space consists of the anatomic dead space and the alveolar dead space. During measurement, the volumes of the breathing valve and mouthpiece apparatus are considered to be in series with the anatomic dead space. This apparatus dead space is usually subtracted from the V_D calculated by the Engoff modification of the Bohr equation:

$$V_D = V_T\,(L) \times \frac{Pa_{CO_2} - P\bar{E}_{CO_2}}{Pa_{CO_2}} - V_{Dm}\,(L)$$

where V_D is subject dead space, V_T is tidal volume, and V_{Dm} is the volume of the apparatus (or valve dead space).

Bradley and Younes,[10] Suwa and Bendixen,[11] and Singleton et al[12] reported that the effective dead space of the valve (the correction term V_{Dm}) may be different from the measured mechanical dead space. The readers are referred to their thorough analyses of the proper correction value under various conditions.

In practice, most reports of V_D during exercise have corrected for apparatus dead space by subtracting the entire mechanical dead space. Any potential error can be minimized if the valve dead space is small and the subject's tidal volume is relatively large compared with V_{Dm}. Valves with large dead spaces may be necessary, however, because they usually offer smaller breathing resistances at high inspiratory and expiratory flows. These high flows would be encountered when studying healthy normal subjects with large tidal volumes during exercise. On the other hand, patients with small tidal volumes will usually not generate high flows during exercise, and the valves with small dead spaces are recommended.

Calculations Used for Breath-by-Breath Analysis

Breath-by-breath methods use the same formulas as for mixed expired gas collection.[9] Conceptually, the expired volume is divided into small sequential samples. The volume of each is determined and, when multiplied by the gas concentrations appropriate for that sample (adjusted for the time difference between the flow and gas concentration signals), gives the volume of CO_2 eliminated or O_2 taken up for that sample. The results are summed and then reported either per breath or per unit time. Thus, the phrase "breath-by-breath" applies to the method of expired gas analysis and data reduction and does not necessarily mean that each breath is individually reported.

If V_E is the sum of all volume exhaled between time 0 and time T, then

$$V_E = \sum_{t=0}^{T} \dot{V}exp\,(t + \Delta t)$$

where $\dot{V}exp\,(t + \Delta t)$ is the volume expired between time t and $(t + \Delta t)$, Δt is a time interval, and T is the total time of expiration for single or multiple breaths.

This is satisfactory if volume is directly measured over small time intervals. If expired flow rather than volume is measured, then

$$V_E = \int_0^T \dot{V}exp(t)dt$$

where $\dot{V}exp(t)$ is the expired flow over the infinitesimally small time interval dt at time t. The volume exhaled over that time is the product $\dot{V}exp(t) \times dt$. In practice, a small constant Δt is substituted for dt, and the mean flow during the time interval $(t + \Delta t)$ is used as $\dot{V}exp(t)$:

$$V_E = \sum_{t=0}^{T} \dot{V}exp\,(t + \Delta t) \times \Delta t$$

where $\dot{V}exp\,(t + \Delta t)$ is the mean flow rate during the time interval $t + \Delta t$. The minute ventilation ($\dot{V}_E$) is the volume per unit time.

In a breath-by-breath system, the volume of CO_2 is calculated by multiplying the instantaneous F_{ECO_2} for each small time interval by the simultaneous expired volume during that interval. These products are then integrated:

$$V_{CO_2} = \int_{t=0}^{T} \dot{V}exp(t)dt \times F_{ECO_2}(t)$$

where $\dot{V}exp(t)dt$ is the instantaneous expired volume, and $F_{ECO_2}(t)$ is the instantaneous expired CO_2 concentration at time t, adjusted for the delay between when the gas is sampled and when the analyzer reads the appropriate concentration. In practice, the small time interval Δt is substituted for dt:

$$V_{CO_2} = \sum_{t=0}^{T} \dot{V}exp(t + \Delta t) \times \Delta t \times F_{ECO_2}(t)$$

where $\dot{V}exp(t + \Delta t)$ is the mean flow for the time period t to $(t + \Delta t)$, $F_{ECO_2}(t)$ is the mean expired CO_2 during this period, and Δt is a small time interval. For the volume of O_2 taken up, the true O_2 difference $[(\Delta F_{O_2})true]$ is substituted for F_{ECO_2} in this equation. The $\dot{V}_{CO_2}$ and $\dot{V}_{O_2}$ are equal to the volume of CO_2 or O_2 divided by the time during exhalation, whether expressed per breath or per minute or other time unit.

An analog-to-digital converter and digital computer perform the necessary multiplications and summations. The respired gas is not, strictly speaking, measured and analyzed continuously, but instead, values are rapidly sampled (eg, every 20 ms). The resultant expired flow versus time curve is, therefore, made up of sequential points sampled at intervals of Δt or at a frequency $f = 1/\Delta t$. The rate of sampling is important because rapid and large changes in expired flow (or gas concentration) may occur during exercise and could be missed if the data are sampled at too slow a rate. Bernard,[13] using generalized simulated curves of expired flow and expired CO_2, found that a sample rate of 30 Hz was adequate during exercise and that sampling rates of 40, 50, and 100 Hz achieved little improvement in fidelity. Beaver et al[14] suggested that a sampling frequency equal to twice the highest frequency occurring in the signal to be measured should be used. They suggested that for human exercise testing, a data sampling frequency of 50 Hz is satisfactory to record flow and mass spectrometer signals.

A serious potential problem deals with time alignment of the appropriate expired flow (or volume) and expired gas concentration because of the appreciable time required for gas transport to and measurement by the gas analyzers. For breath-by-breath analysis, it is essential that the appropriate instantaneous flow rate be multiplied by the proper time-aligned expired gas concentration. Flow rates can be measured accurately and nearly instantaneously. However, gas analyzer measurements cannot with current technology be made without some delay and distortion inherent to the transport of gas to the analyzer and the intrinsic characteristics of the analyzer. The accuracy of a breath-by-breath system is dependent on the ability of the system to match flow rate and appropriate gas concentration prior to integration. Thus, each flow sampled must be stored until the appropriate expired gas concentration value has been determined.

Bernard[13] used simulated curves of expired CO_2 and expired flow to estimate potential error caused by the time delay between measurements of these two variables. Using data from perfectly time-matched hypothetical curves, less than a 5% difference in calculated $\dot{V}CO_2$ was found if the time misalignment was less than or equal to 25 milliseconds. Of importance is that the theoretic sampling rate was 100 Hz, the signals contained random noise, and the product of flow and CO_2 was integrated using the trapezoid rule.

Two factors contribute to the time-alignment problem. Most systems use a capillary tube to draw a continuous expired gas sample into the analyzer. The gas transport time depends on the dimensions of the tube and the flow rate; transport time is on the order of 200 milliseconds. Second, the gas analyzer output itself has an intrinsic response time that further adds to the delay. For infrared CO_2 analyzers, electrochemical O_2 analyzers, and respiratory mass spectrometers, the time constants for exponential response are approximately 50 milliseconds. The result is a delay in the measurement of any instantaneous change in gas concentration at the sampling end of the tubing.

To account for the gas analyzer delay and response time, the transport time plus an additional correction factor are usually used. This function is derived from analysis of the total response of the gas analyzer system. Beaver et al[14] indicated that the most significant wave shape distortion is removed by a total delay correction equal to transport delay plus one time constant and analyzed the magnitude of potential errors. We found that an equal-area method for analyzer delay time adds a one-time-constant delay if the analyzer response curve is exponential and an empirically determined longer delay time if the curve is sigmoidal.[15]

The importance of matching flow rate and appropriate gas concentration cannot be overly stressed for a breath-by-breath system. Although not all investigators agree on the optimal way of dealing with gas analyzer response time, a satisfactory balance among degree of accuracy, speed, and reproducibility can be reached.

REFERENCES

1. Lewis D, Sietsema KE, Casaburi R, Sue DY. Inaccuracy of noninvasive estimates of V_D/V_T in clinical exercise testing. *Chest*. 1994;106:1476-1480.
2. Kim TS, Rahn H, Farhi LE. Estimation of true venous and arterial P_{CO_2} by gas analysis of a single breath. *J Appl Physiol*. 1966;21:1338-1344.
3. Jones NL, Campbell EJM, McHardy GJR, Higgs BE, Clode M. The estimation of carbon dioxide pressure of mixed venous blood during exercise. *Clin Sci*. 1967;32:311-327.
4. Sun XG, Hansen JE, Ting H, et al. Comparison of exercise cardiac output by the Fick principle using oxygen and carbon dioxide. *Chest*. 2000;118:631-640.
5. Sun XG, Hansen JE, Stringer WW, Ting H, Wasserman K. Carbon dioxide pressure-concentration relationship in arterial and mixed venous blood during exercise. *J Appl Physiol (1985)*. 2001;90:1798-1810.
6. Wagner JA, Horvath SM, Dahms TE, Reed S. Validation of open-circuit method for the determination of oxygen consumption. *J Appl Physiol*. 1973;34:859-863.
7. Wilmore JH, Costill DL. Adequacy of the Haldane transformation in the computation of exercise $\dot{V}O_2$ in man. *J Appl Physiol*. 1973;35:85-89.
8. Beaver WL. Water vapor corrections in oxygen consumption calculations. *J Appl Physiol*. 1973;35:928-931.
9. Beaver WL, Wasserman K, Whipp BJ. On-line computer analysis and breath-by-breath graphical display of exercise function tests. *J Appl Physiol*. 1973;34:128-132.
10. Bradley PW, Younes M. Relation between respiratory valve dead space and tidal volume. *J Appl Physiol Respir Environ Exerc Physiol*. 1980;49:528-532.
11. Suwa K, Bendixen HH. Change in P_{aCO_2} with mechanical dead space during artificial ventilation. *J Appl Physiol*. 1960;15:556-562.
12. Singleton GJ, Olsen CR, Smith RL. Correction for mechanical dead space in the calculation of physiological dead space. *J Clin Invest*. 1972;51:2768-2772.
13. Bernard TE. Aspects of on-line digital integration of pulmonary gas transfer. *J Appl Physiol Respir Environ Exerc Physiol*. 1977;43:375-378.
14. Beaver WL, Lamarra N, Wasserman K. Breath-by-breath measurement of true alveolar gas exchange. *J Appl Physiol Respir Environ Exerc Physiol*. 1981;51:1662-1675.
15. Sue DY, Hansen JE, Blais M, Wasserman K. Measurement and analysis of gas exchange during exercise using a programmable calculator. *J Appl Physiol Respir Environ Exerc Physiol*. 1980;49:456-461.

Index

Page numbers followed by an *f* denote figures; page numbers followed by a *t* denote tables.